Leukemia and Lymphoma

Molecular and Therapeutic Insights

A subject collection from *Cold Spring Harbor Perspectives in Medicine*

OTHER SUBJECT COLLECTIONS FROM *COLD SPRING HARBOR PERSPECTIVES IN MEDICINE*

Addiction, Second Edition
Hepatitis C Virus: The Story of a Scientific and Therapeutic Revolution
The PTEN Family
Genetic Counseling: Clinical Practice and Ethical Considerations
Bioelectronic Medicine
Function and Dysfunction of the Cochlea: From Mechanisms to Potential Therapies
Next-Generation Sequencing in Medicine
Prostate Cancer
RAS and Cancer in the 21st Century
Enteric Hepatitis Viruses
Bone: A Regulator of Physiology
Multiple Sclerosis
Cancer Evolution
The Biology of Exercise
Prion Diseases
Tissue Engineering and Regenerative Medicine
Chromatin Deregulation in Cancer
Malaria: Biology in the Era of Eradication
Antibiotics and Antibiotic Resistance

SUBJECT COLLECTIONS FROM *COLD SPRING HARBOR PERSPECTIVES IN BIOLOGY*

Stem Cells: From Biological Principles to Regenerative Medicine
Heart Development and Disease
Cell Survival and Cell Death, Second Edition
Calcium Signaling, Second Edition
Engineering Plants for Agriculture
Protein Homeostasis, Second Edition
Translation Mechanisms and Control
Cytokines
Circadian Rhythms
Immune Memory and Vaccines: Great Debates
Cell–Cell Junctions, Second Edition
Prion Biology
The Biology of the TGF-β Family
Synthetic Biology: Tools for Engineering Biological Systems
Cell Polarity
Cilia
Microbial Evolution
Learning and Memory

Leukemia and Lymphoma

Molecular and Therapeutic Insights

A subject collection from *Cold Spring Harbor Perspectives in Medicine*

EDITED BY

Michael G. Kharas
Memorial Sloan Kettering Cancer Center

Ross L. Levine
Memorial Sloan Kettering Cancer Center

Ari M. Melnick
Weill Cornell Medicine

COLD SPRING HARBOR LABORATORY PRESS
Cold Spring Harbor, New York • www.cshlpress.org

Leukemia and Lymphoma: Molecular and Therapeutic Insights
A subject collection from *Cold Spring Harbor Perspectives in Medicine*
Articles online at perspectivesinmedicine.org

Printed in the United States of America

Executive Editor	Richard Sever
Managing Editor	Maria Smit
Senior Project Manager	Barbara Acosta
Permissions Administrator	Carol Brown
Production Editor	Kathleen Bubbeo
Production Manager/Cover Designer	Denise Weiss
Publisher	John Inglis

Front cover artwork: Illustration showing abundant lymphoblasts in blood—a characteristic of acute lymphoblastic leukemia. (Image used under license from KaterynaKon/Shutterstock.com.)

Library of Congress Cataloging-in-Publication Data

Names: Kharas, Michael G., editor. | Levine, Ross (Ross L.), editor. | Melnick, Ari M., editor.
Title: Leukemia and lymphoma : molecular and therapeutic insights / edited by Michael G. Kharas, Ross L. Levine and Ari M. Melnick.
Description: Cold Spring Harbor, New York : Cold Spring Harbor Laboratory Press, [2020] | Series: Cold Spring Harbor perspectives in medicine | Includes bibliographical references and index. | Summary: "Leukemia and lymphoma are cancers that affect cells of the blood. This book examines the genetic and epigenetic changes in blood cells that lead to these conditions and current treatment strategies"-- Provided by publisher.
Identifiers: LCCN 2019060042 (print) | LCCN 2019060043 (ebook) | ISBN 9781621821427 (hardcover) | ISBN 9781621823056 (epub) | ISBN 9781621823063 (kindle edition)
Subjects: LCSH: Leukemia. | Lymphomas.
Classification: LCC RC633 .L48 2020 (print) | LCC RC633 (ebook) | DDC 616.99/419--dc23
LC record available at https://lccn.loc.gov/2019060042
LC ebook record available at https://lccn.loc.gov/2019060043

10 9 8 7 6 5 4 3 2 1

All World Wide Web addresses are accurate to the best of our knowledge at the time of printing.

For a complete catalog of all Cold Spring Harbor Laboratory Press publications, visit our website at www.cshlpress.org.

Contents

Preface

FROM THE TIME ABERRANT WHITE BLOOD CELLS were first described in the nineteenth century, to the discovery of chromosomal aberrations in the mid-twentieth century, and to the recent explosion of genomic and single-cell analyses, studies of blood cancers have always been at the vanguard of discovery. These milestones changed how we understand normal and malignant hematopoiesis and informed broader understanding of immunology, gene regulation, cancer biology, and targeted therapy.

In this book, we have focused on the biology of cancers of the hematopoietic system, including leukemias and lymphomas. The study of these diseases has laid the foundation for fundamental discoveries in biomedical science and paved the road for translational impact across the spectrum of human cancers. We examine the latest findings and thoughts about the etiology of hematological malignancies, the models used to study them, and the newest paradigms for understanding their biology and developing rationally designed therapies. The development of novel technologies and the accelerated pace of discovery have revealed how remarkably heterogeneous these tumors are and provided significant insight into the normal and malignant physiology of the tissues these tumors affect. This has given us a better appreciation of the significance of cell-context-specific factors and the impact of specific genetic drivers, but at the same time raises many new and ever more complex biological questions.

We assembled experts in myeloid and lymphoid neoplasms to address the key topics in this field. These include studies of the genomic and epigenomic basis of hematopoietic transformation, and how these have led to new insights into how gene regulatory networks are co-opted during transformation and can be leveraged to yield therapeutic benefit. The authors describe in great detail different mechanisms of transformation, both with respect to cell-autonomous processes, including signaling, stem cell biology, and self-renewal, and non-cell-autonomous mechanisms, including immunological activation/escape and interactions with the niche. They describe state-of-the-art preclinical models of hematologic cancers and how these can be used for mechanistic and therapeutic studies. Most importantly, this book illustrates the complexity of hematopoietic and immune system transformation and how new and important concepts relevant to diagnosis and management of leukemia and lymphoma have emerged.

The editors want to thank Barbara Acosta and her Cold Spring Harbor Laboratory Press colleagues for their tireless support and for marshaling this book from conception to completion. We greatly appreciate Barbara's patience, understanding, and organizational skills and her ability to keep the editors and authors on schedule. We apologize in advance if we have failed to include or to cite our colleagues or if we failed to adequately address a topic or concept or missed the latest findings in a specific area. Last, we also want to thank all the authors, contributors, and experts from our laboratories who participated in putting together this volume and ensuring it includes the latest and most exciting findings about leukemia and lymphoma.

MICHAEL G. KHARAS
ROSS L. LEVINE
ARI M. MELNICK

Normal Hematopoiesis Is a Balancing Act of Self-Renewal and Regeneration

Oakley C. Olson,[1] Yoon-A Kang,[1] and Emmanuelle Passegué

Columbia Stem Cell Initiative, Department of Genetics & Development, Columbia University Irving Medical Center, New York, New York 10032, USA

Correspondence: ep2828@cumc.columbia.edu

The hematopoietic system is highly organized to maintain its functional integrity and to meet lifelong organismal demands. Hematopoietic stem cells (HSCs) must balance self-renewal with differentiation and the regeneration of the blood system. It is a complex balancing act between these competing HSC functions. Although highly quiescent at steady state, HSCs become activated in response to inflammatory cytokines and regenerative challenges. This activation phase leads to many intrinsic stresses such as replicative, metabolic, and oxidative stress, which can cause functional decline, impaired self-renewal, and exhaustion of HSCs. To cope with these insults, HSCs use both built-in and emergency-triggered stress-response mechanisms to maintain homeostasis and to defend against disease development. In this review, we discuss how the hematopoietic system operates in steady state and stress conditions, what strategies are used to maintain functional integrity, and how deregulation in the balance between self-renewal and regeneration can drive malignant transformation.

The hematopoietic system is organized in a hierarchical manner, with hematopoietic stem cells (HSCs) sitting at the apex of its differentiation hierarchy. HSCs give rise to progeny transiting through multiple differentiation states, progressing from lineage-biased but still multipotent progenitors to lineage-specific committed progenitors and precursors, ultimately producing all populations of mature blood cells. As an organ, the hematopoietic system is highly plastic and serves a diverse set of biological processes: generating the myeloid and lymphoid cells of the innate and adaptive immune systems to defend the organisms against a host of attacks, making the red blood cells that transport oxygen throughout the body to oxygenate all tissues, and producing the platelets that stop bleeding and orchestrate tissue repair. All these functions are critical for the survival of the organism throughout its life span, and the hematopoietic system has evolved significant levels of regulation and protection to maintain its functional integrity and meet blood production demands.

The hematopoietic system is designed to regenerate continuously, both to maintain ho-

[1]These authors contributed equally to this work.

Cite this article as *Cold Spring Harb Perspect Med* doi: 10.1101/cshperspect.a035519

meostatic replacement of blood cells at steady state and to rapidly increase output to adequately compensate for acute blood loss in the context of physical trauma, infection, and metabolic or toxic stress. This adaptive response requires the hematopoietic system to switch from its steady state, slow production mode to an activated state known as "emergency hematopoiesis." Although emergency hematopoiesis involves adaptive regulation in progenitors, as will be discussed later in the review, this is fundamentally a process that starts at the level of HSCs. HSCs must proliferate and balance two opposing cell-fate decisions, self-renewal and differentiation, to maintain the stem cell compartment and produce all the needed downstream progenitors and mature blood cells. Under homeostatic conditions, HSCs cycle infrequently and are largely in a dormant state known as quiescence (Wilson et al. 2008; Foudi et al. 2009). HSC quiescence serves as a protective mechanism by limiting replicative stress, which can cause the functional decline of HSCs especially on aging (Flach et al. 2014). In response to inflammatory signals that coordinate regeneration, HSCs quickly become activated, proliferate, and expand the needed progenitor compartments to replenish the blood system and produce the required effector cells (Wilson et al. 2008; Sato et al. 2009). When regenerative signaling becomes hyperactivated, differentiation can be prioritized over self-renewal, leading to the loss of the immature stem and progenitor cell (HSPC) compartment. Conversely, in conditions in which differentiation is inhibited and self-renewal is prioritized, as the result of somatic mutation or environmental cues, the HSC compartment becomes hyperplastic at the expense of effective maintenance of blood production. In both cases, the hematopoietic system becomes exhausted, leading to cytopenias and ultimately bone marrow (BM) failures. In the context of malignancies like myeloproliferative neoplasms (MPNs) or acute myeloid leukemia (AML), this regulatory axis is also disrupted but with increased self-renewal and regenerative signaling pathways working in concert to drive leukemic progression. In this review, we discuss how normal hematopoiesis balances regeneration and self-renewal, and how deregulation of these regulatory mechanisms leads to malignant hematopoiesis.

HSC IDENTIFICATION: SELF-RENEWAL AND MULTIPOTENCY

HSCs are defined by multipotency, the ability to differentiate into all lineages of mature blood cells, and the capacity to self-renew for the duration of an organism's life. It is the investigation of these two features that has driven research in the field over the last century and led to the discovery of bona fide HSCs. The earliest conceptual understanding of the BM as a reservoir of self-renewing and multipotent HSCs originates from the first transplant to cure a patient with aplastic anemia (Osgood et al. 1939). Although anemia was previously treated with transfusions, the infusion of BM cells identified the source of blood-producing progenitor cells. Subsequent experimentation revealed that infusion of mouse BM cells could rescue mice from radiation-induced lethality (Jacobson et al. 1951) by restoring both myeloid and lymphoid lineage production (Ford et al. 1956), hence reinforcing the idea of multipotent blood-producing cells. In the 1960s, spleen colony-forming unit (CFU-S) assays provided further evidence for the concept of stem cells. Mice transplanted with syngeneic BM cells formed cellular colonies in the spleen, with differential compositions of myeloid and erythroid cells and self-renewal capacity (Till and McCulloch 1961; Becker et al. 1963). It was also noted at this time that self-renewal and multipotency were related to quiescence (Becker et al. 1965; Bruce et al. 1966).

In the 1980s, with the advance of technologies such as multicolor fluorescence-activated cell sorting (FACS) and monoclonal antibodies, HSCs were prospectively isolated from mouse BM as $Lin^{-}/Thy\text{-}1^{low}/Sca\text{-}1^{+}$ cells and shown to be capable of long-term, multilineage reconstitution in irradiated mice (Muller-Sieburg et al. 1986; Spangrude et al. 1988). Later in the 1990s, single-cell transplantation experiments were performed to truly show the capacity of a single blood-forming HSC to regenerate all hematopoietic lineages (Osawa et al. 1996). The phenotypic characterization of HSCs has considerably progressed with a current consensus on identifying long-term engrafting murine HSCs as $Lin^-/Sca\text{-}1^+/c\text{-}Kit^+/Flk2^-/CD48^-/CD150^+/CD34^-$ BM cells (Cabezas-Wallscheid et al. 2014) and human HSCs as $Lin^-/CD34^+/CD38^-/CD90^+/CD45RA^-$ cord blood and BM cells (Gentles et al. 2010). This significant body of research, conducted during the last century, has defined our understanding of HSC self-renewal and differentiation properties through transplantation assays and has set the stage for further mechanistic investigations of HSC biology.

The immediate downstream progeny of HSCs, the multipotent progenitors (MPPs), produce all hematopoietic lineages but have lost the capacity for extensive self-renewal in transplantation assays, although they retain the ability to maintain long-term blood production in native condition (Busch et al. 2015). The mouse MPP compartment is composed of MPP2 ($Lin^-/Sca\text{-}1^+/c\text{-}Kit^+/Flk2^-/CD48^+/CD150^+/CD34^+$), MPP3 ($Lin^-/Sca\text{-}1^+/c\text{-}Kit^+/Flk2^-/CD48^+/CD150^-/CD34^+$) and MPP4 ($Lin^-/Sca\text{-}1^+/c\text{-}Kit^+/Flk2^+/CD48^+/CD150^-/CD34^+$) populations, which have megakaryocyte, granulocyte-macrophage, and lymphoid lineage-differentiation biases, respectively (Cabezas-Wallscheid et al. 2014; Pietras et al. 2015). These lineage-biased MPPs give rise to more lineage-restricted progenitors such as common myeloid progenitors (CMPs) and common lymphoid progenitors (CLPs). CMPs further differentiate into granulocyte-macrophage progenitors (GMPs) and megakaryocyte-erythroid progenitors (MEPs), which eventually produce all mature myeloid cells (Fig. 1A).

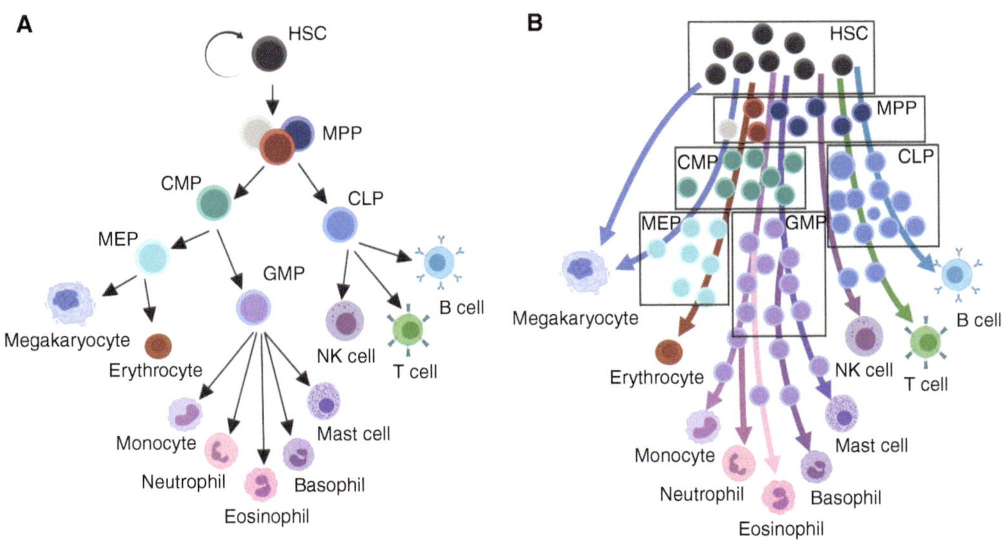

Figure 1. Models of hematopoietic stem cell (HSC) lineage commitment. (*A*) In the classical tree-like model of hematopoietic differentiation, HSCs give rise to multipotent progenitors, which in turn produce lineage-restricted progenitors that ultimately produce all mature hematopoietic cells. This model assumes a relatively uniform developmental and differentiation status at each progenitor stage, and that bifurcating lineage choices occur in either a stochastic manner or in response to instructive cytokines. (*B*) The continuous differentiation model represents the gradual acquisition of lineage restricted features and the presence of transcriptional lineage bias at earlier stages than lineage commitment occurs. Boxes represent progenitor states based on phenotypic markers and illustrate the heterogeneity within each of these populations. MPP, multipotent progenitor; CMP, common myeloid progenitor; CLP, common lymphoid progenitor; MEP, megakaryocyte-erythroid progenitor; GMP, granulocyte-macrophage progenitor.

In response to stress, GMPs form patches in the bone marrow, which function as an amplification compartment, allowing an acute increase of myeloid output (Hérault et al. 2017). This hematopoietic tree-like model of hematopoiesis suggests that HSCs pass through a series of differentiation states with increasingly restricted self-renewal and lineage potentiality (Kondo et al. 1997; Akashi et al. 2000). This model is based on discrete bifurcating cell-fate decisions that restrict potentiality at each relatively homogenous progenitor stage and has guided research and provided the framework for the prospective identification of different multi- and bipotent progenitors by cell surface markers. However, it has become well appreciated that each stem and progenitor population is in fact heterogeneous, and that the majority of HSCs produce a lineage-biased rather than balanced output (Müller-Sieburg et al. 2002, 2004; Dykstra et al. 2007; Morita et al. 2010; Yamamoto et al. 2013). Lineage tracing studies using either polylox (Pei et al. 2017), viral (Naik et al. 2013), or transposon (Sun et al. 2014; Rodriguez-Fraticelli et al. 2018) barcoding strategies to assess the clonal output of single HSCs have gone further to show how heterogenous the HSCs are in terms of lineage bias and output. These approaches have also shown that the megakaryocyte lineage can arise directly from HSCs (Rodriguez-Fraticelli et al. 2018). Collectively, these studies indicate that cell-fate decisions are influenced by cell-intrinsic regulators and are likely occurring at early stages of hematopoietic differentiation. The advent of single-cell technology has clarified these findings by revealing that hematopoietic cells acquire lineage-biased expression in a rather continuous manner (Fig. 1B), and that the classical tree-like model of hematopoiesis represents a semi-artificial segmentation of the data (Pina et al. 2012; Macaulay et al. 2016; Nestorowa et al. 2016; Velten et al. 2017; Karamitros et al. 2018; Tusi et al. 2018). These new differentiation–continuum models of hematopoiesis suggest that differentiation trajectories can be established early on during development, and although these early biases are not immutable to external pressure, they explain, in large part, the bias in lineage output observed in the hematopoietic system (Laurenti and Göttgens 2018).

HSC DEFENSE MECHANISMS: NICHE REGULATION, GENOME MAINTENANCE, AND METABOLIC DORMANCY

The Hematopoietic Stem Cell Niche

To maintain their lifelong functional integrity, HSCs are tightly regulated both in a cell-intrinsic manner and by extrinsic cues from the BM microenvironment known as the BM niche. Much of the regulation of HSC quiescence is controlled by this hypoxic BM microenvironment, in which quiescence-enforcing and self-renewal promoting cytokines are provided by stromal and endothelial niche cells (Schepers et al. 2015; Crane et al. 2017; Wei and Frenette 2018). The c-x-c motif chemokine ligand 12 (CXCL12) and the c-Kit receptor ligand stem cell factor (SCF) have appeared as the most important factors for HSC retention in the niche (Ding et al. 2012). Stromal-derived CXCL12 is also required for HSCs to colonize the BM niche during development (Ara et al. 2003), and following DNA damaging injury from chemotherapy or radiation, CXCL12 expression is increased to promote the migration and repopulation of the BM niche by HSCs (Ponomaryov et al. 2000). Niche cells can also contribute to HSC activation, especially by secreting pro-inflammatory cytokines, and endothelial cells have been shown to sense pathogens and activate HSCs to drive emergency hematopoiesis (Boettcher et al. 2014). In this manner, niche cells work to support HSC maintenance and function, both by maintaining HSC quiescence and self-renewal and by coordinating regeneration in response to physiologic insult. Indeed, hematopoietic function and the niche are so inextricably linked that mutation in the niche compartment is sufficient to drive leukemogenesis (Kode et al. 2014). Although we will include discussion of the BM niche where relevant, as it pertains to HSC function in normal and malignant hematopoiesis, this topic is discussed in depth in a number of recent reviews (see

Schepers et al. 2015; Crane et al. 2017; Wei and Frenette 2018).

DNA Damage and HSC Functional Decline

HSCs reside in the quiescent G_0 state, which serves as the first line of defense against genomic instability, metabolic stress, and functional decline (Wilson et al. 2008; Bakker and Passegué 2013; Chandel et al. 2016). DNA damage and genomic instability can arise from multiple intrinsic and extrinsic sources such as reactive oxygen species (ROS) produced during mitochondrial respiration (Ito and Suda 2014), replication errors and telomere attrition generated during cell division (Rossi et al. 2007), as well as irradiation, ultraviolet (UV), or exposure to genotoxic agents (Biechonski et al. 2017). HSCs use various mechanisms to cope with these intrinsic and environmental stresses to prevent DNA damage accrual. Indeed, an evolutionarily conserved feature of the BM niche is the protection of HSCs from UV (Kapp et al. 2018). HSCs also have high levels of ATP-binding cassette (ABC) transporters to efflux genotoxins and protect from environmental stress (Goodell et al. 1996; Zhou et al. 2002). Replication, however, is the main driver of somatic mutation over the life span (Tomasetti and Vogelstein 2015) and of functional decline in HSCs (Flach et al. 2014). Quiescence protects HSCs from replicative stress, with many studies showing an inverse correlation between proliferative status and engraftment of HSCs, in which dormant cells have the greatest long-term reconstitution potential (Orford and Scadden 2008). Cell cycle regulators such as the retinoblastoma (Rb) family (Viatour et al. 2008), the cyclin D-Cdk4/6 complex (Kozar et al. 2004; Malumbres et al. 2004), and the CIP/KIP family—in particular, p57 (Matsumoto et al. 2011; Zou et al. 2011)—control HSC dormancy in a redundant manner. Interestingly, p53 also regulates HSC quiescence in part by inducing the CIP family member p21 (Asai et al. 2011). Niche factors such as transforming growth factor β1 (TGF-β1) (Scandura et al. 2004; Yamazaki et al. 2009), angiopoietin-1 (Ang-1) (Arai et al. 2004), CXCL12 (Nagasawa et al. 1996), SCF (Thorén et al. 2008), or thrombopoietin (TPO) (Qian et al. 2007) enforce HSC quiescence, either by modulating cell cycle regulators or by promoting DNA damage repair. Additionally, the evolutionarily conserved developmental signaling pathways Wnt, Notch, and Hedgehog (HH) control HSC self-renewal through cell cycle regulation and inhibition of differentiation (Duncan et al. 2005; Trowbridge et al. 2006; Niehrs and Acebron 2012). Ironically, quiescence restricts HSCs to the use of the error-prone nonhomologous end-joining (NHEJ) pathway to repair nonreplicative DNA damage, such as radiation-induced DNA double-strand breaks, which can contribute to mutation and chromosomal instability (Mohrin et al. 2010). Of note, the protective quiescent status of HSCs is unique to adulthood, as fetal and postnatal HSCs are largely cycling (Orkin and Zon 2008; Pietras et al. 2011), which suggest that distinct mechanisms may operate to protect fetal or postnatal HSCs from DNA damage, functional decline, and malignant transformation.

In addition to the tight control of proliferation in HSCs, regulation of ROS, a primary oxidative stress molecule causing nucleotide oxidation and DNA breaks (Sedelnikova et al. 2010), is critical to suppressing the accumulation of DNA damage and HSC functional decline (Yahata et al. 2011). ROS production is regulated in HSCs through a coordinated anti-oxidant response and the suppression of aerobic metabolism (Ito and Suda 2014). HSCs deficient for either the forkhead box protein O (FOXO) transcription factors or nuclear factor erythroid 2-related factor 2 (NRF2), all of which are master regulators of the anti-oxidant response, lose quiescence and have reduced self-renewal capacity (Tothova et al. 2007; Tsai et al. 2013). ROS drives HSCs out of quiescence and impairs self-renewal by activating p38 mitogen-activated protein kinase (MAPK) (Ito et al. 2006). Indeed, not only is ROS itself a mutagen but its accumulation in response to replicative stress and unresolved DNA damage plays an important role in triggering differentiation and the elimination of damaged HSCs (Ito et al. 2004; Yahata et al. 2011). Collectively, these findings show how tightly activation and proliferation are controlled to suppress DNA damage and maintain HSC genome integrity and illustrate how ROS signaling integrates stress signaling and determines cell fate.

Metabolism and HSC Activation

Despite the high vascularity of the BM, direct measurement of oxygen tension indicates a hypoxic microenvironment (Spencer et al. 2014). Hypoxia-inducible factor 1α (HIF1α) is stabilized in HSCs by low oxygen tension, and with myeloid ecotropic viral integration site 1 (MEIS1) regulates quiescent HSC metabolism through the utilization of anaerobic glycolysis rather than mitochondrial oxidative phosphorylation (OXPHOS) (Simsek et al. 2010). Indeed, quiescent HSCs have an abundance of glycolytic metabolites, and a relative absence of tricarboxylic acid cycle (TCA) metabolites (Simsek et al. 2010; Takubo et al. 2013). Maintaining the glycolytic metabolic state is critical to HSC quiescence and mice lacking HIF1α (Takubo et al. 2010) or the glycolytic enzymes pyruvate dehydrogenase kinase 2 (PDK2) and PDK4 (Takubo et al. 2013), which prevent the flux of pyruvate through the TCA cycle, display increased mitochondrial respiration and ROS generation with a concomitant loss of HSC quiescence and reduced self-renewal capacity. Similarly, loss of lactase dehydrogenase (LDH), the terminal enzyme in anaerobic glycolysis, results in a loss of HSCs and long-term BM reconstitution capacity (Wang et al. 2014). Collectively, these studies show the importance of anaerobic glycolysis in maintaining quiescent LT-HSCs.

HSCs have relatively high levels of mitochondria compared with some downstream progenitors, but they are usually small with low activity (Simsek et al. 2010; Norddahl et al. 2011; Ho et al. 2017). The activity of HSC mitochondria is inhibited in part through Sirtuin 7 (SIRT7) and nuclear respiratory factor 1 (NRF1), which suppress the mitochondrial unfolded protein response and metabolic activation (Mohrin et al. 2015). The relatively high, but dormant, mitochondrial content in HSCs likely ensures rapid engagement of OXPHOS to meet the increased energy demands when HSCs activate and proliferate. Indeed, although a metabolic shift to OXPHOS is sufficient to activate HSCs, ongoing oxidative metabolism is required for differentiation, and HSCs deficient for protein tyrosine phosphatase mitochondrial 1 (PTPMT1), a main OXPHOS machinery component, fail to differentiate, leading to rapid hematopoietic failure (Yu et al. 2013). Autophagy is critical for suppressing levels of activated mitochondria and the metabolic switch to OXPHOS, and HSCs with impaired autophagy display increased mitochondria number and ROS with increased proliferation, myeloid bias, and impaired regenerative capacity in transplantation assays (Mortensen et al. 2011; Ho et al. 2017). Phenotypically, this impaired autophagy and increased mitochondrial OXPHOS resemble the main features of aged HSCs (Ho et al. 2017). In Tie2$^+$ HSCs, peroxisome proliferator–activated receptor (PPAR)δ and fatty acid oxidation induce mitophagy and the clearance of mitochondria is critical to HSC self-renewal and expansion (Ito et al. 2016). Thus, a switch from the quiescent glycolytic state to a pro-proliferative/pro-differentiation OXPHOS state is a critical for HSC cell-fate decisions and for balancing HSC self-renewal with regeneration of the hematopoietic system.

Recent studies have uncovered mechanisms by which HSC metabolic status regulates proliferation, differentiation, and self-renewal capacity. Intracellular ROS, a by-product of mitochondrial OXPHOS, appears to function as a rheostat to control HSC response to changing metabolic states through p38 MAPK (Ito et al. 2006; Jang and Sharkis 2007) and p53 (Asai et al. 2011). FOXO3 is also critical in maintaining HSC self-renewal by triggering autophagy in response to nutrient stress (Warr et al. 2013), in addition to its role in suppressing ROS (Miyamoto et al. 2007; Warr et al. 2013). FOXO transcription factors are inhibited by activation of the PI3K–AKT–mTOR signaling pathway, which coordinates HSC proliferation and promotes differentiation in part through regulating mitochondria activity and ROS production (Miyamoto et al. 2007; Tothova et al. 2007). Indeed, the PI3K-negative regulator phosphatase and tensin homolog (PTEN) is required for the maintenance of HSCs, and its loss leads to myeloproliferative disorder and exhaustion of normal HSCs (Yilmaz et al. 2006; Zhang et al. 2006). Similarly, liver kinase B (LKB1), which activates AMPK and negatively regulates the mTOR signaling pathway, also regulates HSC quiescence via a mitochondria-dependent but ROS-independent mechanism (Gan et al. 2010; Gurumurthy et al. 2010; Nakada et al. 2010). Loss of LKB1 leads to the down-regulation of PPARγ coactivators (Gan et al. 2010) and elevates levels of fatty acid metabolites (Gurumurthy et al. 2010). PPAR family members are important regulators of fatty acid oxidation (FAO), which is highly activated in HSCs, and among them PPARδ is highly expressed in HSCs (Ito et al. 2012). PPARδ deletion or pharmacological inhibition impairs FAO and results in HSC exhaustion (Ito et al. 2012). It is proposed that FAO might be a critical source of NADPH and thus serve as a negative regulator of ROS in HSCs, indicating another regulation of HSC self-renewal by the PPAR–FAO metabolic axis (Carracedo et al. 2013). Taken together, HSCs maintain their quiescent metabolic status to ensure self-renewal capacity by suppressing mitochondrial activity and utilizing FAO and deregulation of these pathways exhausts HSCs and leads to BM failure.

Of note, the metabolic switch of HSC activation is not merely a signal driving HSC proliferation and differentiation, it also plays a critical role in the metabolically intensive process of epigenetic remodeling required for differentiation. Upon HSC differentiation, global changes in the DNA methylome occur and these changes are critical to the demethylation and activation of lineage-specific transcriptional programs (Bock et al. 2012; Cabezas-Wallscheid et al. 2014; Farlik et al. 2016). Demethylation of DNA is an energy intensive process requiring ATP, oxygen, and the TCA metabolite α-ketoglutarate (α-KG) and is significantly impaired in a hypoxic and glycolytic metabolic state (Ryall et al. 2015). The DNA demethylase tet methylcytosine dioxygenase 2 (TET2), which requires an active TCA and robust levels of α-KG, is critical to HSC lineage commitment, and its loss leads to impaired differentiation and HSC expansion (Figueroa et al. 2010). The histone demethylase lysine-specific demethylase 1 (LSD1), which uses another OXPHOS metabolite, flavin adenine dinucleotide (FAD), as a cofactor, is also important for normal HSC differentiation and its loss leads to impaired repression of HSPC transcriptional programs during blood cell maturation (Sprüssel et al. 2012; Kerenyi et al. 2013). Therefore, the shift from glycolysis to OXPHOS is crucial to providing the energy and metabolites necessary not only for cellular proliferation but also for the epigenetic remodeling of lineage commitment and differentiation. In this manner, we can understand this stem cell state to be a metabolic ON/OFF switch, which transitions the HSC from its normally protected and self-renewing compartment into a metabolically active cell capable of regenerating the entire blood system.

DEMAND-ADAPTED HEMATOPOIESIS

Lineage Bias and Reprogramming during Emergency Hematopoiesis

Hematopoiesis is a demand-adapted system, which allows the organism to respond to physiological stress and pathogenic challenge in an informed and specific manner. Under steady state conditions, roughly one trillion cells are made in the BM of an adult human on a daily basis (Dancey et al. 1976; Doulatov et al. 2012). The continuous production of immune cells, red blood cells, and platelets is a metabolically intensive process. Therefore, the hematopoietic system tailors its output in a manner that conserves resources and maximizes the production of critical effector cells. Understanding how lineage bias arises from HSC heterogeneity and how it is affected by extrinsic signals is essential to our understanding of hematopoietic regulation by physiological stress. Inflammation can drive demand-adapted hematopoietic response by either activating specific subsets of lineage-biased HSCs or by reprogramming lineage bias in HSPCs more broadly. Indeed, there is evidence that both forms of regulation occur in response to different physiological stressors. TGF-β1 promotes the activation and differentiation of myeloid-biased HSCs (Challen et al. 2010). Conversely, myeloid-biased HSCs have diminished response to the lymphopoietic cytokine interleukin (IL)-7 (Muller-Sieburg et al. 2004). von Willebrand factor (VWF)-expressing HSCs contain quiescent stem cell–like megakaryocyte progenitors, which are activated by acute inflammation to produce only megakaryocytes and restore platelet levels in response to infection or tissue damage (Sanjuan-Pla et al. 2013; Haas et al. 2015). These VWF^+ HSCs express megakaryocyte-specific transcripts, demonstrating intrinsic lineage commitment as early as the stem cell state (Sanjuan-Pla et al. 2013; Haas et al. 2015). In response to platelet depletion alone, these same HSC-like megakaryocyte progenitors become specifically activated in a thrombopoietin-dependent manner, rather than in response to generalized inflammation (Sanjuan-Pla et al. 2013). These studies show that activation of megakaryopoiesis can occur in a targeted manner or as part of a larger emergency hematopoietic response.

Although activation of lineage-biased HSC subpopulations does occur, inflammation generally reprograms the whole HSPC compartment and instructs production of specific lineages. Both IL-1 and M-CSF signaling lead to precocious activation of the myeloid lineage transcription factor PU.1 in HSCs (Mossadegh-Keller et al. 2013; Pietras et al. 2016). In concert with precocious lineage instruction in HSCs, the MPP compartment responds to inflammatory signals in a dynamic manner to alter blood production (Fig. 2). Under steady state conditions, lymphoid-biased MPP4 represents the dominant population relative to myeloid-biased MPP2 and MPP3 (Pietras et al. 2015). However, upon chronic IL-1 exposure, myeloid-biased MPP2 and MPP3 are expanded, and MPP4 output is redirected toward the myeloid lineage (Pietras et al. 2016). This remodeling of the MPP compartment is also evident during regenerative conditions to meet the intense myeloid demand following transplantation (Pietras et al. 2015), suggesting this is a common regenerative mechanism. IL-6 has also been shown to promote myeloid production by reprogramming lymphoid-biased MPP4 to myeloid-biased production (Reynaud et al. 2011). Downstream from the HSPC compartment, rapidly differentiating GMP clusters in the BM fuel mature myeloid cell production during emergency hematopoiesis (Hérault et al. 2017). Although stress-induced changes in lineage bias occur in HSCs and continue at every progenitor stage, the extent to which such bias at the HSC level reprograms downstream progenitors remains an open question.

Inflammatory Signals Drive Hematopoietic Regeneration

The activation of the HSC compartment to trigger emergency hematopoiesis is largely driven by inflammatory cytokines. HSCs rapidly exit quiescence and proliferate in response to a number of inflammatory signals including type I and type II interferons (IFNs) (Essers et al. 2009; Sato et al. 2009; Baldridge et al. 2010), G-CSF (Wilson et al. 2008; Schuettpelz et al. 2014), TPO (Sanjuan-Pla et al. 2013), and IL-1 (Ueda et al. 2009; Pietras et al. 2016; Weisser et al. 2016) to increase regeneration of the blood system. Additionally, HSCs can directly sense pathogen-associated molecular-patterns (PAMPs), such as the toll-like receptor (TLR) ligands LPS and Pam3CSK4 (Nagai et al. 2006; Liu et al. 2015; Takizawa et al. 2017). Much of the functional effects of these inflammatory cytokines are mediated through activation of JAK/STAT, MyD88/NF-κB signaling, and MAPK signaling (Baldridge et al. 2011). Indeed, loss of JAK1 is sufficient to impair regeneration following BM transplant and 5-fluorouracil (5-FU) mediated myeloablation (Kleppe et al. 2017). This is associated with increased HSC quiescence and a loss of responsiveness to type I IFNs and IL-3 signaling (Kleppe et al. 2017). Downstream from the progenitor level, activation of STAT3 is crucial for emergency hematopoiesis, where it controls the proliferative expansion of GMPs in response to G-CSF (McLemore et al. 2001; Panopoulos et al. 2006; Zhang et al. 2010). Although there is significant functional overlap between many of these cytokines in driving emergency hematopoiesis, each of these inflammatory mediators activate HSCs

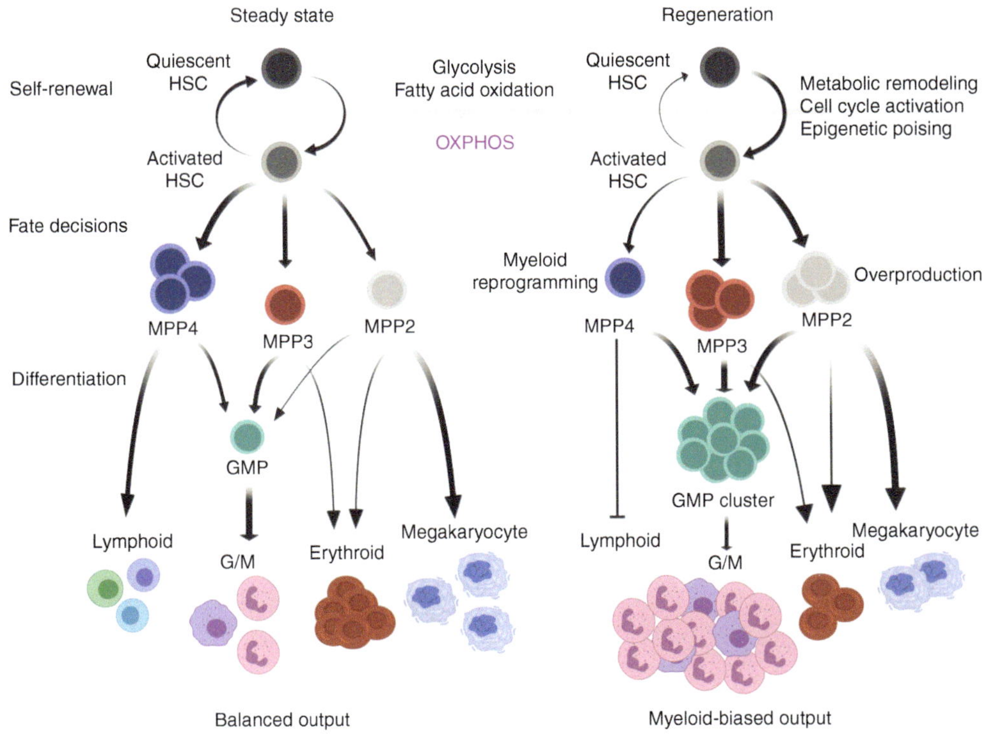

Figure 2. Dynamic alterations to the hematopoietic stem and progenitor cell (HSPC) compartment during regenerative stress. Quiescent hematopoietic stem cells (HSCs) depend on glycolysis and fatty acid oxidation to meet their metabolic needs. Upon activation, HSCs switch to mitochondrial oxidative phosphorylation (OXPHOS). Under steady state conditions, HSCs predominantly produce the lymphoid-biased MPP4. Under regenerative conditions, HSCs overproduce the granulocyte/macrophage (G/M)-biased MPP3 and megakaryocyte-biased MPP2 at the expense of MPP4. Furthermore, MPP4 is reprogrammed toward an almost exclusively myeloid output.

and instruct lineage bias and reprogram differentiation in distinct ways (Schultze et al. 2019). This allows the hematopoietic system to expertly integrate extrinsic signals and efficiently tailor blood production to organismal demand.

Activation of Emergency Hematopoiesis in Response to Pathogens

Emergency hematopoiesis can be further distinguished based on whether the regenerative response is driven by pathogen sensing or sterile inflammation (Manz and Boettcher 2014). This distinction is supported by mechanistic evidence of overlapping but divergent signaling. IL-1 receptor signaling is dispensable for granulopoiesis in response to TLR ligands (Boettcher et al. 2012), whereas it is critical in the context of sterile inflammation such as 5-FU-induced myeloablation (Pietras et al. 2016). In the context of systemic infection, hematopoietic growth factors and cytokines including G-CSF, M-CSF, GM-CSF, IL-3, IL-6, and FLT3 ligand are significantly up-regulated in the circulation (Cheers et al. 1988; Watari et al. 1989; Kawakami et al. 1990; Cebon et al. 1994; Selig and Nothdurft 1995; Tanaka et al. 1996; Presneill et al. 2000). Stromal TLR4/MyD88 signaling is critical for LPS-induced G-CSF secretion and activation of emergency hematopoiesis (Boettcher et al. 2014). However, HSPCs can also directly sense LPS, proliferate, and secrete cytokines through NF-κB signaling, thereby directly initiating emergency hematopoiesis (Zhao et al. 2014a;

Takizawa et al. 2017). Nonhematopoietic pathogen sensing is also necessary for mobilizing immune cells from the BM. In response to circulating TLR ligands, BM niche cells secrete CCL2 to drive mobilization of $Ly6C^{hi}/CCR2^{+}$ inflammatory monocytes into the circulation (Shi et al. 2011). It is believed that homeostatic density-dependent mechanisms sense the number of monocytes and neutrophils available in the BM, either through cell–cell contacts with myeloid cells or through myeloid secreted cytokines, and therefore mobilization of myeloid cells and emptying of these reservoirs stimulates regenerative pathways. Indeed, depletion of neutrophils is sufficient to induce HSC activation and emergency hematopoiesis (Scumpia et al. 2010; Cain et al. 2011; Hérault et al. 2017). Furthermore, clearance of aged and apoptotic neutrophils by BM resident macrophages leads to increased production of G-CSF to promote granulopoiesis and restore homeostasis (Furze and Rankin 2008). Together, emergency programs driven by PAMPs regulate both the production of innate immune cell as well as their release from the BM and, through cross talk with physiological systems throughout the body, coordinate hematopoietic regeneration and prevent the development of neutropenia.

Resolution of Emergency Hematopoiesis

Resolution of emergency hematopoiesis and the return of HSCs to quiescence is critical to hematopoietic system function. TGF-β1 in particular has been shown to be a critical inducer of HSC quiescence (Sitnicka et al. 1996; Batard et al. 2000), and within the BM niche megakaryocytes are the dominant source of TGF-β1 and play an important role in maintaining quiescence under steady state conditions (Zhao et al. 2014b). In response to myeloablative chemotherapy, TGF-β1 secreted by megakaryocytes is critical to resolving hematopoietic regeneration and restoring HSC quiescence (Hérault et al. 2017). In the context of type 1 IFN signaling, the response to acute stimulation causes HSCs to become desensitized and no longer competent to respond to further IFN signaling (Pietras et al. 2014). Similarly, activation of STAT3 during emergency hematopoiesis leads to the up-regulation of its own negative regulator, suppressor of cytokine signaling 3 (SOCS3), which desensitizes the cells to further stimulation and terminates the response (Kimura et al. 2004). The restoration of interferon regulatory factor 8 (IRF8) activity in GMPs is also critical to reestablishing normal function and resolving emergency hematopoiesis (Hu et al. 2016). In addition, it appears that repopulation of mature hematopoietic cells in the BM is required to restore homeostatic conditions as loss of BM neutrophils on its own is sufficient to drive emergency hematopoiesis (Cain et al. 2011; Hérault et al. 2017). Although dispensable for steady state hematopoiesis, Fanconi anemia (FA) pathway proteins are also critical for emergency hematopoiesis responses and the rapid proliferation of GMPs (Hu et al. 2013). In the absence of these proteins, DNA damage leads to TP53-dependent apoptosis, and HSCs become exhausted because of their inability to effectively mount an emergency hematopoiesis response leading to aplastic anemia (Hu et al. 2018). Restoration of cell viability, however, increases the population of mature granulocytes within the BM niche and resolves the regenerative response (Hu et al. 2018). In response to chronic inflammation, the normal regulatory processes that control HSC activation and their return to quiescence can fail. Although HSCs are normally protected from chronic IFN signaling by returning to quiescence (Pietras et al. 2014), when negative regulators of IFN signaling are abrogated, HSCs experience chronic IFN exposure, remain cycling, and eventually exhaust (Hartner et al. 2009; Sato et al. 2009). Similarly, chronic low-level activation of TLR signaling leads to a myeloid bias and loss of reconstitution potential of HSCs in a manner reminiscent of aging (Esplin et al. 2011). Indeed, the phenotypes associated with aging of the hematopoietic system are driven by chronic low-grade inflammation (Kovtonyuk et al. 2016). Collectively, the negative regulators that terminate emergency hematopoiesis are as critical to maintaining HSC function, as the initiators of the regenerative response.

 Cite this article as *Cold Spring Harb Perspect Med* doi: 10.1101/cshperspect.a035519

HEMATOPOIETIC MALIGNANCY

The architecture of the hematopoietic system is inherently tumor-suppressive, with self-renewal capacity restricted to tightly regulate the size of the HSC pool, and unidirectional differentiation leading to the elimination of acquired oncogenic mutation in non-self-renewing cells. Furthermore, the small size of the HSC population and their largely quiescent cell state makes oncogenic mutation events unlikely. However, malignant transformation does occur, with transformed disease-initiating leukemic stem cells (LSCs) acquiring both dysregulated self-renewal and unbalanced or impaired differentiation and often an activated, highly proliferative, regenerative state (Fig. 3). This occurs through the expansion of the HSC population with accumulated somatic mutations that drive proliferation and block differentiation and the acquisition of self-renewal capacity in downstream progenitors (Passegue et al. 2003; Attolini et al. 2010; Altrock et al. 2015). Although the cell of origin remains an active area of research in the hematological malignancy field, the study of steady state and emergency hematopoiesis in native conditions has significant relevance for understanding the events of transformation and their consequences. The mechanisms that regulate HSC quiescence and limit self-renewal are inherently tumor-suppressive and, conversely, those pathways that drive HSC and progenitor expansion in response to stress are oncogenic in the context of malignant transformation. Furthermore, given that emergency hematopoiesis can dynamically alter self-renewal and differentiation phenotypes, reviewing how these processes promote disease initiation and progression during leukemogenesis is of significant value to the study of hematological malignancies.

Dysregulated Self-Renewal in Clonal Hematopoiesis and Malignancy

HSC self-renewal is normally tightly regulated, intrinsically and extrinsically, for the lifelong fitness of the blood system, and mutations causing dysregulation of self-renewal, alone or in conjunction with additional driver mutations, often lead to the development of malignancy. DNA damage associated with replication and mitosis is normally suppressed by HSCs staying largely in a quiescent state and only cycling roughly every 40 weeks in humans (Ito et al. 2004; Rossi et al. 2007; Mohrin et al. 2010; Catlin et al. 2011; Flach et al. 2014). However, upon aging, the toll of replicative stress and the lifelong usage of the error-prone NHEJ DNA repair pathway causes HSCs to accumulate somatic mutations (Mohrin et al. 2010; Flach et al. 2014). When these mutated HSCs acquire increased fitness, they expand in a phenomenon termed age-related clonal hematopoiesis (ARCH) (Young et al. 2016). ARCH is defined as the disproportionate expansion of single HSC clones relative to other clones, without the significant dysplasia or cytopenia associated with myelodysplastic syndromes (MDSs) (Bowman et al. 2018). In this manner, ARCH represents both somatic mutations in HSCs and the clear dysregulation of HSC homeostasis independent of clinically significant effects on hematopoietic output. Studies from either healthy cohorts or patients with cancer, type 2 diabetes, or cardiovascular disease show that ARCH has a clear correlation with aging and development of hematological malignancy, indicating that antecedent ARCH can progress to hematological malignancy. However, the frequency of malignant transformation is very low (~4%) and the relevance of ARCH in malignant transformation is still not fully understood despite the fact that ARCH incidence is higher in cancer patients (Busque et al. 2012; Genovese et al. 2014; Jaiswal et al. 2014, 2017; Xie et al. 2014; Buscarlet et al. 2017; Coombs et al. 2017; Takahashi et al. 2017). An unbiased sequencing study using 2700 germline control blood samples from 11 cancer types identified ARCH-associated recurrent mutations in DNA methyltransferase 3A (*DNMT3A*), *TET2*, Janus kinase 2 (*JAK2*), additional sex-comb like-1 (*ASXL1*), splicing factor 3B subunit 1 (*SF3B1*), protein phosphatase, Mg^{2+}/Mn^{2+}-dependent 1D (*PPM1D*), and tumor protein p53 (*TP53*), which are all known to be mutated in hematological malignancies such as MPN,

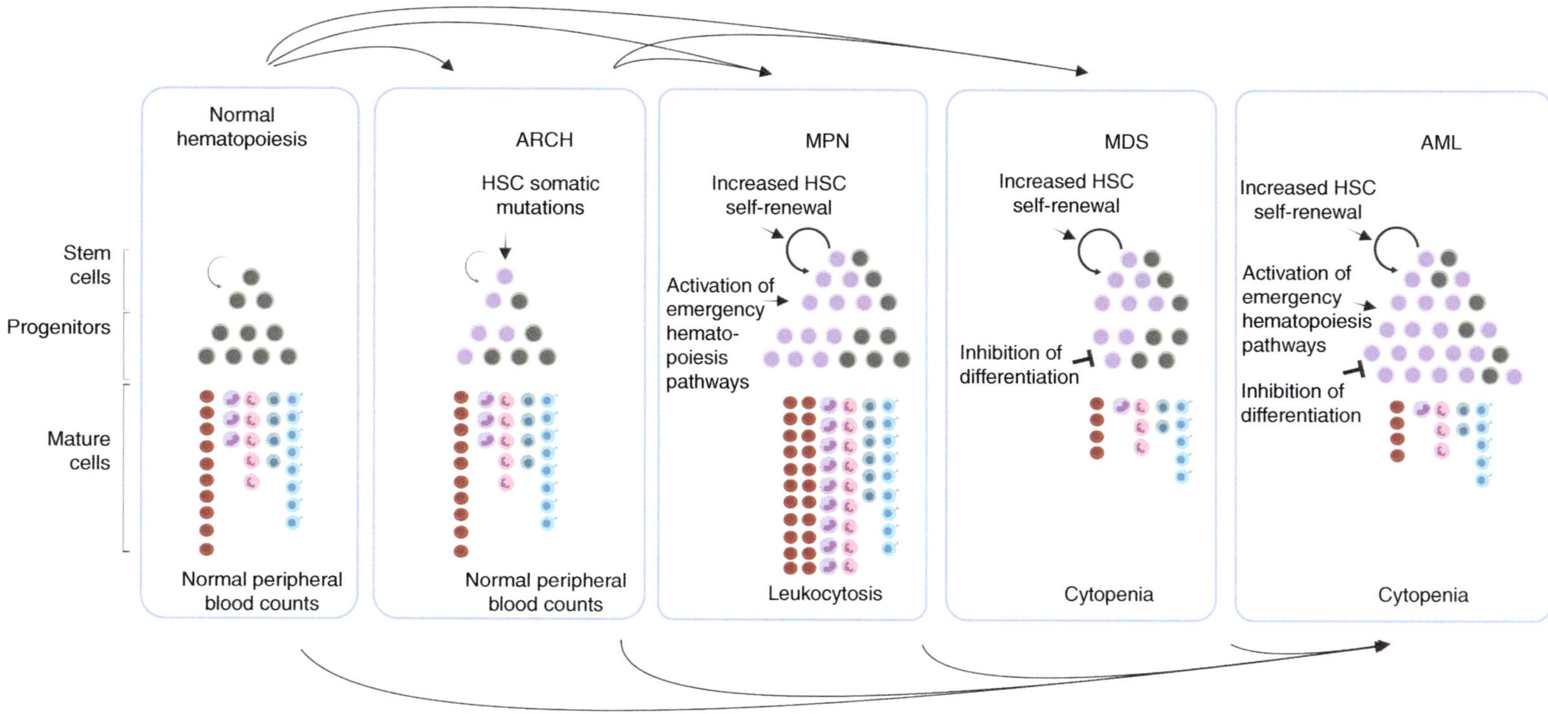

Figure 3. Dysregulation of hematopoietic stem and progenitor cell (HSPC) self-renewal and activation of regenerative pathways during malignant progression. Hematopoietic malignancy arises through the accumulation of mutations that dysregulate self-renewal, inhibit differentiation, and activate proliferation. In age-related clonal hematopoiesis (ARCH), somatic mutations cause the relative expansion of single hematopoietic stem cell (HSC) clones without obvious changes to the hematopoietic system. The accrual of mutations that activate emergency hematopoiesis pathways leads to excessive production of mature cells in myeloproliferative neoplasms (MPNs). In parallel, increased self-renewal and inhibition of differentiation cause dysplasia of the HSPC compartment and mature cell cytopenias in myelodysplastic syndromes (MDSs). In acute myeloid leukemia (AML), both activation of emergency hematopoiesis pathways and inhibition of differentiation combine to drive aggressive proliferation and expansion of leukemic blasts. Although there is evidence that malignant disease can progress in a stepwise manner, MPN, MDS, and AML can also arise de novo from normal hematopoiesis, and ARCH can likely progress directly to AML.

Cite this article as *Cold Spring Harb Perspect Med* doi: 10.1101/cshperspect.a035519

MDS, and AML (Rampal et al. 2014; Xie et al. 2014; Lindsley et al. 2017). In the case of mutations in epigenetic modifiers such as *DNMT3A*, *TET2*, and *ASXL1*, these mutations can provide selective advantages over nonmutated clones by enhancing self-renewal and blocking differentiation (Tadokoro et al. 2007; Moran-Crusio et al. 2011; Quivoron et al. 2011; Abdel-Wahab et al. 2013; Challen et al. 2014). Alternatively, mutations in DNA damage regulators such as *TP53* and *PPM1D* can provide fitness advantage under conditions of genotoxic stress and drive clonal enrichment (Marusyk et al. 2010; Hsu et al. 2018). In this manner, accumulated mutations which favor competitive fitness, either through increased self-renewal or resistance to genotoxic stress, lead to clonal expansion and predisposition to malignant transformation. Indeed, ARCH progression to a lethal MPN and AML can be modeled in the mouse by sequential activation of *DNMT3A* and *NPM1* mutations (Loberg et al. 2019).

Epigenetic modifiers, in particular, are known to regulate HSC self-renewal, and their mutation promotes malignant transformation. Knocking out *DNMT3A/B* in mice results in decreased HSC self-renewal (Tadokoro et al. 2007), and loss of *DNMT3A* alone can drive HSC expansion and both lymphoid and myeloid leukemia upon aging (Challen et al. 2014). Similarly, conditional *TET2* loss-of-function (LOF) mutation also leads to HSPC expansion (Moran-Crusio et al. 2011; Quivoron et al. 2011). HSC metabolism, integral to epigenetic remodeling, is also dysregulated in malignancy. LSCs rely on OXPHOS, resembling activated HSCs and downstream progenitors more than quiescent HSCs (Lagadinou et al. 2013; Wang et al. 2014). Mutations in the TCA enzymes isocitrate dehydrogenase 1 and 2 (*IDH1/2*), lead to the production of the onco-metabolite 2-hydroxygluterate (2HG), which inhibits TET2 and thereby impairs differentiation and increases LSC self-renewal (Dang et al. 2009; Figueroa et al. 2010; Lu et al. 2012). Of note, *IDH1/2* and *TET2* mutations are mutually exclusive, indicating their redundant role in regulating differentiation and self-renewal in malignancy (Figueroa et al. 2010).

The BM niche also has important roles in the development of malignancy through its regulation of LSC self-renewal. Extrinsic signaling pathways controlling HSC self-renewal and differentiation such as Wnt, Notch, and Hh lead to the development of hematological malignancies when their activity is dysregulated. This occurs either through the constitutive activation of the pathways by mutation or epigenetic alteration (Irvine and Copland 2012; Lobry et al. 2014; Staal et al. 2016) or by remodeling the BM niche into a tumor-promoting state (Schepers et al. 2015). Mildly increased Wnt activity enhances HSC repopulating activity (Luis et al. 2011) and the canonical Wnt signaling transducer β-catenin is critical for LSC activity in both chronic myelogenous leukemia (CML) and AML mouse models (Zhao et al. 2007; Wang et al. 2010). Loss of β-catenin can prevent disease onset in a retroviral *HOXA9* and *MEIS1* overexpression model of AML, indicating dysregulated Wnt activity is required for malignancy (Wang et al. 2010). Additionally, a high level of nuclear β-catenin is found in GMPs from blast crisis and an imatinib-resistant CML patient and is shown to engage a self-renewal circuit in GMPs and drive GMP cluster formation in both regenerative and leukemic contexts (Jamieson et al. 2004; Wang et al. 2010; Hérault et al. 2017). Hypermethylation of several Wnt antagonist genes is also observed in the BM of AML patient samples, explaining in part the high Wnt activity in leukemic conditions (Valencia et al. 2009). Notch signaling can be either an oncogene or a tumor suppressor depending on cellular contexts. In a lymphoid malignancy such as T-cell acute lymphoblastic leukemia (T-ALL), B-chronic lymphocytic leukemia (B-CLL), or splenic marginal zone lymphoma, Notch signaling functions as an oncogene, whereas in a myeloid malignancy such as chronic myelomonocytic leukemia (CMML) or AML, it functions as a tumor suppressor (Lobry et al. 2014). LOF mutations in Notch pathway genes are found in CMML patient samples (Klinakis et al. 2011), and reduced Notch activity is observed in AML blast cells (Kannan et al. 2013). Hh signaling is also involved in both myeloid and lymphoid malignancy (Irvine and Copland 2012). Loss of Hh signaling impairs HSC self-renewal and reduces the onset of CML driven by *BCR-ABL*, with sustained activation leading to HSC exhaustion (Zhao et al. 2009). Mutations in Hh pathway genes are also found in T-ALL patients (Burns et al. 2018). Taken together, impaired self-renewal by intrinsically accumulated mutations and/or dysregulated external signaling pathways leads to malignant transformation in a context-dependent manner.

Activation of Regenerative Pathways in Malignancy

In hematological malignancies, mutations conferring clonal fitness advantages, such as *DNMT3A* and *TET2*, often synergize with oncogenic mutations that drive proliferation, thereby driving clonal expansion of transformed malignant LSCs in a manner that disrupts the balancing act between self-renewal and regeneration. The fact that dysregulated HSC self-renewal can result in ARCH without leukemia development further shows the importance of additional regenerative signaling in driving malignant transformation. In fact, *TET2* mutations require microbial-driven inflammatory signals to activate an emergency hematopoietic response and induce preleukemic myeloproliferation, or additional *FLT3*, *JAK2*, or *NRAS* mutations to develop myeloid leukemia (Ortmann et al. 2015; Shih et al. 2015; Kunimoto et al. 2018; Meisel et al. 2018). In adult AML patients, *TET2* mutation co-occurs with *FLT3* mutation along with hypermutation in many loci or with loss of Notch signaling (Lobry et al. 2013; Shih et al. 2015). Similarly, *FLT3* and RAS signaling pathways are comutated with *DNMT3A* (Cancer Genome Atlas Research et al. 2013; Papaemmanuil et al. 2016). Although in normal hematopoiesis HSC self-renewal and continuous proliferation are mutually exclusive, in malignancy LSCs are able to achieve both by dysregulating differentiation.

Oncogenic mutations that drive leukemia often activate pathways involved in hematopoietic regeneration. The BCR-ABL fusion oncogene, a constitutively active tyrosine kinase, interacts with multiple downstream signaling pathways such as JAK/STAT and Ras/MAPK/ERK (Cilloni and Saglio 2012), resulting in the transformation of HSCs in a manner analogous to permanent activation of emergency hematopoiesis. Indeed, GMP clusters, a hallmark of emergency myelopoiesis, can be found in the BM of a CML mouse model (Hérault et al. 2017). *JAK2* mutations are also commonly found in hematologic malignancies and lead to the constitutive activation of regenerative signaling pathways in a ligand-independent manner (Baxter et al. 2005; James et al. 2005; Kralovics et al. 2005; Levine et al. 2005). As discussed in the context of normal hematopoiesis, the chronic activation of regenerative pathways and the increased proliferation of HSCs is detrimental to their genomic stability, and the same is true for LSCs. BCR-ABL-mediated signaling is associated with defective DNA repair and inhibition of apoptosis, leading to additional mutations and further genomic instability, which may in part explain the aggressiveness of advanced blast crisis CML (Calabretta and Perrotti 2004). Similarly, receptor tyrosine kinase *FLT3* internal tandem duplications, found in one-third of AML patients, induce aberrant STAT5 signaling and confer factor-independent proliferation and radio resistance and enhance leukemogenesis in vivo (Hayakawa et al. 2000; Mizuki et al. 2000). Mutations in the key lymphoid transcription factor *IKZF1* found in blast crisis CML, ALL, AML, and MDS also reduce apoptosis, enhance survival, and impair lymphoid differentiation, thereby contributing to leukemogenesis (Mullighan et al. 2008; John and Ward 2011; Gowda et al. 2017). *Nras*^{G12D} promotes HSC survival under ER stress by activating the IRE1α-XBP1 axis through the MAPK pathway and inhibiting IRE1α-XBP1 activation decreases the competitive advantage of *NRAS*^{G12D} HSCs in transplantation (Liu et al. 2019) confirming that mutations altering regenerative capacity can lead to leukemic transformation. Collectively, mutations that dysregulate HSC self-renewal synergize with mutations that drive a regenerative and proliferative response and together transition the hematopoietic system into a state of malignancy.

 Cite this article as *Cold Spring Harb Perspect Med* doi: 10.1101/cshperspect.a035519

CONCLUSION

The hematopoietic system continuously regenerates to meet blood production needs of the organism. For this reason, the protection of HSCs is critical to the lifelong function of the hematopoietic system and this is achieved, in part, through their location in a hypoxic and quiescence-enforcing BM niche microenvironment. The suppression of mitochondrial aerobic respiration in quiescent HSCs, in particular, is an important part of this privileged state. Quiescent HSCs, however, are not invulnerable and the rapid repair of DNA damage through error-prone DNA repair mechanisms makes these cells susceptible to mutation accumulation and functional decline. The activation of HSCs is driven by the metabolic switch to OXPHOS, which controls both the proliferation as well as the epigenetic remodeling and differentiation of HSCs. Indeed, the intersection of metabolism and epigenetics in stem cell biology is an area of active research with the potential to greatly enhance our understanding of hematopoiesis. HSC activation is largely driven by inflammatory cytokines, which coordinate the regenerative response and reprogram the hematopoietic system to produce the required number of mature effector cells for homeostasis and response to physiologic insults. In contrast, much less is known about the return of HSCs to quiescence and the development of quiescence-enforcing therapeutic strategies will be critical to improving hematopoietic function and longevity.

The hematopoietic system normally balance regeneration with HSC self-renewal and, when these two functions are no longer kept at cross purposes, the result is malignancy. New single-cell technologies are set to drive a period of rapid discovery and increase our resolution in the study of HSCs, their multiple cellular states, and the transition between them. This biology is critically relevant for understanding malignancy, and although it was long thought that highly quiescent LSCs drive therapeutic resistance and relapse, it has recently been shown that in fact LSCs become activated in response to the inflammatory environment of therapeutic treatment and initiate a regenerative response (Boyd et al. 2018). This response of LSCs to chemotherapeutic treatment is very similar to that of normal HSCs and shows how our understanding of native hematopoiesis can inform the study and treatment of cancer. With a better understanding of the processes by which normal HSCs return to quiescence, we may in fact be able to develop strategies that enforce quiescence in LSCs and normalize disease. Conversely, our understanding of the mechanisms of HSC activation can be leveraged to develop therapeutic strategies that activate latent reservoirs of quiescent LSCs and enforce their differentiation and exhaustion. Indeed, the success of current therapies likely result from these principles. Redundant and multifactorial signaling pathways that stimulate regeneration allow the body to tailor hematopoietic output with precision. However, in the context of malignancy this redundancy of signaling helps explain why therapeutic development has been so difficult in the context acute leukemias. Further study of normal hematopoiesis will hopefully identify core biology and provide new insight into specific dependencies of hematopoietic regeneration that can serve as therapeutic targets to normalize or eliminate malignant disease.

ACKNOWLEDGMENTS

O.C.O. is supported by National Institutes of Health (NIH) T32HL120826, and Y.-A.K. by a Leukemia & Lymphoma Society (LLS) Special Fellowship. This work was supported by NIH grant 1R35HL135763 to E.P. The authors have no conflicts of interest to disclose.

REFERENCES

Abdel-Wahab O, Gao J, Adli M, Dey A, Trimarchi T, Chung YR, Kuscu C, Hricik T, Ndiaye-Lobry D, Lafave LM, et al. 2013. Deletion of Asxl1 results in myelodysplasia and severe developmental defects in vivo. *J Exp Med* **210:** 2641–2659.

Akashi K, Traver D, Miyamoto T, Weissman IL. 2000. A clonogenic common myeloid progenitor that gives rise to all myeloid lineages. *Nature* **404:** 193–197. doi:10.1038/35004599

Altrock PM, Liu LL, Michor F. 2015. The mathematics of cancer: integrating quantitative models. *Nat Rev Cancer* **15:** 730–745. doi:10.1038/nrc4029

Ara T, Tokoyoda K, Sugiyama T, Egawa T, Kawabata K, Nagasawa T. 2003. Long-term hematopoietic stem cells require stromal cell-derived factor-1 for colonizing bone marrow during ontogeny. *Immunity* **19:** 257–267. doi:10.1016/S1074-7613(03)00201-2

Arai F, Hirao A, Ohmura M, Sato H, Matsuoka S, Takubo K, Ito K, Koh GY, Suda T. 2004. Tie2/angiopoietin-1 signaling regulates hematopoietic stem cell quiescence in the bone marrow niche. *Cell* **118:** 149–161. doi:10.1016/j.cell.2004.07.004

Asai T, Liu Y, Bae N, Nimer SD. 2011. The p53 tumor suppressor protein regulates hematopoietic stem cell fate. *J Cell Physiol* **226:** 2215–2221. doi:10.1002/jcp.22561

Attolini CS, Cheng YK, Beroukhim R, Getz G, Abdel-Wahab O, Levine RL, Mellinghoff IK, Michor F. 2010. A mathematical framework to determine the temporal sequence of somatic genetic events in cancer. *Proc Natl Acad Sci* **107:** 17604–17609. doi:10.1073/pnas.1009117107

Bakker ST, Passegué E. 2013. Resilient and resourceful: genome maintenance strategies in hematopoietic stem cells. *Exp Hematol* **41:** 915–923. doi:10.1016/j.exphem.2013.09.007

Baldridge MT, King KY, Boles NC, Weksberg DC, Goodell MA. 2010. Quiescent haematopoietic stem cells are activated by IFN-γ in response to chronic infection. *Nature* **465:** 793–797. doi:10.1038/nature09135

Baldridge MT, King KY, Goodell MA. 2011. Inflammatory signals regulate hematopoietic stem cells. *Trends Immunol* **32:** 57–65. doi:10.1016/j.it.2010.12.003

Batard P, Monier MN, Fortunel N, Ducos K, Sansilvestri-Morel P, Phan T, Hatzfeld A, Hatzfeld JA. 2000. TGF-β1 maintains hematopoietic immaturity by a reversible negative control of cell cycle and induces CD34 antigen up-modulation. *J Cell Sci* **113:** 383–390.

Baxter EJ, Scott LM, Campbell PJ, East C, Fourouclas N, Swanton S, Vassiliou GS, Bench AJ, Boyd EM, Curtin N, et al. 2005. Acquired mutation of the tyrosine kinase JAK2 in human myeloproliferative disorders. *Lancet* **365:** 1054–1061. doi:10.1016/S0140-6736(05)71142-9

Becker AJ, McCulloch EA, Till JE. 1963. Cytological demonstration of the clonal nature of spleen colonies derived from transplanted mouse marrow cells. *Nature* **197:** 452–454. doi:10.1038/197452a0

Becker AJ, McCulloch EA, Siminovitch L, Till JE. 1965. The effect of differing demands for blood cell production on DNA synthesis by hemopoietic colony-forming cells of mice. *Blood* **26:** 296–308. doi:10.1182/blood.V26.3.296.296

Biechonski S, Yassin M, Milyavsky M. 2017. DNA-damage response in hematopoietic stem cells: an evolutionary trade-off between blood regeneration and leukemia suppression. *Carcinogenesis* **38:** 367–377. doi:10.1093/carcin/bgx002

Bock C, Beerman I, Lien WH, Smith ZD, Gu H, Boyle P, Gnirke A, Fuchs E, Rossi DJ, Meissner A. 2012. DNA methylation dynamics during in vivo differentiation of blood and skin stem cells. *Mol Cell* **47:** 633–647. doi:10.1016/j.molcel.2012.06.019

Boettcher S, Ziegler P, Schmid MA, Takizawa H, van Rooijen N, Kopf M, Heikenwalder M, Manz MG. 2012. Cutting edge: LPS-induced emergency myelopoiesis depends on TLR4-expressing nonhematopoietic cells. *J Immunol* **188:** 5824–5828. doi:10.4049/jimmunol.1103253

Boettcher S, Gerosa RC, Radpour R, Bauer J, Ampenberger F, Heikenwalder M, Kopf M, Manz MG. 2014. Endothelial cells translate pathogen signals into G-CSF-driven emergency granulopoiesis. *Blood* **124:** 1393–1403. doi:10.1182/blood-2014-04-570762

Bowman RL, Busque L, Levine RL. 2018. Clonal hematopoiesis and evolution to hematopoietic malignancies. *Cell Stem Cell* **22:** 157–170. doi:10.1016/j.stem.2018.01.011

Boyd AL, Aslostovar L, Reid J, Ye W, Tanasijevic B, Porras DP, Shapovalova Z, Almakadi M, Foley R, Leber B, et al. 2018. Identification of chemotherapy-induced leukemic-regenerating cells reveals a transient vulnerability of human AML recurrence. *Cancer Cell* **34:** 483–498 e5. doi:10.1016/j.ccell.2018.08.007

Bruce WR, Meeker BE, Valeriote FA. 1966. Comparison of the sensitivity of normal hematopoietic and transplanted lymphoma colony-forming cells to chemotherapeutic agents administered in vivo. *J Natl Cancer Inst* **37:** 233–245.

Burns MA, Liao ZW, Yamagata N, Pouliot GP, Stevenson KE, Neuberg DS, Thorner AR, Ducar M, Silverman EA, Hunger SP, et al. 2018. Hedgehog pathway mutations drive oncogenic transformation in high-risk T-cell acute lymphoblastic leukemia. *Leukemia* **32:** 2126–2137. doi:10.1038/s41375-018-0097-x

Buscarlet M, Provost S, Zada YF, Barhdadi A, Bourgoin V, Lépine G, Mollica L, Szuber N, Dubé MP, Busque L. 2017. *DNMT3A* and *TET2* dominate clonal hematopoiesis and demonstrate benign phenotypes and different genetic predispositions. *Blood* **130:** 753–762. doi:10.1182/blood-2017-04-777029

Busch K, Klapproth K, Barile M, Flossdorf M, Holland-Letz T, Schlenner SM, Reth M, Höfer T, Rodewald HR. 2015. Fundamental properties of unperturbed haematopoiesis from stem cells in vivo. *Nature* **518:** 542–546. doi:10.1038/nature14242

Busque L, Patel JP, Figueroa ME, Vasanthakumar A, Provost S, Hamilou Z, Mollica L, Li J, Viale A, Heguy A, et al. 2012. Recurrent somatic *TET2* mutations in normal elderly individuals with clonal hematopoiesis. *Nat Genet* **44:** 1179–1181. doi:10.1038/ng.2413

Cabezas-Wallscheid N, Klimmeck D, Hansson J, Lipka DB, Reyes A, Wang Q, Weichenhan D, Lier A, von Paleske L, Renders S, et al. 2014. Identification of regulatory networks in HSCs and their immediate progeny via integrated proteome, transcriptome, and DNA methylome analysis. *Cell Stem Cell* **15:** 507–522. doi:10.1016/j.stem.2014.07.005

Cain DW, Snowden PB, Sempowski GD, Kelsoe G. 2011. Inflammation triggers emergency granulopoiesis through a density-dependent feedback mechanism. *PLoS ONE* **6:** e19957. doi:10.1371/journal.pone.0019957

Calabretta B, Perrotti D. 2004. The biology of CML blast crisis. *Blood* **103:** 4010–4022. doi:10.1182/blood-2003-12-4111

Cancer Genome Atlas Research Network, Ley TJ, Miller C, Ding L, Raphael BJ, Mungall AJ, Robertson A, Hoadley K, Triche TJ Jr, Laird PW, et al. 2013. Genomic and epigenomic landscapes of adult de novo acute myeloid leukemia. *N Engl J Med* **368:** 2059–2074. doi:10.1056/NEJMoa1301689

Carracedo A, Cantley LC, Pandolfi PP. 2013. Cancer metabolism: fatty acid oxidation in the limelight. *Nat Rev Cancer* **13:** 227–232. doi:10.1038/nrc3483

Catlin SN, Busque L, Gale RE, Guttorp P, Abkowitz JL. 2011. The replication rate of human hematopoietic stem cells in vivo. *Blood* **117:** 4460–4466. doi:10.1182/blood-2010-08-303537

Cebon J, Layton JE, Maher D, Morstyn G. 1994. Endogenous haemopoietic growth factors in neutropenia and infection. *Br J Haematol* **86:** 265–274. doi:10.1111/j.1365-2141.1994.tb04725.x

Challen GA, Boles NC, Chambers SM, Goodell MA. 2010. Distinct hematopoietic stem cell subtypes are differentially regulated by TGF-β1. *Cell Stem Cell* **6:** 265–278. doi:10.1016/j.stem.2010.02.002

Challen GA, Sun D, Mayle A, Jeong M, Luo M, Rodriguez B, Mallaney C, Celik H, Yang L, Xia Z, et al. 2014. *Dnmt3a* and *Dnmt3b* have overlapping and distinct functions in hematopoietic stem cells. *Cell Stem Cell* **15:** 350–364. doi:10.1016/j.stem.2014.06.018

Chandel NS, Jasper H, Ho TT, Passegué E. 2016. Metabolic regulation of stem cell function in tissue homeostasis and organismal ageing. *Nat Cell Biol* **18:** 823–832. doi:10.1038/ncb3385

Cheers C, Haigh AM, Kelso A, Metcalf D, Stanley ER, Young AM. 1988. Production of colony-stimulating factors (CSFs) during infection: separate determinations of macrophage-, granulocyte-, granulocyte-macrophage-, and multi-CSFs. *Infect Immun* **56:** 247–251.

Cilloni D, Saglio G. 2012. Molecular pathways: BCR-ABL. *Clin Cancer Res* **18:** 930–937. doi:10.1158/1078-0432.CCR-10-1613

Coombs CC, Zehir A, Devlin SM, Kishtagari A, Syed A, Jonsson P, Hyman DM, Solit DB, Robson ME, Baselga J, et al. 2017. Therapy-related clonal hematopoiesis in patients with non-hematologic cancers is common and associated with adverse clinical outcomes. *Cell Stem Cell* **21:** 374–382 e4. doi:10.1016/j.stem.2017.07.010

Crane GM, Jeffery E, Morrison SJ. 2017. Adult haematopoietic stem cell niches. *Nat Rev Immunol* **17:** 573–590. doi:10.1038/nri.2017.53

Dancey JT, Deubelbeiss KA, Harker LA, Finch CA. 1976. Neutrophil kinetics in man. *J Clin Invest* **58:** 705–715. doi:10.1172/JCI108517

Dang L, White DW, Gross S, Bennett BD, Bittinger MA, Driggers EM, Fantin VR, Jang HG, Jin S, Keenan MC, et al. 2009. Cancer-associated IDH1 mutations produce 2-hydroxyglutarate. *Nature* **462:** 739–744. doi:10.1038/nature08617

Ding L, Saunders TL, Enikolopov G, Morrison SJ. 2012. Endothelial and perivascular cells maintain haematopoietic stem cells. *Nature* **481:** 457–462. doi:10.1038/nature10783

Doulatov S, Notta F, Laurenti E, Dick JE. 2012. Hematopoiesis: a human perspective. *Cell Stem Cell* **10:** 120–136. doi:10.1016/j.stem.2012.01.006

Duncan AW, Rattis FM, DiMascio LN, Congdon KL, Pazianos G, Zhao C, Yoon K, Cook JM, Willert K, Gaiano N, et al. 2005. Integration of Notch and Wnt signaling in hematopoietic stem cell maintenance. *Nat Immunol* **6:** 314–322. doi:10.1038/ni1164

Dykstra B, Kent D, Bowie M, McCaffrey L, Hamilton M, Lyons K, Lee SJ, Brinkman R, Eaves C. 2007. Long-term propagation of distinct hematopoietic differentiation programs in vivo. *Cell Stem Cell* **1:** 218–229. doi:10.1016/j.stem.2007.05.015

Esplin BL, Shimazu T, Welner RS, Garrett KP, Nie L, Zhang Q, Humphrey MB, Yang Q, Borghesi LA, Kincade PW. 2011. Chronic exposure to a TLR ligand injures hematopoietic stem cells. *J Immunol* **186:** 5367–5375. doi:10.4049/jimmunol.1003438

Essers MA, Offner S, Blanco-Bose WE, Waibler Z, Kalinke U, Duchosal MA, Trumpp A. 2009. IFNα activates dormant haematopoietic stem cells in vivo. *Nature* **458:** 904–908. doi:10.1038/nature07815

Farlik M, Halbritter F, Müller F, Choudry FA, Ebert P, Klughammer J, Farrow S, Santoro A, Ciaurro V, Mathur A, et al. 2016. DNA methylation dynamics of human hematopoietic stem cell differentiation. *Cell Stem Cell* **19:** 808–822. doi:10.1016/j.stem.2016.10.019

Figueroa ME, Abdel-Wahab O, Lu C, Ward PS, Patel J, Shih A, Li Y, Bhagwat N, Vasanthakumar A, Fernandez HF, et al. 2010. Leukemic *IDH1* and *IDH2* mutations result in a hypermethylation phenotype, disrupt TET2 function, and impair hematopoietic differentiation. *Cancer Cell* **18:** 553–567. doi:10.1016/j.ccr.2010.11.015

Flach J, Bakker ST, Mohrin M, Conroy PC, Pietras EM, Reynaud D, Alvarez S, Diolaiti ME, Ugarte F, Forsberg EC, et al. 2014. Replication stress is a potent driver of functional decline in ageing haematopoietic stem cells. *Nature* **512:** 198–202. doi:10.1038/nature13619

Ford CE, Hamerton JL, Barnes DW, Loutit JF. 1956. Cytological identification of radiation-chimaeras. *Nature* **177:** 452–454. doi:10.1038/177452a0

Foudi A, Hochedlinger K, Van Buren D, Schindler JW, Jaenisch R, Carey V, Hock H. 2009. Analysis of histone 2B-GFP retention reveals slowly cycling hematopoietic stem cells. *Nat Biotechnol* **27:** 84–90. doi:10.1038/nbt.1517

Furze RC, Rankin SM. 2008. The role of the bone marrow in neutrophil clearance under homeostatic conditions in the mouse. *FASEB J* **22:** 3111–3119. doi:10.1096/fj.08-109876

Gan B, Hu J, Jiang S, Liu Y, Sahin E, Zhuang L, Fletcher-Sananikone E, Colla S, Wang YA, Chin L, et al. 2010. Lkb1 regulates quiescence and metabolic homeostasis of haematopoietic stem cells. *Nature* **468:** 701–704. doi:10.1038/nature09595

Genovese G, Kähler AK, Handsaker RE, Lindberg J, Rose SA, Bakhoum SF, Chambert K, Mick E, Neale BM, Fromer M, et al. 2014. Clonal hematopoiesis and blood-cancer risk inferred from blood DNA sequence. *N Engl J Med* **371:** 2477–2487. doi:10.1056/NEJMoa1409405

Gentles AJ, Plevritis SK, Majeti R, Alizadeh AA. 2010. Association of a leukemic stem cell gene expression signature with clinical outcomes in acute myeloid leukemia. *J Am Med Assoc* **304:** 2706–2715. doi:10.1001/jama.2010.1862

Goodell MA, Brose K, Paradis G, Conner AS, Mulligan RC. 1996. Isolation and functional properties of murine hematopoietic stem cells that are replicating in vivo. *J Exp Med* **183:** 1797–1806. doi:10.1084/jem.183.4.1797

Gowda C, Song C, Kapadia M, Payne JL, Hu T, Ding Y, Dovat S. 2017. Regulation of cellular proliferation in acute lymphoblastic leukemia by casein kinase II (CK2) and Ikaros. *Adv Biol Regul* **63:** 71–80. doi:10.1016/j.jbior.2016.09.003

Gurumurthy S, Xie SZ, Alagesan B, Kim J, Yusuf RZ, Saez B, Tzatsos A, Ozsolak F, Milos P, Ferrari F, et al. 2010. The Lkb1 metabolic sensor maintains haematopoietic stem cell survival. *Nature* **468:** 659–663. doi:10.1038/nature09572

Haas S, Hansson J, Klimmeck D, Loeffler D, Velten L, Uckelmann H, Wurzer S, Prendergast AM, Schnell A, Hexel K, et al. 2015. Inflammation-induced emergency megakaryopoiesis driven by hematopoietic stem cell-like megakaryocyte progenitors. *Cell Stem Cell* **17:** 422–434. doi:10.1016/j.stem.2015.07.007

Hartner JC, Walkley CR, Lu J, Orkin SH. 2009. ADAR1 is essential for the maintenance of hematopoiesis and suppression of interferon signaling. *Nat Immunol* **10:** 109–115. doi:10.1038/ni.1680

Hayakawa F, Towatari M, Kiyoi H, Tanimoto M, Kitamura T, Saito H, Naoe T. 2000. Tandem-duplicated Flt3 constitutively activates STAT5 and MAP kinase and introduces autonomous cell growth in IL-3-dependent cell lines. *Oncogene* **19:** 624–631. doi:10.1038/sj.onc.1203354

Hérault A, Binnewies M, Leong S, Calero-Nieto FJ, Zhang SY, Kang YA, Wang X, Pietras EM, Chu SH, Barry-Holson K, et al. 2017. Myeloid progenitor cluster formation drives emergency and leukaemic myelopoiesis. *Nature* **544:** 53–58. doi:10.1038/nature21693

Ho TT, Warr MR, Adelman ER, Lansinger OM, Flach J, Verovskaya EV, Figueroa ME, Passegué E. 2017. Autophagy maintains the metabolism and function of young and old stem cells. *Nature* **543:** 205–210. doi:10.1038/nature21388

Hsu JI, Dayaram T, Tovy A, De Braekeleer E, Jeong M, Wang F, Zhang J, Heffernan TP, Gera S, Kovacs JJ, et al. 2018. *PPM1D* mutations drive clonal hematopoiesis in response to cytotoxic chemotherapy. *Cell Stem Cell* **23:** 700–713 e6. doi:10.1016/j.stem.2018.10.004

Hu L, Huang W, Hjort E, Eklund EA. 2013. Increased Fanconi C expression contributes to the emergency granulopoiesis response. *J Clin Invest* **123:** 3952–3966. doi:10.1172/JCI69032

Hu L, Huang W, Hjort EE, Bei L, Platanias LC, Eklund EA. 2016. The interferon consensus sequence binding protein (Icsbp/Irf8) is required for termination of emergency granulopoiesis. *J Biol Chem* **291:** 4107–4120. doi:10.1074/jbc.M115.681361

Hu L, Huang W, Bei L, Broglie L, Eklund EA. 2018. *TP53* haploinsufficiency rescues emergency granulopoiesis in *FANCC*$^{-/-}$ mice. *J Immunol* **200:** 2129–2139. doi:10.4049/jimmunol.1700931

Irvine DA, Copland M. 2012. Targeting Hedgehog in hematologic malignancy. *Blood* **119:** 2196–2204. doi:10.1182/blood-2011-10-383752

Ito K, Suda T. 2014. Metabolic requirements for the maintenance of self-renewing stem cells. *Nat Rev Mol Cell Biol* **15:** 243–256. doi:10.1038/nrm3772

Ito K, Hirao A, Arai F, Matsuoka S, Takubo K, Hamaguchi I, Nomiyama K, Hosokawa K, Sakurada K, Nakagata N, et al. 2004. Regulation of oxidative stress by ATM is required for self-renewal of haematopoietic stem cells. *Nature* **431:** 997–1002. doi:10.1038/nature02989

Ito K, Hirao A, Arai F, Takubo K, Matsuoka S, Miyamoto K, Ohmura M, Naka K, Hosokawa K, Ikeda Y, et al. 2006. Reactive oxygen species act through p38 MAPK to limit the lifespan of hematopoietic stem cells. *Nat Med* **12:** 446–451. doi:10.1038/nm1388

Ito K, Carracedo A, Weiss D, Arai F, Ala U, Avigan DE, Schafer ZT, Evans RM, Suda T, Lee CH, et al. 2012. A PML-PPAR-δ pathway for fatty acid oxidation regulates hematopoietic stem cell maintenance. *Nat Med* **18:** 1350–1358. doi:10.1038/nm.2882

Ito K, Turcotte R, Cui J, Zimmerman SE, Pinho S, Mizoguchi T, Arai F, Runnels JM, Alt C, Teruya-Feldstein J, et al. 2016. Self-renewal of a purified *Tie*$^{2+}$ hematopoietic stem cell population relies on mitochondrial clearance. *Science* **354:** 1156–1160. doi:10.1126/science.aaf5530

Jacobson LO, Simmons EL, Marks EK, Eldredge JH. 1951. Recovery from radiation injury. *Science* **113:** 510–511. doi:10.1126/science.113.2940.510

Jaiswal S, Fontanillas P, Flannick J, Manning A, Grauman PV, Mar BG, Lindsley RC, Mermel CH, Burtt N, Chavez A, et al. 2014. Age-related clonal hematopoiesis associated with adverse outcomes. *N Engl J Med* **371:** 2488–2498. doi:10.1056/NEJMoa1408617

Jaiswal S, Natarajan P, Silver AJ, Gibson CJ, Bick AG, Shvartz E, McConkey M, Gupta N, Gabriel S, Ardissino D, et al. 2017. Clonal hematopoiesis and risk of atherosclerotic cardiovascular disease. *N Engl J Med* **377:** 111–121. doi:10.1056/NEJMoa1701719

James C, Ugo V, Le Couédic JP, Staerk J, Delhommeau F, Lacout C, Garçon L, Raslova H, Berger R, Bennaceur-Griscelli A, et al. 2005. A unique clonal *JAK2* mutation leading to constitutive signalling causes polycythaemia vera. *Nature* **434:** 1144–1148. doi:10.1038/nature03546

Jamieson CH, Ailles LE, Dylla SJ, Muijtjens M, Jones C, Zehnder JL, Gotlib J, Li K, Manz MG, Keating A, et al. 2004. Granulocyte-macrophage progenitors as candidate leukemic stem cells in blast-crisis CML. *N Engl J Med* **351:** 657–667. doi:10.1056/NEJMoa040258

Jang YY, Sharkis SJ. 2007. A low level of reactive oxygen species selects for primitive hematopoietic stem cells that may reside in the low-oxygenic niche. *Blood* **110:** 3056–3063. doi:10.1182/blood-2007-05-087759

John LB, Ward AC. 2011. The Ikaros gene family: transcriptional regulators of hematopoiesis and immunity. *Mol Immunol* **48:** 1272–1278. doi:10.1016/j.molimm.2011.03.006

Kannan S, Sutphin RM, Hall MG, Golfman LS, Fang W, Nolo RM, Akers LJ, Hammitt RA, McMurray JS, Kornblau SM, et al. 2013. Notch activation inhibits AML growth and survival: a potential therapeutic approach. *J Exp Med* **210:** 321–337. doi:10.1084/jem.20121527

Kapp FG, Perlin JR, Hagedorn EJ, Gansner JM, Schwarz DE, O'Connell LA, Johnson NS, Amemiya C, Fisher DE, Wölfle U, et al. 2018. Protection from UV light is an evolutionarily conserved feature of the haematopoietic niche. *Nature* **558:** 445–448. doi:10.1038/s41586-018-0213-0

Karamitros D, Stoilova B, Aboukhalil Z, Hamey F, Reinisch A, Samitsch M, Quek L, Otto G, Repapi E, Doondeea J, et al. 2018. Single-cell analysis reveals the continuum of human lympho-myeloid progenitor cells. *Nat Immunol* **19:** 85–97. doi:10.1038/s41590-017-0001-2

Kawakami M, Tsutsumi H, Kumakawa T, Abe H, Hirai M, Kurosawa S, Mori M, Fukushima M. 1990. Levels of serum granulocyte colony-stimulating factor in patients with infections. *Blood* **76:** 1962–1964. doi:10.1182/blood.V76.10.1962.1962

Kerenyi MA, Shao Z, Hsu YJ, Guo G, Luc S, O'Brien K, Fujiwara Y, Peng C, Nguyen M, Orkin SH. 2013. Histone demethylase Lsd1 represses hematopoietic stem and progenitor cell signatures during blood cell maturation. *eLife* **2:** e00633. doi:10.7554/eLife.00633

Kimura A, Kinjyo I, Matsumura Y, Mori H, Mashima R, Harada M, Chien KR, Yasukawa H, Yoshimura A. 2004. SOCS3 is a physiological negative regulator for granulopoiesis and granulocyte colony-stimulating factor receptor signaling. *J Biol Chem* **279:** 6905–6910. doi:10.1074/jbc.C300496200

Kleppe M, Spitzer MH, Li S, Hill CE, Dong L, Papalexi E, De Groote S, Bowman RL, Keller M, Koppikar P, et al. 2017. Jak1 integrates cytokine sensing to regulate hematopoietic stem cell function and stress hematopoiesis. *Cell Stem Cell* **21:** 489–501 e7. doi:10.1016/j.stem.2017.08.011

Klinakis A, Lobry C, Abdel-Wahab O, Oh P, Haeno H, Buonamici S, van De Walle I, Cathelin S, Trimarchi T, Araldi E, et al. 2011. A novel tumour-suppressor function for the Notch pathway in myeloid leukaemia. *Nature* **473:** 230–233. doi:10.1038/nature09999

Kode A, Manavalan JS, Mosialou I, Bhagat G, Rathinam CV, Luo N, Khiabanian H, Lee A, Murty VV, Friedman R, et al. 2014. Leukaemogenesis induced by an activating β-catenin mutation in osteoblasts. *Nature* **506:** 240–244. doi:10.1038/nature12883

Kondo M, Weissman IL, Akashi K. 1997. Identification of clonogenic common lymphoid progenitors in mouse bone marrow. *Cell* **91:** 661–672. doi:10.1016/S0092-8674(00)80453-5

Kovtonyuk LV, Fritsch K, Feng X, Manz MG, Takizawa H. 2016. Inflamm-aging of hematopoiesis, hematopoietic stem cells, and the bone marrow microenvironment. *Front Immunol* **7:** 502. doi:10.3389/fimmu.2016.00502

Kozar K, Ciemerych MA, Rebel VI, Shigematsu H, Zagozdzon A, Sicinska E, Geng Y, Yu Q, Bhattacharya S, Bronson RT, et al. 2004. Mouse development and cell proliferation in the absence of D-cyclins. *Cell* **118:** 477–491. doi:10.1016/j.cell.2004.07.025

Kralovics R, Passamonti F, Buser AS, Teo SS, Tiedt R, Passweg JR, Tichelli A, Cazzola M, Skoda RC. 2005. A gain-of-function mutation of *JAK2* in myeloproliferative disorders. *N Engl J Med* **352:** 1779–1790. doi:10.1056/NEJMoa051113

Kunimoto H, Meydan C, Nazir A, Whitfield J, Shank K, Rapaport F, Maher R, Pronier E, Meyer SC, Garrett-Bakelman FE, et al. 2018. Cooperative epigenetic remodeling by *TET2* loss and *NRAS* mutation drives myeloid transformation and MEK inhibitor sensitivity. *Cancer Cell* **33:** 44–59 e8. doi:10.1016/j.ccell.2017.11.012

Lagadinou ED, Sach A, Callahan K, Rossi RM, Neering SJ, Minhajuddin M, Ashton JM, Pei S, Grose V, O'Dwyer KM, et al. 2013. BCL-2 inhibition targets oxidative phosphorylation and selectively eradicates quiescent human leukemia stem cells. *Cell Stem Cell* **12:** 329–341. doi:10.1016/j.stem.2012.12.013

Laurenti E, Göttgens B. 2018. From haematopoietic stem cells to complex differentiation landscapes. *Nature* **553:** 418–426. doi:10.1038/nature25022

Levine RL, Wadleigh M, Cools J, Ebert BL, Wernig G, Huntly BJ, Boggon TJ, Wlodarska I, Clark JJ, Moore S, et al. 2005. Activating mutation in the tyrosine kinase JAK2 in polycythemia vera, essential thrombocythemia, and myeloid metaplasia with myelofibrosis. *Cancer Cell* **7:** 387–397. doi:10.1016/j.ccr.2005.03.023

Lindsley RC, Saber W, Mar BG, Redd R, Wang T, Haagenson MD, Grauman PV, Hu ZH, Spellman SR, Lee SJ, et al. 2017. Prognostic mutations in myelodysplastic syndrome after stem-cell transplantation. *N Engl J Med* **376:** 536–547. doi:10.1056/NEJMoa1611604

Liu A, Wang Y, Ding Y, Baez I, Payne KJ, Borghesi L. 2015. Cutting edge: hematopoietic stem cell expansion and common lymphoid progenitor depletion require hematopoietic-derived, cell-autonomous TLR4 in a model of chronic endotoxin. *J Immunol* **195:** 2524–2528. doi:10.4049/jimmunol.1501231

Liu L, Zhao M, Jin X, Ney G, Yang KB, Peng F, Cao J, Iwawaki T, Del Valle J, Chen X, et al. 2019. Adaptive endoplasmic reticulum stress signalling via IRE1α–XBP1 preserves self-renewal of haematopoietic and pre-leukaemic stem cells. *Nat Cell Biol* **21:** 328–337. doi:10.1038/s41556-019-0285-6

Loberg MA, Bell RK, Goodwin LO, Eudy E, Miles LA, SanMiguel JM, Young K, Bergstrom DE, Levine RL, Schneider RK, et al. 2019. Sequentially inducible mouse models reveal that *Npm1* mutation causes malignant transformation of *Dnmt3a*-mutant clonal hematopoiesis. *Leukemia* **33:** 1635–1649. doi:10.1038/s41375-018-0368-6

Lobry C, Ntziachristos P, Ndiaye-Lobry D, Oh P, Cimmino L, Zhu N, Araldi E, Hu W, Freund J, Abdel-Wahab O, et al. 2013. Notch pathway activation targets AML-initiating cell homeostasis and differentiation. *J Exp Med* **210:** 301–319. doi:10.1084/jem.20121484

Lobry C, Oh P, Mansour MR, Look AT, Aifantis I. 2014. Notch signaling: switching an oncogene to a tumor suppressor. *Blood* **123:** 2451–2459. doi:10.1182/blood-2013-08-355818

Lu C, Ward PS, Kapoor GS, Rohle D, Turcan S, Abdel-Wahab O, Edwards CR, Khanin R, Figueroa ME, Melnick A, et al. 2012. IDH mutation impairs histone demethylation and results in a block to cell differentiation. *Nature* **483:** 474–478. doi:10.1038/nature10860

Luis TC, Naber BA, Roozen PP, Brugman MH, de Haas EF, Ghazvini M, Fibbe WE, van Dongen JJ, Fodde R, Staal FJ. 2011. Canonical wnt signaling regulates hematopoiesis in a dosage-dependent fashion. *Cell Stem Cell* **9:** 345–356. doi:10.1016/j.stem.2011.07.017

Macaulay IC, Svensson V, Labalette C, Ferreira L, Hamey F, Voet T, Teichmann SA, Cvejic A. 2016. Single-cell RNA-sequencing reveals a continuous spectrum of differentiation in hematopoietic cells. *Cell Rep* **14:** 966–977. doi:10.1016/j.celrep.2015.12.082

Malumbres M, Sotillo R, Santamaria D, Galán J, Cerezo A, Ortega S, Dubus P, Barbacid M. 2004. Mammalian cells cycle without the D-type cyclin-dependent kinases Cdk4 and Cdk6. *Cell* **118:** 493–504. doi:10.1016/j.cell.2004.08.002

Manz MG, Boettcher S. 2014. Emergency granulopoiesis. *Nat Rev Immunol* **14:** 302–314. doi:10.1038/nri3660

Marusyk A, Porter CC, Zaberezhnyy V, DeGregori J. 2010. Irradiation selects for p53-deficient hematopoietic progenitors. *PLoS Biol* **8:** e1000324. doi:10.1371/journal.pbio.1000324

Matsumoto A, Takeishi S, Kanie T, Susaki E, Onoyama I, Tateishi Y, Nakayama K, Nakayama KI. 2011. p57 is required for quiescence and maintenance of adult hematopoietic stem cells. *Cell Stem Cell* **9:** 262–271. doi:10.1016/j.stem.2011.06.014

McLemore ML, Grewal S, Liu F, Archambault A, Poursine-Laurent J, Haug J, Link DC. 2001. STAT-3 activation is required for normal G-CSF-dependent proliferation and granulocytic differentiation. *Immunity* **14:** 193–204. doi:10.1016/S1074-7613(01)00101-7

Meisel M, Hinterleitner R, Pacis A, Chen L, Earley ZM, Mayassi T, Pierre JF, Ernest JD, Galipeau HJ, Thuille N, et al. 2018. Microbial signals drive pre-leukaemic myeloproliferation in a *Tet2*-deficient host. *Nature* **557:** 580–584. doi:10.1038/s41586-018-0125-z

Miyamoto K, Araki KY, Naka K, Arai F, Takubo K, Yamazaki S, Matsuoka S, Miyamoto T, Ito K, Ohmura M, et al. 2007. Foxo3a is essential for maintenance of the hematopoietic stem cell pool. *Cell Stem Cell* **1:** 101–112. doi:10.1016/j.stem.2007.02.001

Mizuki M, Fenski R, Halfter H, Matsumura I, Schmidt R, Muller C, Grüning W, Kratz-Albers K, Serve S, Steur C, et al. 2000. Flt3 mutations from patients with acute myeloid leukemia induce transformation of 32D cells mediated by the Ras and STAT5 pathways. *Blood* **96:** 3907–3914. doi:10.1182/blood.V96.12.3907

Mohrin M, Bourke E, Alexander D, Warr MR, Barry-Holson K, Le Beau MM, Morrison CG, Passegué E. 2010. Hematopoietic stem cell quiescence promotes error-prone DNA repair and mutagenesis. *Cell Stem Cell* **7:** 174–185. doi:10.1016/j.stem.2010.06.014

Mohrin M, Shin J, Liu Y, Brown K, Luo H, Xi Y, Haynes CM, Chen D. 2015. Stem cell aging. A mitochondrial UPR-mediated metabolic checkpoint regulates hematopoietic stem cell aging. *Science* **347:** 1374–1377. doi:10.1126/science.aaa2361

Moran-Crusio K, Reavie L, Shih A, Abdel-Wahab O, Ndiaye-Lobry D, Lobry C, Figueroa ME, Vasanthakumar A, Patel J, Zhao X, et al. 2011. *Tet2* loss leads to increased hematopoietic stem cell self-renewal and myeloid transformation. *Cancer Cell* **20:** 11–24. doi:10.1016/j.ccr.2011.06.001

Morita Y, Ema H, Nakauchi H. 2010. Heterogeneity and hierarchy within the most primitive hematopoietic stem cell compartment. *J Exp Med* **207:** 1173–1182. doi:10.1084/jem.20091318

Mortensen M, Watson AS, Simon AK. 2011. Lack of autophagy in the hematopoietic system leads to loss of hematopoietic stem cell function and dysregulated myeloid proliferation. *Autophagy* **7:** 1069–1070. doi:10.4161/auto.7.9.15886

Mossadegh-Keller N, Sarrazin S, Kandalla PK, Espinosa L, Stanley ER, Nutt SL, Moore J, Sieweke MH. 2013. M-CSF instructs myeloid lineage fate in single haematopoietic stem cells. *Nature* **497:** 239–243. doi:10.1038/nature12026

Muller-Sieburg CE, Whitlock CA, Weissman IL. 1986. Isolation of two early B lymphocyte progenitors from mouse marrow: a committed pre-pre-B cell and a clonogenic Thy-1^{lo} hematopoietic stem cell. *Cell* **44:** 653–662. doi:10.1016/0092-8674(86)90274-6

Müller-Sieburg CE, Cho RH, Thoman M, Adkins B, Sieburg HB. 2002. Deterministic regulation of hematopoietic stem cell self-renewal and differentiation. *Blood* **100:** 1302–1309. doi:10.1182/blood.V100.4.1302.h81602001302_1302_1309

Muller-Sieburg CE, Cho RH, Karlsson L, Huang JF, Sieburg HB. 2004. Myeloid-biased hematopoietic stem cells have extensive self-renewal capacity but generate diminished lymphoid progeny with impaired IL-7 responsiveness. *Blood* **103:** 4111–4118. doi:10.1182/blood-2003-10-3448

Mullighan CG, Miller CB, Radtke I, Phillips LA, Dalton J, Ma J, White D, Hughes TP, Le Beau MM, Pui CH, et al. 2008. *BCR-ABL1* lymphoblastic leukaemia is characterized by the deletion of Ikaros. *Nature* **453:** 110–114. doi:10.1038/nature06866

Nagai Y, Garrett KP, Ohta S, Bahrun U, Kouro T, Akira S, Takatsu K, Kincade PW. 2006. Toll-like receptors on hematopoietic progenitor cells stimulate innate immune system replenishment. *Immunity* **24:** 801–812. doi:10.1016/j.immuni.2006.04.008

Nagasawa T, Hirota S, Tachibana K, Takakura N, Nishikawa S, Kitamura Y, Yoshida N, Kikutani H, Kishimoto T. 1996. Defects of B-cell lymphopoiesis and bone-marrow myelopoiesis in mice lacking the CXC chemokine PBSF/SDF-1. *Nature* **382:** 635–638. doi:10.1038/382635a0

Naik SH, Perié L, Swart E, Gerlach C, van Rooij N, de Boer RJ, Schumacher TN. 2013. Diverse and heritable lineage imprinting of early haematopoietic progenitors. *Nature* **496:** 229–232. doi:10.1038/nature12013

Nakada D, Saunders TL, Morrison SJ. 2010. Lkb1 regulates cell cycle and energy metabolism in haematopoietic stem cells. *Nature* **468:** 653–658. doi:10.1038/nature09571

Nestorowa S, Hamey FK, Pijuan Sala B, Diamanti E, Shepherd M, Laurenti E, Wilson NK, Kent DG, Göttgens B. 2016. A single-cell resolution map of mouse hematopoietic stem and progenitor cell differentiation. *Blood* **128:** e20–e31. doi:10.1182/blood-2016-05-716480

Niehrs C, Acebron SP. 2012. Mitotic and mitogenic Wnt signalling. *EMBO J* **31:** 2705–2713. doi:10.1038/emboj.2012.124

Norddahl GL, Pronk CJ, Wahlestedt M, Sten G, Nygren JM, Ugale A, Sigvardsson M, Bryder D. 2011. Accumulating mitochondrial DNA mutations drive premature hematopoietic aging phenotypes distinct from physiological stem cell aging. *Cell Stem Cell* **8:** 499–510. doi:10.1016/j.stem.2011.03.009

Orford KW, Scadden DT. 2008. Deconstructing stem cell self-renewal: genetic insights into cell-cycle regulation. *Nat Rev Genet* **9:** 115–128. doi:10.1038/nrg2269

Orkin SH, Zon LI. 2008. Hematopoiesis: an evolving paradigm for stem cell biology. *Cell* **132:** 631–644. doi:10.1016/j.cell.2008.01.025

Ortmann CA, Kent DG, Nangalia J, Silber Y, Wedge DC, Grinfeld J, Baxter EJ, Massie CE, Papaemmanuil E, Menon S, et al. 2015. Effect of mutation order on myeloproliferative neoplasms. *N Engl J Med* **372:** 601–612. doi:10.1056/NEJMoa1412098

Osawa M, Hanada K, Hamada H, Nakauchi H. 1996. Long-term lymphohematopoietic reconstitution by a single

CD34-low/negative hematopoietic stem cell. *Science* **273:** 242–245. doi:10.1126/science.273.5272.242

Osgood EE, Riddle MC, Mathews TJ. 1939. Aplastic anemia treated with daily transfusions and intravenous marrow; case report. *Ann Intern Med* **13:** 357–367. doi:10.7326/0003-4819-13-2-357

Panopoulos AD, Zhang L, Snow JW, Jones DM, Smith AM, El Kasmi KC, Liu F, Goldsmith MA, Link DC, Murray PJ, et al. 2006. STAT3 governs distinct pathways in emergency granulopoiesis and mature neutrophils. *Blood* **108:** 3682–3690. doi:10.1182/blood-2006-02-003012

Papaemmanuil E, Dohner H, Campbell PJ. 2016. Genomic classification in acute myeloid leukemia. *N Engl J Med* **375:** 900–901. doi:10.1056/NEJMc1608739

Passegue E, Jamieson CH, Ailles LE, Weissman IL. 2003. Normal and leukemic hematopoiesis: are leukemias a stem cell disorder or a reacquisition of stem cell characteristics? *Proc Natl Acad Sci* **100:** 11842–11849. doi:10.1073/pnas.2034201100

Pei W, Feyerabend TB, Rössler J, Wang X, Postrach D, Busch K, Rode I, Klapproth K, Dietlein N, Quedenau C, et al. 2017. *Polylox* barcoding reveals haematopoietic stem cell fates realized in vivo. *Nature* **548:** 456–460. doi:10.1038/nature23653

Pietras EM, Warr MR, Passegué E. 2011. Cell cycle regulation in hematopoietic stem cells. *J Cell Biol* **195:** 709–720. doi:10.1083/jcb.201102131

Pietras EM, Lakshminarasimhan R, Techner JM, Fong S, Flach J, Binnewies M, Passegué E. 2014. Re-entry into quiescence protects hematopoietic stem cells from the killing effect of chronic exposure to type I interferons. *J Exp Med* **211:** 245–262. doi:10.1084/jem.20131043

Pietras EM, Reynaud D, Kang YA, Carlin D, Calero-Nieto FJ, Leavitt AD, Stuart JM, Göttgens B, Passegué E. 2015. Functionally distinct subsets of lineage-biased multipotent progenitors control blood production in normal and regenerative conditions. *Cell Stem Cell* **17:** 35–46. doi:10.1016/j.stem.2015.05.003

Pietras EM, Mirantes-Barbeito C, Fong S, Loeffler D, Kovtonyuk LV, Zhang S, Lakshminarasimhan R, Chin CP, Techner JM, Will B, et al. 2016. Chronic interleukin-1 exposure drives haematopoietic stem cells towards precocious myeloid differentiation at the expense of self-renewal. *Nat Cell Biol* **18:** 607–618. doi:10.1038/ncb3346

Pina C, Fugazza C, Tipping AJ, Brown J, Soneji S, Teles J, Peterson C, Enver T. 2012. Inferring rules of lineage commitment in haematopoiesis. *Nat Cell Biol* **14:** 287–294. doi:10.1038/ncb2442

Ponomaryov T, Peled A, Petit I, Taichman RS, Habler L, Sandbank J, Arenzana-Seisdedos F, Magerus A, Caruz A, Fujii N, et al. 2000. Induction of the chemokine stromal-derived factor-1 following DNA damage improves human stem cell function. *J Clin Invest* **106:** 1331–1339. doi:10.1172/JCI10329

Presneill JJ, Waring PM, Layton JE, Maher DW, Cebon J, Harley NS, Wilson JW, Cade JF. 2000. Plasma granulocyte colony-stimulating factor and granulocyte-macrophage colony-stimulating factor levels in critical illness including sepsis and septic shock: relation to disease severity, multiple organ dysfunction, and mortality. *Crit Care Med* **28:** 2344–2354. doi:10.1097/00003246-200007000-00028

Qian H, Buza-Vidas N, Hyland CD, Jensen CT, Antonchuk J, Månsson R, Thoren LA, Ekblom M, Alexander WS, Jacobsen SE. 2007. Critical role of thrombopoietin in maintaining adult quiescent hematopoietic stem cells. *Cell Stem Cell* **1:** 671–684. doi:10.1016/j.stem.2007.10.008

Quivoron C, Couronné L, Della Valle V, Lopez CK, Plo I, Wagner-Ballon O, Do Cruzeiro M, Delhommeau F, Arnulf B, Stern MH, et al. 2011. *TET2* inactivation results in pleiotropic hematopoietic abnormalities in mouse and is a recurrent event during human lymphomagenesis. *Cancer Cell* **20:** 25–38. doi:10.1016/j.ccr.2011.06.003

Rampal R, Ahn J, Abdel-Wahab O, Nahas M, Wang K, Lipson D, Otto GA, Yelensky R, Hricik T, McKenney AS, et al. 2014. Genomic and functional analysis of leukemic transformation of myeloproliferative neoplasms. *Proc Natl Acad Sci* **111:** E5401–E5410. doi:10.1073/pnas.1407792111

Reynaud D, Pietras E, Barry-Holson K, Mir A, Binnewies M, Jeanne M, Sala-Torra O, Radich JP, Passegué E. 2011. IL-6 controls leukemic multipotent progenitor cell fate and contributes to chronic myelogenous leukemia development. *Cancer Cell* **20:** 661–673. doi:10.1016/j.ccr.2011.10.012

Rodriguez-Fraticelli AE, Wolock SL, Weinreb CS, Panero R, Patel SH, Jankovic M, Sun J, Calogero RA, Klein AM, Camargo FD. 2018. Clonal analysis of lineage fate in native haematopoiesis. *Nature* **553:** 212–216. doi:10.1038/nature25168

Rossi DJ, Bryder D, Seita J, Nussenzweig A, Hoeijmakers J, Weissman IL. 2007. Deficiencies in DNA damage repair limit the function of haematopoietic stem cells with age. *Nature* **447:** 725–729. doi:10.1038/nature05862

Ryall JG, Cliff T, Dalton S, Sartorelli V. 2015. Metabolic reprogramming of stem cell epigenetics. *Cell Stem Cell* **17:** 651–662. doi:10.1016/j.stem.2015.11.012

Sanjuan-Pla A, Macaulay IC, Jensen CT, Woll PS, Luis TC, Mead A, Moore S, Carella C, Matsuoka S, Bouriez Jones T, et al. 2013. Platelet-biased stem cells reside at the apex of the haematopoietic stem-cell hierarchy. *Nature* **502:** 232–236. doi:10.1038/nature12495

Sato T, Onai N, Yoshihara H, Arai F, Suda T, Ohteki T. 2009. Interferon regulatory factor-2 protects quiescent hematopoietic stem cells from type I interferon-dependent exhaustion. *Nat Med* **15:** 696–700. doi:10.1038/nm.1973

Scandura JM, Boccuni P, Massague J, Nimer SD. 2004. Transforming growth factor β-induced cell cycle arrest of human hematopoietic cells requires p57KIP2 up-regulation. *Proc Natl Acad Sci* **101:** 15231–15236. doi:10.1073/pnas.0406771101

Schepers K, Campbell TB, Passegué E. 2015. Normal and leukemic stem cell niches: insights and therapeutic opportunities. *Cell Stem Cell* **16:** 254–267. doi:10.1016/j.stem.2015.02.014

Schuettpelz LG, Borgerding JN, Christopher MJ, Gopalan PK, Romine MP, Herman AC, Woloszynek JR, Greenbaum AM, Link DC. 2014. G-CSF regulates hematopoietic stem cell activity, in part, through activation of Toll-like receptor signaling. *Leukemia* **28:** 1851–1860. doi:10.1038/leu.2014.68

Schultze JL, Mass E, Schlitzer A. 2019. Emerging principles in myelopoiesis at homeostasis and during infection and inflammation. *Immunity* **50:** 288–301. doi:10.1016/j.immuni.2019.01.019

Scumpia PO, Kelly-Scumpia KM, Delano MJ, Weinstein JS, Cuenca AG, Al-Quran S, Bovio I, Akira S, Kumagai Y, Moldawer LL. 2010. Cutting edge: bacterial infection induces hematopoietic stem and progenitor cell expansion in the absence of TLR signaling. *J Immunol* **184:** 2247–2251. doi:10.4049/jimmunol.0903652

Sedelnikova OA, Redon CE, Dickey JS, Nakamura AJ, Georgakilas AG, Bonner WM. 2010. Role of oxidatively induced DNA lesions in human pathogenesis. *Mutat Res* **704:** 152–159. doi:10.1016/j.mrrev.2009.12.005

Selig C, Nothdurft W. 1995. Cytokines and progenitor cells of granulocytopoiesis in peripheral blood of patients with bacterial infections. *Infect Immun* **63:** 104–109.

Shi C, Jia T, Mendez-Ferrer S, Hohl TM, Serbina NV, Lipuma L, Leiner I, Li MO, Frenette PS, Pamer EG. 2011. Bone marrow mesenchymal stem and progenitor cells induce monocyte emigration in response to circulating toll-like receptor ligands. *Immunity* **34:** 590–601. doi:10.1016/j.immuni.2011.02.016

Shih AH, Jiang Y, Meydan C, Shank K, Pandey S, Barreyro L, Antony-Debre I, Viale A, Socci N, Sun Y, et al. 2015. Mutational cooperativity linked to combinatorial epigenetic gain of function in acute myeloid leukemia. *Cancer Cell* **27:** 502–515. doi:10.1016/j.ccell.2015.03.009

Simsek T, Kocabas F, Zheng J, Deberardinis RJ, Mahmoud AI, Olson EN, Schneider JW, Zhang CC, Sadek HA. 2010. The distinct metabolic profile of hematopoietic stem cells reflects their location in a hypoxic niche. *Cell Stem Cell* **7:** 380–390. doi:10.1016/j.stem.2010.07.011

Sitnicka E, Ruscetti FW, Priestley GV, Wolf NS, Bartelmez SH. 1996. Transforming growth factor β1 directly and reversibly inhibits the initial cell divisions of long-term repopulating hematopoietic stem cells. *Blood* **88:** 82–88. doi:10.1182/blood.V88.1.82.82

Spangrude GJ, Heimfeld S, Weissman IL. 1988. Purification and characterization of mouse hematopoietic stem cells. *Science* **241:** 58–62. doi:10.1126/science.2898810

Spencer JA, Ferraro F, Roussakis E, Klein A, Wu J, Runnels JM, Zaher W, Mortensen LJ, Alt C, Turcotte R, et al. 2014. Direct measurement of local oxygen concentration in the bone marrow of live animals. *Nature* **508:** 269–273. doi:10.1038/nature13034

Sprüssel A, Schulte JH, Weber S, Necke M, Händschke K, Thor T, Pajtler KW, Schramm A, König K, Diehl L, et al. 2012. Lysine-specific demethylase 1 restricts hematopoietic progenitor proliferation and is essential for terminal differentiation. *Leukemia* **26:** 2039–2051. doi:10.1038/leu.2012.157

Staal FJ, Famili F, Garcia Perez L, Pike-Overzet K. 2016. Aberrant wnt signaling in leukemia. *Cancers (Basel)* **8:** 78. doi:10.3390/cancers8090078

Sun J, Ramos A, Chapman B, Johnnidis JB, Le L, Ho YJ, Klein A, Hofmann O, Camargo FD. 2014. Clonal dynamics of native haematopoiesis. *Nature* **514:** 322–327. doi:10.1038/nature13824

Tadokoro Y, Ema H, Okano M, Li E, Nakauchi H. 2007. De novo DNA methyltransferase is essential for self-renewal, but not for differentiation, in hematopoietic stem cells. *J Exp Med* **204:** 715–722. doi:10.1084/jem.20060750

Takahashi K, Wang F, Kantarjian H, Doss D, Khanna K, Thompson E, Zhao L, Patel K, Neelapu S, Gumbs C, et al. 2017. Preleukaemic clonal haemopoiesis and risk of therapy-related myeloid neoplasms: a case-control study. *Lancet Oncol* **18:** 100–111. doi:10.1016/S1470-2045(16)30626-X

Takizawa H, Fritsch K, Kovtonyuk LV, Saito Y, Yakkala C, Jacobs K, Ahuja AK, Lopes M, Hausmann A, Hardt WD, et al. 2017. Pathogen-induced TLR4-TRIF innate immune signaling in hematopoietic stem cells promotes proliferation but reduces competitive fitness. *Cell Stem Cell* **21:** 225–240 e5. doi:10.1016/j.stem.2017.06.013

Takubo K, Goda N, Yamada W, Iriuchishima H, Ikeda E, Kubota Y, Shima H, Johnson RS, Hirao A, Suematsu M, et al. 2010. Regulation of the HIF-1α level is essential for hematopoietic stem cells. *Cell Stem Cell* **7:** 391–402. doi:10.1016/j.stem.2010.06.020

Takubo K, Nagamatsu G, Kobayashi CI, Nakamura-Ishizu A, Kobayashi H, Ikeda E, Goda N, Rahimi Y, Johnson RS, Soga T, et al. 2013. Regulation of glycolysis by Pdk functions as a metabolic checkpoint for cell cycle quiescence in hematopoietic stem cells. *Cell Stem Cell* **12:** 49–61. doi:10.1016/j.stem.2012.10.011

Tanaka H, Ishikawa K, Nishino M, Shimazu T, Yoshioka T. 1996. Changes in granulocyte colony-stimulating factor concentration in patients with trauma and sepsis. *J Trauma* **40:** 718–725; discussion 725–726. doi:10.1097/00005373-199605000-00006

Thorén LA, Liuba K, Bryder D, Nygren JM, Jensen CT, Qian H, Antonchuk J, Jacobsen SE. 2008. Kit regulates maintenance of quiescent hematopoietic stem cells. *J Immunol* **180:** 2045–2053. doi:10.4049/jimmunol.180.4.2045

Till JE, McCulloch EA. 1961. A direct measurement of the radiation sensitivity of normal mouse bone marrow cells. *Radiat Res* **14:** 213–222. doi:10.2307/3570892

Tomasetti C, Vogelstein B. 2015. Cancer etiology. Variation in cancer risk among tissues can be explained by the number of stem cell divisions. *Science* **347:** 78–81. doi:10.1126/science.1260825

Tothova Z, Kollipara R, Huntly BJ, Lee BH, Castrillon DH, Cullen DE, McDowell EP, Lazo-Kallanian S, Williams IR, Sears C, et al. 2007. *FoxOs* are critical mediators of hematopoietic stem cell resistance to physiologic oxidative stress. *Cell* **128:** 325–339. doi:10.1016/j.cell.2007.01.003

Trowbridge JJ, Scott MP, Bhatia M. 2006. Hedgehog modulates cell cycle regulators in stem cells to control hematopoietic regeneration. *Proc Natl Acad Sci* **103:** 14134–14139. doi:10.1073/pnas.0604568103

Tsai JJ, Dudakov JA, Takahashi K, Shieh JH, Velardi E, Holland AM, Singer NV, West ML, Smith OM, Young LF, et al. 2013. Nrf2 regulates haematopoietic stem cell function. *Nat Cell Biol* **15:** 309–316. doi:10.1038/ncb2699

Tusi BK, Wolock SL, Weinreb C, Hwang Y, Hidalgo D, Zilionis R, Waisman A, Huh JR, Klein AM, Socolovsky M. 2018. Population snapshots predict early haematopoietic and erythroid hierarchies. *Nature* **555:** 54–60. doi:10.1038/nature25741

Ueda Y, Cain DW, Kuraoka M, Kondo M, Kelsoe G. 2009. IL-1R type I-dependent hemopoietic stem cell proliferation is necessary for inflammatory granulopoiesis and reactive neutrophilia. *J Immunol* **182:** 6477–6484. doi:10.4049/jimmunol.0803961

Valencia A, Roman-Gomez J, Cervera J, Such E, Barragan E, Bolufer P, Moscardo F, Sanz GF, Sanz MA. 2009. Wnt signaling pathway is epigenetically regulated by methylation of Wnt antagonists in acute myeloid leukemia. *Leukemia* **23:** 1658–1666. doi:10.1038/leu.2009.86

Velten L, Haas SF, Raffel S, Blaszkiewicz S, Islam S, Hennig BP, Hirche C, Lutz C, Buss EC, Nowak D, et al. 2017. Human haematopoietic stem cell lineage commitment is a continuous process. *Nat Cell Biol* **19:** 271–281. doi:10.1038/ncb3493

Viatour P, Somervaille TC, Venkatasubrahmanyam S, Kogan S, McLaughlin ME, Weissman IL, Butte AJ, Passegué E, Sage J. 2008. Hematopoietic stem cell quiescence is maintained by compound contributions of the retinoblastoma gene family. *Cell Stem Cell* **3:** 416–428. doi:10.1016/j.stem.2008.07.009

Wang Y, Krivtsov AV, Sinha AU, North TE, Goessling W, Feng Z, Zon LI, Armstrong SA. 2010. The Wnt/β-catenin pathway is required for the development of leukemia stem cells in AML. *Science* **327:** 1650–1653. doi:10.1126/science.1186624

Wang YH, Israelsen WJ, Lee D, Yu VWC, Jeanson NT, Clish CB, Cantley LC, Vander Heiden MG, Scadden DT. 2014. Cell-state-specific metabolic dependency in hematopoiesis and leukemogenesis. *Cell* **158:** 1309–1323. doi:10.1016/j.cell.2014.07.048

Warr MR, Binnewies M, Flach J, Reynaud D, Garg T, Malhotra R, Debnath J, Passegué E. 2013. FoxO3a directs a protective autophagy program in haematopoietic stem cells. *Nature* **494:** 323–327. doi:10.1038/nature11895

Watari K, Asano S, Shirafuji N, Kodo H, Ozawa K, Takaku F, Kamachi S. 1989. Serum granulocyte colony-stimulating factor levels in healthy volunteers and patients with various disorders as estimated by enzyme immunoassay. *Blood* **73:** 117–122. doi:10.1182/blood.V73.1.117.117

Wei Q, Frenette PS. 2018. Niches for hematopoietic stem cells and their progeny. *Immunity* **48:** 632–648. doi:10.1016/j.immuni.2018.03.024

Weisser M, Demel UM, Stein S, Chen-Wichmann L, Touzot F, Santilli G, Sujer S, Brendel C, Siler U, Cavazzana M, et al. 2016. Hyperinflammation in patients with chronic granulomatous disease leads to impairment of hematopoietic stem cell functions. *J Allergy Clin Immunol* **138:** 219–228.e9. doi:10.1016/j.jaci.2015.11.028

Wilson A, Laurenti E, Oser G, van der Wath RC, Blanco-Bose W, Jaworski M, Offner S, Dunant CF, Eshkind L, Bockamp E, et al. 2008. Hematopoietic stem cells reversibly switch from dormancy to self-renewal during homeostasis and repair. *Cell* **135:** 1118–1129. doi:10.1016/j.cell.2008.10.048

Xie M, Lu C, Wang J, McLellan MD, Johnson KJ, Wendl MC, McMichael JF, Schmidt HK, Yellapantula V, Miller CA, et al. 2014. Age-related mutations associated with clonal hematopoietic expansion and malignancies. *Nat Med* **20:** 1472–1478. doi:10.1038/nm.3733

Yahata T, Takanashi T, Muguruma Y, Ibrahim AA, Matsuzawa H, Uno T, Sheng Y, Onizuka M, Ito M, Kato S, et al. 2011. Accumulation of oxidative DNA damage restricts the self-renewal capacity of human hematopoietic stem cells. *Blood* **118:** 2941–2950. doi:10.1182/blood-2011-01-330050

Yamamoto R, Morita Y, Ooehara J, Hamanaka S, Onodera M, Rudolph KL, Ema H, Nakauchi H. 2013. Clonal analysis unveils self-renewing lineage-restricted progenitors generated directly from hematopoietic stem cells. *Cell* **154:** 1112–1126. doi:10.1016/j.cell.2013.08.007

Yamazaki S, Iwama A, Takayanagi S, Eto K, Ema H, Nakauchi H. 2009. TGF-β as a candidate bone marrow niche signal to induce hematopoietic stem cell hibernation. *Blood* **113:** 1250–1256. doi:10.1182/blood-2008-04-146480

Yilmaz OH, Valdez R, Theisen BK, Guo W, Ferguson DO, Wu H, Morrison SJ. 2006. *Pten* dependence distinguishes haematopoietic stem cells from leukaemia-initiating cells. *Nature* **441:** 475–482. doi:10.1038/nature04703

Young AL, Challen GA, Birmann BM, Druley TE. 2016. Clonal haematopoiesis harbouring AML-associated mutations is ubiquitous in healthy adults. *Nat Commun* **7:** 12484. doi:10.1038/ncomms12484

Yu WM, Liu X, Shen J, Jovanovic O, Pohl EE, Gerson SL, Finkel T, Broxmeyer HE, Qu CK. 2013. Metabolic regulation by the mitochondrial phosphatase *PTPMT1* is required for hematopoietic stem cell differentiation. *Cell Stem Cell* **12:** 62–74. doi:10.1016/j.stem.2012.11.022

Zhang J, Grindley JC, Yin T, Jayasinghe S, He XC, Ross JT, Haug JS, Rupp D, Porter-Westpfahl KS, Wiedemann LM, et al. 2006. PTEN maintains haematopoietic stem cells and acts in lineage choice and leukaemia prevention. *Nature* **441:** 518–522. doi:10.1038/nature04747

Zhang H, Nguyen-Jackson H, Panopoulos AD, Li HS, Murray PJ, Watowich SS. 2010. STAT3 controls myeloid progenitor growth during emergency granulopoiesis. *Blood* **116:** 2462–2471. doi:10.1182/blood-2009-12-259630

Zhao C, Blum J, Chen A, Kwon HY, Jung SH, Cook JM, Lagoo A, Reya T. 2007. Loss of β-catenin impairs the renewal of normal and CML stem cells in vivo. *Cancer Cell* **12:** 528–541. doi:10.1016/j.ccr.2007.11.003

Zhao C, Chen A, Jamieson CH, Fereshteh M, Abrahamsson A, Blum J, Kwon HY, Kim J, Chute JP, Rizzieri D, et al. 2009. Hedgehog signalling is essential for maintenance of cancer stem cells in myeloid leukaemia. *Nature* **458:** 776–779. doi:10.1038/nature07737

Zhao JL, Ma C, O'Connell RM, Mehta A, DiLoreto R, Heath JR, Baltimore D. 2014a. Conversion of danger signals into cytokine signals by hematopoietic stem and progenitor cells for regulation of stress-induced hematopoiesis. *Cell Stem Cell* **14:** 445–459. doi:10.1016/j.stem.2014.01.007

Zhao M, Perry JM, Marshall H, Venkatraman A, Qian P, He XC, Ahamed J, Li L. 2014b. Megakaryocytes maintain homeostatic quiescence and promote post-injury regeneration of hematopoietic stem cells. *Nat Med* **20:** 1321–1326. doi:10.1038/nm.3706

Zhou S, Morris JJ, Barnes Y, Lan L, Schuetz JD, Sorrentino BP. 2002. *Bcrp1* gene expression is required for normal numbers of side population stem cells in mice, and confers relative protection to mitoxantrone in hematopoietic cells in vivo. *Proc Natl Acad Sci* **99:** 12339–12344. doi:10.1073/pnas.192276999

Zou P, Yoshihara H, Hosokawa K, Tai I, Shinmyozu K, Tsukahara F, Maru Y, Nakayama K, Nakayama KI, Suda T. 2011. $p57^{Kip2}$ and $p27^{Kip1}$ cooperate to maintain hematopoietic stem cell quiescence through interactions with Hsc70. *Cell Stem Cell* **9:** 247–261. doi:10.1016/j.stem.2011.07.003

Epidemiology and Etiology of Leukemia and Lymphoma

Jordan A. Baeker Bispo,[1] Paulo S. Pinheiro,[2] and Erin K. Kobetz[3]

[1]Department of Public Health Sciences, Miller School of Medicine, University of Miami, Miami, Florida 33136, USA

[2]Sylvester Comprehensive Cancer Center and Department of Public Health Sciences, Miller School of Medicine, University of Miami, Miami, Florida 33136, USA

[3]Sylvester Comprehensive Cancer Center and Department of Medicine, Miller School of Medicine, University of Miami, Miami, Florida 33136, USA

Correspondence: jab549@miami.edu

Available evidence suggests that the incidence of leukemia and lymphoma tends to be higher in highly developed regions of the world and among Whites in the United States. Temporal trends in incidence are dynamic and multifactorial; for instance, the incidence of non-Hodgkin's lymphoma increased around the turn of the century, in part because of the acquired immune deficiency syndrome (AIDS) epidemic. Most leukemias and lymphomas are sporadic and the specific etiology remains elusive. Still, research shows that these malignancies often develop in the context of genetic abnormalities, immunosuppression, and exposure to risk factors like ionizing radiation, carcinogenic chemicals, and oncogenic viruses. The prognosis varies by subtype, with poorer survival outcomes for acute leukemias among adults, and more favorable outcomes for Hodgkin's lymphoma. At a time when specific prevention efforts targeting these malignancies are nonexistent, there is a great need to ensure equitable access to diagnostic services and treatments worldwide.

Hematopoiesis is the highly regulated process by which stem cells differentiate and mature into erythrocytes, megakaryocytes, and immune cells of myeloid, lymphoid, or monocytic lineage in bone marrow or lymphatic tissues. Genetic errors, such as reciprocal chromosomal translocations, chromosomal deletions, point mutations, and epigenetic alterations, can arrest the maturation of stem cells across different stages of hematopoiesis, giving rise to the uncontrolled proliferation of immature, leukemic immune cells. Leukemia refers to the clonal expansion of leukemic cells in the bone marrow, classically resulting in elevated numbers of cells of the affected lineage in circulating blood and, with certain lymphoid malignancies, abnormal cellular proliferation in lymphatic tissue. Lymphomas are neoplasms of well-differentiated B and T lymphocytes, which typically present as malignant masses in lymphatic tissue. Leukemias are generally classified into subtypes defined by cell lineage (lymphocytic or myeloid) and stage of maturation arrest (acute or chronic). Mature lymphoid neoplasms are classified

Cite this article as *Cold Spring Harb Perspect Med* doi: 10.1101/cshperspect.a034819

broadly into three groups: mature B-cell neoplasms, mature T- or natural killer (NK)-cell neoplasms, and Hodgkin's lymphoma (HL). Collectively, B- and T/NK-cell neoplasms comprise non-Hodgkin's lymphomas (NHLs), a heterogeneous group of more than 60 subtypes. HL arises from B cells, but is distinguished from NHL morphologically by the presence of Reed–Sternberg clonal tumor cells, which are large and often multinucleated.

In this review, we discuss the epidemiology and etiology of leukemia (overall and by subtype), NHL, and HL. Our discussion emphasizes racial/ethnic and age-related disparities in disease burden, as illustrated in part by Figure 1 (patterns of disease incidence) and Figure 2 (patterns of 5-yr relative survival). It should be noted that the World Health Organization (WHO) classification for hematopoietic neoplasms is based on cell of origin, and some forms of leukemia and lymphomas are thus considered different presentations of the same disease. Examples include chronic lymphocytic leukemia and small cell lymphoma (a form of mature B-cell lymphoma; CLL/SLL), and acute lymphocytic leukemia and acute precursor B- and T-cell lymphoblastic leukemia/lymphoma (ALL/LBL). Clinically, CLL/SLL is considered a lymphoma. However, population-based cancer surveillance programs typically count CLL/SLL cases as either leukemias or lymphomas depending on whether the cancer cells were found in the bone marrow, blood, or lymph nodes. Here we present CLL/SLL and ALL/LBL as primarily leukemias, recognizing the overlapping classifications.

GLOBAL EPIDEMIOLOGY OF LEUKEMIA

The World Health Organization's International Agency for Research on Cancer (IARC) produces global estimates for all cancers contained in the GLOBOCAN database, using data from mostly high-quality population-based cancer registries worldwide. The Institute for Health Metrics and Evaluation's Global Burden of Disease (GBD) study also produces estimates through modeling techniques that incorporate data from numerous additional sources, including lower-quality cancer registries in countries that are disproportionately low and middle income.

According to GLOBOCAN, leukemia was the 15th most commonly diagnosed cancer and 11th leading cause of cancer mortality worldwide in 2018, accounting for 437,033 incident cancer cases and 309,006 cancer deaths. Globally, the leukemia disease burden is higher among males than females. In 2018, the age-standardized incidence rate for males was 6.1 per 100,000 compared to 4.3 per 100,000 for females. Mortality was also higher in males (4.2 per 100,000) than females (2.8 per 100,000) (Bray et al. 2018). The age distribution of chronic leukemia is generally unimodal, with incidence rates that tend to increase with age. ALL and acute myeloid leukemia (AML), which are important diseases in childhood, accordingly have bimodal age distributions. By GBD estimates, the total number of leukemia cases globally increased by 26% from 2005 to 2015, and population growth and aging accounted for all but 3% of this (Fitzmaurice et al. 2017).

The geographic distribution of leukemia burden is patterned by country-level development, with age-standardized incidence, and mortality higher in more developed countries. The IARC classifies 185 countries in the GLOBOCAN database according to the human development index (HDI), a composite measure of life expectancy, education, and standard of living. In 2018, incidence in high/very high HDI countries substantially exceeded that of low/medium HDI countries (7.5 vs. 4.0 per 100,000 for males; 5.3 vs. 3.0 per 100,000 for females). The same was true for mortality in high/very high HDI countries and low/medium countries (4.5 vs. 3.2 per 100,000 for males; 2.9 vs. 2.4 per 100,000 for females) (Bray et al. 2018).

EPIDEMIOLOGY OF LEUKEMIA IN THE UNITED STATES

In the United States, national trends in leukemia incidence and mortality are monitored using data from state population-based cancer registries, namely through the Surveillance, Epidemiology, and End Results program (SEER),

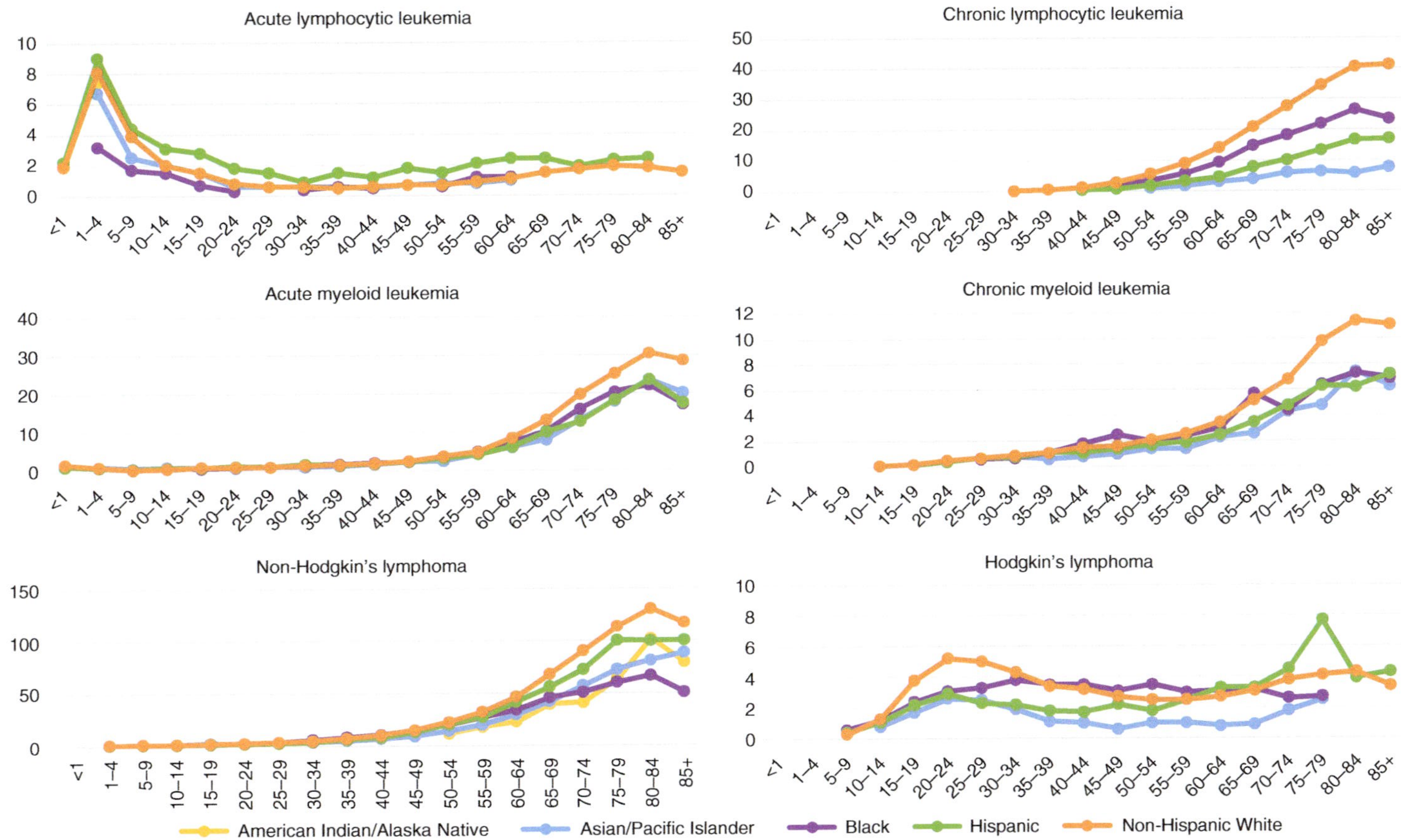

Figure 1. Age-specific incidence rates per 100,000 for leukemia and lymphoma by race/ethnicity, 2011–2015. Data Source: Surveillance, Epidemiology, and End Results Program (SEER; http://seer.cancer.gov/registries/terms.html) 18 areas (San Francisco [SF], Connecticut, Detroit, Hawaii, Iowa, New Mexico, Seattle, Utah, Atlanta [ATL], San Jose–Monterey [JM], Los Angeles [LA], Alaska Native Registry, Rural Georgia [RG], California excluding SF/SJM/LA, Kentucky, Louisiana, New Jersey, and Georgia excluding ATL/RG). Rates are per 100,000 and for 19 age groups (Census P25-1130). Cancer sites are defined using the SEER Site Recode ICD-O-3/World Health Organization (WHO) 2008 Definition. Rates for American Indians/Alaska Natives only include cases that are in a Contract Health Service Delivery Area (CHSDA). Estimates based on 15 or fewer cases are suppressed and not shown.

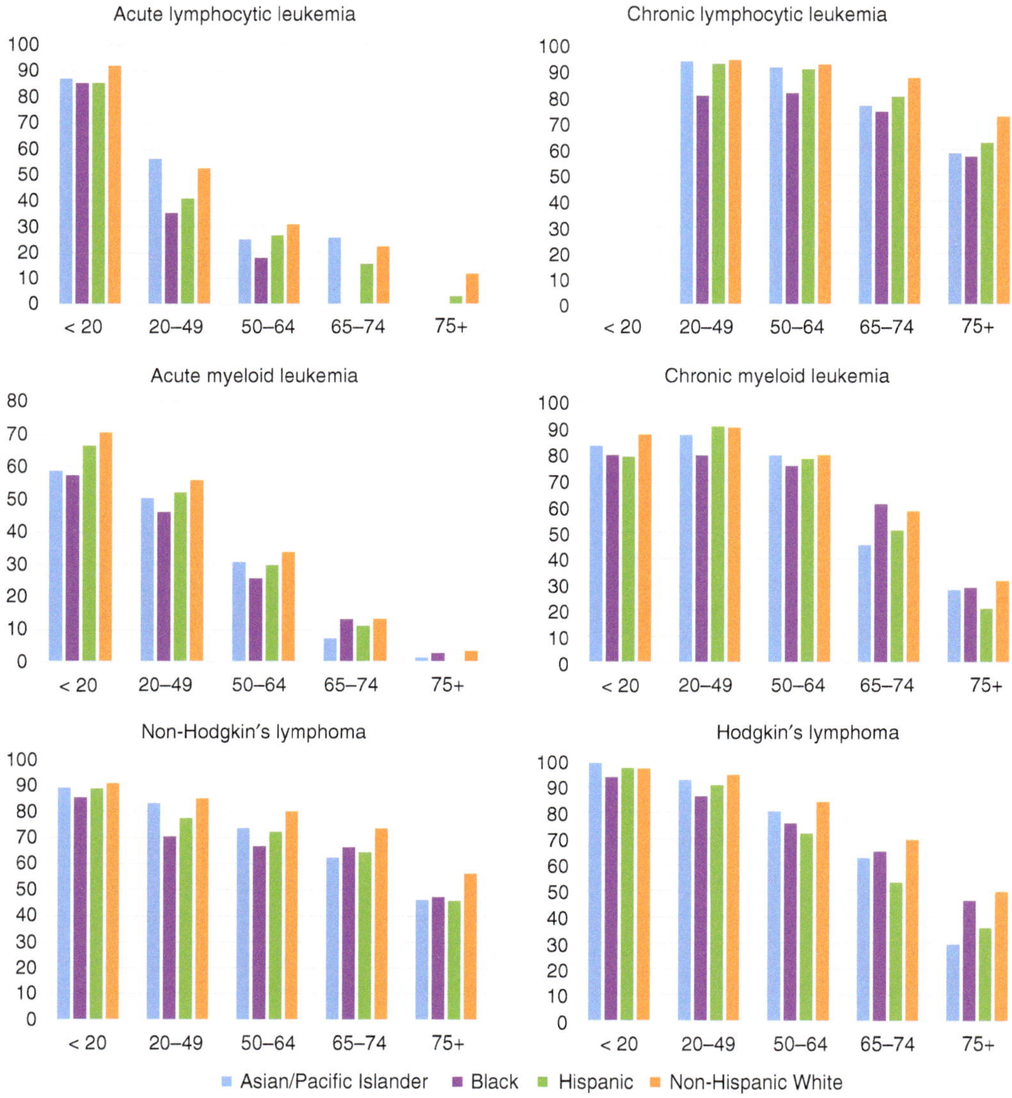

Figure 2. Five-year relative survival proportions for leukemia and lymphoma by race/ethnicity and age, 2008–2014. Data Source: Surveillance, Epidemiology, and End Results Program (SEER; http://seer.cancer.gov/registries/terms.html) 18 areas (San Francisco [SF], Connecticut, Detroit, Hawaii, Iowa, New Mexico, Seattle, Utah, Atlanta [ATL], San Jose18 areas Monterey [SJM], Los Angeles [LA], Alaska Native Registry, Rural Georgia [RG], California excluding SF/SJM/LA, Kentucky, Louisiana, New Jersey and Georgia excluding ATL/RG). The 5-yr survival proportions are calculated using monthly intervals. Cancer sites are defined using the SEER Site Recode ICD-O-3/World Health Organization (WH) 2008 Definition.

and the National Center for Health Statistics. SEER contains high-quality data from 20 regions of the United States, covering 34% of the population. In 2018, leukemia, including CLL, was the 10th most incident cancer in the United States overall, and the seventh leading cause of cancer death. There were an estimated 60,300 incident cases, accounting for 4% of cancer diagnoses in males and 3% in females. Leukemia accounts for 29% of all childhood cancers. The estimated 24,370 leukemia deaths accounted for 4% of cancer deaths among both males and females. Since 2006, the incidence of leukemia has increased by an average of 0.6% per year, whereas mortality has decreased by an annual average of 1.5% (Siegel et al. 2018).

Overall age-adjusted leukemia incidence in the United States tends to be highest in Whites (15 per 100,000), followed by Blacks (11 per 100,000), and Hispanics (10.6 per 100,000). Incidence among Asian/Pacific Islanders (API; 7.8 per 100,000) and American Indian/Alaskan Natives (AIAN; 8.3 per 100,000) is lower by comparison. Similar racial and ethnic patterns hold for age-adjusted mortality rates, which are also higher for Whites (7 per 100,000), Blacks (5.6 per 100,000), and Hispanics (4.8 per 100,000) than API (3.8 per 100,000) and AIAN (3.3 per 100,000). Although incidence and mortality rates are highest among Whites, survival is poorest for Black patients across age strata. Five-year relative survival for patients of <65 yr of age at diagnosis is 73% for Whites and 63% for Blacks. For ages 65 and older, 5-yr relative survival is 50% for Whites and 43% for Blacks (Noone et al. 2017). Importantly, racial/ethnic patterns in leukemia incidence, mortality, and survival vary widely by subtype, as discussed in the sections that follow.

OVERVIEW OF LEUKEMIA RISK FACTORS

Among those exposures most consistently identified as risk factors for leukemia are radiation (therapeutic, occupational, and wartime-related), chemotherapy, family history, genetic syndromes and abnormalities, chemical exposures (e.g., residential and occupational), and lifestyle factors like smoking. Although some exposures have been associated with specific leukemias, the most notable risk factors have an impact on several subtypes. For example, high doses of ionizing atomic bomb radiation among residents of Japan has been associated with increased mortality from all non-CLL leukemias independently (ALL, AML, and CML) (Preston et al. 1994; Richardson et al. 2009; Hsu et al. 2013). Risk of any non-CLL leukemia has been attributed to ionizing radiation exposure in nuclear workers and radiologists prior to 1950 (Mohan et al. 2003; Yoshinaga et al. 2004; Metz-Flamant et al. 2012) and to therapeutic radiation exposure in patients with primary pelvic cancers (Boice et al. 1987; Wright et al. 2010) or benign disorders like cervical polyps and endometrial hyperplasia (Sakata et al. 2012). Occupational exposure to formaldehyde, a chemical used in many building materials, household products, and industrial disinfectants, has demonstrated particularly strong associations with myeloid leukemias (Beane Freeman et al. 2009; Zhang et al. 2009). The mechanisms by which risk factors shared across leukemias promote oncogenic processes likely exhibit commonalities, although detailed discussion of such mechanisms is beyond the scope of this review.

PEDIATRIC LEUKEMIAS

Almost all leukemias in the pediatric population are acute types. ALL is the most commonly diagnosed childhood cancer worldwide. It accounts for ~75% of leukemia cases in children of <15 yr of age, with a peak incidence rate of 7.8 per 100,000 among children 2–4 yr of age in the United States (Noone et al. 2017). Unlike other leukemias, which are more highly incident among Whites, the incidence of pediatric ALL is higher for Hispanics than for other racial and ethnic groups. For Hispanic children of <20 yr of age, ALL incidence was 4.3 per 100,000 in the United States from 2001 to 2014, compared to 3.4 for White, 3.0 for AIAN, 3.2 for API, and 1.9 for Black children (Siegel et al. 2017). These rates have largely remained stable since 2008. AML is the second most common hematologic malignancy in children, with peak incidence in the pediatric population occurring in the first year of life.

The causes of leukemia in pediatric patients remain elusive. Several genetic syndromes and immune disorders are associated with both ALL and AML risk, although most cases are not familial. These include Down syndrome (DS), Li–Fraumeni syndrome, neurofibromatosis, DNA repair deficiency syndromes like Fanconi anemia and Bloom syndrome, and rare inherited bone marrow failure syndromes like Kostmann syndrome, Diamond–Blackfan anemia, dyskeratosis congenita, and Schwachman–Diamond syndrome (Alter 2007; Owen et al. 2008). Approximately 2.1% of individuals with DS develop leukemia by the age of 5, and 2.7% by age 30. Incidence of both ALL and AML among individuals with DS is more than 20-fold that expected in the general population. The magnitude of DS-associated risk for AML is much higher than that for ALL in children of <5 yr of age (short interest ratio (SIR) = 154 vs. SIR = 41), but slightly higher for ALL compared to AML among children and young adults 5–30 yr of age (SIR = 12 vs. SIR = 10) (Hasle et al. 2000).

Pediatric leukemia is also associated with certain therapeutic exposures, such as chemotherapy with alkylating agents and topoisomerase II inhibitors for primary cancers (Hijiya et al. 2009); diagnostic exposures such as ionizing radiation from CT scans (Pearce et al. 2012); and organ transplantation, which may be related to iatrogenic immunosuppression and exposure to oncogenic viruses (Yanik et al. 2017). Several recent studies indicate that environmental exposure to benzene (e.g., via proximity to automobile traffic and factories), elevates AML risk in children (Honoré et al. 2015; Janitz et al. 2017).

Some studies indicate that early immune stimulation (e.g., via exposure to infection) may be protective against ALL (Rudant et al. 2015; Hwee et al. 2018). Using data pooled across 11 studies from the Childhood Leukemia International Consortium, Rudant et al. (2015) reported a 23% reduction in risk of ALL among children who attended day care (a proxy for immune stimulation) in the first year of life, with a trend for lower risks at younger start dates. Several important hypotheses articulate an infectious etiology of ALL. Greaves' *delayed-infection hypothesis,* first outlined in 1988, posits that delayed (e.g., postinfancy) exposure to common infectious agents, for which the immune system is unprepared, elicits an abnormal immune response that triggers ALL (Greaves 1988, 2006). In his model, an initiating genetic event in utero creates a covert preleukemic clone that, upon a second postnatal genetic "hit," progresses to overt leukemia (Greaves 2006). By Kinlen's *population-mixing hypothesis*, also outlined in 1988, childhood leukemia is a rare response to a common, unidentified infection that occurs when an infected population "mixes" with a susceptible, nonimmune population (e.g., urban–rural mixing) (Kinlen 1988, 2012). The *adrenal hypothesis,* more recently proposed by Schmiegelow et al. (2008) postulates that early infection induces the hypothalamus–pituitary–adrenal axis to increase plasma cortisol levels, which may eliminate leukemic and preleukemic cells, and reduces risk of leukemogenesis by suppressing proinflammatory responses. Importantly, not all studies support an infectious etiology of ALL. Designing epidemiologic studies to evaluate these hypotheses is challenging—for example, prospective studies are unfeasible due to the rarity of ALL, and factors like recall bias and temporal ambiguity threaten the validity of retrospective studies (Hwee et al. 2018).

With improvements in recent decades to risk classification and treatments like combination chemotherapies and targeted drug therapies, overall relative survival from ALL is high. Between 1975–1979 and 2003–2009, 5-yr relative survival from pediatric ALL increased dramatically from 57% to a very favorable 90% (Ward et al. 2014). AML also saw major gains during this period (from 21% to 64%), although survival remains less favorable than that for ALL. Numerous studies demonstrate that Black and Hispanic children with ALL historically have suffered worse outcomes than their White and non-Hispanic counterparts (Bhatia et al. 2002; Kadan-Lottick et al. 2003; Pui et al. 2012; Tai et al. 2017). Although survival patterns between White and Black children have converged in recent decades (particularly in children of <15 yr of age), several studies have documented widening disparities for Hispanic children (Wang et al. 2015; Kahn et al. 2016). From 2000 to 2010, ALL mortality among Hispanic children was nearly twice that of Whites (HR = 1.95). Survival disparities may reflect both biologic (e.g., genetic variations associated with ancestry) and socioeconomic (e.g., access to care and treatment adherence) pathways. In one recent study, accounting for the effect of neighborhood socioeconomic status (SES) on hazard of death from ALL reduced the observed racial disparity from HR = 1.43 to HR = 1.22 for Blacks and from HR = 1.63 to HR = 1.40 for Hispanics, respectively, relative to Whites (Kehm et al. 2018). Research on childhood AML has also attributed an elevated risk of death to neighborhood socioeconomic factors—specifically economic and educational disadvantages, housing instability, and immigration-related features (Knoble et al. 2016).

ADULT LEUKEMIAS AND LYMPHOMAS

Acute Myeloid Leukemia

Worldwide, AML occurs with greatest frequency in highly developed regions; age-standardized incidence is highest for both males and females in Australia (2.8 and 2.0 per 100,000), Austria (2.7 and 2.2 per 100,000), and the United Kingdom (2.7 and 2.0 per 100,000) (Miranda-Filho et al. 2018). In the United States, an estimated 19,520 cases of AML were diagnosed in 2018. Beginning in young adulthood, the age distribution of AML incidence is exponentially shaped. SEER data show an especially sharp increase in incidence after 75 yr of age, when the rate nearly doubles that of adults aged 60–74 (209 vs. 109 cases per 1,000,000 person-years) (Dores et al. 2012). AML incidence and mortality are higher among Whites than other racial and ethnic groups. For example, age-adjusted incidence among White males in SEER is 5.4 per 100,000, compared to 4.5 for Blacks and 4.1 for Hispanics (Noone et al. 2017). Mortality rates demonstrate a similar racial pattern (3.8, 2.7, and 2.3 per 100,000 for Whites, Blacks, and Hispanics, respectively), and SEER data indicate that these racial and ethnic trends persist across sex and age groups (Zhao et al. 2018).

The causes of genetic mutations that give rise to most cases of AML are largely unknown. Prominent risk factors evaluated in the literature include radiation therapy, chemotherapy, smoking, and other environmental exposures. Morton et al. (2013) have reported that the number of AML diagnoses among patients who received chemotherapy for a first primary cancer is 4.7 times that expected in the general population. Therapy-related myelodysplasia (MDS)/AML is diagnostically classified by treatment type—namely, alkylating agent/radiation regimens or topoisomerase inhibitor-related regimens—and typically occurs within 10 yr of initial therapy (Bhatia 2013). In an early case-control study of AML in breast cancer patients, Curtis et al. reported relative risks of 2.4 for receipt of radiation treatment alone, 10.0 for alkylating agents, and 17.4 for combined radiation-alkylating agent regimens (Curtis et al. 1992). Saso et al. (2000) also found that the risk of MDS/AML in breast cancer patients treated with alkylating agents was 10-fold that of the general population. Although AML is a relatively rare disease, the absolute excess risk associated with therapy is sizeable (ranging from 5 to 7 excess cases per 100,000 person-years in studies by Howard and colleagues) (Howard et al. 2007, 2008). Another important risk factor for AML in adulthood is smoking. Multiple meta-analysis show elevated risk of AML in smokers. Using data from 23 studies, Fircanis et al. (2014) calculated a 40% and 25% increased risk of AML in current and former smokers, respectively, compared to nonsmokers. Pooling data from nine Japanese cohort studies, Ugai et al. also showed an increased risk of near 40% for current smokers, and a 66% increase for ever-smokers with a history of more than 30 pack-years compared to nonsmokers (Ugai et al. 2018). Although findings for environmental chemical exposures are less consistent, benzene is a well-established risk factor and has been recognized by the IARC as a cause of AML (International Agency for Research on Cancer 1987; Khalade et al. 2010; Carlos-Wallace et al. 2016; Raaschou-Nielsen et al. 2018). Benzene is one of the most widely used chemicals in the United States, and occupational exposure is highest in industries related to rubber, oil refining, shoe manufacturing, and gasoline.

Several genetic abnormalities are associated with AML risk. Although familial AML is rare, AML is considered part of the natural history of rare inherited bone marrow failure syndromes like Kostmann syndrome, Diamond–Blackfan anemia, dyskeratosis congenita, and Schwachman–Diamond syndrome, as well as DNA repair deficiency syndromes like Fanconi anemia and Bloom syndrome (Alter 2007; Owen et al. 2008).

Survival from AML varies substantially by age, with dramatic declines observed for older patients. For those diagnosed before age 65, overall 5-yr relative survival is 45.6%, compared to 7.1% for those diagnosed at age 65 or older (Noone et al. 2017). Despite some studies demonstrating that White patients present with less favorable prognostic profiles than other racial/ethnic groups (namely, lower rates of t(8;21) and acute promyelocytic leukemia), survival outcomes tend to be worst for Black and Hispanic patients (Pulte et al. 2013; Patel et al. 2015b). The survival disparity between Black and White AML patients is especially pronounced for those diagnosed at younger ages (e.g., at <65 yr of age) (Noone et al. 2017) Even after controlling for age and genetic factors, Black race has been associated with increased risk of death relative to Whites (Patel et al. 2012, 2015b). Some of the racial survival disparity may reflect treatment differences; in California, for example, Black race has been associated with lower odds of receiving chemotherapy and transplant (Patel et al. 2015a). Finally, although AML survival has increased for all racial/ethnic groups since 1991–1996, disparities between groups have also increased as gains have favored Whites, particularly at younger ages. For White patients 15–54 yr of age, survival significantly increased by 12.8 percentage points through 2003–2008, whereas gains for other racial and ethnic groups (4.3 percentage points for AA and Hispanics, 7.1 points for API) did not reach statistical significance (Pulte et al. 2013).

Acute Lymphocytic Leukemia

Overall, an estimated 5960 total cases of ALL were diagnosed in the United States in 2018 (Siegel et al. 2018). Whereas the incidence of other leukemias generally increases with age, ALL is distinctly bimodal, with pediatric incidence rates far exceeding those for older age groups. Throughout adulthood, incidence is relatively stable around 1 per 100,000, with an increase to 1.9 per 100,000 among elderly adults aged 80–84 (Noone et al. 2017). Like other leukemias, ALL demonstrates a slight male predominance.

Global incidence patterns for ALL are also unique; whereas other leukemias are patterned by HDI and concentrated in Europe, Northern America, and Australia, ALL incidence is highest in South and Central American countries—namely, Ecuador (2.8 and 3.3 per 100,000 for males and females, respectively), Costa Rica (2.4 and 2.3 per 100,000), and Colombia (2.3 and 2.1 per 100,000) (Miranda-Filho et al. 2018). In the United States, incidence of ALL varies substantially by ethnicity. It is the only leukemia in which incidence, in both pediatric and adult cases, is higher for Hispanics than any other racial or ethnic group.

There are no known causes of ALL. ALL typically arises from noninherited genetic abnormalities. The Philadelphia chromosome, or t(9;22), is the most common chromosomal translocation in adult ALL (present in 25% of cases), and unlike in children it is characterized by a highly aggressive clinical course (Gleissner et al. 2002; Pui et al. 2004; Thomas and Heiblig 2016). Many risk factors for adult ALL are similar to those of pediatric ALL, including chemotherapy (e.g., for primary cancers), ionizing radiation (e.g., therapy-related or atomic bomb exposure), and chemical toxins like benzene. The specific mechanisms of risk for these exposures remain unclear.

Survival from ALL declines with age at diagnosis; 5-yr relative survival is 35.8% for adults 45–54 yr of age, 26.4% for adults 55–64 yr or age, and 16.5% for adults diagnosed at age 65 or older (Noone et al. 2017). When stratified by race and ethnicity, survival is higher for White ALL patients compared to other groups, particularly Black ALL patients. SEER data from 2000 to 2014 indicate that racial survival disparities are more pronounced at younger ages (namely for patients 15–39 yr of age) (Kirtane and Lee 2017). Adult survival disparities have persisted despite Black patients experiencing some of the largest recent improvements in 5-yr survival (e.g., from 24.1% to 43.4% among patients 15–44 yr of age between 1997–2002 and 2003–2008) (Pulte et al. 2013). Hispanic adults, for unclear reasons, also continue to face poorer 5-yr relative survival than White adults and have experienced smaller gains in survival compared to other racial/ethnic groups (Kirtane and Lee 2017).

Chronic Myeloid Leukemia

CML is cytogenetically characterized by the Philadelphia chromosome--a truncation of chromosome 22 resulting from the reciprocal translocation t(9;22)(q32;q11). CML accounts for ~15% of leukemia diagnoses in the United States, or an estimated 8430 new cases in 2018 (Siegel et al. 2018). Incidence increases steadily with age, peaking at 10.3 cases per 100,000 among individuals 80–84 yr of age, although the most frequent age of diagnosis is between 65 and 74 yr of age (comprising 21% of CML diagnoses). Racial and ethnic patterns in CML incidence are more disparate than for other leukemias. In U.S. males, incidence is highest in Whites (2.4 per 100,000) and AI/AN (2.3 per 100,000), whereas for females incidence is highest in Whites and Blacks (1.4 per 100,000) (Noone et al. 2017). Worldwide, there is some variability in CML incidence rates by country, but no clear patterning by HDI. Rates are highest in Australia (1.8 and 1.0 per 100,000 in males and females, respectively), Lithuania (1.6 and 0.9 per 100,000), France (1.7 per 100,000 males), and Uruguay (1.1 per 100,000 females) (Miranda-Filho et al. 2018).

Apart from increasing age, the only known risk factor for CML is exposure to ionizing radiation, which has been described in literature on leukemia among atomic bomb survivors (Heyssel et al. 1960).

CML has a moderate prognosis, with 5-yr relative survival at 68.7% (Noone et al. 2017). Survival from CML underwent drastic improvements after the introduction of the first tyrosine kinase inhibitor (TKI), imatinib mesylate (Gleevec), in 2001. Prior to this, the prognosis was poor, with overall relative survival <50% for patients within 3 yr of diagnosis (Mandal et al. 2013). Although survival has improved across racial and ethnic groups, Mandal et al. found that 3-yr relative survival in the post-imatinib era was nevertheless significantly lower for Black females (80.5%) than White females (90.3%), and that survival gains favored younger patients (<50 yr) over older patients. The reason for racial and ethnic disparities in CML survival have been difficult to identify. Wiggins et al. did not find TKI treatment disparities in the United States by race/ethnicity, SES, urban/rural residence, comorbidity, or insurance status after controlling for age (Wiggins et al. 2010). However, age disparities in survival improvement partially reflected less frequent administration of imatinib regimens in elderly patients.

Chronic Lymphocytic Leukemia/Small Cell Lymphoma

Worldwide, CLL/SLL incidence is highest in countries of very high HDI—namely, Canada and France, where annual rates exceed four new cases per 100,000 males. Incidence is especially low in Asian countries, particularly Japan (0.1 per 100,000), Malaysia (0.1 per 100,000), and the Philippines (0.2 per 100,000). Sex-specific differences are stronger for CLL/SLL than for other leukemias, with incidence among males nearly double that of females, both globally and in the United States (Miranda-Filho et al. 2018).

CLL/SLL is the most common leukemia subtype in the United States, with an estimated 20,940 new cases diagnosed in 2018 (Siegel et al. 2018). Incidence in the United States varies widely by race. The most elevated incidence rates are observed for Whites (5.1 per 100,000) and Blacks (3.6 per 100,000). Incidence is markedly lower, roughly a quarter that of Whites, among the API and AIAN population. Risk of CLL/SLL is strongly age-dependent, with 67% of diagnoses made to individuals older than age 65. Among individuals aged 65 and older, incidence is 26.4 per 100,000; for the oldest age strata (85 and older), incidence is 35.8 per 100,000 (Noone et al. 2017).

Family history of hematologic malignancy is the strongest and most consistent risk factor for CLL/SLL (even if the absolute risk among first-degree relatives is low), implicating common inherited genetic pathways in CLL/SLL pathogenesis. Large-scale studies using data from the Swedish Cancer Registry have demonstrated that relatives of CLL/SLL cases have a 7.5- to

8.5-fold risk of developing CLL/SLL over relatives of controls (Goldin et al. 2004b, 2009). In one of the largest epidemiologic studies on CLL/SLL risk, which pooled data across 13 case-control studies in Europe, North America, and Australia as part of the International Lymphoma Epidemiology Consortium (InterLymph), history of any hematological malignancy among first-degree relatives was associated with a greater than twofold odds of CLL/SLL odds ratio (OR = 2.17) (Slager et al. 2014).

No single germline mutation has been identified as a causal precursor to CLL/SLL (Goldin and Caporaso 2007). Monoclonal B-cell lymphocytosis (MBL), which is more frequent in high-risk CLL/SLL families than the general population, may be an early genetic factor indicative of inherited predisposition (Rawstron et al. 2002; Goldin et al. 2013). Some studies suggest that geographic and racial variability in CLL/SLL incidence and prognosis reflect underlying differences in genetic risk factors between groups. For example, Coombs et al. found that the risk allele frequency of most single nucleotide polymorphisms known to confer risk of CLL/SLL in Whites is not associated with risk among Black CLL/SLL patients (Coombs et al. 2012b). The rarity of CLL/SLL among Asians, both in Asia and abroad, also supports the notion of a strong genetic component to disease risk. Several studies have failed to show differences in rates of CLL/SLL between Asian migrants to the United States (foreign-born) and their U.S.-born descendants, suggesting a limited role for the impact of environmental and lifestyle-related exposures on CLL/SLL risk at the population level (Herrinton et al. 1996; Gale et al. 2000; Pan et al. 2002).

Other exposures evaluated as risk factors for CLL/SLL include medical history, biometric characteristics, lifestyle-related factors, and various environmental, occupational, and chemical exposures. Pooled analyses across InterLymph studies have demonstrated elevated odds of CLL/SLL associated with increasing height (OR = 1.09 per 10 cm), hepatitis C seropositivity (OR = 1.99), residential or occupational history on a farm (OR = 1.20), and occupational history as a hairdresser (OR = 1.77) (Slager et al. 2014). Although studies on chemical exposures are largely inconsistent, the National Institute of Medicine concluded in 2003 that Agent Orange, an dioxin-containing herbicide used in Vietnam, is associated with CLL/SLL in veterans (Institute of Medicine 2009). Protective factors from pooled InterLymph data include history of atopic disorder (OR = 0.85), blood transfusion (OR = 0.79), cigarette smoking (OR = 0.91), and sun exposure (OR = 0.71 for highest quartile compared to lowest) (Slager et al. 2014).

Unlike other leukemias, CLL/SLL generally is considered nonradiogenic. Some researchers challenge this conclusion, particularly in light of evidence on CLL/SLL in Czech uranium miners and those exposed to radiation following the Chernobyl nuclear power plant accident (Řeřicha et al. 2006; Hamblin 2008). Results around occupational and medical radiation exposure are inconsistent overall; however, Silver et al. noted that CLL/SLL risk estimates for irradiated patients in medical cohort studies with >15 yr of follow-up were almost uniformly elevated, albeit nonsignificantly (Silver et al. 2007). The decades-long latency period of CLL/SLL, low case-fatality rate, lack of diagnostic specificity, historical underreporting bias, and difficulty in achieving an adequate sample size are all major challenges in observational studies that examine radiation (and environmental exposures generally) as a risk factor of CLL/SLL (Richardson et al. 2005).

Relative 5-yr survival in the United States overall is high, exceeding 84% (Noone et al. 2017). Both institutional and population-based studies indicate that Black patients have poorer prognostic profiles at diagnosis, and worse survival, than other racial and ethnic groups (Shenoy et al. 2011; Coombs et al. 2012a; Falchi et al. 2013). Pooled data from MD Anderson and Duke University demonstrated that compared to other races combined, Black patients had worse biological and genetic characteristics at diagnosis, including lower hemoglobin and higher β-microglobulin; more frequently presented with unmutated IGHV gene, ZAP70 expression, and chromosome 17p or 11q deletion; more frequently required first-line therapy; and had shorter overall and event-free survival after controlling for prognostic factors (Falchi et al. 2013). Using data from SEER, Shoney et al. also showed that Black CLL/SLL patients are diagnosed at younger ages and suffer worse survival than White patients after controlling for prognostic factors like disease stage, extra-nodal primary site, and B symptoms (HR = 1.67) (Shenoy et al. 2011).

Non-Hodgkin's Lymphomas

By the latest GLOBOCAN estimates, 509,590 new cases of NHL were projected/estimated worldwide in 2018, and 248,724 NHL deaths (Bray et al. 2018). NHL incidence and mortality rates reflect a male predominance (6.7 vs. 4.7 incidence cases per 100,000 for males and females, respectively; 3.3 vs. 2.0 deaths per 100,000). Across countries characterized by very high HDI, the age-standardized incidence estimate for 2018 (9.3 per 100,000) was more than double that of any other HDI level (high HDI = 4.6; medium HDI = 3.4; low HDI = 4.2). Correspondingly, global regions with the highest incidence include Australia and New Zealand (13.3 per 100,000), North America (12.5 per 100,000), Northern Europe (11.5 per 100,000), and Western Europe (10.1 per 100,000). By contrast, incidence of NHL is lowest across Middle and Central Africa (3.0 and 4.0 per 100,000), Central America (4.0 per 100,000), and Eastern and Southeastern Asia (4.9 per 100,000) (Ferlay et al. 2018).

In the United States, NHL accounted for an estimated 74,680 new cancer diagnoses and 19,910 cancer deaths in 2018, making it the seventh most incident cancer and ninth leading cause of cancer mortality. Nearly 90% of all lymphomas in the United States are NHL, but this proportion is reduced at younger ages (62% in children 0–14 yr, 25% in adolescents 15–19 yr) (Ward et al. 2014; Siegel et al. 2018). Diagnosis of NHL is most common in adults 65–74 yr of age (25.6% of all incidence cases) (Noone et al. 2017).

NHLs historically have been classified as indolent or aggressive according to their usual clinical course, despite substantial patient-to-patient variability. Indolent lymphomas include CLL/SLL, low-grade follicular lymphoma, and marginal zone B-cell lymphoma. Aggressive lymphomas include high-grade follicular lymphoma and diffuse large B-cell lymphoma (DLBCL). Burkitt lymphomas (BL) and precursor B- and T-lymphoblastic leukemia/lymphoma are usually highly aggressive. The most common NHL subtype in the United States is DLBCL (32%). Excluding CLL/SLL, the second most common subtype is follicular lymphoma (16%). Less common NHLs include marginal zone lymphoma (9%), mantel cell lymphoma (4%), and Burkitt lymphoma/leukemia (2%) (Teras et al. 2016).

NHL incidence is >50% higher in males than females, although there is considerable variability in the sex ratio by NHL subtype; for example, the male predominance is markedly less pronounced for follicular lymphoma and marginal zone lymphoma incidence ratio (IRR = 1.18 and 1.05, respectively), and stronger for mantel cell and Burkitt lymphoma (IRR = 3.07 and 2.79) (Teras et al. 2016). The strong male predominance of Burkitt lymphoma is likely attributable to its association with human immunodeficiency virus (HIV)/AIDS, which is more prevalent in males than females.

NHL was one of few neoplasms in the United States, and globally, that saw major increases in incidence around the turn of the century. By GBD estimates, the global incidence of NHL rose 23% from 2005 to 2015, with the largest increase in middle social-development index countries (Fitzmaurice et al. 2017). From 1975 to 1991, NHL incidence increased annually by 3.6% in the United States, and nearly doubled between 1975 and 2008, resulting in what has been described as an NHL epidemic (Levine and Hoover 1992; Weisenburger 1994; Bosetti et al. 2008; Shiels et al. 2013). Researchers have hypothesized that the rise in NHL is at least partially attributable to improvements in detection and refinement of the classification system, certain environmental and lifestyle factors, the increasing number of transplant recipients in the population, and the emergence of HIV/AIDS in the early 1980s. NHL (chiefly DLBCL subtypes) is linked etiologically to immunosuppression and considered an AIDS-defining event. Recently, NHL incidence has plateaued, with an annual 0.8% decrease in incidence since 2007 (Noone et al. 2017). Shiels et al. (2013) have suggested that the recent stabilization of NHL rates in the general population is independent of HIV. Among NHL subtypes, decreases in incidence have been most pronounced for CLL/SLL (APC = −2.7% and −2.9% for males and females, respectively, since 2005), and follicular lymphoma (APC = −2.2 for males since 2004, and −3.6% for females since 2007). Rates of DLBCL have remained stable since 2001 (Teras et al. 2016).

NHL incidence and mortality tend to be higher in Whites than other racial/ethnic groups, with some variability in racial and ethnic incidence patterns by subtype. Incidence of B-cell NHL is 7%, 18%, and 72% higher among Whites compared to Blacks, Hispanics, and API, respectively. On the other hand, the incidence of T/NK-cell NHL is 49% higher in Blacks than Whites (Teras et al. 2016)

Lymphomas typically are characterized by chromosomal translocations that are not heritable, and research on NHL etiology most consistently supports a role for infection (predominantly viral) and immunosuppression. Specific pathogens that have been linked to risk of NHL include human herpes virus 8 (Oksenhendler et al. 2002; Deloose et al. 2005), hepatitis C (HCV) (Matsuo et al. 2004; Morton et al. 2014), human T-cell lymphotropic virus (Manns et al. 1993; Cleghorn et al. 1995), and *Helicobacter pylorus* (Parsonnet et al. 1994; Sagaert et al. 2010), among others. In one meta-analysis, the pooled relative risk of NHL associated with HCV infection was 2.5, and the authors estimated that upward of 10% of NHL in areas with high HCV prevalence could be attributed to the infection (Dal Maso and Franceschi 2006). In 2009, the IARC Working Group classified Epstein–Barr virus (EBV), a member of the herpes family, a class 1 carcinogen that causes several NHL subtypes, including Burkitt lymphoma, sinonasal angiocentric T-cell lymphoma, and immunosuppression-related NHL (IARC 2012).

The mechanisms of carcinogenesis for viral exposures vary, but EBV has been the focus of most research. Possible oncogenic properties of EBV include the immortalization of B cells and the encoding of gene products that cause genomic instability, induce cell proliferation, and block apoptosis. Worldwide, EBV infection is ubiquitous; primary infection typically occurs in childhood or adolescence, after which the virus establishes lifelong latency in lymphocytes, with the possibility of reactivation. The carcinogenic potential of EBV frequently arises in the context of sustained immunosuppression or infectious cofactors. For example, there is striking correspondence in the geographic distribution of endemic BL and holoendemic malaria. In tropical zones of subequatorial Africa, endemic BL accounts for 20% of childhood malignancies, and EBV is present in nearly 100% of cases (Orem et al. 2007; Silver et al. 2007). It is generally understood that early coinfection with malaria alters EBV persistence and deteriorates immunoregulatory control of EBV, resulting in a malignant B-cell clone (Rochford et al. 2005; Orem et al. 2007; Chene et al. 2009; Moormann et al. 2011). Several studies support a synergistic effect of malaria and EBV coinfection on risk of childhood BL, with the odds of elevated antibody titers for both EBV and malaria in cases between five to 13 times that of controls (Carpenter et al. 2008; Mutalima et al. 2008).

In individuals with HIV or AIDS, NHL is the second most common malignancy after Kaposi's sarcoma. From 1996 to 2010, incidence of NHL among individuals registered with HIV or AIDS was 193.7 per 100,000 person years, about half of which were DLBCL (Gibson et al. 2014). In one review of population-based studies across the United States, Australia, and Italy, the risk of NHL in individuals with AIDS compared to the general population ranged from 15-fold for low-grade NHL to 400-fold for high-grade NHL (Dal Maso and Franceschi 2003). Incidence of NHL in people with AIDS declined dramatically following the introduction of highly active antiretroviral therapy in 1996. In the United States, the relative risk of NHL in people with AIDS compared to the general population reduced from SIR = 53.2 to SIR = 22.6 between 1990–1995 and 1996–2002 (Engels et al. 2006). In a report by Hernández-Ramírez et al., NHL risks since 1996 have declined significantly for DLBCL and central nervous system NHL, but not BL (Hernández-Ramírez et al. 2017). Nevertheless, incidence of NHL remains elevated for individuals with HIV or AIDS. Analogous to models of malaria as a cofactor in EBV-driven BL pathogenesis, current opinion holds that HIV infection contributes to NHL pathogenesis indirectly through sustained B-cell activation and impaired immunoregulatory control of oncogenic viruses like EBV. Emerging evidence suggests that HIV may also contribute directly through HIV-encoded proteins that enhance B-cell clonogenicity and increase propensity for chromosomal translocations (Dolcetti et al. 2016).

Populations treated with immunosuppressive drugs, including organ transplant recipients and individuals with autoimmune diseases, also experience elevated risk of NHL. In a large cohort study linking 20 years of data from the United States Scientific Registry of Transplants with state and regional cancer registries, Engels et al. reported a more than sevenfold increase in risk of NHL in transplant recipients compared to the general population. Among transplant recipients, an excess of 168.3 cases of NHL per 100,000 person-years could be attributed to transplant (Engels et al. 2011). Relative risks are strongest at younger ages. In a recent registry-linked study on pediatric recipients, 71% of posttransplant malignancies were NHL; risk of NHL in recipients was 212 times that of the general population, and exceeded 300 for recipients of <5 yr of age (Yanik et al. 2017). Data from this study also indicate EBV as a cofactor in pathogenesis. Patients who were seronegative for EBV prior to transplantation had 2.7 times the risk of NHL compared to those already seropositive. Presumably, drug-induced immunosuppression impairs the control of newly acquired EBV infection posttransplant, resulting in heightened risk of the oncogenic effects associated with EBV.

Individuals with autoimmune disorders also experience increased risk of NHL. In their meta-analysis of 20 cohort studies, Zintzaras reported that NHL risk was greatest for patients with Sjögren's syndrome (SIR = 18.8), followed by systemic lupus (SIR = 7.4) and rheumatoid arthritis (SIR = 3.9) (Zintzaras et al. 2005). A pooled analysis of 12 *InterLymph* case-control studies showed more modest effect estimates; Sjögren's syndrome and systemic lupus were associated with 6.5-fold and 2.7-fold odds of NHL, respectively, and both conditions demonstrated significant subtype-specific risk for DLBCL (Ekström Smedby et al. 2008). A large Swedish registry study found that diagnosis with any of 33 autoimmune diseases corresponded to a 60% increase is risk of NHL (Fallah et al. 2014a). The risk of NHL in this population may reflect the effects of sustained inflammatory activity and disease severity over treatment related immunosuppression or EBV infection (Smedby et al. 2006).

Familial aggregation of NHL has been widely reported in the literature. Several large population-based studies in Europe have reported relative risks of NHL near 1.8 for first-degree relatives of individuals with NHL (Altieri et al. 2005; Goldin et al. 2005). It appears that relatives of NHL patients are at highest risk for subtype-concordant malignancy; for example, Goldin et al. (2009) found a 10-fold increase in risk of DLBCL in relatives of DLBCL patients, and a fourfold risk of follicular lymphoma in relatives of follicular lymphoma patients. Despite these associations, the absolute risk attributed to familial predisposition is very modest and does not warrant clinical surveillance of first-degree relatives (Cerhan and Slager 2015).

Research on NHL risks linked to environmental exposures and lifestyle-related factors is largely inconclusive. Although studies generally show no or only modest associations between smoking and NHL overall, pooled data from nine *InterLymph* case-control studies suggest that smoking is positively associated with follicular lymphoma, specifically; the odds of follicular lymphoma were 31% higher in current smokers than nonsmokers, and 45% higher in current heavy smokers (with a history of more than 36 pack-years) (Morton et al. 2005). Researchers have hypothesized that exposure to ultraviolet radiation (UV) may confer NHL risk, but results are inconsistent. Thirty years of prospective data from the Nurses' Health study showed that residing in an area with higher versus lower ambient UV radiation was associated with a 21% increased risk of NHL (Bertrand et al. 2011). Conversely, several studies have found that UV exposure provides a protective effect. In an analysis with data from the California Teachers Study, exposure to residential UV in the highest versus lowest quartile was associated with a 42% decrease in risk of NHL overall, with an even stronger protective effect against DLBCL (relative risk [RR] = 0.36) (Chang et al. 2011). Pooled data from InterLymph studies have also shown a protective effect of recreational sun exposure (Morton et al. 2014). InterLymph analyses do not support a link between BMI as a young adult and NHL risk (Morton et al. 2014); however, a recent meta-analysis of 22 studies by Hidayat and colleagues showed a significant 11% increase in NHL risk per 5 kg/m^2 increase in BMI during early adulthood, and a 21% increase in risk per 10 kg increase in weight (Hidayat et al. 2018). Other important risk factors described in pooled analyses of InterLymph studies include occupational history as a farm worker and exposure to hair dye prior to 1980; additional protective factors include history of atopic diseases, blood transfusion, and alcohol consumption of at least one drink per month (Zhang et al. 2008; Morton et al. 2014).

From 2008 to 2014, the overall 5-yr relative survival in patients diagnosed with NHL was 74.1%, but there is considerable variability by subtype, and survival is typically worse for Black NHL patients than those of other racial and ethnic groups (Noone et al. 2017). Five-year survival tends to be higher for follicular lymphoma (86% and 81% for White and Black males, respectively) and marginal zone lymphomas (89% and 83%), and lower for Burkitt (63% and 47%) and DLBCL (62% and 55%) (Teras et al. 2016).

Hodgkin's Lymphoma

In 2018, HL accounted for an estimated 79,990 incident cancer diagnoses and 26,167 cancer deaths worldwide (Bray et al. 2018). Like NHL, incidence of HL in very high HDI countries (2.1 per 100,000) is more than double that of all other HDI levels. Regions with the most elevated HL incidence rates include Southern, Northern, and Western Europe (2.8, 2.6, and 2.5 per 100,000), Australia and New Zealand (2.5 per 100,000), and North America (2.4 per 100,000). Incidence is lowest across Eastern and Southern Asia, and sub-Saharan Africa (Ferlay et al. 2018). By GBD estimates, the number of new HL diagnoses globally declined by 6.1% after accounting for population growth and changing age structure (Fitzmaurice et al. 2017).

HL comprises roughly 10% of all lymphomas in the United States. In 2018, HL accounted for an estimated 8500 new cancer diagnoses and 1050 cancer deaths (Siegel et al. 2018). Incidence is higher among Whites than other racial and ethnic groups. The age distribution of HL is distinctly bimodal, with peak incidence occurring first among young adults 20–24 yr of age and again among elderly adults 75–79 yr of age (Noone et al. 2017). Most patients diagnosed with HL are of <40 yr of age. In the pediatric context, HL is the most common malignancy in adolescents 15–19 yr of age, accounting for 15% of cancer diagnoses in this age group (Ward et al. 2014). Of note, one large SEER study using 15 years of data observed distinct racial patterns in the age distribution of HL; for Black males, HL incidence remained relatively stable after peaking in early adulthood, and for Hispanics, incidence rose in an exponential form after age 40, with only a small uptick in incidence during early adulthood (Evens et al. 2012).

Clinical features of HL also vary by race and ethnicity in the United States. Several studies have shown that Blacks and Hispanics are more likely than Whites to be diagnosed with HL of mixed cellularity and less likely to be diagnosed with nodular sclerosis HL (the predominant subtype of classic HL in the United States) (Glaser et al. 2008, 2014; Evens et al. 2012; Grubb et al. 2016). Incidence of nodular sclerosis HL reflects a socioeconomic gradient, whereby higher SES is associated with elevated risk (Clarke et al. 2005). EBV-positive HL, which tends to be of mixed cellularity, is more common in Hispanics than Whites, particularly among foreign-born Hispanics, and those diagnosed at younger and older ages (Glaser et al. 2008, 2014).

Family studies indicate that risk of HL, like NHL, shows a familial predisposition. Large

 Cite this article as *Cold Spring Harb Perspect Med* doi: 10.1101/cshperspect.a034819

population-based studies from Sweden and Denmark have reported relative risks ranging from 3.1-fold to 8.8-fold for first-degree relatives of HL patients (Goldin et al. 2004a; Crump et al. 2012). The high concordance of HL in monozygotic, but not dizygotic, twins indicates that genetic factors play an etiologic role in the development of some cases of HL (Mack et al. 1995).

HL pathogenesis likely involves a complex interplay between genetic susceptibility, immune impairment, and environmental exposures. Abnormal immune response to infectious agents may trigger oncogenic processes that cause HL. By the delayed-exposure model of HL etiology, increased exposure to infection at a young age may protect against HL by promoting early maturation of cellular immunity. Markers of early exposure to common childhood pathogens, like day care attendance (Chang et al. 2004b; Rudant et al. 2011) and having older siblings (Chang et al. 2004a; Altieri et al. 2006), typically show a protective effect against HL. Data linking EBV to HL risk also supports an infectious etiology for some HL. EBV infection in adolescence manifests clinically as infectious mononucleosis (IM). Whereas history of infection with chicken pox, measles, mumps, pertussis, and rubella have shown a protective effect against HL, history of IM is associated with increased HL risk in young adults (Alexander et al. 2000; Hjalgrim et al. 2000). Furthermore, IM-related risk appears specific to EBV-positive HL (Hjalgrim et al. 2003).

Immunosuppression is associated with risk of HL, although typically to a smaller magnitude than that for NHL. In a recent study that evaluated cancer outcomes in 448,258 HIV-infected individuals using linked population-based registries, risk of HL was 4.6-fold and 9.4-fold higher for individuals with HIV only and AIDS, respectively (Hernández-Ramírez et al. 2017). An earlier meta-analysis of cohort studies reported 11-fold and fourfold risks of HL in individuals with HIV/AIDS and transplant recipients, respectively. In AIDS patients, nearly 100% of classical HL is EBV-positive and of mixed cellularity histology (Bibas and Antinori 2009). Recently, in a large analysis of linked cancer and transplant registry data in the United States, incidence of HL in pediatric transplants recipients was 19 times that of the general population (Yanik et al. 2017). The risk associated with transplant appears somewhat attenuated (SIR = 3.6) when not restricting to the pediatric population (Engels et al. 2011). Autoimmune diseases characterized by chronic inflammation, like rheumatoid arthritis and systemic lupus, have also been linked to HL, with stronger associations noted for EBV-positive malignancy (Fallah et al. 2014b; Hollander et al. 2015).

Some evidence suggests modest associations between HL and lifestyle factors like smoking and exposure to UV radiation. In a pooled analysis of 12 case-control studies, overall odds of HL in ever smokers were 1.1 times that of never smokers, with higher odds for mixed cellularity HL (OR = 1.6) and EBV-positive HL (OR = 1.8). Risks associated with UV exposure also appear specific to EBV-positive HL, but in the opposite direction; in a pooled analysis of four case-control studies, individuals in the highest category of UV exposure had a 44% reduction in odds of EBV-positive HL compared to those in the lowest category (Monnereau et al. 2013).

Overall, HL has a favorable prognosis; the 5-yr relative survival rate exceeded 88% from 2008 to 2014, and was even higher for individuals younger than 45 yr of age at diagnosis (94%) and pediatric cases (97%) (Ward et al. 2014; Noone et al. 2017). Still, SEER and state-specific registry analyses tend to show poorer survival patterns among Black and Hispanic patients compared to White patients (Keegan et al. 2009, 2016; Grubb et al. 2016). In Grubb's analysis of SEER data, overall survival disparities persisted through 25 years of follow-up after controlling for demographics, stage, histology, and treatment; however, the magnitude of differences was less pronounced for Hispanics, and not significant for Blacks, when considering disease-specific survival versus overall survival (Grubb et al. 2016).

CONCLUDING REMARKS

Leukemias and lymphomas comprise a heterogeneous group of malignancies characterized by the uncontrolled proliferation of cells from predominantly myeloid and lymphoid lineages in hematopoietic and lymphoid tissues. The vast majority of these malignancies are sporadic, and specific etiologic mechanisms remain elusive. Leukemias and lymphomas arise in the context of various host and environmental factors. Host factors include genetic abnormalities (most often chromosomal translocations), rare inherited disorders, and iatrogenic or disease-related immunosuppression. Key environmental factors related to leukemia include ionizing radiation, chemotherapy, and carcinogenic chemicals like benzene. Associations between lymphomas and EBV are suggestive of an infectious etiology for certain subtypes such as Burkitt lymphoma and DLBCL.

Leukemia and lymphoma incidence appear to be highest in highly developed regions across Europe, Northern America, and Australia, and among U.S. Whites. An exception to this is ALL, for which incidence is highest in South and Central American countries, and among Hispanics in the United States. Global comparisons in leukemia and lymphoma incidence are made difficult by limited diagnostic infrastructure in less developed countries. Incidence and mortality rates in part reflect a population's access to the formal health-care system, as well as the availability of medical facilities that support morphological, immunohistochemical, and cytogenetic profiling involved in leukemia diagnosis. These factors likely affect overall global counts of leukemia and lymphoma. Furthermore, they may exaggerate differences in overall incidence between more and less developed regions of the world and particularly limit conclusions about observed global patterns that are subtype-specific.

Survival from leukemia and lymphoma varies widely by subtype, ranging from 27.4% 5-yr relative survival from AML to 84.2% for CLL/SLL and 86.6% for HL. Clearly, new treatments are necessary for poor prognosis malignancies such as ALL and AML among adults both with very low survival. Chemotherapy is the most common treatment modality; additionally, treatment recommendations include radiotherapy, immunotherapy, surgery, and bone marrow or stem cell transplantation depending on the specific disease. Treatment disparities may partially explain poorer survival outcomes among Blacks and Hispanics when compared to their White counterparts. In this regard, equal accessibility to novel treatments, like chimeric antigen receptor T-cell therapy currently being used to treat certain forms of ALL, CLL, and B-cell lymphomas, and precision medicine generally, may be an important focus in the proactive fight against disparities.

Temporal trends in hematologic malignancies are dynamic and sometimes unpredictable, as demonstrated by large global increases in NHL incidence around the turn of the century, because of the HIV epidemic and the increasing number of transplants performed in the developed countries. Understanding and monitoring epidemiologic trends of these malignancies in the context of emerging infections is an important area of research. With the increasing diversity of the United States population, high-quality data from population-based cancer registries, and new data from studies on genetic susceptibility, there is great potential for future research to unlock important discoveries on leukemia and lymphoma etiology and distinguish the relative effects of genetic and environmental risk factors.

ACKNOWLEDGMENTS

The authors thank the Sylvester Comprehensive Cancer Center at the University of Miami, Miller School of Medicine for generously supporting the graduate research assistantship of J.A.B.B.

REFERENCES

Alexander FE, Jarrett RF, Lawrence D, Armstrong AA, Freeland J, Gokhale DA, Kane E, Taylor GM, Wright DH, Cartwright RA. 2000. Risk factors for Hodgkin's disease by Epstein–Barr virus (EBV) status: Prior infection by EBV and other agents. *Br J Cancer* **82:** 1117–1121. doi:10.1054/bjoc.1999.1049

Alter BP. 2007. Diagnosis, genetics, and management of inherited bone marrow failure syndromes. *Hematology Am Soc Hematol Educ Program* **2007:** 29–39.

Altieri A, Bermejo JL, Hemminki K. 2005. Familial risk for non-Hodgkin lymphoma and other lymphoproliferative malignancies by histopathologic subtype: The Swedish

Family-Cancer Database. *Blood* **106:** 668–672. doi:10.1182/blood-2005-01-0140

Altieri A, Castro F, Bermejo JL, Hemminki K. 2006. Number of siblings and the risk of lymphoma, leukemia, and myeloma by histopathology. *Cancer Epidemiol Biomarkers Prev* **15:** 1281–1286. doi:10.1158/1055-9965.EPI-06-0087

Beane Freeman LE, Blair A, Lubin JH, Stewart PA, Hayes RB, Hoover RN, Hauptmann M. 2009. Mortality from lymphohematopoietic malignancies among workers in formaldehyde industries: The National Cancer Institute cohort. *J Natl Cancer Inst* **101:** 751–761. doi:10.1093/jnci/djp096

Bertrand KA, Chang ET, Abel GA, Zhang SM, Spiegelman D, Qureshi AA, Laden F. 2011. Sunlight exposure, vitamin D, and risk of non-Hodgkin lymphoma in the nurses' health study. *Cancer Causes Control* **22:** 1731–1741. doi:10.1007/s10552-011-9849-x

Bhatia S. 2013. Therapy-related myelodysplasia and acute myeloid leukemia. *Semin Oncol* **40:** 666–675. doi:10.1053/j.seminoncol.2013.09.013

Bhatia S, Sather HN, Heerema NA, Trigg ME, Gaynon PS, Robison LL. 2002. Racial and ethnic differences in survival of children with acute lymphoblastic leukemia. *Blood* **100:** 1957–1964. doi:10.1182/blood-2002-02-0395

Bibas M, Antinori A. 2009. EBV and HIV-related lymphoma. *Mediterr J Hematol Infect Dis* **1:** e2009032.

Boice JD Jr, Blettner M, Kleinerman RA, Stovall M, Moloney WC, Engholm G, Austin DF, Bosch A, Cookfair DL, Krementz ET, et al. 1987. Radiation dose and leukemia risk in patients treated for cancer of the cervix. *J Natl Cancer Inst* **79:** 1295–1311.

Bosetti C, Levi F, Ferlay J, Lucchini F, Negri E, La Vecchia C. 2008. Incidence and mortality from non-Hodgkin lymphoma in Europe: The end of an epidemic? *Int J Cancer* **123:** 1917–1923. doi:10.1002/ijc.23722

Bray F, Ferlay J, Soerjomataram I, Siegel RL, Torre LA, Jemal A. 2018. Global cancer statistics 2018: GLOBOCAN estimates of incidence and mortality worldwide for 36 cancers in 185 countries. *CA Cancer J Clin* **68:** 394–424. doi:10.3322/caac.21492

Carlos-Wallace FM, Zhang L, Smith MT, Rader G, Steinmaus C. 2016. Parental, in utero, and early-life exposure to benzene and the risk of childhood leukemia: A meta-analysis. *Am J Epidemiol* **183:** 1–14. doi:10.1093/aje/kwv120

Carpenter LM, Newton R, Casabonne D, Ziegler J, Mbulaiteye S, Mbidde E, Wabinga H, Jaffe H, Beral V. 2008. Antibodies against malaria and Epstein–Barr virus in childhood Burkitt lymphoma: A case-control study in Uganda. *Int J Cancer* **122:** 1319–1323. doi:10.1002/ijc.23254

Cerhan JR, Slager SL. 2015. Familial predisposition and genetic risk factors for lymphoma. *Blood* **126:** 2265–2273. doi:10.1182/blood-2015-04-537498

Chang ET, Montgomery SM, Richiardi L, Ehlin A, Ekbom A, Lambe M. 2004a. Number of siblings and risk of Hodgkin's lymphoma. *Cancer Epidemiol Biomarkers Prev* **13:** 1236–1243.

Chang ET, Zheng T, Weir EG, Borowitz M, Mann RB, Spiegelman D, Mueller NE. 2004b. Childhood social environment and Hodgkin's lymphoma: New findings from a population-based case-control study. *Cancer Epidemiol Biomarkers Prev* **13:** 1361–1370.

Chang ET, Canchola AJ, Cockburn M, Lu Y, Wang SS, Bernstein L, Clarke CA, Horn-Ross PL. 2011. Adulthood residential ultraviolet radiation, sun sensitivity, dietary vitamin D, and risk of lymphoid malignancies in the California teachers study. *Blood* **118:** 1591–1599. doi:10.1182/blood-2011-02-336065

Chene A, Donati D, Orem J, Björkman A, Mbidde ER, Kironde F, Wahlgren M, Bejarano MT. 2009. Endemic Burkitt's lymphoma as a polymicrobial disease: New insights on the interaction between *Plasmodium falciparum* and Epstein–Barr virus. *Semin Cancer Biol* **19:** 411–420. doi:10.1016/j.semcancer.2009.10.002

Clarke CA, Glaser SL, Keegan THM, Stroup A. 2005. Neighborhood socioeconomic status and Hodgkin's lymphoma incidence in California. *Cancer Epidemiol Biomarkers Prev* **14:** 1441–1447. doi:10.1158/1055-9965.EPI-04-0567

Cleghorn FR, Manns A, Falk R, Hartge P, Hanchard B, Jack N, Williams E, Jaffe E, White F, Bartholomew C, et al. 1995. Effect of human T-lymphotropic virus type I infection on non-Hodgkin's lymphoma incidence. *J Natl Cancer Inst* **87:** 1009–1014. doi:10.1093/jnci/87.13.1009

Coombs CC, Falchi L, Weinberg JB, Ferrajoli A, Lanasa MC. 2012a. Chronic lymphocytic leukemia in African Americans. *Leuk Lymphoma* **53:** 2326–2329. doi:10.3109/10428194.2012.698276

Coombs CC, Rassenti LZ, Falchi L, Slager SL, Strom SS, Ferrajoli A, Weinberg JB, Kipps TJ, Lanasa MC. 2012b. Single nucleotide polymorphisms and inherited risk of chronic lymphocytic leukemia among African Americans. *Blood* **120:** 1687–1690. doi:10.1182/blood-2012-02-408799

Crump C, Sundquist K, Sieh W, Winkleby MA, Sundquist J. 2012. Perinatal and family risk factors for Hodgkin's lymphoma in childhood through young adulthood. *Am J Epidemiol* **176:** 1147–1158. doi:10.1093/aje/kws212

Curtis RE, Boice JD Jr, Stovall M, Bernstein L, Greenberg RS, Flannery JT, Schwartz AG, Weyer P, Moloney WC, Hoover RN. 1992. Risk of leukemia after chemotherapy and radiation treatment for breast cancer. *N Engl J Med* **326:** 1745–1751. doi:10.1056/NEJM199206253262605

Dal Maso L, Franceschi S. 2003. Epidemiology of non-Hodgkin lymphomas and other haemolymphopoietic neoplasms in people with AIDS. *Lancet Oncol* **4:** 110–119. doi:10.1016/S1470-2045(03)00983-5

Dal Maso L, Franceschi S. 2006. Hepatitis C virus and risk of lymphoma and other lymphoid neoplasms: A meta-analysis of epidemiologic studies. *Cancer Epidemiol Biomarkers Prev* **15:** 2078–2085. doi:10.1158/1055-9965.EPI-06-0308

Deloose ST, Smit LA, Pals FT, Kersten MJ, van Noesel CJ, Pals ST. 2005. High incidence of Kaposi sarcoma–associated herpesvirus infection in HIV-related solid immunoblastic/plasmablastic diffuse large B-cell lymphoma. *Leukemia* **19:** 851–855. doi:10.1038/sj.leu.2403709

Dolcetti R, Gloghini A, Caruso A, Carbone A. 2016. A lymphomagenic role for HIV beyond immune suppression? *Blood* **127:** 1403–1409. doi:10.1182/blood-2015-11-681411

Dores GM, Devesa SS, Curtis RE, Linet MS, Morton LM. 2012. Acute leukemia incidence and patient survival among children and adults in the United States, 2001–2007. *Blood* **119:** 34–43. doi:10.1182/blood-2011-04-347872

Ekström Smedby K, Vajdic CM, Falster M, Engels EA, Martínez-Maza O, Turner J, Hjalgrim H, Vineis P, Seniori Costantini A, Bracci PM, et al. 2008. Autoimmune disorders and risk of non-Hodgkin lymphoma subtypes: A pooled analysis within the InterLymph Consortium. *Blood* **111:** 4029–4038. doi:10.1182/blood-2007-10-119974

Engels EA, Pfeiffer RM, Goedert JJ, Virgo P, McNeel TS, Scoppa SM, Biggar RJ. 2006. Trends in cancer risk among people with AIDS in the United States 1980–2002. *AIDS* **20:** 1645–1654. doi:10.1097/01.aids.0000238411.75324.59

Engels EA, Pfeiffer RM, Fraumeni JF Jr, Kasiske BL, Israni AK, Snyder JJ, Wolfe RA, Goodrich NP, Bayakly AR, Clarke CA, et al. 2011. Spectrum of cancer risk among US solid organ transplant recipients. *J Am Med Assoc* **306:** 1891–1901. doi:10.1001/jama.2011.1592

Evens AM, Antillón M, Aschebrook-Kilfoy B, Chiu BC. 2012. Racial disparities in Hodgkin's lymphoma: A comprehensive population-based analysis. *Ann Oncol* **23:** 2128–2137. doi:10.1093/annonc/mdr578

Falchi L, Keating MJ, Wang X, Coombs CC, Lanasa MC, Strom S, Wierda WG, Ferrajoli A. 2013. Clinical characteristics, response to therapy, and survival of African American patients diagnosed with chronic lymphocytic leukemia: Joint experience of the MD Anderson Cancer Center and Duke University Medical Center. *Cancer* **119:** 3177–3185. doi:10.1002/cncr.28030

Fallah M, Liu X, Ji J, Försti A, Sundquist K, Hemminki K. 2014a. Autoimmune diseases associated with non-Hodgkin lymphoma: A nationwide cohort study. *Ann Oncol* **25:** 2025–2030. doi:10.1093/annonc/mdu365

Fallah M, Liu X, Ji J, Försti A, Sundquist K, Hemminki K. 2014b. Hodgkin lymphoma after autoimmune diseases by age at diagnosis and histological subtype. *Ann Oncol* **25:** 1397–1404. doi:10.1093/annonc/mdu144

Ferlay J, Ervik M, Lam F, Colombet M, Mery L, Piñeros M, Znaor A, Soerjomataram I, Bray F. 2018. *Global cancer observatory: Cancer today.* International Agency for Research on Cancer, Lyon, France. Available from https://gco.iarc.fr/today, accessed January 10, 2019.

Fircanis S, Merriam P, Khan N, Castillo JJ. 2014. The relation between cigarette smoking and risk of acute myeloid leukemia: an updated meta-analysis of epidemiological studies. *Am J Hematol* **89:** E125–E132. doi:10.1002/ajh.23744

Fitzmaurice C, Allen C, Barber RM, Barregard L, Bhutta ZA, Brenner H, Dicker DJ, Chimed-Orchir O, Dandona R, Dandona L, et al. 2017. Global, regional, and national cancer incidence, mortality, years of life lost, years lived with disability, and disability-adjusted life-years for 32 cancer groups, 1990 to 2015: A systematic analysis for the global burden of disease study. *JAMA Oncol* **3:** 524–548. doi:10.1001/jamaoncol.2017.1747

Gale RP, Cozen W, Goodman MT, Wang FF, Bernstein L. 2000. Decreased chronic lymphocytic leukemia incidence in Asians in Los Angeles county. *Leuk Res* **24:** 665–669. doi:10.1016/S0145-2126(00)00038-2

Gibson TM, Morton LM, Shiels MS, Clarke CA, Engels EA. 2014. Risk of non-Hodgkin lymphoma subtypes in HIV-infected people during the HAART era: A population-based study. *AIDS* **28:** 2313–2318. doi:10.1097/QAD.0000000000000428

Glaser SL, Gulley ML, Clarke CA, Keegan TH, Chang ET, Shema SJ, Craig FE, Digiuseppe JA, Dorfman RF, Mann RB, et al. 2008. Racial/ethnic variation in EBV-positive classical Hodgkin lymphoma in California populations. *Int J Cancer* **123:** 1499–1507. doi:10.1002/ijc.23741

Glaser SL, Clarke CA, Chang ET, Yang J, Gomez SL, Keegan TH. 2014. Hodgkin lymphoma incidence in California Hispanics: Influence of nativity and tumor Epstein–Barr virus. *Cancer Causes Control* **25:** 709–725. doi:10.1007/s10552-014-0374-6

Gleissner B, Gokbuget N, Bartram CR, Janssen B, Rieder H, Janssen JW, Fonatsch C, Heyll A, Voliotis D, Beck J, et al. 2002. Leading prognostic relevance of the BCR-ABL translocation in adult acute B-lineage lymphoblastic leukemia: A prospective study of the German Multicenter Trial Group and confirmed polymerase chain reaction analysis. *Blood* **99:** 1536–1543. doi:10.1182/blood.V99.5.1536

Goldin LR, Caporaso NE. 2007. Family studies in chronic lymphocytic leukaemia and other lymphoproliferative tumours. *Br J Haematol* **139:** 774–779. doi:10.1111/j.1365-2141.2007.06810.x

Goldin LR, Pfeiffer RM, Gridley G, Gail MH, Li X, Mellemkjaer L, Olsen JH, Hemminki K, Linet MS. 2004a. Familial aggregation of Hodgkin lymphoma and related tumors. *Cancer* **100:** 1902–1908. doi:10.1002/cncr.20189

Goldin LR, Pfeiffer RM, Li X, Hemminki K. 2004b. Familial risk of lymphoproliferative tumors in families of patients with chronic lymphocytic leukemia: Results from the Swedish family-cancer database. *Blood* **104:** 1850–1854. doi:10.1182/blood-2004-01-0341

Goldin LR, Landgren O, McMaster ML, Gridley G, Hemminki K, Li X, Mellemkjaer L, Olsen JH, Linet MS. 2005. Familial aggregation and heterogeneity of non-Hodgkin lymphoma in population-based samples. *Cancer Epidemiol Biomarkers Prev* **14:** 2402–2406. doi:10.1158/1055-9965.EPI-05-0346

Goldin LR, Björkholm M, Kristinsson SY, Turesson I, Landgren O. 2009. Elevated risk of chronic lymphocytic leukemia and other indolent non-Hodgkin's lymphomas among relatives of patients with chronic lymphocytic leukemia. *Haematologica* **94:** 647–653. doi:10.3324/haematol.2008.003632

Goldin LR, McMaster ML, Caporaso NE. 2013. Precursors to lymphoproliferative malignancies. *Cancer Epidemiol Biomarkers Prev* **22:** 533–539. doi:10.1158/1055-9965.EPI-12-1348

Greaves MF. 1988. Speculations on the cause of childhood acute lymphoblastic leukemia. *Leukemia* **2:** 120–125.

Greaves M. 2006. Infection, immune responses and the aetiology of childhood leukaemia. *Nat Rev Cancer* **6:** 193–203. doi:10.1038/nrc1816

Grubb WR, Neboori HJ, Diaz AD, Li H, Kwon D, Panoff J. 2016. Racial and ethnic disparities in the pediatric Hodgkin lymphoma population. *Pediatr Blood Cancer* **63:** 428–435. doi:10.1002/pbc.25802

Hamblin TJ. 2008. Have we been wrong about ionizing radiation and chronic lymphocytic leukemia? *Leuk Res* **32:** 523–525. doi:10.1016/j.leukres.2007.08.015

Hasle H, Clemmensen IH, Mikkelsen M. 2000. Risks of leukaemia and solid tumours in individuals with Down's syndrome. *Lancet* **355:** 165–169. doi:10.1016/S0140-6736(99)05264-2

Hernández-Ramírez RU, Shiels MS, Dubrow R, Engels EA. 2017. Cancer risk in HIV-infected people in the USA from 1996 to 2012: A population-based, registry-linkage study. *Lancet HIV* **4:** e495–e504. doi:10.1016/S2352-3018(17)30125-X

Herrinton LJ, Goldoft M, Schwartz SM, Weiss NS. 1996. The incidence of non-Hodgkin's lymphoma and its histologic subtypes in Asian migrants to the United States and their descendants. *Cancer Causes Control* **7:** 224–230. doi:10.1007/BF00051298

Heyssel R, Brill AB, Woodbury LA, Nishimura ET, Ghose T, Hoshino T, Yamasaki M. 1960. Leukemia in Hiroshima atomic bomb survivors. *Blood* **15:** 313–331.

Hidayat K, Li HJ, Shi BM. 2018. Anthropometric factors and non-Hodgkin's lymphoma risk: Systematic review and meta-analysis of prospective studies. *Crit Rev Oncol Hematol* **129:** 113–123. doi:10.1016/j.critrevonc.2018.05.018

Hijiya N, Ness KK, Ribeiro RC, Hudson MM. 2009. Acute leukemia as a secondary malignancy in children and adolescents: Current findings and issues. *Cancer* **115:** 23–35. doi:10.1002/cncr.23988

Hjalgrim H, Askling J, Sorensen P, Madsen M, Rosdahl N, Storm HH, Hamilton-Dutoit S, Eriksen LS, Frisch M, Ekbom A, et al. 2000. Risk of Hodgkin's disease and other cancers after infectious mononucleosis. *J Natl Cancer Inst* **92:** 1522–1528. doi:10.1093/jnci/92.18.1522

Hjalgrim H, Askling J, Rostgaard K, Hamilton-Dutoit S, Frisch M, Zhang JS, Madsen M, Rosdahl N, Konradsen HB, Storm HH, et al. 2003. Characteristics of Hodgkin's lymphoma after infectious mononucleosis. *N Engl J Med* **349:** 1324–1332. doi:10.1056/NEJMoa023141

Hollander P, Rostgaard K, Smedby KE, Chang ET, Amini RM, de Nully Brown P, Glimelius B, Adami HO, Melbye M, Glimelius I, et al. 2015. Autoimmune and atopic disorders and risk of classical Hodgkin's lymphoma. *Am J Epidemiol* **182:** 624–632. doi:10.1093/aje/kwv081

Honoré C, Hémon D, Marquant F, Houot J, Faure L, Roth MH, Goujon S, Clavel J. 2015. Residential proximity to heavy-traffic roads, benzene exposure, and childhood leukemia—The GEOCAP Study, 2002–2007. *Am J Epidemiol* **182:** 685–693. doi:10.1093/aje/kwv111

Howard RA, Gilbert ES, Chen BE, Hall P, Storm H, Pukkala E, Langmark F, Kaijser M, Andersson M, Joensuu H, et al. 2007. Leukemia following breast cancer: An international population-based study of 376,825 women. *Breast Cancer Res Treat* **105:** 359–368. doi:10.1007/s10549-006-9460-0

Howard R, Gilbert E, Lynch CF, Hall P, Storm H, Holowaty E, Pukkala E, Langmark F, Kaijser M, Andersson M, et al. 2008. Risk of leukemia among survivors of testicular cancer: A population-based study of 42,722 patients. *Ann Epidemiol* **18:** 416–421. doi:10.1016/j.annepidem.2008.01.003

Hsu WL, Preston DL, Soda M, Sugiyama H, Funamoto S, Kodama K, Kimura A, Kamada N, Dohy H, Tomonaga M, et al. 2013. The incidence of leukemia, lymphoma and multiple myeloma among atomic bomb survivors: 1950–2001. *Radiat Res* **179:** 361–382. doi:10.1667/RR2892.1

Hwee J, Tait C, Sung L, Kwong JC, Sutradhar R, Pole JD. 2018. A systematic review and meta-analysis of the association between childhood infections and the risk of childhood acute lymphoblastic leukaemia. *Br J Cancer* **118:** 127–137. doi:10.1038/bjc.2017.360

IARC. 2012. *IARC monographs on the evaluation of carcinogenic risks to humans,* No. 100B. Epstein–Barr Virus, Lyon, France

Institute of Medicine. 2009. *Veterans and Agent Orange: Update 2008.* National Academies Press (US). National Academy of Sciences, Washington, D.C.

International Agency for Research on Cancer. 1987. *Benzene: IARC monographs—100f.* International Agency for Research on Cancer, Lyon, France.

Janitz AE, Campbell JE, Magzamen S, Pate A, Stoner JA, Peck JD. 2017. Benzene and childhood acute leukemia in Oklahoma. *Environ Res* **158:** 167–173. doi:10.1016/j.envres.2017.06.015

Kadan-Lottick NS, Ness KK, Bhatia S, Gurney JG. 2003. Survival variability by race and ethnicity in childhood acute lymphoblastic leukemia. *J Am Med Assoc* **290:** 2008–2014. doi:10.1001/jama.290.15.2008

Kahn JM, Keegan THM, Tao L, Abrahão R, Bleyer A, Viny AD. 2016. Racial disparities in the survival of American children, adolescents, and young adults with acute lymphoblastic leukemia, acute myelogenous leukemia, and Hodgkin lymphoma. *Cancer* **122:** 2723–2730. doi:10.1002/cncr.30089

Keegan TH, Clarke CA, Chang ET, Shema SJ, Glaser SL. 2009. Disparities in survival after Hodgkin lymphoma: A population-based study. *Cancer Causes Control* **20:** 1881–1892. doi:10.1007/s10552-009-9382-3

Keegan TH, DeRouen MC, Parsons HM, Clarke CA, Goldberg D, Flowers CR, Glaser SL. 2016. Impact of treatment and insurance on socioeconomic disparities in survival after adolescent and young adult Hodgkin lymphoma: A population-based study. *Cancer Epidemiol Biomarkers Prev* **25:** 264–273. doi:10.1158/1055-9965.EPI-15-0756

Kehm RD, Spector LG, Poynter JN, Vock DM, Altekruse SF, Osypuk TL. 2018. Does socioeconomic status account for racial and ethnic disparities in childhood cancer survival? *Cancer* **124:** 4090–4097. doi:10.1002/cncr.31560

Khalade A, Jaakkola MS, Pukkala E, Jaakkola JJ. 2010. Exposure to benzene at work and the risk of leukemia: A systematic review and meta-analysis. *Environ Health* **9:** 31. doi:10.1186/1476-069X-9-31

Kinlen L. 1988. Evidence for an infective cause of childhood leukaemia: Comparison of a Scottish new town with nuclear reprocessing sites in Britain. *Lancet* **332:** 1323–1327. doi:10.1016/S0140-6736(88)90867-7

Kinlen LJ. 2012. An examination, with a meta-analysis, of studies of childhood leukaemia in relation to population mixing. *Br J Cancer* **107:** 1163–1168. doi:10.1038/bjc.2012.402

Kirtane K, Lee SJ. 2017. Racial and ethnic disparities in hematologic malignancies. *Blood* **130:** 1699–1705. doi:10.1182/blood-2017-04-778225

Knoble NB, Alderfer MA, Hossain MJ. 2016. Socioeconomic status (SES) and childhood acute myeloid leukemia (AML) mortality risk: Analysis of SEER data. *Cancer Epidemiol* **44:** 101–108. doi:10.1016/j.canep.2016.07.007

Levine PH, Hoover R. 1992. The emerging epidemic of non-Hodgkin's lymphoma: Current knowledge regarding etiological factors. *Cancer Epidemiol Biomarkers Prev* **1:** 515–517.

Mack TM, Cozen W, Shibata DK, Weiss LM, Nathwani BN, Hernandez AM, Taylor CR, Hamilton AS, Deapen DM, Rappaport EB. 1995. Concordance for Hodgkin's disease in identical twins suggesting genetic susceptibility to the young-adult form of the disease. *N Engl J Med* **332:** 413–418. doi:10.1056/NEJM199502163320701

Mandal R, Bolt DM, Shah BK. 2013. Disparities in chronic myeloid leukemia survival by age, gender, and ethnicity in pre- and post-imatinib eras in the US. *Acta Oncol* **52:** 837–841. doi:10.3109/0284186X.2012.707784

Manns A, Cleghorn FR, Falk RT, Hanchard B, Jaffe ES, Bartholomew C, Hartge P, Benichou J, Blattner WA. 1993. Role of HTLV-I in development of non-Hodgkin lymphoma in Jamaica and Trinidad and Tobago. The HTLV lymphoma study group. *Lancet* **342:** 1447–1450. doi:10.1016/0140-6736(93)92931-I

Matsuo K, Kusano A, Sugumar A, Nakamura S, Tajima K, Mueller NE. 2004. Effect of hepatitis C virus infection on the risk of non-Hodgkin's lymphoma: A meta-analysis of epidemiological studies. *Cancer Sci* **95:** 745–752. doi:10.1111/j.1349-7006.2004.tb03256.x

Metz-Flamant C, Samson E, Caër-Lorho S, Acker A, Laurier D. 2012. Leukemia risk associated with chronic external exposure to ionizing radiation in a French cohort of nuclear workers. *Radiat Res* **178:** 489–498. doi:10.1667/RR2822.1

Miranda-Filho A, Piñeros M, Ferlay J, Soerjomataram I, Monnereau A, Bray F. 2018. Epidemiological patterns of leukaemia in 184 countries: A population-based study. *Lancet Haematol* **5:** e14–e24. doi:10.1016/S2352-3026(17)30232-6

Mohan AK, Hauptmann M, Freedman DM, Ron E, Matanoski GM, Lubin JH, Alexander BH, Boice JD Jr, Morin Doody M, Linet MS. 2003. Cancer and other causes of mortality among radiologic technologists in the United States. *Int J Cancer* **103:** 259–267. doi:10.1002/ijc.10811

Monnereau A, Glaser SL, Schupp CW, Ekström Smedby K, de Sanjosé S, Kane E, Melbye M, Forétova L, Maynadié M, Staines A, et al. 2013. Exposure to UV radiation and risk of Hodgkin lymphoma: A pooled analysis. *Blood* **122:** 3492–3499. doi:10.1182/blood-2013-04-497586

Moormann AM, Snider CJ, Chelimo K. 2011. The company malaria keeps: How co-infection with Epstein–Barr virus leads to endemic Burkitt lymphoma. *Curr Opin Infect Dis* **24:** 435–441. doi:10.1097/QCO.0b013e328349ac4f

Morton LM, Hartge P, Holford TR, Holly EA, Chiu BC, Vineis P, Stagnaro E, Willett EV, Franceschi S, La Vecchia C, et al. 2005. Cigarette smoking and risk of non-Hodgkin lymphoma: A pooled analysis from the international lymphoma epidemiology consortium (interlymph). *Cancer Epidemiol Biomarkers Prev* **14:** 925–933. doi:10.1158/1055-9965.EPI-04-0693

Morton LM, Dores GM, Tucker MA, Kim CJ, Onel K, Gilbert ES, Fraumeni JF Jr, Curtis RE. 2013. Evolving risk of therapy-related acute myeloid leukemia following cancer chemotherapy among adults in the United States, 1975-2008. *Blood* **121:** 2996–3004. doi:10.1182/blood-2012-08-448068

Morton LM, Slager SL, Cerhan JR, Wang SS, Vajdic CM, Skibola CF, Bracci PM, de Sanjose S, Smedby KE, Chiu BC, et al. 2014. Etiologic heterogeneity among non-Hodgkin lymphoma subtypes: The InterLymph non-Hodgkin lymphoma subtypes project. *J Natl Cancer Inst Monographs* **2014:** 130–144. doi:10.1093/jncimonographs/lgu013

Mutalima N, Molyneux E, Jaffe H, Kamiza S, Borgstein E, Mkandawire N, Liomba G, Batumba M, Lagos D, Gratrix F, et al. 2008. Associations between Burkitt lymphoma among children in Malawi and infection with HIV, EBV and malaria: Results from a case-control study. *PLoS ONE* **3:** e2505. doi:10.1371/journal.pone.0002505

Noone A, Howlader N, Krapcho M, Miller D, Brest A, Yu M, Ruhl J, Tatalovich Z, Mariotto A, Lewis D, et al. 2017. *SEER Cancer Statistics Review, 1975–2015*. National Cancer Institute, Bethesda, Maryland.

Oksenhendler E, Boulanger E, Galicier L, Du MQ, Dupin N, Diss TC, Hamoudi R, Daniel MT, Agbalika F, Boshoff C, et al. 2002. High incidence of Kaposi sarcoma-associated herpesvirus-related non-Hodgkin's lymphoma in patients with HIV infection and multicentric Castleman disease. *Blood* **99:** 2331–2336. doi:10.1182/blood.V99.7.2331

Orem J, Mbidde EK, Lambert B, de Sanjose S, Weiderpass E. 2007. Burkitt's lymphoma in Africa, a review of the epidemiology and etiology. *Afr Health Sci* **7:** 166–175.

Owen C, Barnett M, Fitzgibbon J. 2008. Familial myelodysplasia and acute myeloid leukaemia—A review. *Br J Haematol* **140:** 123–132. doi:10.1111/j.1365-2141.2007.06909.x

Pan JW, Cook LS, Schwartz SM, Weis NS. 2002. Incidence of leukemia in Asian migrants to the United States and their descendants. *Cancer Causes Control* **13:** 791–795. doi:10.1023/A:1020608328969

Parsonnet J, Hansen S, Rodriguez L, Gelb AB, Warnke RA, Jellum E, Orentreich N, Vogelman JH, Friedman GD. 1994. *Helicobacter pylori* infection and gastric lymphoma. *N Engl J Med* **330:** 1267–1271. doi:10.1056/NEJM199405053301803

Patel MI, Ma Y, Mitchell BS, Rhoads KF. 2012. Understanding disparities in leukemia: A national study. *Cancer Causes Control* **23:** 1831–1837. doi:10.1007/s10552-012-0062-3

Patel MI, Ma Y, Mitchell B, Rhoads KF. 2015a. How do differences in treatment impact racial and ethnic disparities in acute myeloid leukemia? *Cancer Epidemiol Biomarkers Prev* **24:** 344–349. doi:10.1158/1055-9965.EPI-14-0963

Patel MI, Ma Y, Mitchell BS, Rhoads KF. 2015b. Age and genetics: How do prognostic factors at diagnosis explain disparities in acute myeloid leukemia? *Am J Clin Oncol* **38:** 159–164. doi:10.1097/COC.0b013e31828d7536

Pearce MS, Salotti JA, Little MP, McHugh K, Lee C, Kim KP, Howe NL, Ronckers CM, Rajaraman P, Sir Craft AW, et al. 2012. Radiation exposure from CT scans in childhood and subsequent risk of leukaemia and brain tumours: A retrospective cohort study. *Lancet* **380:** 499–505. doi:10.1016/S0140-6736(12)60815-0

Preston DL, Kusumi S, Tomonaga M, Izumi S, Ron E, Kuramoto A, Kamada N, Dohy H, Matsuo T, Matsui T, et al. 1994. Cancer incidence in atomic bomb survivors. Part

III: Leukemia, lymphoma and multiple myeloma, 1950-1987. *Radiat Res* **137:** S68–S97. doi:10.2307/3578893

Pui CH, Relling MV, Downing JR. 2004. Acute lymphoblastic leukemia. *N Engl J Med* **350:** 1535–1548. doi:10.1056/NEJMra023001

Pui C-H, Pei D, Pappo AS, Howard SC, Cheng C, Sandlund JT, Furman WL, Ribeiro RC, Spunt SL, Rubnitz JE, et al. 2012. Treatment outcomes in black and white children with cancer: Results from the SEER database and St Jude Children's Research Hospital, 1992 through 2007. *J Clin Oncol* **30:** 2005–2012. doi:10.1200/JCO.2011.40.8617

Pulte D, Redaniel MT, Jansen L, Brenner H, Jeffreys M. 2013. Recent trends in survival of adult patients with acute leukemia: Overall improvements, but persistent and partly increasing disparity in survival of patients from minority groups. *Haematologica* **98:** 222–229. doi:10.3324/haematol.2012.063602

Raaschou-Nielsen O, Hvidtfeldt UA, Roswall N, Hertel O, Poulsen AH, Sørensen M. 2018. Ambient benzene at the residence and risk for subtypes of childhood leukemia, lymphoma and CNS tumor. *Int J Cancer* **143:** 1367–1373. doi:10.1002/ijc.31421

Rawstron AC, Yuille MR, Fuller J, Cullen M, Kennedy B, Richards SJ, Jack AS, Matutes E, Catovsky D, Hillmen P, et al. 2002. Inherited predisposition to CLL is detectable as subclinical monoclonal B-lymphocyte expansion. *Blood* **100:** 2289–2290. doi:10.1182/blood-2002-03-0892

Řeřicha V, Kulich M, Řeřicha R, Shore DL, Sandler DP. 2006. Incidence of leukemia, lymphoma, and multiple myeloma in Czech uranium miners: A case and cohort study. *Environ Health Perspect* **114:** 818–822. doi:10.1289/ehp.8476

Richardson DB, Wing S, Schroeder J, Schmitz-Feuerhake I, Hoffmann W. 2005. Ionizing radiation and chronic lymphocytic leukemia. *Environ Health Perspect* **113:** 1–5. doi:10.1289/ehp.7433

Richardson D, Sugiyama H, Nishi N, Sakata R, Shimizu Y, Grant EJ, Soda M, Hsu WL, Suyama A, Kodama K, et al. 2009. Ionizing radiation and leukemia mortality among Japanese atomic bomb survivors, 1950–2000. *Radiat Res* **172:** 368–382. doi:10.1667/RR1801.1

Rochford R, Cannon MJ, Moormann AM. 2005. Endemic Burkitt's lymphoma: A polymicrobial disease? *Nat Rev Microbiol* **3:** 182–187. doi:10.1038/nrmicro1089

Rudant J, Orsi L, Monnereau A, Patte C, Pacquement H, Landman-Parker J, Bergeron C, Robert A, Michel G, Lambilliotte A, et al. 2011. Childhood Hodgkin lymphoma, non-Hodgkin lymphoma and factors related to the immune system: The Escale Study (SFCE). *Int J Cancer* **129:** 2236–2247. doi:10.1002/ijc.25862

Rudant J, Lightfoot T, Urayama KY, Petridou E, Dockerty JD, Magnani C, Milne E, Spector LG, Ashton LJ, Dessypris N, et al. 2015. Childhood acute lymphoblastic leukemia and indicators of early immune stimulation: A Childhood Leukemia International Consortium study. *Am J Epidemiol* **181:** 549–562. doi:10.1093/aje/kwu298

Sagaert X, Van Cutsem E, De Hertogh G, Geboes K, Tousseyn T. 2010. Gastric MALT lymphoma: A model of chronic inflammation-induced tumor development. *Nat Rev Gastroenterol Hepatol* **7:** 336–346. doi:10.1038/nrgastro.2010.58

Sakata R, Kleinerman RA, Mabuchi K, Stovall M, Smith SA, Weathers R, Wactawski-Wende J, Cookfair DL, Boice JD Jr, Inskip PD. 2012. Cancer mortality following radiotherapy for benign gynecologic disorders. *Radiat Res* **178:** 266–279. doi:10.1667/RR2845.1

Saso R, Kulkarni S, Mitchell P, Treleaven J, Swansbury GJ, Mehta J, Powles R, Ashley S, Kuan A, Powles T. 2000. Secondary myelodysplastic syndrome/acute myeloid leukaemia following mitoxantrone-based therapy for breast carcinoma. *Br J Cancer* **83:** 91–94. doi:10.1054/bjoc.2000.1196

Schmiegelow K, Vestergaard T, Nielsen SM, Hjalgrim H. 2008. Etiology of common childhood acute lymphoblastic leukemia: the adrenal hypothesis. *Leukemia* **22:** 2137–2141. doi:10.1038/leu.2008.212

Shenoy PJ, Malik N, Sinha R, Nooka A, Nastoupil LJ, Smith M, Flowers CR. 2011. Racial differences in the presentation and outcomes of chronic lymphocytic leukemia and variants in the United States. *Clin Lymphoma Myeloma Leuk* **11:** 498–506. doi:10.1016/j.clml.2011.07.002

Shiels MS, Engels EA, Linet MS, Clarke CA, Li J, Hall HI, Hartge P, Morton LM. 2013. The epidemic of non-Hodgkin lymphoma in the United States: Disentangling the effect of HIV, 1992–2009. *Cancer Epidemiol Biomarkers Prev* **22:** 1069–1078. doi:10.1158/1055-9965.EPI-13-0040

Siegel DA, Henley SJ, Li J, Pollack LA, Van Dyne EA, White A. 2017. Rates and trends of pediatric acute lymphoblastic leukemia—United States, 2001–2014. *MMWR Morb Mortal Wkly Rep* **66:** 950–954. doi:10.15585/mmwr.mm6636a3

Siegel RL, Miller KD, Jemal A. 2018. Cancer statistics, 2018. *CA Cancer J Clin* **68:** 7–30. doi:10.3322/caac.21442

Silver SR, Hiratzka SL, Schubauer-Berigan MK, Daniels RD. 2007. Chronic lymphocytic leukemia radiogenicity: A systematic review. *Cancer Causes Control* **18:** 1077–1093. doi:10.1007/s10552-007-9048-y

Slager SL, Benavente Y, Blair A, Vermeulen R, Cerhan JR, Costantini AS, Monnereau A, Nieters A, Clavel J, Call TG, et al. 2014. Medical history, lifestyle, family history, and occupational risk factors for chronic lymphocytic leukemia/small lymphocytic lymphoma: The InterLymph non-Hodgkin lymphoma subtypes project. *J Natl Cancer Inst Monographs* **2014:** 41–51. doi:10.1093/jncimonographs/lgu001

Smedby KE, Baecklund E, Askling J. 2006. Malignant lymphomas in autoimmunity and inflammation: A review of risks, risk factors, and lymphoma characteristics. *Cancer Epidemiol Biomarkers Prev* **15:** 2069–2077. doi:10.1158/1055-9965.EPI-06-0300

Tai EW, Ward KC, Bonaventure A, Siegel DA, Coleman MP. 2017. Survival among children diagnosed with acute lymphoblastic leukemia in the United States, by race and age, 2001 to 2009: Findings from the CONCORD-2 study. *Cancer* **123:** 5178–5189. doi:10.1002/cncr.30899

Teras LR, DeSantis CE, Cerhan JR, Morton LM, Jemal A, Flowers CR. 2016. 2016 US lymphoid malignancy statistics by World Health Organization subtypes. *CA Cancer J Clin* **66:** 443–459. doi:10.3322/caac.21357

Thomas X, Heiblig M. 2016. Diagnostic and treatment of adult Philadelphia chromosome-positive acute lymphoblastic leukemia. *Int J Hematol Oncol* **5:** 77–90. doi:10.2217/ijh-2016-0009

Ugai T, Matsuo K, Oze I, Ito H, Wakai K, Wada K, Nagata C, Nakayama T, Liu R, Kitamura Y, et al. 2018. Smoking and subsequent risk of acute myeloid leukaemia: A pooled analysis of 9 cohort studies in Japan. *Hematol Oncol* **36:** 262–268. doi:10.1002/hon.2457

Wang L, Bhatia S, Gomez SL, Yasui Y. 2015. Differential inequality trends over time in survival among U.S. children with acute lymphoblastic leukemia by race/ethnicity, age at diagnosis, and sex. *Cancer Epidemiol Biomarkers Prev* **24:** 1781–1788. doi:10.1158/1055-9965.EPI-15-0639

Ward E, DeSantis C, Robbins A, Kohler B, Jemal A. 2014. Childhood and adolescent cancer statistics, 2014. *CA Cancer J Clin* **64:** 83–103. doi:10.3322/caac.21219

Weisenburger DD. 1994. Epidemiology of non-Hodgkin's lymphoma: Recent findings regarding an emerging epidemic. *Ann Oncol* **5**(Suppl. 1)**:** S19–S24. doi:10.1093/annonc/5.suppl_1.S19

Wiggins CL, Harlan LC, Nelson HE, Stevens JL, Willman CL, Libby EN, Hromas RA. 2010. Age disparity in the dissemination of imatinib for treating chronic myeloid leukemia. *Am J Med* **123:** 764.e1–764.e9. doi:10.1016/j.amjmed.2010.03.018

Wright JD, St. Clair CM, Deutsch I, Burke WM, Gorrochurn P, Sun X, Herzog TJ. 2010. Pelvic radiotherapy and the risk of secondary leukemia and multiple myeloma. *Cancer* **116:** 2486–2492. doi:10.1002/cncr.25217

Yanik EL, Smith JM, Shiels MS, Clarke CA, Lynch CF, Kahn AR, Koch L, Pawlish KS, Engels EA. 2017. Cancer risk after pediatric solid organ transplantation. *Pediatrics* **139:** e20163893. doi:10.1542/peds.2016-3893

Yoshinaga S, Mabuchi K, Sigurdson AJ, Doody MM, Ron E. 2004. Cancer risks among radiologists and radiologic technologists: Review of epidemiologic studies. *Radiology* **233:** 313–321. doi:10.1148/radiol.2332031119

Zhang Y, Sanjose SD, Bracci PM, Morton LM, Wang R, Brennan P, Hartge P, Boffetta P, Becker N, Maynadie M, et al. 2008. Personal use of hair dye and the risk of certain subtypes of non-Hodgkin lymphoma. *Am J Epidemiol* **167:** 1321–1331. doi:10.1093/aje/kwn058

Zhang L, Steinmaus C, Eastmond DA, Xin XK, Smith MT. 2009. Formaldehyde exposure and leukemia: A new meta-analysis and potential mechanisms. *Mutat Res* **681:** 150–168. doi:10.1016/j.mrrev.2008.07.002

Zhao Y, Wang Y, Ma S. 2018. Racial differences in four leukemia subtypes: Comprehensive descriptive epidemiology. *Sci Rep* **8:** 548. doi:10.1038/s41598-017-19081-4

Zintzaras E, Voulgarelis M, Moutsopoulos HM. 2005. The risk of lymphoma development in autoimmune diseases: A meta-analysis. *Arch Intern Med* **165:** 2337–2344. doi:10.1001/archinte.165.20.2337

Impact of Genetics on Mature Lymphoid Leukemias and Lymphomas

Nathanael G. Bailey[1] **and Kojo S.J. Elenitoba-Johnson**[2]

[1]Division of Hematopathology, Department of Pathology, University of Pittsburgh, Pittsburgh, Pennsylvania 15213, USA

[2]Department of Pathology and Laboratory Medicine, Perelman School of Medicine, University of Pennsylvania, Philadelphia, Pennsylvania 19102, USA

Correspondence: Kojo.Elenitoba-Johnson@uphs.upenn.edu

Recurrent genetic aberrations have long been recognized in mature lymphoid leukemias and lymphomas. As conventional karyotypic and molecular cloning techniques evolved in the 1970s and 1980s, multiple cytogenetic aberrations were identified in lymphomas, often balanced translocations that juxtaposed oncogenes to the immunoglobulin (IG) or T-cell receptor (TR) loci, leading to dysregulation. However, genetic characterization and classification of lymphoma by conventional cytogenetic methods is limited by the infrequent occurrence of recurrent karyotypic abnormalities in many lymphoma subtypes and by the frequent difficulty in growing clinical lymphoma specimens in culture to obtain informative karyotypes. As higher-resolution genomic techniques developed, such as array comparative genomic hybridization and fluorescence in situ hybridization, many recurrent copy number changes were identified in lymphomas, and copy number assessment of interphase cells became part of routine clinical practice for a subset of diseases. Platforms to globally examine mRNA expression led to major insights into the biology of several lymphomas, although these techniques have not gained widespread application in routine clinical settings. With the advent of next-generation sequencing (NGS) techniques in the early 2000s, numerous insights into the genetic landscape of lymphomas were obtained. In contrast to the myeloid malignancies, most common lymphomas exhibit an at least somewhat mutationally complex genome, with few single driver mutations in the majority of patients. However, many recurrently mutated pathways have been identified across lymphoma subtypes, informing targeted therapeutic approaches that are beginning to make meaningful changes in the treatment of lymphoma. In addition to the ability to identify possible therapeutic targets, NGS techniques are highly amenable to the tracking of residual lymphoma following therapy, because of the presence of unique genetic "fingerprints" in lymphoma cells due to V(D)-J recombination at the antigen receptor loci. This review will provide an overview of the impact of novel genetic technologies on lymphoma classification, biology, and therapy.

OVERVIEW OF GENETIC EVENTS IN SELECTED LYMPHOMAS

Lymphoid neoplasms are clonal proliferations of B cells, T cells, or natural killer (NK) cells that may manifest clinically as lymphadenopathy, extranodal tumors, leukemia, or any combination of the three. B-cell lymphomas comprise more than 30 World Health Organization (WHO)-defined entities and account for the majority of all lymphomas (Swerdlow et al.

Cite this article as *Cold Spring Harb Perspect Med* doi: 10.1101/cshperspect.a035444

2017). Different types of B-cell lymphoma are thought to originate from different stages in normal B-cell development (Fig. 1). Certain genetic events are shared in different lymphomas with similar cells of origin (e.g., mutations of chromatin modifiers in germinal center–derived B-cell lymphomas, B-cell receptor [BCR] pathway activation in postgerminal center B-cell lymphomas). T-cell lymphomas are much rarer than B-cell lymphomas, but they are frequently aggressive. Like B-cell lymphomas, some T-cell lymphomas exhibit phenotypic characteristics of physiologic T-cell subsets (Fig. 2). A comprehensive account of lymphoma genetics is outside of the scope of this review; this section will give an overview of genetic events in selected B-cell and T-cell lymphoma entities.

Chronic Lymphocytic Leukemia/Small Lymphocytic Lymphoma

Chronic lymphocytic leukemia/small lymphocytic lymphoma (CLL/SLL) is the most common lymphoid leukemia. CLL/SLL is diagnosed based on characteristic morphologic, clinical, and immunophenotypic characteristics (Rawstron et al. 2018), but it has become clear that the underlying genetics of CLL/SLL are prognostically and therapeutically critical. CLL/SLL may be subdivided into two primary genetic subgroups that each constitute about one-half of cases: those cases that exhibit an unmutated immunoglobulin heavy chain (IGH), and those that harbor a somatic hypermutation of IGH (Damle et al. 1999; Hamblin et al. 1999).

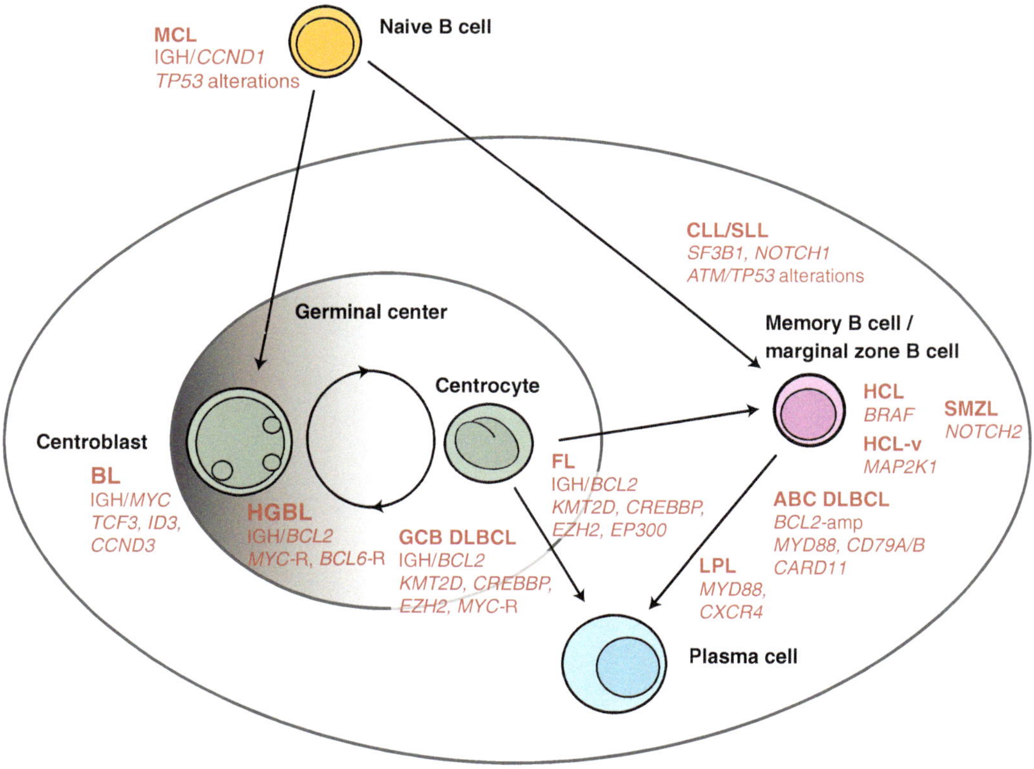

Figure 1. Simplified schematic of B-cell development and the lymphomas thought to originate from specific B-cell developmental stages. Representative frequent and/or clinically relevant genetic alterations are also noted. (MCL) Mantle cell lymphoma, (BL) Burkitt lymphoma, (HGBL) high-grade B-cell lymphoma, (DLBCL) diffuse large B-cell lymphoma, (GCB) germinal center B-cell, (ABC) activated B-cell, (FL) follicular lymphoma, (CLL/SLL) chronic lymphocytic leukemia/small lymphocytic lymphoma, (HCL) hairy cell leukemia, (HCL-v) hairy cell leukemia-variant, (SMZL) splenic marginal zone lymphoma, (LPL) lymphoplasmacytic lymphoma.

Cite this article as *Cold Spring Harb Perspect Med* doi: 10.1101/cshperspect.a035444

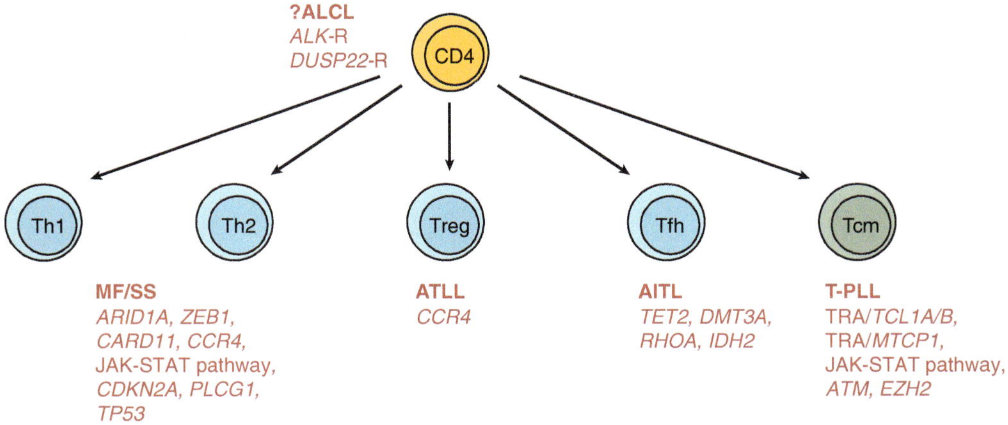

Figure 2. Simplified schematic of $CD4^+$ T-cell subsets and selected corresponding lymphoma subtypes. Because of T-cell plasticity, the association of some of these entities with the subset is somewhat tenuous. Representative frequent and/or clinically relevant genetic alterations are also noted. (ALCL) Anaplastic large cell lymphoma, (MF/SS) mycosis fungoides/Sézary syndrome, (ATLL) adult T-cell leukemia/lymphoma, (AITL) angioimmunoblastic T-cell lymphoma, (T-PLL) T-cell prolymphocytic leukemia, (Th1) T helper type 1, (Th2) T helper type 2, (Treg) regulatory T cell, (Tfh) follicular helper T cell, (Tcm) central memory T cell.

These differences reflect whether the founding neoplastic lymphocyte progressed through a germinal center reaction, eliciting somatic hypermutation through the effect of activation-induced cytidine deaminase (AICDA), or whether the tumor arose either from an antigen-naive lymphocyte or one that encountered antigen through a germinal center–independent mechanism. This genomic distinction has major clinical implications, as patients with unmutated CLL/SLL have worse outcomes than do those with mutated CLL/SLL (Byrd et al. 2006).

CLL/SLL commonly exhibits recurrent structural chromosomal alterations that are amenable to clinical detection by fluorescence in situ hybridization (FISH) and microarray platforms (Döhner et al. 2000). Deletions of 13q are the most common structural alteration in CLL/SLL, occurring in ~55% of patients. 13q deletions encompass *MIR15A* and *MIR16-1*, microRNAs that are important regulators of the antiapoptotic proteins BCL2 and MCL1 (Calin et al. 2008). When present in isolation, patients with 13q deletions have a relatively favorable prognosis. Trisomy 12 is relatively common, although its identification does not lead to specific clinical intervention. It is often associated with atypical phenotypic and/or morphologic characteristics, and so its identification may be diagnostically reassuring in a somewhat unusual case. Deletions of 11q23 (targeting *ATM* and surrounding genes) and 17p (targeting *TP53*) are associated with adverse prognosis in CLL/SLL. *TP53* loss is especially adverse, and its identification has historically been used to direct younger patients to transplant preparation and older patients to agents such as alemtuzumab, as 17p-deleted CLL/SLL patients exhibited especially poor responses to conventional chemoimmunotherapeutic regimens (Gribben 2010; Brown 2018). A new generation of targeted agents such as inhibitors of Bruton tyrosine kinase (BTK), phosphoinositide 3-kinase (PI3K)-δ, and B-cell leukemia/lymphoma 2 (BCL2) have clinical efficacy against this aggressive subset.

Next-generation sequencing (NGS) has allowed identification of numerous recurrently mutated genes in CLL/SLL; although similar to many other lymphomas, there is a long tail of mutated genes, and no single gene is mutated in more than one-half of cases (Puente et al. 2011; Wang et al. 2011; Quesada et al. 2012; Landau et al. 2015). Among the more commonly mutated genes are *SF3B1* (in ~20%), *ATM* (frequently associated with 11q deletion), *TP53* (frequently associated with 17p deletion), and *NOTCH1* (associated with unmutated IGHV). Identification of *TP53* mutations is critical, as they impart a poor prognosis, as does 17p loss, and ~30%–40% of patients with *TP53* mutation do not have 17p losses that are identified by routine FISH testing (Malcikova et al. 2018).

All patients with CLL/SLL should be screened for mutations in *TP53* given its prognostic and therapeutic significance, and FISH studies to identify recurrent copy number changes (such as 17p deletion) are necessary at diagnosis and progression. The mutational status of the CLL should be tested when a patient requires treatment, as fit patients with mutated CLL and without 17p del/*TP53* mutation may exhibit excellent responses to FCR chemotherapy, although alternate approaches are needed for other patients (Eichhorst et al. 2016; Fischer et al. 2016). Ibrutinib has recently been approved as frontline therapy for CLL/SLL in all genetic types; however, ibrutinib resistance can arise in a subset of patients. Some relapses following ibrutinib therapy are mediated by acquired mutations in *BTK*, the target of ibrutinib, or *PLCG2*, which allows for BTK-independent BCR activation (Woyach et al. 2014). Screening for these mutations may be considered for patients with CLL who lose response to ibrutinib.

Mantle Cell Lymphoma

Mantle cell lymphoma (MCL) is a relatively uncommon B-cell lymphoma that, similar to CLL/SLL, typically exhibits expression of the T-cell-associated antigen CD5. Although most often a morphologically indolent-appearing lymphoma, MCL generally exhibits a progressive disease course and is incurable with conventional chemoimmunotherapeutic approaches. MCL is characterized by translocations between chromosomes 11 and 14, causing deregulation of the cyclin D1 (*CCND1*) gene by the IGH enhancer region. The identification of this rearrangement in most cases of MCL contributed to its recognition and acceptance as a distinct lymphoma entity (Banks et al. 1992).

Copy number changes of 13q14, 11q23, and 17p are relatively frequent events in mantle cell lymphoma, targeting regions similar to those lost in CLL/SLL (Beà et al. 1999; Bentz et al. 2000). However, mantle cell lymphomas more frequently manifest more complex karyotypes than are seen in CLL/SLL, although there is no clear clinical indication to routinely test for these copy number changes in MCL. NGS studies have identified recurrent mutations in *CCND1*, *ATM*, *KMT2D (MLL2)*, and *TP53* (Beà et al. 2013; Zhang et al. 2014). *TP53* mutations, in particular, have been associated with poorer outcomes in MCL (Eskelund et al. 2017).

Although *CCND1* translocations are the genetic hallmark of MCL, lymphomas with morphologic and immunophenotypic characteristics of MCL but without detectable *CCND1* translocation or protein expression have been recognized (Yatabe et al. 2000). These so-called *CCND1*$^{-}$ MCL have a gene expression profile similar to that seen in conventional MCL and consistently overexpress *SOX11* (Fu et al. 2005; Mozos et al. 2009). SOX11 is a member of the SOX (sex determining region Y-related HMG-box) proteins and is expressed in ~90% of MCLs, including in early "in situ" disease and in cyclin D1-negative cases (Dictor et al. 2009; Carvajal-Cuenca et al. 2012). It is now recognized that 50% of the cyclin D1-negative cases harbor *CCND2* translocations resulting in juxtaposition with the immunoglobulin genes (Salaverria et al. 2013; Kurita et al. 2016; Martín-Garcia et al. 2018). Additionally, *CCND3* translocations to the immunoglobulin light chain enhancers have also recently been recognized in cyclin D1-negative mantle cell lymphomas (Martín-Garcia et al. 2018).

Although most cases of MCL have a progressive disease course, some cases with a predominantly extranodal disease distribution have been recognized with more indolent clinical behavior. These cases have *CCND1* translocations, tend not to express SOX11, and commonly have hypermutated IGH (as opposed to most MCL with unmutated IGH) (Fernàndez et al. 2010). This disease has been codified in the WHO classification as "leukemic non-nodal MCL." Although generally indolent, some patients with leukemic non-nodal MCL exhibit disease progression, often associated with acquisition of 17p/*TP53* alterations (Carvajal-Cuenca et al. 2012).

 Cite this article as *Cold Spring Harb Perspect Med* doi: 10.1101/cshperspect.a035444

Hairy Cell Leukemia/Splenic Lymphomas

Hairy cell leukemia (HCL) is a rare and clinically indolent mature B-cell leukemia/lymphoma that preferentially involves the spleen, blood, and bone marrow. As opposed to most mature B-cell leukemias that typically present with lymphocytosis, HCL typically manifests with cytopenias, with relatively few circulating neoplastic lymphocytes. HCL cells have characteristic morphologic features and immunophenotypic characteristics (Shao et al. 2013). Until the development of NGS techniques, the genetic basis of HCL was unclear, as few recurrent structural alterations were present in the HCL genome (Forconi et al. 2008). However, in 2011, activating *BRAF* Val600Glu mutations were identified in nearly all cases of HCL (Tiacci et al. 2011). *BRAF* mutations are exceptionally uncommon in other B-cell lymphomas, suggesting this is a relatively specific diagnostic marker for HCL (Tiacci et al. 2011; Arcaini et al. 2012). Rare *BRAF*-negative HCL cases often exhibit preferential usage of IGHV4-34 and frequently have downstream mutations in *MAP2K1* (Waterfall et al. 2014). *BRAF*-mutated HCL may also exhibit loss of wild-type *BRAF* through deletions, along with infrequent mutations of *KMT2C* and *CDKN1B* (Durham et al. 2017).

MAP2K1 mutations are also present in ~30% of HCL variant (HCL-v) cases (Waterfall et al. 2014), a neoplasm with morphologic and immunophenotypic features similar to but distinct from classic HCL, and with poorer responses to single-agent purine analogs. HCL-v cases additionally exhibit recurrent mutations in *CCND3*, *U2AF1*, *ARID1A*, and *TP53* (Waterfall et al. 2014; Durham et al. 2017). The finding of activated MAPK pathways in both HCL and HCL-v unify the pathobiology of these lymphoid leukemias to some degree and point to therapeutic targets in these diseases. Although HCL is relatively well managed by purine analogs, this is not the case for HCL-v. BRAF inhibition has been used successfully in HCL patients in the refractory/relapsed setting (Tiacci et al. 2015), and MEK inhibition has been anecdotally successful in HCL-v (Andritsos et al. 2018).

Splenic Marginal Zone Lymphoma

Splenic marginal zone lymphoma (SMZL) is a low-grade B-cell lymphoma that, like HCL and HCL-v, preferentially involves the blood, bone marrow, and spleen. SMZLs exhibit common karyotypic alterations, with frequent gains of 3 and 3q, gains of 12q, and deletions of 7q and 6q (Salido et al. 2010). *NOTCH2* and *KLF2* are the most frequently mutated genes in SMZL (Kiel et al. 2012; Rossi et al. 2012; Clipson et al. 2015). Both proteins are important regulators of normal marginal zone formation, and they are preferentially mutated in SMZL versus other low-grade B-cell lymphomas. *NOTCH2* and *TP53* mutations are associated with decreased treatment-free survival and overall survival, respectively, in SMZL (Parry et al. 2015; Campos-Martín et al. 2017).

Lymphoplasmacytic Lymphoma

Lymphoplasmacytic lymphoma (LPL) is an indolent B-cell lymphoma typically associated with marrow involvement, some degree of plasmacytic differentiation, and IgM monoclonal gammopathy. Waldenström macroglobulinemia (WM) is defined by the presence of an IgM paraprotein, with >10% marrow involvement by LPL. WM/LPL tumors frequently exhibit loss of 6q, deleting *TNFAIP3* (Braggio et al. 2009). NGS studies identified *MYD88* Leu265Pro mutations in ~90% of patients with LPL (Treon et al. 2012). *MYD88* Leu265Pro mutations are relatively uncommon in other low-grade B-cell lymphomas, although they do rarely occur in SMZL and CLL. Both activating mutations in *MYD88* and deletions of *TNFAIP3* lead to activation of the NF-κB signaling pathway. Patients with *MYD88*-mutated LPL appear very sensitive to BTK inhibition with ibrutinib, but efficacy is diminished in patients with concurrent mutations of *CXCR4* and in the rare *MYD88*-wild type cases (Treon et al. 2015; Dimopoulos et al. 2017).

Follicular Lymphoma

Follicular lymphoma (FL) is the most common indolent B-cell lymphoma in western countries, accounting for ∼20% of all lymphomas worldwide (The Non-Hodgkin's Lymphoma Classification Project 1997). It is composed of germinal center–derived B cells and frequently exhibits a follicular growth pattern. Its genetic hallmark is the translocation of chromosomes 14 and 18, causing the antiapoptotic gene *BCL2* to be upregulated by the IGH enhancer, similar to the *CCND1* rearrangement seen in MCL (Fukuhara et al. 1979; Tsujimoto et al. 1984). IGH/*BCL2* is by itself insufficient to cause lymphoma (Roulland et al. 2006) and requires the presence of additional genetic aberrations. In addition to the t(14;18), FL harbors frequent losses of 1p, 6q, 10q, and 17p, with gains of 1q, 6q, 7, 8q, 12q, 17q, and 18 (Cheung et al. 2009). FL contains several highly recurrent mutations in addition to IGH/*BCL2* fusion. Mutations in chromatin modifiers are particularly frequent, with *KMT2D*, *CREBBP*, *EZH2*, and *EP300* being common mutational targets (Morin et al. 2010, 2011; Pasqualucci et al. 2011). Mutations of chromatin modifiers are present in >90% of FLs, and >70% have mutations in two or more chromatin-modifying genes (Green et al. 2015). In addition to its frequent deletion at chromosome 1p in FL, *TNFRSF14* is commonly mutationally inactivated, and *TNFRSF14* alterations are present in more than one-half of FL cases (Cheung et al. 2010; Launay et al. 2012). Loss of *TNFRSF14* leads to B-cell proliferation through increased BCR signaling and leads to changes in the FL microenvironment that facilitate tumor growth (Boice et al. 2016).

Although FL is an indolent lymphoma, it is generally incurable with conventional immunochemotherapeutic approaches, and transformation to an aggressive B-cell lymphoma is a frequent and clinically devastating event. Several recent studies have explored the underlying genetic basis of transformation in follicular lymphoma. Transformed FL (t-FL) appears to arise from an ancestral clone shared with the dominant FL, rather than as a direct progression of the dominant FL clone. t-FL is enriched for alterations of *MYC*, *CDKN2A/B*, *TP53*, *PIM1*, *EBF1*, and *B2M* (Elenitoba-Johnson et al. 1998; Pasqualucci et al. 2014; Okosun et al. 2014).

A modification of the standard FL international prognostic index (FLIPI) has been proposed that incorporates the presence of mutations in seven commonly mutated genes (m7-FLIPI) (Pastore et al. 2015). In this prognostic model, *EZH2*, *ARID1A*, and *MEF2B* mutations were favorable (particularly *EZH2*), whereas mutations in *EP300*, *FOXO1*, *CREBBP*, and *CARD11* were unfavorable (particularly *EP300* and *FOXO1*). The m7-FLIPI model improved on standard FLIPI risk stratification in FL patients by identifying patients with high-risk FLIPI scores but with favorable outcomes, largely associated with *EZH2* mutation.

Pediatric-type FL (PTFL) is an uncommon and highly indolent lymphoma of germinal center B cells that typically occurs in adolescent males. In contrast to conventional FL, PTFL is less genomically complex, with significantly fewer aberrations and without translocations of *BCL2* or *BCL6*. Like FL, PTFL exhibits frequent losses of 1p/*TNFRSF14* mutations, but mutations of chromatin modifiers are virtually absent, whereas *MAP2K1* mutations are relatively frequent (Louissaint et al. 2016; Schmidt et al. 2016).

Diffuse Large B-Cell Lymphoma

Diffuse large B-cell lymphoma (DLBCL) is the most common lymphoma worldwide (The Non-Hodgkin's Lymphoma Classification Project 1997). The term DLBCL encompasses a genetically diverse group of neoplasms with the common feature of a diffuse proliferation of large, transformed B cells. The heterogeneity of DLBCL was recognized in lymphoma classification systems for decades, but subclassification based on morphologic features is not reproducible among experts and does not clearly associate with outcomes (Harris et al. 1994). In 2000, a landmark study demonstrated that DLBCL could be subdivided into clinically relevant categories based on gene expression as assessed by cDNA microarray analysis (Alizadeh et al. 2000). One large group of DLBCLs exhibited a gene expression profile resembling that of germinal center B cells (GCBs), whereas another exhibited a profile similar to that of

 Cite this article as *Cold Spring Harb Perspect Med* doi: 10.1101/cshperspect.a035444

activated peripheral blood B cells (ABCs). Some cases remained unclassifiable by this approach. Patients with GCB-DLBCL had better outcomes than patients with ABC-DLBCL when treated with CHOP (Rosenwald et al. 2002), and the survival differences persisted with the addition of rituximab to the CHOP regimen (Lenz et al. 2008). Assessment of gene expression signatures has not historically been clinically feasible, and so surrogate immunohistochemical algorithms were developed and implemented clinically (Hans et al. 2004). Newer gene expression technologies, however, hold the promise of robust distinction between ABC- and GCB-DLBCL in routinely processed formalin-fixed, paraffin-embedded material (Scott et al. 2014).

The GCB/ABC paradigm has informed subsequent genetic exploration of DLBCL. Both ABC and GCB subsets exhibit relatively frequent translocations of *BCL6* and mutations of *KMT2D*, *CREBBP*, *EP300*, *B2M*, *TP53*, and *MEF2B*; GCB DLBCL exhibit frequent IGH/*BCL2* translocation, mutations of *EZH2*, and *MYC* translocations; and ABC DLBCL often have alterations of *TNFAIP3*, *CDKN2A/B*, *MYD88*, *PRDM1*, *CD79A/B*, *CARD11*, and frequently exhibit amplification (rather than translocation) of *BCL2* (for review, see Pasqualucci and Dalla-Favera 2015). Many of the mutations identified in ABC-DLBCL lead to chronic active BCR signaling and NF-κB activation, pointing to targetable pathways in this chemoresistant disease (Davis et al. 2010; Ngo et al. 2011).

Recent studies have proposed classifications of DLBCL based on their mutational signatures (Chapuy et al. 2018; Schmitz et al. 2018). Although the studies exhibited some differences in their findings, several common themes emerge, emphasizing that the biologic and clinical heterogeneity of DLBCL cannot be captured with a trichotomous ABC/GCB/other gene expression classification. In both studies, two subgroups were recognized in ABC-DLBCL: One had translocations of *BCL6* and mutations of genes in the *NOTCH2* pathway, suggesting a possible shared cell of origin with MZL, as splenic MZLs frequently harbor *NOTCH2* pathway mutations (Kiel et al. 2012; Rossi et al. 2012) and transformed gastric extranodal MZLs frequently have rearrangements of *BCL6* (Chen et al. 2006; Flossbach et al. 2011).This group was associated with relatively favorable survival in both studies and was also enriched in cases with an unclassifiable gene expression profile (neither clearly ABC or GCB). The other ABC cohort consisted of lymphomas with *MYD88* Leu265Pro mutations and mutations of *CD79B*. This group had an unfavorable prognosis and was enriched for lymphomas with extranodal involvement, concordant with results of previous studies that have identified frequent mutations of *MYD88* in primary extranodal lymphomas such as primary CNS lymphoma, testicular DLBCL, and primary cutaneous DLBCL, leg-type (Pham-Ledard et al. 2014; Chapuy et al. 2016). In both studies, a group of GCB-DLBCL characterized by *BCL2* mutation/rearrangement and mutation of *EZH2* was identified with worse survival than other GCB-DLBCLs. The remaining GCB cases were further characterized by Chapuy and colleagues as commonly having mutations in four linker and four core histone genes, along with *CD83*, *CD58*, *CD70*, *RHOA*, *GNA13*, *SGK1*, *CARD11*, *NFKBIE*, *NFKBIA*, *BRAF*, and *STAT3*, without mutations in chromatin modifiers. Chapuy and colleagues also recognized a *TP53*-mutated cohort with multiple structural chromosomal abnormalities, and Schmitz et al. recognized a small cohort of *NOTCH1*-mutated ABC DBLCL with adverse outcomes.

These efforts point to the biologic complexity of a category that is still classified primarily by its morphologic appearance and that is still treated homogeneously at diagnosis. Although frontline immunochemotherapy for DLBCL has not changed significantly since the introduction of rituximab in the early 2000s, novel agents are now routinely used in the in the relapsed/refractory setting. Particularly favorable responses have been seen in relapsed/refractory ABC DLBCL to agents such as ibrutinib and lenalidomide (Wilson et al. 2015; Czuczman et al. 2017). The specific mutations present in an individual case of DLBCL may better predict response to targeted therapies than the overall gene expression profile, as responses to ibrutinib in ABC DLBCL appear enriched in *MYD88/CD79B* comutated DLBCL cases

(Wilson et al. 2015). The genetic heterogeneity that has been uncovered in DLBCL should inform clinical trials going forward so that possible responses in particular genomic subgroups are not lost.

Burkitt Lymphoma

Burkitt lymphoma (BL) is a highly aggressive mature B-cell neoplasm that arises in different epidemiologic scenarios. Endemic BL is highly associated with EBV infection and occurs in areas with endemic malaria; sporadic BL occurs worldwide and is less frequently associated with EBV; and immunodeficiency-associated BL occurs in patients with immunodeficiency, most commonly HIV infection (Swerdlow et al. 2017). BL is highly aggressive, but curable with intensive chemoimmunotherapy, and its distinction from DLBCL is paramount in adults.

BL is the prototypical example of a lymphoma with a recognized genetic abnormality: extra material on chromosome 14 was first recognized in BL in 1972 (Manolov and Manolova 1972). This material was soon characterized as originating from chromosome 8 (Zech et al. 1976), and the IGH/*MYC* rearrangement was described soon after (Dalla-Favera et al. 1982; Taub et al. 1982). All epidemiologic types of BL are highly associated with translocations of *MYC* to immunoglobulin loci, with only rare *MYC*-fusion-negative cases that may have *MYC* deregulation by alternate mechanisms (Hummel et al. 2006; Leucci et al. 2008). *MYC* translocations are not specific to BL, however, as they are present in a minor subset of DBLCL and in many non-BL high-grade B-cell lymphomas (discussed below). Therefore, accurate diagnosis requires integration of genetic, morphologic, and phenotypic findings. Molecular studies may help distinguish between BL and DLBCL, as aside from *MYC* translocations, BL exhibits few structural alterations, in contrast to DLBCL (Hummel et al. 2006). Sporadic cases of BL exhibit high-frequency mutations of *TCF3* or its negative regulator *ID3*, and oncogenic mutations of *CCND3* are common (Schmitz et al. 2012). EBV-associated endemic BL, in contrast, exhibits less frequent mutations of *TCF3*, *ID3*, and *CCND3*, with more frequent mutations of *ARID1A*, *RHOA*, and *CCNF* (Schmitz et al. 2012; Abate et al. 2015). Many genes commonly mutated in DLBCL are only rarely mutated in BL, such as *EZH2*, *SGK1*, *BCL2*, *CD79B*, and *MYD88*.

High-Grade B-Cell Lymphomas with *MYC* and *BCL2* and/or *BCL6* Rearrangements

High-grade B-cell lymphoma (HGBL) with *MYC* and *BCL2* and/or *BCL6* rearrangements is a category introduced in the 2016 revision of the WHO Classification that encompasses cases that previously would have been classified as "B-cell lymphoma, unclassifiable, with features intermediate between DLBCL and BL." As the name suggests, this category is intended to encompass all mature, aggressive-appearing lymphomas that harbor translocations of *MYC*, along with a translocation of one or both of *BCL2* and *BCL6*. These lymphomas are commonly referred to as "double-hit" lymphomas (DHLs) and have been associated with very poor outcomes when treated with conventional DLBCL therapy (Johnson et al. 2009; Li et al. 2012). They may have Burkitt-like, blastoid, or DLBCL-like morphology. The introduction of this category and its clinical implications has mandated FISH testing for these fusions in most, if not all, cases of large B-cell lymphoma, as strategies that FISH only cases with a GCB phenotype and MYC/BCL2 protein expression miss a large percentage of rearranged cases (Scott et al. 2018). Selection of FISH probes impacts sensitivity of *MYC* rearrangement detection as breaks may occur over several megabases. The most comprehensive methods would rely on application of both break-apart and dual-fusion FISH probes (May et al. 2010; Muñoz-Mármol et al. 2013), although this approach is resource-intensive. Several groups have reported that the *MYC* translocation partner may be prognostically significant, and that lymphomas with nonimmunoglobulin (non-IG) *MYC* translocation partners have better outcomes than those with IG/*MYC* fusions (Johnson et al. 2009; Pedersen et al. 2014; Copie-Bergman et al. 2015; Chong et al. 2018), further complicating possible FISH analysis. The most appropriate regimen for DHL is not clear, but patients benefit from regimens more intensive than standard R-CHOP therapy (Friedberg 2017).

Primary Mediastinal (Thymic) Large B-Cell Lymphoma and Classic Hodgkin Lymphoma

Primary mediastinal (thymic) large B-cell lymphoma (PMBL) is an uncommon genetically distinct subtype of large B-cell lymphoma that occurs in the mediastinum, often in young females. Although it exhibits more robust B-cell antigen expression, PMBL exhibits some morphologic, immunophenotypic, and genetic similarity to classic Hodgkin lymphoma (CHL), which also commonly occurs in the mediastinum in younger patients. Early gene expression profiling studies identified PMBL as distinct from DLBCL more generally, and with shared gene expression features with CHL (Rosenwald et al. 2003; Savage et al. 2003). Later mutational studies have confirmed additional shared features with CHL, including 9p24.1 amplifications involving *JAK2*, *CD274 (PDL1)* and *PDCD1LG2 (PDL2)* (Green et al. 2010); *CIITA* fusions (Steidl et al. 2011); *SOCS1* inactivation (Melzner et al. 2005; Weniger et al. 2006); and *STAT6* mutations (Ritz et al. 2009; Tiacci et al. 2018). Recent studies have identified *IL4R* mutations as another activator of JAK-STAT signaling in PMBL (Viganò et al. 2018a), and these mutations are also present in some cases of DLBCL (Viganò et al. 2018b). Nonmediastinal PMBL have been described, yet they are difficult to confidently diagnose (Yuan et al. 2015). As PMBL is often treated more aggressively than most DLBCLs (Dunleavy et al. 2013), recognition of nonmediastinal PMBL could have clinical implications. Mutational analysis or newer gene expression techniques may assist with this rare diagnosis and could be helpful to support the impression of PMBL when diagnosing a large B-cell lymphoma in the mediastinum (Chong et al. 2018).

Genetic studies of CHL have been historically limited by the relative paucity of the malignant Hodgkin Reed–Sternberg (HRS) cells in most biopsy specimens. However, novel techniques have allowed single-cell interrogation of HRS cells, revealing a mutational profile with significant overlap with PMBL, as discussed above. Copy number alterations of the *PDL1/PDL2* locus are particularly common in CHL, occurring in nearly every lymphoma in one series (Roemer et al. 2016). Amplifications (as opposed to polysomy or low-level copy gain) of *PDL1/PDL2* were associated with decreased progression-free survival and advanced-stage disease in this study and are a likely mechanism for the encouraging clinical responses to immune checkpoint blockade seen in CHL (Ansell et al. 2015). Although relatively few cases of EBV$^+$ CHL have been comprehensively genetically studied, they appear to have a lower mutational burden than EBV$^-$ CHL and contain fewer copy number alterations (Montgomery et al. 2016; Tiacci et al. 2018).

T-Cell Lymphomas

Anaplastic Large Cell Lymphoma

Anaplastic large cell lymphoma (ALCL) is a CD30$^+$ mature T-cell lymphoma that is divided into two primary groups on the basis of its genetic abnormalities: ALCL, ALK-positive (ALK$^+$ ALCL) and ALCL, ALK-negative (ALK$^-$ ALCL). ALK$^+$ ALCL is characterized by the fusion of the tyrosine kinase *ALK* to other genes, most commonly *NPM1* (Le Beau et al. 1989; Rimokh et al. 1989; Morris et al. 1994). This leads to aberrant expression of the ALK protein, easily identifiable by immunohistochemical staining (Pittaluga et al. 1997; Pulford et al. 1997; Falini et al. 1998). ALK expression activates multiple signaling pathways, including JAK-STAT, PI3K-AKT, mTOR, MAPK, and others (for review, see Hallberg and Palmer 2013). Small-molecule inhibitors of ALK, such as crizotinib, have demonstrated clinical efficacy in ALK$^+$ ALCL (Mossé et al. 2017).

ALK$^-$ ALCL, by definition, lacks ALK rearrangement or overexpression. In comparison with ALK$^+$ ALCL, ALK$^-$ ALCL tend to exhibit a somewhat more complex genome, with a higher frequency of chromosomal gains and losses

(Boi et al. 2013). ALK^- ALCL exhibits a heterogeneous clinical course, and emerging evidence demonstrates that outcomes are heavily dependent on the underlying lymphoma genetics. *DUSP22* rearrangements are present in ~30% of ALK^- ALCLs, including cutaneous forms of ALCL (Feldman et al. 2009, 2011; Parrilla Castellar et al. 2014). More rarely, *TP63* rearrangements occur in ALK^- ALCL (Vasmatzis et al. 2012; Parrilla Castellar et al. 2014), and together these translocations identify clinically relevant ALK^- ALCL subgroups. *DUSP22*-rearranged systemic ALK^- ALCL have a favorable prognosis similar to that seen in ALK^+ ALCL, whereas *TP63*-rearranged cases do poorly with conventional chemotherapy (Parrilla Castellar et al. 2014; Pedersen et al. 2017). Other recurrent kinase fusions, such as those involving *TYK2*, occur with less frequency in ALK^- ALCL (Velusamy et al. 2014; Crescenzo et al. 2015) but activate JAK-STAT signaling, whereas mutations of *JAK1* and/or *STAT3* are present in ~20% of cases (Crescenzo et al. 2015). Although the introduction of brentuximab vedotin (an anti-CD30 antibody-drug conjugate) has led to improved therapies in ALK^+ and ALK^- ALCL (Horwitz et al. 2019), the identification of mutationally activated pathways provides alternate drug targets for therapeutic exploration.

T-Cell Prolymphocytic Leukemia

T-cell prolymphocytic leukemia (T-PLL) is a rare mature T-cell leukemia that typically presents with marked lymphocytosis and is associated with poor survival. T-PLL is commonly associated with inv(14) (Malcikova et al. 2018), which juxtaposes the TRA/D locus with the oncogenes *TCL1A* and *TCL1B* (Brito-Babapulle et al. 1987; Russo et al. 1989; Pekarsky et al. 1999). This translocation is analogous to the IG translocations commonly seen in B-cell lymphomas, causing the aberrant expression of *TCL1A/B* owing to its localization near the TRA/D enhancer, leading to increased AKT1 signaling (Pekarsky et al. 2000). Additional common structural events in T-PLL include loss of the *ATM* gene at 11q23 and trisomy 8. In addition to these large-scale genomic events, point mutations in the JAK-STAT pathway are common (Kiel et al. 2014). Recurrent mutations of *JAK1*, *JAK3*, and *STAT5B* are present in ~8%, ~30%, and ~36% of T-PLL cases, respectively. Inactivating mutations and deletions of *EZH2* are additionally present in about one-half of cases (Kiel et al. 2014). Alemtuzumab, an anti-CD52 antibody, has been the mainstay of therapy for T-PLL, but this regimen is not curative and can be associated with significant complications (Dearden 2012). Alternate therapeutic approaches are therefore needed. Although JAK-STAT kinase inhibitors are clinically available, it does not appear that response to JAK-STAT inhibition is readily predictable by mutational status in ex vivo studies (Andersson et al. 2018).

Mycosis Fungoides/Sézary Syndrome

Mycosis fungoides (MF) is the most common cutaneous T-cell lymphoma (CTCL), and it typically exhibits a fairly indolent disease course. However, MF may progress to involve the blood, exhibiting clinical and pathologic overlap with Sézary syndrome (SS), which strictly defined is a de novo aggressive and rare process characterized by erythroderma, lymphadenopathy, and circulating lymphoma cells. MF harbors recurrent mutations of *PLCG1* (Kiel et al. 2015), leading to activation of pathways downstream of the T-cell receptor (Vaqué et al. 2014). *TP53* mutations occur in MF, more commonly in tumor-stage patients than at earlier stages (McGregor et al. 1999). MF exhibits a relatively simple genome (da Silva Almeida et al. 2015), whereas SS exhibits a highly complex genome, typically with numerous copy number changes and structural rearrangements (Choi et al. 2015; da Silva Almeida et al. 2015; Kiel et al. 2015; Wang et al. 2015b). Common mutational/deletional targets in SS include numerous genes involved in epigenetic regulation (*ARID1A*, *ZEB1*, *DMNT3A*, *TET2*, *CREBBP*, and *KMT2D*), components of several signaling pathways (*CARD11*, *CCR4*, *PLCG1*, *BRAF*, *MAKP1*, *JAK1*, *JAK3*, *STAT3*, and *STAT5B*) and tumor suppressors such as *CDKN2A* and *TP53*. CCR4 is a therapeutic target in CTCL, as mogamulizumab, an anti-CCR4 antibody, has recently been Food and Drug Administration (FDA)-approved in the relapsed/refractory setting (Kim et al. 2018). It is not clear that *CCR4* mutational status impacts mogamulizumab response in CTCL, although *CCR4* mutations sensitize to mogamulizumab therapy in the HTLV1-associated adult T-cell leukemia/lymphoma (Sakamoto et al. 2018).

Nodal T Follicular Helper T-Cell Lymphomas

A large group of nodal peripheral T-cell lymphomas exhibit phenotypic characteristics of normal follicular helper T-cells (TFHs). Angioimmunoblastic T-cell lymphomas (AITLs) and follicular T-cell lymphoma (FTCL) are the two main nodal TFH lymphoma subtypes recognized by the WHO classification (Swerdlow et al. 2017). Recent NGS studies have identified recurrent mutations in epigenetic regulators in both AITL and FTCL, contributing to the recognition that these lymphomas exhibit overlapping biologic features, in addition to a largely shared immunophenotype. Both AITL and FTCL exhibit common mutations of *TET2*, *DNMT3A*, and *RHOA* (Lemonnier et al. 2012; Odejide et al. 2014; Palomero et al. 2014; Sakata-Yanagimoto et al. 2014). *IDH2* mutations, in contrast, seem to be restricted to AITL, present in ~20%–30% of cases (Cairns et al. 2012; Odejide et al. 2014; Wang et al. 2015a). The *IDH2* mutations in AITL seem to always target the arginine residue at codon 172, rather than the Arg140 mutations that predominate in acute myeloid leukemia (Marcucci et al. 2010), and in contrast with acute myeloid leukemia, *IDH2* and *TET2* mutations are not mutually exclusive in AITL (Lemonnier et al. 2012). Arg172 mutations lead to greater 2-HG accumulation than do Arg140 mutations (Ward et al. 2013), and *IDH* mutations identify a subset of AITL patients with increased H3K27me3 and hypermethylation of gene promotor regions compared to *IDH*-wild type cases (Wang et al. 2015a). Demethylating agents have demonstrated some clinical efficacy against the lymphoma in AITL patients with concurrent myeloid neoplasms, suggesting that epigenetic modification may be a promising therapeutic approach in AITL (Lemonnier et al. 2018).

Impact of Molecular and Genomic Techniques on Lymphoma Diagnosis and Monitoring

Immunoglobulin/T-Cell Receptor Sequencing

During normal development, lymphocytes undergo somatic V(D)-J recombination of their immunoglobulin (IG) or T-cell receptor (TR) genes. This process generates a genetic "fingerprint" for each unique lymphocyte, as variable numbers of nontemplated nucleotides are inserted at the junctions of the V, D, and J genes, leading to the normal IG and TR repertoire necessary for normal antigen recognition. As lymphomas arise from a single progenitor cell, they exhibit a common, dominant V(D)-J rearrangement, as opposed to a multitude of rearrangements in reactive lymphoproliferations. This phenomenon has long been exploited in the diagnosis of lymphoma, and the detection of monoclonality through assessment of IG or TR diversity through Southern blotting or polymerase chain reaction (PCR) techniques has been a routine ancillary diagnostic technique in hematopathology for decades (van Dongen and Wolvers-Tettero 1991; van Dongen et al. 2003). Routine PCR techniques for monoclonality assessment retain advantages in turnaround time, cost, and ease of analysis. However, using typical capillary electropherograms, the amplified PCR products are separated solely on the basis of size, and each peak in the electropherogram represents the integrated signal of potentially many clones. Although this is not a problem in most cases, this phenomenon can make it difficult to always compare clones between specimens with great confidence and may lead to false-positive calls. Next-generation sequencing (NGS) techniques, on the other hand, generate the sequence itself of each individual V(D)-J read, and reads with shared sequences can be summed to give accurate quantification of each clone present in a specimen.

NGS techniques therefore allow measurement not only of whether a clone is present, but routine determination of hypermutation status and gene family usage, clinically relevant information in common diseases such as CLL/SLL (Byrd et al. 2006; Ghia et al. 2008). NGS techniques allow straightforward and definitive comparison between lymphomas in an individual patient to assess for clonal relatedness, a particularly important determination in the setting of transformation (Rossi et al. 2011). Perhaps the most powerful application of NGS for lymphoid clonality assessment is in the disease monitoring setting. Although minimal residual disease (MRD) testing can be successfully performed with conventional PCR (van der Velden et al. 2007), patient-specific primers are necessary to gain appropriate sensitivity, which is laborious and difficult to implement in most clinical laboratories. As NGS outputs the sequence of each individual read obtained in a specimen, MRD-level detection of lymphoma/leukemia-specific reads can be easily achieved with common primers as long as a sufficiently large number of reads are obtained and the sequence of the diagnostic IG or TR rearrangement is known. This technique has been used for successful disease monitoring in mature lymphomas, acute leukemias, and plasma cell myelomas (Wu et al. 2012; Kurtz et al. 2015; Roschewski et al. 2015; Scherer et al. 2016; Rossi et al. 2017; Perrot et al. 2018; Wood et al. 2018), as the only requirement is the presence of either an IG or TR rearrangement in the neoplastic cells. NGS techniques have recently been FDA-approved in the B-ALL and myeloma MRD setting, and the performance characteristics of the assays compare favorably to that of multiparameter flow cytometry in these diseases.

Clinical Genomics Testing in Lymphoma

Genetic testing in lymphoma has long been performed routinely in the clinical laboratory through comprehensive, but low-resolution, methods such as metaphase karyotyping or through targeted interrogation of specific loci such as through FISH studies. More recently, testing for individual genetic mutations has become common in some circumstances, such as testing for *BRAF* mutations in suspected HCL or *MYD88* mutations in suspected LPL. The recent introduction of high-throughput genomic platforms into the clinical laboratory has made routine extensive genomic characterization of lymphomas feasible, and examples of clinically relevant testing are listed in Table 1.

As discussed previously, recent studies have shown that the traditional, gene expression–based classification of DLBCL (the most com-

Table 1. Examples of genetic biomarkers and possible therapeutic implication in lymphoma entities

Disease	Genetic biomarker	Therapeutic implication
CLL	*TP53* mutation/deletion	Ibrutinib therapy indication
CLL	*BTK* or *PLCG2* mutation	Ibrutinib resistance
LPL	*MYD88* mutation	Reduced ibrutinib response if *MYD88* is not mutated
LPL	*CXCR4* mutation	Reduced ibrutinib response if *CXCR4* is mutated
HCL	*BRAF* mutation	Vemurafenib response
HGBL	*MYC* and *BCL2* and/or *BCL6* rearrangements	R-CHOP is suboptimal therapy
DLBCL	MYD88/CD79B comutation	Increased response to ibrutinib
FL/DLBCL	*EZH2* mutation	EZH2 inhibitors in clinical trials
AITL	*IDH2* mutation	*IDH2* inhibitors in clinical trials
ALCL, ALK^+	*ALK* rearrangement	May respond to crizotinib
ALCL, ALK^-	*DUSP22* rearrangement	May be candidate for less intensive therapy than other ALCL, ALK^-

(CLL) Chronic lymphocytic leukemia, (LPL) lymphoplasmacytic lymphoma, (HCL) hairy cell leukemia, (HGBL) high-grade B-cell lymphoma, (DLBCL) diffuse large B-cell lymphoma, (FL) follicular lymphoma, (AITL) angioimmunoblastic T-cell lymphoma, (ALCL) anaplastic large cell lymphoma, (ALK^+) ALK receptor tyrosine kinase positive, (ALK^-) ALK receptor tyrosine kinase negative.

 Cite this article as *Cold Spring Harb Perspect Med* doi: 10.1101/cshperspect.a035444

mon lymphoma type) into ABC and GCB subtypes is overly simplistic, with prognostically important subsets only identifiable by broad genomic profiling (Chapuy et al. 2018; Schmitz et al. 2018). Emerging data suggest that at least some of these genetic fingerprints predict for response to targeted therapies such as ibrutinib (Wilson et al. 2015), but it is likely that other factors in addition to mutational activation impact therapeutic responses, particularly when targeting pathways that are generally important in lymphoid survival (Phelan et al. 2018). As many mutations are present at relatively low frequency in most lymphoma subtypes, broad testing panels would be necessary to identify rare but potentially targetable lesions, such the infrequent but recurrent mutations of *BRAF* in nodal marginal zone lymphomas (Pillonel et al. 2018). Although examples of genetically directed, targeted therapy remain relatively few in lymphoma, ever-increasing numbers of novel agents are being evaluated in clinical trials, particularly in the setting of relapsed/refractory disease, and comprehensive genetic profiling of lymphomas should be considered in such settings both to identify targets and to identify the determinants of response to novel therapies.

CONCLUSION

NGS technologies have led to an exponential increase in our understanding of the pathogenesis of mature lymphoid leukemias and lymphomas. Although relatively few lymphomas had been associated with karyotypically recognizable abnormalities such as chromosomal translocations, recurrent mutations are now known in virtually every lymphoma subtype. With some exceptions, such as the very high incidence of *BRAF* mutations in HCL, most lymphoma types are not associated with a single highly recurrently mutated gene or recurrent translocation. Rather, lymphomas exhibit mutational complexity, with a long tail of mutations that are present in relatively few patients. However, within this genetic heterogeneity new subgroups have been recognized, possibly with divergent responses to novel therapeutic agents. Our greater understanding of mutational processes in lymphoma holds the promise of better and less toxic therapies for patients with these devastating diseases.

REFERENCES

Abate F, Ambrosio MR, Mundo L, Laginestra MA, Fuligni F, Rossi M, Zairis S, Gazaneo S, De Falco G, Lazzi S, et al. 2015. Distinct viral and mutational spectrum of endemic Burkitt lymphoma. *PLoS Pathog* **11:** e1005158. doi:10.1371/journal.ppat.1005158

Alizadeh AA, Eisen MB, Davis RE, Ma C, Lossos IS, Rosenwald A, Boldrick JC, Sabet H, Yu X, Powell JI, et al. 2000. Distinct types of diffuse large B-cell lymphoma identified by gene expression profiling. *Nature* **403:** 503–511. doi:10.1038/35000501

Andersson EI, Pützer S, Yadav B, Dufva O, Khan S, He L, Sellner L, Schrader A, Crispatzu G, Oleś M, et al. 2018. Discovery of novel drug sensitivities in T-PLL by high-throughput ex vivo drug testing and mutation profiling. *Leukemia* **32:** 774–787. doi:10.1038/leu.2017.252

Andritsos LA, Grieselhuber NR, Anghelina M, Rogers KA, Roychowdhury S, Reeser JW, Timmers CD, Freud AG, Blachly JS, Lucas DM, et al. 2018. Trametinib for the treatment of IGHV4-34, MAP2K1-mutant variant hairy cell leukemia. *Leuk Lymphoma* **59:** 1008–1011. doi:10.1080/10428194.2017.1365853

Ansell SM, Lesokhin AM, Borrello I, Halwani A, Scott EC, Gutierrez M, Schuster SJ, Millenson MM, Cattry D, Freeman GJ, et al. 2015. PD-1 blockade with nivolumab in relapsed or refractory Hodgkin's lymphoma. *New Engl J Med* **372:** 311–319. doi:10.1056/NEJMoa1411087

Arcaini L, Zibellini S, Boveri E, Riboni R, Rattotti S, Varettoni M, Guerrera ML, Lucioni M, Tenore A, Merli M, et al. 2012. The *BRAF* V600E mutation in hairy cell leukemia and other mature B-cell neoplasms. *Blood* **119:** 188–191. doi:10.1182/blood-2011-08-368209

Banks PM, Chan J, Cleary ML, Delsol G, De Wolf-Peeters C, Gatter K, Grogan TM, Harris NL, Isaacson PG, Jaffe ES, et al. 1992. Mantle cell lymphoma. A proposal for unification of morphologic, immunologic, and molecular data. *Am J Surg Pathol* **16:** 637–640. doi:10.1097/00000478-199207000-00001

Beà S, Ribas M, Hernández JM, Bosch F, Pinyol M, Hernández L, García JL, Flores T, González M, López-Guillermo A, et al. 1999. Increased number of chromosomal imbalances and high-level DNA amplifications in mantle cell lymphoma are associated with blastoid variants. *Blood* **93:** 4365–4374.

Beà S, Valdés-Mas R, Navarro A, Salaverria I, Martín-Garcia D, Jares P, Giné E, Pinyol M, Royo C, Nadeu F, et al. 2013. Landscape of somatic mutations and clonal evolution in mantle cell lymphoma. *Proc Natl Acad Sci* **110:** 18250–18255. doi:10.1073/pnas.1314608110

Bentz M, Plesch A, Bullinger L, Stilgenbauer S, Ott G, Müller-Hermelink HK, Baudis M, Barth TF, Möller P, Lichter P, et al. 2000. t(11;14)-positive mantle cell lymphomas exhibit complex karyotypes and share similarities with B-cell chronic lymphocytic leukemia. *Genes Chromosomes Cancer* **27:** 285–294. doi:10.1002/(SICI)1098-2264(200003)27:33.3.CO;2-D

Boi M, Rinaldi A, Kwee I, Bonetti P, Todaro M, Tabbò F, Piva R, Rancoita PM, Matolcsy A, Timar B, et al. 2013. PRDM1/BLIMP1 is commonly inactivated in anaplastic large T-cell lymphoma. *Blood* **122:** 2683–2693. doi:10.1182/blood-2013-04-497933

Boice M, Salloum D, Mourcin F, Sanghvi V, Amin R, Oricchio E, Jiang M, Mottok A, Denis-Lagache N, Ciriello G, et al. 2016. Loss of the HVEM tumor suppressor in lymphoma and restoration by modified CAR-T cells. *Cell* **167:** 405–418.e13. doi:10.1016/j.cell.2016.08.032

Braggio E, Keats JJ, Leleu X, Van Wier S, Jimenez-Zepeda VH, Valdez R, Schop RF, Price-Troska T, Henderson K, Sacco A, et al. 2009. Identification of copy number abnormalities and inactivating mutations in two negative regulators of nuclear factor-κB signaling pathways in Waldenström's macroglobulinemia. *Cancer Res* **69:** 3579–3588. doi:10.1158/0008-5472.CAN-08-3701

Brito-Babapulle V, Pomfret M, Matutes E, Catovsky D. 1987. Cytogenetic studies on prolymphocytic leukemia. II: T cell prolymphocytic leukemia. *Blood* **70:** 926–931. doi:10.1182/blood.V70.4.926.926

Brown JR. 2018. How I treat CLL patients with ibrutinib. *Blood* **131:** 379–386. doi:10.1182/blood-2017-08-764712

Byrd JC, Gribben JG, Peterson BL, Grever MR, Lozanski G, Lucas DM, Lampson B, Larson RA, Caligiuri MA, Heerema NA. 2006. Select high-risk genetic features predict earlier progression following chemoimmunotherapy with fludarabine and rituximab in chronic lymphocytic leukemia: Justification for risk-adapted therapy. *J Clin Oncol* **24:** 437–443. doi:10.1200/JCO.2005.03.1021

Cairns RA, Iqbal J, Lemonnier F, Kucuk C, de Leval L, Jais JP, Parrens M, Martin A, Xerri L, Brousset P, et al. 2012. *IDH2* mutations are frequent in angioimmunoblastic T-cell lymphoma. *Blood* **119:** 1901–1903. doi:10.1182/blood-2011-11-391748

Calin GA, Cimmino A, Fabbri M, Ferracin M, Wojcik SE, Shimizu M, Taccioli C, Zanesi N, Garzon R, Aqeilan RI, et al. 2008. *miR-15a* and *miR-16-1* cluster functions in human leukemia. *Proc Natl Acad Sci* **105:** 5166–5171. doi:10.1073/pnas.0800121105

Campos-Martín Y, Martínez N, Martínez-López A, Cereceda L, Casado F, Algara P, Oscier D, Menarguez FJ, García JF, Piris MA, et al. 2017. Clinical and diagnostic relevance of *NOTCH2*- and *KLF2*-mutations in splenic marginal zone lymphoma. *Haematologica* **102:** e310–e312. doi:10.3324/haematol.2016.161711

Carvajal-Cuenca A, Sua LF, Silva NM, Pittaluga S, Royo C, Song JY, Sargent RL, Espinet B, Climent F, Jacobs SA, et al. 2012. In situ mantle cell lymphoma: Clinical implications of an incidental finding with indolent clinical behavior. *Haematologic* **97:** 270–278. doi:10.3324/haematol.2011.052621

Chapuy B, Roemer MGM, Stewart C, Tan Y, Abo RP, Zhang L, Dunford AJ, Meredith DM, Thorner AR, Jordanova ES, et al. 2016. Targetable genetic features of primary testicular and primary central nervous system lymphomas. *Blood* **127:** 869–881. doi:10.1182/blood-2015-10-673236

Chapuy B, Stewart C, Dunford AJ, Kim J, Kamburov A, Redd RA, Lawrence MS, Roemer MGM, Li AJ, Ziepert M, et al. 2018. Molecular subtypes of diffuse large B cell lymphoma are associated with distinct pathogenic mechanisms and outcomes. *Nat Med* **24:** 679–690. doi:10.1038/s41591-018-0016-8

Chen YW, Hu XT, Liang AC, Au WY, So CC, Wong ML, Shen L, Tao Q, Chu KM, Kwong YL, et al. 2006. High BCL6 expression predicts better prognosis, independent of *BCL6* translocation status, translocation partner, or *BCL6*-deregulating mutations, in gastric lymphoma. *Blood* **108:** 2373–2383. doi:10.1182/blood-2006-05-022517

Cheung KJJ, Shah SP, Steidl C, Johnson N, Relander T, Telenius A, Lai B, Murphy KP, Lam W, Al-Tourah AJ, et al. 2009. Genome-wide profiling of follicular lymphoma by array comparative genomic hybridization reveals prognostically significant DNA copy number imbalances. *Blood* **113:** 137–148. doi:10.1182/blood-2008-02-140616

Cheung KJJ, Johnson NA, Affleck JG, Severson T, Steidl C, Ben-Neriah S, Schein J, Morin RD, Moore R, Shah SP, et al. 2010. Acquired *TNFRSF14* mutations in follicular lymphoma are associated with worse prognosis. *Cancer Res* **70:** 9166–9174. doi:10.1158/0008-5472.CAN-10-2460

Choi J, Goh G, Walradt T, Hong BS, Bunick CG, Chen K, Bjornson RD, Maman Y, Wang T, Tordoff J, et al. 2015. Genomic landscape of cutaneous T cell lymphoma. *Nat Genet* **47:** 1011–1019. doi:10.1038/ng.3356

Chong LC, Ben-Neriah S, Slack GW, Freeman C, Ennishi D, Mottok A, Collinge B, Abrisqueta P, Farinha P, Boyle M, et al. 2018. High-resolution architecture and partner genes of MYC rearrangements in lymphoma with DLBCL morphology. *Blood Adv* **2:** 2755–2765. doi:10.1182/bloodadvances.2018023572

Clipson A, Wang M, de Leval L, Ashton-Key M, Wotherspoon A, Vassiliou G, Bolli N, Grove C, Moody S, Escudero-Ibarz L, et al. 2015. *KLF2* mutation is the most frequent somatic change in splenic marginal zone lymphoma and identifies a subset with distinct genotype. *Leukemia* **29:** 1177–1185. doi:10.1038/leu.2014.330

Copie-Bergman C, Cuillière-Dartigues P, Baia M, Briere J, Delarue R, Canioni D, Salles G, Parrens M, Belhadj K, Fabiani B, et al. 2015. *MYC-IG* rearrangements are negative predictors of survival in DLBCL patients treated with immunochemotherapy: A GELA/LYSA study. *Blood* **126:** 2466–2474. doi:10.1182/blood-2015-05-647602

Crescenzo R, Abate F, Lasorsa E, Tabbo F, Gaudiano M, Chiesa N, Di Giacomo F, Spaccarotella E, Barbarossa L, Ercole E, et al. 2015. Convergent mutations and kinase fusions lead to oncogenic STAT3 activation in anaplastic large cell lymphoma. *Cancer Cell* **27:** 516–532. doi:10.1016/j.ccell.2015.03.006

Czuczman MS, Trněný M, Davies A, Rule S, Linton KM, Wagner-Johnston N, Gascoyne RD, Slack GW, Brousset P, Eberhard DA, et al. 2017. A phase 2/3 multicenter, randomized, open-label study to compare the efficacy and safety of lenalidomide versus investigator's choice in patients with relapsed or refractory diffuse large B-cell lymphoma. *Clin Cancer Res* **23:** 4127–4137. doi:10.1158/1078-0432.CCR-16-2818

Dalla-Favera R, Bregni M, Erikson J, Patterson D, Gallo RC, Croce CM. 1982. Human c-myc onc gene is located on the region of chromosome 8 that is translocated in Burkitt lymphoma cells. *Proc Natl Acad Sci* **79:** 7824–7827. doi:10.1073/pnas.79.24.7824

Damle RN, Wasil T, Fais F, Ghiotto F, Valetto A, Allen SL, Buchbinder A, Budman D, Dittmar K, Kolitz J, et al. 1999. Ig V gene mutation status and CD38 expression as novel prognostic indicators in chronic lymphocytic leukemia. *Blood* **94:** 1840–1847. doi:10.1182/blood.V94.6.1840

da Silva Almeida AC, Abate F, Khiabanian H, Martinez-Escala E, Guitart J, Tensen CP, Vermeer MH, Rabadan R, Ferrando A, Palomero T. 2015. The mutational landscape of cutaneous T cell lymphoma and Sézary syndrome. *Nat Genet* **47:** 1465–1470. doi:10.1038/ng.3442

Davis RE, Ngo VN, Lenz G, Tolar P, Young RM, Romesser PB, Kohlhammer H, Lamy L, Zhao H, Yang Y, et al. 2010. Chronic active B-cell-receptor signalling in diffuse large B-cell lymphoma. *Nature* **463:** 88–92. doi:10.1038/nature08638

Dearden C. 2012. How I treat prolymphocytic leukemia. *Blood* **120:** 538–551. doi:10.1182/blood-2012-01-380139

Dictor M, Ek S, Sundberg M, Warenholt J, György C, Sernbo S, Gustavsson E, Abu-Alsoud W, Wadström T, Borrebaeck C. 2009. Strong lymphoid nuclear expression of *SOX11* transcription factor defines lymphoblastic neoplasms, mantle cell lymphoma and Burkitt's lymphoma. *Haematologica* **94:** 1563–1568. doi:10.3324/haematol.2009.008474

Dimopoulos MA, Trotman J, Tedeschi A, Matous JV, Macdonald D, Tam C, Tournilhac O, Ma S, Oriol A, Heffner LT, et al. 2017. Ibrutinib for patients with rituximab-refractory Waldenström's macroglobulinaemia (iNNOVATE): An open-label substudy of an international, multicentre, phase 3 trial. *Lancet Oncol* **18:** 241–250. doi:10.1016/S1470-2045(16)30632-5

Döhner H, Stilgenbauer S, Benner A, Leupolt E, Kröber A, Bullinger L, Döhner K, Bentz M, Lichter P. 2000. Genomic aberrations and survival in chronic lymphocytic leukemia. *N Engl J Med* **343:** 1910–1916. doi:10.1056/NEJM200012283432602

Dunleavy K, Pittaluga S, Maeda LS, Advani R, Chen CC, Hessler J, Steinberg SM, Grant C, Wright G, Varma G, et al. 2013. Dose-adjusted EPOCH-rituximab therapy in primary mediastinal B-cell lymphoma. *N Engl J Med* **368:** 1408–1416. doi:10.1056/NEJMoa1214561

Durham BH, Getta B, Dietrich S, Taylor J, Won H, Bogenberger JM, Scott S, Kim E, Chung YR, Chung SS, et al. 2017. Genomic analysis of hairy cell leukemia identifies novel recurrent genetic alterations. *Blood* **130:** 1644–1648. doi:10.1182/blood-2017-01-765107

Eichhorst B, Fink AM, Bahlo J, Busch R, Kovacs G, Maurer C, Lange E, Köppler H, Kiehl M, Sökler M, et al. 2016. First-line chemoimmunotherapy with bendamustine and rituximab versus fludarabine, cyclophosphamide, and rituximab in patients with advanced chronic lymphocytic leukaemia (CLL10): An international, open-label, randomised, phase 3, non-inferiority trial. *Lancet Oncol* **17:** 928–942. doi:10.1016/S1470-2045(16)30051-1

Elenitoba-Johnson KSJ, Gascoyne RD, Lim MS, Chhanabai M, Jaffe ES, Raffeld M. 1998. Homozygous deletions at chromosome 9p21 involving p16 and p15 are associated with histologic progression in follicle center lymphoma. *Blood* **91:** 4677–4685. doi:10.1182/blood.V91.12.4677

Eskelund CW, Dahl C, Hansen JW, Westman M, Kolstad A, Pedersen LB, Montano-Almendras CP, Husby S, Freiburhaus C, Ek S, et al. 2017. *TP53* mutations identify younger mantle cell lymphoma patients who do not benefit from intensive chemoimmunotherapy. *Blood* **130:** 1903–1910. doi:10.1182/blood-2017-04-779736

Falini B, Bigerna B, Fizzotti M, Pulford K, Pileri SA, Delsol G, Carbone A, Paulli M, Magrini U, Menestrina F, et al. 1998. ALK expression defines a distinct group of T/null lymphomas ("ALK lymphomas") with a wide morphological spectrum. *Am J Pathol* **153:** 875–886. doi:10.1016/S0002-9440(10)65629-5

Feldman AL, Law M, Remstein ED, Macon WR, Erickson LA, Grogg KL, Kurtin PJ, Dogan A. 2009. Recurrent translocations involving the *IRF4* oncogene locus in peripheral T-cell lymphomas. *Leukemia* **23:** 574–580. doi:10.1038/leu.2008.320

Feldman AL, Dogan A, Smith DI, Law ME, Ansell SM, Johnson SH, Procher JC, Ozsan N, Wieben ED, Eckloff BW, et al. 2011. Discovery of recurrent t(6;7)(p25.3;q32.3) translocations in ALK-negative anaplastic large cell lymphomas by massively parallel genomic sequencing. *Blood* **117:** 915–919. doi:10.1182/blood-2010-08-303305

Fernàndez V, Salamero O, Espinet B, Solé F, Royo C, Navarro A, Camacho F, Beà S, Hartmann E, Amador V, et al. 2010. Genomic and gene expression profiling defines indolent forms of mantle cell lymphoma. *Cancer Res* **70:** 1408–1418. doi:10.1158/0008-5472.CAN-09-3419

Fischer K, Bahlo J, Fink AM, Goede V, Herling CD, Cramer P, Langerbeins P, von Tresckow J, Engelke A, Maurer C, et al. 2016. Long-term remissions after FCR chemoimmunotherapy in previously untreated patients with CLL: Updated results of the CLL8 trial. *Blood* **127:** 208–215. doi:10.1182/blood-2015-06-651125

Flossbach L, Antoneag E, Buck M, Siebert R, Mattfeldt T, Möller P, Barth TF. 2011. *BCL6* gene rearrangement and protein expression are associated with large cell presentation of extranodal marginal zone B-cell lymphoma of mucosa-associated lymphoid tissue. *Int J Cancer* **129:** 70–77. doi:10.1002/ijc.25663

Forconi F, Poretti G, Kwee I, Sozzi E, Rossi D, Rancoita PMV, Capello D, Rinaldi A, Zucca E, Raspadori D, et al. 2008. High density genome-wide DNA profiling reveals a remarkably stable profile in hairy cell leukaemia. *Br J Haematol* **141:** 622–630. doi:10.1111/j.1365-2141.2008.07106.x

Friedberg JW. 2017. How I treat double-hit lymphoma. *Blood* **130:** 590–596. doi:10.1182/blood-2017-04-737320

Fu K, Weisenburger DD, Greiner TC, Dave S, Wright G, Rosenwald A, Chiorazzi M, Iqbal J, Gesk S, Siebert R, et al. 2005. Cyclin D1-negative mantle cell lymphoma: A clinicopathologic study based on gene expression profiling. *Blood* **106:** 4315–4321. doi:10.1182/blood-2005-04-1753

Fukuhara S, Rowley JD, Variakojis D, Golomb HM. 1979. Chromosome abnormalities in poorly differentiated lymphocytic lymphoma. *Cancer Res* **39:** 3119.

Ghia EM, Jain S, Widhopf GF II, Rassenti LZ, Keating MJ, Wierda WG, Gribben JG, Brown JR, Rai KR, Byrd JC, et al. 2008. Use of *IGHV3-21* in chronic lymphocytic leukemia is associated with high-risk disease and reflects antigen-driven, post-germinal center leukemogenic selection. *Blood* **111:** 5101–5108. doi:10.1182/blood-2007-12-130229

Green MR, Monti S, Rodig SJ, Juszczynski P, Currie T, O'Donnell E, Chapuy B, Takeyama K, Neuberg D, Golub TR, et al. 2010. Integrative analysis reveals selective 9p24.1 amplification, increased PD-1 ligand expression, and further induction via JAK2 in nodular sclerosing Hodgkin lymphoma and primary mediastinal large B-cell lymphoma. *Blood* **116:** 3268–3277. doi:10.1182/blood-2010-05-282780

Green MR, Kihira S, Liu CL, Nair RV, Salari R, Gentles AJ, Irish J, Stehr H, Vicente-Dueñas C, Romero-Camarero I, et al. 2015. Mutations in early follicular lymphoma progenitors are associated with suppressed antigen presentation. *Proc Natl Acad Sci* **112:** E1116–E1125. doi:10.1073/pnas.1501199112

Gribben JG. 2010. How I treat CLL up front. *Blood* **115:** 187–197. doi:10.1182/blood-2009-08-207126

Hallberg B, Palmer RH. 2013. Mechanistic insight into ALK receptor tyrosine kinase in human cancer biology. *Nat Rev Cancer* **13:** 685–700. doi:10.1038/nrc3580

Hamblin TJ, Davis Z, Gardiner A, Oscier DG, Stevenson FK. 1999. Unmutated Ig V_H genes are associated with a more aggressive form of chronic lymphocytic leukemia. *Blood* **94:** 1848–1854. doi:10.1182/blood.V94.6.1848

Hans CP, Weisenburger DD, Greiner TC, Gascoyne RD, Delabie J, Ott G, Müller-Hermelink HK, Campo E, Braziel RM, Jaffe ES, et al. 2004. Confirmation of the molecular classification of diffuse large B-cell lymphoma by immunohistochemistry using a tissue microarray. *Blood* **103:** 275–282. doi:10.1182/blood-2003-05-1545

Harris NL, Jaffe ES, Stein H, Banks PM, Chan JK, Cleary ML, Delsol G, De Wolf-Peeters C, Falini B, Gatter KC, et al. 1994. A revised European–American classification of lymphoid neoplasms: A proposal from the International Lymphoma Study Group [see comments]. *Blood* **84:** 1361–1392. doi:10.1182/blood.V84.5.1361.1361

Horwitz S, O'Connor OA, Pro B, Illidge T, Fanale M, Advani R, Bartlett NL, Christensen JH, Morschhauser F, Domingo-Domenech E, et al. 2019. Brentuximab vedotin with chemotherapy for CD30-positive peripheral T-cell lymphoma (ECHELON-2): A global, double-blind, randomised, phase 3 trial. *Lancet* **393:** 229–240. doi:10.1016/S0140-6736(18)32984-2

Hummel M, Bentink S, Berger H, Klapper W, Wessendorf S, Barth TFE, Bernd HW, Cogliatti SB, Dierlamm J, Feller AC, et al. 2006. A biologic definition of Burkitt's lymphoma from transcriptional and genomic profiling. *New Engl J Med* **354:** 2419–2430. doi:10.1056/NEJMoa055351

Johnson NA, Savage KJ, Ludkovski O, Ben-Neriah S, Woods R, Steidl C, Dyer MJ, Siebert R, Kuruvilla J, Klasa R, et al. 2009. Lymphomas with concurrent *BCL2* and *MYC* translocations: The critical factors associated with survival. *Blood* **114:** 2273–2279. doi:10.1182/blood-2009-03-212191

Kiel MJ, Velusamy T, Betz BL, Zhao L, Weigelin HG, Chiang MY, Huebner-Chan DR, Bailey NG, Yang DT, Bhagat G, et al. 2012. Whole-genome sequencing identifies recurrent somatic *NOTCH2* mutations in splenic marginal zone lymphoma. *J Exp Med* **209:** 1553–1565. doi:10.1084/jem.20120910

Kiel MJ, Velusamy T, Rolland D, Sahasrabuddhe AA, Chung F, Bailey NG, Schrader A, Li B, Li JZ, Ozel AB, et al. 2014. Integrated genomic sequencing reveals mutational landscape of T-cell prolymphocytic leukemia. *Blood* **124:** 1460–1472. doi:10.1182/blood-2014-03-559542

Kiel MJ, Sahasrabuddhe AA, Rolland DCM, Velusamy T, Chung F, Schaller M, Bailey NG, Betz BL, Miranda RN, Porcu P, et al. 2015. Genomic analyses reveal recurrent mutations in epigenetic modifiers and the JAK–STAT pathway in Sézary syndrome. *Nat Commun* **6:** 8470. doi:10.1038/ncomms9470

Kim YH, Bagot M, Pinter-Brown L, Rook AH, Porcu P, Horwitz SM, Whittaker S, Tokura Y, Vermeer M, Zinzani PL, et al. 2018. Mogamulizumab versus vorinostat in previously treated cutaneous T-cell lymphoma (MAVORIC): An international, open-label, randomised, controlled phase 3 trial. *Lancet Oncol* **19:** 1192–1204. doi:10.1016/S1470-2045(18)30379-6

Kurita D, Takeuchi K, Kobayashi S, Hojo A, Uchino Y, Sakagami M, Ohtake S, Takahashi H, Miura K, Iriyama N, et al. 2016. A cyclin D1-negative mantle cell lymphoma with an *IGL-CCND2* translocation that relapsed with blastoid morphology and aggressive clinical behavior. *Virchows Arch* **469:** 471–476. doi:10.1007/s00428-016-1995-9

Kurtz DM, Green MR, Bratman SV, Scherer F, Liu CL, Kunder CA, Takahashi K, Glover C, Keane C, Kihira S, et al. 2015. Noninvasive monitoring of diffuse large B-cell lymphoma by immunoglobulin high-throughput sequencing. *Blood* **125:** 3679–3687. doi:10.1182/blood-2015-03-635169

Landau DA, Tausch E, Taylor-Weiner AN, Stewart C, Reiter JG, Bahlo J, Kluth S, Bozic I, Lawrence M, Böttcher S, et al. 2015. Mutations driving CLL and their evolution in progression and relapse. *Nature* **526:** 525–530. doi:10.1038/nature15395

Launay E, Pangault C, Bertrand P, Jardin F, Lamy T, Tilly H, Tarte K, Bastard C, Fest T. 2012. High rate of *TNFRSF14* gene alterations related to 1p36 region in de novo follicular lymphoma and impact on prognosis. *Leukemia* **26:** 559–562. doi:10.1038/leu.2011.266

Le Beau MM, Bitter MA, Larson RA, Doane LA, Ellis ED, Franklin WA, Rubin CM, Kadin ME, Vardiman JW. 1989. The t(2;5)(p23;q35): A recurring chromosomal abnormality in Ki-1-positive anaplastic large cell lymphoma. *Leukemia* **3:** 866–870.

Lemonnier F, Couronné L, Parrens M, Jaïs JP, Travert M, Lamant L, Tournillac O, Rousset T, Fabiani B, Cairns RA, et al. 2012. Recurrent *TET2* mutations in peripheral T-cell lymphomas correlate with T_{FH}-like features and adverse clinical parameters. *Blood* **120:** 1466–1469. doi:10.1182/blood-2012-02-408542

Lemonnier F, Dupuis J, Sujobert P, Tournillhac O, Cheminant M, Sarkozy C, Pelletier L, Marçais A, Robe C, Fataccioli V, et al. 2018. Treatment with 5-azacytidine induces a sustained response in patients with angioimmunoblastic T-cell lymphoma. *Blood* **132:** 2305–2309. doi:10.1182/blood-2018-04-840538

Lenz G, Wright G, Dave SS, Xiao W, Powell J, Zhao H, Xu W, Tan B, Goldschmidt N, Iqbal J, et al. 2008. Stromal gene signatures in large-B-cell lymphomas. *New Engl J Med* **359:** 2313–2323. doi:10.1056/NEJMoa0802885

Leucci E, Cocco M, Onnis A, De Falco G, van Cleef P, Bellan C, van Rijk A, Nyagol J, Byakika B, Lazzi S, et al. 2008. *MYC* translocation-negative classical Burkitt lymphoma cases: An alternative pathogenetic mechanism involving miRNA deregulation. *J Pathol* **216:** 440–450. doi:10.1002/path.2410

Li S, Lin P, Fayad LE, Lennon PA, Miranda RN, Yin CC, Lin E, Medeiros LJ. 2012. B-cell lymphomas with *MYC/8q24* rearrangements and *IGH@BCL2*/t(14;18)(q32;q21): An aggressive disease with heterogeneous histology, germinal center B-cell immunophenotype and poor outcome. *Mod Pathol* **25:** 145–156. doi:10.1038/modpathol.2011.147

Louissaint A, Schafernak KT, Geyer JT, Kovach AE, Ghandi M, Gratzinger D, Roth CG, Paxton CN, Kim S, Namgyal C, et al. 2016. Pediatric-type nodal follicular lymphoma: A biologically distinct lymphoma with frequent MAPK pathway mutations. *Blood* **128:** 1093–1100. doi:10.1182/blood-2015-12-682591

Malcikova J, Tausch E, Rossi D, Sutton LA, Soussi T, Zenz T, Kater AP, Niemann CU, Gonzalez D, Davi F, et al. 2018. ERIC recommendations for *TP53* mutation analysis in chronic lymphocytic leukemia—Update on methodological approaches and results interpretation. *Leukemia* **32:** 1070–1080. doi:10.1038/s41375-017-0007-7

Manolov G, Manolova Y. 1972. Marker band in one chromosome 14 from Burkitt lymphomas. *Nature* **237:** 33–34. doi:10.1038/237033a0

Marcucci G, Maharry K, Wu YZ, Radmacher MD, Mrózek K, Margeson D, Holland KB, Whitman SP, Becker H, Schwind S, et al. 2010. *IDH1* and *IDH2* gene mutations identify novel molecular subsets within de novo cytogenetically normal acute myeloid leukemia: A Cancer and Leukemia Group B Study. *J Clin Oncol* **28:** 2348–2355. doi:10.1200/JCO.2009.27.3730

Martín-Garcia D, Navarro A, Valdés-Mas R, Clot G, Gutiérrez-Abril J, Prieto M, Ribera-Cortada I, Woroniecka R, Rymkiewicz G, Bens S, et al. 2018. *CCND2* and *CCND3* hijack immunoglobulin light chain enhancers in cyclin D1-negative mantle cell lymphoma. *Blood* **133:** 940–951. doi:10.1182/blood-2018-07-862151

May PC, Foot N, Dunn R, Geoghegan H, Neat MJ. 2010. Detection of cryptic and variant IGH-MYC rearrangements in high-grade non-Hodgkin's lymphoma by fluorescence in situ hybridization: Implications for cytogenetic testing. *Cancer Genet Cytogenet* **198:** 71–75. doi:10.1016/j.cancergencyto.2009.12.010

McGregor JM, Crook T, Fraser-Andrews EA, Rozycka M, Crossland S, Brooks L, Whittaker SJ. 1999. Spectrum of p53 gene mutations suggests a possible role for ultraviolet radiation in the pathogenesis of advanced cutaneous lymphomas. *J Invest Dermatol* **112:** 317–321. doi:10.1046/j.1523-1747.1999.00507.x

Melzner I, Bucur AJ, Brüderlein S, Dorsch K, Hasel C, Barth TF, Leithäuser F, Möller P. 2005. Biallelic mutation of *SOCS-1* impairs JAK2 degradation and sustains phospho-JAK2 action in the MedB-1 mediastinal lymphoma line. *Blood* **105:** 2535–2542. doi:10.1182/blood-2004-09-3701

Montgomery ND, Coward WB IV, Johnson S, Yuan J, Gulley ML, Mathews SP, Kaiser-Rogers K, Rao KW, Sanger WG, Sanmann JN, et al. 2016. Karyotypic abnormalities associated with Epstein–Barr virus status in classical Hodgkin lymphoma. *Cancer Genet* **209:** 408–416. doi:10.1016/j.cancergen.2016.08.006

Morin RD, Johnson NA, Severson TM, Mungall AJ, An J, Goya R, Paul JE, Boyle M, Woolcock BW, Kuchenbauer F, et al. 2010. Somatic mutations altering EZH2 (Tyr641) in follicular and diffuse large B-cell lymphomas of germinal-center origin. *Nat Genet* **42:** 181–185. doi:10.1038/ng.518

Morin RD, Mendez-Lago M, Mungall AJ, Goya R, Mungall KL, Corbett RD, Johnson NA, Severson TM, Chiu R, Field M, et al. 2011. Frequent mutation of histone-modifying genes in non-Hodgkin lymphoma. *Nature* **476:** 298–303. doi:10.1038/nature10351

Morris SW, Kirstein MN, Valentine MB, Dittmer KG, Shapiro DN, Saltman DL, Look AT. 1994. Fusion of a kinase gene, *ALK*, to a nucleolar protein gene, *NPM*, in non-Hodgkin's lymphoma. *Science* **263:** 1281–1284. doi:10.1126/science.8122112

Mossé YP, Voss SD, Lim MS, Rolland D, Minard CG, Fox E, Adamson P, Wilner K, Blaney SM, Weigel BJ. 2017. Targeting ALK with Crizotinib in pediatric anaplastic large cell lymphoma and inflammatory myofibroblastic tumor: A Children's Oncology Group Study. *J Clin Oncol* **35:** 3215–3221. doi:10.1200/JCO.2017.73.4830

Mozos A, Royo C, Hartmann E, De Jong D, Baró C, Valera A, Fu K, Weisenburger DD, Delabie J, Chuang SS, et al. 2009. *SOX11* expression is highly specific for mantle cell lymphoma and identifies the cyclin D1-negative subtype. *Haematologica* **94:** 1555. doi:10.3324/haematol.2009.010264

Muñoz-Mármol AM, Sanz C, Tapia G, Marginet R, Ariza A, Mate JL. 2013. *MYC* status determination in aggressive B-cell lymphoma: The impact of FISH probe selection. *Histopathology* **63:** 418–424. doi:10.1111/his.12178

Ngo VN, Young RM, Schmitz R, Jhavar S, Xiao W, Lim KH, Kohlhammer H, Xu W, Yang Y, Zhao H, et al. 2011. Oncogenically active *MYD88* mutations in human lymphoma. *Nature* **470:** 115–119. doi:10.1038/nature09671

Odejide O, Weigert O, Lane AA, Toscano D, Lunning MA, Kopp N, Kim S, van Bodegom D, Bolla S, Schatz JH, et al. 2014. A targeted mutational landscape of angioimmunoblastic T-cell lymphoma. *Blood* **123:** 1293–1296. doi:10.1182/blood-2013-10-531509

Okosun J, Bodor C, Wang J, Araf S, Yang CY, Pan C, Boller S, Cittaro D, Bozek M, Iqbal S, et al. 2014. Integrated genomic analysis identifies recurrent mutations and evolution patterns driving the initiation and progression of follicular lymphoma. *Nat Genet* **46:** 176–181. doi:10.1038/ng.2856

Palomero T, Couronné L, Khiabanian H, Kim MY, Ambesi-Impiombato A, Perez-Garcia A, Carpenter Z, Abate F, Allegretta M, Jaydu JE, et al. 2014. Recurrent mutations in epigenetic regulators, *RHOA* and *FYN* kinase in peripheral T cell lymphomas. *Nat Genet* **46:** 166–170. doi:10.1038/ng.2873

Parrilla Castellar ER, Jaffe ES, Said JW, Swerdlow SH, Ketterling RP, Knudson RA, Sidhu JS, Hsi ED, Karikehalli S, Jiang L, et al. 2014. ALK-negative anaplastic large cell lymphoma is a genetically heterogeneous disease with widely disparate clinical outcomes. *Blood* **124:** 1473–1480. doi:10.1182/blood-2014-04-571091

Parry M, Rose-Zerilli MJJ, Ljungström V, Gibson J, Wang J, Walewska R, Parker H, Parker A, Davis Z, Gardiner A, et al. 2015. Genetics and prognostication in splenic marginal zone lymphoma: Revelations from deep sequencing. *Clin Cancer Res* **21:** 4174–4183. doi:10.1158/1078-0432.CCR-14-2759

Pasqualucci L, Dalla-Favera R. 2015. The genetic landscape of diffuse large B-cell lymphoma. *Semin Hematol* **52:** 67–76. doi:10.1053/j.seminhematol.2015.01.005

Pasqualucci L, Dominguez-Sola D, Chiarenza A, Fabbri G, Grunn A, Trifonov V, Kasper LH, Lerach S, Tang H, Ma J, et al. 2011. Inactivating mutations of acetyltransferase genes in B-cell lymphoma. *Nature* **471:** 189–195. doi:10.1038/nature09730

Pasqualucci L, Khiabanian H, Fangazio M, Vasishtha M, Messina M, Holmes AB, et al. 2014. Genetics of follicular lymphoma transformation. *Cell Rep* **6:** 130–140. doi:10.1016/j.celrep.2013.12.027

Pastore A, Jurinovic V, Kridel R, Hoster E, Staiger AM, Szczepanowski M, Pott C, Kopp N, Murakami M, Horn H, et al. 2015. Integration of gene mutations in risk prognostication for patients receiving first-line immunochemotherapy for follicular lymphoma: A retrospective analysis of a prospective clinical trial and validation in a population-based registry. *Lancet Oncol* **16:** 1111–1122. doi:10.1016/S1470-2045(15)00169-2

Pedersen MØ, Gang AO, Poulsen TS, Knudsen H, Lauritzen AF, Nielsen SL, Klausen TW, Nørgaard P. 2014. MYC translocation partner gene determines survival of patients with large B-cell lymphoma with MYC- or double-hit MYC/BCL2 translocations. *Eur J Haematol* **92:** 42–48. doi:10.1111/ejh.12212

Pedersen MB, Hamilton-Dutoit SJ, Bendix K, Ketterling RP, Bedroske PP, Luoma IM, Sattler CA, Boddicker RL, Bennani NN, Nørgaard P, et al. 2017. *DUSP22* and *TP63* rearrangements predict outcome of ALK-negative anaplastic large cell lymphoma: A Danish cohort study. *Blood* **130:** 554–557. doi:10.1182/blood-2016-12-755496

Pekarsky Y, Hallas C, Isobe M, Russo G, Croce CM. 1999. Abnormalities at 14q32.1 in T cell malignancies involve two oncogenes. *Proc Natl Acad Sci* **96:** 2949–2951. doi:10.1073/pnas.96.6.2949

Pekarsky Y, Koval A, Hallas C, Bichi R, Tresini M, Malstrom S, Russo G, Tsichlis P, Croce CM. 2000. Tcl1 enhances Akt kinase activity and mediates its nuclear translocation. *Proc Natl Acad Sci* **97:** 3028–3033. doi:10.1073/pnas.97.7.3028

Perrot A, Lauwers-Cances V, Corre J, Robillard N, Hulin C, Chretien ML, Dejoie T, Maheo S, Stoppa AM, Pegourie B, et al. 2018. Minimal residual disease negativity using deep sequencing is a major prognostic factor in multiple myeloma. *Blood* **132:** 2456–2464. doi:10.1182/blood-2018-06-858613

Pham-Ledard A, Beylot-Barry M, Barbe C, Leduc M, Petrella T, Vergier B, Martinez F, Cappellen D, Merlio JP, Grange F. 2014. High frequency and clinical prognostic value of MYD88 L265P mutation in primary cutaneous diffuse large B-cell lymphoma, Leg-type. *JAMA Dermatol* **150:** 1173–1179. doi:10.1001/jamadermatol.2014.821

Phelan JD, Young RM, Webster DE, Roulland S, Wright GW, Kasbekar M, Shaffer AL, Ceribelli M, Wang JQ, Schmitz R, et al. 2018. A multiprotein supercomplex controlling oncogenic signalling in lymphoma. *Nature* **560:** 387–391. doi:10.1038/s41586-018-0290-0

Pillonel V, Juskevicius D, Ng CKY, Bodmer A, Zettl A, Jucker D, Dirnhofer S, Tzankov A. 2018. High-throughput sequencing of nodal marginal zone lymphomas identifies recurrent *BRAF* mutations. *Leukemia* **32:** 2412–2426. doi:10.1038/s41375-018-0082-4

Pittaluga S, Wlodarska I, Pulford K, Campo E, Morris SW, Van den Berghe H, De Wolf-Petters C. 1997. The monoclonal antibody ALK1 identifies a distinct morphological subtype of anaplastic large cell lymphoma associated with 2p23/ALK rearrangements. *Am J Pathol* **151:** 343–351.

Puente XS, Pinyol M, Quesada V, Conde L, Ordonez GR, Villamor N, Escaramis G, Jares P, Beà S, González-Díaz M, et al. 2011. Whole-genome sequencing identifies recurrent mutations in chronic lymphocytic leukaemia. *Nature* **475:** 101–105. doi:10.1038/nature10113

Pulford K, Lamant L, Morris SW, Butler LH, Wood KM, Stroud D, Delsol G, Mason DY. 1997. Detection of anaplastic lymphoma kinase (ALK) and nucleolar protein nucleophosmin (NPM)-ALK proteins in normal and neoplastic cells with the monoclonal antibody ALK1. *Blood* **89:** 1394–1404. doi:10.1182/blood.V89.4.1394

Quesada V, Conde L, Villamor N, Ordóñez GR, Jares P, Bassaganyas L, Ramsay AJ, Beà S, Pinyol M, Martínez-Trillos A, et al. 2012. Exome sequencing identifies recurrent mutations of the splicing factor *SF3B1* gene in chronic lymphocytic leukemia. *Nat Genet* **44:** 47–52. doi:10.1038/ng.1032

Rawstron AC, Kreuzer KA, Soosapilla A, Spacek M, Stehlikova O, Gambell P, McIver-Brown N, Villamor N, Psarra K, Arroz M, et al. 2018. Reproducible diagnosis of chronic lymphocytic leukemia by flow cytometry: An European Research Initiative on CLL (ERIC) & European Society for Clinical Cell Analysis (ESCCA) Harmonisation project. *Cytometry B Clin Cytom* **94:** 121–128. doi:10.1002/cyto.b.21595

Rimokh R, Magaud JP, Berger F, Samarut J, Coiffier B, Germain D, Mason DY. 1989. A translocation involving a specific breakpoint (q35) on chromosome 5 is characteristic of anaplastic large cell lymphoma ('Ki-1 lymphoma'). *Br J Haematol* **71:** 31–36. doi:10.1111/j.1365-2141.1989.tb06270.x

Ritz O, Guiter C, Castellano F, Dorsch K, Melzner J, Jais JP, Dubois G, Gaullard P, Moeller P, Leroy K. 2009. Recurrent mutations of the STAT6 DNA binding domain in primary mediastinal B-cell lymphoma. *Blood* **114:** 1236–1242. doi:10.1182/blood-2009-03-209759

Roemer MGM, Advani RH, Ligon AH, Natkunam Y, Redd RA, Homer H, Connelly CF, Sun HH, Daadi SE, Freeman GJ, et al. 2016. *PD-L1* and *PD-L2* genetic alterations define classical Hodgkin lymphoma and predict outcome. *J Clin Oncol* **34:** 2690–2697. doi:10.1200/JCO.2016.66.4482

Roschewski M, Dunleavy K, Pittaluga S, Moorhead M, Pepin F, Kong K, Shovlin M, Jaffe ES, Staudt LM, Lai C, et al. 2015. Circulating tumour DNA and CT monitoring in patients with untreated diffuse large B-cell lymphoma: A correlative biomarker study. *Lancet Oncol* **16:** 541–549. doi:10.1016/S1470-2045(15)70106-3

Rosenwald A, Wright G, Chan WC, Connors JM, Campo E, Fisher RI, Gascoyne RD, Muller-Hermlink HK, Smeland EB, Giltnane JM, et al. 2002. The use of molecular profiling to predict survival after chemotherapy for diffuse large-B-cell lymphoma. *New Engl J Med* **346:** 1937–1947. doi:10.1056/NEJMoa012914

Rosenwald A, Wright G, Leroy K, Yu X, Gaulard P, Gascoyne RD, Chan WC, Zhao T, Haioun C, Greiner TC, et al. 2003. Molecular diagnosis of primary mediastinal B cell lymphoma identifies a clinically favorable subgroup of diffuse large B cell lymphoma related to Hodgkin lymphoma. *J Exp Med* **198:** 851–862. doi:10.1084/jem.20031074

Rossi D, Spina V, Deambrogi C, Rasi S, Laurenti L, Stamatopoulos K, Arcaini L, Lucioni M, Rocque GB, Xu-Monette ZY, et al. 2011. The genetics of Richter syndrome reveals disease heterogeneity and predicts survival after transformation. *Blood* **117:** 3391–3401. doi:10.1182/blood-2010-09-302174

Rossi D, Trifonov V, Fangazio M, Bruscaggin A, Rasi S, Spina V, Monti S, Vaisitti T, Arruga F, Famà R, et al. 2012. The coding genome of splenic marginal zone lymphoma: Activation of *NOTCH2* and other pathways regulating marginal zone development. *J Exp Med* **209:** 1537–1551. doi:10.1084/jem.20120904

Rossi D, Diop F, Spaccarotella E, Monti S, Zanni M, Rasi S, Deambrogi C, Spina V, Bruscaggin A, Favini C, et al. 2017. Diffuse large B-cell lymphoma genotyping on the liquid biopsy. *Blood* **129:** 1947–1957. doi:10.1182/blood-2016-05-719641

Roulland S, Navarro JM, Grenot P, Milili M, Agopian J, Montpellier B, Gauduchon P, Lebailly P, Schiff C, Nadel B. 2006. Follicular lymphoma-like B cells in healthy individuals: A novel intermediate step in early lymphomagenesis. *J Exp Med* **203:** 2425–2431. doi:10.1084/jem.20061292

Russo G, Isobe M, Gatti R, Finan J, Batuman O, Huebner K, Nowell PC, Croce CM. 1989. Molecular analysis of a t(14;14) translocation in leukemic T-cells of an ataxia telangiectasia patient. *Proc Natl Acad Sci* **86:** 602–606. doi:10.1073/pnas.86.2.602

Sakamoto Y, Ishida T, Masaki A, Murase T, Yonekura K, Tashiro Y, Tokunaga M, Utsunomiya A, Ito A, Kusumoto S, et al. 2018. CCR4 mutations associated with superior outcome of adult T-cell leukemia/lymphoma under mogamulizumab treatment. *Blood* **132:** 758–761. doi:10.1182/blood-2018-02-835991

Sakata-Yanagimoto M, Enami T, Yoshida K, Shiraishi Y, Ishii R, Miyake Y, Muto H, Tsuyama N, Sato-Otsubo A, Okuno Y, et al. 2014. Somatic *RHOA* mutation in angioimmunoblastic T cell lymphoma. *Nat Genet* **46:** 171–175. doi:10.1038/ng.2872

Salaverria I, Royo C, Carvajal-Cuenca A, Clot G, Navarro A, Valera A, Song JY, Woroniecka R, Rymkiewicz G, Klapper W, et al. 2013. *CCND2* rearrangements are the most frequent genetic events in cyclin D1^{-} mantle cell lymphoma. *Blood* **121:** 1394–1402. doi:10.1182/blood-2012-08-452284

Salido M, Baró C, Oscier D, Stamatopoulos K, Dierlamm J, Matutes E, Traverse-Glehen A, Berger F, Felman P, Thieblemont C, et al. 2010. Cytogenetic aberrations and their prognostic value in a series of 330 splenic marginal zone B-cell lymphomas: A multicenter study of the Splenic B-Cell Lymphoma Group. *Blood* **116:** 1479–1488. doi:10.1182/blood-2010-02-267476

Savage KJ, Monti S, Kutok JL, Cattoretti G, Neuberg D, De Leval L, Kurtin P, Dal Cin P, Ladd C, Feuerhake F, et al. 2003. The molecular signature of mediastinal large B-cell lymphoma differs from that of other diffuse large B-cell lymphomas and shares features with classical Hodgkin lymphoma. *Blood* **102:** 3871–3879. doi:10.1182/blood-2003-06-1841

Scherer F, Kurtz DM, Newman AM, Stehr H, Craig AF, Esfahani MS, Lovejoy AF, Chabon JJ, Klass DM, Liu CL, et al. 2016. Distinct biological subtypes and patterns of genome evolution in lymphoma revealed by circulating tumor DNA. *Sci Transl Med* **8:** 364ra155. doi:10.1126/scitranslmed.aai8545

Schmidt J, Gong S, Marafioti T, Mankel B, Gonzalez-Farre B, Balagué O, Mozos A, Cabecadas J, van der Walt J, Hoehn D, et al. 2016. Genome-wide analysis of pediatric-type follicular lymphoma reveals low genetic complexity and recurrent alterations of *TNFRSF14* gene. *Blood* **128:** 1101–1111. doi:10.1182/blood-2016-03-703819

Schmitz R, Young RM, Ceribelli M, Jhavar S, Xiao W, Zhang M, Wright G, Shaffer AL, Hodson DJ, Buras E, et al. 2012. Burkitt lymphoma pathogenesis and therapeutic targets from structural and functional genomics. *Nature* **490:** 116–120. doi:10.1038/nature11378

Schmitz R, Wright GW, Huang DW, Johnson CA, Phelan JD, Wang JQ, Roulland S, Kasbekar M, Young RM, Shaffer AL, et al. 2018. Genetics and pathogenesis of diffuse large B-cell lymphoma. *N Engl J Med* **378:** 1396–1407. doi:10.1056/NEJMoa1801445

Scott DW, Wright GW, Williams PM, Lih CJ, Walsh W, Jaffe ES, Rosenwald A, Campo E, Chan WC, Connors JM, et al. 2014. Determining cell-of-origin subtypes of diffuse large B-cell lymphoma using gene expression in formalin-fixed paraffin-embedded tissue. *Blood* **123:** 1214–1217. doi:10.1182/blood-2013-11-536433

Scott DW, King RL, Staiger AM, Ben-Neriah S, Jiang A, Horn H, Mottok A, Farinha P, Slack GW, Ennishi D, et al. 2018. High-grade B-cell lymphoma with *MYC* and *BCL2* and/or *BCL6* rearrangements with diffuse large B-cell lymphoma morphology. *Blood* **131:** 2060–2064. doi:10.1182/blood-2017-12-820605

Shao H, Calvo KR, Grönborg M, Tembhare PR, Kreitman RJ, Stetler-Stevenson M, Yuan CM. 2013. Distinguishing hairy cell leukemia variant from hairy cell leukemia: Development and validation of diagnostic criteria. *Leukemia Res* **37:** 401–409. doi:10.1016/j.leukres.2012.11.021

Steidl C, Shah SP, Woolcock BW, Rui L, Kawahara M, Farinha P, Johnson NA, Zhao Y, Telenius A, Neriah SB, et al. 2011. MHC class II transactivator *CIITA* is a recurrent gene fusion partner in lymphoid cancers. *Nature* **471:** 377–381. doi:10.1038/nature09754

Swerdlow SH, Campo E, Harris NL, Pileri SA, Jaffe ES, Stein H, et al. 2017. *WHO classification of tumours of haematopoietic and lymphoid tissues*. WHO Press, Geneva.

Taub R, Kirsch I, Morton C, Lenoir G, Swan D, Tronick S, Aaronson S, Leder P. 1982. Translocation of the c-myc gene into the immunoglobulin heavy chain locus in human Burkitt lymphoma and murine plasmacytoma cells. *Proc Natl Acad Sci* **79:** 7837–7841. doi:10.1073/pnas.79.24.7837

The Non-Hodgkin's Lymphoma Classification Project [No authors listed]. 1997. A clinical evaluation of the International Lymphoma Study Group classification of non-Hodgkin's lymphoma. *Blood* **89:** 3909–3918. doi:10.1182/blood.V89.11.3909

Tiacci E, Trifonov V, Schiavoni G, Holmes A, Kern W, Martelli MP, Pucciarini A, Bigerna B, Pacini R, Wells VA, et al. 2011. *BRAF* mutations in hairy-cell leukemia. *New Engl J Med* **364:** 2305–2315. doi:10.1056/NEJMoa1014209

Tiacci E, Park JH, De Carolis L, Chung SS, Broccoli A, Scott S, Zaja F, Devlin S, Pulsoni A, Chung YR, et al. 2015. Targeting mutant *BRAF* in relapsed or refractory hairy-cell leukemia. *New Engl J Med* **373:** 1733–1747. doi:10.1056/NEJMoa1506583

Tiacci E, Ladewig E, Schiavoni G, Penson A, Fortini E, Pettirossi V, Wang Y, Rosseto A, Venanzi A, Vlasevska S, et al. 2018. Pervasive mutations of JAK-STAT pathway genes in classical Hodgkin lymphoma. *Blood* **131:** 2454–2465. doi:10.1182/blood-2017-11-814913

Treon SP, Xu L, Yang G, Zhou Y, Liu X, Cao Y, Sheehy P, Manning RJ, Patterson CJ, Tripsas C, et al. 2012. MYD88 L265P somatic mutation in Waldenström's macroglobulinemia. *New Engl J Med* **367:** 826–833. doi:10.1056/NEJMoa1200710

Treon SP, Tripsas CK, Meid K, Warren D, Varma G, Green R, Argyropoulos KV, Yang G, Cao Y, Xu L, et al. 2015. Ibrutinib in previously treated Waldenström's macroglobulinemia. *New Engl J Med* **372:** 1430–1440. doi:10.1056/NEJMoa1501548

Tsujimoto Y, Finger LR, Yunis J, Nowell PC, Croce CM. 1984. Cloning of the chromosome breakpoint of neoplastic B cells with the t(14;18) chromosome translocation. *Science* **226:** 1097–1099. doi:10.1126/science.6093263

van der Velden VH, Cazzaniga G, Schrauder A, Hancock J, Bader P, Panzer-Grumayer ER, Flohr T, Sutton R, Cave H, Madsen HO, et al. 2007. Analysis of minimal residual disease by Ig/TCR gene rearrangements: Guidelines for interpretation of real-time quantitative PCR data. *Leukemia* **21:** 604–611. doi:10.1038/sj.leu.2404586

van Dongen JJ, Wolvers-Tettero IL. 1991. Analysis of immunoglobulin and T cell receptor genes. Part II: Possibilities and limitations in the diagnosis and management of lymphoproliferative diseases and related disorders. *Clin Chim Acta* **198:** 93–174. doi:10.1016/0009-8981(91)90247-A

van Dongen JJ, Langerak AW, Bruggemann M, Evans PA, Hummel M, Lavender FL, Delabesse E, Davi F, Schuuring E, García-Sanz R, et al. 2003. Design and standardization of PCR primers and protocols for detection of clonal immunoglobulin and T-cell receptor gene recombinations in suspect lymphoproliferations: Report of the BIOMED-2 Concerted Action BMH4-CT98-3936. *Leukemia* **17:** 2257–2317. doi:10.1038/sj.leu.2403202

Vaqué JP, Gómez-López G, Monsálvez V, Varela I, Martínez N, Pérez C, Domínguez O, Graña O, Rodríguez-Peralto JL, Rodríguez-Pinilla SM, et al. 2014. *PLCG1* mutations in cutaneous T-cell lymphomas. *Blood* **123:** 2034–2043. doi:10.1182/blood-2013-05-504308

Vasmatzis G, Johnson SH, Knudson RA, Ketterling RP, Braggio E, Fonseca R, Viswanatha DS, Law ME, Kip NS, Ozsan N, et al. 2012. Genome-wide analysis reveals recurrent structural abnormalities of *TP63* and other p53-related genes in peripheral T-cell lymphomas. *Blood* **120:** 2280–2289. doi:10.1182/blood-2012-03-419937

Velusamy T, Kiel MJ, Sahasrabuddhe AA, Rolland D, Dixon CA, Bailey NG, Betz BL, Brown NA, Hristov AC, Wilcox RA, et al. 2014. A novel recurrent *NPM1-TYK2* gene fusion in cutaneous CD30-positive lymphoproliferative disorders. *Blood* **124:** 3768–3771. doi:10.1182/blood-2014-07-588434

Viganò E, Gunawardana J, Mottok A, Van Tol T, Mak K, Chan FC, Chong L, Chavez E, Woolcock B, Takata K, et al. 2018a. Somatic IL4R mutations in primary mediastinal large B-cell lymphoma lead to constitutive JAK-STAT signaling activation. *Blood* **131:** 2036–2046. doi:10.1182/blood-2017-09-808907

Viganò E, Duns G, Ennishi D, Gascoyne RD, Morin RD, Scott DW, Steidl C. 2018b. Recurrent IL4R somatic mutations in diffuse large B-cell lymphoma lead to an altered gene expression profile and changes in tumor microenvironment composition. *Blood* **132:** 669. doi:10.1182/blood-2018-99-110473

Wang L, Lawrence MS, Wan Y, Stojanov P, Sougnez C, Stevenson K, Werner L, Sivachenko A, DeLuca DS, Zhang L, et al. 2011. *SF3B1* and other novel cancer genes in chronic lymphocytic leukemia. *N Engl J Med* **365:** 2497–2506. doi:10.1056/NEJMoa1109016

Wang C, McKeithan TW, Gong Q, Zhang W, Bouska A, Rosenwald A, Gascoyne RD, Wu X, Wang J, Muhammad Z, et al. 2015a. *IDH2*^{R172} mutations define a unique subgroup of patients with angioimmunoblastic T-cell lymphoma. *Blood* **126:** 1741–1752. doi:10.1182/blood-2015-05-644591

Wang L, Ni X, Covington KR, Yang BY, Shiu J, Zhang X, Xi L, Meng Q, Langridge T, Drummond J, et al. 2015b. Genomic profiling of Sézary syndrome identifies alterations of key T cell signaling and differentiation genes. *Nat Genet* **47:** 1426–1434. doi:10.1038/ng.3444

Ward PS, Lu C, Cross JR, Abdel-Wahab O, Levine RL, Schwartz GK, Thompson CB. 2013. The potential for isocitrate dehydrogenase mutations to produce 2-hydroxyglutarate depends on allele specificity and subcellular compartmentalization. *J Biol Chem* **288:** 3804–3815. doi:10.1074/jbc.M112.435495

Waterfall JJ, Arons E, Walker RL, Pineda M, Roth L, Killian JK, Abaan OD, Davis SR, Kreitman RJ, Meltzer PS. 2014. High prevalence of *MAP2K1* mutations in variant and IGHV4-34–expressing hairy-cell leukemias. *Nat Genet* **46:** 8–10. doi:10.1038/ng.2828

Weniger MA, Melzner I, Menz CK, Wegener S, Bucur AJ, Dorsch K, Mattfeldt T, Barth TF, Möller P. 2006. Mutations of the tumor suppressor gene *SOCS-1* in classical Hodgkin lymphoma are frequent and associated with nuclear phospho-STAT5 accumulation. *Oncogene* **25:** 2679–2684. doi:10.1038/sj.onc.1209151

Wilson WH, Young RM, Schmitz R, Yang Y, Pittaluga S, Wright G, Lih CJ, Williams PM, Shaffer AL, Gerecitano J, et al. 2015. Targeting B cell receptor signaling with ibrutinib in diffuse large B cell lymphoma. *Nat Med* **21:** 922–926. doi:10.1038/nm.3884

Wood B, Wu D, Crossley B, Dai Y, Williamson D, Gawad C, Borowitz MJ, Devidas M, Maloney KW, Larsen E, et al. 2018. Measurable residual disease detection by high-throughput sequencing improves risk stratification for pediatric B-ALL. *Blood* **131:** 1350–1359. doi:10.1182/blood-2017-09-806521

Woyach JA, Furman RR, Liu TM, Ozer HG, Zapatka M, Ruppert AS, Xue L, Li DH, Steggerda SM, Versele M, et al. 2014. Resistance mechanisms for the Bruton's tyrosine kinase inhibitor ibrutinib. *New Engl J Med* **370:** 2286–2294. doi:10.1056/NEJMoa1400029

Wu D, Sherwood A, Fromm JR, Winter SS, Dunsmore KP, Loh ML, Greisman HA, Sabath DE, Wood BL, Robins H. 2012. High-throughput sequencing detects minimal residual disease in acute T lymphoblastic leukemia. *Sci Transl Med* **4:** 134ra63.

Yatabe Y, Suzuki R, Tobinai K, Matsuno Y, Ichinohasama R, Okamoto M, Yamagauchi M, Tamaru J, Uike N, Hashimoto Y, et al. 2000. Significance of cyclin D1 overexpression for the diagnosis of mantle cell lymphoma: A clinicopathologic comparison of cyclin D1-positive MCL and cyclin D1-negative MCL-like B-cell lymphoma. *Blood* **95:** 2253–2261.

Yuan J, Wright G, Rosenwald A, Steidl C, Gascoyne RD, Connors JM, Mottok A, Weisenburger DD, Greiner TC, Fu K, et al. 2015. Identification of primary mediastinal large B-cell lymphoma at nonmediastinal sites by gene expression profiling. *Am J Surg Pathol* **39:** 1322–1330. doi:10.1097/PAS.0000000000000473

Zech L, Haglund U, Nilsson K, Klein G. 1976. Characteristic chromosomal abnormalities in biopsies and lymphoid-cell lines from patients with Burkitt and non-Burkitt lymphomas. *Int J Cancer* **17:** 47–56. doi:10.1002/ijc.2910170108

Zhang J, Jima D, Moffitt AB, Liu Q, Czader M, Hsi ED, Fedoriw Y, Dunphy CH, Richards KL, Gill JI, et al. 2014. The genomic landscape of mantle cell lymphoma is related to the epigenetically determined chromatin state of normal B cells. *Blood* **123:** 2988–2996. doi:10.1182/blood-2013-07-517177

Clonal Hematopoiesis and Premalignant Diseases

Justin Kaner,[1] Pinkal Desai,[1] Nuria Mencia-Trinchant,[1] Monica L. Guzman,[1] Gail J. Roboz,[1] and Duane C. Hassane[1,2]

[1]Division of Hematology & Oncology, Weill Cornell Medical College, New York, New York 10065, USA

[2]Caryl and Israel Englander Institute for Precision Medicine, Weill Cornell Medical College, New York, New York 10065, USA

Correspondence: dhassane@med.cornell.edu

Clonal hematopoiesis (CH) arises when mutations in the hematopoietic system confer a fitness advantage to specific clones, thereby favoring their disproportionate growth. The presence of CH increases with age and environmental exposures such as cytotoxic chemotherapy or radiotherapy. The most frequent mutations occur in epigenetic regulators, such as *DNMT3A*, *TET2*, and *ASXL1*, leading to dysregulation of tumor suppressor function, pathogen response, and inflammation. These dysregulated processes elevate risk of overall mortality, cardiovascular disease, and eventual hematologic malignancy (HM). CH is likely acting as an initiating event leading to HM when followed by cooperating mutations. However, further evidence suggests that CH exerts a bystander influence through its pro-inflammatory properties. Delineating the mechanisms that lead to the onset and expansion of CH as well as its contribution to risk of HM is crucial to defining a management and intervention strategy. In this review, we discuss the potential causes, consequences, technical considerations, and possible management strategies for CH in the context of HMs and pre-HMs.

The accumulation of mutations in overtly healthy tissues occurs during normal aging with somatic mosaicism being present from birth (Vilkki et al. 2001; De 2011; Blokzijl et al. 2016; Vattathil and Scheet 2016). Although the majority of these mutations are neutral and do not favor clonal expansion (Martincorena et al. 2017), mutation-driven dominant clones have been observed in nearly all tissues, especially in the hematopoietic system (Bowman et al. 2018). Hematopoietic stem cells (HSCs) initiate hematopoietic development and only seldomly enter into the cell cycle for self-renewal and replication (Catlin et al. 2011), with each HSC acquiring approximately one exonic somatic mutation per decade in a largely stochastic manner (Welch et al. 2012). A subset of these acquired mutations confers a growth advantage (Welch et al. 2012), producing a clonal expansion that has been termed "clonal hematopoiesis" (CH).

Although the genes most commonly mutated in CH are the same genes that drive malignant conditions like myelodysplastic syndrome (MDS) and acute myeloid leukemia (AML),

Cite this article as *Cold Spring Harb Perspect Med* doi: 10.1101/cshperspect.a035675

most persons with CH are overtly healthy and never progress to MDS/AML. Nonetheless, CH is not an inert condition. CH clones have been known to show elevated inflammation, impaired tumor suppressor function, risk of cardiovascular disease (CVD), and risk of eventual hematologic malignancy (HM) (Jaiswal et al. 2014; Xie et al. 2014; Genovese et al. 2015; Rasmussen et al. 2015; Wu et al. 2015). Indeed, CH confers a rate of progression to any HM of 0.5%–1% per year (Jaiswal et al. 2014). This rate of progression is similar to monoclonal gammopathy of undetermined significance (MGUS) and monoclonal B-cell lymphocytosis (MBL) with the notable exception that CH can potentially produce any HM as it can arise in less committed hematopoietic precursors. Recent case-control studies have sought to fine-tune this risk especially in AML (Abelson et al. 2018; Desai et al. 2018). Nonetheless, the certainty of progression to any one condition in any single person is still not absolute given the presence of CH, mutation pattern, and/or any given clinical parameter. Data in model systems have shown that the growth and oncogenic progression of CH mutations may be influenced by extrinsic factors, varying from microbial and inflammatory signals to vitamin C (Cimmino et al. 2017; Cai et al. 2018; Meisel et al. 2018). Thus, the contribution of CH to disease is likely to involve a complex interplay between stochastic molecular events and their interaction with an individual's "exposome" (Wild 2005). Understanding CH mutations in the context of these extrinsic influences will enable development of better predictive models to improve decision-making when CH is detected. Although the cardiovascular risks associated with CH are important and considerable, the present review will focus on presenting what is known about the genetics, risks, and effects of CH in regard to premalignant conditions and hematologic malignancies.

CLONAL HEMATOPOIESIS

CH is functionally defined by the disproportionate growth of hematopoietic clones harboring a common somatic alteration. The first description of CH arose from excess skewing of the 1:1 ratio of maternal to paternal X-inactivation normally observed in women by Gale in 1991 (Lyon 1961; Gale et al. 1991). Subsequent advances in molecular techniques enabled Busque and colleagues, in 1996, to make quantitative assessments showing that neonates and young women had significantly less X-inactivation skewing than women >60 yr old, suggesting that CH is an age-related phenomenon (Busque et al. 1996). Follow-up studies revealed that somatic mutations are the probable underlying drivers of CH with the finding that elderly women with nonrandom X-inactivation were significantly more likely to harbor *TET2* mutations (Busque et al. 2012), which until then had been principally described as a driver event in AML causing epigenetic dysregulation (Delhommeau et al. 2009; Chou et al. 2011; Moran-Crusio et al. 2011). Individuals with CH typically have hematologic parameters that are indistinguishable from normal individuals inclusive of white blood cell count, hemoglobin, red cell distribution width (RDW), and platelets. Notably, the presence of both CH and high RDW synergizes so as to worsen outcomes (Jaiswal et al. 2014). Many groups have shown RDW to be a poor prognostic factor in a variety of settings, suggesting it to be a marker of chronic disease (Baba et al. 2018; Zurauskaite et al. 2018).

MUTATION LANDSCAPE OF CLONAL HEMATOPOIESIS

The most common mutations driving CH occur in the epigenetic modifier genes *DNMT3A*, *TET2*, and *ASXL1* (Jaiswal et al. 2014; Xie et al. 2014; Genovese et al. 2015; Steensma et al. 2015). The prevalence of *DNMT3A* mutations is highest, representing ~45% of all CH mutations. Mutations in *TET2* and *ASXL1* also occur commonly but each represent only 10% or less of all CH mutations (Heuser et al. 2016), although variable coverage of these large tumor suppressor genes on exome/panel-based sequencing suggests the actual mutation frequency may vary in different cohorts. Other less frequent somatic mutations have been shown to occur in *TP53*, *PPM1D*, *JAK2*, *CBL*, and spliceosome genes (Jaiswal et al. 2014; Xie et al. 2014; Geno-

 Cite this article as *Cold Spring Harb Perspect Med* doi: 10.1101/cshperspect.a035675

vese et al. 2015; Steensma et al. 2015; Coombs et al. 2017). Although the genes most commonly mutated in CH are the same genes that drive malignant conditions like MDS and AML, most persons with CH never progress to MDS/AML and otherwise show normal hematologic parameters. These same genes commonly mutated in CH occur as a function of age both in CH (Jaiswal et al. 2014; Genovese et al. 2015) and in overt myeloid neoplasms such as MDS, myeloproliferative neoplasms (MPNs), and AML. Nonetheless, CH is not an inert condition. CH clones have been known to show elevated inflammation, impaired tumor suppressor function, risk of CVD, and risk of eventual HM (Jaiswal et al. 2014; Genovese et al. 2015). Indeed, CH confers a rate of progression to any HM of 0.5%–1% per year (Jaiswal et al. 2014). This rate of progression is similar to MGUS and MBL, with the notable exception that CH can potentially increase risk of any HM as it arises in less-committed hematopoietic precursors. Recent case-control studies have sought to define this risk especially in AML (Abelson et al. 2018; Desai et al. 2018). Nonetheless, the certainty of progression to any one condition in any single person is still not absolute. Data in model systems have shown that the growth and oncogenic penetrance of CH mutations may be influenced by extrinsic factors, such as microbial and inflammatory signals, and nutritional factors like vitamin C (Cimmino et al. 2017; Cai et al. 2018; Meisel et al. 2018). Thus, the contribution of CH to disease is likely to involve a complex interplay between stochastic molecular events and their interaction with an individual's "exposome" (Wild 2005). Understanding CH mutations in the context of these extrinsic influences will enable development of better predictive models to improve decision-making when CH is detected. Although the cardiovascular risks associated with CH are important and considerable and reviewed elsewhere (Sano et al. 2018; Calvillo-Argüelles et al. 2019), the present review will focus on presenting what is known about the genetics, risks, and possible management strategies for CH in the context of premalignant conditions and hematologic malignancies (Fig. 1).

CLONAL HEMATOPOIESIS ELEVATES RISK OF PROGRESSION TO HEMATOLOGIC MALIGNANCIES

Premalignant states are well-established in hematologic malignancies, including MBL as a precursor to chronic lymphocytic leukemia (CLL) and MGUS as a precursor to multiple myeloma (MM), progressing to full disease at a rate of 1% to 2% per year (Kyle et al. 2002; Rawstron et al. 2008). Certain higher-risk presentations of CH can confer similar rates of disease progression. Indeed, Jaiswal and colleagues tested for CH across genes recurrently mutated in myeloid and lymphoid malignancies in the peripheral blood of 17,182 individuals via whole-exome sequencing (WES) at 70× median coverage depth (Jaiswal et al. 2014). Using variant allele fraction (VAF) cutoffs of 3.5% of single-nucleotide variants (SNVs) and 7% for indels, the prevalence of CH increased in an age-dependent manner from 2.5% in the 50–59 age group to 9.5% in the 70–79 age group. The presence of CH in any driver gene increased the risk of HM by >11-fold (hazard ratio [HR]: 11.1, 95% confidence interval [CI] 3.9–33). A large clone size (VAF >10%) further elevated this risk to 49-fold (HR: 49, 95% CI: 21–120). Although the fold change in HM risk is high based on these data, the absolute risk is relatively low with only 4% of individuals with a CH mutation progressing to develop a HM during the study period of 95 mo corresponding to 0.5% per year overall in the presence of any CH. Large clone size (VAF > 10%) elevated the progression rate to 1.0% per year, approaching progression rates similar to MBL or MGUS. All-cause mortality associated with RDW from 1.6 (95% CI: 1.2–2.1) in the absence of CH to 3.7 (95% CI: 2.2–6.5) in the presence of CH when RDW ≥ 14.5%. Similar contemporaneous studies arrived at similar conclusions with regard to risk of progression to HR and rates of elevated CH (Xie et al. 2014; Genovese et al. 2015).

TECHNICAL DEFINITION OF CLONAL HEMATOPOIESIS

Uniform standards for the detection and reporting of CH are absent and urgently needed. Tech-

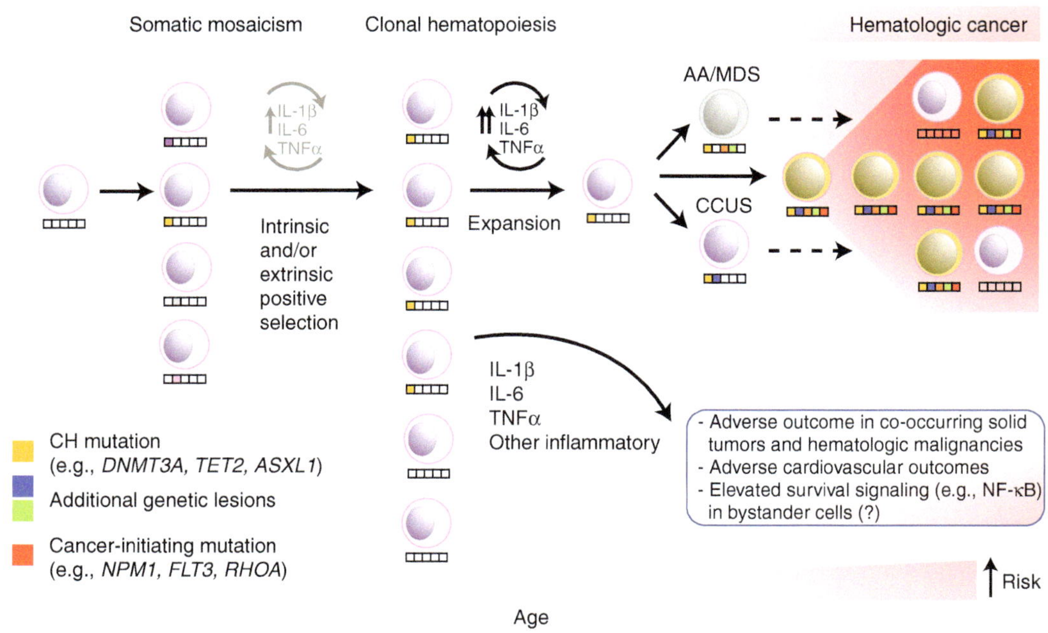

Figure 1. Progression from somatic mosaicism through clonal hematopoiesis (CH) into hematologic malignancy. A combination of intrinsic and/or extrinsic events favors expansion of hematopoietic cells harboring mutations that confer a fitness advantage (e.g., mutations *DNMT3A*, *TET2*, and *ASXL1*) leading to CH. CH is pro-inflammatory and produces a positive-feedback loop that produces conditions favorable for the CH clone's expansion (i.e., its own expansion). Acquisition of subsequent mutations leads to clonal cytopenia of uncertain significance (CCUS), aplastic anemia (AA), or myelodysplastic syndrome (MDS), and other overt hematologic malignancies (e.g., acute myeloid leukemia). Aberrant pro-inflammatory signals also potentially exert a bystander influence on neighboring non-CH cells, thereby favoring adverse outcomes in co-occurring cancers and cardiovascular disease. It is speculated here that the pro-inflammatory environment generated by CH may promote protective survival signaling through pathways such as nuclear factor kappa B (NF-κB). The colored squares under each cell depict indicate somatic mutations. CH mutations are early events and followed by additional genetic lesions, including cooperating cancer mutations. Age increases risk of CH and hematologic malignancies.

nical variations such as read depth, VAF cutoffs, germline variant exclusion criteria, and the breadth of genes interrogated have complicated the comparison of CH rates across cohorts. For example, deep targeted error-corrected sequencing revealed that mutations can be identified in the blood of nearly all persons aged 50–70 at a sensitivity of 0.03% VAF (Young et al. 2016). Although somatic mosaicism in hematopoietic cells is common, the mutations that confer a selective advantage are likely to be most important to the relevance of CH as a clinical condition. To this end, Steensma and colleagues proposed a VAF of >2% in defining CH (Steensma et al. 2015). This cutoff, however, is driven by available technological capacity and limited clinical data. Recent studies have shown elevated risk even at >1% VAF for certain mutation classes (Abelson et al. 2018; Desai et al. 2018). Studies that are scientifically, statistically, and clinically principled are required to establish more formal thresholds.

Overall, the true prevalence of CH is likely underestimated in most studies. For example, whole-exome studies performed at 70×–80× median depth of coverage will only achieve <5% sensitivity for mutations occurring at 2% VAF based on next-generation sequencing (NGS) sensitivity estimates modeled by Shin et al. (2017), thereby missing the vast majority of CH mutations at lower VAF. Earlier whole-exome studies (Jaiswal et al. 2014; Genovese et al. 2015) were also lacking coverage for most coding exons for *TET2* (Genovese et al. 2014; Jaiswal et al. 2014). There is, moreover, an ascertainment bias in the selection of genetic events driving CH in which studies have generally examined small variants related to progression to HM. In an analysis of 11,000 adults of all ages, whole-genome sequencing (WGS) studies by Zink et al. (2017), searching for mutations in candidate and noncandidate driver genes, yielded a significantly higher prevalence of CH than what had previously been reported (Jaiswal et al. 2014; Genovese et al. 2015; Zink et al. 2017). With the inclusion of both leukemia driver mutations and nondriver mutations, ~50% of those 85 and older had evidence of CH in this cohort, compared with ~20% in data from other studies (Jaiswal et al. 2014; Genovese et al. 2015; Zink et al. 2017). More recently, Loh and colleagues showed clonal expansions in which CH is defined by larger-scale mosaic chromosomal alterations (Loh et al. 2018). As consensus forms and depth, uniformity, and breadth of coverage are standardized, the actual prevalence is likely >20%–30% in persons 50 years of age and above based on two recent high-depth studies (Abelson et al. 2018; Desai et al. 2018) as well as data from blood of solid tumor patients derived from MSK-IMPACT (Coombs et al. 2017).

Finally, different terminologies are currently being used to describe similar states of clonal expansion in the absence of cytopenia or dysplastic hematopoiesis. CH and "clonal hematopoiesis of indeterminate potential" (CHIP) roughly refer to the same hematologic process with differing levels of specificity (Bowman et al. 2018). CH has a broader definition as it is inclusive of any disruptive somatic event that attains a fitness advantage exceeding the background level of somatic mosaicism—not necessarily occurring in a HM-associated driver such as DNA structural abnormalities or skewed X-inactivation. The term age-related clonal hematopoiesis (ARCH) emphasizes the age association with the acquisition of such mutations but would seem to exclude CH mutations driven by therapy. In reality, although age is a principle driver, the events driving the expansion of CH clones are unknown in many cases and may arise from prior therapy, chemical, immunological, infectious, and age-related events that initiate and/or select particular clones.

CCUS AND ICUS

Idiopathic cytopenia of undetermined significance (ICUS) was proposed as a classification in 2005 and was defined as persistent cytopenias without evidence of dysplasia in the bone marrow and with normal cytogenetics, in the absence of any secondary cause (Wimazal et al. 2007). The largest study to date on patients determined to meet strict criteria for ICUS showed this entity to be quite rare (10 of 2899 patients over 12 yr) but evolution to MDS was common (6/10) and thus supports the hypothesis that this might actually represent a pre-MDS clinical phase (Steensma 2012). With better diagnostic tools incorporating standard karyotypic and targeted sequencing analyses, diagnosing MDS has become significantly more streamlined (Steensma et al. 2015). There remain, however, large portions of individuals with persistent cytopenias and somatic mutations in the absence of overt dysplasia. These instances of normal marrow morphology, but persistent cytopenias in the presence of somatic mutations, underscore our need for a more inclusive classification system (Jaiswal et al. 2014; Genovese et al. 2015; Steensma et al. 2015). When the term ICUS was derived, the ability to universally sequence patient samples was lacking, and thus it was unclear if this was a clonal process. Although many of the patients in the limited analysis above did eventually develop MDS, it remains unclear whether any of these patients had or developed somatic mutations. In an analysis of a clinical cohort of patients who met criteria for ICUS, between 21% and 33% had CH-associated mutations, and this prevalence was higher than the background rate of CH in an age-matched population (Hall et al. 2014; Kwok et al. 2014). In addition, these clonal cytopenias have a similar prevalence as MDS (Steensma et al. 2015). Yet, it should also be noted that progression of these clonal cytopenias to MDS is not universal, and so they remain distinct entities. Given our better understanding of ICUS and CH, it was proposed that we classify patients meeting criteria for ICUS and harboring CH-associated somatic mutation as CCUS. These entities exist on a spectrum with nonclonal ICUS having a very low progression risk and CCUS having a still low but increased risk of progression to MDS (Steensma et al. 2015).

CLONAL HEMATOPOIESIS IN APLASTIC ANEMIA

CH is a common finding in individuals with aplastic anemia (AA). In a study of 439 patients with AA undergoing immunosuppressive therapy (IST), 47% of patients showed evidence of CH (Yoshizato et al. 2015). Unlike CH in the general population, the predominant mutations were *BCOR/BCORL1*, *PIGA*, *DNMT3A*, and *ASXL1*, accounting for >75% of CH. Mutations in *TET2* were notably underrepresented. Selection pressure in the context of bone marrow failure thus favor patterns of clonal dominance that differ from age-related CH. The prognostic impact in AA varied dependent on the mutation with *PIGA*, *BCOR*, and *BCORL1* mutations predicting better improved overall survival (OS) and progression-free survival (PFS) with immunosuppressive therapy being compared than *TP53*, *DNMT3A*, *JAK2*, and *ASXL1*, showing improved OS (HR: 0.27, 0.09–0.78; $P = 0.016$). *PIGA* and *BCOR/BCORL1* mutations showed clonal attrition over time while *DNMT3A* and *ASXL1* mutations expanded. Despite mutational commonalities with MDS (e.g., *DNMT3A*, *ASXL1*, *RUNX1*, splicing), the average clone size of CH in the AA cohort was lower (<10% VAF) and the clone size substantially rapidly expanded 6 mo post-IST.

Overall, the heightened prevalence of CH mutations that are found in the general population among patients in premalignant states or smoldering disease suggests their causal influence in the stepwise progression to overt leukemias. These findings thus suggest the usage of mutation screening in identifying at-risk persons and, given the high prevalence of CH in the general population, the importance of identifying better methods of predicting who will progress to overt leukemia.

FOUNDER CLONAL HEMATOPOIESIS: KNUDSONIAN PROGRESSION TO LEUKEMIA

Genetics of cancer development are largely modeled around the Knudson "two-hit hypothesis" (Knudson 1971), and the available data suggest that this principle can govern progression from CH to overt leukemia. Accordingly, mutation of epigenetic regulators, such as *DNMT3A*, *TET2*, or *ASXL1*, commonly seen in CH, represent an initial "hit." The ensuing epigenetic remodeling leads to premalignant changes—for example, reduced *GATA2* function leading to impaired differentiation (Madzo et al. 2014; Shih et al. 2015). A subsequent "second hit" promotes progression to overt malignancy. For example, a second-hit mutation in *NPM1* produces AML whereas a second-hit mutation in *RHOA* produces angioimmunoblastic T-cell lymphoma (AITL) (Tiacci et al. 2018). Thus, founder CH mutations show multilineage oncogenic potential that is determined, at least partly, by subsequent oncogenic mutations.

Recent studies from Jan and colleagues and Shlush and colleagues have delineated the clonal trajectory from the early CH-like mutations to overt AML through sequencing of preleukemic stem and progenitor cells (pre-LSCs) (Jan et al. 2012; Shlush et al. 2014). Through single-cell sequencing, Jan and colleagues described a stepwise accumulation of mutations arising initially in pre-LSCs but eventually developing into LSCs and overt AML on acquisition of secondary mutations (*FLT3*-ITD). *FLT3*-ITD was not present in any of the pre-LSCs with several mutations, including *SMC1A*, and *TET2* only present in the pre-LSCs. Similarly, Shlush and colleagues analyzed highly purified HSCs, with progenitor and mature cell fractions from the blood of AML patient fractions and using deep targeted sequencing with a read depth of ~250×, found recurrent *DNMT3A* mutations at high allele frequency but without the co-occurring *NPM1* mutations found in the AML blasts. Consistent with CH and previous mouse model data (Jan et al. 2012; Kim et al. 2013), these *DNMT3A* mutated pre-LSCs showed a self-renewal advantage over nonmutated HSCs in xenografts.

These data together provided support for the presence of pre-LSCs. Further analysis revealed these pre-LSCs exist in remission samples, suggestive of both chemotherapy resistance and cell population poised for relapse (Jan et al. 2012; Shlush et al. 2014).

CH only rarely progresses to AML. Case-control studies from multiple independent teams have sought to better define factors that distinguish CH from pre-AML (Abelson et al. 2018; Desai et al. 2018). Desai and colleagues deeply sequenced banked peripheral blood specimens from the Women's Health Initiative (WHI) study at a median of 9.6 yr before AML diagnosis alongside matched control participants who did not develop AML during an equivalent follow-up period. Overall, mutations were more common in pre-AML cases versus AML-free controls when present at >1% VAF (OR: 4.86, 3.07–7.77; $P = 3.8 \times 10^{-13}$). Particular mutation patterns conferred varying levels of risk when adjusted for age and co-mutations. Multiple mutations in *DNMT3A* or *TET2* were more adverse than single mutations: single *DNMT3A* (OR: 2.11, 1.19–3.75; $P = 0.011$); 2+ *DNMT3A* mutations (OR: 12.6, 3.02–52.92; $P < 0.001$); single *TET2* (OR: 3.29, 1.38–7.83; $P = 0.005$); and 2+ *TET2* (OR: 69.3, 3.76–1280.7; $P < 0.001$). The risk of AML progression for *DNMT3A* and *TET2* mutations was also dependent on allelic fraction with >10% VAF conferring more risk. The converse was true for mutations at any VAF > 1% in *TP53* (OR: 50.9, 2.76–943.01; $P <$ 0.001), *IDH1* or *IDH2* (OR: 29.6, 1.51–582.25; $P < 0.001$), *JAK2* (OR: 5.83, 0.79–43; $P = 0.042$), and spliceosome genes (OR: 7.72, 1.75–34.02, $P = 0.002$). The concurrent study by Abelson and colleagues, using an independent cohort, revealed similar findings with regard to mutation-specific risks. Additionally, subsequent work by Young and colleagues, using a cohort comprised of the Nurses' Health Study and Health Professionals Follow-up Study found a similar elevated risk of AML with mutations at ≥1% VAF (OR: 5.4, 1.8–16.6; $P = 0.003$) as well as elevated risk with *DNMT3A* R882H or R882C variants (OR: 7.3, 1.5–34.7; $P = 0.01$) (Calvillo-Argüelles et al. 2019). All studies found that pre-AML cases were devoid of *FLT3* or *NPM1* mutations with the exception of one case in the study by Desai and colleagues in which longitudinal follow-up at 1-yr postbaseline acquired an *NPM1* mutation followed by AML diagnosis nearly a month later. Abelson and colleagues further developed a predictive model heavily dependent on high RDW as an informative predictor of AML as much as 1 yr before diagnosis from readily available electronic health record data. However, improved sensitivity and specificity are required for a rare disease such as AML. Overall, the data from both studies suggest that, with further study and improved models, a monitoring strategy combining readily available EHR parameters, sensitive mutation testing, and perhaps other molecular parameters, can identify persons at higher risk of progression from CH to HM.

BYSTANDER CLONAL HEMATOPOIESIS: ACTION AT A DISTANCE

The effects of CH on cancer development likely extend beyond the initial genetic hit in the two-hit model of oncogenesis. Preclinical and epidemiological evidence suggests that CH mutations can produce a chronic inflammatory state (Cook et al. 2017; Cull et al. 2017; Fuster et al. 2017; Sano et al. 2018), which is known to be oncogenic and exert prosurvival effects outside the context of CH via multiple mechanisms, including NF-κB activation (Philip et al. 2004). *TET2*-deficient macrophages produce elevated and prolonged expression of pro-inflammatory factors (e.g., IL-1, IL-6, TNFα, CCL-5, CXCL9) (Zhang et al. 2015; Fuster et al. 2017; Cai et al. 2018; Sano et al. 2018). Moreover, hematopoietic cells showing *TET2*-driven CH gain a growth advantage in the presence of an inflammatory environment containing TNF (Abegunde et al. 2018). Thus, CH simultaneously appears to provide an advantage to affected cells under inflammatory conditions while also propagating the inflammation. Cook and colleagues evaluated human serum and found associations between CH mutations and inflammation, revealing elevated IL-6 with *TET2*-driven CH and elevated CCL11 with *DNMT3A*-driven CH. CH of large clone size of >10% presented with elevated TNFα (Cook et al. 2017).

Consistent with this concept, studies of solid tumor and multiple myeloma patients with incidental findings of CH show that CH-positive patients experience worse outcomes (Coombs et al. 2017; Mouhieddine et al. 2018). However, further studies are needed to characterize the inflammatory factors in the serum of these patients and determine if CH-driven signaling is enabling tumor survival or whether tumor-driven inflammation is causing expansion of CH clones or, as is likely, an interplay of both.

CLONAL HEMATOPOIESIS IS ASSOCIATED WITH ADVERSE SOLID TUMOR OUTCOMES

Coombs and colleagues systematically evaluated the impact of CH in solid tumor patients using the MSK-IMPACT panel (Coombs et al. 2017). In a large analysis of ~9000 individuals, ~25% of solid tumor patients had incidental CH and 4.5% harbored mutations in genes typically associated with leukemia and with VAF ≥ 10% (presumptive drivers, CH-PD). Importantly, CH-PD was associated with shorter 24-mo survival: OS: 0.48 (0.40–0.57, 95% CI) with CH-PD versus 0.54 (0.52–0.56, 95% CI) without CH-PD. Cumulative incidence of secondary HM was significantly higher with CH-PD with 3.2% (1.4%–6.2%) of patients with CH-PD progressing to HM within 18 mo versus 0.3% (0.2%–0.6%) of patients without CH-PD ($P < 0.001$). Although the prevalence of CH was higher than previously reported in the general population by previous studies (Jaiswal et al. 2014; Genovese et al. 2015), normalization of sequencing and analytical methodologies is needed to make an accurate comparison given the differences in depth of coverage, limits of detection, and analytics. The study also found that *PPM1D* and *TP53* were associated with prior exposure to chemotherapy and radiotherapy, a finding similar to cohorts of patients with lymphoma and myeloma before ASCT (Abdel-Wahab et al. 2012; Husby et al. 2018; Mouhieddine et al. 2018).

Clonal Hematopoiesis and Risk of Therapy-Related Myeloid Neoplasms

The co-occurrence of CH with other cancers is known to result in worse outcomes in these individuals and an increased risk for treatment related myeloid neoplasms (t-MNs). In a small case-control study, Takahashi and colleagues showed the prognostic impact of CH mutations before receiving chemotherapy or radiation treatment. The HR for development of t-MNs in those with CH as compared with those without CH was 13.7, $P = 0.013$. Additionally, cumulative incidence of t-MNs at 5 yr was significantly higher in patients with CH (30% [95% CI: 16%–51%] vs. 7% [95% CI: 2%–21%], $P = 0.016$) (Takahashi et al. 2017). Given the universally poor outcomes that exist in those that develop t-MNs, close monitoring of blood counts and clone size in individuals with malignancies and co-existing CH could prove to be beneficial, although how to intervene should it become evident that a t-MN is likely requires further investigation and should be performed as part of a clinical trial.

ASSOCIATIONS BETWEEN CH AND MULTIPLE MYELOMA OUTCOMES

Mouhieddine and colleagues evaluated the impact of CH mutations on multiple myeloma (MM) outcomes post-ASCT in the presence and absence of the immunomodulatory (IMiD) agents lenalidomide and pomalidomide (Mouhieddine et al. 2018). HSCs of 629 MM patients were deeply sequenced to nearly 1000× depth of coverage. Overall, having a CH mutation was associated with inferior OS and PFS in MM.

Importantly, the investigators found that the adverse impact of CH seen in MM patients was obviated by IMiD maintenance (lenalidomide, pomalidomide, etc.) therapy after ASCT such that OS and PFS differences were no longer significant. Although a mechanism remains to be described, one possibility is that IMiD therapy is acting via suppression of inflammatory factors normally up-regulated by CH such as TNFα, IL-6, IL-1, and IL-12 (Stahl and Zeidan 2017), thus preventing prosurvival signaling such as NF-κB in the myeloma cells. Given the pleiotropic effects of IMiDs, further study is required to delineate the precise mechanism.

 Cite this article as *Cold Spring Harb Perspect Med* doi: 10.1101/cshperspect.a035675

INHERITED PREDISPOSITION TO CH

Data suggest an inherited risk of CH in some cases, although this does not account for the majority of patients with CH. Zink and colleagues showed that an SNP (rs34002450) in the telomerase reverse transcriptase (*TERT*) was associated with increased CH (OR: 1.37; $P = 7.4 \times 10^{-12}$). In a study of 151,202 individuals with banked blood samples, Loh and colleagues showed several rare mosaic chromosomal alterations (mCA) that were associated with inherited risk for developing CH mutations (Loh et al. 2018).

Other groups have also shown a heritable aspect of CH. In an analysis of 2530 women, *TET2*, but not *DNMT3A*, was shown to have a fairly high risk of heritability as a function of age, between 2.24 and 2.65 times the normal risk in women >55 yr and 65 yr, respectively (Buscarlet et al. 2017). Interestingly, in the allogeneic transplantation setting, matched sibling donors who were donating to a sibling with myeloid disease were more likely to have CH compared with those donating to a sibling with a lymphoid malignancy (19.2% vs. 6.3%).

In addition, an analysis of several young AML patients with high mutational burden and genomic evidence of methylation damage, revealed germline mutations in *MBD4*. It appears that loss-of-function mutations in *MBD4* led to inactivating mutations in *DNMT3A* and acquisition of other high-risk mutations such as *IDH1* and *IDH2*, akin to the process by which CH leads to AML, albeit at an accelerated rate (Sanders et al. 2018). Methyl-binding domain 4 (MBD4) is a DNA glycosylase responsible for the removal of mispaired thymine as a function of base excision repair due to aberrant 5mC deamination.

PRECLINICAL DATA ON MODIFICATION OF CH

Intervention in CH first requires the development of evidence-based guidelines for determining at-risk people who are destined to develop CH-related diseases as well as data to prove that intervention/modification of CH is feasible and will ultimately lead to prevention of disease. Although data thus far suggest an elevated risk of AML mutations in certain genes, high allelic fraction, and multiple mutations, the risk of progression is relatively low (Genovese et al. 2014; Abelson et al. 2018; Desai et al. 2018). There have been several preclinical investigations at possible modes of intervention.

TARGETING HIGH-RISK MUTATIONS IN CH

Inhibitors of *JAK2*, *IDH1*, and *IDH2* are Food and Drug Administration (FDA)-approved targeted therapies with favorable safety profiles. The JAK2 inhibitor ruxolitinib is used in *JAK2*+ myelofibrosis and has been shown to reduce symptom burden while slightly reducing the mutant allele burden (Verstovsek et al. 2012). IDH1 and IDH2 inhibitors ivosidenib and enasidenib respectively, are both approved for use in relapsed/refractory AML (Stein et al. 2017; DiNardo et al. 2018) and are currently being investigated in clinical trials for use in other *IDH1*+ and *IDH2*+ MPNs as well as upfront in AML in combination with induction chemotherapy and in MDS (NCT03839771, NCT03515512, NCT03471260). There are, currently, no clinical trials investigating the safety or efficacy of targeting either *JAK2*, *IDH1*, or *IDH2* in the context of CH. Given the greater tendency of *IDH1/2* and *JAK2* mutations in CH to progress to AML (Desai et al. 2018), targeting these mutations with already approved drugs needs requires investigation, most likely in the context of patients showing abnormal hematological parameters.

Vitamin C to Compensate for TET2 Haploinsufficiency

TET2 mutations exert their effects through altered methylation patterns in affected cells, ultimately leading to CH and possibly MDS or AML. Restoration of normal *TET2* enzymatic function was hypothesized to halt or reverse this process. This hypothesis was tested in a *TET2* knockdown mouse model (Cimmino et al. 2017). Reversible *TET2* knockdown recapitulated the effects of *TET2* deletion, leading to aberrant HSC self-renewal and disease development. In this same mouse model, exogenous vitamin C was shown to promote restoration of normal *TET2* enzymatic function by increasing DNA demethylation in embryonic stem cells and induced pluripotent stem cells leading to enhanced 5-hydroxymethylcytosine (5-hmC) levels (Cimmino et al. 2017). Studies suggesting that this may be true in humans are lacking.

Low Glucose and Metformin

Tet2 protein is destabilized by high glucose levels, a process mediated by the inhibition of AMP-activated protein kinase (AMPK)-dependent phosphorylation of TET2 at serine-99, leading to marked reduction of 5-hydroxymethycytosine levels (Wu et al. 2018). This effect was rescued by metformin in mouse models. Thus, loss of *TET2* enzymatic function via protein destabilization has the potential exacerbate the loss of *TET2* function observed in *TET2*-driven CH, thereby potentiating the effects of CH. Interestingly, large epidemiological analyses have suggested that diabetes is linked to an increased risk for cancer, with type 2 diabetes conferring a 20% increase in HM risk (Gallagher and LeRoith 2015; Lauby-Secretan et al. 2016). Thus, the complex interplay of diabetes and cancer requires further study in the context hematopoiesis.

Inhibition of Inflammation

CH is itself pro-inflammatory and simultaneously confers a fitness advantage under pro-inflammatory conditions (Cook et al. 2017; Cull et al. 2017; Abegunde et al. 2018). Thus, intervening in this pattern of runaway inflammation may mitigate the effects of CH. In CVD, it has already been shown that IL-1 blockade with canakunimab shows improved responsiveness in patients with *TET2*-driven CH (Svensson et al. 2018). In an unrelated preclinical study, Cai and colleagues exposed *TET2* knockout (TET2-KO) mice to inflammatory stress, leading to consistently higher levels of IL-6 being seen in these mice. IL-6 was found to result in hyperactivation of the *SHP2-STAT3* signaling axis and increased expression of anti-apoptotic long noncoding DNA, Morrbid (Cai et al. 2018). Inhibition of IL-6 signaling via knockout of Morrbid or via small-molecule inhibition on the *SHP2-STAT3* pathway with SHP099 or E330 impaired clonal expansion of *TET2* KO HSPCs. Thus, inhibition of IL-6, IL-1, or other pro-inflammatory cytokines using either directed monoclonal antibody or anti-inflammatory small molecules may have the potential for modification of CH and/or mitigating the bystander effects of CH mediated through inflammatory signaling.

CLINICAL FOLLOW-UP OF PATIENTS WITH CLONAL HEMATOPOIESIS

CH is being increasingly detected in patients during workup of cytopenias and as part of tumor genomic reports for both solid and hematologic malignancies. As data on the effect of CH accumulate, there is obvious clinical interest in managing the risks associated with CH. Because CH is associated with increased cardiovascular mortality, the presentation of CH—particularly mutations in *DNMT3A* and *TET2* at high VAFs and/or multiple mutations—should prompt a referral to cardiology for cardiovascular risk assessment and management. The presence of high-risk CH in patients with malignancy (*TP53*, *PPM1D*, clonal complexity, high VAF CH defined as >10% VAF, *DNMT3A*-R882) may influence decisions regarding the use of radiation or chemotherapy in some cases. For example, the presence of these high-risk mutations could prompt a discussion in the setting of autologous transplant if there are alternative therapies available. Regardless, the risks and benefits of either approach needs to be discussed with patients. In the absence of data to support repeat mutation testing, patients with CH should be followed with blood counts only as standard of care and repeat testing of mutations should only be considered as part of a clinical trial or in the context new or worsening cytopenias.

CONCLUDING REMARKS

The prevalence of CH is more common than originally put forward given recent findings from high-depth, high-sensitivity sequencing studies (Young et al. 2016; Coombs et al. 2017; Abelson et al. 2018; Desai et al. 2018; Calvillo-Argüelles et al. 2019; Young et al. 2019). Current evidence suggests mutations of >1% VAF can be of clinical relevance for progression to malignancy (Abelson et al. 2018; Desai et al. 2018; Young et al. 2019). Standardization of methodologies and development of evidence-based guidelines are required to determine detection limits and parameters for identification of clinically significant CH mutations. In addition to providing founding genetic lesions for hematologic cancers, CH is a predictor of adverse risk in existing cancers ranging from solid tumors to multiple myeloma (Coombs et al. 2017; Mouhieddine et al. 2018), suggestive of a CH-driven bystander influence. Further studies are required to ascertain whether this possible bystander influence is mediated through inflammation or by other mechanisms. CH further confers elevated susceptibility to secondary therapy-related HMs (Coombs et al. 2017; Takahashi et al. 2017) and thus potentially impact guidelines for use of radiotherapy and/or chemotherapy in cancer patients who present with CH as a comorbidity.

Preclinical data suggest that CH may be intervened on, although any intervention would require considerable risk–benefit analysis. Preliminary evidence suggests that vitamin C, metformin, and anti-inflammatory agents may represent possible modifying interventions in CH. On further preclinical evaluation and confirmation in CH-focused studies, observational trials may be warranted in humans to test the impact of potential interventions on CH clones — preferably in patients already exposed to these drugs. Regardless, screening of CH in individuals at high risk of myeloid neoplasms could prove to beneficial right now in cancer patients undergoing genotoxic therapy. Overall, management guidelines for CH are urgently needed for both HM and CVD risk. Thus, formation of an international advisory committee of clinical experts, precision medicine specialists, and epidemiological and laboratory medicine experts is required.

ACKNOWLEDGMENTS

We are grateful to members of the Hassane laboratory and Guzman laboratory for useful feedback and discussions. This work is supported in part by Leukemia Fighters and the Sandra and Edward Meyer Cancer Center. We are further thankful to the Caryl & Israel Englander Institute for Precision Medicine for supporting our precision medicine efforts in CH risk prediction and prevention.

REFERENCES

Abdel-Wahab O, Adli M, LaFave LM, Gao J, Hricik T, Shih AH, Pandey S, Patel JP, Chung YR, Koche R, et al. 2012. *ASXL1* mutations promote myeloid transformation through loss of PRC2-mediated gene repression. *Cancer Cell* **22:** 180–193. doi:10.1016/j.ccr.2012.06.032

Abegunde SO, Buckstein R, Wells RA, Rauh MJ. 2018. An inflammatory environment containing TNFα favors *Tet2*-mutant clonal hematopoiesis. *Exp Hematol* **59:** 60–65. doi:10.1016/j.exphem.2017.11.002

Abelson S, Collord G, Ng SWK, Weissbrod O, Mendelson Cohen N, Niemeyer E, Barda N, Zuzarte PC, Heisler L, Sundaravadanam Y, et al. 2018. Prediction of acute myeloid leukaemia risk in healthy individuals. *Nature* **559:** 400–404. doi:10.1038/s41586-018-0317-6

Baba Y, Saito B, Shimada S, Sasaki Y, Murai S, Abe M, Fujiwara S, Arai N, Kawaguchi Y, Kabasawa N, et al. 2018. Association of red cell distribution width with clinical outcomes in myelodysplastic syndrome. *Leuk Res* **67:** 56–59. doi:10.1016/j.leukres.2018.02.004

Blokzijl F, de Ligt J, Jager M, Sasselli V, Roerink S, Sasaki N, Huch M, Boymans S, Kuijk E, Prins P, et al. 2016. Tissue-specific mutation accumulation in human adult stem cells during life. *Nature* **538:** 260–264. doi:10.1038/nature19768

Bowman RL, Busque L, Levine RL. 2018. Clonal hematopoiesis and evolution to hematopoietic malignancies. *Cell Stem Cell* **22:** 157–170. doi:10.1016/j.stem.2018.01.011

Buscarlet M, Provost S, Zada YF, Barhdadi A, Bourgoin V, Lépine G, Mollica L, Szuber N, Dubé MP, Busque L. 2017. *DNMT3A* and *TET2* dominate clonal hematopoiesis and demonstrate benign phenotypes and different genetic predispositions. *Blood* **130:** 753–762. doi:10.1182/blood-2017-04-777029

Busque L, Mio R, Mattioli J, Brais E, Blais N, Lalonde Y, Maragh M, Gilliland DG. 1996. Nonrandom X-inactivation patterns in normal females: Lyonization ratios vary with age. *Blood* **88:** 59–65.

Busque L, Patel JP, Figueroa ME, Vasanthakumar A, Provost S, Hamilou Z, Mollica L, Li J, Viale A, Heguy A, et al. 2012. Recurrent somatic *TET2* mutations in normal elderly individuals with clonal hematopoiesis. *Nat Genet* **44:** 1179–1181. doi:10.1038/ng.2413

Cai Z, Kotzin JJ, Ramdas B, Chen S, Nelanuthala S, Palam LR, Pandey R, Mali RS, Liu Y, Kelley MR, et al. 2018. Inhibition of inflammatory signaling in *Tet2* mutant preleukemic cells mitigates stress-induced abnormalities and clonal hematopoiesis. *Cell Stem Cell* **23:** 833–849 e835. doi:10.1016/j.stem.2018.10.013

Calvillo-Argüelles O, Jaiswal S, Shlush LI, Moslehi JJ, Schimmer A, Barac A, Thavendiranathan P. 2019. Connections between clonal hematopoiesis, cardiovascular disease, and cancer: A review. *JAMA Cardiol* **4:** 380–387. doi:10.1001/jamacardio.2019.0302

Catlin SN, Busque L, Gale RE, Guttorp P, Abkowitz JL. 2011. The replication rate of human hematopoietic stem cells in vivo. *Blood* **117:** 4460–4466. doi:10.1182/blood-2010-08-303537

Chou WC, Chou SC, Liu CY, Chen CY, Hou HA, Kuo YY, Lee MC, Ko BS, Tang JL, Yao M, et al. 2011. *TET2* mutation is an unfavorable prognostic factor in acute myeloid leukemia patients with intermediate-risk cytogenetics. *Blood* **118:** 3803–3810. doi:10.1182/blood-2011-02-339747

Cimmino L, Dolgalev I, Wang Y, Yoshimi A, Martin GH, Wang J, Ng V, Xia B, Witkowski MT, Mitchell-Flack M, et al. 2017. Restoration of TET2 function blocks aberrant self-renewal and leukemia progression. *Cell* **170:** 1079–1095.e20. doi:10.1016/j.cell.2017.07.032

Cook EK, Izukawa T, Young S, Rosen G, Jamali M, Snetsinger B, Johnson D, Bain E, Hilland J, Buckstein J, et al. 2017. Feeding the fire: The comorbid and inflammatory backdrop of clonal hematopoiesis of indeterminate potential (CHIP) by mutation subtype. *Blood* **130:** 426.

Coombs CC, Zehir A, Devlin SM, Kishtagari A, Syed A, Jonsson P, Hyman DM, Solit DB, Robson ME, Baselga J, et al. 2017. Therapy-related clonal hematopoiesis in patients with non-hematologic cancers is common and associated with adverse clinical outcomes. *Cell Stem Cell* **21:** 374–382.e4. doi:10.1016/j.stem.2017.07.010

Cull AH, Snetsinger B, Buckstein R, Wells RA, Rauh MJ. 2017. *Tet2* restrains inflammatory gene expression in macrophages. *Exp Hematol* **55:** 56–70.e13. doi:10.1016/j.exphem.2017.08.001

De S. 2011. Somatic mosaicism in healthy human tissues. *Trends Genet* **27:** 217–223. doi:10.1016/j.tig.2011.03.002

Delhommeau F, Dupont S, Della Valle V, James C, Trannoy S, Massé A, Kosmider O, Le Couedic JP, Robert F, Alberdi A, et al. 2009. Mutation in *TET2* in myeloid cancers. *N Engl J Med* **360:** 2289–2301. doi:10.1056/NEJMoa0810069

Desai P, Mencia-Trinchant N, Savenkov O, Simon MS, Cheang G, Lee S, Samuel M, Ritchie EK, Guzman ML, Ballman KV, et al. 2018. Somatic mutations precede acute myeloid leukemia years before diagnosis. *Nat Med* **24:** 1015–1023. doi:10.1038/s41591-018-0081-z

DiNardo CD, Stein EM, de Botton S, Roboz GJ, Altman JK, Mims AS, Swords R, Collins RH, Mannis GN, Pollyea DA, et al. 2018. Durable remissions with ivosidenib in *IDH1*-mutated relapsed or refractory AML. *N Engl J Med* **378:** 2386–2398. doi:10.1056/NEJMoa1716984

Fuster JJ, MacLauchlan S, Zuriaga MA, Polackal MN, Ostriker AC, Chakraborty R, Wu CL, Sano S, Muralidharan S, Rius C, et al. 2017. Clonal hematopoiesis associated with TET2 deficiency accelerates atherosclerosis development in mice. *Science* **355:** 842–847. doi:10.1126/science.aag1381

Gale RE, Wheadon H, Linch DC. 1991. X-chromosome inactivation patterns using HPRT and PGK polymorphisms in haematologically normal and post-chemotherapy females. *Br J Haematol* **79:** 193–197. doi:10.1111/j.1365-2141.1991.tb04521.x

Gallagher EJ, LeRoith D. 2015. Obesity and diabetes: The increased risk of cancer and cancer-related mortality. *Physiol Rev* **95:** 727–748. doi:10.1152/physrev.00030.2014

Genovese G, Kähler AK, Handsaker RE, Lindberg J, Rose SA, Bakhoum SF, Chambert K, Mick E, Neale BM, Fromer M, et al. 2014. Clonal hematopoiesis and blood-cancer risk inferred from blood DNA sequence. *N Engl J Med* **371:** 2477–2487. doi:10.1056/NEJMoa1409405

Genovese G, Jaiswal S, Ebert BL, McCarroll SA. 2015. Clonal hematopoiesis and blood-cancer risk. *N Engl J Med* **372:** 1071–1072. doi:10.1056/NEJMc1500684

Hall J, Al Hafidh J, Balmert E, Dabbas B, Vaupel C, El Hader C, McGinniss M, Beruti S, Bejar R. 2014. Somatic mutations indicative of clonal hematopoiesis are present in a large fraction of cytopenic patients who lack diagnostic evidence of MDS. *Blood* **124:** 3272.

Heuser M, Thol F, Ganser A. 2016. Clonal hematopoiesis of indeterminate potential. *Dtsch Arztebl Int* **113:** 317–322.

Husby S, Francesco F, Nielsen C, Sorensen B, Baech J, Hansen JW, Gonzalez GGR, Arboe B, Andersen LP, Hastrup EK, et al. 2018. Clinical impact of clonal hematopoiesis after autologous stem cell transplantation for lymphoma: A National Population-Based Cohort Study. *Blood* **132:** 607.

Jaiswal S, Fontanillas P, Flannick J, Manning A, Grauman PV, Mar BG, Lindsley RC, Mermel CH, Burtt N, Chavez A, et al. 2014. Age-related clonal hematopoiesis associated with adverse outcomes. *N Engl J Med* **371:** 2488–2498. doi:10.1056/NEJMoa1408617

Jan M, Snyder TM, Corces-Zimmerman MR, Vyas P, Weissman IL, Quake SR, Majeti R. 2012. Clonal evolution of pre-leukemic hematopoietic stem cells precedes human acute myeloid leukemia. *Sci Transl Med* **4:** 149ra118.

Kim SJ, Zhao H, Hardikar S, Singh AK, Goodell MA, Chen T. 2013. A DNMT3A mutation common in AML exhibits dominant-negative effects in murine ES cells. *Blood* **122:** 4086–4089. doi:10.1182/blood-2013-02-483487

Knudson AG Jr. 1971. Mutation and cancer: Statistical study of retinoblastoma. *Proc Natl Acad Sci* **68:** 820–823. doi:10.1073/pnas.68.4.820

Kwok B, Reddy P, Lin KM, Flamholz R, Yung AN, Dabbas B, McGinniss M, Nahas S, Kines J, Xu Y. 2014. Next-generation sequencing (NGS)-based profiling of idiopathic cytopenia of undetermined significance (ICUS) identifies a subset of patients with genomic similarities to lower-risk myelodysplastic syndrome (MDS). *Blood* **124:** 166.

Kyle RA, Therneau TM, Rajkumar SV, Offord JR, Larson DR, Plevak MF, Melton LJ III. 2002. A long-term study of prognosis in monoclonal gammopathy of undetermined significance. *N Engl J Med* **346:** 564–569. doi:10.1056/NEJMoa01133202

Lauby-Secretan B, Scoccianti C, Loomis D, Grosse Y, Bianchini F, Straif K, International Agency for Research on Cancer Handbook Working Group. 2016. Body fatness and cancer—Viewpoint of the IARC Working Group. *N Engl J Med* **375:** 794–798. doi:10.1056/NEJMsr1606602

Loh PR, Genovese G, Handsaker RE, Finucane HK, Reshef YA, Palamara PF, Birmann BM, Talkowski ME, Bakhoum SF, McCarroll SA, et al. 2018. Insights into clonal haematopoiesis from 8,342 mosaic chromosomal alterations. *Nature* **559:** 350–355. doi:10.1038/s41586-018-0321-x

Lyon MF. 1961. Gene action in the X-chromosome of the mouse (*Mus musculus* L.). *Nature* **190:** 372–373. doi:10.1038/190372a0

Madzo J, Liu H, Rodriguez A, Vasanthakumar A, Sundaravel S, Caces DBD, Looney TJ, Zhang L, Lepore JB, Macrae T, et al. 2014. Hydroxymethylation at gene regulatory regions directs stem/early progenitor cell commitment during erythropoiesis. *Cell Rep* **6:** 231–244. doi:10.1016/j.celrep.2013.11.044

Martincorena I, Raine KM, Gerstung M, Dawson KJ, Haase K, Van Loo P, Davies H, Stratton MR, Campbell PJ. 2017. Universal patterns of selection in cancer and somatic tissues. *Cell* **171:** 1029–1041.e21. doi:10.1016/j.cell.2017.09.042

Meisel M, Hinterleitner R, Pacis A, Chen L, Earley ZM, Mayassi T, Pierre JF, Ernest JD, Galipeau HJ, Thuille N, et al. 2018. Microbial signals drive pre-leukaemic myeloproliferation in a *Tet2*-deficient host. *Nature* **557:** 580–584. doi:10.1038/s41586-018-0125-z

Moran-Crusio K, Reavie L, Shih A, Abdel-Wahab O, Ndiaye-Lobry D, Lobry C, Figueroa ME, Vasanthakumar A, Patel J, Zhao X, et al. 2011. *Tet2* loss leads to increased hematopoietic stem cell self-renewal and myeloid transformation. *Cancer Cell* **20:** 11–24. doi:10.1016/j.ccr.2011.06.001

Mouhieddine TH, Park J, Redd RA, Gibson CJ, Manier S, Nassar AH, Capelletti M, Huynh D, Bustoros M, Sklavenitis-Pistofidis R, et al. 2018. The role of clonal hematopoiesis of indeterminate potential (CHIP) in multiple myeloma: Immunomodulator maintenance post autologous stem cell transplant (ASCT) predicts better outcome. *Blood* **132:** 749.

Philip M, Rowley DA, Schreiber H. 2004. Inflammation as a tumor promoter in cancer induction. *Semin Cancer Biol* **14:** 433–439. doi:10.1016/j.semcancer.2004.06.006

Rasmussen KD, Jia G, Johansen JV, Pedersen MT, Rapin N, Bagger FO, Porse BT, Bernard OA, Christensen J, Helin K. 2015. Loss of *TET2* in hematopoietic cells leads to DNA hypermethylation of active enhancers and induction of leukemogenesis. *Genes Dev* **29:** 910–922. doi:10.1101/gad.260174.115

Rawstron AC, Bennett FL, O'Connor SJ, Kwok M, Fenton JA, Plummer M, de Tute R, Owen RG, Richards SJ, Jack AS, et al. 2008. Monoclonal B-cell lymphocytosis and chronic lymphocytic leukemia. *N Engl J Med* **359:** 575–583. doi:10.1056/NEJMoa075290

Sanders MA, Chew E, Flensburg C, Zeilemaker A, Miller SE, al Hinai AS, Bajel A, Luiken B, Rijken M, McLennan T, et al. 2018. MBD4 guards against methylation damage and germ line deficiency predisposes to clonal hematopoiesis and early-onset AML. *Blood* **132:** 1526–1534. doi:10.1182/blood-2018-05-852566

Sano S, Wang Y, Walsh K. 2018. Clonal hematopoiesis and its impact on cardiovascular disease. *Circ J* **83:** 2–11. doi:10.1253/circj.CJ-18-0871

Shih AH, Jiang Y, Meydan C, Shank K, Pandey S, Barreyro L, Antony-Debre I, Viale A, Socci N, Sun Y, et al. 2015. Mutational cooperativity linked to combinatorial epigenetic gain of function in acute myeloid leukemia. *Cancer Cell* **27:** 502–515. doi:10.1016/j.ccell.2015.03.009

Shin HT, Choi YL, Yun JW, Kim NKD, Kim SY, Jeon HJ, Nam JY, Lee C, Ryu D, Kim SC, et al. 2017. Prevalence and detection of low-allele-fraction variants in clinical cancer samples. *Nat Commun* **8:** 1377. doi:10.1038/s41467-017-01470-y

Shlush LI, Zandi S, Mitchell A, Chen WC, Brandwein JM, Gupta V, Kennedy JA, Schimmer AD, Schuh AC, Yee KW, et al. 2014. Identification of pre-leukaemic haematopoietic stem cells in acute leukaemia. *Nature* **506:** 328–333. doi:10.1038/nature13038

Stahl M, Zeidan AM. 2017. Lenalidomide use in myelodysplastic syndromes: Insights into the biologic mechanisms and clinical applications. *Cancer* **123:** 1703–1713. doi:10.1002/cncr.30585

Steensma DP. 2012. Dysplasia has a differential diagnosis: Distinguishing genuine myelodysplastic syndromes (MDS) from mimics, imitators, copycats and impostors. *Curr Hematol Malig Rep* **7:** 310–320. doi:10.1007/s11899-012-0140-3

Steensma DP, Bejar R, Jaiswal S, Lindsley RC, Sekeres MA, Hasserjian RP, Ebert BL. 2015. Clonal hematopoiesis of indeterminate potential and its distinction from myelodysplastic syndromes. *Blood* **126:** 9–16. doi:10.1182/blood-2015-03-631747

Stein EM, DiNardo CD, Pollyea DA, Fathi AT, Roboz GJ, Altman JK, Stone RM, DeAngelo DJ, Levine RL, Flinn IW, et al. 2017. Enasidenib in mutant *IDH2* relapsed or refractory acute myeloid leukemia. *Blood* **130:** 722–731. doi:10.1182/blood-2017-04-779405

Svensson EC, Madar A, Campbell CD, He Y, Sultan M, Healey ML, D'Aco K, Fernandez A, Wache-Mainer C, Ridker PM, et al. 2018. TET2-driven clonal hematopoiesis predicts enhanced response to canakinumab in the CANTOS Trial: An exploratory analysis. *Circulation* **138:** A15111.

Takahashi K, Wang F, Kantarjian H, Doss D, Khanna K, Thompson E, Zhao L, Patel K, Neelapu S, Gumbs C, et al. 2017. Preleukaemic clonal haemopoiesis and risk of therapy-related myeloid neoplasms: A case-control study. *Lancet Oncol* **18:** 100–111. doi:10.1016/S1470-2045(16)30626-X

Tiacci E, Venanzi A, Ascani S, Marra A, Cardinali V, Martino G, Codoni V, Schiavoni G, Martelli MP, Falini B. 2018. High-risk clonal hematopoiesis as the origin of AITL and *NPM1*-mutated AML. *N Engl J Med* **379:** 981–984. doi:10.1056/NEJMc1806413

Vattathil S, Scheet P. 2016. Extensive hidden genomic mosaicism revealed in normal tissue. *Am J Hum Genet* **98:** 571–578. doi:10.1016/j.ajhg.2016.02.003

Verstovsek S, Mesa RA, Gotlib J, Levy RS, Gupta V, DiPersio JF, Catalano JV, Deininger M, Miller C, Silver RT, et al. 2012. A double-blind, placebo-controlled trial of ruxolitinib for myelofibrosis. *N Engl J Med* **366:** 799–807. doi:10.1056/NEJMoa1110557

Vilkki S, Tsao JL, Loukola A, Poyhonen M, Vierimaa O, Herva R, Aaltonen LA, Shibata D. 2001. Extensive somatic microsatellite mutations in normal human tissue. *Cancer Res* **61:** 4541–4544.

Welch JS, Ley TJ, Link DC, Miller CA, Larson DE, Koboldt DC, Wartman LD, Lamprecht TL, Liu F, Xia J, et al. 2012. The origin and evolution of mutations in acute myeloid leukemia. *Cell* **150:** 264–278. doi:10.1016/j.cell.2012.06.023

Wild CP. 2005. Complementing the genome with an "exposome": The outstanding challenge of environmental exposure measurement in molecular epidemiology. *Cancer Epidemiol Biomarkers Prev* **14:** 1847–1850. doi:10.1158/1055-9965.EPI-05-0456

Wimazal F, Fonatsch C, Thalhammer R, Schwarzinger I, Müllauer L, Sperr WR, Bennett JM, Valent P. 2007. Idiopathic cytopenia of undetermined significance (ICUS) versus low risk MDS: The diagnostic interface. *Leuk Res* **31:** 1461–1468. doi:10.1016/j.leukres.2007.03.015

Wu X, Bekker-Jensen IH, Christensen J, Rasmussen KD, Sidoli S, Qi Y, Kong Y, Wang X, Cui Y, Xiao Z, et al. 2015. Tumor suppressor ASXL1 is essential for the activation of *INK4B* expression in response to oncogene activity and anti-proliferative signals. *Cell Res* **25:** 1205–1218. doi:10.1038/cr.2015.121

Wu D, Hu D, Chen H, Shi G, Fetahu IS, Wu F, Rabidou K, Fang R, Tan L, Xu S, et al. 2018. Glucose-regulated phosphorylation of TET2 by AMPK reveals a pathway linking diabetes to cancer. *Nature* **559:** 637–641. doi:10.1038/s41586-018-0350-5

Xie M, Lu C, Wang J, McLellan MD, Johnson KJ, Wendl MC, McMichael JF, Schmidt HK, Yellapantula V, Miller CA, et al. 2014. Age-related mutations associated with clonal hematopoietic expansion and malignancies. *Nat Med* **20:** 1472–1478. doi:10.1038/nm.3733

Yoshizato T, Dumitriu B, Hosokawa K, Makishima H, Yoshida K, Townsley D, Sato-Otsubo A, Sato Y, Liu D, Suzuki H, et al. 2015. Somatic mutations and clonal hematopoiesis in aplastic anemia. *N Engl J Med* **373:** 35–47. doi:10.1056/NEJMoa1414799

Young AL, Challen GA, Birmann BM, Druley TE. 2016. Clonal haematopoiesis harbouring AML-associated mutations is ubiquitous in healthy adults. *Nat Commun* **7:** 12484. doi:10.1038/ncomms12484

Young AL, Tong RS, Birmann BM, Druley TE. 2019. Clonal haematopoiesis and risk of acute myeloid leukemia. *Haematologica* doi: 10.3324/haematol.2018.215269.

Zhang Q, Zhao K, Shen Q, Han Y, Gu Y, Li X, Zhao D, Liu Y, Wang C, Zhang X, et al. 2015. Tet2 is required to resolve inflammation by recruiting Hdac2 to specifically repress IL-6. *Nature* **525:** 389–393. doi:10.1038/nature15252

Zink F, Stacey SN, Norddahl GL, Frigge ML, Magnusson OT, Jonsdottir I, Thorgeirsson TE, Sigurdsson A, Gudjonsson SA, Gudmundsson J, et al. 2017. Clonal hematopoiesis, with and without candidate driver mutations, is common in the elderly. *Blood* **130:** 742–752. doi:10.1182/blood-2017-02-769869

Zurauskaite G, Meier M, Voegeli A, Koch D, Haubitz S, Kutz A, Bernasconi L, Huber A, Bargetzi M, Mueller B, et al. 2018. Biological pathways underlying the association of red cell distribution width and adverse clinical outcome: Results of a prospective cohort study. *PLoS One* **13:** e0191280. doi:10.1371/journal.pone.0191280

Targeting Immunophenotypic Markers on Leukemic Stem Cells: How Lessons from Current Approaches and Advances in the Leukemia Stem Cell (LSC) Model Can Inform Better Strategies for Treating Acute Myeloid Leukemia (AML)

Kelly Mitchell[1] and Ulrich Steidl[1,2,3,4]

[1]Department of Cell Biology, Albert Einstein College of Medicine, Bronx, New York 10461, USA

[2]Department of Medicine (Oncology), Division of Hemato-Oncology, Albert Einstein College of Medicine–Montefiore Medical Center, Bronx, New York 10461, USA

[3]Albert Einstein Cancer Center, Albert Einstein College of Medicine, Bronx, New York 10461, USA

[4]Institute for Stem Cell and Regenerative Medicine Research, Albert Einstein College of Medicine, Bronx, New York 10461, USA

Correspondence: ulrich.steidl@einstein.yu.edu

Therapies targeting cell-surface antigens in acute myeloid leukemia (AML) have been tested over the past 20 years with limited improvement in overall survival. Recent advances in the understanding of AML pathogenesis support therapeutic targeting of leukemia stem cells as the most promising avenue toward a cure. In this review, we provide an overview of the evolving leukemia stem cell (LSC) model, including evidence of the cell of origin, cellular and molecular disease architecture, and source of relapse in AML. In addition, we explore limitations of current targeted strategies utilized in AML and describe the various immunophenotypic antigens that have been proposed as LSC-directed therapeutic targets. We draw lessons from current approaches as well as from the (pre)-LSC model to suggest criteria that immunophenotypic targets should meet for more specific and effective elimination of disease-initiating clones, highlighting in detail a few targets that we suggest fit these criteria most completely.

Leukemias are hematologic malignancies originating in the bone marrow (BM) that lead to abnormal expansion of white blood cells in an acute or chronic manner. Acute myeloid leukemia (AML) represents around one-third of leukemias and about 10,000 deaths occur yearly in the United States as a result of this disease (Noone et al. 2018). AML is characterized by blocked differentiation and clonal overproliferation of myeloid hematopoietic precursor cells, leading to features of BM failure, and if not treated, results in death within months. Although chemotherapeutic treatments (most commonly cytarabine [ara-C] and anthracyclines) can eliminate detectable leukemic cells in the BM and blood and successfully lead the majority of

Cite this article as *Cold Spring Harb Perspect Med* doi: 10.1101/cshperspect.a036251

patients into remission, most patients still fatally relapse (Ferrara and Schiffer 2013; Döhner et al. 2015), necessitating the discovery of novel approaches for treating AML.

Findings throughout the past 25+ years provide evidence that AML and the closely related "pre-leukemic" myelodysplastic syndromes (MDS) arise from primitive hematopoietic cells that harbor mutations and epigenetic aberrations, initially leading to formation and/or expansion of pre-leukemic cells and ultimately to transformed leukemic stem cells (LSCs) capable of regenerating and maintaining the disease. Experimentally, LSCs are most commonly functionally defined by their ability to initiate and maintain AML in mice. Sequencing studies have provided evidence that these disease-initiating cells are not eliminated by chemotherapy and eventually prompt MDS and AML relapse. Therefore, to achieve permanent cures of AML and MDS and prevent relapse, elimination of LSC is essential. The eradication of pre-LSC (hematopoietic stem cells [HSCs] primed for transformation while retaining the ability to contribute to multilineage differentiation) is also likely necessary. In this review, we will summarize the evolving LSC model and analyze current and prospective strategies for treating AML by targeting LSC populations via aberrantly expressed surface antigens.

THE LEUKEMIA STEM CELL MODEL

Significant evidence has been gathered supporting the existence of LSCs capable of initiating, maintaining, and regenerating AML (for review, see Passegue et al. 2003; Pandolfi et al. 2013; Corces et al. 2017; Thomas and Majeti 2017). To validate this model, several areas have been examined, including (1) the cell of origin for AML, (2) functional heterogeneity in the organization of AML, and (3) contribution of LSCs to relapse.

The Cell of Origin for AML

Initial Evidence from Cytogenetics Studies

Cytogenetic examination of human AML cells provided the first evidence of a stem cell origin in this cancer. The coupling of karyotyping with colony-forming potential assays in primary human AML samples identified cytogenetically abnormal cells that were capable of long-term culture and/or multilineage differentiation, suggesting the presence of these aberrations in stem cells (Hogge et al. 1987; Tamura et al. 1993). In addition, cytogenetic analysis together with immunophenotyping uncovered identical aberrations in bilineage leukemias, supporting the origin of these leukemias as an immature cell with both myeloid and lymphoid potential (Sun et al. 1991; Carbonell et al. 1996; Hyakuna et al. 1998). Finally, cytogenetics coupled with fluorescence-activated cell sorting (FACS) detected chromosomal rearrangements in immunophenotypically defined HSCs and hematopoietic progenitor cells ($CD34^+CD38^-$ and $CD34^+CD38^+$ cells, respectively) in primary MDS and AML samples at diagnosis (Haase et al. 1995, 1997; Feuring-Buske et al. 1999; Nilsson et al. 2000, 2002; Barreyro et al. 2012; Will et al. 2012; Elias et al. 2014; Woll et al. 2014; Shastri et al. 2017) and in the relapse setting (Engel et al. 1999; Diez-Martin et al. 2000).

Early Evidence from Mouse Modeling of Pre-Leukemia

Modeling of frequent molecular changes in MDS/AML in murine models provided important early conceptual insight into pre-leukemic stages at the hematopoietic stem/progenitor level and their functional relevance for leukemia development and maintenance. These studies include reduction in expression of the transcription factor PU.1 (Steidl et al. 2006; Will et al. 2015), overexpression of the MLL-AF9 and CBFβ–SMMHC fusion oncogenes (Kuo et al. 2006; Somervaille and Cleary 2006; Pulikkan and Castilla 2018), and introduction of CEBPα mutations (Kirstetter et al. 2008; Bereshchenko et al. 2009), all resulting in distinct pre-leukemic phases characterized by myeloid-biased HSC, blocked differentiation, and accumulation of immature myeloid or myelomonocytic cells in the BM and blood. AML development occurred in these mice with a latency of 2–6 months, which indicated for the first time that a distinct

Cite this article as *Cold Spring Harb Perspect Med* doi: 10.1101/cshperspect.a036251

pre-leukemic phase with definable cell-intrinsic properties exists, and that stem and immature progenitor cells play a key role in this process. In addition, it was found that some pre-leukemic molecular alterations, such as down-regulation of the transcription factors PU.1 and JunB, remain functionally critical for fully transformed LSC at later stages, which indicated that targeting pre-leukemic/founding aberrations may represent a promising therapeutic avenue (Steidl et al. 2006).

Evidence from Gene Expression Studies

Further support for the HSC origin of AML in humans was initially collected through studies of gene expression in purified cell populations. Gene expression analysis of phenotypic short-term HSCs ($Lin^-CD34^+CD38^-CD90^{low}$) from AML patients identified dysregulated expression of genes in this population such as the JunB and PU.1 transcription factors (Steidl et al. 2006), and the epigenetic regulator SATB1 (Steidl et al. 2007). More broadly, microarray transcriptional profiling studies of immunophenotypically defined HSCs from MDS and AML versus normal BM showed that MDS/AML HSCs exhibit gene expression profiles resembling normal HSCs (Nilsson et al. 2007; Gentles et al. 2010; Eppert et al. 2011), but that multiple specific genes and pathways are dysregulated at the stem cell level such as those involved in apoptosis, adherens junctions, interleukin (IL), Jak-STAT, and interferon (IFN) signaling (Nilsson et al. 2007; Majeti et al. 2009a; Barreyro et al. 2012; Will et al. 2012), suggesting involvement of HSCs in human AML pathogenesis.

Evidence from Sequencing Studies Using Single-Nucleotide Variants as Markers of Subclonality

A logical argument for the stem cell origin of leukemia is that the number of mutations and therefore time required for cellular transformation must occur in a long-lived cell with high proliferative potential, as mutations would not have sufficient time to accumulate in progenitor and more differentiated cells because of their transient nature. Single-colony and single-cell sequencing technologies have allowed for direct evidence of this phenomenon. A cell-surface immunophenotype has been identified ($Lin^-CD34^+CD38^-CD99^-TIM\text{-}3^-$) that distinguishes functionally normal residual HSCs from AML patient samples (as defined by transplantation experiments) (Jan et al. 2011). FACS and targeted sequencing of these normal HSCs from AML patient samples showed that genetic lesions serially accumulate in HSCs, as multiple clones existed in the HSC pool containing the partial spectrum of all mutations seen in AML cells from that patient (Jan et al. 2012). Likewise, whole-exome sequencing on paired diagnosis/remission/relapse AML samples identified that $CD34^+$ progenitors as well as mature cells harbor some of the mutations from the original leukemia at the time of remission (Corces-Zimmerman et al. 2014). The persistence of these mutations in remission indicates that they originate from a stem cell that survived chemotherapy.

An HSC origin is further supported by the detection of the same *DNMT3A* mutations in both the dominant leukemic clone and in normal mature blood cells such as T cells (Shlush et al. 2014). The presence of identical mutations in AML and T cells strongly suggests that the cell of origin in AML is long-lived and has multilineage differentiation potential. In addition, in at least two documented occasions, transplantations performed with donor BM retrospectively determined to harbor a *DNMT3A* mutation resulted in AML in the recipient with a *DNMT3A*-mutant leukemic clone (Yasuda et al. 2014; Hahn et al. 2015). These anecdotal findings suggest an HSC origin as these cells are responsible for long-term repopulation of the immune system.

Single-cell sequencing of $CD34^+CD38^-$ $IL1RAP^+/CD123^+/CD45RA^+$ BM cells from longitudinal MDS and secondary AML samples from individual patients revealed that MDS and AML arise from different but ancestrally related clones, further supporting a stem cell origin for these diseases (Chen et al. 2019). Importantly, the stem cell origin theory has been tested prospectively as well. It was recently shown that a succession of stages ultimately leading to a serially transplantable leukemia could be modeled by creating induced pluripotent stem cells from primary MDS and AML samples with increasing numbers of driver mutations (Kotini et al. 2017).

It has been estimated that HSCs acquire between 1 and 2 exonic mutations per decade, and while most of these do not manifest in clonal expansion or disease, several studies have found that at least 5%–10% of individuals over age 65 have disproportionate expansion of single hematopoietic clones, with the percentage further increasing with age. Detection of mutations associated with myeloid malignancies at a variant allele frequency (VAF) of 2% or greater in the peripheral blood currently defines this phenomenon, termed clonal hematopoiesis (CH) (Genovese et al. 2014; Jaiswal et al. 2014; Xie et al. 2014; Shlush 2018). CH mutations found in BM HSCs and hematopoietic progenitors further hints that CH represents a premalignant event preceding myeloid malignancies (Fig. 1A; Arends et al. 2018).

The nature of the transition from CH to myeloid malignancies is the subject of intense

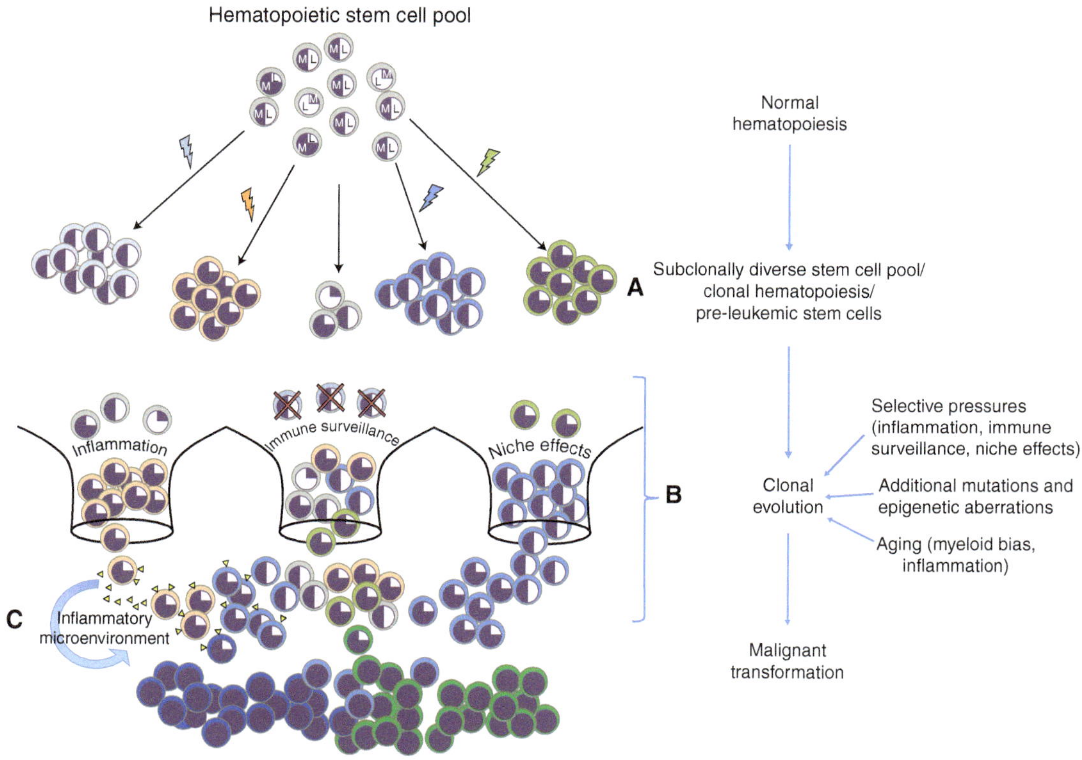

Figure 1. Selective pressure model of acute myeloid leukemia (AML). A proposed model showing transformation of the hematopoietic stem cell (HSC) pool from normal to malignant. "Normal" HSCs are shown in gray. Myeloid (M) and lymphoid (L) biased stem cells are present, as well as unbiased HSCs (represented as equal proportion M and L). Different aberrations such as mutations (colored lightning bolts) are associated with certain HSC subclones that can be detected, for example, by sequencing (clonal hematopoiesis) (*A*). These aberrations can occur in a lineage-biased stem cell or may confer a lineage bias. Selective pressures such as inflammation, immune surveillance, and niche effects may give certain HSC clones an advantage over others (i.e., inflammation gives the clone with an orange mutation a selective advantage over normal HSCs). Clonal evolution is also potentially further driven by additional mutations and aging-associated phenomena such as chronic inflammation and myeloid bias (*B*). For example, an inflammatory microenvironment created by pre-leukemic clones can promote selective expansion of mutated clones over normal HSCs (*C*). Together, these factors can eventually lead to malignant transformation and achievement of clonal dominance of particular stem cell subclones, and consecutive uncontrolled proliferation of leukemic bulk clones (shown as royal blue and bright green cells).

Cite this article as *Cold Spring Harb Perspect Med* doi: 10.1101/cshperspect.a036251

investigation (for review, see Bowman et al. 2018). One study estimated that any detectable CH is associated with an 11-fold greater risk of hematologic cancer and this risk increases to almost 50-fold with a greater clone size (VAF of 10% or greater) (Jaiswal et al. 2014; Steensma et al. 2015; Corces et al. 2017). However, the overall risk for hematologic malignancy in individuals with CH has been estimated to be only 4% (Jaiswal et al. 2014), indicating that further clonal evolution is required for cancer development. Two independent longitudinal analyses detected AML-relevant mutations in whole blood samples several years before AML diagnosis and found that higher mutational burden correlated with increased rates of AML progression (Abelson et al. 2018; Desai et al. 2018). While these studies were not done in BM or in stem-cell-enriched populations, the presence of these mutations years before diagnosis indicates their occurrence in long-lived cells and represents indirect evidence for the accumulation of mutations in HSCs or expansion of HSCs with existing mutations to a detectable limit. It would also be informative, albeit logistically challenging, to perform single-HSC sequencing on these samples to identify co-occurring mutations and their association with development and time-to-development of AML.

Disruption of Hematopoietic Stem Cell Function and Integrity as an Early Step in the Pathogenesis of Myeloid Malignancies

In the BM niche, HSCs are generally maintained in a dormant state with infrequent cell divisions to limit the opportunity for mutations to arise from the byproducts of ATP production (reactive oxygen species [ROS]) or errors during genome replication (Ito et al. 2006; Pietras et al. 2011). Studies have estimated that human HSCs enter the cell cycle on average every 40 weeks (Catlin et al. 2011), implying that there is tight regulation on maintaining HSCs in a noncycling "quiescent" state the vast majority of the time. Accordingly, it has been shown that DNA damage accumulates in HSCs with age, and cell-cycle-associated replication stress contributes to functional impairment in aging HSCs, including reduced proliferative and regenerative capacity (Rossi et al. 2008; Flach et al. 2014).

Although HSCs are usually kept dormant, they must be poised to undergo cell division when an injury or infection cannot be controlled locally. In this case, increased proinflammatory cytokines and Toll-like receptor ligands directly and/or indirectly stimulate hematopoietic stem and progenitor cells (HSPCs) to proliferate and differentiate to regain homeostasis and meet the blood and immune system demands (King and Goodell 2011; Takizawa et al. 2012; Pietras 2017). Different combinations of cytokines and ligands stimulate particular subsets of HSCs to differentiate along specific lineages. For instance, in response to viral infections, IFN-γ is released, promotes differentiation of myeloid-biased HSCs (Matatall et al. 2014) and leads to expression of IL-6 by the BM niche. IL-6 then acts specifically on the multipotent progenitor (MPP) population to regulate hematopoietic output, driving myeloid output at the expense of lymphoid production (Reynaud et al. 2011; Mirantes et al. 2014). Direct cytokine-mediated activation of HSPCs has been demonstrated to be an efficient alternative to cytokine release by mature cells and subsequent paracrine stimulation of HSPCs for rapid myeloid recovery (Zhao et al. 2014).

Although proinflammatory signals can recover homeostasis in acute settings, chronic exposure has been shown to lead to HSC exhaustion and BM failure. For instance, IL-1 exposure in mice resulted in an HSC pool with limited ability to differentiate into nonmyeloid lineages and reduced self-renewal potential as assessed by competitive transplantation (Pietras et al. 2016). Chronic IFN-γ compromised long-term HSC reconstitution capacity after transplantation (Baldridge et al. 2010) and chronic tumor necrosis factor α (TNF-α) has also been shown to inhibit HSC growth and survival, reducing reconstitution ability of human $CD34^+CD38^-$ cells (Baldridge et al. 2011). These drastic effects of chronic inflammation are likely lessened in the endogenous, nontransplant setting where chronic inflammatory signaling and the resultant cytokine microenvironment have been postulated to instead cause continual disruption of HSC quiescence, frequent cell cycling, and an increased probability of accumulating DNA replication-associated mutations (Cohen et al. 1991; Pietras 2017). This idea is supported by studies showing that injection of mice with the double-stranded RNA mimic pI:pC, which mimics viral infection, induces HSCs to exit from quiescence in an IFN-α-receptor-dependent manner and accumulate DNA damage (Pietras et al. 2014; Walter et al. 2015). Similar effects were seen upon chronic LPS exposure (Esplin et al. 2011; Takizawa et al. 2017). In line with this, large epidemiological studies demonstrated that a prior history of infectious disease led to a 1.3-fold increased risk of AML and MDS and a prior history of autoimmune disease was associated with 1.7- and 2.1-fold increased risks for AML and MDS, respectively (Anderson et al. 2009; Kristinsson et al. 2011).

For a malignancy to develop, a mutated HSC conceivably must still retain its ability to sustain itself. Aside from triggering cell cycling and, consequently, mutations in HSCs, chronic inflammation can also act as a selective force and promote expansion of HSCs that are resistant to the detrimental effects of a proinflammatory environment (Fig. 1B). This phenomenon was elegantly shown in a mouse model of pre-leukemic myeloproliferation with variable expressivity. Specifically, upon genetic knockout of *Tet2*, the amount of myeloproliferation seen was positively associated with the presence of bacterial dissemination (potentially because of *Tet2*$^{-/-}$-related intestinal defects), and the presence of bacteria or of TLR agonists were sufficient to cause this myeloproliferation through increased IL-6 secretion. Further, *Tet2*$^{-/-}$ HSPCs were specifically sensitive to IL-6, in part because of up-regulation of the IL-6 receptor compared to *Tet2*$^{+/+}$ HSCs, providing an example of mutated HSCs acquiring properties that give them a competitive advantage in a proinflammatory environment (Meisel et al. 2018). Likewise, in the human setting, HSCs from patients with myeloproliferative neoplasms harboring activating *JAK2* mutations were found to be resistant to suppressive growth signaling from chronic TNF-α stimulation and were clonally selected in this environment (Fleischman et al. 2011; Takizawa et al. 2012; Craver et al. 2018).

Contrastingly, pre-leukemic or CH mutations may foster an inflammatory environment. For instance, although only described in mature hematopoietic cells, Tet2 was shown to repress expression of inflammatory cytokines including IL-1β and IL-6. Loss of function mutations in *Tet2* therefore derepressed these signals and contributed to an inflammatory environment, which in the leukemia setting could promote disease progression (Zhang et al. 2015; Fuster et al. 2017; Jaiswal et al. 2017). CH is also associated with increased risk of diseases with inflammatory components, including coronary heart disease and various cancers (Coombs et al. 2017; Jaiswal et al. 2017); thus, a positive feedback loop between an inflammatory microenvironment and the development of and selection for aberrant HSCs may be a causative factor in AML development (Fig. 1C).

The question remains why certain mutations, such as those providing a proliferative advantage, would necessarily result in myeloid malignancies. One theory for this is the changing capacity and characteristics of HSCs as they age. It is well described in human and mouse hematopoiesis that deficiencies in the adaptive immune system occur with aging. This is accompanied by myeloid skewing, specifically demonstrated by increased myeloid repopulation potential in HSC transplantation experiments from young versus old mice and young versus old human BM specimens (Rossi et al. 2005; Rundberg Nilsson et al. 2016; Yamamoto et al. 2018). Accordingly, the majority of pediatric leukemias are lymphoid, whereas adult leukemias are most frequently myeloid, even when initiated by the same oncogene, for instance t(9;22) (MLL-AF9), suggesting an alteration in the potential of HSCs with age (Meyer et al. 2013). This increased propensity toward myeloid differentiation provides insight into the phenomenon of age-related myeloid malignancies (Fig. 1B), yet the cell-intrinsic mechanisms for this occurrence must still be investigated further. Perhaps an age-related inflammatory environment could provide a link to explain this propensity for myeloid disease.

Functional Heterogeneity in the Organization of AML

The first description of the heterogeneous composition of AML was provided by transplantation of subpopulations of cells from leukemic BM specimens into immunodeficient mice. Whereas $CD34^+CD38^-$ cells were capable of initiating disease in recipient animals, $CD34^-$ cells were not, providing the first indication that all leukemia cells are not created equal, and that a hierarchy exists within a cancer cell population (Lapidot et al. 1994; Bonnet and Dick 1997). These studies were validated in vitro by long-term proliferation and colony output assays of immunophenotypic subpopulations from AML samples (Sutherland et al. 1996). Higher-resolution experiments were done by using lentiviral transduction to mark single cells from AML specimens and performing serial transplantations. These experiments led to the identification of a more complex hierarchy, with subpopulations of cells that were capable of short-term or long-term repopulation, and/or whose repopulation only reached a detectable limit after secondary or tertiary transplantation (indicating initial quiescence). Tracking clones via a lentiviral integration site identified that quiescent long-term leukemia-initiating cells (LICs) gave rise to long-term LICs, which gave rise to short-term LICs, eventually generating bulk tumor cells that lose the ability to self-renew, but are also unable to differentiate, leading to their uncontrolled accumulation (Hope et al. 2004). Of note, expanded studies with a higher number of primary AML specimens have identified that the leukemia-initiating population is not limited to the $CD34^+CD38^-$ immunophenotype and in fact the $CD34^+CD38^+$ and $CD34^-$ populations are also in some cases capable of leukemia initiation (Martelli et al. 2010; Taussig et al. 2010; Goardon et al. 2011; Sarry et al. 2011; Quek et al. 2016). Although these studies have provided pivotal insight into the heterogeneity that exists in AML, the use of xenotransplantation into mice to determine human tumor heterogeneity may select for different functional properties or may underestimate (or overestimate) the actual LSC frequency. These methodological caveats should be kept in mind in our interpretations with regard to the precise architecture of human AML.

Contribution of LSCs to Relapse

LICs have been shown to exhibit stem cell characteristics that contribute to chemotherapy resistance—including quiescence and drug efflux potential (Terpstra et al. 1996; Costello et al. 2000). Indeed, human AML xenograft studies in mice found that certain cell-cycle-quiescent leukemia cells localize in the BM endosteal region, remain after chemotherapy, and can transplant AML to secondary recipients (Ishikawa et al. 2007; Saito et al. 2010). Similarly, sequencing studies have demonstrated that HSCs harboring leukemia-associated mutations persist after standard chemotherapy in AML patients (Miyamoto et al. 2000; Ding et al. 2012; Welch et al. 2012; Corces-Zimmerman et al. 2014). However, in light of evidence that nonleukemic clones expand following induction chemotherapy (Wong et al. 2016), distinguishing CH with a high VAF from incomplete elimination of leukemic clones will be crucial for elucidating the nature of relapse. Considering that it is currently not possible to detect whether chemotherapy has eliminated every leukemic cell because of sensitivity limitations in minimal residual disease (MRD) detection (Hourigan et al. 2017; Hollein et al. 2018), whether relapse is being driven by residual LSCs (dominant or minor subclones), by chemotherapy-induced mutations that lead to drug resistance, or by chemotherapy-induced clonal evolution of pre-LSCs, is not entirely clear (Jan and Majeti 2013), but current evidence supports the former (Corces et al. 2017; Shlush et al. 2017). Specifically, sequencing of paired diagnosis and relapse samples has demonstrated several cases of minor subclones at diagnosis that present as the dominant subclone at relapse (Parkin et al. 2013; Corces-Zimmerman et al. 2014; Shlush et al. 2017). Because of detection limits of sequencing, even in studies where new subclones appeared at relapse (Ding et al. 2012; Corces-Zimmerman et al. 2014), it cannot be ruled out that these clones were present in low frequency at diagnosis and expanded after chemotherapy.

Until more sensitive techniques are available, it may not become entirely clear what the nature of relapse is. Despite these limitations, the suspected stem cell origin of AML relapse suggests that eradication of both malignant and premalignant HSPC, but not necessarily HSCs in a CH stage, holds promise for achieving lasting cures. Thus, an ideal therapeutic target should be present not only on LSC-enriched populations at diagnosis, but also in the relapse setting, and with expression during complete remission being predictive of relapse.

PRESENT AND FUTURE STRATEGIES FOR TARGETING LSCs IN AML

Associated Limitations of Current Targeted Approaches in AML

In AML, heterogeneity in the cellular compartment of origin and the varied mutational spectrum across patients have challenged the identification of commonly dysregulated pathways that are relevant in the initiation and maintenance of the disease (Sarry et al. 2011; Papaemmanuil et al. 2016). Sequencing studies have determined that AML is genetically complex, with patients typically having multiple driver mutations, and despite there being overlap in these mutations, no single genetic aberration is found in more than 35% of patients (Papaemmanuil et al. 2016). Thus, a treatment designed to eliminate cells carrying a particular mutation will likely only be relevant in a minority of patients. Further, individual patients have high intratumor heterogeneity; any detected mutation is usually only present in a subset of tumor cells and focusing a therapeutic strategy on a particular mutation may leave many subclones (especially smaller ones) unaccounted for (Ding et al. 2012; Welch et al. 2012; Parkin et al. 2013; Chen et al. 2019). For this reason, several groups have sought to identify common characteristics of leukemia cells across AMLs with different genetic profiles—most notably cell-surface protein markers—that might be exploited for therapeutic targeting in most patients (Jordan et al. 2000b; Majeti et al. 2009b). Three of the most commonly sought-after targets in AML cells are CD33, FLT3, and CD123, but clinically, toxicities caused by lack of specificity of expression and resistance mechanisms are presenting considerable challenges.

CD33

Currently, the only approved immunotherapy in AML is gemtuzumab ozogamicin, an anti-CD33 antibody conjugated to a cytotoxic derivative of calicheamicin (Sievers et al. 1999, 2001), but this treatment has been on and off the market because of hematologic and nonhematologic toxicities (Baron and Wang 2018). In 2017, it was reapproved for use at lower doses in combination with chemotherapy and as a single agent in patients not eligible for intensive chemotherapy or with relapsed/refractory AML (Amadori et al. 2010; Castaigne et al. 2012). Whereas CD33 is often expressed on LSC-enriched populations (Griffin et al. 1984; Hauswirth et al. 2007; Sadovnik et al. 2017), hematopoietic toxicity of anti-CD33 treatments relate to its expression on normal hematopoietic cells, including HSCs (Taussig et al. 2005; Kikushige et al. 2010; Sadovnik et al. 2017; Haubner et al. 2019). Several creative approaches are being tested to circumvent this toxicity. For instance, a bispecific antibody targeting CD47 and CD33 was developed and reported to be effective in an AML xenograft model (Boyd-Kirkup et al. 2017). Another approach under development is the use of CRISPR-Cas9 technology to delete CD33 in HSCs and subsequent use of anti-CD33 targeting approaches such as CAR T cells to eliminate leukemic cells (Kim et al. 2018).

FLT3

FLT3, or CD135, is a highly sought-after therapeutic target in AML because of the substantial fraction of patients harboring activating mutations in this gene (up to 35%) (Gilliland and Griffin 2002; Patel et al. 2012; Papaemmanuil et al. 2016). In-frame length polymorphisms (resulting from internal tandem duplications) in the juxtamembrane domain of *FLT3* (*FLT3*-ITD) were discovered in AML patients in 1996, and led to a constitutively active kinase by destabilizing the inhibitory functions of this domain (Chan 2011). *FLT3* mutations are demonstrated to be driving mutations in leukemogenesis (Lee et al. 2005; Schessl et al. 2005; Kim et al. 2008; Mallardo et al. 2013), but detection of minor leukemic subclones with *FLT3*-ITD mutations indicate it is preferentially a late event (Corces-Zimmerman et al. 2014; Shouval et al. 2014). Targeted sequencing of single-LSC-derived colonies has resolved the likely order of acquisition of mutations in several patients, concluding that FLT3 mutations occur late, as they never occur as the sole aberration but only co-occur with other leukemia-relevant mutations (Jan et al. 2012). Meanwhile, sequencing of residual normal HSC-derived colonies showed that *FLT3* mutations never occur in these cells (Jan et al. 2012; Corces-Zimmerman et al. 2014), and *FLT3* mutations are not found in CH (Abelson et al. 2018; Desai et al. 2018), suggesting they are not early, or pre-leukemic events. In addition, *FLT3* mutations are often gained or lost between diagnosis and relapse, further evidence that they are not a part of the founding AML clone (Krönke et al. 2013; Corces-Zimmerman et al. 2014; Shlush et al. 2014; Shouval et al. 2014).

Over 60 clinical trials have been conducted to test FLT3 inhibitors alone or in combination therapy in AML. Currently, only midostaurin has FDA approval for treatment of AML patients with *FLT3*-ITD mutations in combination with standard induction therapy, as it modestly improved event-free and overall survival in clinical trials (Stone et al. 2017). Although most *FLT3*-ITD subclones are sensitive to tyrosine kinase inhibitor (TKI) treatment, particularly circulating leukemic cells, BM leukemic cells are not effectively eliminated and MRD often contains *FLT3*-ITD$^+$ cells. Studies of samples from patients who relapsed while under treatment with the TKI quizartinib have uncovered resistance mechanisms. These include suboptimal pharmacokinetics and pharmacodynamics of TKIs, acquisition of additional mutations in *FLT3* (commonly in the kinase domain) leading to decreased inhibitor efficacy (Alvarado et al. 2014; Ghiaur and Levis 2017; Smith et al. 2017), and activation of compensatory signaling pathways, including stromal-derived fibroblast growth factor and CXCL12, which lead to activation of mitogen-activating protein kinases (MAPKs) and Bcl2 family survival pathways (Yang et al. 2014; Traer et al. 2016; Ghiaur and Levis 2017; Smith et al. 2017). In addition, high FLT3 ligand levels in the BM that occur during chemotherapy have been proposed to stimulate FLT3-ITD$^+$ cells through their remaining FLT3 wild-type (WT) copy, facilitating cell survival amid quizartinib treatment, which preferentially targets the mutated receptor (Sato et al. 2011; Yang et al. 2014; Chen et al. 2016; Taylor et al. 2017).

Elimination of MRD is not apparent under the use of FLT3 inhibitors because of one or many of these mechanisms, and the findings that FLT3 mutations are not early events in leukemogenesis may be the driving reason behind their limited sustained efficacy. Whereas proposed immunotherapeutic approaches (Reiter et al. 2018) may prevent some mechanisms of resistance by eliminating any FLT3-expressing leukemic cells, expression on normal HSCs (Sadovnik et al. 2017) will likely prevent progression of this tactic to wider use in the treatment and cure of AML.

CD123

Several studies have reported high expression of CD123 (IL-3Rα) on CD34$^+$CD38$^-$ populations from AML samples (Jordan et al. 2000a; Munoz et al. 2001; Graf et al. 2004; Yalcintepe et al. 2006; Sadovnik et al. 2017). The expression of CD123 on normal HSPC is somewhat conflicting. Most analyses of CD123 protein expression by flow cytometry in normal human hematopoietic cells have reported that CD123 is expressed on a low–mid proportion of normal BM CD34$^+$ cells, attributed to expression on myeloid progenitors (common myeloid and granulocyte-macrophage progenitors [CMPs and GMPs]), but with no expression on CD34$^+$CD38$^-$ cells (Sato et al. 1993; Jordan et al. 2000a; Munoz et al. 2001; Graf et al. 2004). However, other studies have detected expression in HSCs (Taussig et al. 2005; van Rhenen et al. 2007a; Sadovnik et al. 2017; Haubner et al. 2019) and when side population (SP) stem cells from normal BM were analyzed, CD123 was detected in up to 82% of SP cells with a median of 27% (Moshaver et al. 2008). CD123 was also highly expressed in $CD34^+CD38^-$ cells in regenerating BM, which may be particularly relevant for patients undergoing chemotherapy (van Rhenen et al. 2007a).

CD123 targeting by monoclonal antibodies has been modestly effective in preclinical models, at least in part via inhibition of IL-3 signaling and Fc-mediated recruitment and cell killing by innate immune effector cells (Jin et al. 2009). Several CD123-directed agents have been tested in phase I/II clinical trials, with results awaited (NCT02113982, NCT02152956, NCT02715011 (suspended), NCT02730312, NCT02848248 (terminated). The CD123 monoclonal antibody talacotuzumab reached a phase III clinical trial to be tested in combination with decitabine in patients with AML not eligible for intensive chemotherapy, but was discontinued (NCT02472145), and another phase II clinical trial with talacotuzumab as a monotherapy (NCT02992860) was terminated because of risk to patients. Toxicity to normal HSPC may limit whether CD123-directed therapies will progress to clinical approval (Thomas and Majeti 2017), particularly given the importance of IL-3 for hematopoietic cell viability and proliferation (Barreda et al. 2004).

Considerations for Prospective LSC Targets

Advances in the LSC model imply conditions that therapeutic targets in AML should meet. For instance, studying the cell of origin and architecture of AML indicate that a $Lin^-CD34^+CD38^-CD90^-$ immunophenotype is most characteristic of LICs, thus proteins expressed on this population in AML samples have therapeutic promise. Further, studies of the subclonal composition of relapse suggest that the timing in which a target is expressed in the transformation process should be of high importance. Toxicities associated with current targeted therapies reinforce the importance of minimal expression on normal tissues and hint at the benefits and drawbacks associated with different classes of biopharmaceutical agents. These and other considerations are detailed below.

Immunophenotype

Several proteins expressed on immunophenotypically defined LSCs have been discovered by transcriptional profiling and subsequent validation of protein overexpression in HSC-enriched populations ($CD34^+CD38^-$ cells) from AML versus normal BM samples. Tables 1 and 2 list these targets, expression on LSC-enriched populations and in normal tissues, described functions in AML, and exploration of targeting strategies. The immunophenotypic populations profiled in many studies are somewhat heterogeneous, containing only a fraction of true LSCs; thus, there have been efforts to improve immunophenotypic enrichment of LSCs. Studies coupling immunophenotyping of AML samples and xenotransplantation have identified that LSC populations in over 90% of cases bear a $Lin^-CD34^+CD38^-CD90^-$ immunophenotype (Goardon et al. 2011; Thomas and Majeti 2017). Ideally, a therapeutic target for AML should be highly expressed in this compartment to increase accuracy and reduce targeting irrelevant populations that may contain many normal clones. TIM-3, IL1RAP, and CD96 have been specifically shown to be up-regulated in this population in AML specimens (Jan et al. 2011; Barreyro et al. 2012). Aside from intratumor heterogeneity, contamination with some normal HSPC has not been fully avoided by most profiling approaches. Most studies have hence analyzed mixed populations of leukemic and normal stem cells, leaving unexplored whether expression is fully specific to leukemic cells or to some extent reflects a systemic feature of (otherwise normal) HSPC in a leukemic microenvironment. Transplantation studies combining index FACS sorting and single-clone sequencing can potentially improve this by identifying which surface markers are in fact marking stem cells that are part of the leukemic clone(s) (Jan et al. 2011), keeping in mind that xenograft models leave room for "false negatives" such as LSCs or relevant pre-leukemic clones that do not engraft into immunodeficient mice for various reasons.

Expression on Normal HSC and Other Tissues

As demonstrated by toxicities associated with CD33- and CD123-directed therapies, the expression (albeit often lower) of LSC antigens on normal HSC complicates the therapeutic efficacy of many otherwise potent targets. Therefore, studies have sought to identify markers of LSCs that truly distinguish them from normal HSCs to minimize off-tumor, on-target toxicity. Some LSC antigens found to be absent from normal BM HSC include CD32, CLL-1, and IL1RAP (see Tables 1 and 2 for relevant references), so developing therapies against these proteins may result in reduced toxicity. Although some studies have detected its expression on normal HSC, TIM-3 expression has been demonstrated to distinguish residual, normal HSCs from LSCs in AML patient specimens using xenotransplantation (Jan et al. 2011), providing evidence of a strong therapeutic window for this target as well. Minimal expression of therapeutic targets on normal HSC and hematopoietic progenitors is particularly important for immunotherapeutic approaches as cells with any expression of the target may be eliminated. Along these lines, an ideal therapeutic target should be minimally expressed in normal tissues, particularly those that are vital.

Timing in AML Pathogenesis

A relationship between the order of mutations in AML and whether these mutations predict relapse has begun to be established. As *DNMT3A*, *TET2*, and *ASXL1* mutations (which often occur early and are associated with CH) detected in MRD were found not to be predictive of relapse while mutations in *NPM1* were predictive (Jongen-Lavrencic et al. 2018), mutations acquired after the initial CH stage in leukemogenesis may be better markers of MRD than CH markers. Likewise, immunophenotypic markers expressed after the CH stage may be more efficient and less toxic therapeutic targets than early markers whose expression may occur on nondiseased, clonal hematopoietic cells. One indication that aberrant expression of a target commonly occurs in this timeframe is if expression predicts relapse when detected at the complete remission/MRD stage; this has been shown to be the case for CLL-1 (van Rhenen et al. 2007b). It has been proposed that FLT3 mutations may be useful in MRD diagnosis because of their presence only on frank, leukemic clones (Corces et al. 2017); however, the limited efficacy of FLT3 targeting in AML suggests that very late hits in the leukemic progression may not be ideal targets either. Therefore, a target that is not commonly expressed on cells only harboring CH-associated mutations but that is expressed in later pre-leukemic stages may be most efficient at eliminating malignant and relevant premalignant stem cells while sparing normal hematopoietic clones. Whereas the order of genetic hits in AML has been elucidated by various model systems and methods, future studies should monitor the timing of aberrant cell-surface protein expression on LSCs throughout the process of leukemic transformation. For instance, the expression of potential LSC targets could be measured by flow cytometry in serial samples collected from patients progressing from CH to AML, and in cells harboring progressive numbers of leukemia-relevant driver mutations.

Target Functionality

Aside from differential expression on leukemic versus normal HSCs, functionality is also prudent for an LSC target. Whereas, in principle, certain targeted therapies such as immunotherapeutic approaches do not depend on a target having a cancer cell-intrinsic function to be effective, without functionality, down-regulation or mutation of the target, could readily lead to resistance to any type of therapeutic agent (Fig. 2A). Functionality also provides an opportunity for a larger therapeutic window in the case that a therapeutic target is expressed in normal HSPC or other tissues; if a leukemic cell is more dependent on the target for cell survival than a normal cell, a targeting strategy that inhibits the target's function could be preferentially cytotoxic to the leukemic cells while sparing normal cells (Fig. 2B). CD44, CD47, TIM-3, CLL-1, and IL1RAP have been found to play a functional role in AML cells, while the roles of many other LSC targets have yet to be explored (Tables 1 and 2).

Table 1. Antigens expressed on LSC-enriched populations with limited specificity or functionality

Gene	Evidence as a leukemic stem marker	Described function in AML?	Investigation of targeting strategies in AML	Expression in normal tissues[a]
CD9	Protein expressed on AML $CD34^+CD38^-$ cells in 75%–90% of patients, expressed on normal BM $CD34^+CD38^-$ cells in 50%–75% of healthy donors (Sadovnik et al. 2017) Protein up-regulation on $CD34^+CD19^-CD13^+/CD33^+$ AML versus normal BM cells in 29% of patients, expression persists at relapse (Coustan-Smith et al. 2018) Protein expression correlated with failure of induction therapy (Wu et al. 2016)	Not described	N/A	Ubiquitous
IL2RA (*CD25*)	Protein up-regulation on $CD34^+CD38^-$ AML versus normal BM or CB cells in ~25% of samples; no expression on normal $CD34^+CD38^-CD133^+$ BM cells (Saito et al. 2010; de Boer et al. 2018) Protein expressed on AML $CD34^+CD38^-$ cells in 50%–75% of patients, expressed on normal BM $CD34^+CD38^-$ cells in 15%–50% of healthy donors (Herrmann et al. 2014; Sadovnik et al. 2017) Protein expression correlates with treatment failure (Terwijn et al. 2009; Cerny et al. 2013; Allan et al. 2018)	Not described	Phase I clinical trial: NCT02588092 (Flynn et al. 2016; Madhumathi et al. 2017)	Hematopoietic (some HSCs, activated T cells, activated B cells, basophils) (Vincenti et al. 1998; Brisslert et al. 2006; Saito et al. 2010)
FCGR2A (*CD32*)	Protein up-regulation on $CD34^+CD38^-$ AML versus normal BM or CB cells in ~34% of samples; expression on $<2\%$ of normal $CD34^+CD38^-CD133^+$ BM cells (Saito et al. 2010) Protein expression distinguishes leukemic versus normal $CD34^+CD38^-$ cells (Ho et al. 2016) Protein up-regulation on $CD34^+CD19^-CD13^+/CD33^+$ AML versus normal BM cells in 31% of patients; expression persists at relapse (Coustan-Smith et al. 2018)	Not described	N/A	Hematopoietic (macrophages, B cells)
CD44	Protein expression on $CD34^+CD38^-$ AML cells in all patients analyzed (Florian et al. 2006; Sadovnik et al. 2017) Protein up-regulation on $CD34^+CD19^-CD13^+/CD33^+$ AML versus normal BM cells in 35% of patients; expression persists at relapse (Coustan-Smith et al. 2018)	Homing, engraftment, proliferation, and cell survival signaling (Jin et al. 2006; Hertweck et al. 2011)	Phase I clinical trial: NCT01641250 (Song et al. 2004; Jin et al. 2006; Quéré et al. 2011)	Ubiquitous (Liu and Jiang 2006)

Cite this article as *Cold Spring Harb Perspect Med* doi: 10.1101/cshperspect.a036251

	Some protein expression on normal BM $CD34^{+}CD38^{-}$ and $CD34^{+}CD38^{+}$ cells (Reuss-Borst et al. 1992; Liesveld et al. 1994; Jin et al. 2006; Liu and Jiang 2006; Sadovnik et al. 2017)			
CD47	Significant protein up-regulation on AML $lymphoid^{-}CD34^{+}CD38^{-}CD90^{-}$ cells versus normal BM HSC ($lymphoid^{-}CD34^{+}CD38^{-}CD90^{+}$) and MPP ($lymphoid^{-}CD34^{+}CD38^{-}CD90^{-}CD45RA^{-}$); some protein expression on normal BM HSC and MPP (Majeti et al. 2009b) Protein expressed on AML $CD34^{+}CD38^{-}$ cells in >90% of patients, expressed on normal BM $CD34^{+}CD38^{-}$ cells in >90% of healthy donors (Sadovnik et al. 2017) Expressed on 100% of normal BM $CD34^{+}$ cells (de Boer et al. 2018) No significant protein up-regulation on $CD34^{+}CD19^{-}CD13^{+}/CD33^{+}$ AML versus normal BM cells (Coustan-Smith et al. 2018)	CD47-SIRPα interaction inhibits phagocytosis by macrophages (Jaiswal et al. 2009)	Phase I clinical trials: NCT02641002 (terminated), NCT02663518, NCT02678338, NCT03248479 (Majeti et al. 2009b; for review, see Murata et al. 2018)	Ubiquitous (Majeti et al. 2009b)
CD52 (Campath-1)	Protein up-regulation on $CD45^{+}CD34^{+}CD38^{-}$ MDS and AML cells versus AML complete remission samples (Blatt et al. 2014) Protein expressed on AML $CD34^{+}CD38^{-}$ cells in 50%–75% of patients, expressed on normal BM $CD34^{+}CD38^{-}$ cells in 50%–75% of healthy donors (Sadovnik et al. 2017) Protein up-regulation on $CD34^{+}CD19^{-}CD13^{+}/CD33^{+}$ AML versus normal BM cells in 35% of patients; expression persists at relapse (Coustan-Smith et al. 2018) Some protein expression on normal BM $CD34^{+}CD38^{-}$ cells (Olweus et al. 1994)	Not described	Saito et al. 2011; Blatt et al. 2014	Not described
CD93	Protein up-regulation on $CD34^{+}CD38^{-}$ AML versus normal BM or CB in ~7% of samples (Saito et al. 2010) Specific protein expression on $CD34^{+}CD38^{-}$ MLL-rearranged AML cells versus non-MLL-rearranged AML cells; absence of protein expression on $CD34^{+}CD38^{-}$ CB cells; increased leukemia initiating frequency in $CD34^{+}CD38^{-}CD93^{+}$ versus $CD34^{+}CD38^{-}CD93^{-}$ AML (MLL-AF9) cells (Iwasaki et al. 2015)	Not described	Iwasaki et al. 2015	Hematopoietic (platelets, neutrophils, monocytes, macrophages, some B-cell precursors, some dendritic and NK cells, HSCs); microglia; endothelial cells (Fonseca et al. 2001;

Continued

Table 1. *Continued*

Gene	Evidence as a leukemic stem marker	Described function in AML?	Investigation of targeting strategies in AML	Expression in normal tissues[a]
	Protein expressed on AML $CD34^+CD38^-$ cells in 75%–90% of patients, expressed on normal BM $CD34^+CD38^-$ cells in 50%–75% of healthy donors (Sadovnik et al. 2017) Protein expression on 99% of CB $Lin^-CD34^+CD38^-$ cells (Danet et al. 2002) Protein up-regulation on $CD34^+CD19^-CD13^+/CD33^+$ AML versus normal BM cells in 15% of patients, expression persists at relapse (Coustan-Smith et al. 2018)			Danet et al. 2002; McGreal et al. 2002)
CD96 (tactile)	Significant protein up-regulation on $CD34^+CD38^-$ AML versus normal BM cells (Gramatzki et al. 1998; Kikushige et al. 2010; Du et al. 2015) Significant protein up-regulation on $CD34^+CD38^-$ AML cells (specifically $CD90^-$) compared to normal $Lin^-CD34^+CD38^-$ BM cells in 2/3 of AML samples examined; >85% of $CD34^+CD38^-CD96^+$ AML cells did not express lineage markers; increased leukemia initiating frequency in $CD34^+CD38^-CD96^+$ versus $CD34^+CD38^-CD96^-$ AML cells (Hosen et al. 2007) Expressed on 5%–20% of normal BM $CD34^+CD38^-$ cells (Hosen et al. 2007) Protein expressed on AML $CD34^+CD38^-$ cells in 15%–50% of patients, expressed on normal BM $CD34^+CD38^-$ cells in <15% of healthy donors (Sadovnik et al. 2017)	Potential inhibitory role in immune function (for review, see Georgiev et al. 2018)	Mohseni Nodehi et al. 2012; Kellner et al. 2013	Hematopoietic (T cells, NK cells, some HSCs); epithelial (mucosal, vascular) (Perna et al. 2017)

	Protein up-regulation on CD34$^+$CD19$^-$CD13$^+$/CD33$^+$ AML versus normal BM cells in 49% of patients; expression persists at relapse (Coustan-Smith et al. 2018) Complete remission rate lower in patients with higher percentage of CD34$^+$CD38$^-$CD96$^+$ cells (Du et al. 2015); high expression associated with poorer overall survival (Jiang et al. 2017)			
CD99	Protein expression distinguishes functionally normal from leukemia-initiating Lin$^-$CD34$^+$CD38$^-$ cells in AML samples (Jan et al. 2012) CD99$^-$CD34$^+$CD38$^-$ AML cells lack leukemia-relevant mutations and have multilineage potential (Chung et al. 2017) Expressed on 100% of normal BM CD34$^+$ cells (de Boer et al. 2018) Protein overexpression on CD34$^+$CD19$^-$CD13$^+$/CD33$^+$ AML versus normal BM cells in 26% of patients (Coustan-Smith et al. 2018)	Not described	Chung et al. 2017	Ubiquitous
ADGRG1 (*GPR56*)	Protein highly expressed on AML cells that positively engrafted in immunodeficient mice; protein expressed on healthy CD34$^+$ cells (Pabst et al. 2016) Ectopic expression of Gpr56 significantly accelerated HOXA9-induced leukemogenesis in mice (Daria et al. 2016)	Not described	Daria et al. 2016; Saha et al. 2018	Hematopoietic (cytotoxic T cells, NK cells); epithelial (lung, GI tract, epidermal cells, reproductive and endocrine tissues); hepatocytes; kidney cells

AML, Acute myeloid leukemia; BM, bone marrow; CB, cord blood; GI, gastrointestinal; HSC, hematopoietic stem cell; MPP, multipotent progenitor; NK, natural killer.

[a]Expression data was gathered from Human Protein Atlas (Uhlen et al. 2015), Proteomics Database (Kim et al. 2014), and Human Proteome Map (Wilhelm et al. 2014), as well as the noted references.

Table 2. Functional LSC targets with no expression on normal/functional HSC

Gene	Evidence as a leukemic stem marker	Described function in AML?	Investigation of targeting strategies	Expression in normal tissues[a]
HAVCR2 (*CD366*, *TIM-3*)	Significant protein up-regulation on $CD34^+CD38^-$ AML versus normal BM cells; no expression on normal HSC (Kikushige et al. 2010; Haubner et al. 2019) Protein up-regulation on $CD34^+CD19^-CD13^+$/$CD33^+$ AML versus normal BM cells in 41% of patients; expression persists at relapse (Coustan-Smith et al. 2018) Significantly higher expression on lymphoid$^-$$CD34^+CD38^-CD90^-$ AML versus lymphoid$^-$$CD34^+CD38^-CD90^+$ normal BM cells; lymphoid$^-$$CD34^+$TIM-$3^+$ AML cells gave rise to leukemia in immunodeficient mice, whereas lymphoid$^-$$CD34^+$TIM-$3^-$ did not; expression on ~30% of normal BM lymphoid$^-$$CD34^+CD38^-$ cells (Jan et al. 2011) TIM-3 expression marks functional LSCs and distinguishes leukemic versus normal $CD34^+CD38^-$ cells (Ho et al. 2016)	Galactin-9-mediated signal transduction leading to MCL-1 expression and cell survival (Kikushige et al. 2015)	Kikushige et al. 2010	Hematopoietic (monocytes, some NK cells, GMPs) (Haubner et al. 2019)
CLEC12A (*CD371*, *CLL-1*)	Protein expression on $CD34^+CD38^-$ AML cells; absence of protein expression on normal BM, regenerating BM, and mobilized peripheral blood $CD34^+CD38^-$ cells (Bakker et al. 2004; van Rhenen et al. 2007a,b; Kikushige et al. 2010; Sadovnik et al. 2017; Bill et al. 2018; de Boer et al. 2018; Haubner et al. 2019)	Potential negative regulation of immune system (Han et al. 2004; Marshall et al. 2004; Chen et al. 2006; Gagné et al. 2013; Neumann et al. 2014)	Phase I clinical trial: NCT03038230 (Zhao et al. 2010; Lu et al. 2014; Laborda et al. 2017; Leong et al. 2017; Tashiro et al. 2017; Jiang et al. 2018; Wang et al. 2018; Zheng et al. 2019; for review, see Morsink et al. 2019)	Hematopoietic (myeloid) (Bakker et al. 2004; Perna et al. 2017; Haubner et al. 2019)

	$FSC^{low}SSC^{low}CD38^{low}$ side population cells from AML patients were 2%–100% positive for CLL-1 and cytogenetically abnormal, $FSC^{low}SSC^{low}CD38^{low}$ side population cells from normal BM were 0%–4% positive for CLL-1 (Moshaver et al. 2008) $CD34^+CD38^-CLL\text{-}1^+$ cells gave rise to leukemia in immunodeficient mice, protein expression persists in remission and relapse (van Rhenen et al. 2007b)			
IL1RAP	Significant protein overexpression on AML versus normal $Lin^-CD34^+CD38^-$ BM cells; IL1RAP protein is absent from normal $Lin^-CD34^+CD38^-$ cells; cytogenetically abnormal cells were contained in the $IL1RAP^+$ fraction of AML specimens (Barreyro et al. 2012) Increased IL1RAP expression on AML $CD34^+CD38^-$ cells versus normal BM $CD34^+CD38^-$ cells (Askmyr et al. 2013) IL1RAP protein expression distinguishes leukemic versus normal $CD34^+CD38^-$ cells (Ho et al. 2016) Protein expressed on $CD34^+CD38^-$ AML cells in 50%–75% of all AML samples and absent from normal $CD34^+CD38^-$ cells (Jaras et al. 2010; Sadovnik et al. 2017; de Boer et al. 2018) Protein expression persists in relapse (Ho et al. 2016; de Boer et al. 2018)	Facilitates IL-1 and receptor tyrosine kinase signaling (Ågerstam et al. 2015; Mitchell et al. 2018)	Askmyr et al. 2013; Ågerstam et al. 2015; Mitchell et al. 2018	Hematopoietic (monocytes/ macrophages, lowly expressed on myeloid progenitors, lymphocytes, NK cells, and mast cells) (Jaras et al. 2010); epithelial (lowly expressed in GI tract, reproductive, and endocrine tissues) (Ågerstam et al. 2015); lowly expressed on skin fibroblasts and keratinocytes

AML, Acute myeloid leukemia; BM, bone marrow; HSC, hematopoietic stem cell; CB, cord blood; GI, gastrointestinal; MPP, multipotent progenitor; NK, natural killer; GMP, granulocyte-macrophage progenitor; IL, interleukin.

[a]Expression data was gathered from Human Protein Atlas (Uhlen et al. 2015), Proteomics Database (Kim et al. 2014), and Human Proteome Map (Wilhelm et al. 2014), as well as the noted references.

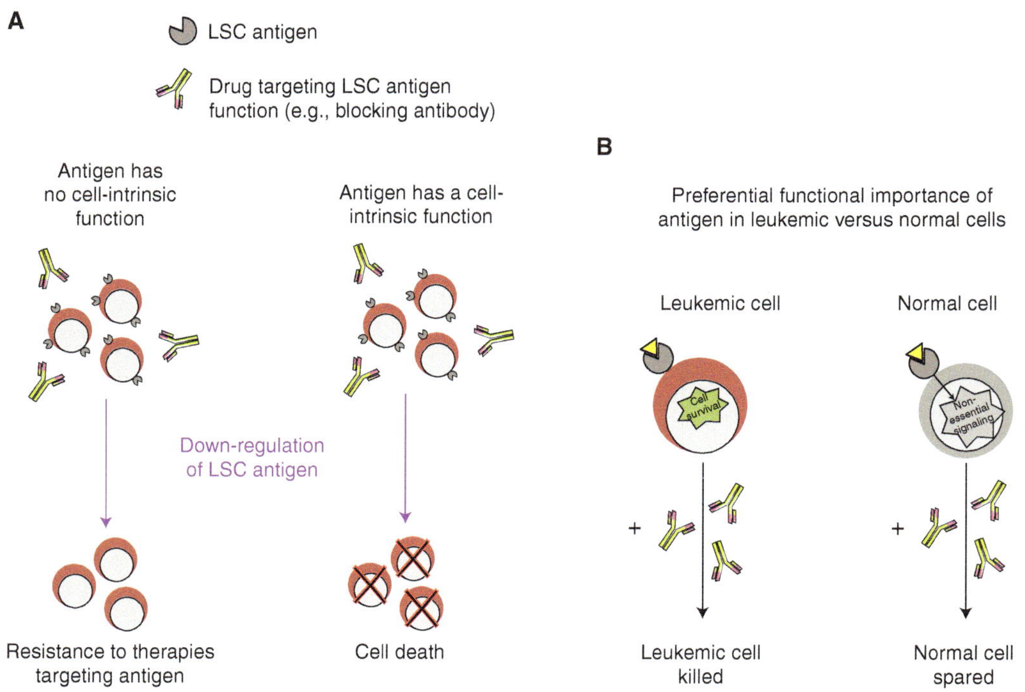

Figure 2. Importance of target functionality for therapeutic targeting. (*A*) If a therapeutic target does not have a cell-intrinsic function in leukemic cells, leukemic cells may be able to escape elimination by the drug through down-regulating the target. (*B*) If a target provides essential signaling in leukemic cells but is dispensable for normal cells, even normal cells expressing the target could be spared by a drug that inhibits the target's function (but would likely be eliminated with an immunotherapeutic approach or antibody–drug conjugate).

Targeting Strategy

Target function and relative expression in leukemic and normal cells are important factors for determining which therapeutic modality will create a proper balance between elimination of leukemic cells and sparing of normal cells. A direct targeting approach (such as a blocking antibody or small molecule inhibitor) may reduce on-target off-tumor toxicity in the presence of lower levels of antigen on normal HSPC than on LSCs or preferential dependence of leukemic versus normal cells on the antigen for cell survival. For instance, if a normal cell expresses the target but is not reliant on it for its function, this cell could be spared by a direct targeting approach but would be killed by an immunotherapeutic approach or antibody–drug conjugate (Fig. 2B). In addition, while immunotherapeutic approaches (such as CAR T cells, bispecific T-cell engager antibodies, and antibodies capable of Fc-mediated recruitment) in other hematologic malignancies have shown effectiveness in eliminating cells with even minimal expression of the relevant target (Cheson and Leonard 2008; June and Sadelain 2018), patients with AML often have aberrant immune responses, thus, antileukemic immune activation may not be effective (Le Dieu et al. 2009). It may therefore be important to explore AML therapies with mechanisms of action dominated by direct targeting and functional inhibition for this reason as well.

Of the LSC therapeutic targets that have been proposed, three targets that best fit the criteria described above are TIM-3, CLL-1, and IL1RAP.

TIM-3

TIM-3 protein was found to be significantly up-regulated on lymphoid^{-}CD34^{+}CD38^{-}CD90^{-}

AML versus lymphoid$^-$CD34$^+$CD38$^-$CD90$^+$ normal BM cells (Jan et al. 2011), and more broadly in CD34$^+$CD38$^-$ (Kikushige et al. 2010; Ho et al. 2016) and myeloid CD34$^+$ cells (Coustan-Smith et al. 2018) in AML versus normal BM samples. TIM-3 has been shown to identify CD34$^+$ AML cells with leukemia initiating activity upon xenotransplantation (Kikushige et al. 2010; Jan et al. 2011; Ho et al. 2016).

There is conflicting data on the expression of TIM-3 in normal HSCs. One study found expression on ~30% of normal BM lymphoid$^-$ CD34$^+$CD38$^-$ cells, but further showed that within this population, TIM-3$^-$ cells contributed to significantly increased multilineage engraftment in immunocompromised mice than TIM-3$^+$ cells, leading to the conclusion that functional HSCs are primarily TIM-3$^-$ (Jan et al. 2011). However, other studies found no TIM-3 expression on normal BM CD34$^+$CD38$^-$ cells (Kikushige et al. 2010; Haubner et al. 2019). TIM-3 expression is restricted to the hematopoietic system, within which TIM-3 is only expressed on monocytes and a fraction of natural killer cells and GMPs (Kikushige et al. 2010; Haubner et al. 2019).

A TIM-3-directed monoclonal antibody reduced engraftment of primary AML cells in immunodeficient mice and minimized AML engraftment upon secondary transplantation, indicating LSCs were targeted. Normal CD34$^+$ cord blood cells were not affected in similar xenograft/antibody experiments. The authors attributed the effects on AML cells to antibody-dependent cell-mediated cytotoxicity (ADCC) and complement-dependent cytotoxicity (CDC) (Kikushige et al. 2010).

TIM-3 has been described to be a receptor for a molecule secreted by AML cells, galactin-9 (Gal-9). Kikushige and colleagues demonstrated that TIM-3 activation by Gal-9 led to activation of Akt, ERK, and NF-κB, and to nuclear translocation of β-catenin in primary AML cells. They also showed that Gal-9 is functionally important for LSCs as antibody-mediated neutralization of Gal-9 reduced engraftment of CD34$^+$ AML cells in xenograft models (including the CD34$^+$ CD38$^-$ population) but did not affect engraftment of normal human cord blood cells (Kikushige et al. 2015). Finally, because expression of TIM-3 persists at relapse in most patients, these cells are likely part of a therapy-refractory clone (Ho et al. 2016; Coustan-Smith et al. 2018).

CLL-1

Expression of CLL-1 has been reported on CD34$^+$CD38$^-$ as well as FSC^{low}SSC^{low}CD38^{low} SP AML cells by several groups; meanwhile, expression is absent on these populations in normal BM, on regenerating BM CD34$^+$CD38$^-$ cells, and on mobilized peripheral blood CD34$^+$CD38$^-$ cells (Bakker et al. 2004; van Rhenen et al. 2007a,b; Moshaver et al. 2008; Kikushige et al. 2010; Sadovnik et al. 2017; Bill et al. 2018; de Boer et al. 2018; Haubner et al. 2019). Further, CLL-1$^+$ AML cells were found to be cytogenetically abnormal (Moshaver et al. 2008) and CD34$^+$CD38$^-$CLL-1$^+$ AML cells gave rise to leukemia in immunodeficient mice (van Rhenen et al. 2007b).

CLL-1 expression has only been detected in the hematopoietic system (Bakker et al. 2004), where it is expressed by some normal myeloid cells, including monocytes, macrophages, dendritic cells, granulocytes, and myeloid precursors (primarily GMPs, but also on a smaller percentage on CMPs and megakaryocyte–erythrocyte progenitors) (Bakker et al. 2004; Perna et al. 2017; Bill et al. 2018; de Boer et al. 2018; Haubner et al. 2019). No significant increase in CLL-1 expression was found in immunophenotypic myeloid progenitors in AML versus normal samples (Coustan-Smith et al. 2018; de Boer et al. 2018) and expression of CLL-1 is lower in LSCs compared to bulk AML cells and normal mature myeloid cells (de Boer et al. 2018). These may be important caveats for therapeutic targeting of this protein.

Several CLL-1-directed therapies have been developed that lead to cytotoxicity in AML cell lines and primary AML cells, as well as in AML cell line xenografts, while sparing normal HSCs (for a review, see Morsink et al. 2019). These include monoclonal antibodies (Zhao et al. 2010), antibody–drug conjugates (Jiang et al. 2018; Zheng et al. 2019), CLL-1/CD3 bispecific antibodies (Lu et al. 2014; Leong et al. 2017), and anti-CLL-1 CAR T cells (Laborda et al. 2017; Tashiro et al. 2017; Wang et al. 2018). A CLL-1/CD3 bispecific antibody (MCLA-117) is being tested in a phase I clinical trial in patients with AML (NCT03038230), as is a compound CLL-1/CD33 CAR T-cell therapy (Liu et al. 2018).

Given the high expression of CLL-1 in monocytes and granulocytes, CLL-1-directed therapies may have toxicity issues. This is evidenced by studies showing that only bispecific antibodies with low (vs. high) affinity for T cells were tolerated in preclinical trials in monkeys (Leong et al. 2017), and CLL-1 antibody–drug conjugates and CAR T cells were cytotoxic to mature normal myeloid cells (Tashiro et al. 2017; Zheng et al. 2019). CAR T approaches against this target must incorporate a suicide system for safety reasons (Tashiro et al. 2017). It will be important to test the relative functional relevance of CLL-1 in these normal cell types versus AML cells to determine whether a strategy that blocks the function of CLL-1 instead of recruiting the immune system might limit toxicity. In this light, studies on CLL-1 (Clec12a) knockout mice provide some encouragement. Although the number of *Clecl12a*$^{-/-}$ mice born is lower than Mendelian ratios, once born, *Clecl12a*$^{-/-}$ mice have no major abnormalities, a normal life span, and no signs of disease. These mice show normal cellularity in hematopoietic organs and no changes in frequency of mature hematopoietic cells compared to WT mice (Neumann et al. 2014). These studies suggest a broadly nonessential role of CLL-1.

Although a specific role for CLL-1 has not been studied in leukemia or cancer in general, studies in normal hematopoietic cells indicate it plays a role in negative regulation of the immune system. For instance, CLL-1 was found to physically associate with the signaling phosphatases SHP-1 and SHP-2, inhibiting activation of immune cells through a cytoplasmic inhibitory motif (Han et al. 2004; Marshall et al. 2004). CLL-1 was shown to be involved in Toll-like receptor and T-cell activation pathways (such as CD40L) through regulating cytokine production (Chen et al. 2006). It was also found that CLL-1 dampens immune responses triggered by damage-associated molecular patterns (Gagné et al. 2013; Neumann et al. 2014). Together, these studies suggest that CLL-1 normally inhibits some inflammatory processes, and suggest the role of CLL-1 in leukemia could be to modulate immune responses as an immune-evasion mechanism.

Lastly, CLL-1 expression persists in remission and relapse in most patients, implying CLL-1 is part of a chemotherapy-resistant clone (van Rhenen et al. 2007b; Coustan-Smith et al. 2018; Haubner et al. 2019). Specifically, CLL-1 expression on $CD34^{+}CD38^{-}$ cells at complete remission was associated with relapse in several patients and more strongly correlated with relapse than did standard MRD detection by leukemia-associated (immune) phenotype expression. Furthermore, lasting remissions occurred in patients with low or absent CLL-1 expression in the stem cell population at complete remission (van Rhenen et al. 2007b).

IL1RAP

IL1RAP gene expression was specifically shown to be significantly up-regulated in AML $Lin^{-}CD34^{+}CD38^{-}CD90^{-}$ cells (a population highly enriched for LSCs; Goardon et al. 2011) compared to this population in age-matched healthy BM samples (Barreyro et al. 2012). Multiple additional studies have identified IL1RAP as a target for LSC-directed therapy in AML based on its surface expression in HSC-enriched populations from AML specimens (Askmyr et al. 2013; Bonardi et al. 2013; Ho et al. 2016; Sadovnik et al. 2017).

IL1RAP protein expression is absent from normal HSCs (Jaras et al. 2010; Barreyro et al. 2012; Ho et al. 2016; Sadovnik et al. 2017; de Boer et al. 2018), but is present in mature cells of the immune system, primarily monocytes and macrophages, and to a lesser extent lymphocytes, natural killer cells, and mast cells. It is lowly expressed on some myeloid progenitors as well (Jaras et al. 2010; Barreyro et al. 2012; de Boer et al. 2018). It is known that the canonical ligand for the IL1RAP/IL-1 receptor complex, IL-1β, acts on epithelial cells, fibroblasts, keratinocytes, endothelial cells, muscle cells, and neurons (Striz 2017); thus, IL1RAP may be

 Cite this article as *Cold Spring Harb Perspect Med* doi: 10.1101/cshperspect.a036251

expressed in these tissues, at least in the inflammatory setting. Protein array data confirms low IL1RAP expression in some of these tissues (Kim et al. 2014; Wilhelm et al. 2014; Ågerstam et al. 2015; Uhlen et al. 2015). Toxicity in these cell types would be important to monitor if IL1RAP-directed therapies move forward. However, given that total body *Il1rap*$^{-/-}$ mice do not have overt abnormalities, and *Il1rap*$^{-/-}$ BM is capable of complete and long-term (>20 wk) reconstitution of lymphoid and myeloid hematopoietic cells (Mitchell et al. 2018), on-target, off-tumor toxicity may be limited.

Several groups have targeted IL1RAP in AML using different strategies. Some have focused on the utility of IL1RAP as a surface label and target for immune effector cells in AML. For instance, an IL1RAP-directed monoclonal antibody significantly reduced leukemic burden in BM and spleens of mice transplanted with *MLL-AF9* and activated *NRAS* cotransduced cord blood cells as well as mice transplanted with primary AML cells, with effects attributed to natural killer cell ADCC activity (Ågerstam et al. 2015). These studies have led to testing of an IL1RAP-directed antibody in a phase I clinical trial (CANFOUR trial) where dose escalation will first be tested in patients with solid malignant tumors (NCT03267316). Jiang and colleagues showed in a xenograft of the AML cell line EOL-1 that several different IL1RAP-directed monoclonal antibodies completely eliminated AML engraftment in BM and blood. These antibodies induced CDC of primary AML blasts when incubated with cells and complement in vitro (Jiang et al. 2016). Additionally, an IL1RAP/CD3 bispecific antibody is in development, and both in vivo and in vitro effects on the MV4;11 AML cell line were presented at the 2017 American Society of Hematology meeting (Meng et al. 2017).

The functional importance of IL1RAP in leukemic cells has also been tested. shRNA-mediated knockdown of IL1RAP in primary AML cells led to reduced clonogenic growth and in AML cell lines led to reduced engraftment in immunodeficient mice. In addition, IL1RAP-directed antibodies increased apoptosis of primary AML cells in the absence of immune effector cells but spared normal hematopoietic cells. These IL1RAP-directed antibodies nearly eliminated leukemic cells in the BM in AML cell line xenografts. Finally, *Il1rap* loss impaired LSC function/frequency in MLL-AF9-driven AML. These studies imply that IL1RAP is functionally important for growth and survival of AML cells (Mitchell et al. 2018).

Specific functions of IL1RAP in AML cells have been recently explored. IL1RAP antibodies inhibited IL-1-induced AML cell growth (Ågerstam et al. 2015) and signaling (Mitchell et al. 2018) in vitro. In MLL-AF9 AML, shRNA-mediated knockdown of IL1RAP led to reduced degradation of the WT MLL protein, which normally competes with the MLL-AF9 fusion; thus, IL1RAP targeting reduced MLL-AF9 occupancy and aberrant transcription (Liang et al. 2017). Whereas the canonical role of IL1RAP is to facilitate signaling through the IL-1 pathway, several lines of evidence suggest that IL1RAP has alternative or at least additional mechanisms in AML. *FLT3 WT* and *FLT3* mutant AML cells were found to be differentially sensitive to IL1RAP antibody-mediated inhibition, which led to studies demonstrating that IL1RAP modulates FLT3 ligand-mediated signaling and that growth and these two proteins physically interact. This relationship was also demonstrated for the receptor tyrosine kinase c-KIT (Mitchell et al. 2018). Thus, AML cells may use up-regulation of IL1RAP as a way to amplify multiple signaling pathways involved in cell survival and proliferation.

High *IL1RAP* expression in AML correlates with poor prognosis (Barreyro et al. 2012; de Boer et al. 2018), and IL1RAP expression persists at relapse (de Boer et al. 2018). IL1RAP expression may be associated with the acquisition of certain mutations, as it was found to mark genetically distinct AML subclones such as those with *NRAS* mutations (de Boer et al. 2018). In monosomy 7 AML patient samples, the clone size of IL1RAP^{+} AML HSPCs included and exceeded that of cells bearing the chromosomal aberration, suggesting IL1RAP overexpression preceded loss of chromosome 7, potentially marking a pre-leukemic cell population. The timing of IL1RAP overexpression in leukemic transformation should be further explored in future studies.

CONCLUDING REMARKS

For AML patients over the age of 65, which represent the majority (Noone et al. 2018), the 5-year overall survival is currently only estimated to be ∼14%, and has improved marginally in the last 45 years (Mokdad et al. 2017; Lancet 2018). In recent years, therapeutic advances leading to improved patient outcomes in AML are a result of the optimization of existing drugs rather than the use of novel therapeutics (Fernandez et al. 2009; Lancet et al. 2017; Wei and Tiong 2017). Clearly, improved and more specific treatments are necessary in this disease, yet a universal antigen that fits all criteria for an ideal LSC target has been challenging to find.

Because of their lack of expression on normal HSC and minimal expression/essentiality on other normal tissues, their functional importance in AML cells, and persistent expression at relapse, we would propose TIM-3, CLL-1, and IL1RAP as the most promising current therapeutic targets to safely eliminate LSCs. Recent findings appear to favor the development of direct targeting strategies against these targets to reduce toxicities and minimize potential resistance mechanisms (Fig. 2). In addition, while CD25 only marks LSCs in a fraction of patients, it appears to be a strong predictor of relapse and may represent another potent drug target in a smaller population of patients.

Although targeting a common immunophenotypic antigen at the stem/progenitor cell level is a potential means to overcoming the daunting genetic complexity, inter- and intrapatient heterogeneity of AML, therapies may still need to be tailored to distinct molecular subtypes of AML, and, accordingly, more studies will be required to relate mutational profiles to cell-surface expression of putative LSC antigens in larger cohorts of patients. Targeting several antigens to eliminate leukemic cells that persist at remission may be necessary (Haubner et al. 2019). Overall, advances in our understanding of AML pathogenesis provide insight into the improvement of LSC-targeted therapies in AML: continued development of the LSC model, including further understanding of the progression from CH to pre-leukemia and AML, hold promise in informing better targets and therapeutic agents for the treatment and cure of AML.

REFERENCES

Abelson S, Collord G, Ng SWK, Weissbrod O, Mendelson Cohen N, Niemeyer E, Barda N, Zuzarte PC, Heisler L, Sundaravadanam Y, et al. 2018. Prediction of acute myeloid leukaemia risk in healthy individuals. *Nature* **559:** 400–404. doi:10.1038/s41586-018-0317-6

Ågerstam H, Karlsson C, Hansen N, Sandén C, Askmyr M, von Palffy S, Högberg C, Rissler M, Wunderlich M, Juliusson G, et al. 2015. Antibodies targeting human IL1RAP (IL1R3) show therapeutic effects in xenograft models of acute myeloid leukemia. *Proc Natl Acad Sci* **112:** 10786–10791. doi:10.1073/pnas.1422749112

Allan JN, Roboz GJ, Askin G, Ritchie E, Scandura J, Christos P, Hassane DC, Guzman ML. 2018. CD25 expression and outcomes in older patients with acute myelogenous leukemia treated with plerixafor and decitabine. *Leuk Lymphoma* **59:** 821–828. doi:10.1080/10428194.2017.1352089

Alvarado Y, Kantarjian HM, Luthra R, Ravandi F, Borthakur G, Garcia-Manero G, Konopleva M, Estrov Z, Andreeff M, Cortes JE. 2014. Treatment with FLT3 inhibitor in patients with *FLT3*-mutated acute myeloid leukemia is associated with development of secondary *FLT3*-tyrosine kinase domain mutations. *Cancer* **120:** 2142–2149. doi:10.1002/cncr.28705

Amadori S, Suciu S, Selleslag D, Stasi R, Alimena G, Baila L, Rizzoli V, Borlenghi E, Gaidano G, Magro D, et al. 2010. Randomized trial of two schedules of low-dose gemtuzumab ozogamicin as induction monotherapy for newly diagnosed acute myeloid leukaemia in older patients not considered candidates for intensive chemotherapy. A phase II study of the EORTC and GIMEMA leukaemia groups (AML-19). *Br J Haematol* **149:** 376–382. doi:10.1111/j.1365-2141.2010.08095.x

Anderson LA, Pfeiffer RM, Landgren O, Gadalla S, Berndt SI, Engels EA. 2009. Risks of myeloid malignancies in patients with autoimmune conditions. *Br J Cancer* **100:** 822–828. doi:10.1038/sj.bjc.6604935

Arends CM, Galan-Sousa J, Hoyer K, Chan W, Jäger M, Yoshida K, Seemann R, Noerenberg D, Waldhueter N, Fleischer-Notter H, et al. 2018. Hematopoietic lineage distribution and evolutionary dynamics of clonal hematopoiesis. *Leukemia* **32:** 1908–1919. doi:10.1038/s41375-018-0047-7

Askmyr M, Agerstam H, Hansen N, Gordon S, Arvanitakis A, Rissler M, Juliusson G, Richter J, Jaras M, Fioretos T. 2013. Selective killing of candidate AML stem cells by antibody targeting of IL1RAP. *Blood* **121:** 3709–3713. doi:10.1182/blood-2012-09-458935

Bakker AB, van den Oudenrijn S, Bakker AQ, Feller N, van Meijer M, Bia JA, Jongeneelen MA, Visser TJ, Bijl N, Geuijen CA, et al. 2004. C-type lectin-like molecule-1: A novel myeloid cell surface marker associated with acute

 Cite this article as *Cold Spring Harb Perspect Med* doi: 10.1101/cshperspect.a036251

myeloid leukemia. *Cancer Res* **64:** 8443–8450. doi:10.1158/0008-5472.CAN-04-1659

Baldridge MT, King KY, Boles NC, Weksberg DC, Goodell MA. 2010. Quiescent haematopoietic stem cells are activated by IFN-γ in response to chronic infection. *Nature* **465:** 793–797. doi:10.1038/nature09135

Baldridge MT, King KY, Goodell MA. 2011. Inflammatory signals regulate hematopoietic stem cells. *Trends Immunol* **32:** 57–65. doi:10.1016/j.it.2010.12.003

Baron J, Wang ES. 2018. Gemtuzumab ozogamicin for the treatment of acute myeloid leukemia. *Expert Rev Clin Pharmacol* **11:** 549–559. doi:10.1080/17512433.2018.1478725

Barreda DR, Hanington PC, Belosevic M. 2004. Regulation of myeloid development and function by colony stimulating factors. *Dev Comp Immunol* **28:** 509–554. doi:10.1016/j.dci.2003.09.010

Barreyro L, Will B, Bartholdy B, Zhou L, Todorova TI, Stanley RF, Ben-Neriah S, Montagna C, Parekh S, Pellagatti A, et al. 2012. Overexpression of IL-1 receptor accessory protein in stem and progenitor cells and outcome correlation in AML and MDS. *Blood* **120:** 1290–1298. doi:10.1182/blood-2012-01-404699

Bereshchenko O, Mancini E, Moore S, Bilbao D, Månsson R, Luc S, Grover A, Jacobsen SE, Bryder D, Nerlov C. 2009. Hematopoietic stem cell expansion precedes the generation of committed myeloid leukemia-initiating cells in C/EBPα mutant AML. *Cancer Cell* **16:** 390–400. doi:10.1016/j.ccr.2009.09.036

Bill M, van Kooten Niekerk PB, Woll PS, Laine Herborg L, Stidsholt Roug A, Hokland P, Nederby L. 2018. Mapping the CLEC12A expression on myeloid progenitors in normal bone marrow; implications for understanding CLEC12A-related cancer stem cell biology. *J Cell Mol Med* **22:** 2311–2318. doi:10.1111/jcmm.13519

Blatt K, Herrmann H, Hoermann G, Willmann M, Cerny-Reiterer S, Sadovnik I, Herndlhofer S, Streubel B, Rabitsch W, Sperr WR, et al. 2014. Identification of campath-1 (CD52) as novel drug target in neoplastic stem cells in 5q-patients with MDS and AML. *Clin Cancer Res* **20:** 3589–3602. doi:10.1158/1078-0432.CCR-13-2811

Bonardi F, Fusetti F, Deelen P, van Gosliga D, Vellenga E, Schuringa JJ. 2013. A proteomics and transcriptomics approach to identify leukemic stem cell (LSC) markers. *Mol Cell Proteomics* **12:** 626–637. doi:10.1074/mcp.M112.021931

Bonnet D, Dick JE. 1997. Human acute myeloid leukemia is organized as a hierarchy that originates from a primitive hematopoietic cell. *Nat Med* **3:** 730–737. doi:10.1038/nm0797-730

Bowman RL, Busque L, Levine RL. 2018. Clonal hematopoiesis and evolution to hematopoietic malignancies. *Cell Stem Cell* **22:** 157–170. doi:10.1016/j.stem.2018.01.011

Boyd-Kirkup J, Thakkar D, Brauer P, Zhou J, Chng WJ, Ingram PJ. 2017. HMBD004, a novel anti-CD47xCD33 bispecific antibody displays potent anti-tumor effects in pre-clinical models of AML. *Blood* **130:** 1378–1378.

Brisslert M, Bokarewa M, Larsson P, Wing K, Collins LV, Tarkowski A. 2006. Phenotypic and functional characterization of human $CD25^+$ B cells. *Immunology* **117:** 548–557. doi:10.1111/j.1365-2567.2006.02331.x

Carbonell F, Swansbury J, Min T, Matutes E, Farahat N, Buccheri V, Morilla R, Secker-Walker L, Catovsky D. 1996. Cytogenetic findings in acute biphenotypic leukaemia. *Leukemia* **10:** 1283–1287.

Castaigne S, Pautas C, Terré C, Raffoux E, Bordessoule D, Bastie JN, Legrand O, Thomas X, Turlure P, Reman O, et al. 2012. Effect of gemtuzumab ozogamicin on survival of adult patients with de-novo acute myeloid leukaemia (ALFA-0701): A randomised, open-label, phase 3 study. *Lancet* **379:** 1508–1516. doi:10.1016/S0140-6736(12)60485-1

Catlin SN, Busque L, Gale RE, Guttorp P, Abkowitz JL. 2011. The replication rate of human hematopoietic stem cells in vivo. *Blood* **117:** 4460–4466. doi:10.1182/blood-2010-08-303537

Cerny J, Yu H, Ramanathan M, Raffel GD, Walsh WV, Fortier N, Shanahan L, O'Rourke E, Bednarik J, Barton B, et al. 2013. Expression of CD25 independently predicts early treatment failure of acute myeloid leukaemia (AML). *Br J Haematol* **160:** 262–266. doi:10.1111/bjh.12109

Chan PM. 2011. Differential signaling of Flt3 activating mutations in acute myeloid leukemia: A working model. *Protein Cell* **2:** 108–115. doi:10.1007/s13238-011-1020-7

Chen CH, Floyd H, Olson NE, Magaletti D, Li C, Draves K, Clark EA. 2006. Dendritic-cell-associated C-type lectin 2 (DCAL-2) alters dendritic-cell maturation and cytokine production. *Blood* **107:** 1459–1467. doi:10.1182/blood-2005-08-3264

Chen F, Ishikawa Y, Akashi A, Naoe T, Kiyoi H. 2016. Co-expression of wild-type FLT3 attenuates the inhibitory effect of FLT3 inhibitor on FLT3 mutated leukemia cells. *Oncotarget* **7:** 47018–47032. doi:10.18632/oncotarget.10147

Chen J, Kao YR, Sun D, Todorova TI, Reynolds D, Narayanagari SR, Montagna C, Will B, Verma A, Steidl AU. 2019. Myelodysplastic syndrome progression to acute myeloid leukemia at the stem cell level. *Nat Med* **25:** 103–110. doi:10.1038/s41591-018-0267-4

Cheson BD, Leonard JP. 2008. Monoclonal antibody therapy for B-cell non-Hodgkin's lymphoma. *N Engl J Med* **359:** 613–626. doi:10.1056/NEJMra0708875

Chung SS, Eng WS, Hu W, Khalaj M, Garrett-Bakelman FE, Tavakkoli M, Levine RL, Carroll M, Klimek VM, Melnick AM, et al. 2017. CD99 is a therapeutic target on disease stem cells in myeloid malignancies. *Sci Transl Med* **9:** eaaj2025. doi:10.1126/scitranslmed.aaj2025

Cohen SM, Purtilo DT, Ellwein LB. 1991. Ideas in pathology. Pivotal role of increased cell proliferation in human carcinogenesis. *Mod Pathol* **4:** 371–382.

Coombs CC, Zehir A, Devlin SM, Kishtagari A, Syed A, Jonsson P, Hyman DM, Solit DB, Robson ME, Baselga J, et al. 2017. Therapy-related clonal hematopoiesis in patients with non-hematologic cancers is common and associated with adverse clinical outcomes. *Cell Stem Cell* **21:** 374–382.e4. doi:10.1016/j.stem.2017.07.010

Corces MR, Chang HY, Majeti R. 2017. Preleukemic hematopoietic stem cells in human acute myeloid leukemia. *Front Oncol* **7:** 263. doi:10.3389/fonc.2017.00263

Corces-Zimmerman MR, Hong WJ, Weissman IL, Medeiros BC, Majeti R. 2014. Preleukemic mutations in human acute myeloid leukemia affect epigenetic regulators and persist in remission. *Proc Natl Acad Sci* **111:** 2548–2553. doi:10.1073/pnas.1324297111

Costello RT, Mallet F, Gaugler B, Sainty D, Arnoulet C, Gastaut JA, Olive D. 2000. Human acute myeloid eukemia CD34$^+$/CD38$^-$ progenitor cells have decreased sensitivity to chemotherapy and Fas-induced apoptosis, reduced immunogenicity, and impaired dendritic cell transformation capacities. *Cancer Res* **60:** 4403–4411.

Coustan-Smith E, Song G, Shurtleff S, Yeoh AE, Chng WJ, Chen SP, Rubnitz JE, Pui CH, Downing JR, Campana D. 2018. Universal monitoring of minimal residual disease in acute myeloid leukemia. *JCI Insight* **3:** 98561. doi:10.1172/jci.insight.98561

Craver BM, El Alaoui K, Scherber RM, Fleischman AG. 2018. The critical role of inflammation in the pathogenesis and progression of myeloid malignancies. *Cancers (Basel)* **10:** E104. doi:10.3390/cancers10040104

Danet GH, Luongo JL, Butler G, Lu MM, Tenner AJ, Simon MC, Bonnet DA. 2002. C1qRp defines a new human stem cell population with hematopoietic and hepatic potential. *Proc Natl Acad Sci* **99:** 10441–10445. doi:10.1073/pnas.162104799

Daria D, Kirsten N, Muranyi A, Mulaw M, Ihme S, Kechter A, Hollnagel M, Bullinger L, Döhner K, Döhner H, et al. 2016. GPR56 contributes to the development of acute myeloid leukemia in mice. *Leukemia* **30:** 1734–1741. doi:10.1038/leu.2016.76

de Boer B, Prick J, Pruis MG, Keane P, Imperato MR, Jaques J, Brouwers-Vos AZ, Hogeling SM, Woolthuis CM, Nijk MT, et al. 2018. Prospective isolation and characterization of genetically and functionally distinct AML subclones. *Cancer Cell* **34:** 674–689.e8. doi:10.1016/j.ccell.2018.08.014

Desai P, Mencia-Trinchant N, Savenkov O, Simon MS, Cheang G, Lee S, Samuel M, Ritchie EK, Guzman ML, Ballman KV, et al. 2018. Somatic mutations precede acute myeloid leukemia years before diagnosis. *Nat Med* **24:** 1015–1023. doi:10.1038/s41591-018-0081-z

Diez-Martin JL, Buno I, Llamas P, Gosalvez J, Lopez-Fernandez C, Polo N, Regidor C. 2000. Fluorescence in situ hybridization evaluation of minimal residual disease on stem-cell harvests. *Cancer Detect Prev* **24:** 169–172.

Ding L, Ley TJ, Larson DE, Miller CA, Koboldt DC, Welch JS, Ritchey JK, Young MA, Lamprecht T, McLellan MD, et al. 2012. Clonal evolution in relapsed acute myeloid leukaemia revealed by whole-genome sequencing. *Nature* **481:** 506–510. doi:10.1038/nature10738

Döhner H, Weisdorf DJ, Bloomfield CD. 2015. Acute myeloid leukemia. *N Engl J Med* **373:** 1136–1152. doi:10.1056/NEJMra1406184

Du W, Hu Y, Lu C, Li J, Liu W, He Y, Wang P, Cheng C, Hu YU, Huang S, et al. 2015. Cluster of differentiation 96 as a leukemia stem cell-specific marker and a factor for prognosis evaluation in leukemia. *Mol Clin Oncol* **3:** 833–838. doi:10.3892/mco.2015.552

Elias HK, Schinke C, Bhattacharyya S, Will B, Verma A, Steidl U. 2014. Stem cell origin of myelodysplastic syndromes. *Oncogene* **33:** 5139–5150. doi:10.1038/onc.2013.520

Engel H, Drach J, Keyhani A, Jiang S, Van NT, Kimmel M, Sanchez-Williams G, Goodacre A, Andreeff M. 1999. Quantitation of minimal residual disease in acute myelogenous leukemia and myelodysplastic syndromes in complete remission by molecular cytogenetics of progenitor cells. *Leukemia* **13:** 568–577. doi:10.1038/sj.leu.2401359

Eppert K, Takenaka K, Lechman ER, Waldron L, Nilsson B, van Galen P, Metzeler KH, Poeppl A, Ling V, Beyene J, et al. 2011. Stem cell gene expression programs influence clinical outcome in human leukemia. *Nat Med* **17:** 1086–1093. doi:10.1038/nm.2415

Esplin BL, Shimazu T, Welner RS, Garrett KP, Nie L, Zhang Q, Humphrey MB, Yang Q, Borghesi LA, Kincade PW. 2011. Chronic exposure to a TLR ligand injures hematopoietic stem cells. *J Immunol* **186:** 5367–5375. doi:10.4049/jimmunol.1003438

Fernandez HF, Sun Z, Yao X, Litzow MR, Luger SM, Paietta EM, Racevskis J, Dewald GW, Ketterling RP, Bennett JM, et al. 2009. Anthracycline dose intensification in acute myeloid leukemia. *N Engl J Med* **361:** 1249–1259. doi:10.1056/NEJMoa0904544

Ferrara F, Schiffer CA. 2013. Acute myeloid leukaemia in adults. *Lancet* **381:** 484–495. doi:10.1016/S0140-6736(12)61727-9

Feuring-Buske M, Haase D, Buske C, Hiddemann W, Wörmann B. 1999. Clonal chromosomal abnormalities in the stem cell compartment of patients with acute myeloid leukemia in morphological complete remission. *Leukemia* **13:** 386–392. doi:10.1038/sj.leu.2401300

Flach J, Bakker ST, Mohrin M, Conroy PC, Pietras EM, Reynaud D, Alvarez S, Diolaiti ME, Ugarte F, Forsberg EC, et al. 2014. Replication stress is a potent driver of functional decline in ageing haematopoietic stem cells. *Nature* **512:** 198–202. doi:10.1038/nature13619

Fleischman AG, Aichberger KJ, Luty SB, Bumm TG, Petersen CL, Doratotaj S, Vasudevan KB, LaTocha DH, Yang F, Press RD, et al. 2011. TNFα facilitates clonal expansion of JAK2V617F positive cells in myeloproliferative neoplasms. *Blood* **118:** 6392–6398. doi:10.1182/blood-2011-04-348144

Florian S, Sonneck K, Hauswirth AW, Krauth MT, Schernthaner GH, Sperr WR, Valent P. 2006. Detection of molecular targets on the surface of CD34$^+$/CD38$^-$ stem cells in various myeloid malignancies. *Leuk Lymphoma* **47:** 207–222. doi:10.1080/10428190500272507

Flynn MJ, Zammarchi F, Tyrer PC, Akarca AU, Janghra N, Britten CE, Havenith CE, Levy JN, Tiberghien A, Masterson LA, et al. 2016. ADCT-301, a pyrrolobenzodiazepine (PBD) dimer-containing antibody-drug conjugate (ADC) targeting CD25-expressing hematological malignancies. *Mol Cancer Ther* **15:** 2709–2721. doi:10.1158/1535-7163.MCT-16-0233

Fonseca MI, Carpenter PM, Park M, Palmarini G, Nelson EL, Tenner AJ. 2001. C1qR(P), a myeloid cell receptor in blood, is predominantly expressed on endothelial cells in human tissue. *J Leukoc Biol* **70:** 793–800.

Fuster JJ, MacLauchlan S, Zuriaga MA, Polackal MN, Ostriker AC, Chakraborty R, Wu CL, Sano S, Muralidharan S, Rius C, et al. 2017. Clonal hematopoiesis associated with TET2 deficiency accelerates atherosclerosis development in mice. *Science* **355:** 842–847. doi:10.1126/science.aag1381

Gagné V, Marois L, Levesque JM, Galarneau H, Lahoud MH, Caminschi I, Naccache PH, Tessier P, Fernandes MJ. 2013. Modulation of monosodium urate crystal-induced responses in neutrophils by the myeloid inhibitory C-type lectin-like receptor: Potential therapeutic implications. *Arthritis Res Ther* **15:** R73. doi:10.1186/ar4250

Genovese G, Kähler AK, Handsaker RE, Lindberg J, Rose SA, Bakhoum SF, Chambert K, Mick E, Neale BM, Fromer M, et al. 2014. Clonal hematopoiesis and blood-cancer risk inferred from blood DNA sequence. *N Engl J Med* **371:** 2477–2487. doi:10.1056/NEJMoa1409405

Gentles AJ, Plevritis SK, Majeti R, Alizadeh AA. 2010. Association of a leukemic stem cell gene expression signature with clinical outcomes in acute myeloid leukemia. *JAMA* **304:** 2706–2715. doi:10.1001/jama.2010.1862

Georgiev H, Ravens I, Papadogianni G, Bernhardt G. 2018. Coming of age: CD96 emerges as modulator of immune responses. *Front Immunol* **9:** 1072. doi:10.3389/fimmu.2018.01072

Ghiaur G, Levis M. 2017. Mechanisms of resistance to FLT3 inhibitors and the role of the bone marrow microenvironment. *Hematol Oncol Clin North Am* **31:** 681–692. doi:10.1016/j.hoc.2017.04.005

Gilliland DG, Griffin JD. 2002. The roles of FLT3 in hematopoiesis and leukemia. *Blood* **100:** 1532–1542. doi:10.1182/blood-2002-02-0492

Goardon N, Marchi E, Atzberger A, Quek L, Schuh A, Soneji S, Woll P, Mead A, Alford KA, Rout R, et al. 2011. Coexistence of LMPP-like and GMP-like leukemia stem cells in acute myeloid leukemia. *Cancer Cell* **19:** 138–152. doi:10.1016/j.ccr.2010.12.012

Graf M, Hecht K, Reif S, Pelka-Fleischer R, Pfister K, Schmetzer H. 2004. Expression and prognostic value of hemopoietic cytokine receptors in acute myeloid leukemia (AML): Implications for future therapeutical strategies. *Eur J Haematol* **72:** 89–106. doi:10.1046/j.0902-4441.2003.00184.x

Gramatzki M, Ludwig WD, Burger R, Moos P, Rohwer P, Grunert C, Sendler A, Kalden JR, Andreesen R, Henschke F, et al. 1998. Antibodies TC-12 ("unique") and TH-111 (CD96) characterize T-cell acute lymphoblastic leukemia and a subgroup of acute myeloid leukemia. *Exp Hematol* **26:** 1209–1214.

Griffin JD, Linch D, Sabbath K, Larcom P, Schlossman SF. 1984. A monoclonal antibody reactive with normal and leukemic human myeloid progenitor cells. *Leuk Res* **8:** 521–534. doi:10.1016/0145-2126(84)90001-8

Haase D, Feuring-Buske M, Konemann S, Fonatsch C, Troff C, Verbeek W, Pekrun A, Hiddemann W, Wormann B. 1995. Evidence for malignant transformation in acute myeloid leukemia at the level of early hematopoietic stem cells by cytogenetic analysis of $CD34^+$ subpopulations. *Blood* **86:** 2906–2912.

Haase D, Feuring-Buske M, Schäfer C, Schoch C, Troff C, Gahn B, Hiddemann W, Wormann B. 1997. Cytogenetic analysis of $CD34^+$ subpopulations in AML and MDS characterized by the expression of CD38 and CD117. *Leukemia* **11:** 674–679. doi:10.1038/sj.leu.2400638

Hahn CN, Ross DM, Feng J, Beligaswatte A, Hiwase DK, Parker WT, Ho M, Zawitkowski M, Ambler KL, Cheetham GD, et al. 2015. A tale of two siblings: Two cases of AML arising from a single pre-leukemic DNMT3A mutant clone. *Leukemia* **29:** 2101–2104. doi:10.1038/leu.2015.67

Han Y, Zhang M, Li N, Chen T, Zhang Y, Wan T, Cao X. 2004. KLRL1, a novel killer cell lectinlike receptor, inhibits natural killer cell cytotoxicity. *Blood* **104:** 2858–2866. doi:10.1182/blood-2004-03-0878

Haubner S, Perna F, Köhnke T, Schmidt C, Berman S, Augsberger C, Schnorfeil FM, Krupka C, Lichtenegger FS, Liu X, et al. 2019. Coexpression profile of leukemic stem cell markers for combinatorial targeted therapy in AML. *Leukemia* **33:** 64–74.

Hauswirth AW, Florian S, Printz D, Sotlar K, Krauth MT, Fritsch G, Schernthaner GH, Wacheck V, Selzer E, Sperr WR, et al. 2007. Expression of the target receptor CD33 in $CD34^+/CD38^-/CD123^+$ AML stem cells. *Eur J Clin Invest* **37:** 73–82. doi:10.1111/j.1365-2362.2007.01746.x

Herrmann H, Sadovnik I, Cerny-Reiterer S, Rulicke T, Stefanzl G, Willmann M, Hoermann G, Bilban M, Blatt K, Herndlhofer S, et al. 2014. Dipeptidylpeptidase IV (CD26) defines leukemic stem cells (LSC) in chronic myeloid leukemia. *Blood* **123:** 3951–3962. doi:10.1182/blood-2013-10-536078

Hertweck MK, Erdfelder F, Kreuzer KA. 2011. CD44 in hematological neoplasias. *Ann Hematol* **90:** 493–508. doi:10.1007/s00277-011-1161-z

Ho TC, LaMere M, Stevens BM, Ashton JM, Myers JR, O'Dwyer KM, Liesveld JL, Mendler JH, Guzman M, Morrissette JD, et al. 2016. Evolution of acute myelogenous leukemia stem cell properties after treatment and progression. *Blood* **128:** 1671–1678. doi:10.1182/blood-2016-02-695312

Hogge DE, Shannon KM, Kalousek DK, Schonberg S, Schaffner V, Zoger S, Eaves CJ, Eaves AC. 1987. Juvenile monosomy 7 syndrome: Evidence that the disease originates in a pluripotent hemopoietic stem cell. *Leuk Res* **11:** 705–709. doi:10.1016/0145-2126(87)90006-3

Hollein A, Jeromin S, Meggendorfer M, Fasan A, Nadarajah N, Kern W, Haferlach C, Haferlach T. 2018. Minimal residual disease (MRD) monitoring and mutational landscape in AML with RUNX1-RUNX1T1: A study on 134 patients. *Leukemia* **32:** 2270–2274. doi:10.1038/s41375-018-0086-0

Hope KJ, Jin L, Dick JE. 2004. Acute myeloid leukemia originates from a hierarchy of leukemic stem cell classes that differ in self-renewal capacity. *Nat Immunol* **5:** 738–743. doi:10.1038/ni1080

Hosen N, Park CY, Tatsumi N, Oji Y, Sugiyama H, Gramatzki M, Krensky AM, Weissman IL. 2007. CD96 is a leukemic stem cell-specific marker in human acute myeloid leukemia. *Proc Natl Acad Sci* **104:** 11008–11013. doi:10.1073/pnas.0704271104

Hourigan CS, Gale RP, Gormley NJ, Ossenkoppele GJ, Walter RB. 2017. Measurable residual disease testing in acute myeloid leukaemia. *Leukemia* **31:** 1482–1490. doi:10.1038/leu.2017.113

Hyakuna N, Naritomi K, Ito E. 1998. Retrospective analysis of clonality and detection of residual disease in myeloid leukemia by FISH on long-term stored bone marrow smears. *Acta Paediatr Jpn* **40:** 318–323. doi:10.1111/j.1442-200X.1998.tb01939.x

Ishikawa F, Yoshida S, Saito Y, Hijikata A, Kitamura H, Tanaka S, Nakamura R, Tanaka T, Tomiyama H, Saito N, et al. 2007. Chemotherapy-resistant human AML stem cells home to and engraft within the bone-marrow endosteal region. *Nat Biotechnol* **25:** 1315–1321. doi:10.1038/nbt1350

Ito K, Hirao A, Arai F, Takubo K, Matsuoka S, Miyamoto K, Ohmura M, Naka K, Hosokawa K, Ikeda Y, et al. 2006. Reactive oxygen species act through p38 MAPK to limit the lifespan of hematopoietic stem cells. *Nat Med* **12:** 446–451. doi:10.1038/nm1388

Iwasaki M, Liedtke M, Gentles AJ, Cleary ML. 2015. CD93 marks a non-quiescent human leukemia stem cell population and is required for development of MLL-rearranged acute myeloid leukemia. *Cell Stem Cell* **17:** 412–421. doi:10.1016/j.stem.2015.08.008

Jaiswal S, Jamieson CH, Pang WW, Park CY, Chao MP, Majeti R, Traver D, van Rooijen N, Weissman IL. 2009. CD47 is upregulated on circulating hematopoietic stem cells and leukemia cells to avoid phagocytosis. *Cell* **138:** 271–285. doi:10.1016/j.cell.2009.05.046

Jaiswal S, Fontanillas P, Flannick J, Manning A, Grauman PV, Mar BG, Lindsley RC, Mermel CH, Burtt N, Chavez A, et al. 2014. Age-related clonal hematopoiesis associated with adverse outcomes. *N Engl J Med* **371:** 2488–2498. doi:10.1056/NEJMoa1408617

Jaiswal S, Natarajan P, Silver AJ, Gibson CJ, Bick AG, Shvartz E, McConkey M, Gupta N, Gabriel S, Ardissino D, et al. 2017. Clonal hematopoiesis and risk of atherosclerotic cardiovascular disease. *N Engl J Med* **377:** 111–121. doi:10.1056/NEJMoa1701719

Jan M, Majeti R. 2013. Clonal evolution of acute leukemia genomes. *Oncogene* **32:** 135–140. doi:10.1038/onc.2012.48

Jan M, Chao MP, Cha AC, Alizadeh AA, Gentles AJ, Weissman IL, Majeti R. 2011. Prospective separation of normal and leukemic stem cells based on differential expression of TIM3, a human acute myeloid leukemia stem cell marker. *Proc Natl Acad Sci* **108:** 5009–5014. doi:10.1073/pnas.1100551108

Jan M, Snyder TM, Corces-Zimmerman MR, Vyas P, Weissman IL, Quake SR, Majeti R. 2012. Clonal evolution of preleukemic hematopoietic stem cells precedes human acute myeloid leukemia. *Sci Transl Med* **4:** 149ra118. doi:10.1126/scitranslmed.3004315

Jaras M, Johnels P, Hansen N, Agerstam H, Tsapogas P, Rissler M, Lassen C, Olofsson T, Bjerrum OW, Richter J, et al. 2010. Isolation and killing of candidate chronic myeloid leukemia stem cells by antibody targeting of IL-1 receptor accessory protein. *Proc Natl Acad Sci* **107:** 16280–16285. doi:10.1073/pnas.1004408107

Jiang P, Liu BY, Huang J, Lu J, Sharmili R, Mishra M, Zhao X, Lin J, Hsi ED, Junutula JR. 2016. Targeting acute myeloid leukemia via anti-IL1RAP antibodies. In *Proceedings of the 107th Annual Meeting of the American Association for Cancer Research*. American Association for Cancer Research, New Orleans, LA.

Jiang Y, Xu P, Yao D, Chen X, Dai H. 2017. CD33, CD96 and death associated protein kinase (DAPK) expression are associated with the survival rate and/or response to the chemotherapy in the patients with acute myeloid leukemia (AML). *Med Sci Monit* **23:** 1725–1732. doi:10.12659/MSM.900305

Jiang YP, Liu BY, Zheng Q, Panuganti S, Chen R, Zhu J, Mishra M, Huang J, Dao-Pick T, Roy S, et al. 2018. CLT030, a leukemic stem cell-targeting CLL1 antibody-drug conjugate for treatment of acute myeloid leukemia. *Blood Adv* **2:** 1738–1749. doi:10.1182/bloodadvances.2018020107

Jin L, Hope KJ, Zhai Q, Smadja-Joffe F, Dick JE. 2006. Targeting of CD44 eradicates human acute myeloid leukemic stem cells. *Nat Med* **12:** 1167–1174. doi:10.1038/nm1483

Jin L, Lee EM, Ramshaw HS, Busfield SJ, Peoppl AG, Wilkinson L, Guthridge MA, Thomas D, Barry EF, Boyd A, et al. 2009. Monoclonal antibody-mediated targeting of CD123, IL-3 receptor α chain, eliminates human acute myeloid leukemic stem cells. *Cell Stem Cell* **5:** 31–42. doi:10.1016/j.stem.2009.04.018

Jongen-Lavrencic M, Grob T, Hanekamp D, Kavelaars FG, Al Hinai A, Zeilemaker A, Erpelinck-Verschueren CAJ, Gradowska PL, Meijer R, Cloos J, et al. 2018. Molecular minimal residual disease in acute myeloid leukemia. *N Engl J Med* **378:** 1189–1199. doi:10.1056/NEJMoa1716863

Jordan CT, Upchurch D, Szilvassy SJ, Guzman ML, Howard DS, Pettigrew AL, Meyerrose T, Rossi R, Grimes B, Rizzieri DA, et al. 2000a. The interleukin-3 receptor α chain is a unique marker for human acute myelogenous leukemia stem cells. *Leukemia* **14:** 1777–1784. doi:10.1038/sj.leu.2401903

Jordan CT, Upchurch D, Szilvassy SJ, Guzman ML, Howard DS, Pettigrew AL, Meyerrose T, Rossi R, Grimes B, Rizzieri DA, et al. 2000b. The interleukin-3 receptor α chain is a unique marker for human acute myelogenous leukemia stem cells. *Leukemia* **14:** 1777–1784. doi:10.1038/sj.leu.2401903

June CH, Sadelain M. 2018. Chimeric antigen receptor therapy. *N Engl J Med* **379:** 64–73. doi:10.1056/NEJMra1706169

Kellner C, Peipp M, Schub N, Humpe A, Gramatzki M. 2013. Targeting CD96 for antibody based elimination of leukemic stem cells in AML: A new strategy in stem cell transplantation. *Blood* **122:** 3972.

Kikushige Y, Shima T, Takayanagi S, Urata S, Miyamoto T, Iwasaki H, Takenaka K, Teshima T, Tanaka T, Inagaki Y, et al. 2010. TIM-3 is a promising target to selectively kill acute myeloid leukemia stem cells. *Cell Stem Cell* **7:** 708–717. doi:10.1016/j.stem.2010.11.014

Kikushige Y, Miyamoto T, Yuda J, Jabbarzadeh-Tabrizi S, Shima T, Takayanagi S, Niiro H, Yurino A, Miyawaki K, Takenaka K, et al. 2015. A TIM-3/Gal-9 autocrine stimulatory loop drives self-renewal of human myeloid leukemia stem cells and leukemic progression. *Cell Stem Cell* **17:** 341–352. doi:10.1016/j.stem.2015.07.011

Kim HG, Kojima K, Swindle CS, Cotta CV, Huo Y, Reddy V, Klug CA. 2008. FLT3-ITD cooperates with inv(16) to promote progression to acute myeloid leukemia. *Blood* **111:** 1567–1574. doi:10.1182/blood-2006-06-030312

Kim MS, Pinto SM, Getnet D, Nirujogi RS, Manda SS, Chaerkady R, Madugundu AK, Kelkar DS, Isserlin R, Jain S, et al. 2014. A draft map of the human proteome. *Nature* **509:** 575–581. doi:10.1038/nature13302

Kim MY, Yu KR, Kenderian SS, Ruella M, Chen S, Shin TH, Aljanahi AA, Schreeder D, Klichinsky M, Shestova O, et al. 2018. Genetic inactivation of CD33 in hematopoietic stem cells to enable CAR T cell immunotherapy for acute myeloid leukemia. *Cell* **173:** 1439–1453.e19. doi:10.1016/j.cell.2018.05.013

King KY, Goodell MA. 2011. Inflammatory modulation of HSCs: Viewing the HSC as a foundation for the immune response. *Nat Rev Immunol* **11:** 685–692. doi:10.1038/nri3062

Kirstetter P, Schuster MB, Bereshchenko O, Moore S, Dvinge H, Kurz E, Theilgaard-Monch K, Mansson R, Pedersen TA, Pabst T, et al. 2008. Modeling of C/EBPα mutant acute myeloid leukemia reveals a common expression signature of committed myeloid leukemia-initiating cells. *Cancer Cell* **13:** 299–310. doi:10.1016/j.ccr.2008.02.008

Kotini AG, Chang CJ, Chow A, Yuan H, Ho TC, Wang T, Vora S, Solovyov A, Husser C, Olszewska M, et al. 2017. Stage-specific human induced pluripotent stem cells map the progression of myeloid transformation to transplantable leukemia. *Cell Stem Cell* **20:** 315–328.e7. doi:10.1016/j.stem.2017.01.009

Kristinsson SY, Björkholm M, Hultcrantz M, Derolf AR, Landgren O, Goldin LR. 2011. Chronic immune stimulation might act as a trigger for the development of acute myeloid leukemia or myelodysplastic syndromes. *J Clin Oncol* **29:** 2897–2903. doi:10.1200/JCO.2011.34.8540

Krönke J, Bullinger L, Teleanu V, Tschürtz F, Gaidzik VI, Kühn MWM, Rücker FG, Holzmann K, Paschka P, Kapp-Schwörer S, et al. 2013. Clonal evolution in relapsed *NPM1*-mutated acute myeloid leukemia. *Blood* **122:** 100–108. doi:10.1182/blood-2013-01-479188

Kuo YH, Landrette SF, Heilman SA, Perrat PN, Garrett L, Liu PP, Le Beau MM, Kogan SC, Castilla LH. 2006. Cbfβ-SMMHC induces distinct abnormal myeloid progenitors able to develop acute myeloid leukemia. *Cancer Cell* **9:** 57–68. doi:10.1016/j.ccr.2005.12.014

Laborda E, Mazagova M, Shao S, Wang X, Quirino H, Woods AK, Hampton EN, Rodgers DT, Kim CH, Schultz PG, et al. 2017. Development of a chimeric antigen receptor targeting C-type lectin-like molecule-1 for human acute myeloid leukemia. *Int J Mol Sci* **18:** E2259. doi:10.3390/ijms18112259

Lancet JE. 2018. Is the overall survival for older adults with AML finally improving? *Best Pract Res Clin Haematol* **31:** 387–390. doi:10.1016/j.beha.2018.09.005

Lancet JE, Rizzieri D, Schiller GJ, Stuart RK, Kolitz JE, Solomon SR, Newell LF, Erba HP, Uy GL, Ryan R, et al. 2017. Overall survival (OS) with CPX-351 versus 7+3 in older adults with newly diagnosed, therapy-related acute myeloid leukemia (tAML): Subgroup analysis of a phase III study. *J Clin Oncol* **35:** 7035–7035. doi:10.1200/JCO.2017.35.15_suppl.7035

Lapidot T, Sirard C, Vormoor J, Murdoch B, Hoang T, Caceres-Cortes J, Minden M, Paterson B, Caligiuri MA, Dick JE. 1994. A cell initiating human acute myeloid leukaemia after transplantation into SCID mice. *Nature* **367:** 645–648. doi:10.1038/367645a0

Le Dieu R, Taussig DC, Ramsay AG, Mitter R, Miraki-Moud F, Fatah R, Lee AM, Lister TA, Gribben JG. 2009. Peripheral blood T cells in acute myeloid leukemia (AML) patients at diagnosis have abnormal phenotype and genotype and form defective immune synapses with AML blasts. *Blood* **114:** 3909–3916. doi:10.1182/blood-2009-02-206946

Lee BH, Williams IR, Anastasiadou E, Boulton CL, Joseph SW, Amaral SM, Curley DP, Duclos N, Huntly BJ, Fabbro D, et al. 2005. FLT3 internal tandem duplication mutations induce myeloproliferative or lymphoid disease in a transgenic mouse model. *Oncogene* **24:** 7882–7892. doi:10.1038/sj.onc.1208933

Leong SR, Sukumaran S, Hristopoulos M, Totpal K, Stainton S, Lu E, Wong A, Tam L, Newman R, Vuillemenot BR, et al. 2017. An anti-CD3/anti-CLL-1 bispecific antibody for the treatment of acute myeloid leukemia. *Blood* **129:** 609–618. doi:10.1182/blood-2016-08-735365

Liang K, Volk AG, Haug JS, Marshall SA, Woodfin AR, Bartom ET, Gilmore JM, Florens L, Washburn MP, Sullivan KD, et al. 2017. Therapeutic targeting of MLL degradation pathways in MLL-rearranged leukemia. *Cell* **168:** 59–72.e13. doi:10.1016/j.cell.2016.12.011

Liesveld JL, Dipersio JF, Abboud CN. 1994. Integrins and adhesive receptors in normal and leukemic $CD34^+$ progenitor cells: Potential regulatory checkpoints for cellular traffic. *Leuk Lymphoma* **14:** 19–28. doi:10.3109/10428199409049647

Liu J, Jiang G. 2006. CD44 and hematologic malignancies. *Cell Mol Immunol* **3:** 359–365.

Liu F, Pinz K, Ma Y, Wada M, Chen K, Ma G, Su Y, Zhang S, He G, Ma Y. 2018. First-in-human CLL1-CD33 compound CAR T cells as a two-pronged approach for the treatment of refractory acute myeloid leukemia. In *European Hematology Association Congress 23*, Stockholm, Sweden.

Lu H, Zhou Q, Deshmukh V, Phull H, Ma J, Tardif V, Naik RR, Bouvard C, Zhang Y, Choi S, et al. 2014. Targeting human C-type lectin-like molecule-1 (CLL1) with a bispecific antibody for immunotherapy of acute myeloid leukemia. *Angew Chem Int Ed Engl* **53:** 9841–9845. doi:10.1002/anie.201405353

Madhumathi J, Sridevi S, Verma RS. 2017. CD25 targeted therapy of chemotherapy resistant leukemic stem cells using DR5 specific TRAIL peptide. *Stem Cell Res* **19:** 65–75. doi:10.1016/j.scr.2017.01.001

Majeti R, Becker MW, Tian Q, Lee TL, Yan X, Liu R, Chiang JH, Hood L, Clarke MF, Weissman IL. 2009a. Dysregulated gene expression networks in human acute myelogenous leukemia stem cells. *Proc Natl Acad Sci* **106:** 3396–3401. doi:10.1073/pnas.0900089106

Majeti R, Chao MP, Alizadeh AA, Pang WW, Jaiswal S, Gibbs KD Jr, van Rooijen N, Weissman IL. 2009b. CD47 is an adverse prognostic factor and therapeutic antibody target on human acute myeloid leukemia stem cells. *Cell* **138:** 286–299. doi:10.1016/j.cell.2009.05.045

Mallardo M, Caronno A, Pruneri G, Raviele PR, Viale A, Pelicci PG, Colombo E. 2013. $NPMc^+$ and FLT3_ITD mutations cooperate in inducing acute leukaemia in a novel mouse model. *Leukemia* **27:** 2248–2251. doi:10.1038/leu.2013.114

Marshall AS, Willment JA, Lin HH, Williams DL, Gordon S, Brown GD. 2004. Identification and characterization of a novel human myeloid inhibitory C-type lectin-like receptor (MICL) that is predominantly expressed on granulocytes and monocytes. *J Biol Chem* **279:** 14792–14802. doi:10.1074/jbc.M313127200

Martelli MP, Pettirossi V, Thiede C, Bonifacio E, Mezzasoma F, Cecchini D, Pacini R, Tabarrini A, Ciurnelli R, Gionfriddo I, et al. 2010. CD34$^+$ cells from AML with mutated NPM1 harbor cytoplasmic mutated nucleophosmin and generate leukemia in immunocompromised mice. *Blood* **116:** 3907–3922. doi:10.1182/blood-2009-08-238899

Matatall KA, Shen CC, Challen GA, King KY. 2014. Type II interferon promotes differentiation of myeloid-biased hematopoietic stem cells. *Stem Cells* **32:** 3023–3030. doi:10.1002/stem.1799

McGreal EP, Ikewaki N, Akatsu H, Morgan BP, Gasque P. 2002. Human C1qRp is identical with CD93 and the mNI-11 antigen but does not bind C1q. *J Immunol* **168:** 5222–5232. doi:10.4049/jimmunol.168.10.5222

Meisel M, Hinterleitner R, Pacis A, Chen L, Earley ZM, Mayassi T, Pierre JF, Ernest JD, Galipeau HJ, Thuille N, et al. 2018. Microbial signals drive pre-leukaemic myeloproliferation in a Tet2-deficient host. *Nature* **557:** 580–584. doi:10.1038/s41586-018-0125-z

Meng W, Del Real M, Wei G, Hernandez R, Marcucci E, Lin A, Mcdonald T, Zhao D, Wu H, Carlesso N, et al. 2017. Anti-IL1RAP/CD3 bispecific Antibody (BsAb) is a promising novel and effective therapy for acute myeloid leukemia (AML). *Blood* **130:** 1361–1361.

Meyer C, Hofmann J, Burmeister T, Groger D, Park TS, Emerenciano M, Pombo de Oliveira M, Renneville A, Villarese P, Macintyre E, et al. 2013. The MLL recombinome of acute leukemias in 2013. *Leukemia* **27:** 2165–2176. doi:10.1038/leu.2013.135

Mirantes C, Passegué E, Pietras EM. 2014. Pro-inflammatory cytokines: Emerging players regulating HSC function in normal and diseased hematopoiesis. *Exp Cell Res* **329:** 248–254. doi:10.1016/j.yexcr.2014.08.017

Mitchell K, Barreyro L, Todorova TI, Taylor SJ, Antony-Debré I, Narayanagari SR, Carvajal LA, Leite J, Piperdi Z, Pendurti G, et al. 2018. IL1RAP potentiates multiple oncogenic signaling pathways in AML. *J Exp Med* **215:** 1709–1727. doi:10.1084/jem.20180147

Miyamoto T, Weissman IL, Akashi K. 2000. AML1/ETO-expressing nonleukemic stem cells in acute myelogenous leukemia with 8;21 chromosomal translocation. *Proc Natl Acad Sci* **97:** 7521–7526. doi:10.1073/pnas.97.13.7521

Mohseni Nodehi S, Repp R, Kellner C, Bräutigam J, Staudinger M, Schub N, Peipp M, Gramatzki M, Humpe A. 2012. Enhanced ADCC activity of affinity maturated and Fc-engineered mini-antibodies directed against the AML stem cell antigen CD96. *PLoS ONE* **7:** e42426. doi:10.1371/journal.pone.0042426

Mokdad AH, Dwyer-Lindgren L, Fitzmaurice C, Stubbs RW, Bertozzi-Villa A, Morozoff C, Charara R, Allen C, Naghavi M, Murray CJ. 2017. Trends and patterns of disparities in cancer mortality among US counties, 1980–2014. *JAMA* **317:** 388–406. doi:10.1001/jama.2016.20324

Morsink LM, Walter RB, Ossenkoppele GJ. 2019. Prognostic and therapeutic role of CLEC12A in acute myeloid leukemia. *Blood Rev* **34:** 26–33. doi:10.1016/j.blre.2018.10.003

Moshaver B, van Rhenen A, Kelder A, van der Pol M, Terwijn M, Bachas C, Westra AH, Ossenkoppele GJ, Zweegman S, Schuurhuis GJ. 2008. Identification of a small subpopulation of candidate leukemia-initiating cells in the side population of patients with acute myeloid leukemia. *Stem Cells* **26:** 3059–3067. doi:10.1634/stemcells.2007-0861

Munoz L, Nomdedeu JF, Lopez O, Carnicer MJ, Bellido M, Aventin A, Brunet S, Sierra J. 2001. Interleukin-3 receptor α chain (CD123) is widely expressed in hematologic malignancies. *Haematologica* **86:** 1261–1269.

Murata Y, Saito Y, Kotani T, Matozaki T. 2018. CD47-signal regulatory protein α signaling system and its application to cancer immunotherapy. *Cancer Sci* **109:** 2349–2357. doi:10.1111/cas.13663

Neumann K, Castiñeiras-Vilariño M, Höckendorf U, Hannesschläger N, Lemeer S, Kupka D, Meyermann S, Lech M, Anders HJ, Kuster B, et al. 2014. Clec12a is an inhibitory receptor for uric acid crystals that regulates inflammation in response to cell death. *Immunity* **40:** 389–399. doi:10.1016/j.immuni.2013.12.015

Nilsson L, Astrand-Grundstrom I, Arvidsson I, Jacobsson B, Hellstrom-Lindberg E, Hast R, Jacobsen SE. 2000. Isolation and characterization of hematopoietic progenitor/stem cells in 5q-deleted myelodysplastic syndromes: Evidence for involvement at the hematopoietic stem cell level. *Blood* **96:** 2012–2021.

Nilsson L, Astrand-Grundstrom I, Anderson K, Arvidsson I, Hokland P, Bryder D, Kjeldsen L, Johansson B, Hellstrom-Lindberg E, Hast R, et al. 2002. Involvement and functional impairment of the CD34$^+$CD38-Thy$^-$1$^+$ hematopoietic stem cell pool in myelodysplastic syndromes with trisomy 8. *Blood* **100:** 259–267.

Nilsson L, Eden P, Olsson E, Mansson R, Astrand-Grundstrom I, Strombeck B, Theilgaard-Monch K, Anderson K, Hast R, Hellstrom-Lindberg E, et al. 2007. The molecular signature of MDS stem cells supports a stem-cell origin of 5q myelodysplastic syndromes. *Blood* **110:** 3005–3014. doi:10.1182/blood-2007-03-079368

Noone AM, Howlader N, Krapcho M, Miller D, Brest A YM, Ruhl J, Tatalovich Z, Mariotto A, Lewis DR, Chen HS, Feuer EJ, Cronin KA. 2018. *SEER Cancer Statistics Review, 1975–2015*. National Cancer Institute, Bethesda, MD. https://seer.cancer.gov/csr/1975_2016

Olweus J, Lund-Johansen F, Terstappen LW. 1994. Expression of cell surface markers during differentiation of CD34$^+$, CD38$^{-/lo}$ fetal and adult bone marrow cells. *Immunomethods* **5:** 179–188. doi:10.1006/immu.1994.1054

Pabst C, Bergeron A, Lavallee VP, Yeh J, Gendron P, Norddahl GL, Krosl J, Boivin I, Deneault E, Simard J, et al. 2016. GPR56 identifies primary human acute myeloid leukemia cells with high repopulating potential in vivo. *Blood* **127:** 2018–2027. doi:10.1182/blood-2015-11-683649

Pandolfi A, Barreyro L, Steidl U. 2013. Concise review: Preleukemic stem cells: Molecular biology and clinical implications of the precursors to leukemia stem cells. *Stem Cells Transl Med* **2:** 143–150. doi:10.5966/sctm.2012-0109

Papaemmanuil E, Gerstung M, Bullinger L, Gaidzik VI, Paschka P, Roberts ND, Potter NE, Heuser M, Thol F, Bolli N, et al. 2016. Genomic classification and prognosis in acute myeloid leukemia. *N Engl J Med* **374:** 2209–2221. doi:10.1056/NEJMoa1516192

Parkin B, Ouillette P, Li Y, Keller J, Lam C, Roulston D, Li C, Shedden K, Malek SN. 2013. Clonal evolution and devolution after chemotherapy in adult acute myelogenous leukemia. *Blood* **121:** 369–377. doi:10.1182/blood-2012-04-427039

Passegue E, Jamieson CH, Ailles LE, Weissman IL. 2003. Normal and leukemic hematopoiesis: Are leukemias a stem cell disorder or a reacquisition of stem cell characteristics? *Proc Natl Acad Sci* **100:** 11842–11849. doi:10.1073/pnas.2034201100

Patel JP, Gonen M, Figueroa ME, Fernandez H, Sun Z, Racevskis J, Van Vlierberghe P, Dolgalev I, Thomas S, Aminova O, et al. 2012. Prognostic relevance of integrated genetic profiling in acute myeloid leukemia. *N Engl J Med* **366:** 1079–1089. doi:10.1056/NEJMoa1112304

Perna F, Berman SH, Soni RK, Mansilla-Soto J, Eyquem J, Hamieh M, Hendrickson RC, Brennan CW, Sadelain M. 2017. Integrating proteomics and transcriptomics for systematic combinatorial chimeric antigen receptor therapy of AML. *Cancer Cell* **32:** 506–519.e5. doi:10.1016/j.ccell.2017.09.004

Pietras EM. 2017. Inflammation: A key regulator of hematopoietic stem cell fate in health and disease. *Blood* **130:** 1693–1698. doi:10.1182/blood-2017-06-780882

Pietras EM, Warr MR, Passegué E. 2011. Cell cycle regulation in hematopoietic stem cells. *J Cell Biol* **195:** 709–720. doi:10.1083/jcb.201102131

Pietras EM, Lakshminarasimhan R, Techner JM, Fong S, Flach J, Binnewies M, Passegué E. 2014. Re-entry into quiescence protects hematopoietic stem cells from the killing effect of chronic exposure to type I interferons. *J Exp Med* **211:** 245–262. doi:10.1084/jem.20131043

Pietras EM, Mirantes-Barbeito C, Fong S, Loeffler D, Kovtonyuk LV, Zhang S, Lakshminarasimhan R, Chin CP, Techner JM, Will B, et al. 2016. Chronic interleukin-1 exposure drives haematopoietic stem cells towards precocious myeloid differentiation at the expense of self-renewal. *Nat Cell Biol* **18:** 607–618. doi:10.1038/ncb3346

Pulikkan JA, Castilla LH. 2018. Preleukemia and leukemia-initiating cell activity in inv(16) acute myeloid leukemia. *Front Oncol* **8:** 129. doi:10.3389/fonc.2018.00129

Quek L, Otto GW, Garnett C, Lhermitte L, Karamitros D, Stoilova B, Lau IJ, Doondeea J, Usukhbayar B, Kennedy A, et al. 2016. Genetically distinct leukemic stem cells in human $CD34^{-}$ acute myeloid leukemia are arrested at a hemopoietic precursor-like stage. *J Exp Med* **213:** 1513–1535. doi:10.1084/jem.20151775

Quéré R, Andradottir S, Brun AC, Zubarev RA, Karlsson G, Olsson K, Magnusson M, Cammenga J, Karlsson S. 2011. High levels of the adhesion molecule CD44 on leukemic cells generate acute myeloid leukemia relapse after withdrawal of the initial transforming event. *Leukemia* **25:** 515–526. doi:10.1038/leu.2010.281

Reiter K, Polzer H, Krupka C, Maiser A, Vick B, Rothenberg-Thurley M, Metzeler KH, Dorfel D, Salih HR, Jung G, et al. 2018. Tyrosine kinase inhibition increases the cell surface localization of FLT3-ITD and enhances FLT3-directed immunotherapy of acute myeloid leukemia. *Leukemia* **32:** 313–322. doi:10.1038/leu.2017.257

Reuss-Borst MA, Buhring HJ, Klein G, Müller CA. 1992. Adhesion molecules on $CD34^{+}$ hematopoietic cells in normal human bone marrow and leukemia. *Ann Hematol* **65:** 169–174. doi:10.1007/BF01703110

Reynaud D, Pietras E, Barry-Holson K, Mir A, Binnewies M, Jeanne M, Sala-Torra O, Radich JP, Passegué E. 2011. IL-6 controls leukemic multipotent progenitor cell fate and contributes to chronic myelogenous leukemia development. *Cancer Cell* **20:** 661–673. doi:10.1016/j.ccr.2011.10.012

Rossi DJ, Bryder D, Zahn JM, Ahlenius H, Sonu R, Wagers AJ, Weissman IL. 2005. Cell intrinsic alterations underlie hematopoietic stem cell aging. *Proc Natl Acad Sci* **102:** 9194–9199. doi:10.1073/pnas.0503280102

Rossi DJ, Jamieson CH, Weissman IL. 2008. Stems cells and the pathways to aging and cancer. *Cell* **132:** 681–696. doi:10.1016/j.cell.2008.01.036

Rundberg Nilsson A, Soneji S, Adolfsson S, Bryder D, Pronk CJ. 2016. Human and murine hematopoietic stem cell aging is associated with functional impairments and intrinsic megakaryocytic/erythroid bias. *PLoS ONE* **11:** e0158369. doi:10.1371/journal.pone.0158369

Sadovnik I, Herrmann H, Eisenwort G, Blatt K, Hoermann G, Mueller N, Sperr WR, Valent P. 2017. Expression of CD25 on leukemic stem cells in $BCR-ABL1^{+}$ CML: Potential diagnostic value and functional implications. *Exp Hematol* **51:** 17–24. doi:10.1016/j.exphem.2017.04.003

Saha HR, Kaneda-Nakashima K, Shimosaki S, Suekane A, Sarkar B, Saito Y, Ogoh H, Nakahata S, Inoue K, Watanabe T, et al. 2018. Suppression of GPR56 expression by pyrrole-imidazole polyamide represents a novel therapeutic drug for AML with high EVI1 expression. *Sci Rep* **8:** 13741. doi:10.1038/s41598-018-32205-8

Saito Y, Kitamura H, Hijikata A, Tomizawa-Murasawa M, Tanaka S, Takagi S, Uchida N, Suzuki N, Sone A, Najima Y, et al. 2010. Identification of therapeutic targets for quiescent, chemotherapy-resistant human leukemia stem cells. *Sci Transl Med* **2:** 17ra9. doi:10.1126/scitranslmed.3000349

Saito Y, Nakahata S, Yamakawa N, Kaneda K, Ichihara E, Suekane A, Morishita K. 2011. CD52 as a molecular target for immunotherapy to treat acute myeloid leukemia with high EVI1 expression. *Leukemia* **25:** 921–931. doi:10.1038/leu.2011.36

Sarry JE, Murphy K, Perry R, Sanchez PV, Secreto A, Keefer C, Swider CR, Strzelecki AC, Cavelier C, Recher C, et al. 2011. Human acute myelogenous leukemia stem cells are rare and heterogeneous when assayed in NOD/SCID/IL2Rγc-deficient mice. *J Clin Invest* **121:** 384–395. doi:10.1172/JCI41495

Sato N, Caux C, Kitamura T, Watanabe Y, Arai K, Banchereau J, Miyajima A. 1993. Expression and factor-dependent modulation of the interleukin-3 receptor subunits on human hematopoietic cells. *Blood* **82:** 752–761.

Sato T, Yang X, Knapper S, White P, Smith BD, Galkin S, Small D, Burnett A, Levis M. 2011. FLT3 ligand impedes the efficacy of FLT3 inhibitors in vitro and in vivo. *Blood* **117:** 3286–3293. doi:10.1182/blood-2010-01-266742

Schessl C, Rawat VP, Cusan M, Deshpande A, Kohl TM, Rosten PM, Spiekermann K, Humphries RK, Schnittger S, Kern W, et al. 2005. The AML1-ETO fusion gene and the FLT3 length mutation collaborate in inducing acute leukemia in mice. *J Clin Invest* **115:** 2159–2168. doi:10.1172/JCI24225

Shastri A, Will B, Steidl U, Verma A. 2017. Stem and progenitor cell alterations in myelodysplastic syndromes.

Blood **129:** 1586–1594. doi:10.1182/blood-2016-10-696062

Shlush LI. 2018. Age-related clonal hematopoiesis. *Blood* **131:** 496–504. doi:10.1182/blood-2017-07-746453

Shlush LI, Zandi S, Mitchell A, Chen WC, Brandwein JM, Gupta V, Kennedy JA, Schimmer AD, Schuh AC, Yee KW, et al. 2014. Identification of pre-leukaemic haematopoietic stem cells in acute leukaemia. *Nature* **506:** 328–333. doi:10.1038/nature13038

Shlush LI, Mitchell A, Heisler L, Abelson S, Ng SWK, Trotman-Grant A, Medeiros JJF, Rao-Bhatia A, Jaciw-Zurakowsky I, Marke R, et al. 2017. Tracing the origins of relapse in acute myeloid leukaemia to stem cells. *Nature* **547:** 104–108. doi:10.1038/nature22993

Shouval R, Shlush LI, Yehudai-Resheff S, Ali S, Pery N, Shapiro E, Tzukerman M, Rowe JM, Zuckerman T. 2014. Single cell analysis exposes intratumor heterogeneity and suggests that FLT3-ITD is a late event in leukemogenesis. *Exp Hematol* **42:** 457–463. doi:10.1016/j.exphem.2014.01.010

Sievers EL, Appelbaum FR, Spielberger RT, Forman SJ, Flowers D, Smith FO, Shannon-Dorcy K, Berger MS, Bernstein ID. 1999. Selective ablation of acute myeloid leukemia using antibody-targeted chemotherapy: A phase I study of an anti-CD33 calicheamicin immunoconjugate. *Blood* **93:** 3678–3684.

Sievers EL, Larson RA, Stadtmauer EA, Estey E, Löwenberg B, Dombret H, Karanes C, Theobald M, Bennett JM, Sherman ML, et al. 2001. Efficacy and safety of gemtuzumab ozogamicin in patients with CD33-positive acute myeloid leukemia in first relapse. *J Clin Oncol* **19:** 3244–3254. doi:10.1200/JCO.2001.19.13.3244

Smith CC, Paguirigan A, Jeschke GR, Lin KC, Massi E, Tarver T, Chin CS, Asthana S, Olshen A, Travers KJ, et al. 2017. Heterogeneous resistance to quizartinib in acute myeloid leukemia revealed by single-cell analysis. *Blood* **130:** 48–58. doi:10.1182/blood-2016-04-711820

Somervaille TC, Cleary ML. 2006. Identification and characterization of leukemia stem cells in murine MLL-AF9 acute myeloid leukemia. *Cancer Cell* **10:** 257–268. doi:10.1016/j.ccr.2006.08.020

Song G, Liao X, Zhou L, Wu L, Feng Y, Han ZC. 2004. HI44a, an anti-CD44 monoclonal antibody, induces differentiation and apoptosis of human acute myeloid leukemia cells. *Leuk Res* **28:** 1089–1096. doi:10.1016/j.leukres.2004.02.005

Steensma DP, Bejar R, Jaiswal S, Lindsley RC, Sekeres MA, Hasserjian RP, Ebert BL. 2015. Clonal hematopoiesis of indeterminate potential and its distinction from myelodysplastic syndromes. *Blood* **126:** 9–16. doi:10.1182/blood-2015-03-631747

Steidl U, Rosenbauer F, Verhaak RG, Gu X, Ebralidze A, Otu HH, Klippel S, Steidl C, Bruns I, Costa DB, et al. 2006. Essential role of Jun family transcription factors in PU.1 knockdown-induced leukemic stem cells. *Nat Genet* **38:** 1269–1277. doi:10.1038/ng1898

Steidl U, Steidl C, Ebralidze A, Chapuy B, Han HJ, Will B, Rosenbauer F, Becker A, Wagner K, Koschmieder S, et al. 2007. A distal single nucleotide polymorphism alters long-range regulation of the PU.1 gene in acute myeloid leukemia. *J Clin Invest* **117:** 2611–2620. doi:10.1172/JCI30525

Stone RM, Mandrekar SJ, Sanford BL, Laumann K, Geyer S, Bloomfield CD, Thiede C, Prior TW, Döhner K, Marcucci G, et al. 2017. Midostaurin plus chemotherapy for acute myeloid leukemia with a *FLT3* mutation. *N Engl J Med* **377:** 454–464. doi:10.1056/NEJMoa1614359

Striz I. 2017. Cytokines of the IL-1 family: Recognized targets in chronic inflammation underrated in organ transplantations. *Clin Sci* **131:** 2241–2256. doi:10.1042/CS20170098

Sun GX, Wormsley S, Sparkes RS, Naeim F, Gale RP. 1991. Where does transformation occur in acute leukemia? *Leuk Res* **15:** 1183–1189. doi:10.1016/0145-2126(91)90188-Y

Sutherland HJ, Blair A, Zapf RW. 1996. Characterization of a hierarchy in human acute myeloid leukemia progenitor cells. *Blood* **87:** 4754–4761.

Takizawa H, Boettcher S, Manz MG. 2012. Demand-adapted regulation of early hematopoiesis in infection and inflammation. *Blood* **119:** 2991–3002. doi:10.1182/blood-2011-12-380113

Takizawa H, Fritsch K, Kovtonyuk LV, Saito Y, Yakkala C, Jacobs K, Ahuja AK, Lopes M, Hausmann A, Hardt WD, et al. 2017. Pathogen-induced TLR4-TRIF innate immune signaling in hematopoietic stem cells promotes proliferation but reduces competitive fitness. *Cell Stem Cell* **21:** 225–240.e5. doi:10.1016/j.stem.2017.06.013

Tamura S, Kanamaru A, Takemoto Y, Kakishita E, Nagai K. 1993. Clonal evolutions during long-term cultures of bone marrow from de novo acute myeloid leukaemia with trilineage myelodysplasia and with myelodysplastic remission marrow. *Br J Haematol* **84:** 219–226. doi:10.1111/j.1365-2141.1993.tb03055.x

Tashiro H, Sauer T, Shum T, Parikh K, Mamonkin M, Omer B, Rouce RH, Lulla P, Rooney CM, Gottschalk S, et al. 2017. Treatment of acute myeloid leukemia with T cells expressing chimeric antigen receptors directed to C-type lectin-like molecule 1. *Mol Ther* **25:** 2202–2213. doi:10.1016/j.ymthe.2017.05.024

Taussig DC, Pearce DJ, Simpson C, Rohatiner AZ, Lister TA, Kelly G, Luongo JL, Danet-Desnoyers GA, Bonnet D. 2005. Hematopoietic stem cells express multiple myeloid markers: Implications for the origin and targeted therapy of acute myeloid leukemia. *Blood* **106:** 4086–4092. doi:10.1182/blood-2005-03-1072

Taussig DC, Vargaftig J, Miraki-Moud F, Griessinger E, Sharrock K, Luke T, Lillington D, Oakervee H, Cavenagh J, Agrawal SG, et al. 2010. Leukemia-initiating cells from some acute myeloid leukemia patients with mutated *nucleophosmin* reside in the $CD34^-$ fraction. *Blood* **115:** 1976–1984. doi:10.1182/blood-2009-02-206565

Taylor SJ, Duyvestyn JM, Dagger SA, Dishington EJ, Rinaldi CA, Dovey OM, Vassiliou GS, Grove CS, Langdon WY. 2017. Preventing chemotherapy-induced myelosuppression by repurposing the FLT3 inhibitor quizartinib. *Sci Transl Med* **9:** eaam8060. doi:10.1126/scitranslmed.aam8060

Terpstra W, Ploemacher RE, Prins A, van Lom K, Pouwels K, Wognum AW, Wagemaker G, Lowenberg B, Wielenga JJ. 1996. Fluorouracil selectively spares acute myeloid leukemia cells with long-term growth abilities in immunodeficient mice and in culture. *Blood* **88:** 1944–1950.

Terwijn M, Feller N, van Rhenen A, Kelder A, Westra G, Zweegman S, Ossenkoppele G, Schuurhuis GJ. 2009. Interleukin-2 receptor α-chain (CD25) expression on leukaemic blasts is predictive for outcome and level of residual disease in AML. *Eur J Cancer* **45:** 1692–1699. doi:10.1016/j.ejca.2009.02.021

Thomas D, Majeti R. 2017. Biology and relevance of human acute myeloid leukemia stem cells. *Blood* **129:** 1577–1585. doi:10.1182/blood-2016-10-696054

Traer E, Martinez J, Javidi-Sharifi N, Agarwal A, Dunlap J, English I, Kovacsovics T, Tyner JW, Wong M, Druker BJ. 2016. FGF2 from marrow microenvironment promotes resistance to FLT3 inhibitors in acute myeloid leukemia. *Cancer Res* **76:** 6471–6482. doi:10.1158/0008-5472.CAN-15-3569

Uhlen M, Fagerberg L, Hallstrom BM, Lindskog C, Oksvold P, Mardinoglu A, Sivertsson A, Kampf C, Sjostedt E, Asplund A, et al. 2015. Proteomics. Tissue-based map of the human proteome. *Science* **347:** 1260419. doi:10.1126/science.1260419

van Rhenen A, Moshaver B, Kelder A, Feller N, Nieuwint AW, Zweegman S, Ossenkoppele GJ, Schuurhuis GJ. 2007a. Aberrant marker expression patterns on the $CD34^+CD38^-$ stem cell compartment in acute myeloid leukemia allows to distinguish the malignant from the normal stem cell compartment both at diagnosis and in remission. *Leukemia* **21:** 1700–1707. doi:10.1038/sj.leu.2404754

van Rhenen A, van Dongen GA, Kelder A, Rombouts EJ, Feller N, Moshaver B, Stigter-van Walsum M, Zweegman S, Ossenkoppele GJ, Jan Schuurhuis G. 2007b. The novel AML stem cell associated antigen CLL-1 aids in discrimination between normal and leukemic stem cells. *Blood* **110:** 2659–2666. doi:10.1182/blood-2007-03-083048

Vincenti F, Kirkman R, Light S, Bumgardner G, Pescovitz M, Halloran P, Neylan J, Wilkinson A, Ekberg H, Gaston R, et al. 1998. Interleukin-2-receptor blockade with daclizumab to prevent acute rejection in renal transplantation. Daclizumab triple therapy study group. *N Engl J Med* **338:** 161–165. doi:10.1056/NEJM199801153380304

Walter D, Lier A, Geiselhart A, Thalheimer FB, Huntscha S, Sobotta MC, Moehrle B, Brocks D, Bayindir I, Kaschutnig P, et al. 2015. Exit from dormancy provokes DNA-damage-induced attrition in haematopoietic stem cells. *Nature* **520:** 549–552. doi:10.1038/nature14131

Wang J, Chen S, Xiao W, Li W, Wang L, Yang S, Wang W, Xu L, Liao S, Liu W, et al. 2018. CAR-T cells targeting CLL-1 as an approach to treat acute myeloid leukemia. *J Hematol Oncol* **11:** 7. doi:10.1186/s13045-017-0553-5

Wei AH, Tiong IS. 2017. Midostaurin, enasidenib, CPX-351, gemtuzumab ozogamicin, and venetoclax bring new hope to AML. *Blood* **130:** 2469–2474. doi:10.1182/blood-2017-08-784066

Welch JS, Ley TJ, Link DC, Miller CA, Larson DE, Koboldt DC, Wartman LD, Lamprecht TL, Liu F, Xia J, et al. 2012. The origin and evolution of mutations in acute myeloid leukemia. *Cell* **150:** 264–278. doi:10.1016/j.cell.2012.06.023

Wilhelm M, Schlegl J, Hahne H, Gholami AM, Lieberenz M, Savitski MM, Ziegler E, Butzmann L, Gessulat S, Marx H, et al. 2014. Mass-spectrometry-based draft of the human proteome. *Nature* **509:** 582–587. doi:10.1038/nature13319

Will B, Zhou L, Vogler TO, Ben-Neriah S, Schinke C, Tamari R, Yu Y, Bhagat TD, Bhattacharyya S, Barreyro L, et al. 2012. Stem and progenitor cells in myelodysplastic syndromes show aberrant stage-specific expansion and harbor genetic and epigenetic alterations. *Blood* **120:** 2076–2086. doi:10.1182/blood-2011-12-399683

Will B, Vogler TO, Narayanagari S, Bartholdy B, Todorova TI, da Silva Ferreira M, Chen J, Yu Y, Mayer J, Barreyro L, et al. 2015. Minimal PU.1 reduction induces a preleukemic state and promotes development of acute myeloid leukemia. *Nat Med* **21:** 1172–1181. doi:10.1038/nm.3936

Woll PS, Kjallquist U, Chowdhury O, Doolittle H, Wedge DC, Thongjuea S, Erlandsson R, Ngara M, Anderson K, Deng Q, et al. 2014. Myelodysplastic syndromes are propagated by rare and distinct human cancer stem cells in vivo. *Cancer Cell* **25:** 794–808. doi:10.1016/j.ccr.2014.03.036

Wong TN, Miller CA, Klco JM, Petti A, Demeter R, Helton NM, Li T, Fulton RS, Heath SE, Mardis ER, et al. 2016. Rapid expansion of preexisting nonleukemic hematopoietic clones frequently follows induction therapy for de novo AML. *Blood* **127:** 893–897. doi:10.1182/blood-2015-10-677021

Wu S, Yang S, Zhu L, Wang Y, Zhang Y, Zhou J, Li D. 2016. Prognosis of patients with de novo acute myeloid leukemia resistant to initial induction chemotherapy. *Am J Med Sci* **351:** 473–479. doi:10.1016/j.amjms.2016.02.034

Xie M, Lu C, Wang J, McLellan MD, Johnson KJ, Wendl MC, McMichael JF, Schmidt HK, Yellapantula V, Miller CA, et al. 2014. Age-related mutations associated with clonal hematopoietic expansion and malignancies. *Nat Med* **20:** 1472–1478. doi:10.1038/nm.3733

Yalcintepe L, Frankel AE, Hogge DE. 2006. Expression of interleukin-3 receptor subunits on defined subpopulations of acute myeloid leukemia blasts predicts the cytotoxicity of diphtheria toxin interleukin-3 fusion protein against malignant progenitors that engraft in immunodeficient mice. *Blood* **108:** 3530–3537. doi:10.1182/blood-2006-04-013813

Yamamoto R, Wilkinson AC, Ooehara J, Lan X, Lai CY, Nakauchi Y, Pritchard JK, Nakauchi H. 2018. Large-scale clonal analysis resolves aging of the mouse hematopoietic stem cell compartment. *Cell Stem Cell* **22:** 600–607.e4. doi:10.1016/j.stem.2018.03.013

Yang X, Sexauer A, Levis M. 2014. Bone marrow stroma-mediated resistance to FLT3 inhibitors in FLT3-ITD AML is mediated by persistent activation of extracellular regulated kinase. *Br J Haematol* **164:** 61–72. doi:10.1111/bjh.12599

Yasuda T, Ueno T, Fukumura K, Yamato A, Ando M, Yamaguchi H, Soda M, Kawazu M, Sai E, Yamashita Y, et al. 2014. Leukemic evolution of donor-derived cells harboring IDH2 and DNMT3A mutations after allogeneic stem cell transplantation. *Leukemia* **28:** 426–428. doi:10.1038/leu.2013.278

Zhang Q, Zhao K, Shen Q, Han Y, Gu Y, Li X, Zhao D, Liu Y, Wang C, Zhang X, et al. 2015. Tet2 is required to resolve inflammation by recruiting Hdac2 to specifically repress IL-6. *Nature* **525:** 389–393. doi:10.1038/nature15252

Zhao X, Singh S, Pardoux C, Zhao J, Hsi ED, Abo A, Korver W. 2010. Targeting C-type lectin-like molecule-1 for antibody-mediated immunotherapy in acute myeloid leukemia. *Haematologica* **95:** 71–78. doi:10.3324/haematol.2009.009811

Zhao JL, Ma C, O'Connell RM, Mehta A, DiLoreto R, Heath JR, Baltimore D. 2014. Conversion of danger signals into cytokine signals by hematopoietic stem and progenitor cells for regulation of stress-induced hematopoiesis. *Cell Stem Cell* **14:** 445–459. doi:10.1016/j.stem.2014.01.007

Zheng B, Yu SF, Del Rosario G, Leong SR, Lee GY, Vij R, Chiu CPC, Liang WC, Wu Y, Chalouni C, et al. 2019. An anti-CLL-1 antibody-drug conjugate for the treatment of acute myeloid leukemia. *Clin Cancer Res* **25:** 1358–1368. doi:10.1158/1078-0432.CCR-18-0333

Epigenetic Mechanisms in Leukemias and Lymphomas

Cihangir Duy, Wendy Béguelin, and Ari Melnick

Department of Medicine, Weill Cornell Medicine, New York, New York 10021, USA
Correspondence: web2002@med.cornell.edu; amm2014@med.cornell.edu

Although we are just beginning to understand the mechanisms that regulate the epigenome, aberrant epigenetic programming has already emerged as a hallmark of hematologic malignancies including acute myeloid leukemia (AML) and B-cell lymphomas. Although these diseases arise from the hematopoietic system, the epigenetic mechanisms that drive these malignancies are quite different. Yet, in all of these tumors, somatic mutations in transcription factors and epigenetic modifiers are the most commonly mutated set of genes and result in multilayered disruption of the epigenome. Myeloid and lymphoid neoplasms generally manifest epigenetic allele diversity, which contributes to tumor cell population fitness regardless of the underlying genetics. Epigenetic therapies are emerging as one of the most promising new approaches for these patients. However, effective targeting of the epigenome must consider the need to restore the various layers of epigenetic marks, appropriate biological end points, and specificity of therapeutic agents to truly realize the potential of this modality.

Epigenetic instructions are the equivalent of software programs that instruct cellular phenotypes, including those of tumor cells. Along these lines, it has been shown that aberrant epigenetic programming occurs universally in hematologic malignancies, and somatic mutations in genes encoding epigenetic modifiers and transcription factors are the most abundant class of genetic lesions in these tumors. Therefore, hematological malignancies provide an excellent viewpoint for exploring how the many layers of epigenetic mechanisms interact to mediate transformed phenotypes. Herein, we focus on, and provide the basis to compare and contrast, epigenetic mechanisms underlying pathogenesis of acute myeloid leukemia (AML) and the common lymphomas derived from germinal center (GC) B cells.

EPIGENETIC MECHANISMS IN AML

Aberrant Cytosine Methylation Profiles Are a Hallmark of AML

A significant subset of recurrent mutations in AML affect epigenetic modifications of DNA and/or histones (Fig. 1) (Abbas et al. 2010; Marcucci et al. 2010, 2012; Paschka et al. 2010; Hollink et al. 2011; Shen et al. 2011; Gaidzik et al. 2012; Patel et al. 2012; Weissmann et al. 2012;

Cite this article as *Cold Spring Harb Perspect Med* doi: 10.1101/cshperspect.a034959

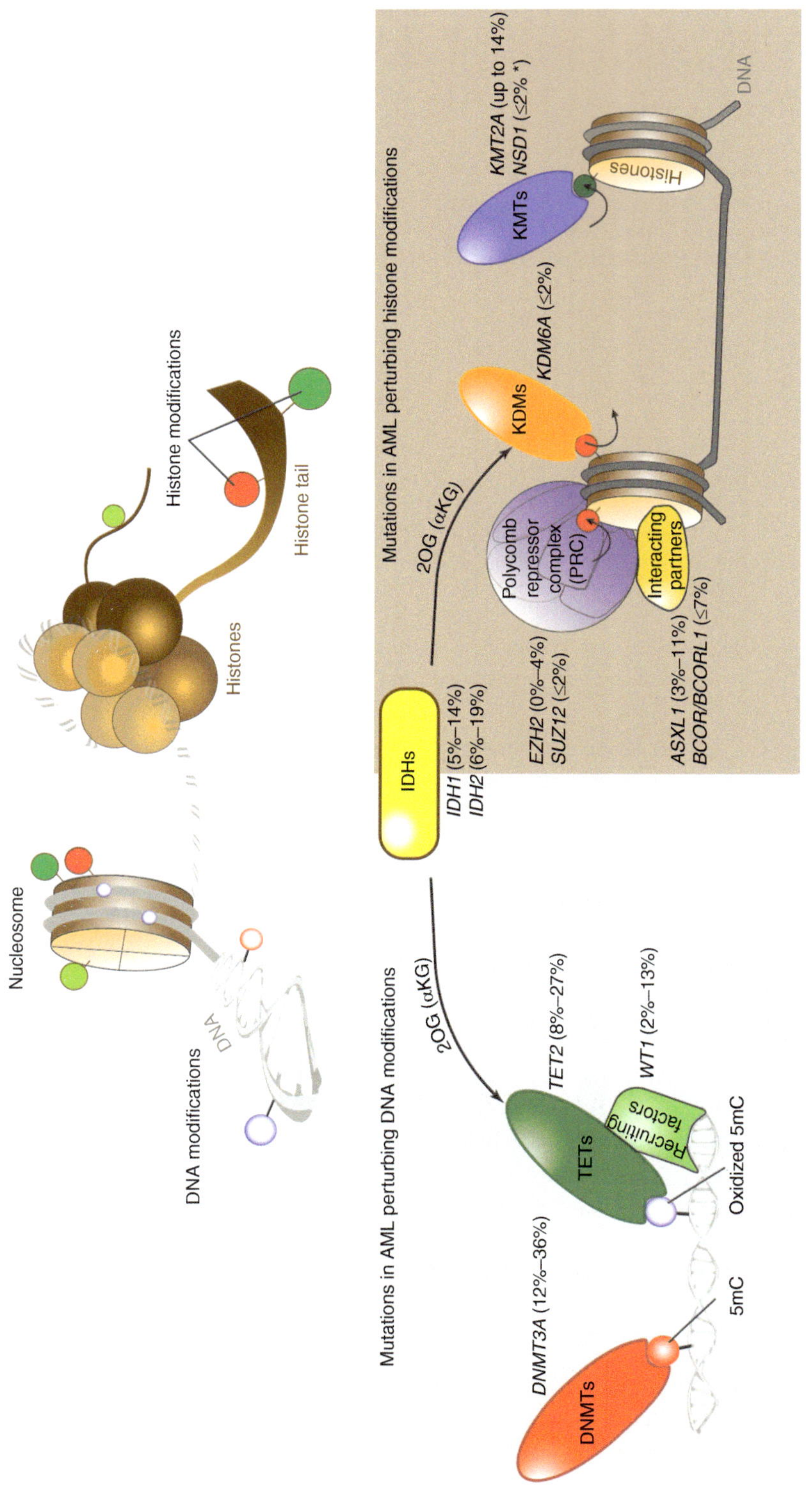

Figure 1. Frequent mutations of epigenetic regulators in acute myeloid leukemia (AML). *Upper* panel illustrates epigenetic modifications on the DNA and histone layer of the epigenome. *Lower* panel shows gene mutations that impact DNA and/or histone modifications in at least 1% of AML cases. Ranges of reported mutation frequency are indicated in parentheses (Abbas et al. 2010; Marcucci et al. 2010, 2012; Paschka et al. 2010; Hollink et al. 2011; Shen et al. 2011; Gaidzik et al. 2012; Patel et al. 2012; Weissmann et al. 2012; Cancer Genome Atlas Research 2013; Gao et al. 2013; Metzeler et al. 2016; Papaemmanuil et al. 2016; Terada et al. 2018). The asterisk indicates frequency in adult AML. KMT, lysine methyltransferase; KDM, lysine demethylase; 2OG, 2-oxoglutarate, also called α-ketoglutarate (αKG).

Cancer Genome Atlas Research 2013; Gao et al. 2013; Metzeler et al. 2016; Papaemmanuil et al. 2016; Terada et al. 2018). Cytosine methylation (5mC) is critical for gene silencing, imprinting, X-chromosome inactivation, genome stability, and cell fate determination (Bird 2002). Tissue-specific 5mC patterns are established primarily by de novo DNA methyltransferases DNMT3A and DNMT3B (Okano et al. 1999) and are subsequently maintained by DNMT1 in a replication-dependent manner (Fig. 2A) (Robert et al. 2003). CpG islands (CGIs), comprising <10% of all CpGs, are found in ~70% of promoters and are predominantly unmethylated, whereas a majority of remaining CpGs (60%–80%) are methylated in human cells (Saxonov et al. 2006; Smith and Meissner 2013). Disruption of cytosine methylation patterning at gene promoters is a hallmark of AML and is clearly linked to aberrant gene silencing (Figueroa et al. 2010b; Cancer Genome Atlas Research 2013). However, more recent studies indicate that critical 5mC changes in AML are also present at gene enhancers, in which their effects on gene expression are more nuanced (Glass et al. 2017). Importantly, 5mC profiles allow AMLs to be classified into biologically defined subtypes with distinct clinical outcomes (Figueroa et al. 2010a,b). Some of these profiles are linked to specific somatic mutations, whereas others are independent of mutations and are dependent on underlying disease-driving mechanisms such as overexpression of EVI1 (Lugthart et al. 2011) or silencing of myeloid lineage transcription factors such as CEBPα (Figueroa et al. 2009). Importantly, a subset of genes appears to be almost universally aberrantly methylated and silenced in AML patients regardless of somatic mutations (Figueroa et al. 2010b). It is possible that these epigenetic alleles are "epi-drivers" that are required for normal hematopoietic cells to manifest a leukemic phenotype in cooperation with somatic mutations and may explain why AMLs manifest relatively few genetic lesions. 5mC redistribution plays a critical role in myeloid differentiation (Bröske et al. 2009; Ji et al. 2010; Bock et al. 2012) and might be prone to disruption by such epi-drivers.

AMLs Feature Highly Recurrent Mutations of Proteins That Modify Cytosine Residues

DNMT3A Mutations

Most mutant *DNMT3A* AML show either a heterozygous missense (R882H/C) mutation that affects the catalytic domain or truncating mutations (Cancer Genome Atlas Research 2013; Yang et al. 2015). R882 hotspot mutations impair DNMT3A methyltransferase activity and are linked to hypomethylation at specific CpGs (Russler-Germain et al. 2014). *Dnmt3a* knockout mice manifest severe differentiation block and enhanced self-renewal potential of hematopoietic stem cells (HSCs) (Challen et al. 2011). This is associated with DNA hypomethylation at borders of so-called "canyons" at regulatory regions of self-renewal genes (Jeong et al. 2014) consisting of large hypomethylated regions that contain histone activating marks (H3K4me3), repressive marks (H3K27me3), or both (Xie et al. 2013; Jeong et al. 2014). Noncompetitive transplantation experiments reveal that loss of DNMT3A predisposes murine HSCs to malignant transformation (Mayle et al. 2015), consistent with findings in humans, in which *DNMT3A* mutations establish a reservoir of preleukemic stem cells that can evolve to AML (Shlush et al. 2014). In addition, mutant $DNMT3A^{R882}$ impairs chromatin remodeling and nucleosome eviction during chemotherapy, conferring resistance against anthracyclines that could explain the poor prognosis of $DNMT3A^{mut}$ AML (Ley et al. 2010; Shen et al. 2011; Guryanova et al. 2016).

Somatic Mutations of TET2 *in AML*

Removal of 5mC is initiated by members of the ten-eleven translocation (TET) family of dioxygenases through successive oxidization of 5mC to 5-hydroxymethylcytosine (5hmC), 5-formylcytosine (5fC), and 5-carboxylcytosine (5caC) (Fig. 2A) (Tahiliani et al. 2009; He et al. 2011; Ito et al. 2011). Apart from DNA demethylation by passive dilution following cell replication, 5fC and 5caC can be actively excised by thymine-DNA glycosylase (TDG) and repaired by the base excision repair (BER) pathway to regen-

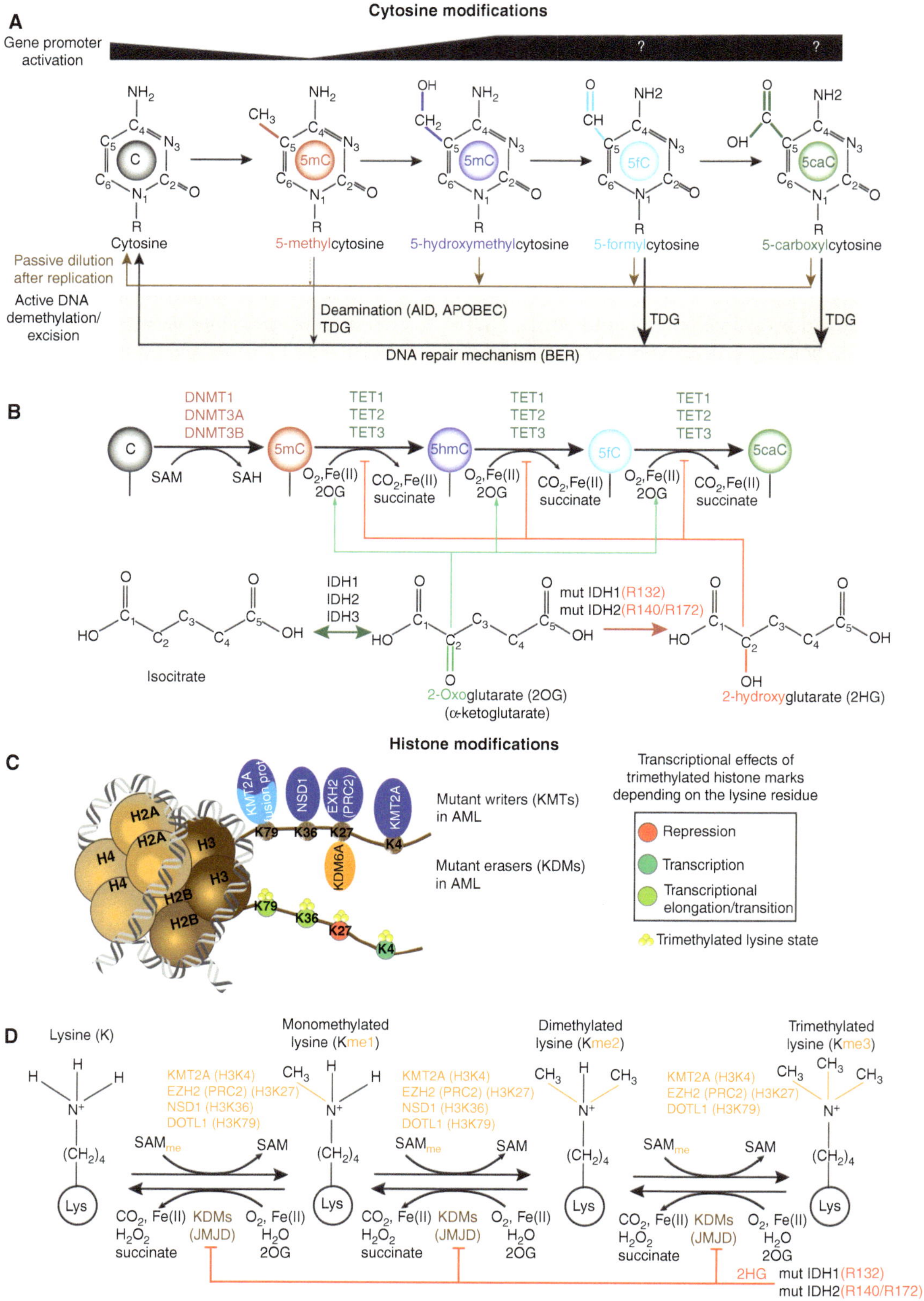

Figure 2. (*See legend on following page.*)

erate unmodified cytosines (Maiti and Drohat 2011; Rasmussen and Helin 2016). In addition, activation-induced cytidine deaminase (AID) and APOBEC can deaminate 5mC but not 5hmC, contributing to 5mC erasure (Fig. 2A) (Nabel et al. 2012). Recent findings suggest that genomic 5hmC might also play an active role as an epigenetic mark that regulates transcription through modulation of chromatin accessibility and recruitment/hinderance of specific factors (e.g., MBD proteins binds to 5hmC DNA with weaker affinity than to 5mC DNA) (Hashimoto et al. 2012; Shen et al. 2013; Bachman et al. 2014; Ngo et al. 2016). In murine embryonic stem cells (ESCs), 5hmC function is involved in maintaining the active state of gene enhancers (Hon et al. 2014). Importantly, TET2 is primarily localized at CpG-sparse distal regulatory elements, suggesting a main function in enhancer regulation (Rasmussen et al. 2019). In agreement with this, deletion of TET2 in hematopoietic cells reduces 5hmC primarily at enhancers leading to down-regulation of tumor-suppressor genes (Rasmussen et al. 2015; Duy et al. 2019). *TET2* is frequently mutated in AML, largely by frameshift or nonsense mutations (Chou et al. 2011; Weissmann et al. 2012). Loss of TET2 impairs differentiation and increases self-renewal potential of HSCs but requires cooperating mutations such as FLT3-ITD for full leukemic transformation (Delhommeau et al. 2009; Moran-Crusio et al. 2011; Quivoron et al. 2011; Shih et al. 2015). Notably, loss of TET2 alone has little effect on 5mC, but TET2 can synergistically induce DNA hypermethylation in the presence of a cooperating oncogene such as FLT3-ITD (Shih et al. 2015). Transformed cells derived from *Tet2*-deleted *Flt3*-ITD mice or human AML cells show DNA hypermethylation and suppression of GATA2, a hematopoietic master regulator, whose reconstitution impaires leukemia growth (Shih et al. 2015; Duy et al. 2019). Recruitment of TET2 to chromatin depends on transcription factors such as WT1 (Rampal et al. 2014; Wang et al. 2015). TET2 functions as a tumor suppressor in AML and requires the interaction with WT1 to suppress leukemia growth (Rampal et al. 2014; Wang et al. 2015). Overexpression of WT1 increased global levels of 5hmC, whereas reduced 5hmC levels were observed when WT1 was silenced. Recurrent missense mutations of TET2 can compromise its binding to WT1 and thereby fail to inhibit leukemia proliferation (Wang et al. 2015). Finally, loss of TET2 inactivates enhancers not only by reducing 5hmC but also through reduced enhancer histone marks such H3K4me1 mediated through LSD1 (KDM1A) (Duy et al. 2019). Hence, loss of TET2 impairs multiple layers of the epigenome.

Figure 2. Epigenetic features and perturbations in acute myeloid leukemia (AML). (*A*) Diagram showing the structure of methylated cytosine (5mC) and oxidized mCs (5hmC, 5fC, 5caC) as well as their transcriptional association at promoters. Active DNA demethylation is indicated by black arrows below modified cytosines. 5fC and 5caC can be excised directly by the thymine DNA glycosylase (TDG), resulting in an abasic site that is eventually replaced with unmethylated cytosine by the base excision repair (BER) machinery. Activation-induced cytidine deaminase (AID) or APOBEC can deaminated 5mC to thymine that is subsequently removed by TDG and repaired by BER. On the other hand, passive demethylation (brown arrows) is an alternative process that can occur through dilution following cell replication. DNMT1 can directly replicate the 5mC pattern onto the newly synthesized daughter strand unlike the pattern of oxidized mCs. (For review, see Rasmussen and Helin 2016.) (*B*) Enzymatic processes involved in cytosine methylation and oxidation of 5mC. DNMTs catalyze the addition of a methyl group to cytosine using *S*-adenosyl methionine (SAM) as methyl donor. Ten-eleven translocation (TET) proteins oxidize methylated cytosines to 5hmC, 5fC, and 5caC in an iterative manner using 2OG (αKG) as cosubstrate. Mutant IDH1/2 generates 2HG that inhibits competitively the enzymatic activity of TET proteins. (*C*) Nucleosome model shows lysine substrate residues on histone H3 for writers (KMTs) and erasers (KDMs) that are found mutated in AML. Chromosomal translocations involving KMT2A (KMT2A-re) often result in fusion proteins that associate with the H3K79 histone methyltransferase DOT1L. (*D*) Enzymatic processes of lysine (de)methylation for selected KMTs. Besides TET proteins, 2HG can also impair the enzymatic activity Jumonji domain (JMJD)-containing KDMs.

Somatic Mutations of IDH1 *and* IDH2

AML somatic mutations in the *IDH1* and *IDH2* genes are virtually always heterozygous and affect IDH1 on R132 or IDH2 on the R140, R172 residues (Mardis et al. 2009; Abbas et al. 2010; Paschka et al. 2010). IDH1 (cytosolic protein) and IDH2 (mitochondrial protein) are metabolic enzymes that catalyze the interconversion of isocitrate to α-ketoglutarate (αKG) (Fig. 2B). αKG is necessary for oxidation of 5mC by TET enzymes (Fig. 2B). IDH1/2 hotspot mutations yield an enzymatic gain of function that instead favors the synthesis and accumulation of (R)-2-hydroxyglutarate (2HG) (Dang et al. 2009; Gross et al. 2010; Ward et al. 2011). 2HG competitively inhibits αKG-dependent dioxygenases such as TET enzymes and the Jumonji domain histone lysine demethylases, resulting in loss of 5hmC, gain of 5mC, and gain of histone methylation (Fig. 2B,C) (Figueroa et al. 2010a; Chowdhury et al. 2011; Xu et al. 2011; Lu et al. 2012; Rampal et al. 2014). Mutant IDH1/2 impairs HSC differentiation and it is notable that IDH1/2 mutations are almost entirely mutually exclusive with TET2 mutations in AML, suggesting that their effects on 5hmC and/or 5mC are dominant transforming effects in myeloid cells (Figueroa et al. 2010a). However, unlike *Tet2* knockout mice, mutant $IDH1^{R132}$ knock-in mice show reduced long-term (LT) HSCs and an altered DNA damage response caused by down-regulation of the ATM kinase independent of TET2 (Inoue et al. 2016). It was proposed that ATM down-regulation was mediated by 2HG inhibition of KDM4, resulting in a repressive chromatin environment suppressing ATM (Inoue et al. 2016). Moreover, 2HG can impair all TET enzymes, thereby causing a more pleiotropic effect than just mutant TET2 alone. Indeed, IDH^{mut} AML shows a greater DNA hypermethylation phenotype than $TET2^{mut}$ AML (Rampal et al. 2014). Altogether, this suggests that the leukemogenic mechanisms are not equivalent and may contribute to different therapeutic responses of IDH^{mut} AML compared to $TET2^{mut}$ (Patel et al. 2012; Duy et al. 2019). Moreover, IDH^{mut} and $DNMT3A^{mut}$ AMLs feature opposing cytosine methylation profiles, and double-mutant *IDH1/DNMT3A* AML show almost complete loss of these profiles, thus questioning the relevance of DNA methylation (Glass et al. 2017). How these mutations cooperate is still unknown, but double-mutant IDH1/DNMT3A AML features up-regulation of RAS signatures and unique sensitivity to MEK inhibition ex vivo relative to AMLs with either single mutation (Glass et al. 2017).

Somatic Mutation of Chromatin Modifiers in AML

Loss-of-function and missense mutations have been reported in core components of the Polycomb repressive complex 2 (PRC2) *SUZ12* and *EZH2*, which trimethylates histone H3 lysine 27 (H3K27me3) to induce transcriptional repression (Figs. 1 and 2C,D) (Ernst et al. 2010, 2012; Cancer Genome Atlas Research 2013). PRC2 induces stable silencing of early development genes, as well as transiently repressed bivalent chromatin promoters (H3K4me3, H3K27me3) (Margueron and Reinberg 2011). This complexity is exemplified by the finding that *Ezh2* deletion preceding transduction of oncogenes like MLL-AF9 or AML1-ETO9a accelerates leukemia progression, whereas deletion of *Ezh2* in already established AMLs with these oncogenes had the opposite effect and, in this case, attenuated disease progression (Basheer et al. 2019). Thus, EZH2 has a tumor-suppressive function at initiation of AML but a tumor-supportive one in maintenance of AML. Epigenetic changes induced by impaired function of PRC2 allows AML cells to tolerate increased stress including chemotherapy treatment (Göllner et al. 2017; Duy and Melnick 2018; Maganti et al. 2018). PRC2 functions can also be disrupted in the presence of inactivating somatic mutations in *ASXL1*, which directs PRC2 to target loci (Fig. 1) (Abdel-Wahab et al. 2012). Disrupting mutations in *BCOR* and *BCORL1* have been reported and likely impact Polycomb-like complexes (Grossmann et al. 2011; Metzeler et al. 2016; Chittock et al. 2017). Mutations in KDM6A (UTX), which demethylates H3K27me3, have been reported in a small cohort of AML (Figs. 1 and 2D) (Cancer Genome Atlas Research

2013; Metzeler et al. 2016). Knockout of UTX induces spontaneous AML and results primarily in bidirectional changes of H3K27Ac as well as chromatin remodeling that is associated with inactivation of tumor-suppressive GATA programs and activation of oncogenic ETS programs (Gozdecka et al. 2018).

The histone methyltransferase KMT2A (MLL) is frequently mutated by partial tandem duplications (PTDs) or chromosomal rearrangements, the latter resulting in loss of the catalytic SET domain (Caligiuri et al. 1998; Grimwade et al. 2001; Krivtsov and Armstrong 2007). KMT2A methylates H3K4, which plays a role in the formation and activity of enhancers and promoters (Fig. 2C,D) (Ernst et al. 2011). The duplicated region in MLL-PTD includes the CXXC domain, which preferentially binds to nonmethylated CpGs (Schichman et al. 1994; Birke et al. 2002) that can potentially perturb coordination with DNA methylation. Mice with *MLL-PTD* show dysregulation of homeobox (*Hox*) gene expression but require additional mutations such as the Flt3-ITD for full leukemogenesis (Dorrance et al. 2008; Zorko et al. 2012). MLL rearrangements (KMT2A-re) result frequently in fusion with genes encoding super elongation complex proteins like AF9, AF10, and ENL (Krivtsov and Armstrong 2007). This complex associates with the histone methyltransferase DOT1L that targets H3K79 (Fig. 2C,D). MLL-transformed AML samples show aberrant H3K79 methylation, leading to ongoing expression of *Hox* genes. The NSD1 H3K36 histone methyltransferase is sometimes fused with NUP98, which could affect several gene regulatory functions (Fig. 2C,D) (Wagner and Carpenter 2012).

An additional layer of epigenetic regulation in AML is conferred by the 3D conformation of chromatin that brings distant genes into spatial proximity with each other or that forms loops between enhancers and promoters (Kagey et al. 2010). Many of these interactions are mediated by the cohesin complex, a ring-like structure composed of *SMC1A, SMC3, RAD21*, and *STAG1/STAG2*. The cohesin complex is responsible for connecting sister chromatids, regulation of transcription, and DNA repair (Haarhuis et al. 2014; Kim et al. 2016). Mutations in the cohesin complex are found between 6% and 18% in AML (Ding et al. 2012; Cancer Genome Atlas Research 2013; Kon et al. 2013; Thol et al. 2014; Thota et al. 2014; Tsai et al. 2017) and induce expansion of hematopoietic stem/progenitor cells and impair myeloid differentiation (Mullenders et al. 2015; Viny et al. 2015; Tothova et al. 2017). ASXL1 also interacts with the cohesin complex for proper gene regulation and might indicate a potential role in chromatin conformation (Li et al. 2017).

Epigenetic Therapy of AML

Targeting Specific Epigenetic Mechanisms

Aberrant DNA hypermethylation can be removed by DNMT inhibitors (DNMTi) (Fig. 3A) (Jones and Baylin 2007), although these drugs have pleiotropic effects and impact methylation on a genome-wide level. Specific inhibitors were recently developed against mutant IDH1/2 (AG120/AG221) and show a promising overall response rate of ~40% in patients with relapsed/refractory IDH-mutant AML (Stein et al. 2017; DiNardo et al. 2018); however, their impact on epigenetic reprogramming and remodeling in patient samples remains to be delineated. Despite the initial response to IDH inhibitors, multiple drug resistance pathways have been reported including isoform switching between mutant IDH1 and mutant IDH2, second-site target mutations, co-occurring NRAS mutations, and selection of ancestral or terminal clones (Amatangelo et al. 2017; Harding et al. 2018; Intlekofer et al. 2018; Quek et al. 2018). Although protein loss (e.g., truncating *TET2* mutations) cannot be targeted directly, approaches to compensate its function present an option. This has been shown with vitamin C, which enhances the catalytic activity of the residual wild-type TET proteins and suppresses leukemia growth (Fig. 3A) (Cimmino et al. 2017). A related approach was proposed for mutant DNMT3A by increasing intracellular levels of SAM (Fig. 3A) (Adema et al. 2017).

Targeting Epigenetic Mechanisms on Histones

LSD1 has emerged as a promising therapeutic target in AML (Fig. 3B) (Harris et al. 2012;

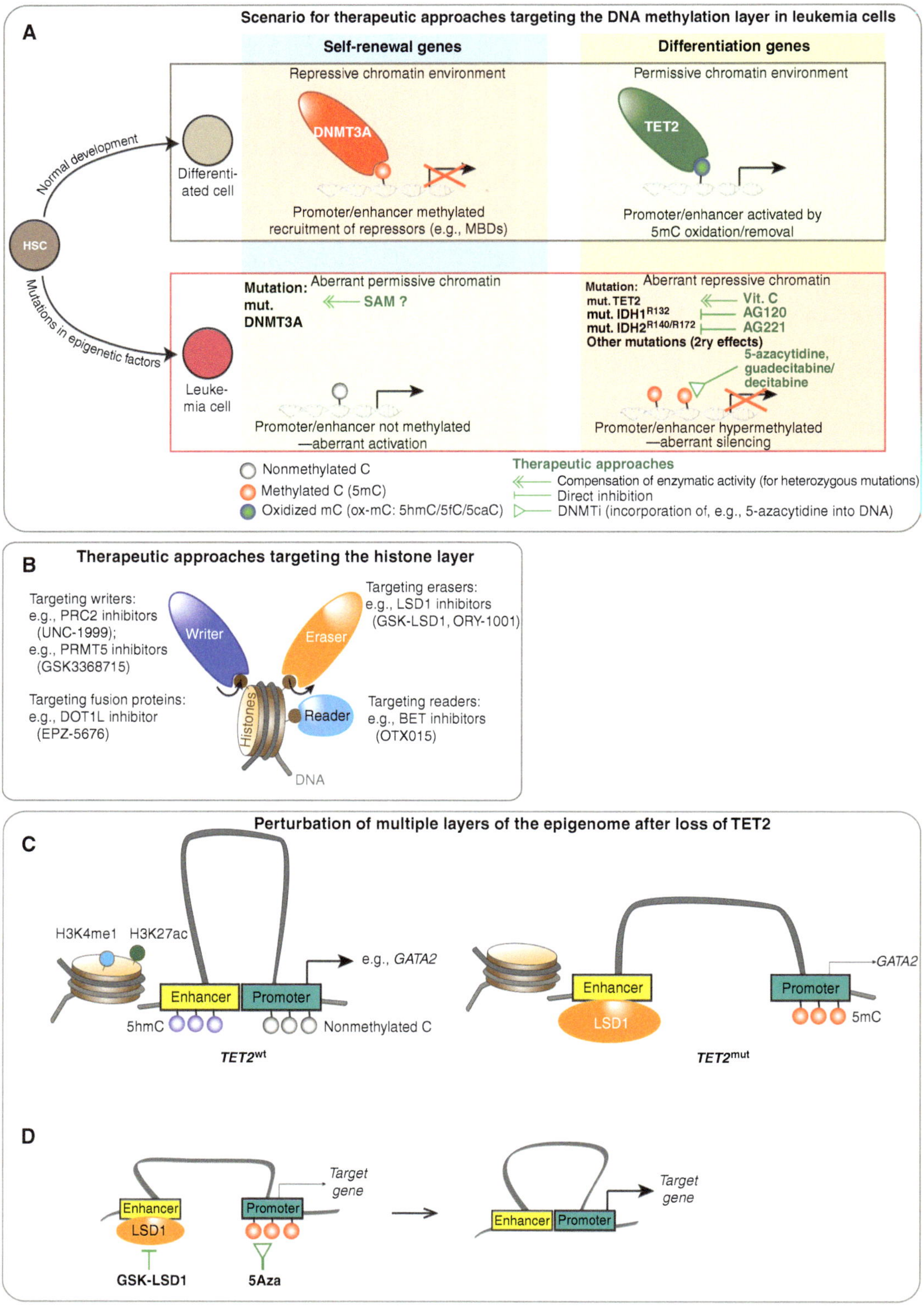

Figure 3. (*See legend on following page.*)

Schenk et al. 2012; McGrath et al. 2016; Maes et al. 2018). LSD1 inhibitors (LSD1i) present also another option in *TET2*^{mut} AML, in which it reverses aberrant repression of LSD1-inactivating enhancers (Duy et al. 2019). Moreover, inhibition of LSD1 can overcome nongenetic acquired drug resistance against BET inhibitors by modulating enhancer dependencies of key survival genes, showing further the critical role of enhancers in drug tolerance in AML (Bell et al. 2019). BET proteins can bind to acetylated lysines on histones (Fig. 3B) and facilitate transcriptional activation and promoter–enhancer interactions (Florence and Faller 2001; Wu and Chiang 2007). BRD4, a BET family member, has been implicated in AML, perhaps linked to maintaining MYC expression (Zuber et al. 2011). The role of PRC2 (EZH2) in AML is complex and not clear (Duy and Melnick 2018; Basheer et al. 2019). The use of UNC1999, a dual inhibitor of EZH1/2, impaired the growth of *MLL*(*KMT2A*)-rearranged leukemia cell lines suggesting that inhibition of PRC2 is detrimental in these leukemias (Fig. 3B) (Xu et al. 2015). Inhibition of DOT1L (EPZ-5676) also targets *MLL*-rearranged AML (Fig. 3B) (Chen et al. 2016). In addition, inhibition of protein arginine methyltransferase 1 (PRMT1) and 5 (PRMT5) displays an antileukemic effect in certain AMLs (Fig. 3B) (Shia et al. 2012; Tarighat et al. 2016; Fedoriw et al. 2019). Overall, it is important to note that all these histone-regulating proteins are not frequently mutated or overexpressed in AML and also play distinct roles in normal cells. Thus, targeting these factors requires a careful approach in a therapeutic window that will preferentially interfere with key nononcogene dependencies underlying the malignant program of AML.

Epigenetic Combination Therapy

Because the epigenome consists of many functionally interdependent mechanisms, it is inherently challenging to fully correct aberrant epigenetic programming by hitting only a single epigenetic target. This consideration may explain in part the relatively modest activity of epigenetic therapies to date (Fennell et al. 2019). Combining epigenetic therapies is chal-

Figure 3. Epigenetic therapy and combination therapy targeting cooperating layers of the epigenome in acute myeloid leukemia (AML). (*A*) Scenario illustrating the effect of distinct epigenetic mutations (indicated in bold letters) in leukemia cells versus normal differentiated cells derived from hematopoietic stem cells (HSCs). Epigenetic therapy and strategies targeting aberrant DNA methylation are shown by green lines. Loss of DNA methylation at self-renewal genes in *DNMT3A*^{mut} AML may be potentially reversible by increasing intracellular levels of SAM (methyl donor). Loss of TET2 function can be compensated with vitamin C treatment. Specific inhibitors (AG120, AG221) against mutant IDH1/2 can block production of the TET inhibitor 2HG. Direct DNA hypermethylation (mutant TET2 or IDH1/2) or indirect hypermethylation due to secondary effects from other disease-driving mutations can be treated with DNMT inhibitors like 5-azacytidine or guadecitabine/decitabine (Issa et al. 2015; Gardin and Dombret 2017). (*B*) Drugs to target histone-modifying enzymes (writers+erasers) as well as readers (e.g., BET inhibitors) that are critical for AML maintenance and present vulnerabilities of the disease. Specific LSD1 inhibitors include GSK-LSD1 and ORY-1001 (Mohammad et al. 2015; Maes et al. 2018). Although PRC2 is deleted in a subset of AML, other AML subtypes such as *KMT2A*-re (*MLL*-rearranged) leukemias depend on functional PRC2. UNC1999, a dual inhibitor of EZH1/2 EZH1/2, impaired the growth of KMT2A-re in preclinical studies (Xu et al. 2015). DOT1L inhibitors (e.g., EPZ-5676) were also developed to target *KMT2A*(*MLL*)-re AML (Chen et al. 2016). The BRD 2/3/4 inhibitor OTX015 induces apoptosis in a variety of AMLs (Coudé et al. 2015). Inhibition of PRMT1 and PRMT5 show an antileukemia effect in distinct AMLs (Shia et al. 2012; Tarighat et al. 2016; Fedoriw et al. 2019). (*C*) Scheme illustrating the disruption of multiple layers of the epigenome in *TET2*^{mut} cells. Loss of *TET2* facilitates recruitment of the H3K4me1/2 histone demethylase LSD1 that inactivates enhancers at target genes. In addition, loss of TET2 results in promoter methylation at target genes such as *GATA2*. (*D*) Concept of targeting cooperating layers of the epigenome at enhancers and promoters in *TET2*^{mut} AML to reconstitute enhancer–promoter interactions. Removal of 5mC promoter methylation by 5Aza treatment combined with LSD1 inhibition (GSK-LSD1) facilitates interactions of the LSD1-occupied enhancer and its target promoter, resulting in up-regulation of target genes like *GATA2*.

lenging, however, because they may antagonize in vivo, such as occurred with the combination of DNMT inhibitors (DNMTi) + histone deacetylase inhibitors (HDACi) in AML patients (Prebet et al. 2014), and certain compounds such as HDACi have profoundly pleiotropic effects and hence significant toxicity in humans. Moreover, because little is known yet about how epigenetic mechanisms play into AML, it is difficult to predict which patients might respond to a given therapy, with rare exceptions such as HDACi. On the other hand, it is difficult to assess the efficacy of epigenetic therapies in the laboratory because AML cell lines do not reflect the genetic and epigenetic spectrum of AML cases. However, recent studies deploying organoid type cultures of primary AML cells are better suited to test epigenetic agents, many of which mediate their effects through slow and gradual effects. The unexpected enhanced activity of LSD1i+DNMTi against TET2 leukemia was discovered through such an approach, in which a large cohort of genetically characterized primary AMLs were screened using an organoid system (Duy et al. 2019). In $TET2^{mut}$ AML, full activation of aberrantly silenced tumor suppressors such as GATA2 could only be restored by simultaneously reversing gene promoter hypermethylation using DNMTi and restoring active enhancer marks for the same genes using LSD1i (because loss of TET2/5hmC results in LSD1-mediated enhancer repression; Fig. 3C,D).

Combination of Epigenetic with Nonepigenetic Drugs

AML mutations in nonepigenetic factors (e.g., FLT3) provide a rationale to combine epigenetic with specific nonepigenetic drugs. Supporting this, combination of DNMTi and FLT3 inhibitors improved therapeutic response in *FLT3-ITD*-mutant AML (Ravandi et al. 2013; Muppidi et al. 2015; Strati et al. 2015; Chang et al. 2016; Shih et al. 2017). Also, combination of DNMTi with drugs targeting nonmutant proteins like BCL2 (venetoclax) improved therapeutic efficacy particularly in elderly patients with AML (Tsao et al. 2012; Bogenberger et al. 2015; Shih et al. 2017; Aldoss et al. 2018; DiNardo et al. 2019). However, it is unclear whether this combination therapy is driven by epigenetic effects or rather by partial DNA damage caused by DNMTi treatment that results in apoptosis in leukemia cells after inhibition of BCL2. Because DNMTis also show immunomodulatory effects like induction of PD-1 and IFN-γ signaling, clinical trials exploring the combination of DNMTi with immune checkpoint inhibitor (ICI) drugs (e.g., nivolumab) are underway (Daver et al. 2019). Although CTLA-4 and PD-1 immune checkpoint drugs have revolutionized the management of certain cancer types like melanoma (Postow et al. 2015; Robert et al. 2015), other cancer types (e.g., pancreatic cancer) remain unaffected by ICI drugs (Brahmer et al. 2012). Given that the mutational burden of AML is one of the lowest compared with other cancers (Lawrence et al. 2013), the recognition of AML cells by the immune system is presumably less efficient compared with cancers with high mutational burden such as melanoma.

EPIGENETIC MECHANISMS IN B-CELL MALIGNANCIES

Most Lymphomas Arise from GC B Cells, Which Are Epigenetically Programmed to Resemble Tumor Cells

B-cell lymphomas arise from a wide variety of functionally distinct B-cell subsets to yield a bewildering number of lymphoma subtypes. Some of the more common B-cell neoplasms, their mutations, and their cell of origin are depicted in Figure 4. However, a majority of B-cell lymphomas (diffuse large B-cell lymphomas [DLBCLs] and follicular lymphomas [FLs]) arise from B cells transiting the GC reaction, which will be the focus of this section. GCs are transient structures that form in response to T-cell-dependent antigen (Hatzi and Melnick 2014). Naive B cells are epigenetically "primed"—that is, feature active chromatin marks—to induce expression of genes required for plasma cell differentiation, on receiving activation signals. However, after T-cell-directed activation, a subset of naive B cells is able to transiently silence these terminal differentiation genes and instead migrate within

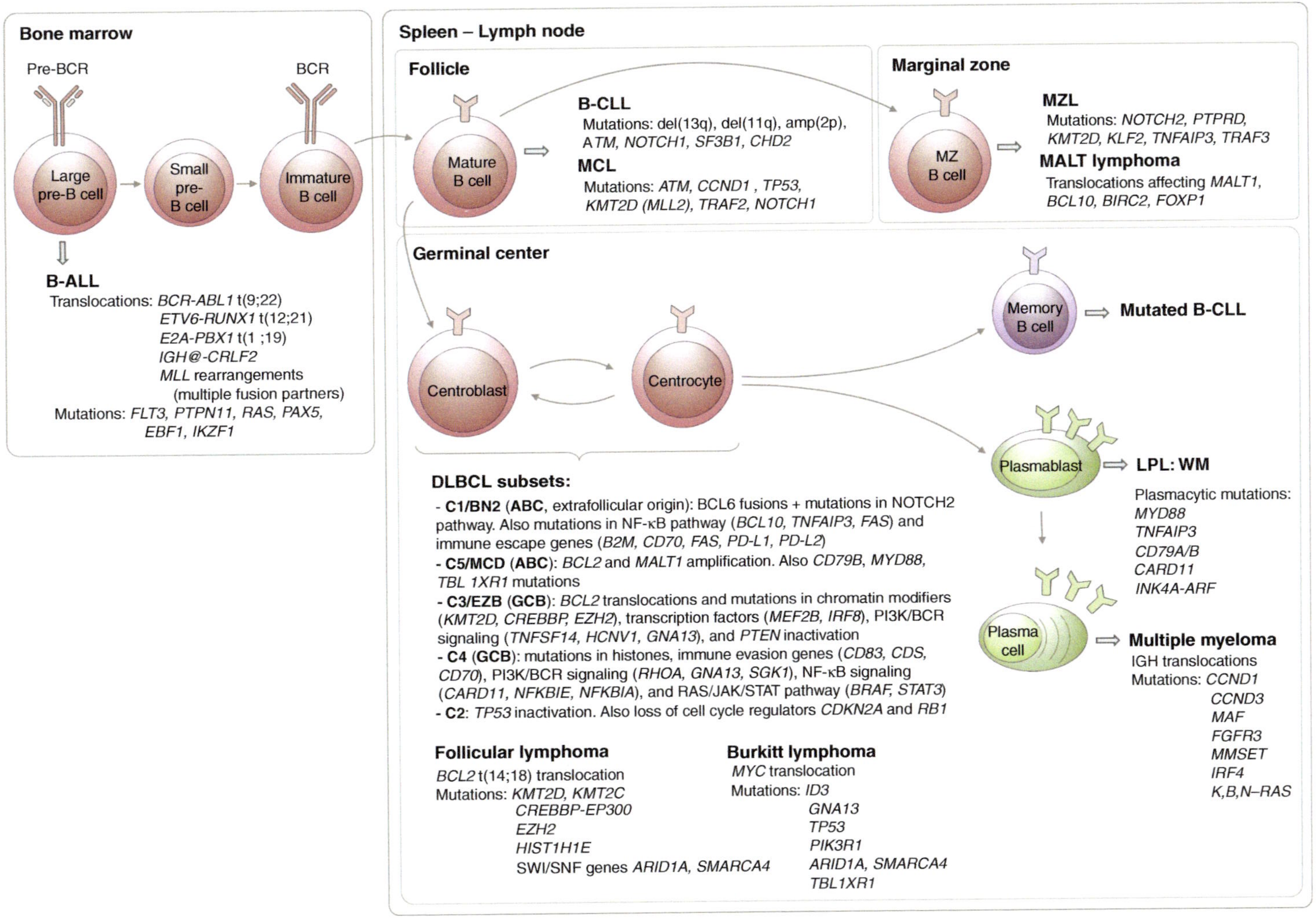

Figure 4. (*See legend on following page.*)

lymphoid follicles to form nests of highly proliferative GC B cells called "centroblasts," which undergo somatic hypermutation of their immunoglobulin genes because of the actions of AICDA. After several rounds of division these GC B cells stop proliferating and compete to interact with a limiting number of T follicular helper (TFH) cells to survive. These nonproliferating GC B cells are called "centrocytes," and interact with TFH cells through a number of receptor–ligand processes collectively called the "immune synapse" (Papa and Vinuesa 2018). Only the few GC B cells that generate high-affinity B-cell receptors interact strongly with TFH cells and can then restore their original epigenetic programming to differentiate into plasma or memory B cells or undergo further somatic hypermutation. However, the vast majority of GC B cells undergo apoptosis (Fig. 5A) (Mesin et al. 2016).

Importantly, the phenotype of GC B cells features many hallmarks that are considered pathognomonic for cancer (Hanahan and Weinberg 2011). These include (1) sustained proliferation and self-renewal (through repression of

---

Figure 4. Frequent mutations during B-cell development. In the bone marrow, rearrangements of the immunoglobulin genes of B-cell precursors to form a B-cell receptor (BCR) generate DNA breaks that are occasionally resolved aberrantly, leading to chromosomal translocations (Fugmann et al. 2000). These are the most common genetic alterations in B-precursor acute lymphoblastic leukemia (B-ALL) (Mullighan 2012). The most frequent mature B-cell neoplasms that have their origin outside the germinal center (GC) are B-cell chronic lymphocytic leukemia (B-CLL), mantle cell lymphoma (MCL), marginal zone lymphoma (MZL), and mucosa-associated lymphoid tissue (MALT) lymphoma. B-CLL and MCL differ in their molecular pathways, genomic alterations, and clinical behavior, being more aggressive in naive-like- than memory-like-derived tumors. The pathogenesis of the two malignancies involves the BCR signaling, tumor cell microenvironment interactions, genomic alterations, and epigenome modifications (Zhang et al. 2014; Landau et al. 2015). MALT lymphoma is the commonest MZL type and presents recurrent chromosomal translocations, which usually lead to activation of the NF-κB pathway. Nodal and splenic MZLs share recurrent mutations affecting the Notch pathway and the transcription factor *KLF2*, but differ for the inactivation of two tumor-suppressor genes, detected exclusively (*PTPRD*) or much more commonly (*KMT2D/MLL2*) in the nodal type (Rossi et al. 2012; Spina et al. 2016). The presence of immunoglobulin mutations is evidence that the cell of origin of the tumor passed through the GC microenvironment. Follicular lymphomas, Burkitt lymphomas, and DLBCLs express GC B cell signature genes. In the GC, two molecular processes remodel DNA: immunoglobulin class switch recombination (CSR) and somatic hypermutation (SHM), mechanisms that predispose to chromosomal translocations and mutations (Muramatsu et al. 2000). DLBCL is a clinically and genetically heterogeneous disease and accounts for 35% of non-Hodgkin lymphomas. Based on transcriptional profiles, DLBCL is further classified into activated B-cell (ABC) and germinal center B-cell (GCB) subtypes (Alizadeh et al. 2000; Rosenwald et al. 2002). ABC-DLBCLs derive from B cells that are committed to plasmablastic differentiation (Victora et al. 2012). These tumors have increased NF-κB activity, genetic alterations in NF-κB modifiers and components of the BCR pathway, and perturbed terminal B-cell differentiation (Lenz et al. 2008; Ngo et al. 2011). GCB-DLBCLs originate from light-zone GC B cells (Alizadeh et al. 2000; Victora et al. 2012). These tumors have frequent alterations in chromatin-modifying enzymes, PI3 K signaling, and genetic alterations of *BCL2* (Pfeifer et al. 2013; Basso and Dalla-Favera 2015). Modifications in these pathways could favor epigenetic reprogramming and escape from cellular immunity. Recent genomic profiles have identified sub-ABC and GCB-DLBCL clusters: C1-C5 in one study (of which two are GCB-, two are ABC-subtypes, and the fifth is mostly characterized by genomic instability and *TP53* mutations) (Chapuy et al. 2018), BN2, MCD, N1 (mostly ABC), and EZB (mostly GCB) in a different study (Schmitz et al. 2018). Follicular lymphoma (FL) is characterized by a unique histology in which tumor B cells form follicle-like structures with large numbers of nonmalignant immune cells infiltrating within the follicular and interfollicular regions (Kridel et al. 2012). The most frequent genetic event is the t(14;18) translocation that places *BCL2* under control of the immunoglobulin heavy-chain enhancer, which occurs in 90% of FL patients. Mutations in epigenetic modifiers (*KMT2D*, *CREBBP*, and *EZH2*) are also a hallmark of FL (Green 2018). These mutations result in altering normal B-cell differentiation programs and impeding GC exit (Green et al. 2015). Burkitt lymphoma is characterized by deregulation of the *MYC* gene through its translocation to one of the immunoglobulin loci (Love et al. 2012). LPL, lymphoplasmacytic lymphoma; WM, Waldenstrom macroglobulinemia.

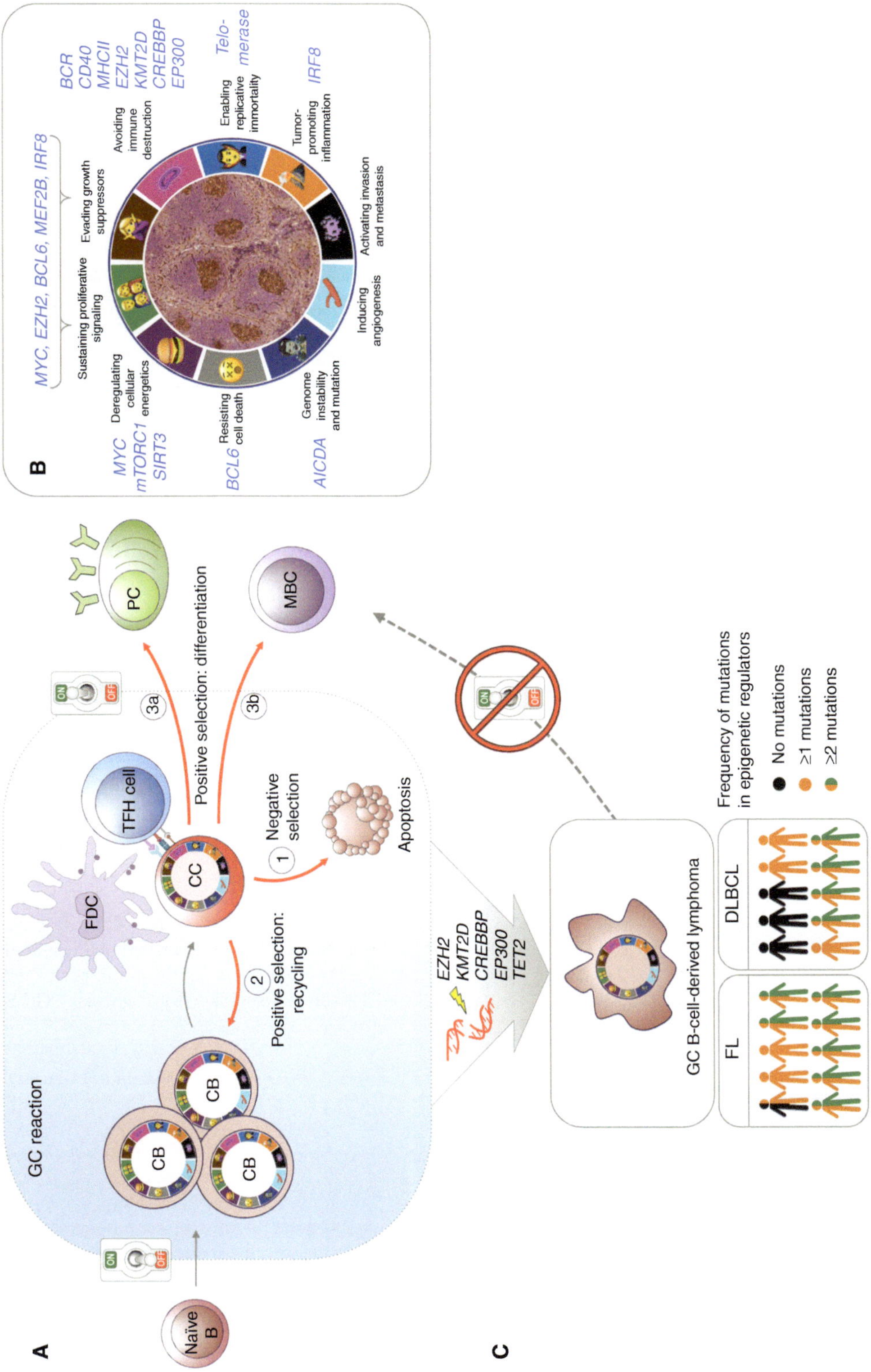

Figure 5. *(See legend on following page.)*

cell cycle checkpoint genes) (Phan and Dalla-Favera 2004; Phan et al. 2005; Cato et al. 2011; Béguelin et al. 2013, 2017); (2) potential immortalization (induction of telomerase) (Hu et al. 1997; Herrera et al. 2000; Norrback et al. 2001); (3) silencing of DNA damage checkpoint genes (repression of *ATR*, *CHEK1*, and *TP53*) (Phan and Dalla-Favera 2004; Ranuncolo et al. 2007, 2008); (4) genome instability and mutagenesis (caused by AICDA) (Muramatsu et al. 2000; McHeyzer-Williams et al. 2015; Teater et al. 2018); (5) resistance to cell death (induction of stress response pathways) (Cerchietti et al. 2009; Fernando et al. 2019); (6) deregulated energetics (efficient anaplerosis to support massive growth needs) (Doughty et al. 2006; Jellusova et al. 2017; Waters et al. 2018); (7) blockade of terminal differentiation (Béguelin et al. 2013, 2016); and (8) evasion from immune surveillance (down-regulation of antigen presentation and immune synapse genes) (Fig. 5B) (Basso et al. 2004; Good-Jacobson et al. 2010).

However, unlike cancer cells in which the transformed phenotype is primarily irreversible and caused by somatic mutations, in GC B cells this phenotype is solely induced through epigenetic reprogramming, which is reversible once B cells exit from the GC reaction (Bunting et al. 2016; Rivas and Melnick 2019). One of the more prominent epigenetic features of the GC reaction is the transient silencing of promoters and enhancers for genes involved in proliferation checkpoints, BCR signaling, CD40 signaling, interferon response, antigen presentation, and plasma cell differentiation (Béguelin et al. 2013, 2016; Hatzi et al. 2013; Ortega-Molina et al. 2015; Jiang et al. 2017). Most of this effect is coordinated by the transcriptional repressor BCL6, which is induced in the GC reaction and silenced on GC exit. Many of the mutations occurring in DLBCL and FL result in strengthening this effect (Fig. 5C).

Somatic Mutations in Epigenetic Modifiers Are a Hallmark of GC-Derived B-Cell Lymphomas

More than 70% of the genes mutated in DLBCL and FL are epigenetic modifiers and components of transcription factor complexes (Green et al. 2015; Ortega-Molina et al. 2015; Reddy et al. 2017; Chapuy et al. 2018; Schmitz et al. 2018). These include the H3K4 methyltransferase *KMT2D*, the H3 acetyltransferases *CREBBP* and *EP300*, the H3K27 methyltransferase *EZH2*, and *TET2*. Approximately 95% of FL patients manifest at least one of these mutations (Green et al. 2015), as do a majority of patients with GCB-DLBCL (Reddy et al. 2017; Chapuy et al. 2018; Schmitz et al. 2018). Each one of these genes is required to either establish the GC phenotype or to facilitate exit from the GC reaction. All are acquired early during pathogenesis and are considered founder mutations (Green et al. 2015; Pasqualucci and Dalla-Favera 2015). Mutations in *TET2* are the earliest and only DLBCL

Figure 5. Vulnerable points of germinal center (GC) B cells that give advantage to lymphomagenesis. (*A*) Chromatin-based epigenetic switches transiently poise the active plasma/memory B-cell program to enable the GC phenotype to emerge in a reversible manner. Cell fate decisions during a normal GC reaction: (1) negatively selected centrocytes (CC) undergo apoptosis; positively selected centrocytes may (2) recycle to centroblast (CB) and reenter the dark zone, or (3) differentiate to (3a) plasma cells (PC) or (3b) memory B cells (MBC). (*B*) GC B cells feature the typical hallmarks of transformed cells through epigenetic mechanisms, without requiring somatic mutations. This "pseudo-malignant" state can be reversed to normal state also through epigenetic switching mechanisms. (Sketch adapted from Hanahan and Weinberg 2011.) An immunohistochemistry (IHC) picture of GCs identified with peanut agglutinin (PNA) stain in a murine splenic section is shown in the middle. (*C*) Mutations in epigenetic modifiers maintain B cells in the GC phenotype, allowing the development of GC-derived B-cell lymphomas. Although mutations of one or more chromatin modifier genes occur within 96% of follicular lymphoma (FL) and ~70% diffuse B-cell lymphoma (DLBCL) patients, 76% FL, and ~40% DLBCL cases feature at least two mutations in epigenetic regulators (Green et al. 2015; Ortega-Molina et al. 2015; Reddy et al. 2017; Chapuy et al. 2018; Schmitz et al. 2018).

mutations that originate in HSCs (Quivoron et al. 2011; Dominguez et al. 2018).

Wild-Type and Mutant EZH2 in the GC Reaction

EZH2 is induced and required for the formation of GC B cells (Velichutina et al. 2010; Béguelin et al. 2013; Caganova et al. 2013), where it deposits the H3K27me3 mark at active promoters (marked with H3K4me3) to form bivalent chromatin (Béguelin et al. 2013). The H3K27me3 mark then attracts the repressive Polycomb-like BCOR complex (Béguelin et al. 2016). However, a second tether is needed for BCOR recruitment and is provided by BCL6 (Huynh et al. 2000; Ghetu et al. 2008; Béguelin et al. 2016). This EZH2-BCOR-BCL6 combinatorial tethering process explains how EZH2 represses GC context-specific target genes, thanks to DNA sequence-specific binding of BCL6. Heterozygous somatic mutation of *EZH2* occurs in up to 30% of FL and GCB-DLBCL patients and primarily affects the EZH2 SET (histone methyltransferase) domain at residue Y641 (Morin et al. 2010; Bödör et al. 2013; Okosun et al. 2014; Reddy et al. 2017). Unlike AML, in which *EZH2* mutations result in loss of function, these mutations confer a gain of function that makes EZH2 more efficient at H3K27 trimethylation, but less efficient at H3K27 monomethylation (Sneeringer et al. 2010; Yap et al. 2011; McCabe et al. 2012). Mice engineered to express heterozygous mutant *Ezh2* in GC B cells develop hyperplasia and B-cell lymphoma (Béguelin et al. 2013, 2016). This may be a consequence of more profound and less reversible silencing of EZH2 target genes involved in cell cycle checkpoints and GC exit. In contrast homozygous expression of mutant *Ezh2* phenocopies the *EZH2* knockout phenotype, showing that the WT *EZH2* allele is required to cooperate with the mutant allele (Béguelin et al. 2016).

Somatic Mutations of CREBBP and EP300

These often manifest as missense mutations that inactivate their histone acetyltransferase domain, or truncations leading to loss of the allele (Cerchietti et al. 2010; Morin et al. 2011; Pasqualucci et al. 2011; Green et al. 2015; Jiang et al. 2017). *CREBBP* and *EP300* maintain H3K27 acetylation mark at enhancers for genes involved in immune synapse and antigen presentation functions in B cells (Jiang et al. 2017). However, during the GC reaction BCL6 toggles these enhancers to a poised configuration by recruiting the SMRT/HDAC3 complex (Hatzi et al. 2013) (different than the function of BCL6 at promoters with BCOR and EZH2). CREBBP and p300 reactivate these enhancers when B cells are induced to exit the GC reaction. However, their loss-of-function mutation in lymphoma impairs this function and results in unopposed repression of these genes by HDAC3 and biological dependence on this protein (Jiang et al. 2017; Mondello et al. 2019). Loss of *CREBBP* or *EP300* in GC B cells accelerates lymphomagenesis in mice (Garcia-Ramírez et al. 2017; Hashwah et al. 2017; Jiang et al. 2017; Zhang et al. 2017). The MHC class II genes are critical CREBBP targets that are aberrantly and persistently silenced by HDAC3 in *CREBBP*-mutant lymphoma cells (Hashwah et al. 2017; Jiang et al. 2017; Zhang et al. 2017).

Somatic Mutations of KMT2D

KMT2D has functions analogous to *CREBBP* in maintaining H3K4 monomethylation of gene enhancers in B cells. During the GC reaction, BCL6 represses KMT2D regulated enhancers in part through direct recruitment of LSD1, which in turn recruits the CoREST complex (Hatzi et al. 2019). In B cells, exiting the GC reaction KMT2D is required to enable the functionality of enhancers that normally respond to CD40 and BCR signaling. Lack of KMT2D leads to aberrant repression of these genes, failure of B cells to differentiate and exit the GC reaction, and eventually lymphomagenesis (Ortega-Molina et al. 2015; Zhang et al. 2015).

TET2 Mutations in the GC Context

TET2 mutations in DLBCL are similar in nature to those occurring in myeloid neoplasms (Quivoron et al. 2011). Loss of *TET2* in GC B cells results in loss of enhancer 5hmC including at the *PRDM1* locus, which is a master regulator of plasma cell differentiation. In addition, there is repression of many of the same genes that are normally induced by CREBBP on GC exit. Indeed, *TET2* and *CREBBP* mutations are generally mutually exclusive, suggesting they represent a similar pathogenic hit. Along these lines, *TET2* loss of function results in failure of CREBBP to mediate H3K27 acetylation at gene enhancers and makes lymphoma cells biologically dependent on HDAC3 (Dominguez et al. 2018).

The Immune Synapse as a Focal Point for Epigenetic Deregulation in Lymphoma

Reversion of the GC B-cell phenotype is essential to immune homeostasis. This effect is largely dependent on the immune synapse and interaction with TFH and follicular dendritic cells, involving CD40, BCR, MHC class II, IL21, and other signaling pathways (Fig. 6A) (Papa and Vinuesa 2018). Through unknown signals, the immune synapse reverses the poised state of gene promoters and enhancers driven by BCL6 with BCOR, EZH2, HDAC3, and LSD1 during the GC reaction. This is impaired by somatic mutations of *EZH2*, *CREBBP*, *EP300*, *KMT2D*, and *TET2*. Mutant *EZH2* mediates aberrant silencing of cell cycle checkpoint inhibitors, MHC I and MHC II, and other GC exit genes (Béguelin et al. 2013; Ennishi et al. 2019). *CREBBP*, *KMT2D*, *EP300*, and *TET2* loss of function disables enhancers that respond to CD40, BCR, and MHC class II genes (Ortega-Molina et al. 2015; Zhang et al. 2015, 2017; Hashwah et al. 2017; Jiang et al. 2017; Dominguez et al. 2018). Thus, the primary effect of epigenetic founder mutations in DLBCL and FL is mostly about "maintaining" GC B cells in an inherently oncogenic state by suppressing their ability to interface with the immune microenvironment. This also likely explains how mutant GC B cells evade immune surveillance to give rise to DLBCLs and FLs (Nicholas et al. 2016). Moreover, it is possible that aberrant immune synapse interactions with mutant GC B cells could epigenetically reprogram components of the immune microenvironment to form a lymphoma-permissive cell niche (Fig. 6B).

Cytosine Methylation Patterning in Lymphomagenesis

Unlike the case of AML, 5mC patterning is not established as a driver of disease pathogenesis in GC-derived lymphomas. To date, DNA methylation profiling studies in DLBCL and FL have failed to identify robust and specific patterns of cytosine methylation indicative of underlying pathogenesis or with links to particular somatic mutations, with the possible exception of *TET2*. As compared with naive B cells, human and murine GC B cells manifest a characteristic hypomethylation signature (Dominguez et al. 2015, 2018; Teater et al. 2018). This appears to most likely represent a genomic "scar" effect of AICDA-mediated cytosine deamination of methylated residues that are replaced with unmethylated cytosines during replication, because *AICDA* knockout GC B cells fail to manifest this phenotype (Dominguez et al. 2015). Maintenance of DNA methylation is clearly important because, as expected, reduction of DNMT1 levels in mice severely impair GC formation (Shaknovich et al. 2011). DNA methylation profiling studies in cohorts of DLBCL patients have shown that progressive shifting of 5mC distribution from the normal GC pattern is linked to inferior clinical outcomes (Chambwe et al. 2014). Moreover, aberrant methylation and silencing of genes such as *SMAD1* have been causally linked to chemotherapy resistance in DLBCL and can be overcome by administering DNA methyltransferase inhibitors (Clozel et al. 2013).

The Role of Epigenetic Therapy in GC-Derived Lymphomas

Nonspecific Epigenetic Therapies

The most experience to date with "epigenetic" therapy in lymphoma involves first-generation, pan-HDAC inhibitors. By and large these stud-

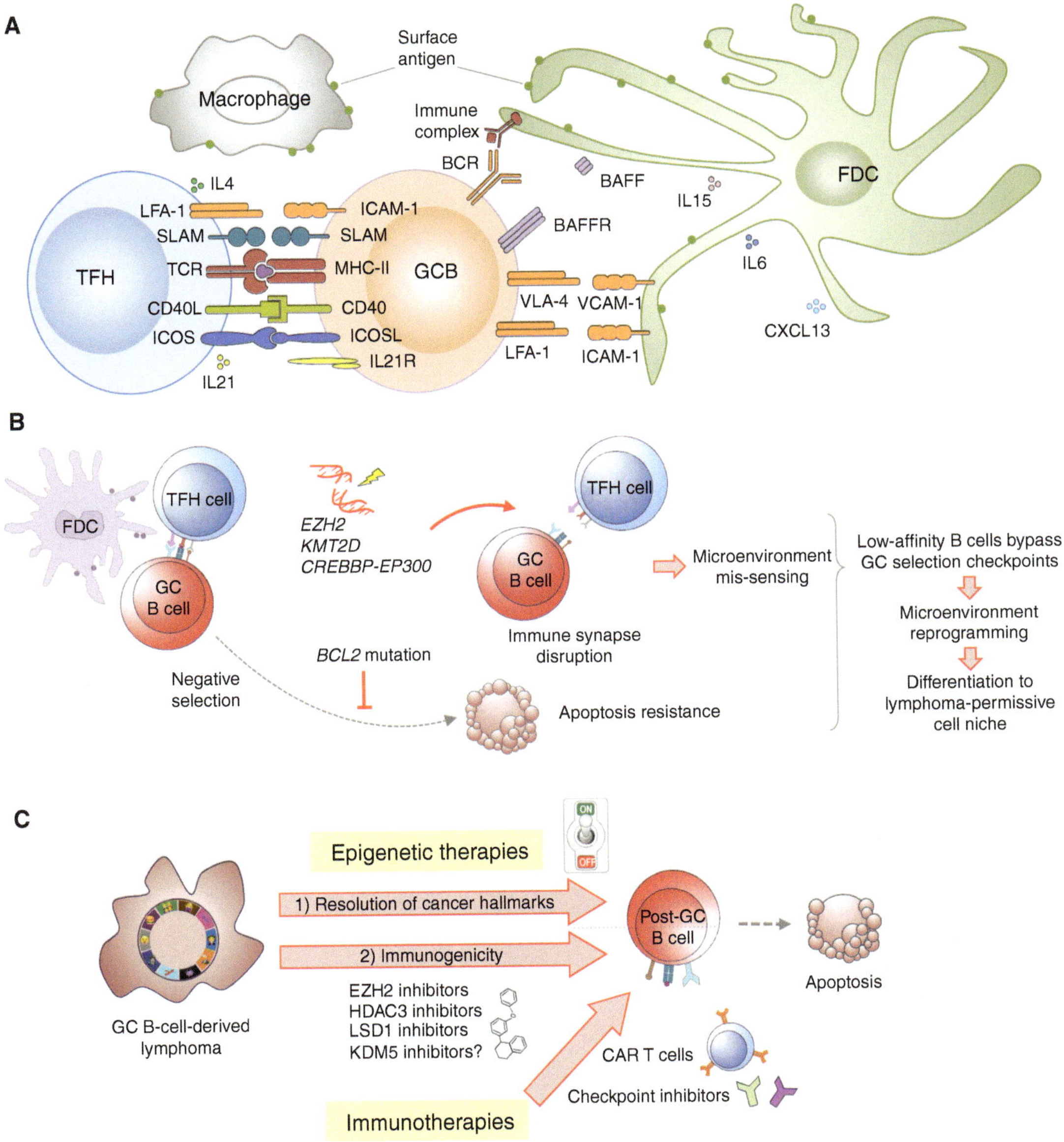

Figure 6. The immune synapse and epigenetic therapy. Like germinal center (GC) B cells, the microenvironment in B-cell malignancies is crucial for the provision of survival and proliferation signals. (*A*) In both cases, normal GC B cells and malignant B cells interact with T cells, dendritic cells, macrophages, and lymphoid stromal cells (follicular dendritic cells) (Papa and Vinuesa 2018). (*B*) Mutations in epigenetic regulators and oncogenes such as *BCL2* allow low-affinity B cells to survive, leading to the initiation of a prosurvival, immunosuppressive microenvironment in the lymphoid tissue. (*C*) Although epigenetic therapy can overcome the effect of founder mutations, the microenvironment makes critical contributions to both disease progression and drug resistance/disease relapse. The combination of epigenetic therapy with checkpoint inhibitor therapy can lead to potent antilymphoma effects.

ies have been disappointing (Sermer et al. 2019). This may not be entirely surprising because these drugs are pleiotropic in their actions, have toxic side effects and there are no definitive, causal data indicating that they affect lymphoma cells through a particular epigenetic effect. The one bright spot has been in the setting of T-cell lymphomas, albeit for unknown biological reasons. BET inhibitors, which block binding of BRD4 to acetylated lysines, have shown toxicity against lymphoma cells in laboratory models but modest effects in patients (Chapuy et al. 2013; Amorim et al. 2016). On the other hand, DNMTis are well-tolerated in lymphoma patients in combination with chemo-immunotherapy and yielded favorable outcomes in phase I/II studies (Clozel et al. 2013). DNMTis were shown to reverse chemotherapy resistance in patients through the ex vivo study of sequential lymphoma biopsies obtained on patients enrolled in DNMTi trials (Clozel et al. 2013), warranting the expansion of these studies into the phase III setting.

Precision Epigenetic Therapy

Given the specific role of aberrant epigenetic modifiers in DLBCL and FL, there is great interest to deploy therapeutic agents that could reverse these effects. The only such approach to reach the clinic are EZH2 inhibitors, based on the strong rationale that EZH2 is essential to GC B cells and its mutant forms further enhance dependency on EZH2. Early clinical trials (albeit in patients with aggressive disease) show that EZH2i are well-tolerated and confer a significant clinical benefit (Gulati et al. 2018). Although there are a number of PRC2 inhibitors moving into clinical trials, most data available to date come from studies of the selective EZH2 inhibitor tazemetostat. A phase I, dose-escalation study in DLBCL patients previously treated with R-CHOP (NCT02889523) reported favorable safety results. However, in April 2018, the Food and Drug Administration (FDA) placed a temporary hold on the enrollment of new U.S. patients into this clinical trial because of a pediatric patient who developed a T-cell lymphoma while taking the drug. Another phase II clinical trial enrolls subjects with DLBCL and FL for the determination of efficacy and safety of tazemetostat monotherapy in combination with prednisolone (NCT01897571). For FL, it was reported that tazemetostat achieved objective response rates of 71% in patients with EZH2 mutations and 33% in patients with wild-type EZH2. These data are encouraging because the patients enrolled in this study had already undergone at least two previous therapies.

Despite achieving this milestone, there are currently no biomarkers that can predict whether a given patient will be responsive nor is the optimal timing and duration of dosing established. The fact that DLBCLs with *EZH2* mutations manifest silencing of MHC I, MHC II, and reduced infiltrating CD4 and CD8 cells has pointed toward a potential immunomodulatory effect of EZH2i (Ennishi et al. 2019). However, it will be necessary to assess whether EZH2i might suppress antitumor immunity, given that PRC2 also plays critical roles in T-cell activation.

Because *CREBBP*- and *TET2*-mutant DLBCLs are addicted to HDAC3, there is a rationale for deploying selective HDAC3i to the clinic. HDAC3 has been biochemically purified as a component of the SMRT complex, >90% of which is bound with BCL6 in lymphoma B cells, pointing to the likely highly selective impact of HDAC3 inhibitors (Hatzi et al. 2013). Indeed, treatment of DLBCL cell lines or primary patient specimens with HDAC3i resulted in strong induction of MHC class II and triggered T-cell-mediated killing of lymphoma cells (Mondello et al. 2019). In contrast to pan-HDACis, HDAC3is lack toxicity against hematopoietic and T cells (Mondello et al. 2019) and hence represent a promising approach to restore T-cell-mediated immune surveillance against *CREBBP*-mutant DLBCL or FL cells. In the case of *KMT2D*-mutant lymphomas, there may be a rationale for targeting LSD1, although it would be required to use compounds that degrade LSD1 because purely enzymatic inhibition of this histone demethylase is insufficient to counteract its full affect in suppressing KMT2D target genes (Hatzi et al. 2019). It is also proposed that compounds that target the KDM5 family of H3K4 demethylases might also offer selective activity in the setting of *KMT2D*-mutant patients (Mondello et al. 2018).

Although these more precise epigenetic therapies represent a logical and promising opportunity, their most effective use will be in combination regimens, especially with immunotherapies. The success of immunotherapies such as checkpoint inhibitors and even CAR T cells is generally mixed in the setting of FL and DLBCL, perhaps linked to their epigenetic down-regulation of genes needed for B cells to effectively interface with T cells. Epigenetic therapies that reverse these effects might potently synergize with these immunotherapy modalities (Fig. 6C).

EPIGENETIC ALLELES, CLONAL EVOLUTION, AND THERAPY RESISTANCE IN HEME MALIGNANCIES

AMLs and lymphoma are composed of genetically distinct clones, and clonal complexity is linked to inferior clinical outcome, presumably because this endows tumors with greater population fitness. Because 5mC patterning is maintained with 1000-fold less fidelity than genome sequencing during replication, there is far more opportunity to develop clonal variance in epigenetic marks than in genetic composition. Indeed, foci of CpGs with variable methylation with populations of cells were identified by two initial studies (Hansen et al. 2011; Shaknovich et al. 2011), one in solid tumor cells and one in normal GC B cells. Epigenetic heterogeneity in GC B cells was considered as a possible precursor to malignant transformation: Perhaps sampling of epigenetic states during the GC reaction could yield selection advantages and the formation of premalignant clonal precursor cells (Shaknovich et al. 2011). Indeed, the first study of epigenetic heterogeneity was performed in GC-derived lymphomas (FL and DLBCL) and showed more severe 5mC heterogeneity in these tumors as compared with GC B cells (De et al. 2013). The extent of 5mC heterogeneity was associated with shorter survival, suggesting that it contributes to lymphoma population fitness (De et al. 2013).

Linking together the concepts of epigenetic heterogeneity and tumor clonality, several groups developed the concept of "epigenetic alleles," defined as the DNA methylation status of groups of four consecutive CpGs present on the same DNA strand (Li et al. 2016). Analysis of DLBCL patients indicated that epigenetic allele diversity is linked to risk for relapse (Pan et al. 2015). Relapsed DLBCLs showed selection epigenetic allele states, which suggests that particular 5mC patterns were best suited to tolerate exposure to chemotherapy (Pan et al. 2015). Epigenetic allele studies in CLL also showed a link between 5mC diversity and outcome (Landau et al. 2014). Loci that manifested epigenetic allele diversity in CLL patients were also associated with deregulated transcription, providing further evidence that epigenetic heterogeneity has functional implications (Landau et al. 2014). Notably, 5mC heterogeneity in the context of normal GC B cells and GC-derived lymphomas was shown to be caused at least in part by AICDA (Dominguez et al. 2015; Teater et al. 2018). This is likely due to stochastic deamination of 5mCs in B cells, which eventually leads to AICDA dose-dependent 5mC heterogeneity (Dominguez et al. 2015; Teater et al. 2018).

A large-scale integrative analysis of exomes, whole-genome sequencing, methylomes, and transcriptomes in matched paired AML specimens showed that epigenetic allele diversity was an independent risk factor for time to relapse and, most remarkably, was completely independent of genetic clonality (Li et al. 2016). Genes linked to promoters with epigenetic allele diversity manifested diversity in their transcriptional output, and after relapse there was also evidence of selection for distinct epigenetic clonal states (Li et al. 2016). Taken together, epigenetic allele diversity or 5mC heterogeneity have emerged as critically important biological features of lymphoid and myeloid neoplasms that cannot be predicted based on tumor genetics. It is intriguing to speculate that DNMT inhibitors might actually suppress epigenetic clonal diversity, perhaps explaining in part how these drugs enhance the effect of chemotherapy drugs in AMLs and DLBCLs.

CONCLUDING REMARKS

It is evident that epigenetic mechanisms play a fundamental role in the pathogenesis of hematologic malignancies. However, as of yet, we only have a very superficial view of the depth and breadth of epigenetic mechanisms and very few therapeutic approaches that are amenable for clinical translation. We need to dig deeper into how epigenetic marks connect with each other and the role of novel layers of the epigenome. It is also necessary to consider the potential for epigenetic heterogeneity among these layers and within given patients. There is a need to understand bidirectional epigenetic programming between tumor and microenvironment and the host immune system, and how epigenetic drugs could have beneficial or deleterious effects on these various cellular compartments. This is an important and richly rewarding avenue of research that will require concerted effort to truly harness from the therapeutic standpoint.

ACKNOWLEDGMENTS

A.M. is supported by National Cancer Institute (NCI) R35 CA220499, NCI 1UG CA233332, NCI R01 CA198089, the Leukemia & Lymphoma Society (LLS) TRP 6572-19, LLS SCOR 7013-17, the Follicular Lymphoma Consortium, and the Chemotherapy Foundation. W.B. is supported through LLS SCOR 7012-16, LLS TRP 6572-19, and NCI R35 CA220499, C.D. is a recipient of the LLS Fellow Award LLS 5486 and is supported by NCI R01 CA198089.

REFERENCES

Abbas S, Lugthart S, Kavelaars FG, Schelen A, Koenders J, Zeilemaker A, van Putten WJL, Rijneveld A, Löwenberg B, Valk PJM. 2010. Acquired mutations in the genes encoding IDH1 and IDH2 both are recurrent aberrations in acute myeloid leukemia (AML): prevalence and prognostic value. *Blood* **116:** 2122–2126. doi:10.1182/blood-2009-11-250878

Abdel-Wahab O, Adli M, LaFave LM, Gao J, Hricik T, Shih AH, Pandey S, Patel JP, Chung YR, Koche R, et al. 2012. *ASXL1* mutations promote myeloid transformation through loss of PRC2-mediated gene repression. *Cancer Cell* **22:** 180–193. doi:10.1016/j.ccr.2012.06.032

Adema V, Balasubramanian SK, Hirsch CM, Przychodzen BP, Phillips JG, Lindner D, Radivoyevitch T, Mukherjee S, Nazha A, Carraway HE, et al. 2017. Novel therapeutic targets for *DNMT3A* mutant myeloid neoplasms. *Blood* **130:** 106. doi:10.1182/blood-2017-05-786277

Aldoss I, Yang D, Aribi A, Ali H, Sandhu K, Al Malki MM, Mei M, Salhotra A, Khaled S, Nakamura R, et al. 2018. Efficacy of the combination of venetoclax and hypomethylating agents in relapsed/refractory acute myeloid leukemia. *Haematologica* **103:** e404–e407. doi:10.3324/haematol.2018.188094

Alizadeh AA, Eisen MB, Davis RE, Ma C, Lossos IS, Rosenwald A, Boldrick JC, Sabet H, Tran T, Yu X, et al. 2000. Distinct types of diffuse large B-cell lymphoma identified by gene expression profiling. *Nature* **403:** 503–511. doi:10.1038/35000501

Amatangelo MD, Quek L, Shih A, Stein EM, Roshal M, David MD, Marteyn B, Farnoud NR, de Botton S, Bernard OA, et al. 2017. Enasidenib induces acute myeloid leukemia cell differentiation to promote clinical response. *Blood* **130:** 732–741. doi:10.1182/blood-2017-04-779447

Amorim S, Stathis A, Gleeson M, Iyengar S, Magarotto V, Leleu X, Morschhauser F, Karlin L, Broussais F, Rezai K, et al. 2016. Bromodomain inhibitor OTX015 in patients with lymphoma or multiple myeloma: a dose-escalation, open-label, pharmacokinetic, phase 1 study. *Lancet Haematol* **3:** e196–e204. doi:10.1016/S2352-3026(16)00021-1

Bachman M, Uribe-Lewis S, Yang X, Williams M, Murrell A, Balasubramanian S. 2014. 5-Hydroxymethylcytosine is a predominantly stable DNA modification. *Nat Chem* **6:** 1049–1055. doi:10.1038/nchem.2064

Basheer F, Giotopoulos G, Meduri E, Yun H, Mazan M, Sasca D, Gallipoli P, Marando L, Gozdecka M, Asby R, et al. 2019. Contrasting requirements during disease evolution identify EZH2 as a therapeutic target in AML. *J Exp Med* **216:** 966–981. doi:10.1084/jem.20181276

Basso K, Dalla-Favera R. 2015. Germinal centres and B cell lymphomagenesis. *Nat Rev Immunol* **15:** 172–184. doi:10.1038/nri3814

Basso K, Klein U, Niu H, Stolovitzky GA, Tu Y, Califano A, Cattoretti G, Dalla-Favera R. 2004. Tracking CD40 signaling during germinal center development. *Blood* **104:** 4088–4096. doi:10.1182/blood-2003-12-4291

Béguelin W, Popovic R, Teater M, Jiang Y, Bunting KL, Rosen M, Shen H, Yang SN, Wang L, Ezponda T, et al. 2013. EZH2 is required for germinal center formation and somatic EZH2 mutations promote lymphoid transformation. *Cancer Cell* **23:** 677–692. doi:10.1016/j.ccr.2013.04.011

Béguelin W, Teater M, Gearhart MD, Calvo Fernández MT, Goldstein RL, Cárdenas MG, Hatzi K, Rosen M, Shen H, Corcoran CM, et al. 2016. EZH2 and BCL6 cooperate to assemble CBX8-BCOR complex to repress bivalent promoters, mediate germinal center formation and lymphomagenesis. *Cancer Cell* **30:** 197–213. doi:10.1016/j.ccell.2016.07.006

Béguelin W, Rivas MA, Calvo Fernandez MT, Teater M, Purwada A, Redmond D, Shen H, Challman MF, Elemento O, Singh A, et al. 2017. EZH2 enables germinal centre formation through epigenetic silencing of CDKN1A and an Rb-E2F1 feedback loop. *Nat Commun* **8:** 877. doi:10.1038/s41467-017-01029-x

Bell CC, Fennell KA, Chan YC, Rambow F, Yeung MM, Vassiliadis D, Lara L, Yeh P, Martelotto LG, Rogiers A, et al. 2019. Targeting enhancer switching overcomes non-genetic drug resistance in acute myeloid leukaemia. *Nat commun* **10:** 2723. doi:10.1038/s41467-019-10652-9

Bird A. 2002. DNA methylation patterns and epigenetic memory. *Genes Dev* **16:** 6–21. doi:10.1101/gad.947102

Birke M, Schreiner S, Garcia-Cuéllar MP, Mahr K, Titgemeyer F, Slany RK. 2002. The MT domain of the proto-oncoprotein MLL binds to CpG-containing DNA and discriminates against methylation. *Nucleic Acids Res* **30:** 958–965. doi:10.1093/nar/30.4.958

Bock C, Beerman I, Lien WH, Smith ZD, Gu H, Boyle P, Gnirke A, Fuchs E, Rossi DJ, Meissner A. 2012. DNA methylation dynamics during in vivo differentiation of blood and skin stem cells. *Mol Cell* **47:** 633–647. doi:10.1016/j.molcel.2012.06.019

Bödör C, Grossmann V, Popov N, Okosun J, O'Riain C, Tan K, Marzec J, Araf S, Wang J, Lee AM, et al. 2013. EZH2 mutations are frequent and represent an early event in follicular lymphoma. *Blood* **122:** 3165–3168. doi:10.1182/blood-2013-04-496893

Bogenberger JM, Delman D, Hansen N, Valdez R, Fauble V, Mesa RA, Tibes R. 2015. Ex vivo activity of BCL-2 family inhibitors ABT-199 and ABT-737 combined with 5-azacytidine in myeloid malignancies. *Leuk Lymphoma* **56:** 226–229. doi:10.3109/10428194.2014.910657

Brahmer JR, Tykodi SS, Chow LQ, Hwu WJ, Topalian SL, Hwu P, Drake CG, Camacho LH, Kauh J, Odunsi K, et al. 2012. Safety and activity of anti-PD-L1 antibody in patients with advanced cancer. *N Engl J Med* **366:** 2455–2465. doi:10.1056/NEJMoa1200694

Bröske AM, Vockentanz L, Kharazi S, Huska MR, Mancini E, Scheller M, Kuhl C, Enns A, Prinz M, Jaenisch R, et al. 2009. DNA methylation protects hematopoietic stem cell multipotency from myeloerythroid restriction. *Nat Genet* **41:** 1207–1215. doi:10.1038/ng.463

Bunting KL, Soong TD, Singh R, Jiang Y, Béguelin W, Poloway DW, Swed BL, Hatzi K, Reisacher W, Teater M, et al. 2016. Multi-tiered reorganization of the genome during B cell affinity maturation anchored by a germinal center-specific locus control region. *Immunity* **45:** 497–512. doi:10.1016/j.immuni.2016.08.012

Caganova M, Carrisi C, Varano G, Mainoldi F, Zanardi F, Germain PL, George L, Alberghini F, Ferrarini L, Talukder AK, et al. 2013. Germinal center dysregulation by histone methyltransferase EZH2 promotes lymphomagenesis. *J Clin Invest* **123:** 5009–5022. doi:10.1172/JCI70626

Caligiuri MA, Strout MP, Lawrence D, Arthur DC, Baer MR, Yu F, Knuutila S, Mrozek K, Oberkircher AR, Marcucci G, et al. 1998. Rearrangement of ALL1 (MLL) in acute myeloid leukemia with normal cytogenetics. *Cancer Res* **58:** 55–59.

Cancer Genome Atlas Research Network. 2013. Genomic and epigenomic landscapes of adult de novo acute myeloid leukemia. *N Engl J Med* **368:** 2059–2074. doi:10.1056/NEJMoa1301689

Cato MH, Chintalapati SK, Yau IW, Omori SA, Rickert RC. 2011. Cyclin D3 is selectively required for proliferative expansion of germinal center B cells. *Mol Cell Biol* **31:** 127–137. doi:10.1128/MCB.00650-10

Cerchietti LC, Lopes EC, Yang SN, Hatzi K, Bunting KL, Tsikitas LA, Mallik A, Robles AI, Walling J, Varticovski L, et al. 2009. A purine scaffold Hsp90 inhibitor destabilizes BCL-6 and has specific antitumor activity in BCL-6-dependent B cell lymphomas. *Nat Med* **15:** 1369–1376. doi:10.1038/nm.2059

Cerchietti LC, Hatzi K, Caldas-Lopes E, Yang SN, Figueroa ME, Morin RD, Hirst M, Mendez L, Shaknovich R, Cole PA, et al. 2010. BCL6 repression of *EP300* in human diffuse large B cell lymphoma cells provides a basis for rational combinatorial therapy. *J Clin Invest* **120:** 4569–4582. doi:10.1172/JCI42869

Challen GA, Sun D, Jeong M, Luo M, Jelinek J, Berg JS, Bock C, Vasanthakumar A, Gu H, Xi Y, et al. 2011. Dnmt3a is essential for hematopoietic stem cell differentiation. *Nat Genet* **44:** 23–31. doi:10.1038/ng.1009

Chambwe N, Kormaksson M, Geng H, De S, Michor F, Johnson NA, Morin RD, Scott DW, Godley LA, Gascoyne RD, et al. 2014. Variability in DNA methylation defines novel epigenetic subgroups of DLBCL associated with different clinical outcomes. *Blood* **123:** 1699–1708. doi:10.1182/blood-2013-07-509885

Chang E, Ganguly S, Rajkhowa T, Gocke CD, Levis M, Konig H. 2016. The combination of FLT3 and DNA methyltransferase inhibition is synergistically cytotoxic to FLT3/ITD acute myeloid leukemia cells. *Leukemia* **30:** 1025–1032. doi:10.1038/leu.2015.346

Chapuy B, McKeown MR, Lin CY, Monti S, Roemer MG, Qi J, Rahl PB, Sun HH, Yeda KT, Doench JG, et al. 2013. Discovery and characterization of super-enhancer-associated dependencies in diffuse large B cell lymphoma. *Cancer Cell* **24:** 777–790. doi:10.1016/j.ccr.2013.11.003

Chapuy B, Stewart C, Dunford AJ, Kim J, Kamburov A, Redd RA, Lawrence MS, Roemer MGM, Li AJ, Ziepert M, et al. 2018. Molecular subtypes of diffuse large B cell lymphoma are associated with distinct pathogenic mechanisms and outcomes. *Nat Med* **24:** 679–690. doi:10.1038/s41591-018-0016-8

Chen C, Zhu H, Stauffer F, Caravatti G, Vollmer S, Machauer R, Holzer P, Möbitz H, Scheufler C, Klumpp M, et al. 2016. Discovery of novel Dot1L inhibitors through a structure-based fragmentation approach. *ACS Med Chem Lett* **7:** 735–740. doi:10.1021/acsmedchemlett.6b00167

Chittock EC, Latwiel S, Miller TC, Müller CW. 2017. Molecular architecture of Polycomb repressive complexes. *Biochem Soc Trans* **45:** 193–205. doi:10.1042/BST20160173

Chou WC, Chou SC, Liu CY, Chen CY, Hou HA, Kuo YY, Lee MC, Ko BS, Tang JL, Yao M, et al. 2011. *TET2* mutation is an unfavorable prognostic factor in acute myeloid leukemia patients with intermediate-risk cytogenetics. *Blood* **118:** 3803–3810. doi:10.1182/blood-2011-02-339747

Chowdhury R, Yeoh KK, Tian YM, Hillringhaus L, Bagg EA, Rose NR, Leung IK, Li XS, Woon EC, Yang M, et al. 2011. The oncometabolite 2-hydroxyglutarate inhibits histone lysine demethylases. *EMBO Rep* **12:** 463–469. doi:10.1038/embor.2011.43

Cimmino L, Dolgalev I, Wang Y, Yoshimi A, Martin GH, Wang J, Ng V, Xia B, Witkowski MT, Mitchell-Flack M, et al. 2017. Restoration of TET2 function blocks aberrant self-renewal and leukemia progression. *Cell* **170:** 1079–1095.e20. doi:10.1016/j.cell.2017.07.032

Clozel T, Yang S, Elstrom RL, Tam W, Martin P, Kormaksson M, Banerjee S, Vasanthakumar A, Culjkovic B, Scott DW, et al. 2013. Mechanism-based epigenetic chemosensitization therapy of diffuse large B-cell lymphoma. *Cancer Discov* **3:** 1002–1019. doi:10.1158/2159-8290.CD-13-0117

Coudé M-M, Braun T, Berrou J, Dupont M, Bertrand S, Masse A, Raffoux E, Itzykson R, Delord M, Riveiro ME, et al. 2015. BET inhibitor OTX015 targets BRD2 and BRD4 and decreases c-MYC in acute leukemia cells. *Oncotarget* **6:** 17698–17712.

Dang L, White DW, Gross S, Bennett BD, Bittinger MA, Driggers EM, Fantin VR, Jang HG, Jin S, Keenan MC, et al. 2009. Cancer-associated IDH1 mutations produce 2-hydroxyglutarate. *Nature* **462:** 739–744. doi:10.1038/nature08617

Daver N, Garcia-Manero G, Basu S, Boddu PC, Alfayez M, Cortes JE, Konopleva M, Ravandi-Kashani F, Jabbour E, Kadia T, et al. 2019. Efficacy, safety, and biomarkers of response to azacitidine and nivolumab in relapsed/refractory acute myeloid leukemia: a nonrandomized, open-label, phase II study. *Cancer Discov* **9:** 370–383. doi:10.1158/2159-8290.CD-18-0774

De S, Shaknovich R, Riester M, Elemento O, Geng H, Kormaksson M, Jiang Y, Woolcock B, Johnson N, Polo JM, et al. 2013. Aberration in DNA methylation in B-cell lymphomas has a complex origin and increases with disease severity. *PLoS Genet* **9:** e1003137. doi:10.1371/journal.pgen.1003137

Delhommeau F, Dupont S, Valle VD, James C, Trannoy S, Massé A, Kosmider O, Le Couedic JP, Robert F, Alberdi A, et al. 2009. Mutation in *TET2* in myeloid cancers. *N Engl J Med* **360:** 2289–2301. doi:10.1056/NEJMoa0810069

DiNardo CD, Stein EM, de Botton S, Roboz GJ, Altman JK, Mims AS, Swords R, Collins RH, Mannis GN, Pollyea DA, et al. 2018. Durable remissions with ivosidenib in *IDH1*-mutated relapsed or refractory AML. *N Engl J Med* **378:** 2386–2398. doi:10.1056/NEJMoa1716984

DiNardo CD, Pratz K, Pullarkat V, Jonas BA, Arellano M, Becker PS, Frankfurt O, Konopleva M, Wei AH, Kantarjian HM, et al. 2019. Venetoclax combined with decitabine or azacitidine in treatment-naive, elderly patients with acute myeloid leukemia. *Blood* **133:** 7–17. doi:10.1182/blood-2018-08-868752

Ding L, Ley TJ, Larson DE, Miller CA, Koboldt DC, Welch JS, Ritchey JK, Young MA, Lamprecht T, McLellan M, et al. 2012. Clonal evolution in relapsed acute myeloid leukaemia revealed by whole-genome sequencing. *Nature* **481:** 506–510. doi:10.1038/nature10738

Dominguez PM, Teater M, Chambwe N, Kormaksson M, Redmond D, Ishii J, Vuong B, Chaudhuri J, Melnick A, Vasanthakumar A, et al. 2015. DNA methylation dynamics of germinal center B cells are mediated by AID. *Cell Rep* **12:** 2086–2098. doi:10.1016/j.celrep.2015.08.036

Dominguez PM, Ghamlouch H, Rosikiewicz W, Kumar P, Beguelin W, Fontan L, Rivas MA, Pawlikowska P, Armand M, Mouly E, et al. 2018. TET2 deficiency causes germinal center hyperplasia, impairs plasma cell differentiation, and promotes B-cell lymphomagenesis. *Cancer Discov* **8:** 1632–1653.

Dorrance AM, Liu S, Chong A, Pulley B, Nemer D, Guimond M, Yuan W, Chang D, Whitman SP, Marcucci G, et al. 2008. The *Mll* partial tandem duplication: differential, tissue-specific activity in the presence or absence of the wild-type allele. *Blood* **112:** 2508–2511. doi:10.1182/blood-2008-01-134338

Doughty CA, Bleiman BF, Wagner DJ, Dufort FJ, Mataraza JM, Roberts MF, Chiles TC. 2006. Antigen receptor-mediated changes in glucose metabolism in B lymphocytes: role of phosphatidylinositol 3-kinase signaling in the glycolytic control of growth. *Blood* **107:** 4458–4465. doi:10.1182/blood-2005-12-4788

Duy C, Melnick A. 2018. Untangling the role of Polycomb complexes in chemotherapy resistance. *Cancer Discov* **8:** 1348–1351. doi:10.1158/2159-8290.CD-18-1080

Duy C, Teater M, Garrett-Bakelman FE, Lee TC, Meydan C, Glass JL, Li M, Hellmuth JC, Mohammad HP, Smitheman KN, et al. 2019. Rational targeting of cooperating layers of the epigenome yields enhanced therapeutic efficacy against AML. *Cancer Discov* **9:** 872–889. doi:10.1158/2159-8290.CD-19-0106

Ennishi D, Takata K, Béguelin W, Duns G, Mottok A, Farinha P, Bashashati A, Saberi S, Boyle M, Meissner B, et al. 2019. Molecular and genetic characterization of MHC deficiency identifies EZH2 as therapeutic target for enhancing immune recognition. *Cancer Discov* **9:** 546–563. doi:10.1158/2159-8290.CD-18-1090

Ernst T, Chase AJ, Score J, Hidalgo-Curtis CE, Bryant C, Jones AV, Waghorn K, Zoi K, Ross FM, Reiter A, et al. 2010. Inactivating mutations of the histone methyltransferase gene *EZH2* in myeloid disorders. *Nat Genet* **42:** 722–726. doi:10.1038/ng.621

Ernst J, Kheradpour P, Mikkelsen TS, Shoresh N, Ward LD, Epstein CB, Zhang X, Wang L, Issner R, Coyne M, et al. 2011. Mapping and analysis of chromatin state dynamics in nine human cell types. *Nature* **473:** 43–49. doi:10.1038/nature09906

Ernst T, Pflug A, Rinke J, Ernst J, Bierbach U, Beck JF, Hochhaus A, Gruhn B. 2012. A somatic *EZH2* mutation in childhood acute myeloid leukemia. *Leukemia* **26:** 1701–1703. doi:10.1038/leu.2012.16

Fedoriw A, Rajapurkar SR, O'Brien S, Gerhart SV, Mitchell LH, Adams ND, Rioux N, Lingaraj T, Ribich SA, Pappalardi MB, et al. 2019. Anti-tumor activity of the type I PRMT inhibitor, GSK3368715, synergizes with PRMT5 inhibition through MTAP loss. *Cancer Cell* **36:** 100–114.e25. doi:10.1016/j.ccell.2019.05.014

Fennell KA, Bell CC, Dawson MA. 2019. Epigenetic therapies in acute myeloid leukemia: where to from here? *Blood* **134:** 1891–1901. doi:10.1182/blood.2019003262

Fernando TM, Marullo R, Pera Gresely B, Phillip JM, Yang SN, Lundell-Smith G, Torregroza I, Ahn H, Evans T, Győrffy B, et al. 2019. BCL6 evolved to enable stress tolerance in vertebrates and is broadly required by cancer cells to adapt to stress. *Cancer Discov* **9:** 662–679. doi:10.1158/2159-8290.CD-17-1444

Figueroa ME, Wouters BJ, Skrabanek L, Glass J, Li Y, Erpelinck-Verschueren CA, Langerak AW, Löwenberg B, Fazzari M, Greally JM, et al. 2009. Genome-wide epigenetic analysis delineates a biologically distinct immature acute leukemia with myeloid/T-lymphoid features. *Blood* **113:** 2795–2804. doi:10.1182/blood-2008-08-172387

Figueroa ME, Abdel-Wahab O, Lu C, Ward PS, Patel J, Shih A, Li Y, Bhagwat N, Vasanthakumar A, Fernandez HF, et al. 2010a. Leukemic IDH1 and IDH2 mutations result in a hypermethylation phenotype, disrupt TET2 function, and impair hematopoietic differentiation. *Cancer Cell* **18:** 553–567. doi:10.1016/j.ccr.2010.11.015

Figueroa ME, Lugthart S, Li Y, Erpelinck-Verschueren C, Deng X, Christos PJ, Schifano E, Booth J, van Putten W, Skrabanek L, et al. 2010b. DNA methylation signatures identify biologically distinct subtypes in acute myeloid leukemia. *Cancer Cell* **17:** 13–27. doi:10.1016/j.ccr.2009.11.020

Florence B, Faller DV. 2001. You bet-cha: a novel family of transcriptional regulators. *Front Biosci* **6:** D1008–D1018.

Fugmann SD, Lee AI, Shockett PE, Villey IJ, Schatz DG. 2000. The RAG proteins and V(D)J recombination: complexes, ends, and transposition. *Annu Rev Immunol* **18:** 495–527. doi:10.1146/annurev.immunol.18.1.495

Gaidzik VI, Paschka P, Späth D, Habdank M, Köhne CH, Germing U, von Lilienfeld-Toal M, Held G, Horst HA, Haase D, et al. 2012. *TET2* mutations in acute myeloid leukemia (AML): results from a comprehensive genetic and clinical analysis of the AML study group. *J Clin Oncol* **30:** 1350–1357. doi:10.1200/JCO.2011.39.2886

Gao J, Aksoy BA, Dogrusoz U, Dresdner G, Gross B, Sumer SO, Sun Y, Jacobsen A, Sinha R, Larsson E, et al. 2013. Integrative analysis of complex cancer genomics and clinical profiles using the cBioPortal. *Sci Signal* **6:** l1.

Garcia-Ramírez I, Tadros S, González-Herrero I, Martin-Lorenzo A, Rodriguez-Hernández G, Moore D, Ruiz-Roca L, Blanco O, Alonso-López D, Rivas JL, et al. 2017. *Crebbp* loss cooperates with *Bcl2* overexpression to promote lymphoma in mice. *Blood* **129:** 2645–2656. doi:10.1182/blood-2016-08-733469

Gardin C, Dombret H. 2017. Hypomethylating agents as a therapy for AML. *Curr Hematol Malig Rep* **12:** 1–10. doi:10.1007/s11899-017-0363-4

Ghetu AF, Corcoran CM, Cerchietti L, Bardwell VJ, Melnick A, Privé GG. 2008. Structure of a BCOR corepressor peptide in complex with the BCL6 BTB domain dimer. *Mol Cell* **29:** 384–391. doi:10.1016/j.molcel.2007.12.026

Glass JL, Hassane D, Wouters BJ, Kunimoto H, Avellino R, Garrett-Bakelman FE, Guryanova OA, Bowman R, Redlich S, Intlekofer AM, et al. 2017. Epigenetic identity in AML depends on disruption of nonpromoter regulatory elements and is affected by antagonistic effects of mutations in epigenetic modifiers. *Cancer Discov* **7:** 868–883. doi:10.1158/2159-8290.CD-16-1032

Göllner S, Oellerich T, Agrawal-Singh S, Schenk T, Klein HU, Rohde C, Pabst C, Sauer T, Lerdrup M, Tavor S, et al. 2017. Loss of the histone methyltransferase EZH2 induces resistance to multiple drugs in acute myeloid leukemia. *Nat Med* **23:** 69–78. doi:10.1038/nm.4247

Good-Jacobson KL, Szumilas CG, Chen L, Sharpe AH, Tomayko MM, Shlomchik MJ. 2010. PD-1 regulates germinal center B cell survival and the formation and affinity of long-lived plasma cells. *Nat Immunol* **11:** 535–542. doi:10.1038/ni.1877

Gozdecka M, Meduri E, Mazan M, Tzelepis K, Dudek M, Knights AJ, Pardo M, Yu L, Choudhary JS, Metzakopian E, et al. 2018. UTX-mediated enhancer and chromatin remodeling suppresses myeloid leukemogenesis through noncatalytic inverse regulation of ETS and GATA programs. *Nat Genet* **50:** 883–894. doi:10.1038/s41588-018-0114-z

Green MR. 2018. Chromatin modifying gene mutations in follicular lymphoma. *Blood* **131:** 595–604. doi:10.1182/blood-2017-08-737361

Green MR, Kihira S, Liu CL, Nair RV, Salari R, Gentles AJ, Irish J, Stehr H, Vicente-Dueñas C, Romero-Camarero I, et al. 2015. Mutations in early follicular lymphoma progenitors are associated with suppressed antigen presentation. *Proc Natl Acad Sci* **112:** E1116–E1125. doi:10.1073/pnas.1501199112

Grimwade D, Walker H, Harrison G, Oliver F, Chatters S, Harrison CJ, Wheatley K, Burnett AK, Goldstone AH. 2001. The predictive value of hierarchical cytogenetic classification in older adults with acute myeloid leukemia (AML): analysis of 1065 patients entered into the United Kingdom Medical Research Council AML11 trial. *Blood* **98:** 1312–1320. doi:10.1182/blood.V98.5.1312

Gross S, Cairns RA, Minden MD, Driggers EM, Bittinger MA, Jang HG, Sasaki M, Jin S, Schenkein DP, Su SM, et al. 2010. Cancer-associated metabolite 2-hydroxyglutarate accumulates in acute myelogenous leukemia with isocitrate dehydrogenase 1 and 2 mutations. *J Exp Med* **207:** 339–344. doi:10.1084/jem.20092506

Grossmann V, Tiacci E, Holmes AB, Kohlmann A, Martelli MP, Kern W, Spanhol-Rosseto A, Klein HU, Dugas M, Schindela S, et al. 2011. Whole-exome sequencing identifies somatic mutations of *BCOR* in acute myeloid leukemia with normal karyotype. *Blood* **118:** 6153–6163. doi:10.1182/blood-2011-07-365320

Gulati N, Béguelin W, Giulino-Roth L. 2018. Enhancer of zeste homolog 2 (EZH2) inhibitors. *Leuk Lymphoma* **59:** 1574–1585. doi:10.1080/10428194.2018.1430795

Guryanova OA, Shank K, Spitzer B, Luciani L, Koche RP, Garrett-Bakelman FE, Ganzel C, Durham BH, Mohanty A, Hoermann G, et al. 2016. *DNMT3A* mutations promote anthracycline resistance in acute myeloid leukemia via impaired nucleosome remodeling. *Nat Med* **22:** 1488–1495. doi:10.1038/nm.4210

Haarhuis JH, Elbatsh AM, Rowland BD. 2014. Cohesin and its regulation: on the logic of X-shaped chromosomes. *Dev Cell* **31:** 7–18. doi:10.1016/j.devcel.2014.09.010

Hanahan D, Weinberg RA. 2011. Hallmarks of cancer: the next generation. *Cell* **144:** 646–674. doi:10.1016/j.cell.2011.02.013

Hansen KD, Timp W, Bravo HC, Sabunciyan S, Langmead B, McDonald OG, Wen B, Wu H, Liu Y, Diep D, et al. 2011. Increased methylation variation in epigenetic domains across cancer types. *Nat Genet* **43:** 768–775. doi:10.1038/ng.865

Harding JJ, Lowery MA, Shih AH, Schvartzman JM, Hou S, Famulare C, Patel M, Roshal M, Do RK, Zehir A, et al. 2018. Isoform switching as a mechanism of acquired resistance to mutant isocitrate dehydrogenase inhibition. *Cancer Discov* **8:** 1540–1547. doi:10.1158/2159-8290.CD-18-0877

Harris WJ, Huang X, Lynch JT, Spencer GJ, Hitchin JR, Li Y, Ciceri F, Blaser JG, Greystoke BF, Jordan AM, et al. 2012. The histone demethylase KDM1A sustains the oncogenic potential of MLL-AF9 leukemia stem cells. *Cancer Cell* **21:** 473–487. doi:10.1016/j.ccr.2012.03.014

Hashimoto H, Liu Y, Upadhyay AK, Chang Y, Howerton SB, Vertino PM, Zhang X, Cheng X. 2012. Recognition and potential mechanisms for replication and erasure of cytosine hydroxymethylation. *Nucleic Acids Res* **40:** 4841–4849. doi:10.1093/nar/gks155

Hashwah H, Schmid CA, Kasser S, Bertram K, Stelling A, Manz MG, Müller A. 2017. Inactivation of CREBBP expands the germinal center B cell compartment, downregulates MHCII expression and promotes DLBCL growth. *Proc Natl Acad Sci* **114:** 9701–9706. doi:10.1073/pnas.1619555114

Hatzi K, Melnick A. 2014. Breaking bad in the germinal center: how deregulation of BCL6 contributes to lymphomagenesis. *Trends Mol Med* **20:** 343–352. doi:10.1016/j.molmed.2014.03.001

Hatzi K, Jiang Y, Huang C, Garrett-Bakelman F, Gearhart MD, Giannopoulou EG, Zumbo P, Kirouac K, Bhaskara S, Polo JM, et al. 2013. A hybrid mechanism of action for BCL6 in B cells defined by formation of functionally distinct complexes at enhancers and promoters. *Cell Rep* **4:** 578–588. doi:10.1016/j.celrep.2013.06.016

Hatzi K, Geng H, Doane AS, Meydan C, LaRiviere R, Cardenas M, Duy C, Shen H, Vidal MNC, Baslan T, et al. 2019. Histone demethylase LSD1 is required for germinal center formation and BCL6-driven lymphomagenesis. *Nat Immunol* **20:** 86–96. doi:10.1038/s41590-018-0273-1

He YF, Li BZ, Li Z, Liu P, Wang Y, Tang Q, Ding J, Jia Y, Chen Z, Li L, et al. 2011. Tet-mediated formation of 5-carboxylcytosine and its excision by TDG in mammalian DNA. *Science* **333:** 1303–1307. doi:10.1126/science.1210944

Herrera E, Martinez-A C, Blasco MA. 2000. Impaired germinal center reaction in mice with short telomeres. *EMBO J* **19:** 472–481. doi:10.1093/emboj/19.3.472

Hollink IH, van den Heuvel-Eibrink MM, Arentsen-Peters ST, Pratcorona M, Abbas S, Kuipers JE, van Galen JF, Beverloo HB, Sonneveld E, Kaspers GJ, et al. 2011. *NUP98/NSD1* characterizes a novel poor prognostic group in acute myeloid leukemia with a distinct *HOX* gene expression pattern. *Blood* **118:** 3645–3656. doi:10.1182/blood-2011-04-346643

Hon GC, Song CX, Du T, Jin F, Selvaraj S, Lee AY, Yen CA, Ye Z, Mao SQ, Wang BA, et al. 2014. 5mC oxidation by Tet2 modulates enhancer activity and timing of transcriptome reprogramming during differentiation. *Mol Cell* **56:** 286–297. doi:10.1016/j.molcel.2014.08.026

Hu BT, Lee SC, Marin E, Ryan DH, Insel RA. 1997. Telomerase is up-regulated in human germinal center B cells in vivo and can be re-expressed in memory B cells activated in vitro. *J Immunol* **159:** 1068–1071.

Huynh KD, Fischle W, Verdin E, Bardwell VJ. 2000. BCoR, a novel corepressor involved in BCL-6 repression. *Genes Dev* **14:** 1810–1823.

Inoue S, Li WY, Tseng A, Beerman I, Elia AJ, Bendall SC, Lemonnier F, Kron KJ, Cescon DW, Hao Z, et al. 2016. Mutant IDH1 downregulates ATM and alters DNA repair and sensitivity to DNA damage independent of TET2. *Cancer Cell* **30:** 337–348. doi:10.1016/j.ccell.2016.05.018

Intlekofer AM, Shih AH, Wang B, Nazir A, Rustenburg AS, Albanese SK, Patel M, Famulare C, Correa FM, Takemoto N, et al. 2018. Acquired resistance to IDH inhibition through trans or cis dimer-interface mutations. *Nature* **559:** 125–129. doi:10.1038/s41586-018-0251-7

Issa JJ, Roboz G, Rizzieri D, Jabbour E, Stock W, O'Connell C, Yee K, Tibes R, Griffiths EA, Walsh K, et al. 2015. Safety and tolerability of guadecitabine (SGI-110) in patients with myelodysplastic syndrome and acute myeloid leukaemia: a multicentre, randomised, dose-escalation phase 1 study. *Lancet Oncol* **16:** 1099–1110. doi:10.1016/S1470-2045(15)00038-8

Ito S, Shen L, Dai Q, Wu SC, Collins LB, Swenberg JA, He C, Zhang Y. 2011. Tet proteins can convert 5-methylcytosine to 5-formylcytosine and 5-carboxylcytosine. *Science* **333:** 1300–1303. doi:10.1126/science.1210597

Jellusova J, Cato MH, Apgar JR, Ramezani-Rad P, Leung CR, Chen C, Richardson AD, Conner EM, Benschop RJ, Woodgett JR, et al. 2017. GSK3 is a metabolic checkpoint regulator in B cells. *Nat Immunol* **18:** 303–312. doi:10.1038/ni.3664

Jeong M, Sun D, Luo M, Huang Y, Challen GA, Rodriguez B, Zhang X, Chavez L, Wang H, Hannah R, et al. 2014. Large conserved domains of low DNA methylation maintained by Dnmt3a. *Nat Genet* **46:** 17–23. doi:10.1038/ng.2836

Ji H, Ehrlich LIR, Seita J, Murakami P, Doi A, Lindau P, Lee H, Aryee MJ, Irizarry RA, Kim K, et al. 2010. Comprehensive methylome map of lineage commitment from haematopoietic progenitors. *Nature* **467:** 338–342. doi:10.1038/nature09367

Jiang Y, Ortega-Molina A, Geng H, Ying HY, Hatzi K, Parsa S, McNally D, Wang L, Doane AS, Agirre X, et al. 2017. *CREBBP* inactivation promotes the development of HDAC3-dependent lymphomas. *Cancer Discov* **7:** 38–53. doi:10.1158/2159-8290.CD-16-0975

Jones PA, Baylin SB. 2007. The epigenomics of cancer. *Cell* **128:** 683–692. doi:10.1016/j.cell.2007.01.029

Kagey MH, Newman JJ, Bilodeau S, Zhan Y, Orlando DA, van Berkum NL, Ebmeier CC, Goossens J, Rahl PB, Levine SS, et al. 2010. Mediator and cohesin connect gene expression and chromatin architecture. *Nature* **467:** 430–435. doi:10.1038/nature09380

Kim JS, He X, Orr B, Wutz G, Hill V, Peters JM, Compton DA, Waldman T. 2016. Intact cohesion, anaphase, and chromosome segregation in human cells harboring tumor-derived mutations in *STAG2*. *PLoS Genet* **12:** e1005865. doi:10.1371/journal.pgen.1005865

Kon A, Shih LY, Minamino M, Sanada M, Shiraishi Y, Nagata Y, Yoshida K, Okuno Y, Bando M, Nakato R, et al. 2013. Recurrent mutations in multiple components of the cohesin complex in myeloid neoplasms. *Nat Genet* **45:** 1232–1237. doi:10.1038/ng.2731

Kridel R, Sehn LH, Gascoyne RD. 2012. Pathogenesis of follicular lymphoma. *J Clin Invest* **122:** 3424–3431. doi:10.1172/JCI63186

Krivtsov AV, Armstrong SA. 2007. *MLL* translocations, histone modifications and leukaemia stem-cell development. *Nat Rev Cancer* **7:** 823–833. doi:10.1038/nrc2253

Landau DA, Clement K, Ziller MJ, Boyle P, Fan J, Gu H, Stevenson K, Sougnez C, Wang L, Li S, et al. 2014. Locally disordered methylation forms the basis of intratumor methylome variation in chronic lymphocytic leukemia. *Cancer Cell* **26:** 813–825. doi:10.1016/j.ccell.2014.10.012

Landau DA, Tausch E, Taylor-Weiner AN, Stewart C, Reiter JG, Bahlo J, Kluth S, Bozic I, Lawrence M, Böttcher S, et al. 2015. Mutations driving CLL and their evolution in progression and relapse. *Nature* **526:** 525–530. doi:10.1038/nature15395

Lawrence MS, Stojanov P, Polak P, Kryukov GV, Cibulskis K, Sivachenko A, Carter SL, Stewart C, Mermel CH, Roberts SA, et al. 2013. Mutational heterogeneity in cancer and the search for new cancer-associated genes. *Nature* **499:** 214–218. doi:10.1038/nature12213

Lenz G, Davis RE, Ngo VN, Lam L, George TC, Wright GW, Dave SS, Zhao H, Xu W, Rosenwald A, et al. 2008. Oncogenic *CARD11* mutations in human diffuse large B cell lymphoma. *Science* **319:** 1676–1679. doi:10.1126/science.1153629

Ley TJ, Ding L, Walter MJ, McLellan MD, Lamprecht T, Larson DE, Kandoth C, Payton JE, Baty J, Welch J, et al. 2010. *DNMT3A* mutations in acute myeloid leukemia. *N Engl J Med* **363:** 2424–2433. doi:10.1056/NEJMoa1005143

Li S, Garrett-Bakelman FE, Chung SS, Sanders MA, Hricik T, Rapaport F, Patel J, Dillon R, Vijay P, Brown AL, et al. 2016. Distinct evolution and dynamics of epigenetic and genetic heterogeneity in acute myeloid leukemia. *Nat Med* **22:** 792–799. doi:10.1038/nm.4125

Li Z, Zhang P, Yan A, Guo Z, Ban Y, Li J, Chen S, Yang H, He Y, Li J, et al. 2017. ASXL1 interacts with the cohesin complex to maintain chromatid separation and gene expression for normal hematopoiesis. *Sci Adv* **3:** e1601602. doi:10.1126/sciadv.1601602

Love C, Sun Z, Jima D, Li G, Zhang J, Miles R, Richards KL, Dunphy CH, Choi WW, Srivastava G, et al. 2012. The genetic landscape of mutations in Burkitt lymphoma. *Nat Genet* **44:** 1321–1325. doi:10.1038/ng.2468

Lu C, Ward PS, Kapoor GS, Rohle D, Turcan S, Abdel-Wahab O, Edwards CR, Khanin R, Figueroa ME, Melnick A, et al. 2012. IDH mutation impairs histone demethylation and results in a block to cell differentiation. *Nature* **483:** 474–478. doi:10.1038/nature10860

Lugthart S, Figueroa ME, Bindels E, Skrabanek L, Valk PJ, Li Y, Meyer S, Erpelinck-Verschueren C, Greally J, Lowenberg B, et al. 2011. Aberrant DNA hypermethylation signature in acute myeloid leukemia directed by EVI1. *Blood* **117:** 234–241. doi:10.1182/blood-2010-04-281337

Maes T, Mascaró C, Tirapu I, Estiarte A, Ciceri F, Lunardi S, Guibourt N, Perdones A, Lufino MMP, Somervaille TCP, et al. 2018. ORY-1001, a potent and selective covalent KDM1A inhibitor, for the treatment of acute leukemia. *Cancer Cell* **33:** 495–511.e12. doi:10.1016/j.ccell.2018.02.002

Maganti HB, Jrade H, Cafariello C, Manias Rothberg JL, Porter CJ, Yockell-Lelièvre J, Battaion HL, Khan ST, Howard JP, Li Y, et al. 2018. Targeting the MTF2–MDM2 axis sensitizes refractory acute myeloid leukemia to chemotherapy. *Cancer Discov* **8:** 1376–1389. doi:10.1158/2159-8290.CD-17-0841

Maiti A, Drohat AC. 2011. Thymine DNA glycosylase can rapidly excise 5-formylcytosine and 5-carboxylcytosine: potential implications for active demethylation of CpG sites. *J Biol Chem* **286:** 35334–35338. doi:10.1074/jbc.C111.284620

Marcucci G, Maharry K, Wu YZ, Radmacher MD, Mrózek K, Margeson D, Holland KB, Whitman SP, Becker H, Schwind S, et al. 2010. *IDH1* and *IDH2* gene mutations identify novel molecular subsets within de novo cytogenetically normal acute myeloid leukemia: a Cancer and Leukemia Group B study. *J Clin Oncol* **28:** 2348–2355. doi:10.1200/JCO.2009.27.3730

Marcucci G, Metzeler KH, Schwind S, Becker H, Maharry K, Mrozek K, Radmacher MD, Kohlschmidt J, Nicolet D, Whitman SP, et al. 2012. Age-related prognostic impact of different types of *DNMT3A* mutations in adults with primary cytogenetically normal acute myeloid leukemia. *J Clin Oncol* **30:** 742–750. doi:10.1200/JCO.2011.39.2092

Mardis ER, Ding L, Dooling DJ, Larson DE, McLellan MD, Chen K, Koboldt DC, Fulton RS, Delehaunty KD, McGrath SD, et al. 2009. Recurring mutations found by sequencing an acute myeloid leukemia genome. *N Engl J Med* **361:** 1058–1066. doi:10.1056/NEJMoa0903840

Margueron R, Reinberg D. 2011. The Polycomb complex PRC2 and its mark in life. *Nature* **469:** 343–349. doi:10.1038/nature09784

Mayle A, Yang L, Rodriguez B, Zhou T, Chang E, Curry CV, Challen GA, Li W, Wheeler D, Rebel VI, et al. 2015. *Dnmt3a* loss predisposes murine hematopoietic stem cells to malignant transformation. *Blood* **125:** 629–638. doi:10.1182/blood-2014-08-594648

McCabe MT, Graves AP, Ganji G, Diaz E, Halsey WS, Jiang Y, Smitheman KN, Ott HM, Pappalardi MB, Allen KE, et al. 2012. Mutation of A677 in histone methyltransferase EZH2 in human B-cell lymphoma promotes hypertrimethylation of histone H3 on lysine 27 (H3K27). *Proc Natl Acad Sci* **109:** 2989–2994. doi:10.1073/pnas.1116418109

McGrath JP, Williamson KE, Balasubramanian S, Odate S, Arora S, Hatton C, Edwards TM, O'Brien T, Magnuson S, Stokoe D, et al. 2016. Pharmacological inhibition of the histone lysine demethylase KDM1A suppresses the growth of multiple acute myeloid leukemia subtypes. *Cancer Res* **76:** 1975–1988. doi:10.1158/0008-5472.CAN-15-2333

McHeyzer-Williams LJ, Milpied PJ, Okitsu SL, McHeyzer-Williams MG. 2015. Class-switched memory B cells remodel BCRs within secondary germinal centers. *Nat Immunol* **16:** 296–305. doi:10.1038/ni.3095

Mesin L, Ersching J, Victora GD. 2016. Germinal center B cell dynamics. *Immunity* **45:** 471–482. doi:10.1016/j.immuni.2016.09.001

Metzeler KH, Herold T, Rothenberg-Thurley M, Amler S, Sauerland MC, Görlich D, Schneider S, Konstandin NP, Dufour A, Bräundl K, et al. 2016. Spectrum and prognostic relevance of driver gene mutations in acute myeloid leukemia. *Blood* **128:** 686–698. doi:10.1182/blood-2016-01-693879

Mohammad HP, Smitheman KN, Kamat CD, Soong D, Federowicz KE, Van Aller GS, Schneck JL, Carson JD, Liu Y, Butticello M, et al. 2015. A DNA hypomethylation signature predicts antitumor activity of LSD1 inhibitors in SCLC. *Cancer Cell* **28:** 57–69. doi:10.1016/j.ccell.2015.06.002

Mondello P, Toska E, Teater M, Fontan L, Durant M, Casalena G, De Stanchina E, Inghirami G, Baselga J, Weill Melnick A. 2018. Targeting KDM5 demethylases counteracts KMT2D loss of function in diffuse large B-cell lymphoma. In *AACR advances in malignant lymphoma*, Boston. AACR, Philadelphia.

Mondello P, Tadros S, Teater M, Fontan L, Chang A, Jain N, Singh S, Ma MCJ, Yang H, Toska E, et al. 2019. Selective inhibition of HDAC3 targets synthetic vulnerabilities and activates immune surveillance in lymphoma. *Cancer Discov.* doi:10.1158/2159-8290.CD-19-0116

Moran-Crusio K, Reavie L, Shih A, Abdel-Wahab O, Ndiaye-Lobry D, Lobry C, Figueroa ME, Vasanthakumar A, Patel J, Zhao X, et al. 2011. *Tet2* loss leads to increased hematopoietic stem cell self-renewal and myeloid transformation. *Cancer Cell* **20:** 11–24. doi:10.1016/j.ccr.2011.06.001

Morin RD, Johnson NA, Severson TM, Mungall AJ, An J, Goya R, Paul JE, Boyle M, Woolcock BW, Kuchenbauer F, et al. 2010. Somatic mutations altering EZH2 (Tyr641) in follicular and diffuse large B-cell lymphomas of germinal-center origin. *Nat Genet* **42:** 181–185. doi:10.1038/ng.518

Morin RD, Mendez-Lago M, Mungall AJ, Goya R, Mungall KL, Corbett RD, Johnson NA, Severson TM, Chiu R, Field M, et al. 2011. Frequent mutation of histone-modifying genes in non-Hodgkin lymphoma. *Nature* **476:** 298–303. doi:10.1038/nature10351

Mullenders J, Aranda-Orgilles B, Lhoumaud P, Keller M, Pae J, Wang K, Kayembe C, Rocha PP, Raviram R, Gong Y, et al. 2015. Cohesin loss alters adult hematopoietic stem cell homeostasis, leading to myeloproliferative neoplasms. *J Exp Med* **212:** 1833–1850. doi:10.1084/jem.20151323

Mullighan CG. 2012. Molecular genetics of B-precursor acute lymphoblastic leukemia. *J Clin Invest* **122:** 3407–3415. doi:10.1172/JCI61203

Muppidi MR, Portwood S, Griffiths EA, Thompson JE, Ford LA, Freyer CW, Wetzler M, Wang ES. 2015. Decitabine and sorafenib therapy in *FLT-3* ITD-mutant acute myeloid leukemia. *Clin Lymphoma Myeloma Leuk* **15:** S73–S79. doi:10.1016/j.clml.2015.02.033

Muramatsu M, Kinoshita K, Fagarasan S, Yamada S, Shinkai Y, Honjo T. 2000. Class switch recombination and hypermutation require activation-induced cytidine deaminase (AID), a potential RNA editing enzyme. *Cell* **102:** 553–563. doi:10.1016/S0092-8674(00)00078-7

Nabel CS, Jia H, Ye Y, Shen L, Goldschmidt HL, Stivers JT, Zhang Y, Kohli RM. 2012. AID/APOBEC deaminases disfavor modified cytosines implicated in DNA demethylation. *Nat Chem Biol* **8:** 751–758. doi:10.1038/nchembio.1042

Ngo VN, Young RM, Schmitz R, Jhavar S, Xiao W, Lim KH, Kohlhammer H, Xu W, Yang Y, Zhao H, et al. 2011. Oncogenically active *MYD88* mutations in human lymphoma. *Nature* **470:** 115–119. doi:10.1038/nature09671

Ngo TT, Yoo J, Dai Q, Zhang Q, He C, Aksimentiev A, Ha T. 2016. Effects of cytosine modifications on DNA flexibility and nucleosome mechanical stability. *Nat Commun* **7:** 10813. doi:10.1038/ncomms10813

Nicholas NS, Apollonio B, Ramsay AG. 2016. Tumor microenvironment (TME)-driven immune suppression in B cell malignancy. *Biochim Biophys Acta* **1863:** 471–482. doi:10.1016/j.bbamcr.2015.11.003

Norrback KF, Hultdin M, Dahlenborg K, Osterman P, Carlsson R, Roos G. 2001. Telomerase regulation and telomere dynamics in germinal centers. *Eur J Haematol* **67:** 309–317. doi:10.1034/j.1600-0609.2001.00588.x

Okano M, Bell DW, Haber DA, Li E. 1999. DNA methyltransferases Dnmt3a and Dnmt3b are essential for de novo methylation and mammalian development. *Cell* **99:** 247–257. doi:10.1016/S0092-8674(00)81656-6

Okosun J, Bödör C, Wang J, Araf S, Yang CY, Pan C, Boller S, Cittaro D, Bozek M, Iqbal S, et al. 2014. Integrated genomic analysis identifies recurrent mutations and evolution patterns driving the initiation and progression of follicular lymphoma. *Nat Genet* **46:** 176–181. doi:10.1038/ng.2856

Ortega-Molina A, Boss IW, Canela A, Pan H, Jiang Y, Zhao C, Jiang M, Hu D, Agirre X, Niesvizky I, et al. 2015. The histone lysine methyltransferase KMT2D sustains a gene expression program that represses B cell lymphoma development. *Nat Med* **21:** 1199–1208. doi:10.1038/nm.3943

Pan H, Jiang Y, Boi M, Tabbò F, Redmond D, Nie K, Ladetto M, Chiappella A, Cerchietti L, Shaknovich R, et al. 2015. Epigenomic evolution in diffuse large B-cell lymphomas. *Nat Commun* **6:** 6921. doi:10.1038/ncomms7921

Papa I, Vinuesa CG. 2018. Synaptic interactions in germinal centers. *Front Immunol* **9:** 1858. doi:10.3389/fimmu.2018.01858

Papaemmanuil E, Gerstung M, Bullinger L, Gaidzik VI, Paschka P, Roberts ND, Potter NE, Heuser M, Thol F, Bolli N, et al. 2016. Genomic classification and prognosis in acute myeloid leukemia. *N Engl J Med* **374:** 2209–2221. doi:10.1056/NEJMoa1516192

Paschka P, Schlenk RF, Gaidzik VI, Habdank M, Krönke J, Bullinger L, Späth D, Kayser S, Zucknick M, Götze K, et al. 2010. *IDH1* and *IDH2* mutations are frequent genetic alterations in acute myeloid leukemia and confer adverse prognosis in cytogenetically normal acute myeloid leukemia with *NPM1* mutation without *FLT3* internal tandem duplication. *J Clin Oncol* **28:** 3636–3643. doi:10.1200/JCO.2010.28.3762

Pasqualucci L, Dalla-Favera R. 2015. The genetic landscape of diffuse large B-cell lymphoma. *Semin Hematol* **52:** 67–76. doi:10.1053/j.seminhematol.2015.01.005

Pasqualucci L, Dominguez-Sola D, Chiarenza A, Fabbri G, Grunn A, Trifonov V, Kasper LH, Lerach S, Tang H, Ma J, et al. 2011. Inactivating mutations of acetyltransferase genes in B-cell lymphoma. *Nature* **471:** 189–195. doi:10.1038/nature09730

Patel JP, Gönen M, Figueroa ME, Fernandez H, Sun Z, Racevskis J, Van Vlierberghe P, Dolgalev I, Thomas S, Aminova O, et al. 2012. Prognostic relevance of integrated genetic profiling in acute myeloid leukemia. *N Engl J Med* **366:** 1079–1089. doi:10.1056/NEJMoa1112304

Pfeifer M, Grau M, Lenze D, Wenzel SS, Wolf A, Wollert-Wulf B, Dietze K, Nogai H, Storek B, Madle H, et al. 2013. PTEN loss defines a PI3K/AKT pathway-dependent germinal center subtype of diffuse large B-cell lymphoma. *Proc Natl Acad Sci* **110:** 12420–12425. doi:10.1073/pnas.1305656110

Phan RT, Dalla-Favera R. 2004. The *BCL6* proto-oncogene suppresses p53 expression in germinal-centre B cells. *Nature* **432:** 635–639. doi:10.1038/nature03147

Phan RT, Saito M, Basso K, Niu H, Dalla-Favera R. 2005. BCL6 interacts with the transcription factor Miz-1 to suppress the cyclin-dependent kinase inhibitor p21 and cell cycle arrest in germinal center B cells. *Nat Immunol* **6:** 1054–1060. doi:10.1038/ni1245

Postow MA, Chesney J, Pavlick AC, Robert C, Grossmann K, McDermott D, Linette GP, Meyer N, Giguere JK, Agarwala SS, et al. 2015. Nivolumab and ipilimumab versus ipilimumab in untreated melanoma. *N Engl J Med* **372:** 2006–2017. doi:10.1056/NEJMoa1414428

Prebet T, Sun Z, Figueroa ME, Ketterling R, Melnick A, Greenberg PL, Herman J, Juckett M, Smith MR, Malick L, et al. 2014. Prolonged administration of azacitidine with or without entinostat for myelodysplastic syndrome and acute myeloid leukemia with myelodysplasia-related changes: results of the US Leukemia Intergroup trial E1905. *J Clin Oncol* **32:** 1242–1248. doi:10.1200/JCO.2013.50.3102

Quek L, David MD, Kennedy A, Metzner M, Amatangelo M, Shih A, Stoilova B, Quivoron C, Heiblig M, Willekens C, et al. 2018. Clonal heterogeneity of acute myeloid leukemia treated with the IDH2 inhibitor enasidenib. *Nature Med* **24:** 1167–1177. doi:10.1038/s41591-018-0115-6

Quivoron C, Couronne L, Della Valle V, Lopez CK, Plo I, Wagner-Ballon O, Do Cruzeiro M, Delhommeau F, Arnulf B, Stern MH, et al. 2011. TET2 inactivation results in pleiotropic hematopoietic abnormalities in mouse and is a recurrent event during human lymphomagenesis. *Cancer Cell* **20:** 25–38. doi:10.1016/j.ccr.2011.06.003

Rampal R, Alkalin A, Madzo J, Vasanthakumar A, Pronier E, Patel J, Li Y, Ahn J, Abdel-Wahab O, Shih A, et al. 2014. DNA hydroxymethylation profiling reveals that *WT1* mutations result in loss of TET2 function in acute myeloid leukemia. *Cell Rep* **9:** 1841–1855. doi:10.1016/j.celrep.2014.11.004

Ranuncolo SM, Polo JM, Dierov J, Singer M, Kuo T, Greally J, Green R, Carroll M, Melnick A. 2007. Bcl-6 mediates the germinal center B cell phenotype and lymphomagenesis through transcriptional repression of the DNA-damage sensor ATR. *Nat Immunol* **8:** 705–714. doi:10.1038/ni1478

Ranuncolo SM, Polo JM, Melnick A. 2008. BCL6 represses CHEK1 and suppresses DNA damage pathways in normal and malignant B-cells. *Blood Cells Mol Dis* **41:** 95–99. doi:10.1016/j.bcmd.2008.02.003

Rasmussen KD, Helin K. 2016. Role of TET enzymes in DNA methylation, development, and cancer. *Genes Dev* **30:** 733–750. doi:10.1101/gad.276568.115

Rasmussen KD, Jia G, Johansen JV, Pedersen MT, Rapin N, Bagger FO, Porse BT, Bernard OA, Christensen J, Helin K. 2015. Loss of *TET2* in hematopoietic cells leads to DNA hypermethylation of active enhancers and induction of leukemogenesis. *Genes Dev* **29:** 910–922. doi:10.1101/gad.260174.115

Rasmussen KD, Berest I, Kebetaler S, Nishimura K, Simon-Carrasco L, Vassiliou GS, Pedersen MT, Christensen J, Zaugg JB, Helin K. 2019. TET2 binding to enhancers facilitates transcription factor recruitment in hematopoietic cells. *Genome Res* **29:** 564–575. doi:10.1101/gr.239277.118

Ravandi F, Alattar ML, Grunwald MR, Rudek MA, Rajkhowa T, Richie MA, Pierce S, Daver N, Garcia-Manero G, Faderl S, et al. 2013. Phase 2 study of azacytidine plus sorafenib in patients with acute myeloid leukemia and FLT-3 internal tandem duplication mutation. *Blood* **121:** 4655–4662. doi:10.1182/blood-2013-01-480228

Reddy A, Zhang J, Davis NS, Moffitt AB, Love CL, Waldrop A, Leppa S, Pasanen A, Meriranta L, Karjalainen-Lindsberg ML, et al. 2017. Genetic and functional drivers of diffuse large B cell lymphoma. *Cell* **171:** 481–494.e15. doi:10.1016/j.cell.2017.09.027

Rivas MA, Melnick AM. 2019. Role of chromosomal architecture in germinal center B cells and lymphomagenesis. *Curr Opin Hematol* **26:** 294–302. doi:10.1097/MOH.0000000000000505

Robert MF, Morin S, Beaulieu N, Gauthier F, Chute IC, Barsalou A, MacLeod AR. 2003. DNMT1 is required to maintain CpG methylation and aberrant gene silencing in human cancer cells. *Nat Genet* **33:** 61–65. doi:10.1038/ng1068

Robert C, Schachter J, Long GV, Arance A, Grob JJ, Mortier L, Daud A, Carlino MS, McNeil C, Lotem M, et al. 2015. Pembrolizumab versus ipilimumab in advanced melanoma. *N Engl J Med* **372:** 2521–2532. doi:10.1056/NEJMoa1503093

Rosenwald A, Wright G, Chan WC, Connors JM, Campo E, Fisher RI, Gascoyne RD, Muller-Hermelink HK, Smeland EB, Giltnane JM, et al. 2002. The use of molecular profiling to predict survival after chemotherapy for diffuse large-B-cell lymphoma. *N Engl J Med* **346:** 1937–1947. doi:10.1056/NEJMoa012914

Rossi D, Trifonov V, Fangazio M, Bruscaggin A, Rasi S, Spina V, Monti S, Vaisitti T, Arruga F, Famà R, et al. 2012. The coding genome of splenic marginal zone lymphoma: activation of *NOTCH2* and other pathways regulating marginal zone development. *J Exp Med* **209:** 1537–1551. doi:10.1084/jem.20120904

Russler-Germain DA, Spencer DH, Young MA, Lamprecht TL, Miller CA, Fulton R, Meyer MR, Erdmann-Gilmore P, Townsend RR, Wilson RK, et al. 2014. The R882H DNMT3A mutation associated with AML dominantly inhibits wild-type DNMT3A by blocking its ability to form active tetramers. *Cancer Cell* **25:** 442–454. doi:10.1016/j.ccr.2014.02.010

Saxonov S, Berg P, Brutlag DL. 2006. A genome-wide analysis of CpG dinucleotides in the human genome distinguishes two distinct classes of promoters. *Proc Natl Acad Sci* **103:** 1412–1417. doi:10.1073/pnas.0510310103

Schenk T, Chen WC, Göllner S, Howell L, Jin L, Hebestreit K, Klein HU, Popescu AC, Burnett A, Mills K, et al. 2012. Inhibition of the LSD1 (KDM1A) demethylase reactivates the all-trans-retinoic acid differentiation pathway in acute myeloid leukemia. *Nat Med* **18:** 605–611. doi:10.1038/nm.2661

Schichman SA, Caligiuri MA, Gu Y, Strout MP, Canaani E, Bloomfield CD, Croce CM. 1994. *ALL-1* partial duplication in acute leukemia. *Proc Natl Acad Sci* **91:** 6236–6239. doi:10.1073/pnas.91.13.6236

Schmitz R, Wright GW, Huang DW, Johnson CA, Phelan JD, Wang JQ, Roulland S, Kasbekar M, Young RM, Shaffer AL, et al. 2018. Genetics and pathogenesis of diffuse large B-cell lymphoma. *N Engl J Med* **378:** 1396–1407. doi:10.1056/NEJMoa1801445

Sermer D, Pasqualucci L, Wendel HG, Melnick A, Younes A. 2019. Emerging epigenetic-modulating therapies in lymphoma. *Nat Rev Clin Oncol* **16:** 494–507. doi:10.1038/s41571-019-0190-8

Shaknovich R, Cerchietti L, Tsikitas L, Kormaksson M, De S, Figueroa ME, Ballon G, Yang SN, Weinhold N, Reimers M, et al. 2011. DNA methyltransferase 1 and DNA methylation patterning contribute to germinal center B-cell differentiation. *Blood* **118:** 3559–3569. doi:10.1182/blood-2011-06-357996

Shen Y, Zhu YM, Fan X, Shi JY, Wang QR, Yan XJ, Gu ZH, Wang YY, Chen B, Jiang CL, et al. 2011. Gene mutation patterns and their prognostic impact in a cohort of 1185 patients with acute myeloid leukemia. *Blood* **118:** 5593–5603. doi:10.1182/blood-2011-03-343988

Shen L, Wu H, Diep D, Yamaguchi S, D'Alessio AC, Fung HL, Zhang K, Zhang Y. 2013. Genome-wide analysis reveals TET- and TDG-dependent 5-methylcytosine oxidation dynamics. *Cell* **153:** 692–706. doi:10.1016/j.cell.2013.04.002

Shia W-J, Okumura AJ, Yan M, Sarkeshik A, Lo M-C, Matsuura S, Komeno Y, Zhao X, Nimer SD, Yates JR III, et al. 2012. PRMT1 interacts with AML1-ETO to promote its transcriptional activation and progenitor cell proliferative potential. *Blood* **119:** 4953–4962. doi:10.1182/blood-2011-04-347476

Shih AH, Jiang Y, Meydan C, Shank K, Pandey S, Barreyro L, Antony-Debre I, Viale A, Socci N, Sun Y, et al. 2015. Mutational cooperativity linked to combinatorial epigenetic gain of function in acute myeloid leukemia. *Cancer Cell* **27:** 502–515. doi:10.1016/j.ccell.2015.03.009

Shih AH, Meydan C, Shank K, Garrett-Bakelman FE, Ward PS, Intlekofer AM, Nazir A, Stein EM, Knapp K, Glass J, et al. 2017. Combination targeted therapy to disrupt aberrant oncogenic signaling and reverse epigenetic dysfunction in *IDH2*- and *TET2*-mutant acute myeloid leukemia. *Cancer Discov* **7:** 494–505. doi:10.1158/2159-8290.CD-16-1049

Shlush LI, Zandi S, Mitchell A, Chen WC, Brandwein JM, Gupta V, Kennedy JA, Schimmer AD, Schuh AC, Yee KW, et al. 2014. Identification of pre-leukaemic haematopoietic stem cells in acute leukaemia. *Nature* **506:** 328–333. doi:10.1038/nature13038

Smith ZD, Meissner A. 2013. DNA methylation: roles in mammalian development. *Nat Rev Genet* **14:** 204–220. doi:10.1038/nrg3354

Sneeringer CJ, Scott MP, Kuntz KW, Knutson SK, Pollock RM, Richon VM, Copeland RA. 2010. Coordinated activities of wild-type plus mutant EZH2 drive tumor-associated hypertrimethylation of lysine 27 on histone H3 (H3K27) in human B-cell lymphomas. *Proc Natl Acad Sci* **107:** 20980–20985. doi:10.1073/pnas.1012525107

Spina V, Khiabanian H, Messina M, Monti S, Cascione L, Bruscaggin A, Spaccarotella E, Holmes AB, Arcaini L, Lucioni M, et al. 2016. The genetics of nodal marginal zone lymphoma. *Blood* **128:** 1362–1373. doi:10.1182/blood-2016-02-696757

Stein EM, DiNardo CD, Pollyea DA, Fathi AT, Roboz GJ, Altman JK, Stone RM, DeAngelo DJ, Levine RL, Flinn IW, et al. 2017. Enasidenib in mutant *IDH2* relapsed or refractory acute myeloid leukemia. *Blood* **130:** 722–731. doi:10.1182/blood-2017-04-779405

Strati P, Kantarjian H, Ravandi F, Nazha A, Borthakur G, Daver N, Kadia T, Estrov Z, Garcia-Manero G, Konopleva M, et al. 2015. Phase I/II trial of the combination of midostaurin (PKC412) and 5-azacytidine for patients with acute myeloid leukemia and myelodysplastic syndrome. *Am J Hematol* **90:** 276–281. doi:10.1002/ajh.23924

Tahiliani M, Koh KP, Shen Y, Pastor WA, Bandukwala H, Brudno Y, Agarwal S, Iyer LM, Liu DR, Aravind L, et al. 2009. Conversion of 5-methylcytosine to 5-hydroxymethylcytosine in mammalian DNA by MLL partner TET1. *Science* **324:** 930–935. doi:10.1126/science.1170116

Tarighat SS, Santhanam R, Frankhouser D, Radomska HS, Lai H, Anghelina M, Wang H, Huang X, Alinari L, Walker A, et al. 2016. The dual epigenetic role of PRMT5 in acute myeloid leukemia: gene activation and repression via histone arginine methylation. *Leukemia* **30:** 789–799. doi:10.1038/leu.2015.308

Teater M, Dominguez PM, Redmond D, Chen Z, Ennishi D, Scott DW, Cimmino L, Ghione P, Chaudhuri J, Gascoyne RD, et al. 2018. AICDA drives epigenetic heterogeneity and accelerates germinal center-derived lymphomagenesis. *Nat Commun* **9:** 222. doi:10.1038/s41467-017-02595-w

Terada K, Yamaguchi H, Ueki T, Usuki K, Kobayashi Y, Tajika K, Gomi S, Kurosawa S, Saito R, Furuta Y, et al. 2018. Usefulness of *BCOR* gene mutation as a prognostic factor in acute myeloid leukemia with intermediate cytogenetic prognosis. *Genes Chromosomes Canc* **57:** 401–408. doi:10.1002/gcc.22542

Thol F, Bollin R, Gehlhaar M, Walter C, Dugas M, Suchanek KJ, Kirchner A, Huang L, Chaturvedi A, Wichmann M, et al. 2014. Mutations in the cohesin complex in acute myeloid leukemia: clinical and prognostic implications. *Blood* **123:** 914–920. doi:10.1182/blood-2013-07-518746

Thota S, Viny AD, Makishima H, Spitzer B, Radivoyevitch T, Przychodzen B, Sekeres MA, Levine RL, Maciejewski JP. 2014. Genetic alterations of the cohesin complex genes in myeloid malignancies. *Blood* **124:** 1790–1798. doi:10.1182/blood-2014-04-567057

Tothova Z, Krill-Burger JM, Popova KD, Landers CC, Sievers QL, Yudovich D, Belizaire R, Aster JC, Morgan EA, Tsherniak A, et al. 2017. Multiplex CRISPR/Cas9-based genome editing in human hematopoietic stem cells models clonal hematopoiesis and myeloid neoplasia. *Cell Stem Cell* **21:** 547–555.e8. doi:10.1016/j.stem.2017.07.015

Tsai CH, Hou HA, Tang JL, Kuo YY, Chiu YC, Lin CC, Liu CY, Tseng MH, Lin TY, Liu MC, et al. 2017. Prognostic impacts and dynamic changes of cohesin complex gene mutations in de novo acute myeloid leukemia. *Blood Cancer J* **7:** 663. doi:10.1038/s41408-017-0022-y

Tsao T, Shi Y, Kornblau S, Lu H, Konoplev S, Antony A, Ruvolo V, Qiu YH, Zhang N, Coombes KR, et al. 2012. Concomitant inhibition of DNA methyltransferase and BCL-2 protein function synergistically induce mitochondrial apoptosis in acute myelogenous leukemia cells. *Ann Hematol* **91:** 1861–1870. doi:10.1007/s00277-012-1537-8

Velichutina I, Shaknovich R, Geng H, Johnson NA, Gascoyne RD, Melnick AM, Elemento O. 2010. EZH2-mediated epigenetic silencing in germinal center B cells contributes to proliferation and lymphomagenesis. *Blood* **116:** 5247–5255. doi:10.1182/blood-2010-04-280149

Victora GD, Dominguez-Sola D, Holmes AB, Deroubaix S, Dalla-Favera R, Nussenzweig MC. 2012. Identification of human germinal center light and dark zone cells and their relationship to human B-cell lymphomas. *Blood* **120:** 2240–2248. doi:10.1182/blood-2012-03-415380

Viny AD, Ott CJ, Spitzer B, Rivas M, Meydan C, Papalexi E, Yelin D, Shank K, Reyes J, Chiu A, et al. 2015. Dose-dependent role of the cohesin complex in normal and malignant hematopoiesis. *J Exp Med* **212:** 1819–1832. doi:10.1084/jem.20151317

Wagner EJ, Carpenter PB. 2012. Understanding the language of Lys36 methylation at histone H3. *Nat Rev Mol Cell Biol* **13:** 115–126. doi:10.1038/nrm3274

Wang Y, Xiao M, Chen X, Chen L, Xu Y, Lv L, Wang P, Yang H, Ma S, Lin H, et al. 2015. WT1 recruits TET2 to regulate its target gene expression and suppress leukemia cell proliferation. *Mol Cell* **57:** 662–673. doi:10.1016/j.molcel.2014.12.023

Ward PS, Cross JR, Lu C, Weigert O, Abel-Wahab O, Levine RL, Weinstock DM, Sharp KA, Thompson CB. 2011. Identification of additional IDH mutations associated with oncometabolite R(-)-2-hydroxyglutarate production. *Oncogene* **31:** 2491–2498. doi:10.1038/onc.2011.416

Waters LR, Ahsan FM, Wolf DM, Shirihai O, Teitell MA. 2018. Initial B cell activation induces metabolic reprogramming and mitochondrial remodeling. *iScience* **5:** 99–109. doi:10.1016/j.isci.2018.07.005

Weissmann S, Alpermann T, Grossmann V, Kowarsch A, Nadarajah N, Eder C, Dicker F, Fasan A, Haferlach C, Haferlach T, et al. 2012. Landscape of *TET2* mutations in acute myeloid leukemia. *Leukemia* **26:** 934–942. doi:10.1038/leu.2011.326

Wu SY, Chiang CM. 2007. The double bromodomain-containing chromatin adaptor Brd4 and transcriptional regulation. *J Biol Chem* **282:** 13141–13145. doi:10.1074/jbc.R700001200

Xie W, Schultz MD, Lister R, Hou Z, Rajagopal N, Ray P, Whitaker JW, Tian S, Hawkins RD, Leung D, et al. 2013. Epigenomic analysis of multilineage differentiation of human embryonic stem cells. *Cell* **153:** 1134–1148. doi:10.1016/j.cell.2013.04.022

Xu W, Yang H, Liu Y, Yang Y, Wang P, Kim SH, Ito S, Yang C, Wang P, Xiao MT, et al. 2011. Oncometabolite 2-hydroxyglutarate is a competitive inhibitor of α-ketoglutarate-dependent dioxygenases. *Cancer Cell* **19:** 17–30. doi:10.1016/j.ccr.2010.12.014

Xu B, On DM, Ma A, Parton T, Konze KD, Pattenden SG, Allison DF, Cai L, Rockowitz S, Liu S, et al. 2015. Selective inhibition of EZH2 and EZH1 enzymatic activity by a small molecule suppresses *MLL*-rearranged leukemia. *Blood* **125:** 346–357. doi:10.1182/blood-2014-06-581082

Yang L, Rau R, Goodell MA. 2015. DNMT3A in haematological malignancies. *Nat Rev Cancer* **15:** 152–165. doi:10.1038/nrc3895

Yap DB, Chu J, Berg T, Schapira M, Cheng SW, Moradian A, Morin RD, Mungall AJ, Meissner B, Boyle M, et al. 2011. Somatic mutations at EZH2 Y641 act dominantly through a mechanism of selectively altered PRC2 catalytic activity, to increase H3K27 trimethylation. *Blood* **117:** 2451–2459. doi:10.1182/blood-2010-11-321208

Zhang J, Jima D, Moffitt AB, Liu Q, Czader M, Hsi ED, Fedoriw Y, Dunphy CH, Richards KL, Gill JI, et al. 2014. The genomic landscape of mantle cell lymphoma is related to the epigenetically determined chromatin state of normal B cells. *Blood* **123:** 2988–2996. doi:10.1182/blood-2013-07-517177

Zhang J, Dominguez-Sola D, Hussein S, Lee JE, Holmes AB, Bansal M, Vlasevska S, Mo T, Tang H, Basso K, et al. 2015. Disruption of KMT2D perturbs germinal center B cell development and promotes lymphomagenesis. *Nat Med* **21:** 1190–1198. doi:10.1038/nm.3940

Zhang J, Vlasevska S, Wells VA, Nataraj S, Holmes AB, Duval R, Meyer SN, Mo T, Basso K, Brindle PK, et al. 2017. The CREBBP acetyltransferase is a haploinsufficient tumor suppressor in B-cell lymphoma. *Cancer Discov* **7:** 322–337. doi:10.1158/2159-8290.CD-16-1417

Zorko NA, Bernot KM, Whitman SP, Siebenaler RF, Ahmed EH, Marcucci GG, Yanes DA, McConnell KK, Mao C, Kalu C, et al. 2012. *Mll* partial tandem duplication and *Flt3* internal tandem duplication in a double knock-in mouse recapitulates features of counterpart human acute myeloid leukemias. *Blood* **120:** 1130–1136. doi:10.1182/blood-2012-03-415067

Zuber J, Shi J, Wang E, Rappaport AR, Herrmann H, Sison EA, Magoon D, Qi J, Blatt K, Wunderlich M, et al. 2011. RNAi screen identifies Brd4 as a therapeutic target in acute myeloid leukaemia. *Nature* **478:** 524–528. doi:10.1038/nature10334

RNA Regulators in Leukemia and Lymphoma

Camila Prieto and Michael G. Kharas

Molecular Pharmacology Program, Memorial Sloan Kettering Cancer Center, New York, New York 10065, USA
Correspondence: kharasm@mskcc.org

Posttranscriptional regulation of mRNA is a powerful and tightly controlled process in which cells command the integrity, diversity, and abundance of their protein products. RNA-binding proteins (RBPs) are the principal players that control many intermediary steps of posttranscriptional regulation. Recent advances in this field have discovered the importance of RBPs in hematological diseases. Herein we will review a number of RBPs that have been determined to play critical functions in leukemia and lymphoma. Furthermore, we will discuss the potential therapeutic strategies that are currently being studied to specifically target RBPs in these diseases.

The integrity, diversity, and abundance of the cell's protein products are largely controlled through posttranscriptional regulation, consisting of many intermediary steps between transcription and translation. This highly coordinated process includes nascent RNAs undergoing alternative splicing, editing, polyadenylation, capping, 3′ end formation, and nucleocytoplasmic transport to the ribosome before being translated and ultimately degraded (Hong 2017; Pereira et al. 2017). Posttranscriptional regulation is primarily controlled by RNA-binding proteins (RBPs) and small RNAs that predominantly bind to specific elements located in the untranslated regions (UTRs) of target mRNAs.

Large-scale quantitative methods have revealed at least 1500 distinct eukaryotic RBPs belonging to a variety of functional families and with the ability to bind and regulate thousands of transcripts (Gerstberger et al. 2014). This diversity seems to have increased during evolution in correlation with the rise in the number of introns (Glisovic et al. 2008). RBPs bind to specific mRNA sequences or structures to recruit and form functional complexes with other molecules to modulate gene expression (Table 1). These dynamic ribonucleoprotein (RNP) complexes dictate how the transcript is processed, where it is localized, and if or when it is translated.

The first step of posttranscriptional regulation occurs when these RNP complexes are formed in the nucleus as transcription progresses. Alternative splicing, the process in which introns are removed from the pre-mRNA and the remaining exons are ligated, is carried out by the spliceosome. The spliceosome is a macromolecule complex consisting of five small nuclear ribonucleoproteins (snRNPs) and small nuclear RNAs, and includes the RBPs SF3B1, SRSF2, and U2AF1 (Graveley and Maniatis 1998; Schaal and Maniatis 1999; Chen and Man-

Cite this article as *Cold Spring Harb Perspect Med* doi: 10.1101/cshperspect.a034967

Table 1. RNA-binding proteins (RBPs) have the ability to bind and regulate a myriad of transcripts

RBP	mRNA mechanistic basis	Putative targets	Role in leukemia and lymphoma	Carcinogenic potential
Splicing factor 3 subunit b1 (SF3B1), Serine arginine-rich splicing factor 2 (SRSF2), U2 small nuclear RNA auxiliary factor 1 (U2AF1)	Splicing; mRNA processing	Enhancer of zeste 2 Polycomb repressive complex 2 subunit (EZH2)	Mutated in myelodysplastic syndrome (MDS), myeloproliferative neoplasms (MPN), and leukemia; mutations are mutually exclusive; mutations in *SRSF2* and *U2AF1* resulted in elevated R loops and replication stress	Proto-oncogenic
RNA-binding motif protein 39 (RBM39)	Splicing	BMI1; MYB; GATA2	Overexpressed in acute myeloid leukemia (AML); depletion resulted in RNA splicing changes in AML	Proto-oncogenic
Methyltransferase-like 3 (METTL3)	RNA methylation (m^6A writer)	MYC; MYB; BCL2; phosphatase and tensin homolog (PTEN)	Overexpressed in leukemia; depletion resulted in induced differentiation, increased apoptosis, and delayed leukemogenesis in vivo	Proto-oncogenic
RNA-binding motif protein 15 (RBM15)	Splicing; mRNA export; RNA methylation (m^6A adaptor protein)	Suppressor of hairless [Su(H); human homolog (RBPJ); SET domain containing 1B protein (SETD1B)	MKL fusion partner in acute megakaryoblastic leukemia (AMKL); AMKL in non-Down syndrome infants has poor prognosis	Proto-oncogenic
LIN28A	miRNA processing	*let-7* family members	Overexpression in OCI-AML3 resulted in cell cycle arrest and differentiation	Tumor-suppressor
LIN28B	miRNA processing	*let-7* family members; *miR-150*	Overexpressed in peripheral T-cell lymphoma (PTCL), blast crisis chronic myeloid leukemia (BC-CML), and	Proto-oncogenic

Continued

Table 1. *Continued*

RBP	mRNA mechanistic basis	Putative targets	Role in leukemia and lymphoma	Carcinogenic potential
			AP-CML; overexpression in mice led to lymphoma and PTCL; promoted AML cell proliferation; MYC up-regulated its expression	
Human antigen R (HuR)	mRNA stability; mRNA translation; pre-mRNA processing	Eukaryotic initiation factor 4E (eIF4E)	Overexpressed in M4 AML; promoted tumorigenesis	Proto-oncogenic
eIF4E	mRNA translation by binding to 5′ cap; mRNA transport	Cyclin D1	Overexpressed in M4/M5 AML and BC-AML; accelerated lymphomagenesis	Proto-oncogenic
Eukaryotic initiation factor 4A (eIF4A)	mRNA translation	MYC; MYB; NOTCH; CDK6; BCL2	Promoted T-cell acute lymphoblastic leukemia (T-ALL) development in vivo	Proto-oncogenic
Insulin-like growth factor 2 mRNA-binding protein 1 (IGF2BP1)	mRNA stability; mRNA localization; mRNA translation		Overexpressed in Hodgkin's lymphoma, B-cell lymphoma, and ETV6/RUNX1-positive leukemia	Proto-oncogenic
Insulin-like growth factor 2 mRNA-binding protein 3 (IGF2BP3)	mRNA stability; mRNA localization; mRNA translation	IGF2; MYC; CDK6	Overexpressed in lymphomas, mixed-lineage leukemia (MLL)-AF4-positive leukemia, and BCR/ABL1-positive acute lymphoblastic leukemia (ALL); dysregulated in B-cell acute lymphoblastic leukemia (B-ALL)	Proto-oncogenic

Continued

Table 1. *Continued*

RBP	mRNA mechanistic basis	Putative targets	Role in leukemia and lymphoma	Carcinogenic potential
Insulin-like growth factor-binding protein 7 (IGFBP7)			Low expression correlates with poor prognosis in AML; suppressed tumorigenesis; low expression in leukemia stem cells (LSCs)	Tumor-suppressor
Musashi RNA-binding protein 2 (MSI2)	mRNA translation	MYC; homeobox A9 (HOXA9); IKAROS family zinc finger 2 (IKZF2); Tetrespanin-3 (TSPAN3); FMS-like tyrosine kinase 3 (FLT3); branched-chain amino acid aminotransferase 1 (BCAT1)	Fusion partner; overexpressed in chronic lymphocytic leukemia (CLL), adult B-ALL, T-ALL, MDS, CML, and AML; required for leukemia progression	Proto-oncogenic
Synaptotagmin-binding, cytoplasmic RNA-interacting protein (SYNCRIP)	mRNA translation	HOXA9	Promoted leukemogenesis in AML; tumor suppressor in T-ALL with 6q deletion	Proto-oncogenic and tumor-suppressor
Heterogeneous nuclear ribonucleoprotein K (hnRNPK)	mRNA metabolism	MYC; p21; CCAAT-enhancer-binding protein (C/EBP)	Depletion in BCR/ABL transformed cells resulted in impaired leukemogenesis; reduced expression in AML patients with 6q deletion; *Hnrnpk* haploinsufficient mice developed a myeloproliferative phenotype and lymphoma	Proto-oncogenic and tumor-suppressor

Cite this article as *Cold Spring Harb Perspect Med* doi: 10.1101/cshperspect.a034967

ley 2009). After splicing, the mature mRNA is further associated with RBPs and exported out of the nucleus. Upon localization to the cytoplasm, additional RBPs bind to and dictate the fate of the mRNA. Some RBPs, including human antigen R (HuR) and IGF2BP3, stabilize the mRNA and protect it from rapid turnover (Brennan and Steitz 2001; Bell et al. 2013; Wurth and Gebauer 2015). Other RBPs, such as Musashi RNA-binding protein 2 (MSI2), enhance the translation of their mRNA targets (Park et al. 2015). Yet other RBPs drive efficient translation, such as the heterotrimeric complex eIF4F, which consists of the subunits eIF4E, eIF4A, and eIF4G. This complex is responsible for regulating cap-dependent translation initiation by binding to the mRNA 5′ cap and unwinding the mRNA 5′ UTR secondary structure to create a binding site for ribosomes (Fig. 1; Table 1; Parsyan et al. 2011).

For the large repertoire of RBPs, one would expect an equal amount of diversity in structures with the ability to recognize mRNA. Yet, RBPs often contain one or multiple highly conserved RNA-binding domains (RBDs), consisting of 60–100 amino acids. RBDs provide specificity for the RBPs to bind to their target mRNAs and allow the functional classification of RBPs into families. Although there are more than 40 RBDs identified, some of the most well-characterized include RNA recognition motif (RRM), K-homology (KH) domain, RGG (Arg-Gly-Gly) box, Sm domain, DEAD/DEAH box, Zinc finger (ZF) domain, double stranded RNA-binding domain (dsRBD), cold-shock domain (CSD), and Piwi/Argonaute/Zwille (PAZ) domain. RBPs containing different combinations of RBDs have increased flexibility to bind numerous mRNAs with different specificities and affinities (Lunde et al. 2007; Glisovic et al. 2008; Hong

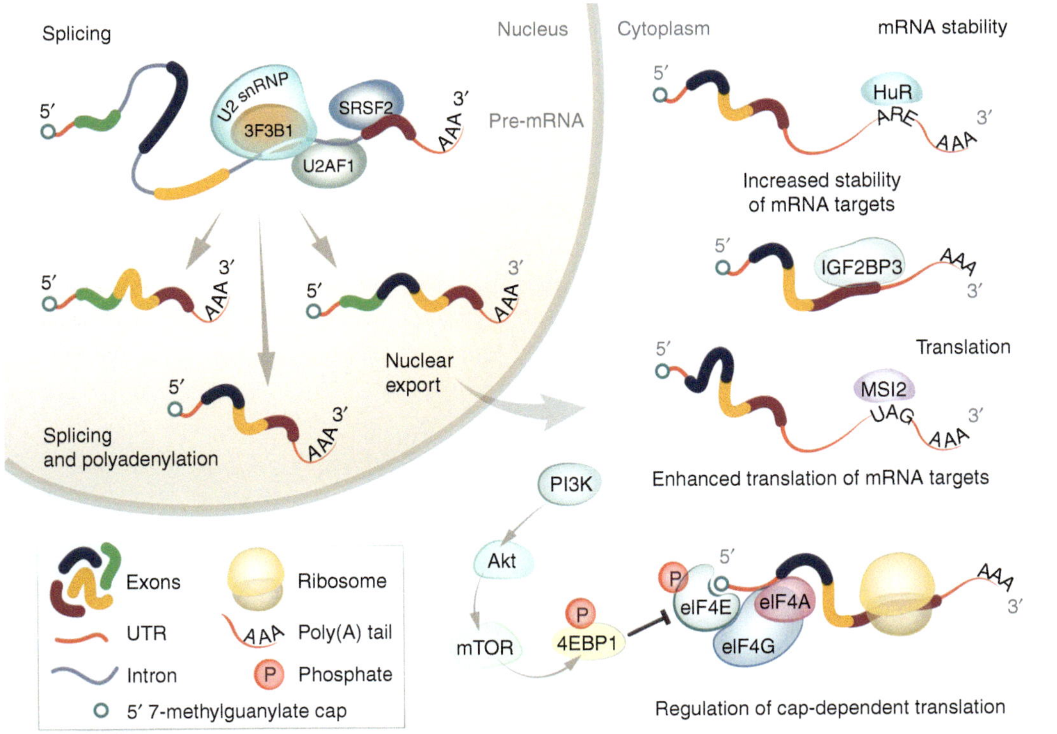

Figure 1. Overview of the main cellular stages of posttranscriptional regulation. A general pathway for several of the many intermediary steps of posttranscriptional regulation, including some RNA-binding proteins (RBPs) demonstrated to be involved in controlling these steps. The steps highlighted include splicing, nucleocytoplasmic transport, mRNA stability, and translation.

2017). Yet, many RBPs lack these characterized RBDs and instead are composed of low complexity, intrinsically disordered regions, allowing them to associate with mRNA in a highly flexible and adaptable manner (Wurth and Gebauer 2015; Pereira et al. 2017).

With this central role in the regulation of the gene expression program, it follows that dysregulation of RBPs can lead to disease, including cancer (Lukong et al. 2008; Cooper et al. 2009; Darnell 2010). Although cytogenetic aberrations and alterations to signaling pathways have been well-studied in cancer, the mechanisms of posttranscriptional regulation have only recently come to the forefront of scientific investigation. Aberrant expression and mutations of RBPs have been reported in numerous cancer types, with several RBPs being identified as important players in leukemia and lymphoma (Kechavarzi and Janga 2014). This review will cover RNA regulators that are dysregulated in leukemia and lymphoma and explore their potential as therapeutic targets.

RNA-BINDING PROTEINS IN LEUKEMIA AND LYMPHOMA

RBPs Regulating Splicing

Splicing Factors SF3B1, SRSF2, and U2AF1

One of the steps integral to posttranscriptional regulation is mRNA splicing. mRNA splicing is a crucial contributor to the integrity and diversity of final protein products and is accomplished by spliceosomes. Spliceosomes are formed by five snRNPs and small nuclear RNAs. They function by removing introns from the primary transcript, the pre-mRNA, and ligating the remaining flanking exons to generate mature mRNA. Alternative splicing increases genomic diversity by altering the mRNA by using alternative 5′ and 3′ splice sites or retaining introns and unconventional exons. Because RNA splicing is very conserved in eukaryotic cells, alterations to this pathway can lead to disease, including leukemia and lymphoma (Chen and Manley 2009).

In hematological diseases, genomic studies have identified somatic mutations in many classes of genes, including splicing factors. Similarly, advances in exome sequencing have revealed mutations in spliceosomal genes most commonly occurring in myelodysplastic syndrome (MDS), myeloproliferative neoplasms (MPN), acute myeloid leukemia (AML), chronic lymphcytic leukemia (CLL), and chronic myelomonocytic leukemia (CMML) (Malcovati et al. 2011; Papaemmanuil et al. 2011; Wang et al. 2011; Yoshida et al. 2011; Graubert et al. 2012; Quesada et al. 2012; Visconte et al. 2012a). The most commonly mutated genes are splicing factor 3 subunit b1 (*SF3B1*), serine arginine-rich splicing factor 2 (*SRSF2*), and U2 small nuclear RNA auxiliary factor 1 (*U2AF1*); this review will concentrate primarily on SF3B1 and SRSF2 (Visconte et al. 2012b). Recurrent mutations in those genes are the most common genetic alterations in MDS patients. They occur as heterozygous point mutations in specific residues and are mutually exclusive with one another. However, the importance of these significant mutational occurrences and how they mechanistically contribute to tumorigenesis are just beginning to be investigated.

SF3B1, a component of the SF3B complex, is part of the U2-small nuclear ribonucleoprotein (U2snRNP) complex and responsible for binding to the exon–intron junction at the 3′ splice site. The SF3B1 protein consists of an amino-terminal domain involved in protein–RNA and protein–protein interactions and a carboxy-terminal region of 22 HEAT domains (Huntingtin, elongation factor 3, protein phosphatase 2A, and the yeast PI3-kinase TOR1). *SF3B1* mutations were identified in 20% of patients with MDS, 19% with MDS/MPN, and 5.3% with AML. These mutations occur most frequently in the fourth, fifth, and sixth HEAT domains and are associated with overall better survival and lower risk of evolution into AML (Malcovati et al. 2011; Papaemmanuil et al. 2011). *SF3B1* mutations were also found in 81% of patients with two MDS subtypes: refractory anemia with ring sideroblasts (RAR) and refractory cytopenia with multilineage dysplasia and ring sideroblasts (RCMD-RS). These patients exhibited ring sideroblasts, mitochondrial iron deposits, and significantly better overall survival, consistent with previous literature (Visconte

 Cite this article as *Cold Spring Harb Perspect Med* doi: 10.1101/cshperspect.a034967

et al. 2012a; Malcovati et al. 2015). Interestingly, a *Sf3b1* heterozygous knockout mice model displayed the same ring sideroblast phenotype. Additionally, SF3B1 depletion in K562 cells resulted in down-regulation of U2-type intron splicing (Visconte et al. 2012c). Contrarily, *SF3B1* mutations were identified in 15% of CLL patients that exhibited more aggressive disease (Wang et al. 2011; Quesada et al. 2012).

The *SRSF2* gene belongs to the serine/arginine-rich (SR) family of pre-mRNA splicing factors, contains an RRM and an arginine and serine–rich domain, and is important for constitutive and alternative splicing (Graveley and Maniatis 1998; Schaal and Maniatis 1999; Liu et al. 2000). *SRSF2* mutations occur in CMML and advanced forms of MDS, and unlike *SF3B1* mutations, they predict shorter survival (Yoshida et al. 2011; Makishima et al. 2012; Meggendorfer et al. 2012; Papaemmanuil et al. 2013). Conditional knockout of SRSF2 in the thymus caused a T-cell maturation defect by affecting the alternative splicing of CD45 (lymphocyte common antigen), a known receptor tyrosine phosphatase involved in thymocyte development (Wang et al. 2001).

More recently, several studies have attempted to untangle the role of these splicing factor mutations in vivo, suggesting that these mutations alter RNA splicing preferences distinct from those observed upon wild-type protein loss (Lee and Abdel-Wahab 2016). *Srsf2*(P95H) mice displayed multilineage dysplasia, and this *Srsf2* mutation altered SRSF2's specific exonic splicing enhancer motifs recognition, leading to the missplicing and nonsense-mediated decay of the hematopoietic regulator *enhancer of zeste 2 polycomb repressive complex 2 subunit* (*EZH2*) (Kim et al. 2015; Kon et al. 2018). *Sf3b1*(K700E) mice developed erythroid defects, possibly because of abnormal 3′ splice-site selection (Obeng et al. 2016). Last, transgenic *U2af1*(S34F) mice exhibited altered hematopoiesis, with pre-mRNA splicing changes in hematopoietic progenitor cells (Shirai et al. 2015). As mentioned, these mutations occur in a heterozygous manner, consistent with research demonstrating the synthetic lethality between murine *Sf3b1* and *Srsf2* mutations in vivo and the necessity for a wild-type gene copy (Fei et al. 2016; Lee et al. 2016, 2018). Strikingly, each of these splicing factor mutations seems to affect splicing distinctly, yet they all cause the same phenotype. One paper noted that these mutations might all contribute to MDS via R-loop formation, in which mutations in *SRSF2* and *U2AF1* resulted in elevated R loops and replication stress (Chen et al. 2018). Despite these recent advances, questions still remain concerning whether these splicing factor mutations are the main drivers of the disease, if other converging mechanisms exist, and if synergy with other types of mutations drive disease progression.

RBM39

RNA-binding motif protein 39 (RBM39; also known as CAPER-α) is a known splicing factor that has been shown to interact with other splicing factors, such as SF3B1 and U2AF65, and cause splicing changes when depleted (Imai et al. 1993; Loerch et al. 2014; Stepanyuk et al. 2016; Han et al. 2017; Uehara et al. 2017). Furthermore, RBM39 function has been linked to malignant progression, and its expression is up-regulated in several cancers, including small cell lung carcinoma, breast cancer, and colorectal adenoma (Bangur et al. 2002; Mercier et al. 2009; Sillars-Hardebol et al. 2012; Chai et al. 2014). More recently, RBM39 was identified as one of the top candidates to be selectively required in AML from a comprehensive clustered regularly interspaced short palindromic repeats/CRISPR-associated protein 9 (CRISPR/Cas9) domain-focused screen targeting RBDs of 490 RBPs. Increasing its significance in hematological malignancies, *RBM39* was also found to be up-regulated in AML patients compared to normal hematopoietic cells, based on transcriptome analysis of The Cancer Genome Atlas (TCGA) (Wang et al. 2019).

Because RBM39 was found to be required in AML, a CRISPR/Cas9 domain screen was used to further analyze RBM39 essential protein domains by targeting its three RRM domains and its SR region. sgRNAs targeting RRM1 and RRM2 were more selectively depleted, and targeting these two domains delayed leukemogenesis in vivo. Thus, these data suggest that the requirement of RBM39 in AML relies on its RNA-binding activity of specific RBDs. Mechanistically, in AML RBM39 was demonstrated to interact with numerous proteins associated with the spliceosome, including SF3B1, and ribosome biogenesis, which is consistent with previous studies demonstrating the interactions of RBM39 with splicing factors. RBM39 was also determined to interact with 15 RBPs that exhibited strong essentiality in the CRISPR/Cas9 domain–focused screen. Moreover, loss of RBM39 resulted in RNA splicing changes, the most predominant being changes in cassette exon inclusion and exclusion. Interestingly, RBM39 depletion led to aberrant splicing of the homeobox A9 (HOXA9) targets *BMI1* and *MYB* and, subsequently, to their down-regulation as a result of nonsense-medicated decay (NMD) (Wang et al. 2019).

In summary, these data suggest that RBM39 and its RBP network are required for AML survival, and by therapeutically targeting this RBM39 network, the changes of AML splicing can also be exploited.

RBPs Regulating RNA Modifications

METTL3 & m^{6}A Modifications

Posttranscriptional modifications of mRNAs have recently been elucidated as an additional layer in the regulation of gene expression, even though they were observed decades ago (Desrosiers et al. 1974; Rottman et al. 1974). In mRNA, N^6-methyladenosine (m^{6}A) is the most abundant posttranscriptional modification and is involved in various aspects of mRNA metabolism, such as mRNA decay, export, and translation (Cantara et al. 2011; Meyer et al. 2012; Machnicka et al. 2013; Zheng et al. 2013; Linder et al. 2015). m^{6}A marks are dynamically added by "writers," removed by "erasers," and recognized by "readers."

The "writer" complex consists of methyltransferase-like 3 (METTL3) and methyltransferase-like 14 (METTL14) and is responsible for adding the methyl group to mRNAs. The "writer" complex is also made up of adaptor proteins that lead the METTL3-METTL14 complex to particular mRNAs. Wilms tumor 1–associated protein (WTAP) was the first adaptor protein identified. Other adaptor proteins include RNA-binding motif protein 15 (RBM15), its paralog RBM15B, and KIAA1429. m^{6}A demethylases, known as "erasers," include fat mass and obesity associated (FTO) and AlkB homolog 5 (ALKBH5). The m^{6}A "readers" bind either directly or indirectly to the RNAs; these include the YT521-B homology (YTH) family proteins, hnRNP proteins, and eukaryotic initiation factor 3 (EIF3). They have been reviewed comprehensively, so this review will briefly describe the current findings regarding the role of FTO and METTL3 in AML (Dai et al. 2018; Vu et al. 2019).

First, a study determined that FTO is highly expressed in several subtypes of AML, and its depletion increased m^{6}A levels, induced apoptosis, and delayed leukemogenesis (Li et al. 2017). In contrast, certain mutant isocitrate dehydrogenase 1 or 2 (IDH1/2) AML cases demonstrate inhibition of FTO, leading to increased m^{6}A levels. Consistently, another study observed that IDH1/2 mutant cells had increased m^{6}A levels, likely because of inhibited FTO (Elkashef et al. 2017). Last, the metabolite R-2-hydroxyglutarate (R-2HG) was shown to have antileukemic activity, by directly inhibiting FTO activity and increasing m^{6}A levels in non-IDH-mutant lines (Su et al. 2018). Therefore, additional studies are necessary to further explore the context-dependent role of FTO in AML with attention to the mutational backgrounds.

Meanwhile, two studies found METTL3 to be essential in myeloid leukemia. METTL3 mRNA and protein were found to be highly expressed in human leukemia cell lines, which correlated with high m^{6}A levels. METTL3 depletion resulted in induced differentiation, increased apoptosis, cell cycle arrest, and delayed leukemogenesis in vivo (Barbieri et al. 2017; Vu et al. 2017a). One study showed that although METTL3 depletion increased m^{6}A-marked transcripts, these transcripts had reduced translation. Some of these METTL3-regulated targets included MYC, BCL2, and phosphatase and tensin homolog (PTEN), which regulate cell survival and differentiation (Vu et al. 2017a).

 Cite this article as *Cold Spring Harb Perspect Med* doi: 10.1101/cshperspect.a034967

The other study found METTL3 to bind chromatin, in particular to the transcriptional start site of active genes that have the CAATT-box binding protein CEBPZ binding motif. Interestingly, METTL3 induced m^6A marks on the mRNA transcript of these genes, enhancing their translation (Barbieri et al. 2017). More recently, two additional studies noted the key role METTL3 plays in hematopoietic stem cell (HSC) self-renewal, in which deletion of *Mettl3* resulted in altered differentiation of HSCs. Both studies identified *Myc* as a direct target of RNA methylation in HSCs with differential effects on either mRNA stability or translation in HSCs (Cheng et al. 2019; Lee et al. 2019).

METTL14, WTAP, and the m^6A reader YTHDF2 have also been implicated as oncogenes in leukemia. METTL14 depletion resulted in increased differentiation and reduced proliferation of AML, which is the same phenotype as seen with loss of METTL3. Mechanistically, this study found that METTL14 regulates mRNA targets *MYB* and *MYC* through m^6A and affects their mRNA stability and translation (Weng et al. 2018). Loss of WTAP also decreased proliferation and increased myeloid differentiation of AML cells (Bansal et al. 2014). YTHDF2 was found to be overexpressed in human AML and to be required for disease survival in murine and human AML. This study also determined that loss of YTHDF2 decreased the half-life of m^6A transcripts, including the tumor necrosis factor receptor *Tnfrsf2* (Paris et al. 2019). Altogether, these studies strongly demonstrate critical roles for the "writer" complex and at least one m^6A reader in leukemia and support their potential as therapeutic targets. As METTL3 and METTL14 are the two components of the "writer" complex and their depletion in AML resulted in similar phenotypes, therapeutically targeting these two proteins will likely be redundant. However, targeting the m^6A "readers," such as YTHDF2, could be an alternative approach to target the m^6A network.

RBM15

The RNA-binding motif protein 15 (RBM15; also known as OTT1) belongs to the split end (SPEN) family of proteins, which is characterized by three amino-terminal RRMs and a Spen paralog and ortholog carboxy-terminal domain (SPOC) (Wiellette et al. 1999). In *Drosophila* development, SPEN proteins control neuronal cell fate by regulating the expression of suppressor of hairless (Su(H); human homolog is RBPJ), a key transcriptional regulator involved in Notch signaling (Kuang et al. 2000). Similarly, RBM15 is required for normal embryonic development and HSC function (Raffel et al. 2007). Mechanistically, RBM15 has been observed to regulate both mRNA export and transcription (Hiriart et al. 2005; Uranishi et al. 2009; Zolotukhin et al. 2009).

RBM15 was first identified in leukemia as one of the two genes involved in the t(1;22) translocation of acute megakaryoblastic leukemia (AMKL), a heterogeneous subtype of AML compromising about 10% of childhood AML. This chromosomal rearrangement results in an in-frame fusion of *RBM15* to megakaryoblastic leukemia 1 (MKL1), with the fusion gene containing nearly the full-length coding regions of both genes. AMKL in non–Down syndrome infants has poor prognosis with a median survival of only eight months, and, importantly, this translocation is specific to this disease (Ma et al. 2001).

A knock-in mouse model of the RBM15-MKL1 fusion resulted in abnormal fetal and adult hematopoiesis. Fetal liver *RBM15-MKL1* $\text{Lineage}^{\text{Low}}$ Sca1^{+} c-Kit^{+} stem and progenitor (LSK) cells demonstrated increased colony-forming efficiency because of increased multipotent myeloid progenitors, revealing aberrant differentiation of HSCs toward the megakaryotic lineage. RBM15-MKL1, in cooperation with an activating mutation of the thrombopoietin receptor myeloproliferative leukemia virus gene (MPL), MPL^{W515L}, induced AMKL with low frequency in adult mice, with infiltration of the bone marrow, spleen, liver, and kidney with a mixture of immature megakaryocytic and erythroid elements. Additionally, RBM15-MKL1 expression deregulated the transcriptional activity of the Notch signaling pathway transcription factor RBPJ, which is consistent with previous literature describing a role for SPEN proteins in

Notch signaling (Mercher et al. 2009). Moreover, RBM15 inhibited myeloid differentiation in the 32DWT18 myeloid precursor cell line through its interaction with RBPJ and, consequently, Notch signaling stimulation (Ma et al. 2007).

Another study revealed that RBM15-MKL1 associates with the histone methyltransferase SET domain containing 1B protein (SETD1B) through its SPOC domain. Forced expression of RBM15-MKL1 in murine megakaryotic leukemic cells resulted in enhanced proliferation in a SPOC domain–dependent manner, suggesting that the interaction between the RBM15-MKL1 fusion protein and SETD1B was required for transformation (Lee and Skalnik 2012). Moreover, RBM15 is a component of the RNA methylation "writer" complex. These data suggest an important role for RBM15 in leukemia and hematopoiesis; however, more research is necessary to delineate if these phenotypes are through a m^6A-dependent pathway.

RBPs Regulating Noncoding RNAs

LIN28

The gene *lin-28* was originally identified as a heterochronic gene required for normal development in *Caenorhabditis elegans* (Moss et al. 1997). The two mammalian RBP homologs, *LIN28A* and *LIN28B,* share 69% amino acid sequence identity, and their role in developmental processes has been well-studied (Guo et al. 2006). Interestingly, LIN28A is one of the four factors, along with octamer-binding transcription factor 4 (OCT4), SRY-box 2 (SOX2), and NANOG, necessary to reprogram human somatic cells into induced pluripotent cells (Yu et al. 2007). The LIN28 proteins function by blocking the biogenesis of *let-7* micro-RNAs (miRNA)s, which are 18- to 24-nucleotide RNAs that regulate the stability and translation of their target RNAs. By binding to the terminal loop of pre-*let-7* miRNAs, LIN28 proteins facilitate the recruitment of terminal uridylyl transferase 4 (TUT4), which leads to the addition of uracil residues. This uridylation inhibits Dicer processing of pre-*let-7* and decreases levels of mature *let-7* (Heo et al. 2009). The *let-7* family of miRNAs act as tumor suppressors, as repression of *let-7* enhances the expression of its targets, which include known oncogenes. For example, *let-7* regulates targets such as cell cycle promoting genes, high mobility group AT-hook 2 (HMGA2), Kirsten rat sarcoma viral oncogene homolog (KRAS), and MYC, providing evidence for the role of LIN28 proteins in malignancies (Roush and Slack 2008; Chang et al. 2009).

LIN28A or LIN28B overexpression has been found in ~15% of human malignancies with LIN28B expression being associated with poorly differentiated and aggressive tumors, such as colon and ovarian cancers (Viswanathan et al. 2009; King et al. 2011). Furthermore, *LIN28B* is overexpressed in peripheral T-cell lymphoma (PTCL) patient samples compared to activated $CD4^+$ cells (Beachy et al. 2012). *LIN28B* expression was demonstrated to increase dramatically in BC-CML and accelerated phase CML as compared with chronic phase (CP) CML. Interestingly, in these patient samples *LIN28B* expression also correlates with reduced let-7 transcripts and increased HMGA2 expression, suggesting that LIN28B drives CML progression through *let-7* pathways (Viswanathan et al. 2009). Elevated *LIN28B* expression was also identified in about half of juvenile myelomonocytic leukemia patients, defining a novel fetal-like disease subgroup. Consistently, this subgroup also had reduced *let-7* levels (Helsmoortel et al. 2016).

Mouse models overexpressing LIN28B developed lymphoma, as well as neuroblastoma, liver, and colorectal cancers (Beachy et al. 2012; Molenaar et al. 2012; Madison et al. 2013; Nguyen et al. 2014). Conversely, expression of LIN28A in a transgenic mouse resulted in developmental alterations, such as increased body and organ size (Zhu et al. 2010). Thus, these studies suggest that LIN28B might be sufficient to drive malignant transformation. Consistent with this hypothesis, overexpression of LIN28B in the hematopoietic compartment resulted in an aggressive and fatal PTCL in vivo with mice developing lymphadenopathy and

Cite this article as *Cold Spring Harb Perspect Med* doi: 10.1101/cshperspect.a034967

splenomegaly. LIN28B expression led to reduced *let-7* expression, increased *interleukin 6* (*IL6*) and c-*Myc* levels, and nuclear factor-κB (NF-κB) activation. NF-κB activation in turn resulted in enhanced transcription of *Lin28b*, leading to a positive-feedback loop exacerbating the disease (Iliopoulos et al. 2010; Beachy et al. 2012).

Several different studies have also noted a link between c-Myc and LIN28B. In a B-cell lymphoma model, MYC was demonstrated to directly up-regulate LIN28B expression by binding to the *Lin28b* promotor, leading to reduced *let-7* expression and impaired cell proliferation (Chang et al. 2009). In mixed-lineage leukemia (MLL)-associated leukemia, MLL fusion proteins drive MYC expression, leading to increased LIN28B. LIN28B can repress miR-150 precursors processing, which is also suppressed in AML (Jiang et al. 2012). Furthermore, *LIN28B* was found to be differentially expressed in MLL fusion protein transformed cell lines, correlating with *c-Myc* expression. LIN28B negatively regulated miR-150 and to a weaker extent *let-7g*, consistent with previous studies. Because *let-7* repressed c-Myc, *let-7g* down-regulation due to increased LIN28B expression maintained *c-Myc* levels (Chen et al. 2016).

As further evidence of the LIN28B role in leukemia, depletion of LIN28B in AML resulted in decreased cell proliferation and colony formation and cell cycle arrest. Conversely, overexpression of LIN28B promoted cell proliferation and increased tumorigenicity. Depletion of LIN28B resulted in a decrease of insulin-like growth factor 2 mRNA-binding protein 1 (IGF2BP1), which was found to be regulated in a let-7-dependent mechanism and will be discussed later in the text (Zhou et al. 2017a). In another study, LIN28B was identified to be up-regulated by protein tyrosine phosphatase of regenerating liver 3 (PRL-3), which is up-regulated in AML patients (Zhou et al. 2017b).

Altogether these data suggest a requirement for LIN28B in lymphoma and leukemia through the regulation of *let-7* and c-Myc pathways. Interestingly, a recent study suggests that LIN28A may act as a tumor suppressor, as overexpression of LIN28A in the OCI-AML3 cell line resulted in cell cycle arrest and myeloid differentiation (De Luca et al. 2017). Thus, further studies investigating the dichotomy of these two LIN28 proteins could prove useful for a deeper understanding of how they function in hematological malignancies.

RBPs Regulating mRNA Stability and Translation

HuR

Human antigen R (HuR) is a member of the human embryonic abnormal vision family of proteins, and although other members of this family are expressed exclusively in neuronal tissues, HuR is ubiquitously expressed (Akamatsu et al. 1999; Lu and Schneider 2004). Upon stimulation, HuR translocates to the cytoplasm, where it regulates the mRNA stability and translation of a number of transcripts by binding to U- or AU-rich elements (AREs) within 3′ UTRs (Brennan and Steitz 2001; Wurth and Gebauer 2015). HuR can also bind to introns or the 5′ UTR of some mRNAs, suggesting that HuR may have a role in precursor mRNA (pre-mRNA) processing (Mukherjee et al. 2011). It has been suggested that HuR stabilizes mRNAs by interfering with the binding of ARE-binding proteins or miRNAs, but the extent of interplay between HuR and miRNAs remains unclear (Lebedeva et al. 2011).

HuR is essential for postnatal hematopoiesis as global deletion induced atrophy of the spleen, thymus, and lymph nodes with reduction of lymphoid, myeloid, and erythroid progenitors in the bone marrow (Ghosh et al. 2009). In regard to malignant hematopoiesis, HuR is overexpressed in the M4 subtype of AML, which correlates with high expression levels of eukaryotic initiation factor 4E (eIF4E), an essential translation factor that will be discussed later in the text (Topisirovic et al. 2009b). Furthermore, HuR and eIF4E collaborate to sustain tumorigenesis as HuR promotes eIF4E expression by increasing the stability of its transcripts. In turn, eIF4E stimulates the translation of pro-oncogenic targets that are also stabilized by HuR (Topisirovic et al. 2009a). These data suggest an important role for HuR in normal and malignant hematopoiesis, but further studies elucidating how HuR regulates mRNA stability or processing are needed.

eIF4F Protein Complex

The well-characterized eukaryotic initiation factor 4F (eIF4F) is a heterotrimeric protein complex consisting of three subunits: the cap-binding protein eIF4E, the DEAD-box RNA helicase eIF4A, and the scaffold protein eIF4G. The eIF4F complex promotes eukaryotic translation initiation by mediating the mRNA 5′ cap function. The mRNA 5′ cap structure is an important aspect of cap-dependent translation regulation as it has important roles in RNA metabolism, including splicing, 3′ end processing, nucleocytoplasmic transport stability, and translation. Functionally, eIF4F binds to mRNA through the interaction of eIF4E to the mRNA 5′ 7-methyl guanosine (m^7G) cap and eIF4G to the mRNA. eIF4A then unwinds the mRNA 5′ UTR secondary structure to create a binding site for the eukaryotic small ribosomal subunit (40S) (Parsyan et al. 2011). To note, mRNAs with extensive 5′ secondary structure have poor translation, so binding of eIF4E to the cap as well as the role of eIF4A are critical for their translation (Sonenberg and Gingras 1998). As eIF4E is the component that directly binds to the 5′ cap, most studies have focused on this key participant and its regulation.

Regulation of eIF4E is mostly accomplished by phosphorylation, as phosphorylated eIF4E has higher binding affinity to the 5′ cap and increases translation rates (Minich et al. 1994). Additionally, eIF4E-binding protein 1 (4EBP1) prevents the assembly of eIF4F by competing with eIF4G for the binding to eIF4E. Phosphorylation of 4EBP1 causes its dissociation with eIF4E, thus stimulating cap-dependent translation (Haghighat et al. 1995). Moreover, the phosphoinositide 3-OH kinase (PI3K) pathway is the major regulator of 4EBP1 phosphorylation. Activation of the downstream protein kinase B (AKT) by phosphorylation activates mammalian target of rapamycin complex 1 (mTOR), which in turn phosphorylates ribosomal protein S6 kinase (p70S6K) and 4EBP1 (Gingras et al. 1998; Wendel et al. 2004). Interestingly, oncogenic transformation by AKT is dependent on its phosphorylation of p70S6K and 4EBP1, and thus regulation of translation initiation through eIF4E (Aoki et al. 2001).

The dysregulation of eIF4E has been described in several malignancies. eIF4E was observed to accelerate lymphomagenesis in a manner similar to AKT, displaying a high proliferation-to-apoptosis ratio and a resistance to chemotherapy. Unlike AKT-driven lymphomas, these eIF4E-lymphomas were derived from a more mature B-cell type and were resistant to the combination of chemotherapy and mTOR inhibitor rapamycin in vivo, possibly because eIF4E acts downstream of mTOR (Wendel et al. 2004). eIF4E is also overexpressed in FAB M4/M5 primary AML and BC-CML patient samples but not in M1/M2 AML, acute lymphoblastic leukemia (ALL), or CP-CML patient samples. Furthermore, elevated eIF4E blocked monocytic and granulocytic differentiation, contributing to leukemogenesis. Interestingly in these AML and CP-CML, eIF4E contributed to leukemogenesis through its role in mRNA transport (Topisirovic et al. 2003). Similarly, a number of previous studies have described a role for nuclear eIF4E in promoting the cytoplasmic transport of specific mRNAs through its 5′ cap-binding activity (Lejbkowicz et al. 1992; Strudwick and Borden 2002).

Similar to eIF4E, eIF4A was determined to accelerate T-cell acute lymphoblastic leukemia (T-ALL) development in vivo. Transcriptome-scale ribosome footprinting revealed that eIF4A-dependent transcripts contain the 12-nucleotide guanine quartet $(CGG)_4$ motif or a similar but shorter 9-nucleotide motif, which form RNA G-quadruplex structures. Thus, eIF4A is necessary for the translation of mRNAs containing G-quadruplexes in their 5′ UTRs, such as *MYC*, *MYB*, *NOTCH*, *cyclin-dependent kinase 6* (*CDK6*), and *BCL2* transcripts (Wolfe et al. 2014).

Altogether, these data propose that the translation initiation factor eIF4F, consisting of eIF4E, eIF4A, and eIF4G, plays an important role in maintaining the translation of a wide

 Cite this article as *Cold Spring Harb Perspect Med* doi: 10.1101/cshperspect.a034967

variety of crucial leukemia and lymphoma oncogenes and transcription factors.

IGF2BPs and IGFBPs

The insulin-like growth factor 2 mRNA-binding protein family (IGF2BPs) consists of three structurally and functionally related paralogs: IG2BP1, IGF2BP2, and IGF2BP3. These three proteins contain two amino-terminal RRMs and four carboxy-terminal KH domains. Additionally, these proteins are highly similar at the protein level, sharing >56% amino acid sequence identity. IGF2BP1 and IGF2BP3 share an even higher similarity of 73% homology, suggesting that the proteins play similar biochemical functions. These cytoplasmic RBPs bind to their target mRNAs to form ribonucleoprotein complexes (mRNPs), affecting the localization, stability, and translation of their target mRNAs (Bell et al. 2013). In vitro studies have demonstrated that IGF2BPs bind to their target mRNAs through their KH domains, whereas their RRMs could be involved in the stabilization of mRNPs with surprisingly long half-lives (Farina et al. 2003; Nielsen et al. 2004). These stable mRNPs allow for "long-distance" transport and transient storage of their target mRNAs. Studies have observed that signaling events, such as phosphorylation of IGF2BPs, are likely to be involved in the controlled release of their target mRNAs leading to mRNA decay or protein synthesis (Hüttelmaier et al. 2005; Git et al. 2009; Dai et al. 2011). IGF2BPs are involved in important aspects of cell function, such as metabolism, proliferation, and differentiation. IGF2BP1 and IGF2BP3 are oncofetal proteins, being highly expressed during embryogenesis and in many cancers. Although many studies highlight their significance and prognostic ability in epithelial and soft tissue tumors, their role in malignant hematopoiesis remains to be completely understood (Stoskus et al. 2011; Bell et al. 2013; Lederer et al. 2014).

IGF2BP expression has been extensively studied in lymphomas; immunohistochemical analyses demonstrated high expression in positive classical or lymphocyte-predominant Hodgkin lymphomas. One study noted that IGF2BP1 is highly expressed in Hodgkin's lymphoma, as well as various B-cell lymphomas (Natkunam et al. 2007). However, IGF2BP3 seems to be the predominant paralog expressed in primary lymphomas, based on reverse transcription–polymerase chain reaction (RT-PCR) analyses of a small lymphoma cohort. Furthermore, IGF2BP3 expression was also observed in a small percentage of AML samples (Natkunam et al. 2007; King et al. 2009; Navarro et al. 2012; Tang et al. 2013; Lederer et al. 2014). Another study determined that IGF2BP1 is overexpressed in ETV6/RUNX1-postive leukemia, whereas IGF2BP3 is overexpressed in MLL/AF4-positive leukemia. Additionally, IGF2BP3 has also been shown to be a marker of disease aggressiveness in BCR/ABL1-postive ALL (Stoskus et al. 2011). IGF2BP3 is one of the most dysregulated genes in MLL-translocated B-cell acute lymphoblastic leukemia (B-ALL) and is essential for B-ALL cell survival. Because of the difficulty in raising paralog-specific antibodies, these immunohistochemical analyses of IGF3BP1 and IGF2BP3 expression should be carefully evaluated and further studies are needed to confirm their expression patterns in hematological malignancies (Bell et al. 2013).

Depletion of IGF2BP3 in a human CML cell line resulted in reduced cell growth, enhanced γ-irradiation-induced apoptosis, and reduced IGF2 expression. Mechanistically, IGF2BP3 was demonstrated to bind to the 5′ UTR of *IGF2* and promote its translation (Liao et al. 2005, 2011). IGF2BP3 has also been found to bind to the 3′ UTRs of other target transcripts, which include oncogenes *c-Myc* and *CDK6*, and to maintain the translation of these targets. IGF2BP3 overexpression led to enhanced expression of MYC and CDK6 in B-ALL cells as well as hematopoietic progenitor cells in vivo (Palanichamy et al. 2016). However, there is a lack of studies on the mechanistic function of IGF2BP1 in lymphomas. Further studies are needed for a comprehensive identification of shared and unique targets bound and regulated by IGF2BP1 and IGF2BP3 in malignant hematopoiesis.

The insulin-like growth factor-binding protein family (IGFBPs) regulate insulin-like growth factor 1 and 2 (IGF1 and IGF2) availability as well as their binding to the IGF1 receptor (IGF1R). A recent study implicated IGFBP7 as a tumor suppressor in AML. Previous work established that IGFBP7 inhibits IGF1 and IGF2 from binding to IGF1R in breast cancer, thus suppressing IGF1R signaling and tumor cell growth (Evdokimova et al. 2012). Consistent with this finding, low *IGFBP7* expression correlates with poor prognosis in patients with AML or hepatocellular carcinoma (Tomimaru et al. 2012; Verhagen et al. 2018). Additionally, overexpression of IGFBP7 induced apoptosis and G_2 cell cycle arrest in AML cells (Verhagen et al. 2014). More recently, *IGFBP7* was found to be differentially expressed in leukemia stem cells (LSCs) and HSCs, in which LSCs were characterized by low *IGFBP7* expression. Moreover, overexpression of IGFBP7 in primary AML cells resulted in decreased cell survival and increased differentiation and chemotherapy sensitivity. Importantly, forced IGFBP7 expression did not affect HSC survival (Verhagen et al. 2018).

Overall, these data suggest a requirement for IGF2BP3 in lymphoma and leukemia through the 3′ UTR regulation of its target transcripts, MYC and CDK6. However, the role that IGF2BP3's related paralog IGF2BP1 plays in malignant hematopoiesis remains unclear. Additionally, IGFBP7 seems to act as a tumor suppressor in leukemia, yet its mechanism remains unstudied.

MSI2

The Musashi RNA-binding protein 2 (MSI2) belongs to the mammalian Musashi family RBPs. The two mammalian *Msi* genes, *Msi1* and *Msi2*, have essential roles as oncoproteins in various tumor types, but have been most extensively studied in colorectal cancers and hematopoietic malignancies. MSI1 and MSI2 share high homology and are characterized by two tandem RRMs and a carboxy-terminal polyA binding protein association domain. They both have similar binding specificities to target RNAs containing a minimum UAG sequence present in the 3′ UTR. Once bound, MSI interacts with the poly(A) binding proteins and competes for eIF4G, leading to the inhibition of translation (Kawahara et al. 2008). The Msi family has also been implicated in controlling polyadenylation of specific mRNAs in *Xenopus* oocytes and alternative splicing in photoreceptor cells and neurons, suggesting that their role is not solely limited to inhibition of translation (Charlesworth et al. 2006; Murphy et al. 2016).

In hematopoietic malignancies, the significance of *MSI2* was first identified in several BC-CML patients harboring the *MSI2-HOXA9* translocation (Barbouti et al. 2003). Later, *MSI2-EVI* rearrangement was found in myeloid leukemia patients (De Weer et al. 2008) and a *PAX5-MSI2* fusion was recently observed in B-ALL (Wang et al. 2017). Yet, it remains unclear if and how these MSI2 fusions contribute to disease development or progression.

Additionally, *MSI2* expression is elevated in CLL, adult B-ALL, T-ALL, MDS, and AML. *MSI2* is up-regulated during disease progression in MDS and CML, and expression levels correlate with poor clinical prognosis in most of these hematological malignancies (adult B-ALL, MDS, CML, and AML) (Ito et al. 2010; Kharas et al. 2010; Pereira et al. 2012; Thol et al. 2013; Ho et al. 2016; Taggart et al. 2016).

Besides its expression in patients, functional studies using several leukemic mouse models have shown a requirement for MSI2 in leukemic progression and stem cell renewal. In a BC-CML model, deletion or depletion of MSI2 resulted in reduced leukemogenesis and forced MSI2 expression drove a more aggressive CML (Kharas et al. 2010). Similarly, MSI2 deletion led to a reversal of MDS phenotypes, and forced expression of MSI2 drove MPN and MDS/AML in a NUP98-HOXD13 mouse model (Taggart et al. 2016). Depletion of MSI2 in human AML and BC-CML cell lines resulted in reduced proliferation and increased apoptosis (Kharas et al. 2010; Kharas and Lengner 2017). MSI2 was also found to be required in maintaining AML LSCs in an MLL-AF9 AML murine model (Park et al. 2015).

Mechanistically, MSI has been linked to Notch signaling as MSI1 has been identified to repress the translation of NUMB, and MSI2 overexpression resulted in decreased NUMB in CML cells (Ito et al. 2010). In a murine leukemia model, MSI2 was determined to maintain the mixed-lineage leukemia self-renewal program by binding to the transcripts encoding *IKAROS family zinc finger 2* (*IKZF2*), *HOXA9*, and *MYC* and promoting their translation (Park et al. 2015). Other studies reported Tetrespanin-3 (TSPAN3), FMS-like tyrosine kinase 3 (FLT3), and branched-chain amino acid aminotransferase 1 (BCAT1) as direct MSI2 targets in AML and BC-CML cells (Kwon et al. 2015; Hattori et al. 2017a, b).

Altogether, these studies determine a crucial functional role for MSI2 in leukemia. Although MSI2 direct targets have started to be studied, further genome-wide target analysis will advance our knowledge of MSI2 downstream targets and their functions.

SYNCRIP

Synaptotagmin-binding, cytoplasmic RNA-interacting protein (SYNCRIP), also known as heterogeneous nuclear ribonucleoprotein Q (hnRNPQ), has three tandem RRMs and has been implicated in regulating RNA processing and protein (Grosset et al. 2000; Mizutani et al. 2000; Cho et al. 2007; Stohr et al. 2008). Previous studies have also suggested that SYNCRIP plays a role in neuronal morphogenesis (Chen et al. 2012; Xing et al. 2012). Regarding malignant hematopoiesis, a pooled in vivo shRNA screening of the MSI2 interactome identified SYNCRIP as a MSI2 protein interactor and a novel regulator of leukemia. SYNCRIP was found to be required for the survival of murine leukemia cells in vitro and in vivo but dispensable for normal hematopoiesis. Similarly, depletion of SYNCRIP in human leukemia cells resulted in decreased cell proliferation, induction of apoptosis, and increased differentiation. Mechanistically, SYNCRIP was found to coregulate the LSC gene expression program with MSI2 by binding to MSI2 mRNA targets *IKZF2*, *MYC*, and *HOXA9*. Furthermore, SYNCRIP was determined to directly regulate the translation of HOXA9, while overexpression of HOXA9 partially rescued the SYNCRIP-depletion phenotype (Vu et al. 2017b).

Conversely, SYNCRIP was identified in another study as a tumor suppressor in T-ALL with chromosome 6q deletion. 6q deletion led to the silencing of both *SYNCRIP* and *small nucleolar RNA host gene 5* (*SNHG5*), a noncoding snoRNA. This dual silencing accelerated leukemogenesis and decreased ribosome and mitochondrial activities (Gachet et al. 2018). Together, these recent studies highlight SYNCRIP as both an oncogene and a tumor suppressor, yet additional studies are needed to determine whether its role is disease-specific and elucidate its mechanism in each context.

hnRNPK

Heterogeneous nuclear ribonucleoprotein K (hnRNPK) is a nucleocytoplasmic shuttling protein, which regulates gene transcription and mRNA metabolism upon binding to DNA or RNA. One study noted that the $p210^{BCR/ABL}$ oncoprotein elevated hnRNPK expression by enhancing *hnRNPK* transcription and mRNA stability. hnRNPK depletion and interference with its translation activity in these BCR/ABL-transformed cells decreased cell proliferation and impaired leukemogenesis in vivo, in part through the translational regulation of *MYC* (Notari et al. 2006).

A more recent study implicated hnRNPK as a haploinsufficient tumor suppressor in hematologic malignancies. AML patients harboring a 9q deletion were found to have reduced *HNRNPK* expression. *Hnrnpk* haploinsufficient mice had reduced survival and were prone to develop hematologic malignancies, with increased genomic instability. Sixty-two percent of mice displayed a myeloproliferative phenotype, whereas 31% of mice developed lymphomas. Mechanistically, this study suggested that hnRNPK reduction reduced *p21* mRNA expression, down-regulated CCAAT-enhancer-binding protein (C/EBP) and mRNA levels, and activated signal transducer and activator of transcription 3 (STAT3) signaling, regulating proliferation and differentiation pathways. Importantly, chromatin immunoprecipitation

(ChIP) assays demonstrated that hnRNPK directly interacted with *p21* and *C/EBPα/C/EBPβ*, whereas RNA immunoprecipitation revealed an interaction between hnRNPK and *C/EBPα* mRNA. Thus, these data suggest that hnRNPK regulates cellular differentiation through the C/EBP pathways and proliferation through the p21/p53 and JAK/STAT pathways (Gallardo et al. 2015).

These studies implicate hnRNPK as both a tumor suppressor and an oncogene. Further studies will be needed to elucidate whether its role as a tumor suppressor is dependent on 9q deletion in AML or if it is disease-specific, as well if its role is dependent on its RNA- or DNA-binding ability.

THERAPEUTICS

Therapeutic Targeting of the Spliceosome

During splicing, the spliceosome component U2snRNP binds to the pre-mRNA via the interaction of its branchpoint-binding region and the branchpoint sequence in the intron. This binding is a crucial step in the formation of the catalytic center of the spliceosome. SF3B1, part of the U2snRNP complex, recognizes the pre-mRNA intron branchpoint and cross-links to sequences both 5′ and 3′ of the branchpoint to facilitate this binding. Several bacterially derived products and their analogs target SF3B, resulting in blocking spliceosome assembly (Bonnal et al. 2012). These original products, including pladienolides and herboxidienes, were chemically unstable (Lee and Abdel-Wahab 2016). Further studies resulted in the development of the chemically stable analogs spliceostatin A (SSA), E7017, and sudemycins (Kaida et al. 2007; Kotake et al. 2007; Fan et al. 2011).

SSA binds to the SF3B complex, preventing its interaction with the pre-mRNA intron and destabilizing the spliceosome assembly (Corrionero et al. 2011). The inhibitor E7107 also targets the SF3B complex and prevents the conformational change of U2snRNP that exposes its branchpoint-binding region, thus blocking spliceosome formation as well (Folco et al. 2011). At first, it was unclear which component of the SF3B complex these compounds targets. However, a recent functional genetic study on human colorectal cell lines that acquired resistance to pladienolide B determined that these compounds bind SF3B1. Even with this mechanistic understanding, additional research is needed to determine the transcriptome-wide effects of these compounds. Recent efforts have demonstrated that in vivo E7107 treatment resulted in changes to all classes of alternative splicing events, but further preclinical studies are necessary to fully predict the effects of these compounds (Lee et al. 2016).

Therapeutic Targeting of RBM39

Anticancer sulfonamides were recently determined to selectively degrade RBM39 through the recruitment of RBM39 to DCAF15, an adaptor protein for the CUL4/Ddb1 E3 ubiquitin ligase. This interaction led to the polyubiquitination and proteasomal degradation of RBM39. These sulfonamides include indisulam (also known as E7070), E7820, and chloroquinoxaline sulfonamide (Han et al. 2017; Uehara et al. 2017). Of note, *DCAF15* was determined to be elevated in AML patient samples compared to hematopoietic progenitors. In vivo administration of indisulam in two AML cell line xenograft models extended survival and led to degradation of RBM39. Additionally, indisulam-treated patient-derived xenografts (PDXs) showed reduced leukemia burden. In contrast, both C57/B6 mice and immunocompromised mice transplanted with CD-CD34^{+} cells showed no significant hematological effects, highlighting the differential effects of RBM39 loss on AML compared to normal hematopoietic cells (Wang et al. 2019).

Given the importance of change-in-function mutations in splicing factors SF3B1 and U2AF1 in AML and MDS and the interaction of RBM39 with both SF3B1 and U2AF1, it would follow that spliceosomal mutant AML cell lines were found to be the most sensitive cells to sulfonamides among many AML subtypes. Interestingly, AML cell lines with elevated expression of *DCAF15* also had increased sensitivity to sulfonamides. RBM39 degradation was consistent among cell lines with or without the spliceosomal mutations, suggesting that the increased sensitivity of the spliceosomal mutant cells was due to their dependency on wild-type splicing function. Additionally, RBM39 degradation via E7820 treatment resulted in enhanced aberrant splicing and reduced expression of HOXA9 target genes *BMI1* and *MYB*, as well as *GATA2*, in spliceosomal mutant AML compared to its wild-type counterparts. Several RBPs were also found to be aberrantly spliced upon RBM39 degradation, supporting the idea of targeting the RBM39 RBP network (Wang et al. 2019).

Previously, sulfonamides had shown low rates of antitumor efficacy, which could be due to the fact that biomarkers of response were unknown (Owa et al. 1999; Supuran 2003). Together, these data suggest that the presence of spliceosomal mutations and elevated DCAF15 expression are good biomarkers to respond to sulfonamide treatment. Currently, indisulam combined with chemotherapy is in phase II clinical trials in patients with refractory or relapsed myeloid malignancies (Assi et al. 2018). Whereas indisulam is administered intravenously, E7820 is administered orally and has been tested as a highly effective second-generation sulfonamide in phase II clinical trials for solid tumors (Milojkovic Kerklaan et al. 2016). Thus, this study suggests further clinical investigation of E7820 in patients with myeloid malignancies with the proper biomarkers, and indeed, a multicenter clinical trial using E7820 is currently being planned (Wang et al. 2019).

Therapeutic Targeting of LIN28

Ongoing studies have been focusing on finding a small-molecule inhibitor of the LIN28/let-7 interaction. One study used a protein/RNA fluorescence resonance energy transfer (FRET) assay to identify a small-molecule inhibitor, which blocked the LIN28/let-7 interaction and rescued let-7 processing and function (Roos et al. 2016). Another study used fluorescence polarization to identify two small-molecule inhibitors for the LIN28 domains implicated in let-7 interactions. TPEN destabilizes the zinc-knuckle domain of LIN28, while LI17 binds to the cold shock domain of LIN28 to block LIN28's suppression of let-7 in leukemia cells (Wang et al. 2018). Although more drug development is required, it is also important to understand how these small molecules relate to genetic perturbation.

Therapeutic Targeting of Cap-Dependent Translation

As mentioned previously, phosphorylation of 4EBP1 by mTOR allows for the release of eIF4E, and, consequently, the proper binding of eIF4E to eIF4G and the assembly if the translation initiation complex. Hence, eIF4E is an attractive target for therapeutic inhibition. The small-molecule inhibitor 4EGI-1 binds to eIF4E, preventing its interaction to eIF4G and inhibiting cap-dependent translation. Surprisingly, 4EGI-1 also enhances the binding of eIF4E to 4EBP1 (Moerke et al. 2007). Meanwhile, the antiviral drug ribavirin mimics the m^7G cap structure, allowing it to bind and block eIF4E from its association to mRNA (Kentsis et al. 2004, 2005; Tan et al. 2008). In a phase II clinical trial of M4/M5 AML patients, ribavirin led to complete remission in one patient, partial remissions in two patients, and stable disease in four patients. Ribavirin caused the relocalization of eIF4E from the nucleus to the cytoplasm, and, interestingly, resistance to ribavirin occurred when eIF4E localized to the nucleus once again (Assouline et al. 2009).

Another therapeutic target in this pathway is mTOR, as its inhibition would prevent phosphorylation of 4EBP1 and p70S6K. Rapamycin and its analogs, RAD001 and CCI-779, block mTOR activity through an allosteric mechanism. Rapamycin binds to FK-binding protein 12 (FKBP12), and, subsequently, this complex inhibits the FKBP-rapamycin-binding (FRB) domain of mTOR. Rapamycin can restore normal HSC function and deplete LSCs; however, rapamycin is an incomplete mTOR inhibitor, as it only partially reduces 4EBP1 phosphorylation (Yilmaz et al. 2006). Although rapamycin strongly inhibits p70S6K activity, 4EBP1 recovers phosphorylation ability within hours of drug treatment (Choo et al. 2008; Kuo et al. 2011). A second-generation inhibitor, PP242, competes against ATP to bind mTOR's catalytic site and strongly blocks 4EBP1 phosphorylation. These findings demonstrated that PP242, unlike rapamycin, results in human leukemia cell death and delay of leukemic progression in vivo (Janes et al. 2010).

More recently, inhibition of another component of the translation initiation factor has been promising. Silvestrol inhibits eIF4A, thus blocking cap-dependent translation. Treatment with silvestrol led to cell death in primary human T-ALL samples, cell lines, and murine T-ALLs in vitro. Similarly, silvestrol also delayed tumor growth in vivo. By targeting eIF4A, silvestrol drastically decreased the expression of eIF4A target transcripts, such as *MYC*, *NOTCH*, and *BCL2* (Wolfe et al. 2014). Altogether, these findings support the potential to clinically develop small-molecule inhibitors of these RBPs.

Therapeutic Targeting of MSI2

A previous fluorescent polarization screen identified several small molecules with the ability to inhibit the RNA-binding activity of MSI (Minuesa et al. 2014). More recently, one of these small molecules, Ro 08-2750 (Ro), was characterized as an MSI RNA-competitive inhibitor. This study determined that Ro binds to MSI2 RRM1, reduces the proliferation of human AML cells, and decreases the binding of MSI2 to its mRNA targets as well as their protein expression (Minuesa et al. 2019). Overall, these data demonstrate the ability to therapeutically target MSI2 in leukemia.

CONCLUSION AND FUTURE DIRECTIONS

Posttranscriptional regulation is a tightly controlled process that allows cells to dictate the integrity, diversity, and supply of proteins. As highlighted herein, RBPs play a crucial role in all steps of this regulatory process and their dysregulation can result in hematopoietic malignancies (Fig. 2). Our increased knowledge in the identification of a greater number of these dysregulated RBPs, as well as their role in leukemia and lymphoma, has garnered excitement and increased interest in this emerging field. Furthermore, advances in sequencing technology and novel techniques to survey the riboproteome are expanding our understanding of the players involved in posttranscriptional regulation.

RBPs coordinate the fates of multiple mRNAs, but the principles underlying these interactions remain poorly understood. Questions remain regarding how RBPs achieve binding specificity and how they interact and compete with other RBPs. Moreover, the specific mRNA sequences bound by RBPs remain to be fully identified and their cell context specificity remains unknown. Cross-linking technologies coupled with sequencing (cross-linking immunoprecipitation [CLIP], photoactivatable ribonucleoside-enhanced cross-linking immunoprecipitation [PAR-CLIP], and high-throughput sequencing of RNA isolated by cross-linking immunoprecipitation [HITS-CLIP]) have been effective in discovering novel RBP targets but have limitations. A new technique, targets of RBPs identified by editing (TRIBE), has recently been developed and allows for the capture of RBP targets without the limitation of a large quantity of cells or specific RBP antibodies (McMahon et al. 2016; Hong 2017). Additionally, TRIBE allows for insight of RBP targets in rare subsets of cells, such as LSCs. Further studies are necessary to augment our knowledge of how these dynamic and multifunctional proteins modulate the gene expression program and disease.

Besides discovering how these RBPs regulate gene expression and malignancies, the identity of critical RBPs remain unknown. Several studies have recently suggested the importance of an RBP network in hematological malignancies. One study identified several RBPs that are essential for AML survival through a CRISPR/Cas9 RBD domain screen. Many of these have yet to be studied in the context of hematological malignancies, including *DHX37*, *PABPN1*, *ZFP36L2*, *TRA2B*, *SRSF10*, *HNRNPH1*, and *SUPT6H*. Comparing the CRISPR/Cas9 screen to identical screens in T-ALL, melanoma, and lung adenocarcinoma identified these RBPs as preferentially required in AML. Critically, the importance of

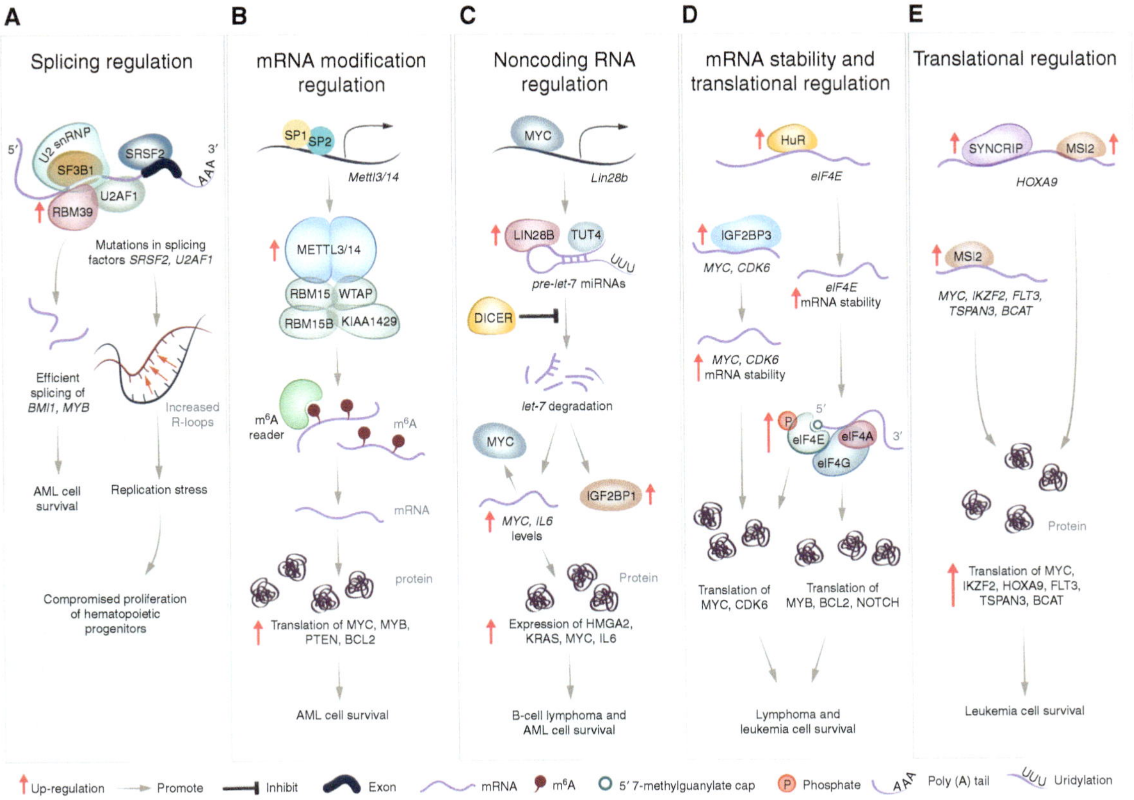

Figure 2. RNA-binding proteins (RBPs) are essential players in leukemia and lymphoma. Overview of the main RBPs and their regulatory pathways discussed in this review. (*A*) Mutations in splicing factors *SRSF2* and *U2AF1* contribute to the myelodysplastic syndrome (MDS) through elevated R loops and replication stress. In human acute myeloid leukemia (AML) cells, RNA-binding motif protein 39 (RBM39) interacts with the spliceosome, including splicing factor 3 subunit b1 (SF3B1), and elevated RBM39 expression maintains efficient splicing of homeobox A9 (*HOXA9*) targets *BMI1* and *MYB*, resulting in enhanced cell survival. (*B*) In human leukemia cells, high expression of methyltransferase-like 3 (METTL3) and methyltransferase-like 14 (METTL14) increases global N^6-methyladenosine (m^6A levels). Increased m^6A on target genes *MYC*, *MYB*, *PTEN*, and *BCL2* promotes their translation, which results in enhanced cell survival. (*C*) In B-cell lymphoma, MYC binds to the *Lin28b* promoter, which drives elevated LIN28B expression. LIN28B binds to the terminal loop of pre-*let-7* microRNAs (miRNAs) and recruits terminal uridylyl transferase 4 (TUT4), leading to the uridylation and degradation of pre-*let-7* miRNAs. Decreased levels of mature *let-7* miRNAs result in increased levels of *IL6* and *MYC* mRNA and elevated levels of high mobility group AT-hook 2 (HMGA2), Kirsten rat sarcoma viral oncogene homolog (KRAS), MYC, and IL6, resulting in enhanced cell survival. (*D*) In AML, overexpression of human antigen R (HuR) leads to increased stability of *eIF4E* transcripts and increased expression of eukaryotic initiation factor 4E (eIF4E). In lymphoma, elevated eIF4E expression results in efficient translation of MYC, cyclin-dependent kinase 6 (CDK6), MYB, BCL2, and NOTCH. Insulin-like growth factor 2 mRNA-binding protein 3 (IGF2BP3) is highly expressed in lymphomas and leukemias, and in B-ALL cells, IGF2BP3 binds to the 3′ UTR of target transcripts, including *MYC* and *CDK6*, increases their stability, and maintains their efficient translation. (*E*) Musashi RNA-binding protein 2 (MSI2) and synaptotagmin-binding, cytoplasmic RNA-interacting protein (SYNCRIP) are highly expressed in leukemia and they coregulate the LSC gene expression program through the regulation of *HOXA9* translation. MSI2 also binds to the transcripts *MYC*, *IKZF2*, *FLT3*, *TSPAN3*, and *BCAT* and promotes their translation, which results in increased cell survival.

an RBP network in AML was highlighted as RBM39 was found to interact with several of these essential RBPs and loss of RBM39 resulted in aberrant splicing of some of these same RBPs (Wang et al. 2019). Similarly, a pooled in vivo shRNA screen of the MSI2 interactome identified novel RBP regulators of leukemia, such as *HNRNPA3*, *HNRNPR*, and *MYBBP1A*, and suggested that a dysregulated RBP network is required for leukemia survival. Thus, further studies aimed to uncover the function of these RBPs are necessary (Vu et al. 2017b).

In summary, we emphasize the importance of understanding the regulation of the riboproteome to uncover novel targets and mechanisms that drive hematological malignancies. Future studies will be instrumental for uncovering the identity of essential RBPs, their RBP targets, and the relationship between these RBPs in hematological malignancies.

ACKNOWLEDGMENTS

We would like to acknowledge Sun Mi Park and Diu Nguyen from the Kharas laboratory for their critical reading of the manuscript and invaluable insights. We apologize in advance for any possible omissions due to space constraints or a failure to cite published work.

REFERENCES

Akamatsu W, Okano HJ, Osumi N, Inoue T, Nakamura S, Sakakibara SI, Miura M, Matsuo N, Darnell RB, Okano H. 1999. Mammalian ELAV-like neuronal RNA-binding proteins HuB and HuC promote neuronal development in both the central and the peripheral nervous systems. *Proc Natl Acad Sci* **96:** 9885–9890. doi:10.1073/pnas.96.17.9885

Aoki M, Blazek E, Vogt PK. 2001. A role of the kinase mTOR in cellular transformation induced by the oncoproteins P3k and Akt. *Proc Natl Acad Sci* **98:** 136–141. doi:10.1073/pnas.98.1.136

Assi R, Kantarjian HM, Kadia TM, Pemmaraju N, Jabbour E, Jain N, Daver N, Estrov Z, Uehara T, Owa T, et al. 2018. Final results of a phase 2, open-label study of indisulam, idarubicin, and cytarabine in patients with relapsed or refractory acute myeloid leukemia and high-risk myelodysplastic syndrome. *Cancer* **124:** 2758–2765. doi:10.1002/cncr.31398

Assouline S, Culjkovic B, Cocolakis E, Rousseau C, Beslu N, Amri A, Caplan S, Leber B, Roy D, Miller WH Jr, et al. 2009. Molecular targeting of the oncogene eIF4E in acute myeloid leukemia (AML): A proof-of-principle clinical trial with ribavirin. *Blood* **114:** 257–260. doi:10.1182/blood-2009-02-205153

Bangur CS, Switzer A, Fan L, Marton MJ, Meyer MR, Wang T. 2002. Identification of genes over-expressed in small cell lung carcinoma using suppression subtractive hybridization and cDNA microarray expression analysis. *Oncogene* **21:** 3814–3825. doi:10.1038/sj.onc.1205480

Bansal H, Yihua Q, Ganapathy S, Proia D, Penalva L, Uren P, Suresh U, Carew J, Karnad A, Weitman S, et al. 2014. WTAP is a novel oncogenic protein in acute myeloid leukemia. *Leukemia* **28:** 1171–1174. doi:10.1038/leu.2014.16

Barbieri I, Tzelepis K, Pandolifini L, Shi J, Millán-Zambrano G, Robson SC, Aspris D, Migliori V, Bannister AJ, Han N, et al. 2017. Promoter-bound METTL3 maintains myeloid leukaemia by m^6A-dependent translation control. *Nature* **552:** 126–131. doi:10.1038/nature24678

Barbouti A, Ho M, Johansson B, Lassen C, Nilsson P, Hagemeijer A, Mitelman F, Fioretos T. 2003. A novel gene, *MSI2*, encoding a putative RNA-binding protein is recurrently rearranged at disease progression of chronic myeloid leukemia and forms a fusion gene with *HOXA9* as a result of the cryptic t(7;17)(p15;q23). *Cancer Res* **63:** 1202–1206.

Beachy SH, Onozawa M, Chung YJ, Slape C, Bilke S, Francis P, Pineda M, Walker RL, Meltzer P, Aplan PD. 2012. Enforced expression of Lin28b leads to impaired T-cell development, release of inflammatory cytokines, and peripheral T-cell lymphoma. *Blood* **120:** 1048–1059. doi:10.1182/blood-2012-01-401760

Bell JL, Wächter K, Mühleck B, Pazaitis N, Köhn M, Lederer M, Hüttelmaier S. 2013. Insulin-like growth factor 2 mRNA-binding proteins (IGF2BPs): posttranscriptional drivers of cancer progression? *Cell Mol Life Sci* **70:** 2657–2675. doi:10.1007/s00018-012-1186-z

Bonnal S, Vigevani L, Valcárcel J. 2012. The spliceosome as a target of novel antitumour drugs. *Nat Rev Drug Discov* **11:** 847–859. doi:10.1038/nrd3823

Brennan CM, Steitz JA. 2001. HuR and mRNA stability. *Cell Mol Life Sci* **58:** 266–277. doi:10.1007/PL00000854

Cantara WA, Crain PF, Rozenski J, McCloskey JA, Harris KA, Zhang X, Vendeix FAP, Fabris D, Agris PF. 2011. The RNA modification database, RNAMDB: 2011 update. *Nucleic Acids Res* **39:** D195–D201. doi:10.1093/nar/gkq1028

Chai Y, Liu X, Dai L, Li Y, Liu M, Zhang JY. 2014. Overexpression of HCC1/CAPERα may play a role in lung cancer carcinogenesis. *Tumor Biol* **35:** 6311–6317. doi:10.1007/s13277-014-1819-y

Chang TC, Zeitels LR, Hwang HW, Chivukula RR, Wentzel EA, Dews M, Jung J, Gao P, Dang CV, Beer MA, et al. 2009. Lin-28B transactivation is necessary for Myc-mediated let-7 repression and proliferation. *Proc Natl Acad Sci* **106:** 3384–3389. doi:10.1073/pnas.0808300106

Charlesworth A, Wilczynska A, Thampi P, Cox LL, Macnicol AM. 2006. Musashi regulates the temporal order of mRNA translation during *Xenopus* oocyte maturation. *EMBO J* **25:** 2792–2801. doi:10.1038/sj.emboj.7601159

Chen M, Manley JL. 2009. Mechanisms of alternative splicing regulation: Insights from molecular and genomics approaches. *Nat Rev Mol Cell Biol* **10:** 741–754. doi:10.1038/nrm2777

Chen HH, Yu HI, Chiang WC, Lin YD, Shia BC, Tarn WY. 2012. hnRNP Q regulates Cdc42-mediated neuronal morphogenesis. *Mol Cell Biol* **32:** 2224–2238. doi:10.1128/MCB.06550-11

Chen L, Sun Y, Wang J, Jiang H, Muntean AG. 2016. Differential regulation of the c-Myc/Lin28 axis discriminates subclasses of rearranged MLL leukemia. *Oncotarget* **7:** 25208–25223.

Chen L, Chen JY, Huang YJ, Gu Y, Qiu J, Qian H, Shao C, Zhang X, Hu J, Li H, et al. 2018. The augmented R-loop is a unifying mechanism for myelodysplastic syndromes induced by high-risk splicing factor mutations. *Mol Cell* **69:** 412–425.e6. doi:10.1016/j.molcel.2017.12.029

Cheng Y, Luo H, Izzo F, Pickering BF, Nguyen D, Myers R, Schurer A, Gourkanti S, Bruning JC, Vu LP, et al. 2019. m^6A RNA methylation maintains hematopoietic stem cell identity and symmetric commitment. *Cell Rep* **28:** 1703–1716.e6. doi:10.1016/j.celrep.2019.07.032

Cho S, Park SM, Kim TD, Kim JH, Kim KT, Jang SK. 2007. BiP internal ribosomal entry site activity is controlled by heat-induced interaction of NSAP1. *Mol Cell Biol* **27:** 368–383. doi:10.1128/MCB.00814-06

Choo AY, Yoon S, Kim SG, Roux PP, Blenis J. 2008. Rapamycin differentially inhibits S6Ks and 4E-BP1 to mediate cell-type-specific repression of mRNA translation. *Proc Natl Acad Sci* **105:** 17414–17419. doi:10.1073/pnas.0809136105

Cooper TA, Wan L, Dreyfuss G. 2009. RNA and disease. *Cell* **136:** 777–793. doi:10.1016/j.cell.2009.02.011

Corrionero A, Miñana B, Valcarcel J. 2011. Reduced fidelity of branch point recognition and alternative splicing induced by the antitumor drug spliceostatin A. *Genes Dev* **25:** 445–459. doi:10.1101/gad.2014311

Dai N, Rapley J, Angel M, Yanik FM, Blower MD, Avruch J. 2011. mTOR phosphorylates IMP2 to promote IGF2 mRNA translation by internal ribosomal entry. *Genes Dev* **25:** 1159–1172. doi:10.1101/gad.2042311

Dai D, Wang H, Zhu L, Jin H, Wang X. 2018. N6-methyladenosine links RNA metabolism to cancer progression. *Cell Death Dis* **9:** 124. doi:10.1038/s41419-017-0129-x

Darnell RB. 2010. RNA regulation in neurologic disease and cancer. *Cancer Res Treat* **42:** 125–129. doi:10.4143/crt.2010.42.3.125

De Luca L, Trino S, Laurenzana I, Tagliaferri D, Falco G, Grieco V, Bianchino G, Nozza F, Campia V, D'Alessio F, et al. 2017. Knockdown of *miR-128a* induces *Lin28a* expression and reverts myeloid differentiation blockage in acute myeloid leukemia. *Cell Death Dis* **8:** e2849. doi:10.1038/cddis.2017.253

Desrosiers R, Friderici K, Rottman F. 1974. Identification of methylated nucleosides in messenger RNA from Novikoff hepatoma cells. *Proc Natl Acad Sci* **71:** 3971–3975. doi:10.1073/pnas.71.10.3971

De Weer A, Speleman F, Cauwelier B, Van Roy N, Yigit N, Verhasselt B, De Moerloose B, Benoit Y, Noens L, Selleslag D, et al. 2008. *EVI1* overexpression in t(3;17) positive myeloid malignancies results from juxtaposition of *EVI1* to the *MSI2* locus at 17q22. *Haematologica* **93:** 1903–1907. doi:10.3324/haematol.13192

Elkashef SM, Lin AP, Myers J, Sill H, Jiang D, Dahia PLM, Aguiar RCT. 2017. IDH mutation, competitive inhibition of FTO, and RNA methylation. *Cancer Cell* **31:** 619–620. doi:10.1016/j.ccell.2017.04.001

Evdokimova V, Tognon CE, Benatar T, Yang W, Krutikov K, Pollak M, Sorensen PHB, Seth A. 2012. IGFBP7 binds to the IGF-1 receptor and blocks its activation by insulin-like growth factors. *Sci Signal* **5:** ra92. doi:10.1126/scisignal.2003184

Fan L, Lagisetti C, Edwards CC, Webb TR, Potter PM. 2011. Sudemycins, novel small molecule analogues of FR901464, induce alternative gene splicing. *ACS Chem Biol* **6:** 582–589.

Farina KL, Hüttelmaier S, Musunuru K, Darnell R, Singer RH. 2003. Two ZBP1 KH domains facilitate β-actin mRNA localization, granule formation, and cytoskeletal attachment. *J Cell Biol* **160:** 77–87. doi:10.1083/jcb.200206003

Fei DL, Motowski H, Chatrikhi R, Prasad S, Yu J, Gao S, Kielkopf CL, Bradley RK, Varmus H. 2016. Wild-type U2AF1 antagonizes the splicing program characteristic of U2AF1-mutant tumors and is required for cell survival. *PLoS Genet* **12:** 1–26.

Folco EG, Coil KE, Reed R. 2011. The antitumor drug E7107 reveals an essential role for SF3b in remodeling U2 snRNP to expose the branch point-binding region. *Genes Dev* **25:** 440–444. doi:10.1101/gad.2009411

Gachet S, El-Chaar T, Avran D, Genesca E, Catez F, Quentin S, Delord M, Thérizols G, Briot D, Meunier G, et al. 2018. Deletion 6q drives T-cell leukemia progression by ribosome modulation. *Cancer Discov* **8:** 1614–1631. doi:10.1158/2159-8290.CD-17-0831

Gallardo M, Lee HJ, Zhang X, Bueso-Ramos C, Pageon LR, McArthur M, Multani A, Nazha A, Manshouri T, Parker-Thornburg J, et al. 2015. hnRNP K is a haploinsufficient tumor suppressor that regulates proliferation and differentiation programs in hematologic malignancies. *Cancer Cell* **28:** 486–499. doi:10.1016/j.ccell.2015.09.001

Gerstberger S, Hafner M, Tuschl T. 2014. A census of human RNA-binding proteins. *Nat Rev Genet* **15:** 829–845. doi:10.1038/nrg3813

Ghosh M, Aguila HL, Michaud J, Ai Y, Wu MT, Hemmes A, Ristimaki A, Guo C, Furneaux H, Hla T. 2009. Essential role of the RNA-binding protein HuR in progenitor cell survival in mice. *J Clin Invest* **119:** 3530–3543. doi:10.1172/JCI38263

Gingras A, Kennedy SG, O'Leary MA, Sonenberg N, Hay N. 1998. 4E-BP1, a repressor of mRNA translation, is phosphorylated and inactivated by the Akt(PKB) signaling pathway. *Genes Dev* **12:** 502–513. doi:10.1101/gad.12.4.502

Git A, Allison R, Perdiguero E, Nebreda AR, Houliston E, Standart N. 2009. Vg1RBP phosphorylation by Erk2 MAP kinase correlates with the cortical release of Vg1 mRNA during meiotic maturation of *Xenopus* oocytes. *RNA* **15:** 1121–1133. doi:10.1261/rna.1195709

Glisovic T, Bachorik JL, Yong J, Dreyfuss G. 2008. RNA-binding proteins and post-transcriptional gene regulation. *FEBS Lett* **582:** 1977–1986. doi:10.1016/j.febslet.2008.03.004

Graubert TA, Shen D, Ding L, Okeyo-Owuor T, Lunn CL, Shao J, Krysiak K, Harris CC, Koboldt DC, Larson DE, et al. 2012. Recurrent mutations in the *U2AF1* splicing factor in myelodysplastic syndromes. *Nat Genet* **44:** 53–57. doi:10.1038/ng.1031

Graveley BR, Maniatis T. 1998. Arginine/serine-rich domains of SR proteins can function as activators of pre-mRNA splicing. *Mol Cell* **1:** 765–771. doi:10.1016/S1097-2765(00)80076-3

Grosset C, Chen CYA, Xu N, Sonenberg N, Jacquemin-Sablon H, Shyu AB. 2000. A mechanism for translationally coupled mRNA turnover: Interaction between the poly(A) tail and a *c-fos* RNA coding determinant via a protein complex. *Cell* **103:** 29–40. doi:10.1016/S0092-8674(00)00102-1

Guo Y, Chen Y, Ito H, Watanabe A, Ge X, Kodama T, Aburatani H. 2006. Identification and characterization of lin-28 homolog B (LIN28B) in human hepatocellular carcinoma. *Gene* **384:** 51–61. doi:10.1016/j.gene.2006.07.011

Haghighat A, Mader S, Pause A, Sonenberg N. 1995. Repression of cap-dependent translation by 4E-binding protein 1: Competition with p220 for binding to eukaryotic initiation factor-4E. *EMBO J* **14:** 5701–5709. doi:10.1002/j.1460-2075.1995.tb00257.x

Han T, Goralski M, Gaskill N, Capota E, Kim J, Ting TC, Xie Y, Williams NS, Nijhawan D. 2017. Anticancer sulfonamides target splicing by inducing RBM39 degradation via recruitment to DCAF15. *Science* **356:** eaal3755.

Hattori A, McSkimming D, Kannan N, Ito T. 2017a. RNA binding protein MSI2 positively regulates FLT3 expression in myeloid leukemia. *Leuk Res* **54:** 47–54. doi:10.1016/j.leukres.2017.01.015

Hattori A, Tsunoda M, Konuma T, Kobayashi M, Nagy T, Glushka J, Tayyari F, McSkimming D, Kannan N, Tojo A, et al. 2017b. Cancer progression by reprogrammed BCAA metabolism in myeloid leukaemia. *Nature* **545:** 500–504. doi:10.1038/nature22314

Helsmoortel HH, Bresolin S, Lammens T, Cavé H, Noellke P, Caye A, Ghazavi F, de Vries A, Hasle H, Labarque V, et al. 2016. *LIN28B* overexpression defines a novel fetal-like subgroup of juvenile myelomonocytic leukemia. *Blood* **127:** 1163–1172. doi:10.1182/blood-2015-09-667808

Heo I, Joo C, Kim YK, Ha M, Yoon MJ, Cho J, Yeom KH, Han J, Kim VN. 2009. TUT4 in concert with Lin28 suppresses microRNA biogenesis through pre-microRNA uridylation. *Cell* **138:** 696–708. doi:10.1016/j.cell.2009.08.002

Hiriart E, Gruffat H, Buisson M, Mikaelian I, Keppler S, Meresse P, Mercher T, Bernard OA, Sergeant A, Manet E. 2005. Interaction of the Epstein-Barr virus mRNA export factor EB2 with human Spen proteins SHARP, OTT1, and a novel member of the family, OTT3, links Spen proteins with splicing regulation and mRNA export. *J Biol Chem* **280:** 36935–36945. doi:10.1074/jbc.M501725200

Ho TC, Taggart J, Kharas MG. 2016. MUSASHI-2 duels in myelodysplastic syndromes. *Cell Cycle* **15:** 1799–1800. doi:10.1080/15384101.2016.1176401

Hong S. 2017. RNA binding protein as an emerging therapeutic target for cancer prevention and treatment. *J Cancer Prev* **22:** 203–210. doi:10.15430/JCP.2017.22.4.203

Hüttelmaier S, Zenklusen D, Lederer M, Dictenberg J, Lorenz M, Meng XH, Bassell GJ, Condeelis J, Singer RH. 2005. Spatial regulation of β-actin translation by Src-dependent phosphorylation of ZBP1. *Nature* **438:** 512–515. doi:10.1038/nature04115

Iliopoulos D, Jaeger SA, Hirsch HA, Bulyk ML, Struhl K. 2010. STAT3 activation of miR-21 and miR-181b-1 via PTEN and CYLD are part of the epigenetic switch linking inflammation to cancer. *Mol Cell* **39:** 493–506. doi:10.1016/j.molcel.2010.07.023

Imai H, Chan EKL, Kiyosawa K, Fu XD, Tan EM. 1993. Novel nuclear autoantigen with splicing factor motifs identified with antibody from hepatocellular carcinoma. *J Clin Invest* **92:** 2419–2426. doi:10.1172/JCI116848

Ito T, Kwon HY, Zimdahl B, Congdon KL, Blum J, Lento WE, Zhao C, Lagoo A, Gerrard G, Foroni L, et al. 2010. Regulation of myeloid leukaemia by the cell-fate determinant Musashi. *Nature* **466:** 765–768. doi:10.1038/nature09171

Janes MR, Limon JJ, So L, Chen J, Lim RJ, Chavez MA, Vu C, Lilly MB, Mallya S, Ong ST, et al. 2010. Effective and selective targeting of Ph^+ leukemia cells using a TORC1/2 kinase inhibitor. *Nat Med* **16:** 205–213. doi:10.1038/nm.2091

Jiang X, Huang H, Li Z, Li Y, Wang X, Gurbuxani S, Chen P, He C, You D, Zhang S, et al. 2012. Blockade of miR-150 maturation by *MLL*-fusion/MYC/LIN-28 is required for *MLL*-associated leukemia. *Cancer Cell* **22:** 524–535. doi:10.1016/j.ccr.2012.08.028

Kaida D, Motoyoshi H, Tashiro E, Nojima T, Hagiwara M, Ishigami K, Watanabe H, Kitahara T, Yoshida T, Nakajima H, et al. 2007. Spliceostatin A targets SF3b and inhibits both splicing and nuclear retention of pre-mRNA. *Nat Chem Biol* **3:** 576–583.

Kawahara H, Imai T, Imataka H, Tsujimoto M, Matsumoto K, Okano H. 2008. Neural RNA-binding protein Musashi1 inhibits translation initiation by competing with eIF4G for PABP. *J Cell Biol* **181:** 639–653. doi:10.1083/jcb.200708004

Kechavarzi B, Janga SC. 2014. Dissecting the expression landscape of RNA-binding proteins in human cancers. *Genome Biol* **15:** R14. doi:10.1186/gb-2014-15-1-r14

Kentsis A, Topisirovic I, Culjkovic B, Shao L, Borden KLB. 2004. Ribavirin suppresses eIF4E-mediated oncogenic transformation by physical mimicry of the 7-methyl guanosine mRNA cap. *Proc Natl Acad Sci* **101:** 18105–18110.

Kentsis A, Volpon L, Topisirovic I, Soll CE, Culjkovic B, Shao L, Borden KLB. 2005. Further evidence that ribavirin interacts with eIF4E. *RNA* **11:** 1762–1766. doi:10.1261/rna.2238705

Kharas MG, Lengner CJ. 2017. Stem cells, cancer, and MUSASHI in blood and guts. *Trends Cancer* **3:** 347–356. doi:10.1016/j.trecan.2017.03.007

Kharas MG, Lengner CJ, Al-Shahrour F, Bullinger L, Ball B, Zaidi S, Morgan K, Tam W, Paktinat M, Okabe R, et al. 2010. Musashi-2 regulates normal hematopoiesis and promotes aggressive myeloid leukemia. *Nat Med* **16:** 903–908. doi:10.1038/nm.2187

Kim E, Ilagan JO, Liang Y, Daubner GM, Lee SCW, Ramakrishnan A, Li Y, Chung YR, Micol JB, Murphy ME, et al. 2015. *SRSF2* mutations contribute to myelodysplasia by mutant-specific effects on exon recognition. *Cancer Cell* **27:** 617–630. doi:10.1016/j.ccell.2015.04.006

King RL, Pasha T, Roullet MR, Zhang PJ, Bagg A. 2009. IMP-3 is differentially expressed in normal and neoplastic lymphoid tissue. *Hum Pathol* **40:** 1699–1705. doi:10.1016/j.humpath.2009.05.003

King C, Cuatrecasas M, Castells A, Sepulveda A, Lee JS, Rustgi AK. 2011. Lin28b promotes colon cancer progression and metastasis. *Cancer Res* **71:** 4260–4268. doi:10.1158/0008-5472.CAN-10-4637

Kon A, Yamazaki S, Nannya Y, Kataoka K, Ota Y, Nakagawa MM, Yoshida K, Shiozawa Y, Morita M, Yoshizato T, et al. 2018. Physiological *Srsf2* P95H expression causes impaired hematopoietic stem cell functions and aberrant RNA splicing in mice. *Blood* **131:** 621–635. doi:10.1182/blood-2017-01-762393

Kotake Y, Sagane K, Owa T, Mimori-kiyosue Y, Shimizu H, Uesugi M, Ishihama Y, Iwata M, Mizui Y. 2007. Splicing factor SF3b as a target of the antitumor natural product pladienolide. *Nat Chem Biol* **3:** 570–575.

Kuang B, Wu SC, Shin Y, Luo L, Kolodziej P. 2000. split ends encodes large nuclear proteins that regulate neuronal cell fate and axon extension in the *Drosophila* embryo. *Development* **1529:** 1517–1529.

Kuo SH, Hsu CH, Chen LT, Lu YS, Lin CH, Yeh PY, Jeng HJ, Gao M, Yeh KH, Cheng AL. 2011. Lack of compensatory pAKT activation and eIF4E phosphorylation of lymphoma cells towards mTOR inhibitor, RAD001. *Eur J Cancer* **47:** 1244–1257. doi:10.1016/j.ejca.2011.01.003

Kwon HY, Bajaj J, Ito T, Blevins A, Konuma T, Weeks J, Lytle NK, Koechlein CS, Rizzieri D, Chuah C, et al. 2015. Tetraspanin 3 is required for the development and propagation of acute myelogenous leukemia. *Cell Stem Cell* **17:** 152–164. doi:10.1016/j.stem.2015.06.006

Lebedeva S, Jens M, Theil K, Schwanhäusser B, Selbach M, Landthaler M, Rajewsky N. 2011. Transcriptome-wide analysis of regulatory interactions of the RNA-binding protein HuR. *Mol Cell* **43:** 340–352. doi:10.1016/j.molcel.2011.06.008

Lederer M, Bley N, Schleifer C, Hüttelmaier S. 2014. The role of the oncofetal IGF2 mRNA-binding protein 3 (IGF2BP3) in cancer. *Semin Cancer Biol* **29:** 3–12. doi:10.1016/j.semcancer.2014.07.006

Lee SCW, Abdel-Wahab O. 2016. Therapeutic targeting of splicing in cancer. *Nat Med* **22:** 976–986. doi:10.1038/nm.4165

Lee JH, Skalnik DG. 2012. Rbm15-Mkl1 interacts with the Setd1b histone H3-Lys4 methyltransferase via a SPOC domain that is required for cytokine-independent proliferation. *PLoS ONE* **7:** 27–29.

Lee SCW, Dvinge H, Kim E, Cho H, Micol JB, Chung YR, Durham BH, Yoshimi A, Kim YJ, Thomas M, et al. 2016. Modulation of splicing catalysis for therapeutic targeting of leukemia with mutations in genes encoding spliceosomal proteins. *Nat Med* **22:** 672–678. doi:10.1038/nm.4097

Lee SCW, North K, Kim E, Jang E, Obeng E, Lu SX, Liu B, Inoue D, Yoshimi A, Ki M, et al. 2018. Synthetic lethal and convergent biological effects of cancer-associated spliceosomal gene mutations. *Cancer Cell* **34:** 225–241.e8. doi:10.1016/j.ccell.2018.07.003

Lee H, Bao S, Qian Y, Geula S, Leslie J, Zhang C, Hanna JH, Ding L. 2019. Stage-specific requirement for *Mettl3*-dependent m^6A mRNA methylation during haematopoietic stem cell differentiation. *Nat Cell Biol* **21:** 700–709. doi:10.1038/s41556-019-0318-1

Lejbkowicz F, Goyer C, Darveaut A, Neron S, Lemieux R, Sonenberg N. 1992. A fraction of the mRNA 5′ cap-binding protein, eukaryotic initiation factor 4E, localizes to the nucleus. *Proc Natl Acad Sci* **89:** 9612–9616. doi:10.1073/pnas.89.20.9612

Li Z, Weng H, Su R, Weng X, Zuo Z, Li C, Huang H, Nachtergaele S, Dong L, Hu C, et al. 2017. FTO plays an oncogenic role in acute myeloid leukemia as a N^6-methyladenosine RNA demethylase. *Cancer Cell* **31:** 127–141. doi:10.1016/j.ccell.2016.11.017

Liao B, Hu Y, Herrick DJ, Brewer G. 2005. The RNA-binding protein IMP-3 is a translational activator of insulin-like growth factor II leader-3 mRNA during proliferation of human K562 leukemia cells. *J Biol Chem* **280:** 18517–18524. doi:10.1074/jbc.M500270200

Liao B, Hu Y, Brewer G. 2011. RNA-binding protein insulin-like growth factor mRNA-binding protein 3 (IMP-3) promotes cell survival via insulin-like growth factor II signaling after ionizing radiation. *J Biol Chem* **286:** 31145–31152. doi:10.1074/jbc.M111.263913

Linder B, Grozhik AV, Olarerin-George AO, Meydan C, Mason CE, Jaffrey SR. 2015. Single-nucleotide-resolution mapping of m^6A and m^6Am throughout the transcriptome. *Nat Methods* **12:** 767–772. doi:10.1038/nmeth.3453

Liu H-X, Chew SL, Cartegni L, Zhang MQ, Krainer AR. 2000. Exonic splicing enhancer motif recognized by human SC35 under splicing conditions. *Mol Cell Biol* **20:** 1063–1071. doi:10.1128/MCB.20.3.1063-1071.2000

Loerch S, Maucuer A, Manceau V, Green MR, Kielkopf CL. 2014. Cancer-relevant splicing factor CAPERα engages the essential splicing factor SF3b155 in a specific ternary complex. *J Biol Chem* **289:** 17325–17337. doi:10.1074/jbc.M114.558825

Lu JY, Schneider RJ. 2004. Tissue distribution of AU-rich mRNA-binding proteins involved in regulation of mRNA decay. *J Biol Chem* **279:** 12974–12979. doi:10.1074/jbc.M310433200

Lukong KE, Chang KW, Khandjian EW, Richard S. 2008. RNA-binding proteins in human genetic disease. *Trends Genet* **24:** 416–425. doi:10.1016/j.tig.2008.05.004

Lunde BM, Moore C, Varani G. 2007. RNA-binding proteins: Modular design for efficient function. *Nat Rev Mol Cell Biol* **8:** 479–490. doi:10.1038/nrm2178

Ma Z, Morris SW, Valentine V, Herbrick JA, Cui X, Bouman D, Li Y, Mehta PK, Nizetic D, Kaneko Y, et al. 2001. Fusion of two novel genes, *RBM15* and *MKL1*, in the t(1;22)(p13;q13) of acute megakaryoblastic leukemia. *Nat Genet* **28:** 220–221. doi:10.1038/90054

Ma X, Renda MJ, Wang L, Cheng E, Niu C, Morris SW, Chi AS, Krause DS. 2007. *Rbm15* modulates Notch-induced transcriptional activation and affects myeloid differentiation. *Mol Cell Biol* **27:** 3056–3064. doi:10.1128/MCB.01339-06

Machnicka MA, Milanowska K, Oglou OO, Purta E, Kurkowska M, Olchowik A, Januszewski W, Kalinowski S, Dunin-Horkawicz S, Rother KM, et al. 2013. MODOMICS: A database of RNA modification pathways—2013 update. *Nucleic Acids Res* **41:** D262–D267. doi:10.1093/nar/gks1007

Madison B, Liu Q, Zhong X, Hahn CM, Lin N, Emmet M, Stanger BZ, Rustgi AK. 2013. LIN28B promotes growth and tumorigenesis of the intestinal epithelium primarily via Let-7. *Cancer Res* **73:** 2233–2245.

Makishima H, Visconte V, Sakaguchi H, Jankowska AM, Kar SA, Jerez A, Przychodzen B, Bupathi M, Guinta K, Afable MG, et al. 2012. Mutations in the spliceosome machinery, a novel and ubiquitous pathway in leukemogenesis. *Blood* **119:** 3203–3210. doi:10.1182/blood-2011-12-399774

Malcovati L, Papaemmanuil E, Bowen DT, Boultwood J, Della Porta MG, Pascutto C, Travaglino E, Groves MJ, Godfrey AL, Ambaglio I, et al. 2011. Clinical significance of *SF3B1* mutations in myelodysplastic syndromes and myelodysplastic/myeloproliferative neoplasms. *Blood* **118:** 6239–6246. doi:10.1182/blood-2011-09-377275

Malcovati L, Karimi M, Papaemmanuil E, Ambaglio I, Jädersten M, Jansson M, Elena C, Gallì A, Walldin G, Della Porta MG, et al. 2015. *SF3B1* mutation identifies a distinct subset of myelodysplastic syndrome with ring sideroblasts. *Blood* **126:** 233–241. doi:10.1182/blood-2015-03-633537

McMahon AC, Rahman R, Jin H, Shen JL, Fieldsend A, Luo W, Rosbash M. 2016. TRIBE: Hijacking an RNA-editing enzyme to identify cell-specific targets of RNA-binding proteins. *Cell* **165:** 742–753. doi:10.1016/j.cell.2016.03.007

Meggendorfer M, Roller A, Haferlach T, Eder C, Dicker F, Grossmann V, Kohlmann A, Alpermann T, Yoshida K, Ogawa S, et al. 2012. *SRSF2* mutations in 275 cases with chronic myelomonocytic leukemia (CMML). *Blood* **120:** 3080–3088. doi:10.1182/blood-2012-01-404863

Mercher T, Raffel GD, Moore SA, Cornejo MG, Baudry-bluteau D, Cagnard N, Jesneck JL, Pikman Y, Cullen D, Williams IR, et al. 2009. The OTT-MAL fusion oncogene activates RBPJ-mediated transcription and induces acute megakaryoblastic leukemia in a knockin mouse model. *J Clin Invest* **119:** 852–864.

Mercier I, Casimiro MC, Zhou J, Wang C, Plymire C, Bryant KG, Daumer KM, Sotgia F, Bonuccelli G, Witkiewicz AK, et al. 2009. Genetic ablation of caveolin-1 drives estrogen-hypersensitivity and the development of DCIS-like mammary lesions. *Am J Pathol* **174:** 1172–1190. doi:10.2353/ajpath.2009.080882

Meyer KD, Saletore Y, Zumbo P, Elemento O, Mason CE, Jaffrey SR. 2012. Comprehensive analysis of mRNA methylation reveals enrichment in 3′ UTRs and near stop codons. *Cell* **149:** 1635–1646. doi:10.1016/j.cell.2012.05.003

Milojkovic Kerklaan B, Slater S, Flynn M, Greystoke A, Witteveen PO, Megui-Roelvink M, de Vos F, Dean E, Reyderman L, Ottesen L, et al. 2016. A phase I, dose escalation, pharmacodynamic, pharmacokinetic, and food-effect study of α2 integrin inhibitor E7820 in patients with advanced solid tumors. *Invest New Drugs* **34:** 329–337. doi:10.1007/s10637-016-0344-9

Minich WB, Balasta ML, Goss DJ, Rhoads RE. 1994. Chromatographic resolution of in vivo phosphorylated and nonphosphorylated eukaryotic translation initiation factor eIF-4E: increased cap affinity of the phosphorylated form. *Proc Natl Acad Sci* **91:** 7668–7672. doi:10.1073/pnas.91.16.7668

Minuesa G, Antczak C, Shum D, Radu C, Bhinder B, Li Y, Djaballah H, Kharas MG. 2014. A 1536-well fluorescence polarization assay to screen for modulators of the MUSASHI family of RNA-binding proteins. *Comb Chem High Throughput Screen* **17:** 596–609. doi:10.2174/1386207317666140609122714

Minuesa G, Albanese SK, Xie W, Kazansky Y, Worroll D, Chow A, Schurer A, Park S, Rotsides CZ, Taggart J, et al. 2019. Small-molecule targeting of MUSASHI RNA-binding activity in acute myeloid leukemia. *Nat Commun* **10:** 1–15. doi:10.1038/s41467-019-10523-3

Mizutani A, Fukuda M, Ibata K, Shiraishi Y, Mikoshiba K. 2000. SYNCRIP, a cytoplasmic counterpart of heterogeneous nuclear ribonucleoprotein R, interacts with ubiquitous synaptotagmin isoforms. *J Biol Chem* **275:** 9823–9831. doi:10.1074/jbc.275.13.9823

Moerke NJ, Aktas H, Chen H, Cantel S, Reibarkh MY, Fahmy A, Gross JD, Degterev A, Yuan J, Chorev M, et al. 2007. Small-molecule inhibition of the interaction between the translation initiation factors eIF4E and eIF4G. *Cell* **128:** 257–267.

Molenaar JJ, Domingo-Fernández R, Ebus ME, Lindner S, Koster J, Drabek K, Mestdagh P, Van Sluis P, Valentijn LJ, Van Nes J, et al. 2012. LIN28B induces neuroblastoma and enhances MYCN levels via *let-7* suppression. *Nat Genet* **44:** 1199–1206. doi:10.1038/ng.2436

Moss EG, Lee RC, Ambros V. 1997. The cold shock domain protein LIN-28 controls developmental timing in *C. elegans* and is regulated by the *lin-4* RNA. *Cell* **88:** 637–646. doi:10.1016/S0092-8674(00)81906-6

Mukherjee N, Corcoran DL, Nusbaum JD, Reid DW, Georgiev S, Hafner M, Ascano M, Tuschl T, Ohler U, Keene JD. 2011. Integrative regulatory mapping indicates that the RNA-binding protein HuR couples pre-mRNA processing and mRNA stability. *Mol Cell* **43:** 327–339. doi:10.1016/j.molcel.2011.06.007

Murphy D, Cieply B, Carstens R, Ramamurthy V, Stoilov P, Desplan C. 2016. The Musashi 1 controls the splicing of photoreceptor-specific exons in the vertebrate retina. *PLoS Genet* **12:** e1006256. doi:10.1371/journal.pgen.1006256

Natkunam Y, Vainer G, Chen J, Zhao S, Marinelli RJ, Hammer AS, Hamilton-Dutoit S, Pikarsky E, Amir G, Levy R, et al. 2007. Expression of the RNA-binding protein VICKZ in normal hematopoietic tissues and neoplasms. *Haematologica* **92:** 176–183. doi:10.3324/haematol.10724

Navarro A, Trapp V, Hartmann EM, Beà S, Campo E, Ott G, Rosenwald A. 2012. Increased tumor cell proliferation in mantle cell lymphoma is associated with elevated insulin-like growth factor 2 mRNA-binding protein 3 expression. *Mod Pathol* **25:** 1227–1235. doi:10.1038/modpathol.2012.84

Nguyen LH, Robinton DA, Seligson MT, Wu L, Li L, Rakheja D, Comerford SA, Ramezani S, Sun X, Parikh MS, et al. 2014. *Lin28b* is sufficient to drive liver cancer and necessary for its maintenance in murine models. *Cancer Cell* **26:** 248–261. doi:10.1016/j.ccr.2014.06.018

Nielsen J, Kristensen MA, Willemoës M, Nielsen FC, Christiansen J. 2004. Sequential dimerization of human zipcode-binding protein IMP1 on RNA: A cooperative mechanism providing RNP stability. *Nucleic Acids Res* **32:** 4368–4376. doi:10.1093/nar/gkh754

Notari M, Neviani P, Santhanam R, Blaser BW, Chang JS, Galietta A, Willis AE, Roy DC, Caligiuri MA, Marcucci G, et al. 2006. A MAPK/HNRPK pathway controls BCR/

ABL oncogenic potential by regulating MYC mRNA translation. *Blood* **107:** 2507–2516. doi:10.1182/blood-2005-09-3732

Obeng EA, Chappell RJ, Seiler M, Chen MC, Campagna DR, Schmidt PJ, Schneider RK, Lord AM, Wang L, Gambe RG, et al. 2016. Physiologic expression of Sf3b1^{K700E} causes impaired erythropoiesis, aberrant splicing, and sensitivity to therapeutic spliceosome modulation. *Cancer Cell* **30:** 404–417. doi:10.1016/j.ccell.2016.08.006

Owa T, Yoshino H, Okauchi T, Yoshimatsu K, Ozawa Y, Sugi NH, Nagasu T, Koyanagi N, Kitoh K. 1999. Discovery of novel antitumor sulfonamides targeting G1 phase of the cell cycle. *J Med Chem* **42:** 3789–3799. doi:10.1021/jm9902638

Palanichamy JK, Tran TM, Howard JM, Contreras JR, Fernando TR, Sterne-Weiler T, Katzman S, Toloue M, Yan W, Basso G, et al. 2016. RNA-binding protein IGF2BP3 targeting of oncogenic transcripts promotes hematopoietic progenitor proliferation. *J Clin Invest* **126:** 1495–1511. doi:10.1172/JCI80046

Papaemmanuil E, Cazzola M, Boultwood J, Malcovati L, Vyas P, Bowen D, Pellagatti A, Wainscoat JS, Hellstrom-Lindberg E, Gambacorti-Passerini C, et al. 2011. Somatic *SF3B1* mutation in myelodysplasia with ring sideroblasts. *N Engl J Med* **365:** 1384–1395. doi:10.1056/NEJMoa1103283

Papaemmanuil , Gerstung M, Malcovati L, Tauro S, Gundem G, Van Loo P, Yoon CJ, Ellis P, Wedge DC, Pellagatti A, et al. 2013. Clinical and biological implications of driver mutations in myelodysplastic syndromes. *Blood* **122:** 3616–3627. doi:10.1182/blood-2013-08-518886

Paris J, Morgan M, Campos J, Spencer GJ, Shmakova A, Ivanova I, Mapperley C, Lawson H, Wotherspoon DA, Sepulveda C, et al. 2019. Targeting the RNA m^{6}A reader YTHDF2 selectively compromises cancer stem cells in acute myeloid leukemia. *Cell Stem Cell* **25:** 137–148.e6. doi:10.1016/j.stem.2019.03.021

Park S, Gönen M, Vu L, Minuesa G, Tivnan P, Barlowe TS, Taggart J, Lu Y, Deering RP, Hacohen N, et al. 2015. Musashi2 sustains the mixed-lineage leukemia–driven stem cell regulatory program. *J Clin Invest* **125:** 1286–1298. doi:10.1172/JCI78440

Parsyan A, Svitkin Y, Shahbazian D, Gkogkas C, Lasko P, Merrick WC, Sonenberg N. 2011. mRNA helicases: The tacticians of translational control. *Nat Rev Mol Cell Biol* **12:** 235–245. doi:10.1038/nrm3083

Pereira JKN, Traina F, Machado-Neto JA, Duarte AdSS, Lopes MR, Saad ST, Favaro P. 2012. Distinct expression profiles of *MSI2* and *NUMB* genes in myelodysplastic syndromes and acute myeloid leukemia patients. *Leuk Res* **36:** 1300–1303. doi:10.1016/j.leukres.2012.06.010

Pereira B, Billaud M, Almeida R. 2017. RNA-binding proteins in cancer: Old players and new actors. *Trends Cancer* **3:** 506–528. doi:10.1016/j.trecan.2017.05.003

Quesada V, Ramsay AJ, Lopez-Otin C. 2012. Chronic lymphocytic leukemia with *SF3B1* mutation. *N Engl J Med* **366:** 2530. doi:10.1056/NEJMc1204033

Raffel GD, Mercher T, Shigematsu H, Williams IR, Cullen DE, Akashi K, Bernard OA, Gilliland DG. 2007. *Ott1* (*Rbm15*) has pleiotropic roles in hematopoietic development. *Proc Natl Acad Sci* **104:** 6001–6006. doi:10.1073/pnas.0609041104

Roos M, Pradère U, Ngondo RP, Behera A, Allegrini S, Civenni G, Zagalak JA, Marchand J-R, Menzi M, Towbin H, et al. 2016. A small-molecule inhibitor of Lin28. *ACS Chem Biol* **11:** 2773–2781. doi:10.1021/acschembio.6b00232

Rottman F, Shatkin AJ, Perry RP. 1974. Sequences containing methylated nucleotides at the 5′ termini of messenger RNAs: Possible implications for processing. *Cell* **3:** 197–199. doi:10.1016/0092-8674(74)90131-7

Roush S, Slack FJ. 2008. The *let-7* family of microRNAs. *Trends Cell Biol* **18:** 505–516. doi:10.1016/j.tcb.2008.07.007

Schaal TD, Maniatis T. 1999. Multiple distinct splicing enhancers in the protein-coding sequences of a constitutively spliced pre-mRNA. *Mol Cell Biol* **19:** 261–273. doi:10.1128/MCB.19.1.261

Shirai CL, Ley JN, White BS, Kim S, Tibbitts J, Shao J, Ndonwi M, Wadugu B, Duncavage EJ, Okeyo-Owuor T, et al. 2015. Mutant U2AF1 expression alters hematopoiesis and pre-mRNA splicing in vivo. *Cancer Cell* **27:** 631–643. doi:10.1016/j.ccell.2015.04.008

Sillars-Hardebol AH, Carvalho B, Beliën JAM, De Wit M, Delis-Van Diemen PM, Tijssen M, Van De Wiel MA, Pontén F, Meijer GA, Fijneman RJA. 2012. *CSE1L*, *DIDO1* and *RBM39* in colorectal adenoma to carcinoma progression. *Cell Oncol* **35:** 293–300. doi:10.1007/s13402-012-0088-2

Sonenberg N, Gingras A. 1998. The mRNA 5′ cap-binding protein eIF4E and control of cell growth. *Curr Opin Cell Biol* **10:** 268–275. doi:10.1016/S0955-0674(98)80150-6

Stepanyuk GA, Serrano P, Peralta E, Farr CL, Axelrod HL, Geralt M, Das D, Chiu H-J, Jaroszewski L, Deacon AM, et al. 2016. UHM–ULM interactions in the RBM39–U2AF65 splicing-factor complex. *Acta Crystallogr D Biol Crystallogr* **72:** 497–511. doi:10.1107/S2059798316001248

Stohr N, Buchmeier S, Kohn M, Lederer M, Baude A, Huttelmaier S, Wahle E, Weidensdorfer D, Schierhorn A. 2008. Control of c-myc mRNA stability by IGF2BP1-associated cytoplasmic RNPs. *RNA* **15:** 104–115. doi:10.1261/rna.1175909

Stoskus M, Gineikiene E, Valceckiene V, Valatkaite B, Pileckyte R, Griskevicius L. 2011. Identification of characteristic *IGF2BP* expression patterns in distinct B-ALL entities. *Blood Cells Mol Dis* **46:** 321–326. doi:10.1016/j.bcmd.2011.02.005

Strudwick S, Borden KLB. 2002. The emerging roles of translation factor eIF4E in the nucleus. *Differentiation* **70:** 10–22. doi:10.1046/j.1432-0436.2002.700102.x

Su R, Dong L, Li C, Nachtergaele S, Wunderlich M, Qing Y, Deng X, Wang Y, Weng X, Hu C, et al. 2018. R-2HG exhibits anti-tumor activity by targeting FTO/m^{6}A/MYC/CEBPA signaling. *Cell* **172:** 90–105.e23. doi:10.1016/j.cell.2017.11.031

Supuran CT. 2003. Indisulam: An anticancer sulfonamide in clinical development. *Expert Opin Investig Drugs* **12:** 283–287. doi:10.1517/13543784.12.2.283

Taggart J, Ho T, Amin E, Xu H, Barlowe TS, Perez AR, Durham BH, Tivnan P, Okabe R, Chow A, et al. 2016. MSI2 is required for maintaining activated myelodysplastic syndrome stem cells. *Nat Commun* **7:** 10739. doi:10.1038/ncomms10739

Tan K, Culjkovic B, Amri A, Borden KLB. 2008. Ribavirin targets eIF4E dependent Akt survival signaling. *Biochem Biophys Res Commun* **375:** 341–345. doi:10.1016/j.bbrc.2008.07.163

Tang H, Wei Q, Ge J, Jian W, Liu J, Zhong L, Fu B, Zhao T. 2013. IMP3 as a supplemental diagnostic marker for Hodgkin lymphoma. *Hum Pathol* **44:** 2167–2172. doi:10.1016/j.humpath.2013.04.011

Thol F, Winschel C, Sonntag A, Damm F, Wagner K, Chaturvedi A, Göhring G, Schlegelberger B, Lübbert M, Fiedler W, et al. 2013. Prognostic significance of expression levels of stem cell regulators *MSI2* and *NUMB* in acute myeloid leukemia. *Ann Hematol* **92:** 315–323. doi:10.1007/s00277-012-1637-5

Tomimaru Y, Eguchi H, Wada H, Kobayashi S, Marubashi S, Tanemura M, Umeshita K, Kim T, Wakasa K, Doki Y, et al. 2012. IGFBP7 downregulation is associated with tumor progression and clinical outcome in hepatocellular carcinoma. *Int J Cancer* **130:** 319–327. doi:10.1002/ijc.25994

Topisirovic I, Guzman ML, McConnell MJ, Licht JD, Culjkovic B, Neering SJ, Jordan CT, Borden KLB. 2003. Aberrant eukaryotic translation initiation factor 4E-dependent mRNA transport impedes hematopoietic differentiation and contributes to leukemogenesis. *Mol Cell Biol* **23:** 8992–9002. doi:10.1128/MCB.23.24.8992-9002.2003

Topisirovic I, Siddiqui N, Borden KLB. 2009a. The eukaryotic translation initiation factor 4E (eIF4E) and HuR RNA operons collaboratively regulate the expression of survival and proliferative genes. *Cell Cycle* **8:** 959–964. doi:10.4161/cc.8.7.8093

Topisirovic I, Siddiqui N, Orolicki S, Skrabanek LA, Tremblay M, Hoang T, Borden KLB. 2009b. Stability of eukaryotic translation initiation factor 4E mRNA is regulated by HuR, and this activity is dysregulated in cancer. *Mol Cell Biol* **29:** 1152–1162. doi:10.1128/MCB.01532-08

Uehara T, Minoshima Y, Sagane K, Sugi NH, Mitsuhashi KO, Yamamoto N, Kamiyama H, Takahashi K, Kotake Y, Uesugi M, et al. 2017. Selective degradation of splicing factor CAPERα by anticancer sulfonamides. *Nat Chem Biol* **13:** 675–680. doi:10.1038/nchembio.2363

Uranishi H, Zolotukhin AS, Lindtner S, Warming S, Zhang G, Bear J, Copeland NG, Jenkins NA, Pavlakis GN, Felber BK. 2009. The RNA-binding motif protein 15B (RBM15B/OTT3) acts as cofactor of the nuclear export receptor NXF1. *J Biol Chem* **284:** 26106–26116. doi:10.1074/jbc.M109.040113

Verhagen HJMP, De Leeuw DC, Roemer MGM, Denkers F, Pouwels W, Rutten A, Celie PH, Ossenkoppele GJ, Schuurhuis GJ, Smit L. 2014. IGFBP7 induces apoptosis of acute myeloid leukemia cells and synergizes with chemotherapy in suppression of leukemia cell survival. *Cell Death Dis* **5:** e1300.

Verhagen HJMP, van Gils N, Martiañez T, van Rhenen A, Rutten A, Denkers F, de Leeuw DC, Smit MA, Tsui ML, de Vos Klootwijk LLE, et al. 2018. IGFBP7 induces differentiation and loss of survival of human acute myeloid leukemia stem cells without affecting normal hematopoiesis. *Cell Rep* **25:** 3021–3035.e5. doi:10.1016/j.celrep.2018.11.062

Visconte V, Makishima H, Jankowska A, Szpurka H, Traina F, Jerez A, O'Keefe C, Rogers HJ, Sekeres MA, Maciejewski JP, et al. 2012a. SF3B1, a splicing factor is frequently mutated in refractory anemia with ring sideroblasts. *Leukemia* **26:** 542–545. doi:10.1038/leu.2011.232

Visconte V, Makishima H, Maciejewski JP, Tiu RV. 2012b. Emerging roles of the spliceosomal machinery in myelodysplastic syndromes and other hematological disorders. *Leukemia* **26:** 2447–2454. doi:10.1038/leu.2012.130

Visconte V, Rogers HJ, Singh J, Barnard J, Bupathi M, Traina F, McMahon J, Makishima H, Szpurka H, Jankowska A, et al. 2012c. *SF3B1* haploinsufficiency leads to formation of ring sideroblasts in myelodysplastic syndromes. *Blood* **120:** 3173–3186. doi:10.1182/blood-2012-05-430876

Viswanathan SR, Powers JT, Einhorn W, Hoshida Y, Ng TL, Toffanin S, O'Sullivan M, Lu J, Phillips LA, Lockhart VL, et al. 2009. Lin28 promotes transformation and is associated with advanced human malignancies. *Nat Genet* **41:** 843–848. doi:10.1038/ng.392

Vu LP, Pickering BF, Cheng Y, Zaccara S, Nguyen D, Minuesa G, Chou T, Chow A, Saletore Y, MacKay M, et al. 2017a. The N^6-methyladenosine (m^6A)-forming enzyme METTL3 controls myeloid differentiation of normal hematopoietic and leukemia cells. *Nat Med* **23:** 1369–1376. doi:10.1038/nm.4416

Vu LP, Prieto C, Amin EM, Chhangawala S, Krivtsov A, Calvo-Vidal MN, Chou T, Chow A, Minuesa G, Park SM, et al. 2017b. Functional screen of MSI2 interactors identifies an essential role for SYNCRIP in myeloid leukemia stem cells. *Nat Genet* **49:** 866–875. doi:10.1038/ng.3854

Vu LP, Cheng Y, Kharas MG. 2019. The biology of m^6A RNA methylation in normal and malignant hematopoiesis. *Cancer Discov* **9:** 25–33. doi:10.1158/2159-8290.CD-18-0959

Wang HY, Xu X, Ding JH, Bermingham JR, Fu XD. 2001. SC35 plays a role in T cell development and alternative splicing of CD45. *Mol Cell* **7:** 331–342. doi:10.1016/S1097-2765(01)00181-2

Wang L, Lawrence MS, Wan Y, Stojanov P, Sougnez C, Stevenson K, Werner L, Sivachenko A, DeLuca DS, Zhang L, et al. 2011. *SF3B1* and other novel cancer genes in chronic lymphocytic leukemia. *N Engl J Med* **365:** 2497–2506. doi:10.1056/NEJMoa1109016

Wang K, Sanchez-Martin M, Wang X, Knapp KM, Koche R, Vu L, Nahas MK, He J, Hadler M, Stein EM, et al. 2017. Patient-derived xenotransplants can recapitulate the genetic driver landscape of acute leukemias. *Leukemia* **31:** 151–158. doi:10.1038/leu.2016.166

Wang L, Rowe RG, Jaimes A, Yu C, Nam Y, Pearson DS, Zhang J, Xie X, Marion W, Heffron GJ, et al. 2018. Small-molecule inhibitors disrupt let-7 oligouridylation and release the selective blockade of let-7 processing by LIN28. *Cell Rep* **23:** 3091–3101. doi:10.1016/j.celrep.2018.04.116

Wang E, Lu SX, Pastore A, Chen X, Imig J, Chun-Wei Lee S, Hockemeyer K, Ghebrechristos YE, Yoshimi A, Inoue D, et al. 2019. Targeting an RNA-binding protein network in acute myeloid leukemia. *Cancer Cell* **35:** 369–384.e7. doi:10.1016/j.ccell.2019.01.010

Wendel H-G, De Stanchina E, Fridman JS, Malina A, Ray S, Kogan S, Cordon-Cardo C, Pelletier J, Lowe SW. 2004. Survival signalling by Akt and eIF4E in oncogenesis and cancer therapy. *Nature* **428:** 332–337. doi:10.1038/nature02369

Weng H, Huang H, Wu H, Qin X, Zhao BS, Dong L, Shi H, Skibbe J, Shen C, Hu C, et al. 2018. METTL14 inhibits hematopoietic stem/progenitor differentiation and promotes leukemogenesis via mRNA m^6A modification. *Cell Stem Cell* **22:** 191–205.e9. doi:10.1016/j.stem.2017.11.016

Wiellette EL, Harding KW, Mace KA, Ronshaugen MR, Wang FY, Mcginnis W. 1999. spen encodes an RNP motif protein that interacts with Hox pathways to repress the development of head-like sclerites in the *Drosophila* trunk. *Development* **126:** 5373–5385.

Wolfe AL, Singh K, Zhong Y, Drewe P, Rajasekhar VK, Sanghvi VR, Mavrakis KJ, Jiang M, Roderick JE, Van der Meulen J, et al. 2014. RNA G-quadruplexes cause eIF4A-dependent oncogene translation in cancer. *Nature* **513:** 65–70. doi:10.1038/nature13485

Wurth L, Gebauer F. 2015. RNA-binding proteins, multifaceted translational regulators in cancer. *Biochim Biophys Acta* **1849:** 881–886. doi:10.1016/j.bbagrm.2014.10.001

Xing L, Yao X, Williams KR, Bassell GJ. 2012. Negative regulation of RhoA translation and signaling by hnRNP-Q1 affects cellular morphogenesis. *Mol Biol Cell* **23:** 1500–1509. doi:10.1091/mbc.e11-10-0867

Yilmaz H, Valdez R, Theisen BK, Guo W, Ferguson DO, Wu H, Morrison SJ. 2006. *Pten* dependence distinguishes haematopoietic stem cells from leukaemia-initiating cells. *Nature* **441:** 475–482. doi:10.1038/nature04703

Yoshida K, Sanada M, Shiraishi Y, Nowak D, Nagata Y, Yamamoto R, Sato Y, Sato-Otsubo A, Kon A, Nagasaki M, et al. 2011. Frequent pathway mutations of splicing machinery in myelodysplasia. *Nature* **478:** 64–69. doi:10.1038/nature10496

Yu J, Vodyanik MA, Smuga-Otto K, Antosiewicz-Bourget J, Frane JL, Tian S, Nie J, Jonsdottir GA, Ruotti V, Stewart R, et al. 2007. Induced pluripotent stem cell lines derived from human somatic cells. *Science* **318:** 1917–1920. doi:10.1126/science.1151526

Zheng G, Dahl JA, Niu Y, Fedorcsak P, Huang CM, Li CJ, Vågbø CB, Shi Y, Wang WL, Song SH, et al. 2013. ALKBH5 is a mammalian RNA demethylase that impacts RNA metabolism and mouse fertility. *Mol Cell* **49:** 18–29. doi:10.1016/j.molcel.2012.10.015

Zhou J, Bi C, Ching YQ, Chooi J, Lu X, Quah JY, Toh SH, Chan Z, Tan TZ, Chong PSY, et al. 2017a. Inhibition of LIN28B impairs leukemia cell growth and metabolism in acute myeloid leukemia. *J Hematol Oncol* **10:** 138. doi:10.1186/s13045-017-0507-y

Zhou J, Chan ZL, Bi C, Lu X, Chong PSY, Chooi JY, Cheong LL, Liu SC, Ching YQ, Zhou Y, et al. 2017b. LIN28B activation by PRL-3 promotes leukemogenesis and a stem cell–like transcriptional program in AML. *Mol Cancer Res* **15:** 294–303. doi:10.1158/1541-7786.MCR-16-0275-T

Zhu H, Shah S, Shyh-Chang N, Shinoda G, Einhorn WS, Viswanathan SR, Takeuchi A, Grasemann C, Rinn JL, Lopez MF, et al. 2010. *Lin28a* transgenic mice manifest size and puberty phenotypes identified in human genetic association studies. *Nat Genet* **42:** 626–630. doi:10.1038/ng.593

Zolotukhin AS, Uranishi H, Lindtner S, Bear J, Pavlakis GN, Felber BK. 2009. Nuclear export factor RBM15 facilitates the access of DBP5 to mRNA. *Nucleic Acids Res* **37:** 7151–7162. doi:10.1093/nar/gkp782

Oncogenic Mechanisms and Therapeutic Targeting of Metabolism in Leukemia and Lymphoma

Maximilian Stahl,[1] Zachary D. Epstein-Peterson,[1] and Andrew M. Intlekofer

Department of Medicine and Human Oncology & Pathogenesis Program, Memorial Sloan Kettering Cancer Center, New York, New York 10065, USA

Correspondence: intlekoa@mskcc.org

Leukemias and lymphomas acquire the capacity for unrestrained cell growth and proliferation in conjunction with loss of responsiveness to molecular programs that promote terminal differentiation. Malignant cells generate the building blocks required for rapid cell division through both increased acquisition of nutrients from the environment and reprogrammed intermediary metabolism to shunt these molecules into producing the protein, lipids, and nucleic acids that comprise cell biomass. These accelerated metabolic processes require energy in the form of ATP and reducing equivalents in the form of NADPH, which power biosynthetic reactions and buffer oxidative stress encountered by the metabolically active cancer cell. Cancer-associated metabolic alterations can also promote accumulation or depletion of specific metabolites that directly regulate cell fate and function, thereby coupling metabolic reprogramming to dedifferentiation and stemness. This review will focus on the mechanisms by which leukemia and lymphoma cells rewire cellular metabolism to support: (1) bioenergetics, (2) biomass accumulation, (3) redox balance, and (4) differentiation blockade. We will further highlight examples of how specific pathways of leukemia and lymphoma metabolism confer therapeutic vulnerabilities that can be targeted to inhibit growth or promote differentiation.

At a fundamental level, cancer is a problem of hijacked cellular metabolism (Vander Heiden et al. 2009). Normally, metazoan cells require "permission" from growth factors, cytokines, hormones, or antigen/costimulatory receptors to increase nutrient uptake. All cancers, including leukemias and lymphomas, acquire the capacity for cell-autonomous uptake of nutrients that circumvents normal regulatory mechanisms (Palm and Thompson 2017). Such unrestricted nutrient uptake is critical to build the cellular biomass (protein, lipids, nucleic acids) necessary for rapid cell doubling (Fig. 1). Because the availability of specific nutrients in the environment does not precisely match the necessary outputs, cancer cells must rewire metabolic circuits to rapidly convert available nutrients into precursor metabolites

[1]These authors contributed equally to this work.

Cite this article as *Cold Spring Harb Perspect Med* doi: 10.1101/cshperspect.a035477

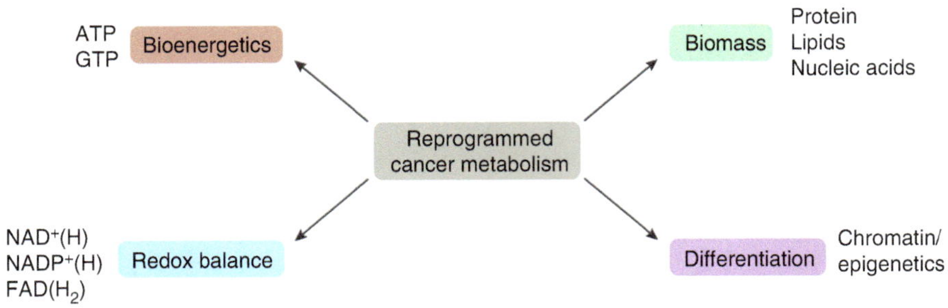

Figure 1. Key functions of reprogrammed cancer metabolism. Leukemias and lymphomas reprogram cellular metabolism to meet the anabolic demands of malignant growth and proliferation. Glycolysis and mitochondrial oxidative phosphorylation provide energy in the form of ATP and GTP (Bioenergetics). Metabolic intermediates are shunted into biosynthetic pathways that produce the protein, lipids, and nucleic acids required for cell doubling and division (Biomass). Malignant cells require increased regeneration of NAD^+ to enable oxidative biosynthetic reactions (e.g., nucleotides), as well as increased production of NADPH to fuel reductive biosynthetic reactions (e.g., lipids) and buffer oxidative stress (redox balance). Deregulation of specific metabolites or metabolic pathways can also disrupt chromatin marks, resulting in impaired differentiation and/or enhanced self-renewal (differentiation). (ATP) Adenosine triphosphate, (GTP) guanosine triphosphate, (NAD) nicotinamide adenine dinucleotide, (NADP) nicotinamide adenine dinucleotide phosphate, (FAD) flavin adenine dinucleotide.

that can be used to synthesize the macromolecules that comprise cell biomass. This intensive metabolic activity requires energy in the form of adenosine triphosphate (ATP) and reducing equivalents in the form of nicotinamide adenine dinucleotide phosphate (NADPH) to fuel biosynthetic reactions (Fig. 1).

As first described by Otto Warburg almost 100 years ago, most cancer cells rapidly ferment glucose to lactate regardless of oxygen availability (Warburg 1924, 1956). A high rate of glycolysis by cancer cells serves at least two important functions, which are often difficult to dissociate mechanistically: (1) ATP production and (2) generation of precursor molecules and reducing equivalents required for biosynthesis of macromolecules (Fig. 2; Vander Heiden et al. 2009). Surprisingly, the limited amount of ATP (maximum of 2 ATP per glucose) generated by glycolysis can be sufficient to support cell proliferation in highly glycolytic cancer cells without a requirement for additional ATP generated by mitochondrial oxidative phosphorylation (OXPHOS) (Birsoy et al. 2015; Sullivan et al. 2015). Running glycolysis at a high rate appears to necessitate the Warburg effect, which drives conversion of pyruvate to lactate by lactate dehydrogenase (LDH) in order to rapidly regenerate the cytosolic NAD^+ required to maintain glycolytic flux. However, despite the ability of glycolysis to provide adequate ATP, mitochondrial electron transport remains essential for virtually all cancer cells in order to regenerate the electron acceptors (NAD^+) required for macromolecular biosynthesis (Hosios and Vander Heiden 2018). Moreover, certain cancer cells without high glycolytic flux, including leukemic stem cells and a subset of diffuse large B-cell lymphoma (DLBCL), appear to be particularly dependent on OXPHOS, which may be related to their preferential oxidation of alternative fuels that can only generate ATP through the mitochondria (Caro et al. 2012; Ye et al. 2016; Jones et al. 2018).

Proliferating cells must double their biomass in order to divide, which requires assembling all of the proteins, lipids, and nucleic acids that comprise the cell (Fig. 1; Hosios et al. 2016). A subset of carbohydrates, amino acids, lipids, and nucleotides can be acquired from the microenvironment for direct incorporation into macromolecules, However, a major function of cancer metabolism involves conversion of available nutrients, such as glucose and glutamine, into metabolic intermediates that can be directed into macromolecular biosynthetic pathways (Fig. 2;

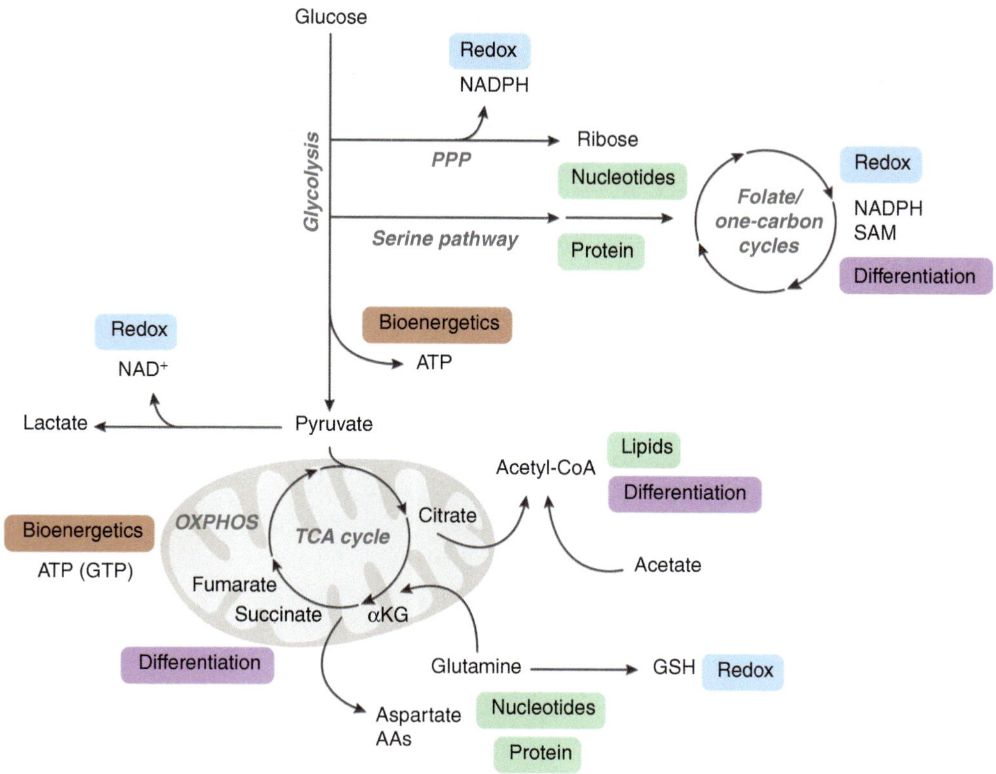

Figure 2. Simplified overview of metabolic pathways in leukemia and lymphoma. Altered and/or enhanced glycolysis, pentose phosphate pathway (PPP), serine biosynthetic pathway, folate/one-carbon cycles, tricarboxylic acid (TCA) cycle, oxidative phosphorylation (OXPHOS), lipid synthesis, and amino acid (AA) metabolism support bioenergetics (red), biomass accumulation (green), redox balance (blue), and differentiation blockade (purple). Most precursors, products, cofactors, and enzymes are intentionally absent for simplicity. (ATP) Adenosine triphosphate, (GTP) guanosine triphosphate, (NAD) nicotinamide adenine dinucleotide, (NADPH) nicotinamide adenine dinucleotide phosphate, (SAM) *S*-adenosyl methionine, (αKG) alpha-ketoglutarate, (GSH) reduced glutathione.

Vander Heiden and DeBerardinis 2017). Glycolytic intermediates provide a key pool of substrates for biosynthetic reactions: The pentose phosphate shunt produces ribose sugars for nucleotide biosynthesis; dihydroxyacetone phosphate can be converted into glycerol for lipid biosynthesis; serine biosynthesis from 3-phosphoglycerate operates in conjunction with the folate pathway to form one-carbon units for nucleotide production; and multiple glycolytic intermediates can be used for the synthesis of nonessential amino acids. Moreover, glucose-or-acetate-derived acetyl-CoA functions as a key building block for fatty acid and cholesterol biosynthesis.

Analogous to enhanced glucose consumption and glycolytic flux, most leukemias and lymphomas exhibit increased uptake and consumption of glutamine, or glutaminolysis (Fig. 2; Wise and Thompson 2010). Glutamine serves as a nitrogen donor for nucleotide synthesis and for transamination reactions to generate nonessential amino acids. Likewise, glutamine-derived aspartate functions as a key building block for nucleotide biosynthesis (Wise and Thompson 2010). Glutamine also serves as a carbon backbone to generate nonessential amino acids and glutathione, an exchange factor for the import of essential amino acids from the environment, a key anaplerotic substrate to maintain pools of tricarboxylic acid (TCA) cycle intermediates, and an alternative source of acetyl-CoA for lipid biosynthesis via reductive carboxylation. In addition, glutamine and glucose together supply hexosamine biosynthesis for N- and O-linked glycosylation reactions.

Many of the common oncogenic pathways in leukemia and lymphoma (and other cancers) coordinate proliferation with reprogramming of cellular metabolism to meet the anabolic demands of growth and cell division. MYC oncoproteins are frequently overexpressed in leukemias and lymphomas through variety of mechanisms, including enhancer hijacking (Bahr et al. 2018; Schuijers et al. 2018), NOTCH1 activation (Sanchez-Martin and Ferrando 2017), or chromosomal translocations (Altman and Dang 2012). MYC exerts pleiotropic metabolic effects by promoting glucose uptake, glycolytic flux, glutamine uptake, glutaminolysis, nucleotide biosynthesis, lipid synthesis, and mitochondrial and ribosomal biogenesis (Stine et al. 2015). Likewise, RAS pathway activation enhances glucose uptake, increases flux through glycolysis and the nonoxidative pentose phosphate pathway, and promotes macropinocytosis of proteins/lipids that can be metabolized in lysosomes (Kimmelman 2015). Many genetic alterations in leukemias and lymphomas lead to constitutive PI3K/AKT/TOR pathway activation, enhancing glucose uptake, glycolytic flux, amino acid uptake, acetyl-CoA production, and synthesis of lipids and nucleotides (Saxton and Sabatini 2017). Additional leukemia- and lymphoma-specific genetic alterations that reprogram metabolism will be discussed throughout the review where relevant.

Redox balance refers to the relative availability of electron donors (NADH, $FADH_2$, NADPH) and electron acceptors (NAD^+, FAD, $NADP^+$) to perform reduction and oxidation reactions, respectively (Fig. 1). In simplistic terms, cancer cells must maintain sufficient supplies of NADPH and NAD^+ to meet the redox demands of anabolic proliferative metabolism (Hosios and Vander Heiden 2018). NADPH serves a crucial role in regenerating reduced glutathione and other antioxidants that can buffer oxidative damage from reactive oxygen species (ROS) (Sullivan and Chandel 2014). In addition, NADPH functions as an electron donor for key biosynthetic reactions such as lipid synthesis. NADPH can be produced by the oxidative pentose phosphate pathway, isocitrate dehydrogenase enzymes, malic enzyme, or serine-driven one-carbon metabolism in conjunction with the folate pathway (Fan et al. 2014). The relative importance of each source of NADPH varies depending on the cellular context. For example, RAS activation promotes NADPH production via malic enzyme, whereas loss of p53 enhances NADPH production through malic enzyme and the oxidative pentose phosphate pathway (Jiang et al. 2011, 2013; Son et al. 2013). The redox requirements for biosynthetic reactions have been an area of intense investigation in recent years (Hosios and Vander Heiden 2018). Emerging evidence demonstrates that NAD^+ can often be limiting for tumor growth, given its essential function in the biosynthesis of macromolecules (e.g., nucleic acids), which are more oxidized than glucose itself (Garcia-Bermudez et al. 2018; Sullivan et al. 2018; Diehl et al. 2019). Because aerobic glycolysis is redox neutral, glycolysis alone provides no means to generate the "extra" oxidized NAD^+ molecules required for macromolecular biosynthesis. This necessitates some degree of mitochondrial electron transport chain (ETC) activity to eliminate the excess electrons produced during glycolysis by reduction of molecular oxygen to water, which is coupled to regeneration of NAD^+ (Birsoy et al. 2015; Sullivan et al. 2015).

To sustain continuous proliferation, cancer cells or subpopulations of cancer stem-like cells must also avoid terminal differentiation (Fig. 1; Intlekofer and Finley 2019). In both leukemia and lymphoma, impaired differentiation frequently results from genetic alterations in chromatin-modifying enzymes (Feinberg et al. 2016). The discovery of somatic isocitrate dehydrogenase (*IDH*) mutations and the oncometabolite 2-hydroxyglutarate (2HG) demonstrated that aberrant regulation of specific metabolites or metabolic pathways can directly drive dedifferentiation and "stemness" through inhibitory effects on chromatin-modifying enzymes (Fig. 3; Losman and Kaelin 2013). Whereas succinate, fumarate, and 2HG can inhibit demethylation reactions, deposition of methyl marks requires *S*-adenosyl-methionine (SAM) produced by the interlinked methionine and folate cycles (Locasale 2013). Likewise, acetyl-CoA derived from glucose, fatty acids, or free acetate regulates acetylation of histones and other proteins, which can influence gene expression and cell differentiation states (Kinnaird et al. 2016). As will be discussed below, recent discoveries have revealed unexpected new connections between the differentiation state of leukemias and lymphomas with the metabolism of branched chain amino acids, alpha-ketoglutarate, cholesterol, and nucleic acids. Thus, the push and pull to meet anabolic proliferative demands can have downstream effects on metabolites and metabolic pathways that influence chromatin dynamics and cell fate decisions.

Given the breadth of diversity within leukemias and the more than 70 different kinds of lymphoma with distinct cells of origin and lineage-specific metabolic networks, it is difficult to make generalizations that apply to all cases. For example, the metabolic features of aggressive acute leukemias and lymphomas differ substantially from indolent, chronic variants. Notably, even among acute leukemias, there are major

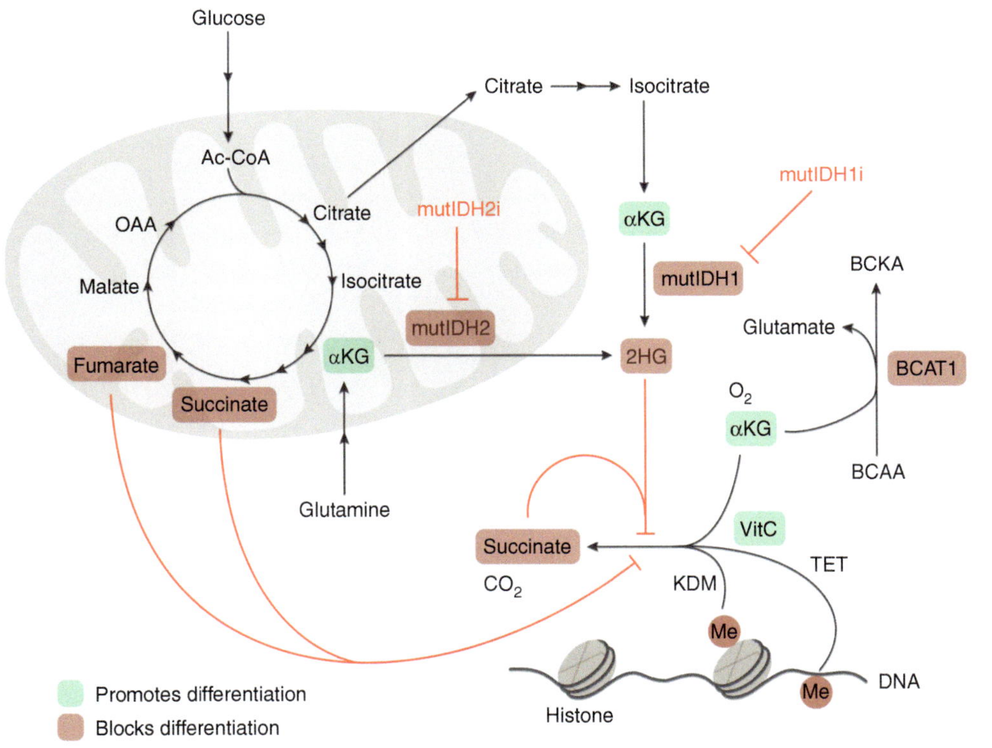

Figure 3. Metabolic inputs into demethylation reactions. Alpha-ketoglutarate (αKG), vitamin C (VitC)/ascorbate, and oxygen (O_2) are required for the demethylation of histones and DNA by histone lysine demethylases (KDM) and ten-eleven-translocation (TET) enzymes, respectively. Fumarate, succinate, and 2-hydroxyglutarate (2HG) inhibit demethylases, resulting in accumulation of repressive methyl marks and impaired cell differentiation. Mutations in isocitrate dehydrogenase 1 or 2 (mutIDH1 or mutIDH2*)* result in enhanced production of 2HG, which can be suppressed by isoform-specific inhibitors (mutIDH1i/mutIDH2i). Overexpression of branched chain amino acid transaminase 1 (BCAT1) results in excessive transfer of α-amino groups from branched chain amino acids (BCAA) to αKG, depletion of αKG, decreased demethylase activity, and impaired differentiation. (OAA) Oxaloacetate, (Me) methyl mark, (BCKA) branched-chain alpha-keto acid.

differences in the metabolic states of myeloid and lymphoid leukemias, with lymphocyte-specific transcriptional programs conferring an energy-poor metabolic state that must be surmounted for transformation and progression (Müschen 2019). Nonetheless, reprogrammed cancer metabolism generally serves at least four important needs of the cancer cell: (1) bioenergetics, (2) biomass accumulation, (3) redox balance, and (4) differentiation blockade (Fig. 1). In this review, we will discuss these hallmarks of cancer metabolism with a focus on leukemia and lymphoma, highlight their clinical relevance, and outline potential strategies for therapeutic targeting.

LEUKEMIA BIOENERGETICS

Glycolysis

Increased glycolysis is a well-recognized hallmark of leukemias (Fig. 2; Boag et al. 2006; Herst et al. 2011; Chen et al. 2014). Oncogenic pathways, such as RAS, MYC, and PI3K/ATK/TOR each induce expression of glucose transporters and glycolytic enzymes and increase glycolytic flux in a wide variety of cancer types, including leukemia and lymphoma (Shim et al. 1997; Osthus et al. 2000; Yun et al. 2009; Coloff et al. 2011; Ying et al. 2012; Poulain et al. 2017). In addition, leukemia-specific genetic alterations, such as BCR-ABL fusions or FLT3 alterations, enhance glycolytic flux and confer oncogenic dependence on glycolysis (Gottschalk et al. 2004; Liu et al. 2014; Ju et al. 2017). Genetic ablation or pharmacologic inhibition of glycolytic machinery, such as glucose transporters, lactate dehydrogenase A (LDHA), or pyruvate kinase M2 (PKM2), can deplete ATP levels, induce cell death, and/or impair proliferation of leukemia cells (Xu et al. 2005; Liu et al. 2014; Wang et al. 2014).

Notably, the B-cell lineage harbors an intrinsic transcriptional program driven by PAX5 and IKZF that suppresses access to glucose and keeps B cells in a relatively energy-poor state compared to myeloid cells (Chan et al. 2017; Martín-Lorenzo et al. 2018; Xiao et al. 2018). Progression of B-cell acute lymphoblastic leukemia (ALL) is associated with genetic events leading to the loss of these transcription factors to allow for increased glucose import, enhanced glycolytic flux, and elevated levels of ATP (Mullighan et al. 2007, 2008; Chan et al. 2017). Interestingly, *PTEN* deletion in B-cell ALL results in enhanced glucose uptake coupled with excessive kinase activation leading to depletion of cellular ATP stores and cell death, thereby conferring a unique oncogenic dependence on PTEN in B-lineage leukemias (Shojaee et al. 2016).

The importance of glycolysis for leukemogenesis and progression is also evident at the level of systemic glucose metabolism. Epidemiologic studies have identified a direct correlation between hyperglycemia and poor response to chemotherapy in ALL (Weiser et al. 2004). Strikingly, acute myeloid leukemia (AML) was shown to induce production of insulin-like growth factor binding protein 1 (IGFBP1) by adipocytes, resulting in systemic insulin resistance, hyperglycemia, and increased glucose availability for the leukemia cells; interventions aimed at reducing hyperglycemia were able to inhibit leukemic progression (Ye et al. 2018b). Likewise, fasting prevented initiation and progression of B- and T-cell ALL via up-regulation of leptin signaling, which exerted a tumor-suppressive effect (Lu et al. 2017). In contrast, a ketogenic diet accelerated leukemic progression in experimental models of AML (Hopkins et al. 2018). This suggests that different dietary strategies to limit systemic glucose availability may have lineage-specific utility or be counteracted by other poorly understood pro-leukemic effects.

The highly glycolytic phenotype of leukemia cells might result in a limited supply of glucose within the bone marrow microenvironment, as significantly lower glucose levels have been measured in leukemic bone marrow compared to peripheral blood (Tiziani et al. 2013). As one strategy to adapt to an insufficient glucose supply, AML cells were shown to enhance fructose uptake by increasing transcription and expression of the GLUT5 fructose transporter, which correlated with inferior survival (Chen et al. 2016). This is of particular importance as high fructose corn syrup, commonly used as a sweetener in processed foods, has been shown to enhance intestinal tumor growth in mice (Goncalves et al. 2019). Of note, pharmacologic inhibition of fructose uptake by AML cells inhibited leukemia growth and synergized with cytarabine chemotherapy (Chen et al. 2016).

Therapeutic targeting of aerobic glycolysis in leukemia has shown minimal success to date. Although 2-deoxyglucose (2-DG) is a useful experimental tool that can inhibit glycolysis and synergize with cytarabine chemotherapy in vitro, it cannot be employed clinically because the high dose of 2-DG required to achieve target inhibition in vivo results in hypoglycemia, as well as cardiac and red blood cell toxicities (Larrue et al. 2015). Furthermore, although highly glycolytic cells appear to be most susceptible to traditional cytotoxic chemotherapies, rare leukemia cell populations dependent on OXPHOS grow out under the pressure of chemotherapy and mediate therapy resistance and relapse (Fig. 4; Farge et al. 2017). More promising results have been shown in AML by targeting altered mitochondrial metabolism, as will be discussed below.

Oxidative Phosphorylation

In contrast to Warburg's initial hypothesis, it is now well established that mitochondrial oxidative phosphorylation (OXPHOS) is essential for leukemia survival and proliferation. Inhibiting mitochondrial function by disrupting mitochondrial protein synthesis (Škrtić et al. 2011), mitochondrial DNA replication (Liyanage et al. 2017), or mitochondrial protein degradation (Cole et al. 2015) effectively kills leukemia stem cells (LSCs) (Fig. 4). The antimicrobial tigecycline was demonstrated to inhibit mitochondrial translation, resulting in selective elimination of leukemia stem and progenitor cells but not their normal counterparts (Škrtić et al. 2011). Likewise, inhibiting mitochondrial DNA replication in leukemia cell lines and primary AML cells disrupted OXPHOS and induced cell death (Liyanage et al. 2017). The mitochondrial protease ClpP was identified as an important regulator of OXPHOS and mitochondrial metabolism in leukemia cells but not normal cells (Cole et al. 2015). Puzzlingly, although AML cells possess a higher mitochondrial mass compared to normal hematopoietic cells,

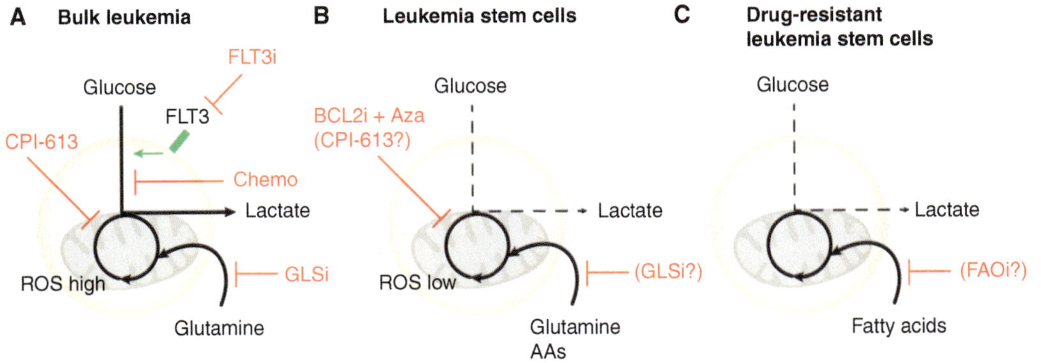

Figure 4. Metabolic vulnerabilities of bulk leukemia and leukemia stem cells. (*A*) Rapidly dividing bulk leukemia cells exhibit high glycolytic activity and high levels of reactive oxygen species (ROS), whereas (*B*) quiescent leukemia stem cells exhibit low levels of ROS and depend on mitochondrial oxidation of alternative fuels, such as amino acids (AAs) or fatty acids. Cytotoxic chemotherapies (Chemo) and inhibitors of mutant fms-like tyrosine kinase 3 (FLT3i) target highly glycolytic bulk leukemia cells, but leukemia stem cells are resistant to these therapies and contribute to disease relapse. (*B*) Mitochondrial metabolism of leukemia stem cells can be targeted by BCL-2 inhibition (BCL2i) in combination with DNA hypomethylating agents, such as azacitidine (Aza). (*C*) Leukemia stem cells can develop therapeutic resistance by changing their mitochondrial fuel source from AAs to fatty acids. Novel metabolic targeted therapeutics such as inhibitors of glutamine metabolism (GLSi), TCA cycle enzymes (CPI-613), or fatty acid oxidation (FAOi) are under investigation in clinical trials.

this does not seem to correspond with an enhanced capacity for respiratory chain complex activity (Sriskanthadevan et al. 2015).

Selective utilization of OXPHOS has also been identified as a key feature of AML cells that are resistant to cytotoxic chemotherapy (Fig. 4; Farge et al. 2017; Baccelli et al. 2019). AML cells resistant to cytarabine treatment in mouse xenografts were found to be primarily reliant on OXPHOS for their survival (Farge et al. 2017), and ETC inhibitors were selectively toxic to a distinct subset of chemotherapy-resistant AML (Baccelli et al. 2019). Furthermore, OXPHOS was demonstrated to be required for tyrosine kinase inhibitor (TKI)-resistant chronic myeloid leukemia (CML) stem cells; inhibition of mitochondrial protein translation with tigecycline in combination with TKIs was able to eliminate these resistant stem cells (Kuntz et al. 2017).

Several recent publications have shown that disrupting OXPHOS by targeting mitochondrial ETC has therapeutic potential in AML. Targeting the ETC complex I with the small-molecule inhibitor IACS-010759 resulted in potent inhibition of proliferation and induction of apoptosis in vitro and improved leukemia-specific survival in mouse models of AML (Molina et al. 2018). These promising preclinical findings resulted in a phase I clinical trial of IACS-010759 for patients with relapsed and treatment-refractory AML (NCT02882321). Additionally, the ERBB2 inhibitor mubritinib, which was recently shown to inhibit ETC complex I activity, exerted significant antileukemic activity against chemotherapy-resistant AML cells with OXPHOS hyperactivity (Baccelli et al. 2019).

The therapeutic benefit achieved by targeting OXPHOS in AML has further been demonstrated by the recently U.S. Federal Drug Administration (FDA)-approved combination of the BCL2 inhibitor venetoclax with the DNA hypomethylating agent azacitidine (DiNardo et al. 2019). This drug combination, which results in unprecedented high response rates, was recently shown to eliminate LSCs by targeting mitochondrial OXPHOS (Fig. 4; Lagadinou et al. 2013; Pollyea et al. 2018; DiNardo et al. 2019). Mechanistically, venetoclax in combination with azacitidine appears to inhibit ETC complex II activity by disrupting glutathionylation of succinate dehydrogenase (Pollyea et al. 2018). It was further demonstrated that venetoclax can directly inhibit ETC complex I (Sharon et al. 2019). Additionally, disrupted heme biosynthesis could potentiate venetoclax-induced apoptosis through the loss of ETC activity (Lin et al. 2019). Further clinical evidence for the importance of the ETC in mediating sensitivity of leukemia cells to venetoclax + azacitidine comes from the observation that *IDH* mutations induce a dependence on BCL2, likely explaining the especially high response rates of *IDH*-mutated AML to this treatment combination (Chan et al. 2015). Mutant IDH-derived 2HG, among many other effects, inhibited the activity of cytochrome *c* oxidase (COX) in the ETC, thereby lowering the mitochondrial threshold to trigger apoptosis upon BCL2 inhibition (Chan et al. 2015).

An alternative strategy to inhibit mitochondrial metabolism is to directly interfere with the activity of the TCA cycle. Glutamine depletion or inhibition of glutamine metabolism by blocking the rate-limiting enzyme glutaminase impairs TCA anaplerosis and blocks OXPHOS (Fig. 4; Emadi 2015; Jacque et al. 2015; Matre et al. 2016; Gallipoli et al. 2018; Gregory et al. 2018). The lipoic acid analog CPI-613 is a first-in-class TCA cycle inhibitor purported to disrupt lipoylation of pyruvate dehydrogenase (PDH) and α-KG dehydrogenase (OGDH) (Stuart et al. 2014). CPI-613 showed modest activity in early-phase clinical trials in patients with advanced hematological malignancies (Pardee et al. 2014) and AML (Pardee et al. 2018). CPI-613 is currently being tested in combination with chemotherapy for patients with relapsed/refractory AML in randomized phase III clinical trial (NCT03504410).

Fatty Acid Oxidation

Fatty acid oxidation (FAO) provides electron donors NADH and $FADH_2$ to ETC complex I and complex II, respectively, and produces acetyl-CoA, which can be oxidized in the TCA cycle or deposited on histones for regulation of gene expression (Carracedo et al. 2013; Ye et al. 2016; Farge et al. 2017). FAO has been shown to mediate resistance to a variety of antileukemic agents (Fig. 4; German et al. 2016; Jones et al. 2018). Chemotherapy-resistant CML LSCs were demonstrated to induce lipolysis in the gonadal adipose tissue niche and capture free fatty acids through increased expression of the fatty acid transporter CD36 (Ye et al. 2016). Utilizing patient-derived xenograft models of primary human AML, it was shown that the cytarabine-resistant residual AML cells were characterized by high OXPHOS activity, increased FAO, and up-regulated CD36 expression; inhibiting FAO induced an energetic shift toward low OXPHOS status and significantly augmented the antileukemic effects of cytarabine (Farge et al. 2017). Notably, whereas newly diagnosed AML exhibited impressively high response rates to venetoclax + azacitidine, response rates in relapsed/refractory AML were much lower (DiNardo et al. 2019; Bewersdorf et al. 2020). One possible explanation for this observation could be differences in the metabolism of LSCs at diagnosis versus at time of disease relapse (Jones et al. 2018). Treatment-naive LSCs exhibited dependence on amino acid uptake for OXPHOS maintenance and could not up-regulate FAO metabolism to preserve TCA cycle activity, whereas LSCs from patients at the time of relapse were able to compensate for the loss of amino acids by rewiring their metabolism toward FAO (Jones et al. 2018). Several different inhibitors of FAO have exhibited promising activity in preclinical AML models. Inhibition of FAO with the carnitine palmitoyltransferase 1 (CPT1) inhibitor etomoxir induced apoptosis in AML cells, which was synergistic with the BCL2 inhibitor ABT-731 and cytarabine (Samudio et al. 2010). Likewise, a novel CPT1b inhibitor ST1326 (Teglicar) demonstrated significant activity against both AML cell lines and primary samples, in conjunction with a more favorable safety profile (Ricciardi et al. 2015).

LEUKEMIA BIOMASS

Amino Acids

Asparaginase exploits the unusual dependency of ALL cells on exogenous supply of the nonessential amino acid asparagine and represents of the best-known metabolic dependencies in cancer (Clavell et al. 1986; Akagi et al. 2006; Williams et al. 2020). Compared to ALL cells, AML cells demonstrate reduced sensitivity to asparagine depletion, and asparaginase is not part of standard therapeutic regimens in AML. Asparaginase resistance in AML appears to be attributable to both variable expression levels of asparagine synthetase (ASNS) levels in AML cells as well as production of cathepsin B, a protease that inactivates L-asparaginase, by mesenchymal stromal cells and monocytes/macrophages in the bone marrow microenvironment of AML cells (Michelozzi et al. 2019). Additionally, bone marrow adipocytes have been shown mediate resistance to asparaginase by producing glutamine that can be captured by AML cells (Ehsanipour et al. 2013). However, there has been an intense search for other amino acid dependencies in AML and glutamine, arginine, and cysteine have been shown to represent potential metabolic dependencies in AML, as will be discussed below.

Inhibition of glutamine utilization in leukemia cells by genetic or pharmacological targeting of glutaminase exerted potent antileukemic activity, which could be augmented by chemotherapy (Fig. 4; Jacque et al. 2015). Although FLT3 inhibitors potently down-regulated glycolysis in myeloid leukemia cells, glutamine metabolism remained unaffected (Gallipoli et al. 2018). However, combining FLT3 inhibitors with the glutaminase inhibitor CB-839 resulted in synergistic antileukemic activity (Gallipoli et al. 2018; Gregory et al. 2018). Furthermore, inhibition of glutaminase depleted cellular stores of reduced glutathione, leading to increased mitochondrial ROS and synergistic toxicity when combined with arsenic trioxide (Gregory et al. 2019) or venetoclax (Emadi 2015; Jacque et al. 2015). Likewise, glutaminase inhibition synergized with NOTCH inhibition in T-ALL, although this effect could be counteracted by *PTEN* loss, which induced a switch to a hyperglycolytic state (Herranz et al. 2015). As an alternative strategy, genetic or pharmacological inhibition of the amino acid transporter ASCT2, whose preferred substrate is glutamine, blocked TOR signaling and induced apoptosis in MLL-

AF9-driven leukemia cells (Ni et al. 2019). These preclinical findings prompted several clinical trials attempting to target glutamine metabolism in myeloid neoplasms, either alone or in combination with other agents (NCT02071927; NCT03047993) (Wang et al. 2015b).

Arginine is important for the synthesis of protein, nitric oxide, polyamines, and other amino acids, such as glutamate and proline; cells can either import arginine or synthesize it from citrulline by utilizing argininosuccinate synthetase-1 (ASS1) (Szlosarek 2014). A subgroup of AML lacks ASS1 expression and relies on the import of arginine, potentially conferring susceptibility to arginine deprivation therapy (Miraki-Moud et al. 2015). Moreover, AML with overexpression of ecotropic virus integration site 1 protein (EVI1) relies on a functional creatine kinase pathway, which in turn depends on sufficient supply of arginine, to maintain cytosolic ATP levels and mitochondrial OXPHOS activity (Fenouille et al. 2017). Arginine-depleting enzymes, arginine deiminase (ADI-PEG 20) and arginase (BCT-100), demonstrated antileukemic activity in AML models with low or absent expression levels of ASS1 (Miraki-Moud et al. 2015; Mussai et al. 2015). However, when ADI-PEG20 was tested in a phase II trial in RR-AML patients, only 9.5% of patients achieved a complete response despite almost all pretreatment tumor samples showing ASS1 deficiency (NCT01910012) (Tsai et al. 2017). Somewhat counterintuitively to the above described dependence of AML blasts on arginine for proliferation, AML blasts have also been shown to secrete arginase II leading to inhibition of arginine-dependent T cells and immune evasion (Mussai et al. 2013).

The combination of venetoclax + azacitidine was shown to decrease amino acid uptake in LSCs, which were uniquely reliant on amino acid metabolism for OXPHOS and survival (Fig. 4; Jones et al. 2018). Whereas the bulk population of leukemia cells were able to adapt to amino acid starvation by increasing FAO to supply TCA cycle intermediates and energy, LSCs appeared to be more metabolically inflexible and unable to compensate for the decreased amino acid uptake induced by venetoclax + azacitidine (Jones et al. 2018). Subsequent studies demonstrated that cysteine was particularly important for the viability of LSCs (Jones et al. 2019). Depletion of cysteine resulted in impaired glutathione synthesis, loss of glutathionylation of succinate dehydrogenase A, impaired ETC complex II activity, and cell death (Jones et al. 2019).

Lipids

Rapidly dividing leukemia cells need to meet the high demand for phospholipids, cholesterol, and triglycerides required for the synthesis of cell membrane structures (Currie et al. 2013). Apoptosis of AML cells can be induced by inhibiting the lipogenic enzymes fatty acid synthase (FASN) and stearoyl CoA desaturase 1 (SCD1) (Pizer et al. 1996; Khanim et al. 2009; Southam et al. 2015). However, in a phase I trial testing combination of lipid-regulating bezafibrate and the sex hormone medroxyprogesterone acetate, which was shown to inhibit SCD1, only one of 19 patients with AML achieved a partial response (Murray et al. 2010).

Several studies have focused on redeploying statins as anticancer therapy after an antileukemic effect of statin drugs was recognized early on in AML (Newman et al. 1994; Clutterbuck et al. 1998; Dimitroulakos et al. 2000). Statins inhibit HMG-CoA reductase, the rate-limiting enzyme of the mevalonate pathway that produces cholesterol, ubiquinone, dolichol, and geranylgeranyl/farnesyl pyrophosphate (Wong et al. 2002). Although some early-phase nonrandomized clinical trials showed some encouraging response rates when combining pravastatin with idarubicin and cytarabine in patients with relapsed/refractory AML, a similar trial in the up-front treatment setting was unable to confirm these results (Kornblau et al. 2007; Shadman et al. 2015; Advani et al. 2018). It is possible the differential activity was due to alterations in cholesterol and lipid metabolism induced by prior chemotherapy, as described above (Kornblau et al. 2007; Shadman et al. 2015; Farge et al. 2017; Advani et al. 2018). Recently, statins were shown to prime leukemia and lymphoma cells for venetoclax-mediated apoptosis via suppressed protein geranylgeranylation, resulting in induction of the proapoptotic protein p53 up-regulated modulator of apoptosis (PUMA) (Lee et al. 2018). In a retrospective multivariate regression analysis of three studies examining venetoclax in patients with chronic lymphocytic leukemia (CLL), statins were associated with significantly increased odds of attaining a complete response (OR 2.68, $P = 0.0054$) (Lee et al. 2018).

Nucleotides

Mitochondrial electron transport function plays a vital role in regenerating NAD^+ to enable aspartate production and nucleotide biosynthesis (Birsoy et al. 2015; Sullivan et al. 2015, 2018; Garcia-Bermudez et al. 2018). The sensitivity to ETC inhibition varied across cancer cell lines, with cell lines resistant to ETC inhibition being able to maintain aspartate levels by import through the aspartate-glutamate transporter SLC1A3 (Garcia-Bermudez et al. 2018). Because ETC inhibition is under investigation as a promising antileukemic therapy (venetoclax and IACS-01075), the ability of a leukemic cell to maintain aspartate levels in response to ETC inhibition may determine sensitivity to this treatment strategy. Indeed, antileukemic activity of IACS-01075 was associated with reduced aspartate production and impaired nucleotide biosynthesis (Molina et al. 2018).

Antimetabolites, which mimic purines (e.g., fludarabine, 6-MP) or pyrimidines (e.g., cytarabine) required for DNA synthesis or interfere with folate-dependent nucleotide synthesis (e.g., methotrexate), represent the oldest effective treatments for leukemia (Farber and Diamond 1948). Modern genetic studies have confirmed the importance of nucleotide biosynthesis in leukemia. For example, ablation of methylenetetrahydrofolate dehydrogenase-cyclohydrolase 2 (MTHFD2), a key enzyme in the one-carbon folate metabolism and purine synthesis, inhibited leukemic growth and promoted differentiation of AML blasts in vivo (Pikman et al. 2016). Thiopurine-resistant ALL acquired gain-of-function mutations in the enzyme NT5C2, which facilitates removal of toxic nucleotide intermediates that build up in the context of thiopurine treatment; notably, NTC52 mutations created a new vulnerability to inosine-5′-monophosphate dehydrogenase (IMPDH) inhibition (Meyer et al. 2013; Tzoneva et al. 2013, 2018; Dieck et al. 2018). Utilizing a large drug screening approach, inhibition of dihydro-orotate dehydrogenase (DHODH) with brequinar sodium was found to inhibit leukemia growth by promoting myeloid differentiation of AML blasts (Sykes et al. 2016). DHODH is a mitochondrial enzyme that catalyzes the ubiquinone-mediated conversion of dihydro-orotate to orotate in the pyrimidine biosynthetic pathway. Based on this promising preclinical activity, multiple DHODH inhibitors are being tested in early phase clinical trials for a variety of myeloid malignancies (Sykes et al. 2016; Ladds et al. 2018; Wu et al. 2018b; Cao et al. 2019; Christian et al. 2019).

LEUKEMIA REDOX

Conventional chemotherapy induces redox stress in the form of ROS (Trachootham et al. 2009). Significant differences in ROS levels distinguish the rapidly dividing bulk population of leukemia cells from quiescent LSCs, which have been proposed to drive chemotherapy resistance and relapse (Lagadinou et al. 2013). Functionally defined LSCs exhibited relatively low levels of ROS, increased BCL2 expression, and dependence on OXPHOS for survival (Lagadinou et al. 2013). Treatment of AML LSCs with the BCL2 inhibitor venetoclax in combination with azacitidine resulted in depletion of cysteine and the antioxidant glutathione, leading to increased ROS levels and disruption of ETC complex II function (Pollyea et al. 2018; DiNardo et al. 2019; Jones et al. 2019). Alternative strategies to disrupt cysteine metabolism can deplete intracellular pools of reduced glutathione, increased ROS, and blocked growth of CLL (Zhang et al. 2012; Cramer et al. 2017). Likewise, targeting the pentose phosphate pathway, an important source of NADPH for buffering oxidative stress, displayed antileukemic activity toward chemoresistant AML (Bhanot et al. 2017; Poulain et al. 2017).

LEUKEMIA DIFFERENTIATION

The discovery of leukemia-associated mutations in IDH enzymes provided seminal insights into the interplay between metabolism, epigenetics, and differentiation (Dang et al. 2009; Mardis et al. 2009; Ward et al. 2010). Mutant IDH enzymes lose normal enzyme function and gain the ability to produce the oncometabolite 2HG. 2HG inhibits the function of αKG-dependent chromatin-modifying enzymes, resulting in blockade of myeloid differentiation (Fig. 3; Figueroa et al. 2010; Lu et al. 2012; Turcan et al. 2012; Rohle et al. 2013; Wang et al. 2013; Yen et al. 2017). In addition, 2HG can inhibit the function of enzymes involved in RNA demethylation, DNA repair, hypoxia-inducible factor (HIF) stability, collagen maturation, and intermediary metabolism (Koivunen et al. 2012; Chan et al. 2015; Fu et al. 2015; Wang et al. 2015c; Sulkowski et al. 2017, 2020; McBrayer et al. 2018; Su et al. 2018). Because some of effects of 2HG can be tumor-suppressive, the net effect of *IDH* mutations and 2HG in a given cell lineage likely depends on the balance of oncogenic and tumor-suppressive activities (Elkashef et al. 2017; Ye et al. 2018a). Importantly, small-molecule inhibitors of mutant IDH enzymes can suppress 2HG production, restore myeloid differentiation, and induce clinical responses in ∼40% of patients with relapsed/refractory *IDH*-mutant AML, leading to their recent FDA approvals for this indication (Fig. 3; Stein et al. 2017; DiNardo et al. 2018).

The branched chain amino acid amino transferase 1 (BCAT1) also influences αKG levels and has been shown to regulate leukemogenesis and leukemia cell differentiation (Hattori et al. 2017; Raffel et al. 2017). In AML, overexpression of BCAT1 caused excessive transfer of α-amino groups from branched chain amino acids (BCAAs) to αKG, resulting in depletion of αKG stores, DNA hypermethylation, and impaired myeloid differentiation (Fig. 3; Raffel et al. 2017). This BCAT1-mediated mechanism can mimic the epigenetic effects of 2HG in *IDH*-wild-type AML. In contrast, in CML blast crisis, overexpression of BCAT1 promoted excessive conversion of branched chain keto acids to BCAAs, which promoted leukemogenesis through TOR activation (Hattori et al. 2017).

Vitamin C, or ascorbate, functions as an essential cofactor for a variety of αKG- and Fe^{2+}-dependent enzymes, including TET enzymes involved in DNA demethylation (Fig. 3; Cimmino et al. 2018). Vitamin C promoted enhanced TET activity, promoted DNA demethylation, and restored differentiation in models of myeloid leukemia (Agathocleous et al. 2017; Cimmino et al. 2017). Vitamin C may also act by depleting glutathione and increasing ROS levels (Yun et al. 2015). It remains unclear whether vitamin C could be used clinically—for example, as a preventative strategy in TET2-mutant clonal hematopoiesis (Huijskens et al. 2016). Notably, prior attempts to use vitamin C as an antineoplastic agent were not successful (Moertel et al. 1985), but more recent work suggests that vitamin C may be effective in *KRAS/RAF*-mutant cancers (Yun et al. 2015). The vitamin B6 pathway was also recently identified as a metabolic dependence in AML; perturbation of the pathway with isoniazid resulted in antileukemic activity in vivo (Chen et al. 2020).

LYMPHOMA BIOENERGETICS

Glycolysis

Enhanced glycolysis in lymphoma is evident from the utility of fluorodeoxyglucose positron emission tomography (FDG PET) scans for staging and response assessment and the use of blood LDH levels for prognostication (Seam et al. 2007; Sehn et al. 2007). The degree of glucose uptake, as measured by FDG avidity, effectively distinguishes indolent and aggressive forms of lymphoma (Noy et al. 2009). Aggressive forms of B-cell lymphoma exhibit aberrant overexpression of MYC, either through chromosomal translocations or transcriptional deregulation (Stine et al. 2015). Numerous studies have demonstrated that MYC enhances glycolytic flux through direct transactivation of glucose transporters (GLUT1), glycolytic enzymes (e.g., PFK, enolase), and LDHA (Shim et al. 1997; Osthus et al. 2000). In a model of Burkitt lymphoma with inducible control of MYC expression, MYC drove Warburg-like aerobic glycolysis with increased glucose consumption and lactate production (Le et al. 2012). This effect of MYC was counteracted by the activity of the energy-stress kinase AMPK, as deletion of AMPK accelerated MYC-induced lymphomagenesis (Faubert et al. 2013). Both PI3K/AKT/TOR and NF-κB signaling can cooperate with MYC to enhance GLUT1 transporter expression and transport to the cell surface (Sommermann et al. 2011; Bhatt et al. 2012; Broecker-Preuss et al. 2017). Epstein–Barr virus (EBV)-driven lymphomagenesis is characterized by an initial energy-poor state sustained by autophagy with progression of disease associated with up-regulation of the GLUT1 transporter and increased glycolytic flux (Bhatt et al. 2012; McFadden et al. 2016). In addition, targeting glucose uptake and/or glycolysis was demonstrated to abolish MCL-1 expression and overcome resistance to BCL2 inhibitors in DLBCL (Coloff et al. 2011).

The glycolytic enzyme glyceraldehyde 3-phosphate dehydrogenase (GAPDH) has been identified as a metabolic marker of aggressive DLBCL, irrespective of MYC expression (Chiche et al. 2015). Despite having more aggressive pathologic features, DLBCL with high expression of GAPDH predicted for better outcomes in response to R-CHOP chemotherapy (Chiche et al. 2019). In contrast, GAPDH-low DLBCL produced less ATP from glycolysis, preferentially used mitochondrial OXPHOS, and exhibited higher TOR activity. Several patients with GAPDH-low DLBCL responded to a combination of metabolic agents, including asparaginase, temsirolimus (TOR inhibitor), and metformin (ETC complex I inhibitor). In contrast to GAPDH, overexpression of glycolytic enzyme hexokinase 2 (HK2) was shown to mediate therapeutic resistance in DLBCL and ablation of HK2 inhibited lymphoma growth (Gu et al. 2018). Interestingly, the histone deacetylase (HDAC) inhibitor panobinostat was shown to diminish HK2 expression and restore platinum chemosensitivity in DLBCL cells (Nakajima et al. 2019).

Diabetes has been associated with increased risk of non-Hodgkin lymphoma (NHL), possibly because of increased glucose availability for lymphoma cells (Mitri et al. 2008; Castillo et al. 2012). Compounds targeting glucose uptake pathways in cancer cells have yet to demonstrate viability for clinical practice as a result of unacceptably low target specificity (Montrose and Galluzzi 2019). However, emerging evidence suggests that glucocorticoids may act, at least in part, through inhibition of glucose uptake by malignant lymphoid cells (Holleman et al. 2004; Hulleman et al. 2009; Chan et al. 2017).

Oxidative Phosphorylation

Numerous studies have demonstrated that DLBCL can be segregated into distinct subtypes based on mitochondrial OXPHOS activity (Fig. 5; Monti et al. 2005; Caro et al. 2012). Mechanistic studies found that the OXPHOS subset of DLBCL had increased activity of and dependence on mitochondrial FAO. Intriguingly, when B-cell receptor (BCR) signaling was inhibited in other subtypes of DLBCL, there was a shift from glycolysis to increased FAO, suggesting that this might represent a metabolic mechanism of adaptation and/or resistance to targeted therapies in DLBCL (Fig. 5; Caro et al. 2012). Recent investigations demonstrated that the genes involved in OXPHOS (e.g., ETC complexes I, III, IV, V) were largely dependent on MYC for translation (Singh et al. 2019). Another line of evidence supports a role for glutamine-dependent OXPHOS as a mediator of ibrutinib resistance in mantle cell lymphoma (MCL), potentially driven by MYC and TOR activity (Lee et al. 2019; Zhang et al. 2019a). Ibrutinib-resistant MCL was uniquely dependent on glutamine uptake and glutaminolysis; disruption of glutamine metabolism or ETC complex I increased ROS, induced energetic stress, and overcame resistance to ibrutinib. Enhanced OXPHOS was recently identified as a mechanism of resistance to the BCL2 inhibitor venetoclax in lymphoma, and treatment with ETC inhibitors restored sensitivity to venetoclax (Chukkapalli et al. 2018; Guièze et al. 2019).

LYMPHOMA BIOMASS

Amino Acids

MYC drives glutamine uptake and glutaminolysis (Stine et al. 2015). In MYC-driven lymphomas, MYC-induced expression of the glutamine

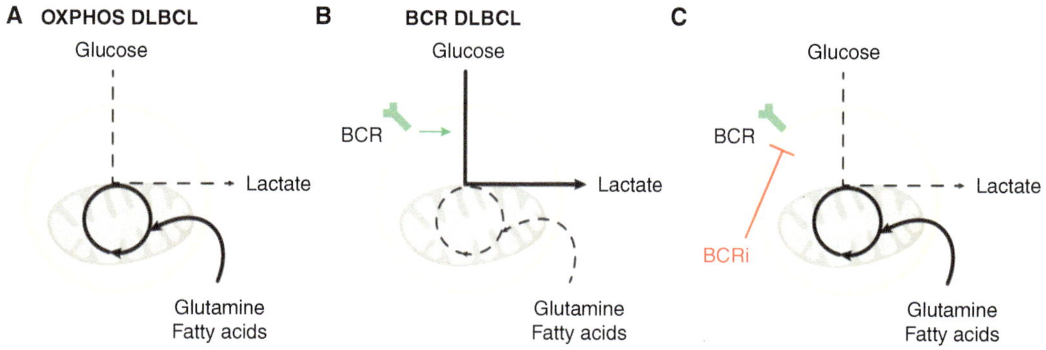

Figure 5. Metabolic subtypes of diffuse large B cell lymphoma (DLBCL). Gene expression and metabolic profiling distinguishes subtypes of DLBCL based on activity of and dependency on mitochondrial oxidative phosphorylation (OXPHOS). (*A*) OXPHOS DLBCL exhibits relatively low glycolytic flux and enhanced mitochondrial oxidation of glutamine and fatty acids. (*B*) B-cell receptor (BCR) DLBCL exhibits enhanced glycolytic flux and limited mitochondrial OXPHOS. (*C*) Inhibition of BCR signaling (BCRi) in BCR DLBCL results in decreased glycolysis and increased mitochondrial OXPHOS as a putative adaptive response.

transporters SLC7A5 and SLC1A5 and relieved microRNA-mediated inhibition of glutaminase expression (Gao et al. 2009). Glutamine deprivation depleted TCA cycle intermediates, ATP, and glutathione, resulting in lymphoma cell death (Gao et al. 2009). Likewise, in MYC-driven Burkitt lymphoma, glutamine deprivation activated the integrated stress response (e.g., GCN2-elF2α, ATF4) and proapoptotic pathways (e.g., PUMA, NOXA, BAX) (Qing et al. 2012). Additional evidence demonstrated that DLBCL requires the mitochondrial lysine deacetylase SIRT3 to maintain glutamine flux into the TCA cycle via glutamate dehydrogenase (Li et al. 2019).

In addition to *MYC*, direct mutations in genes that mediate amino acid sensing have been identified in follicular lymphoma (FL) (Okosun et al. 2016; Ying et al. 2016). Approximately 17% of patients with FL harbored mutations in *RRAGC*, which encodes for RagC. RagC normally forms a complex with Ragulator, V-ATPase, and SLC38A9 to activate TOR in response to amino acids. Lymphoma-associated *RRAGC* mutants aberrantly activated TOR even in conditions of amino acid deprivation, relieved dependency on activation/stimulation signals from CD4$^+$ T cells, and conferred heightened sensitivity to TOR inhibitors (Ortega-Molina et al. 2019; Wang et al. 2019a). FL also harbors mutations in *ATP6V1B2* (V-ATPase subunit) or deletions of *SESTRIN1* (negative regulator of TOR), which analogously function to stimulate aberrant TOR activity (Oricchio et al. 2017; Ortega-Molina et al. 2019; Wang et al. 2019a).

Analogous to its application in ALL, asparaginase demonstrates selective activity for natural killer (NK)-cell lymphoma, a relatively rare and aggressive form of EBV-driven lymphoma that depends on exogenous asparagine for survival (Chien et al. 2015; d'Amore et al. 2015). Asparagine depletion activated the integrated stress response (GCN2/elF2α/ATF4) and suppressed TOR activity, but failure to activate ATF-mediated ASNS expression and increase asparaginase synthesis resulted in cell death (Bunpo et al. 2009; Ye et al. 2010; Chien et al. 2015). Response to asparaginase was further associated with proteolytic cleavage of BCL2A1, which converted it from an antiapoptotic to a proapoptotic factor (Chien et al. 2015). Loss of critical genes involved in polyamine metabolism (AMD1, eIF5A) was shown to promote lymphomagenesis, suggesting that metabolism of amino acids in the urea cycle can exert tumor-suppressive effects in some lymphomas (Scuoppo et al. 2012).

Lipids

Up-regulated lipid synthesis has been observed across a range of lymphoma types, which can create a therapeutic vulnerability to fatty acid synthase inhibitors (Bhatt et al. 2012). Lipid droplets have long been recognized as a pathologic hallmark of Burkitt lymphoma, the prototypical MYC-driven cancer (Morrish et al. 2010; Ambrosio et al. 2012; Eberlin et al. 2014). Mechanistically, MYC induces the transcription factor sterol-regulated element-binding protein (SREBP1) and cooperates with SREBP1 to drive expression of key enzymes involved in fatty acid synthesis, fatty acid elongation, and phospholipid synthesis; these effects were coordinated with MYC-induced glycolysis and glutaminolysis to provide acetyl-CoA building blocks for lipid synthesis (Southam et al. 2015; Gouw et al. 2019). Similarly, MYC was shown to induce phosphocholine synthesis in DLBCL through transcriptional activation of PCYT1A (Xiong et al. 2017). Inhibition of lipid synthesis impaired growth of MYC-dependent lymphomas (Xiong et al. 2017; Gouw et al. 2019). Cholesterol metabolism offers a potential vulnerability for some lymphomas. For example, ALK^+ anaplastic large cell lymphoma (ALCL) lacks expression of squalene monooxygenase (SQLE), which catalyzes the rate-limiting step of cholesterol synthesis (Garcia-Bermudez et al. 2019). Thus, ALK^+ ALCL cells were functionally auxotrophic for exogenous cholesterol and inhibition of cholesterol import was a therapeutic vulnerability. Interestingly, loss of SQLE was suggested to confer a fitness advantage by allowing accumulation of squalene, which could block ferroptotic cell death in response oxidative stress (Garcia-Bermudez et al. 2019).

Nucleotides

Nucleotide synthesis represents another therapeutic vulnerability in lymphomas, as evidenced by the long-standing use of methotrexate and pralatrexate in these diseases. Targeted inhibition of serine hydroxymethyltransferases 1 and 2 (SHMT1/2), key enzymes in serine-driven one-carbon folate metabolism, impeded purine biosynthesis, disrupted DNA/histone methylation, and arrested B-cell lymphoma proliferation; concurrent glycine restriction and/or inhibition of glycine uptake augmented this effect (Ducker et al. 2017; Parsa et al. 2020). EBV-driven lymphomas exhibit increased uptake of serine and glycine and enhanced metabolic flux through the one-carbon folate pathway for nucleotide biosynthesis (Wang et al. 2019b, 2019c). These effects appear to be driven by the EBV protein EBNA2, and targeting one-carbon folate metabolism via inhibition of SHTM1/2 markedly decreased EBV-driven B-cell lymphoproliferation.

LYMPHOMA REDOX

Increased ETC activity created a potential metabolic vulnerability from mitochondrial ROS, such that OXPHOS DLBCL cells were particularly sensitive to depletion of antioxidants (Norberg et al. 2017). In a variety of B- and T-cell lymphoma lines, inhibition of ETC complex I by metformin or other agents increased ROS and impaired mitochondrial oxygen consumption (Khan et al. 2019). Mitochondrial ROS stabilized hypoxia-inducible factor (HIF) and increased glycolytic flux and glucose dependence; concomitant ablation of HIF induced cell death (Khan et al. 2019). Ferroptosis, a form of programmed cell death triggered by lipid peroxidation, could be induced in DLBCL cells by targeted inhibition of the cystine-glutamine antiporter xCT (Zhang et al. 2019b). In ALCL, oxidative stress induced a reversion to a more stem-like state driven by activation of the WNT/β-catenin signaling; inhibiting WNT signaling reversed this effect and overcame chemoresistance (Wu et al. 2018a). In B-cell lymphomas and leukemias, the pentose phosphate pathway was shown to play a critical role in generating NADPH to buffer oxidative stress. For this reason, B-cell malignancies exhibited a unique dependency on the phosphatase PP2A, which inhibits PFK2B, limits production of fructose-2,6-bisphosphate, and ensures adequate glycolytic flux through glucose-6-phosphate dehydrogenase (G6PD) and the pentose phosphate shunt (Xiao et al. 2018). This created a therapeutic vulnerability such that combined inhibition of PP2A and G6PD dramatically depleted NADPH and glutathione pools, increased ROS, and synergized in lymphoma cell killing.

LYMPHOMA DIFFERENTIATION

Of all lymphoid malignancies, only angioimmunoblastic T-cell lymphoma (AITL) exhibits recurrent mutations in IDH enzymes (Cairns et al. 2012; Wang et al. 2015a). *IDH2*-mutant AITL exhibited decreased 5-hydoxymethylcytosine and increased 5-methylcytosine because of inhibition of TET enzymes by the oncometabolite 2HG. Likewise, histone methylation was enhanced in *IDH2*-mutant versus wild-type cases. In mouse models, *IDH2* mutations were shown to impair T lymphocyte development and differentiation, decreasing thymocyte numbers and skewing mature T cells toward memory phenotypes (Lemonnier et al. 2016). This suggests that *IDH2* mutations may cause an arrest in T-cell development, analogous to the stemness promoting effects of *IDH* mutations in AML. Enzymes that regulate TCA cycle metabolites have also been explored in DLBCL, in which 9% of 69 tumor samples were shown to have loss-of-function mutations of the 2HG-disposal enzyme D2HGDH (Lin et al. 2015). Loss of D2HGDH was associated with increased 2HG and decreased αKG levels, which increased repressive methylation of histones and DNA. However, further work is needed to determine whether 2HG metabolism offers a viable therapeutic target in lymphomas.

CONCLUDING REMARKS

We have described how leukemias and lymphomas rewire metabolism to support rapid cell growth and proliferation and, in some cases, couple this to dedifferentiation and self-renewal. Investigations into blood cancer metabolism have led to promising new therapies that target mitochondrial oxidative function, mutant IDH enzymes, pyrimidine biosynthesis, or serine production. Furthermore, long-standing metabolically targeted therapies such as methotrexate remain cornerstones of treatment for many patients with leukemias and lymphomas. As novel therapies advance further in clinical development with concurrent laboratory-based studies, important new insights will be made into the mechanisms by which targeting cancer cell metabolism can exert pleotropic downstream effects. For example, it remains unclear how targeting specific metabolic pathways apparently involved in biosynthetic processes triggers differentiation in leukemia, such as DHODH.

Of particular interest are those metabolically targeted therapies that can specifically target cancer stem cells, which are hypothesized to drive resistance to conventional treatments and contribute to disease relapses. Why LSCs appear to be particularly dependent on mitochondrial oxidative metabolism remains unclear. It is possible that these cancer stem cells reside in microenvironmental niches with restricted access to glucose, necessitating the use of alternative fuels such as amino acids or fatty acids that can only generate ATP through mitochondrial oxidation. Because LSCs are not highly proliferative, they might not depend on the high glycolytic flux and Warburg-like metabolism required for rapidly doubling biomass. This would also make them inherently resistant to most conventional therapies that target macromolecular biosynthetic pathways, in particular nucleic acid biosynthesis and DNA replication. However, to truly understand the metabolic state of LSCs, new technologies that allow for in situ assessments of metabolite levels, metabolic flux, and mitochondrial function will be required.

Another emerging realm of importance is the complex interplay between cancer cell metabolism, the tumor microenvironment, and antitumor immune responses. For example, 2HG and lactate have been demonstrated to disrupt antitumor T-cell differentiation (Brand et al. 2016; Xia et al. 2017; Bunse et al. 2018), whereas lactate can also promote differentiation of suppressive macrophages (Colegio et al. 2014). Likewise, tumor microenvironmental factors, such as hypoxia and acidic pH, can disrupt T-cell differentiation and function (Eil et al. 2016). In addition to the emerging roles of lactate and other metabolites as immunoregulatory molecules, new in vivo metabolic tracing methodologies revealed the surprising discovery that circulating lactate functions as the major mitochondrial fuel for most normal and malignant cells (Hensley et al. 2016; Hui et al. 2017). Although these findings have yet to be confirmed in blood cancers, it is conceivable that the unique dependency of LSCs on OXPHOS could, at least in part, be related to preferential oxidation of lactate.

Otto Warburg's early intuition regarding the importance of tumor metabolism has been validated by the recent explosion of scientific discoveries in this area. Nonetheless, significant work remains to successfully translate these discoveries into therapies that improve outcomes for patients. Future efforts will focus on identifying cancer-specific metabolic dependencies, such that targeting of these pathways does not cause prohibitive toxicities toward normal cells. These endeavors will require sophisticated new techniques to unravel complex and dynamically changing metabolic programs within specific cell populations in vivo. Despite the complexity of cancer metabolism and the challenges associated with manipulating these processes for therapeutic benefit, the future of metabolism research in leukemia and lymphoma appears bright. To paraphrase Anthelme Brillat-Savarin, who in 1825 wrote in his celebrated book *The Physiology of Taste*, "Tell me what you eat and I will tell you what you are"; indeed, investigating the metabolic circuitry of leukemia and lymphoma cells will both provide fundamental insights about cancer biology and guide development of novel therapeutic approaches to improve outcomes for these diseases.

ACKNOWLEDGMENTS

We thank Lydia Finley, Santosh Vardhana, and Juanma Schvartzman for helpful discussions. M.S. is supported by the Conquer Cancer Foundation of ASCO Young Investigator Award. Z.D.E.-P. is supported by the American Association for Cancer Research–AstraZeneca Lymphoma Research Fellowship. A.M.I. is supported by the National Institutes of Health (NIH)/National Cancer Institute (NCI) (K08 CA201483, R37 CA251543), Burroughs Wellcome Fund (CAMS 1015584), Damon Runyon Cancer Research Foundation (CI 95-18), Leukemia & Lymphoma Society (SCOR 7011-16), Starr Cancer Consortium, Geoffrey Beene Cancer Research Foundation, Cycle for Survival, Susan & Peter Solomon Divisional Genomics Program, and Steven A. Greenberg Fund. The authors are also grateful for support from the Memorial Sloan Kettering Cancer Center Support Grant (NIH P30 CA008748).

Disclosures: A.M.I. previously consulted for Foundation Medicine, Inc.

REFERENCES

Advani AS, Li H, Michaelis LC, Medeiros BC, Liedtke M, List AF, O'Dwyer K, Othus M, Erba HP, Appelbaum FR. 2018. Report of the relapsed/refractory cohort of SWOG S0919: A phase 2 study of idarubicin and cytarabine in combination with pravastatin for acute myelogenous leukemia (AML). *Leuk Res* **67:** 17–20. doi:10.1016/j.leukres.2018.01.021

Agathocleous M, Meacham CE, Burgess RJ, Piskounova E, Zhao Z, Crane GM, Cowin BL, Bruner E, Murphy MM, Chen W, et al. 2017. Ascorbate regulates haematopoietic stem cell function and leukaemogenesis. *Nature* **549:** 476–481. doi:10.1038/nature23876

Akagi T, Yin D, Kawamata N, Bartram CR, Hofmann WK, Wolf I, Miller CW, Koeffler HP. 2006. Methylation analysis of asparagine synthetase gene in acute lymphoblastic leukemia cells. *Leukemia* **20:** 1303–1306. doi:10.1038/sj.leu.2404216

Altman BJ, Dang CV. 2012. Normal and cancer cell metabolism: Lymphocytes and lymphoma. *FEBS J* **279:** 2598–2609. doi:10.1111/j.1742-4658.2012.08651.x

Ambrosio MR, Piccaluga PP, Ponzoni M, Rocca BJ, Malagnino V, Onorati M, De Falco G, Calbi V, Ogwang M, Naresh KN, et al. 2012. The alteration of lipid metabolism in Burkitt lymphoma identifies a novel marker: Adipophilin. *PLoS One* **7:** e44315. doi:10.1371/journal.pone.0044315

Baccelli I, Gareau Y, Lehnertz B, Gingras S, Spinella JF, Corneau S, Mayotte N, Girard S, Frechette M, Blouin-Chagnon V, et al. 2019. Mubritinib targets the electron transport chain complex I and reveals the landscape of OXPHOS dependency in acute myeloid leukemia. *Cancer Cell* **36:** 84–99.e8. doi:10.1016/j.ccell.2019.06.003

Bahr C, von Paleske L, Uslu VV, Remeseiro S, Takayama N, Ng SW, Murison A, Langenfeld K, Petretich M, Scognamiglio R, et al. 2018. A *Myc* enhancer cluster regulates normal and leukaemic haematopoietic stem cell hierarchies. *Nature* **553:** 515–520. doi:10.1038/nature25193

Bewersdorf JP, Giri S, Wang R, Williams RT, Tallman MS, Zeidan AM, Stahl M. 2020. Venetoclax as monotherapy and in combination with hypomethylating agents or low dose cytarabine in relapsed and treatment refractory acute myeloid leukemia: A systematic review and meta-analysis. *Haematologica* doi:10.3324/haematol.2019.242826.

Bhanot H, Weisberg EL, Reddy MM, Nonami A, Neuberg D, Stone RM, Podar K, Salgia R, Griffin JD, Sattler M. 2017. Acute myeloid leukemia cells require 6-phosphogluconate dehydrogenase for cell growth and NADPH-dependent metabolic reprogramming. *Oncotarget* **8:** 67639–67650. doi:10.18632/oncotarget.18797

Bhatt AP, Jacobs SR, Freemerman AJ, Makowski L, Rathmell JC, Dittmer DP, Damania B. 2012. Dysregulation of fatty acid synthesis and glycolysis in non-Hodgkin lymphoma. *Proc Natl Acad Sci* **109:** 11818–11823. doi:10.1073/pnas.1205995109

Birsoy K, Wang T, Chen WW, Freinkman E, Abu-Remaileh M, Sabatini DM. 2015. An essential role of the mitochondrial electron transport chain in cell proliferation is to enable aspartate synthesis. *Cell* **162:** 540–551. doi:10.1016/j.cell.2015.07.016

Boag JM, Beesley AH, Firth MJ, Freitas JR, Ford J, Hoffmann K, Cummings AJ, de Klerk NH, Kees UR. 2006. Altered glucose metabolism in childhood pre-B acute lymphoblastic leukaemia. *Leukemia* **20:** 1731–1737. doi:10.1038/sj.leu.2404365

Brand A, Singer K, Koehl GE, Kolitzus M, Schoenhammer G, Thiel A, Matos C, Bruss C, Klobuch S, Peter K, et al. 2016. LDHA-associated lactic acid production blunts tumor immunosurveillance by T and NK cells. *Cell Metab* **24:** 657–671. doi:10.1016/j.cmet.2016.08.011

Broecker-Preuss M, Becher-Boveleth N, Bockisch A, Dührsen U, Müller S. 2017. Regulation of glucose uptake in lymphoma cell lines by c-MYC- and PI3K-dependent signaling pathways and impact of glycolytic pathways on cell viability. *J Transl Med* **15:** 158. doi:10.1186/s12967-017-1258-9

Bunpo P, Dudley A, Cundiff JK, Cavener DR, Wek RC, Anthony TG. 2009. GCN2 protein kinase is required to activate amino acid deprivation responses in mice treated with the anti-cancer agent L-asparaginase. *J Biol Chem* **284:** 32742–32749. doi:10.1074/jbc.M109.047910

Bunse L, Pusch S, Bunse T, Sahm F, Sanghvi K, Friedrich M, Alansary D, Sonner JK, Green E, Deumelandt K, et al. 2018. Suppression of antitumor T cell immunity by the oncometabolite (R)-2-hydroxyglutarate. *Nat Med* **24:** 1192–1203. doi:10.1038/s41591-018-0095-6

Cairns RA, Iqbal J, Lemonnier F, Kucuk C, de Leval L, Jais JP, Parrens M, Martin A, Xerri L, Brousset P, et al. 2012. *IDH2* mutations are frequent in angioimmunoblastic T-cell lymphoma. *Blood* **119:** 1901–1903. doi:10.1182/blood-2011-11-391748

Cao L, Weetall M, Trotta C, Cintron K, Ma J, Kim MJ, Furia B, Romfo C, Graci JD, Li W, et al. 2019. Targeting of hematologic malignancies with PTC299, a novel potent inhibitor of dihydroorotate dehydrogenase with favorable pharmaceutical properties. *Mol Cancer Ther* **18:** 3–16. doi:10.1158/1535-7163.MCT-18-0863

Caro P, Kishan AU, Norberg E, Stanley IA, Chapuy B, Ficarro SB, Polak K, Tondera D, Gounarides J, Yin H, et al. 2012. Metabolic signatures uncover distinct targets in molecular subsets of diffuse large B cell lymphoma. *Cancer Cell* **22:** 547–560. doi:10.1016/j.ccr.2012.08.014

Carracedo A, Cantley LC, Pandolfi PP. 2013. Cancer metabolism: Fatty acid oxidation in the limelight. *Nat Rev Cancer* **13:** 227–232. doi:10.1038/nrc3483

Castillo JJ, Mull N, Reagan JL, Nemr S, Mitri J. 2012. Increased incidence of non-Hodgkin lymphoma, leukemia, and myeloma in patients with diabetes mellitus type 2: A meta-analysis of observational studies. *Blood* **119:** 4845–4850. doi:10.1182/blood-2011-06-362830

Chan SM, Thomas D, Corces-Zimmerman MR, Xavy S, Rastogi S, Hong WJ, Zhao F, Medeiros BC, Tyvoll DA, Majeti R. 2015. Isocitrate dehydrogenase 1 and 2 mutations induce BCL-2 dependence in acute myeloid leukemia. *Nat Med* **21:** 178–184. doi:10.1038/nm.3788

Chan LN, Chen Z, Braas D, Lee JW, Xiao G, Geng H, Cosgun KN, Hurtz C, Shojaee S, Cazzaniga V, et al. 2017. Metabolic gatekeeper function of B-lymphoid transcription factors. *Nature* **542:** 479–483. doi:10.1038/nature21076

Chen WL, Wang JH, Zhao AH, Xu X, Wang YH, Chen TL, Li JM, Mi JQ, Zhu YM, Liu YF, et al. 2014. A distinct glucose metabolism signature of acute myeloid leukemia with prognostic value. *Blood* **124:** 1645–1654. doi:10.1182/blood-2014-02-554204

Chen WL, Wang YY, Zhao A, Xia L, Xie G, Su M, Zhao L, Liu J, Qu C, Wei R, et al. 2016. Enhanced fructose utilization mediated by *SLC2A5* is a unique metabolic feature of acute myeloid leukemia with therapeutic potential. *Cancer Cell* **30:** 779–791. doi:10.1016/j.ccell.2016.09.006

Chen CC, Li B, Millman SE, Chen C, Li X, Morris J, Mayle A, Ho YJ, Loizou E, Liu H, et al. 2020. Vitamin B6 addiction in acute myeloid leukemia. *Cancer Cell* **37:** 71–84.e7. doi:10.1016/j.ccell.2019.12.002

Chiche J, Pommier S, Beneteau M, Mondragon L, Meynet O, Zunino B, Mouchotte A, Verhoeyen E, Guyot M, Pagès G, et al. 2015. GAPDH enhances the aggressiveness and the vascularization of non-Hodgkin's B lymphomas via NF-κB-dependent induction of HIF-1α. *Leukemia* **29:** 1163–1176. doi:10.1038/leu.2014.324

Chiche J, Reverso-Meinietti J, Mouchotte A, Rubio-Patiño C, Mhaidly R, Villa E, Bossowski JP, Proics E, Grima-Reyes M, Paquet A, et al. 2019. GAPDH expression predicts the response to R-CHOP, the tumor metabolic status, and the response of DLBCL patients to metabolic inhibitors. *Cell Metab* **29:** 1243–1257.e10. doi:10.1016/j.cmet.2019.02.002

Chien WW, Le Beux C, Rachinel N, Julien M, Lacroix CE, Allas S, Sahakian P, Cornut-Thibaut A, Lionnard L, Kucharczak J, et al. 2015. Differential mechanisms of asparaginase resistance in B-type acute lymphoblastic leukemia and malignant natural killer cell lines. *Sci Rep* **5:** 8068. doi:10.1038/srep08068

Christian S, Merz C, Evans L, Gradl S, Seidel H, Friberg A, Eheim A, Lejeune P, Brzezinka K, Zimmermann K, et al. 2019. The novel dihydroorotate dehydrogenase (DHODH) inhibitor BAY 2402234 triggers differentiation and is effective in the treatment of myeloid malignancies. *Leukemia* **33:** 2403–2415. doi:10.1038/s41375-019-0461-5

Chukkapalli V, Gordon LI, Venugopal P, Borgia JA, Karmali R. 2018. Metabolic changes associated with metformin potentiates Bcl-2 inhibitor, Venetoclax, and CDK9 inhibitor, BAY1143572 and reduces viability of lymphoma cells. *Oncotarget* **9:** 21166–21181. doi:10.18632/oncotarget.24989

Cimmino L, Dolgalev I, Wang Y, Yoshimi A, Martin GH, Wang J, Ng V, Xia B, Witkowski MT, Mitchell-Flack M, et al. 2017. Restoration of TET2 function blocks aberrant self-renewal and leukemia progression. *Cell* **170:** 1079–1095.e20. doi:10.1016/j.cell.2017.07.032

Cimmino L, Neel BG, Aifantis I. 2018. Vitamin C in stem cell reprogramming and cancer. *Trends Cell Biol* **28:** 698–708. doi:10.1016/j.tcb.2018.04.001

Clavell LA, Gelber RD, Cohen HJ, Hitchcock-Bryan S, Cassady JR, Tarbell NJ, Blattner SR, Tantravahi R, Leavitt P, Sallan SE. 1986. Four-agent induction and intensive asparaginase therapy for treatment of childhood acute lymphoblastic leukemia. *N Engl J Med* **315:** 657–663. doi:10.1056/NEJM198609113151101

Clutterbuck RD, Millar BC, Powles RL, Newman A, Catovsky D, Jarman M, Millar JL. 1998. Inhibitory effect of simvastatin on the proliferation of human myeloid leukaemia cells in severe combined immunodeficient (SCID) mice. *Br J Haematol* **102:** 522–527. doi:10.1046/j.1365-2141.1998.00783.x

Cole A, Wang Z, Coyaud E, Voisin V, Gronda M, Jitkova Y, Mattson R, Hurren R, Babovic S, Maclean N, et al. 2015. Inhibition of the mitochondrial protease ClpP as a therapeutic strategy for human acute myeloid leukemia. *Cancer Cell* **27:** 864–876. doi:10.1016/j.ccell.2015.05.004

Colegio OR, Chu NQ, Szabo AL, Chu T, Rhebergen AM, Jairam V, Cyrus N, Brokowski CE, Eisenbarth SC, Phillips GM, et al. 2014. Functional polarization of tumour-associated macrophages by tumour-derived lactic acid. *Nature* **513:** 559–563. doi:10.1038/nature13490

Coloff JL, Macintyre AN, Nichols AG, Liu T, Gallo CA, Plas DR, Rathmell JC. 2011. Akt-dependent glucose metabolism promotes Mcl-1 synthesis to maintain cell survival and resistance to Bcl-2 inhibition. *Cancer Res* **71:** 5204–5213. doi:10.1158/0008-5472.CAN-10-4531

Cramer SL, Saha A, Liu J, Tadi S, Tiziani S, Yan W, Triplett K, Lamb C, Alters SE, Rowlinson S, et al. 2017. Systemic depletion of L-cyst(e)ine with cyst(e)inase increases reactive oxygen species and suppresses tumor growth. *Nat Med* **23:** 120–127. doi:10.1038/nm.4232

Currie E, Schulze A, Zechner R, Walther TC, Farese RV Jr. 2013. Cellular fatty acid metabolism and cancer. *Cell Metab* **18:** 153–161. doi:10.1016/j.cmet.2013.05.017

d'Amore F, Gaulard P, Trümper L, Corradini P, Kim WS, Specht L, Bjerregaard Pedersen M, Ladetto M, ESMO Guidelines Committee. 2015. Peripheral T-cell lymphomas: ESMO Clinical Practice Guidelines for diagnosis, treatment and follow-up. *Ann Oncol* **26:** v108–v115. doi:10.1093/annonc/mdv201

Dang L, White DW, Gross S, Bennett BD, Bittinger MA, Driggers EM, Fantin VR, Jang HG, Jin S, Keenan MC, et al. 2009. Cancer-associated IDH1 mutations produce 2-hydroxyglutarate. *Nature* **462:** 739–744. doi:10.1038/nature08617

Dieck CL, Tzoneva G, Forouhar F, Carpenter Z, Ambesi-Impiombato A, Sánchez-Martín M, Kirschner-Schwabe R, Lew S, Seetharaman J, Tong L, et al. 2018. Structure and mechanisms of NT5C2 mutations driving thiopurine resistance in relapsed lymphoblastic leukemia. *Cancer Cell* **34:** 136–147.e6. doi:10.1016/j.ccell.2018.06.003

Diehl FF, Lewis CA, Fiske BP, Vander Heiden MG. 2019. Cellular redox state constrains serine synthesis and nucleotide production to impact cell proliferation. *Nat Metab* **1:** 861–867. doi:10.1038/s42255-019-0108-x

Dimitroulakos J, Thai S, Wasfy GH, Hedley DW, Minden MD, Penn LZ. 2000. Lovastatin induces a pronounced differentiation response in acute myeloid leukemias. *Leuk Lymphoma* **40:** 167–178. doi:10.3109/10428190009054894

DiNardo CD, Stein EM, de Botton S, Roboz GJ, Altman JK, Mims AS, Swords R, Collins RH, Mannis GN, Pollyea D, et al. 2018. Durable remissions with Ivosidenib in *IDH1*-mutated relapsed or refractory AML. *N Engl J Med* **378:** 2386–2398. doi:10.1056/NEJMoa1716984

DiNardo CD, Pratz K, Pullarkat V, Jonas BA, Arellano M, Becker PS, Frankfurt O, Konopleva M, Wei AH, Kantarjian H, et al. 2019. Venetoclax combined with decitabine or azacitidine in treatment-naive, elderly patients with acute myeloid leukemia. *Blood* **133:** 7–17. doi:10.1182/blood-2018-08-868752

Ducker GS, Ghergurovich JM, Mainolfi N, Suri V, Jeong SK, Hsin-Jung Li S, Friedman A, Manfredi MG, Gitai Z, Kim H, et al. 2017. Human SHMT inhibitors reveal defective glycine import as a targetable metabolic vulnerability of diffuse large B-cell lymphoma. *Proc Natl Acad Sci* **114:** 11404–11409. doi:10.1073/pnas.1706617114

Eberlin LS, Gabay M, Fan AC, Gouw AM, Tibshirani RJ, Felsher DW, Zare RN. 2014. Alteration of the lipid profile in lymphomas induced by MYC overexpression. *Proc Natl Acad Sci* **111:** 10450–10455. doi:10.1073/pnas.1409778111

Ehsanipour EA, Sheng X, Behan JW, Wang X, Butturini A, Avramis VI, Mittelman SD. 2013. Adipocytes cause leukemia cell resistance to L-asparaginase via release of glutamine. *Cancer Res* **73:** 2998–3006. doi:10.1158/0008-5472.CAN-12-4402

Eil R, Vodnala SK, Clever D, Klebanoff CA, Sukumar M, Pan JH, Palmer DC, Gros A, Yamamoto TN, Patel SJ, et al. 2016. Ionic immune suppression within the tumour microenvironment limits T cell effector function. *Nature* **537:** 539–543. doi:10.1038/nature19364

Elkashef SM, Lin AP, Myers J, Sill H, Jiang D, Dahia PLM, Aguiar RCT. 2017. IDH mutation, competitive inhibition of FTO, and RNA methylation. *Cancer Cell* **31:** 619–620. doi:10.1016/j.ccell.2017.04.001

Emadi A. 2015. Exploiting AML vulnerability: Glutamine dependency. *Blood* **126:** 1269–1270. doi:10.1182/blood-2015-07-659508

Fan J, Ye J, Kamphorst JJ, Shlomi T, Thompson CB, Rabinowitz JD. 2014. Quantitative flux analysis reveals folate-dependent NADPH production. *Nature* **510:** 298–302. doi:10.1038/nature13236

Farber S, Diamond LK. 1948. Temporary remissions in acute leukemia in children produced by folic acid antagonist, 4-aminopteroyl-glutamic acid (Aminopterin). *N Engl J Med* **238:** 787–793. doi:10.1056/NEJM194806032382301

Farge T, Saland E, de Toni F, Aroua N, Hosseini M, Perry R, Bosc C, Sugita M, Stuani L, Fraisse M, et al. 2017. Chemotherapy-resistant human acute myeloid leukemia cells are not enriched for leukemic stem cells but require oxidative metabolism. *Cancer Discov* **7:** 716–735. doi:10.1158/2159-8290.CD-16-0441

Faubert B, Boily G, Izreig S, Griss T, Samborska B, Dong Z, Dupuy F, Chambers C, Fuerth BJ, Viollet B, et al. 2013. AMPK is a negative regulator of the Warburg effect and suppresses tumor growth in vivo. *Cell Metab* **17:** 113–124. doi:10.1016/j.cmet.2012.12.001

Feinberg AP, Koldobskiy MA, Göndör A. 2016. Epigenetic modulators, modifiers and mediators in cancer aetiology and progression. *Nat Rev Genet* **17:** 284–299. doi:10.1038/nrg.2016.13

Fenouille N, Bassil CF, Ben-Sahra I, Benajiba L, Alexe G, Ramos A, Pikman Y, Conway AS, Burgess MR, Li Q, et al. 2017. The creatine kinase pathway is a metabolic vulnerability in EVI1-positive acute myeloid leukemia. *Nat Med* **23:** 301–313. doi:10.1038/nm.4283

Figueroa ME, Abdel-Wahab O, Lu C, Ward PS, Patel J, Shih A, Li Y, Bhagwat N, Vasanthakumar A, Fernandez HF, et al. 2010. Leukemic IDH1 and IDH2 mutations result in a hypermethylation phenotype, disrupt TET2 function, and impair hematopoietic differentiation. *Cancer Cell* **18:** 553–567. doi:10.1016/j.ccr.2010.11.015

Fu X, Chin RM, Vergnes L, Hwang H, Deng G, Xing Y, Pai MY, Li S, Ta L, Fazlollahi F, et al. 2015. 2-Hydroxyglutarate inhibits ATP synthase and mTOR signaling. *Cell Metab* **22:** 508–515. doi:10.1016/j.cmet.2015.06.009

Gallipoli P, Giotopoulos G, Tzelepis K, Costa ASH, Vohra S, Medina-Perez P, Basheer F, Marando L, Di Lisio L, Dias JML, et al. 2018. Glutaminolysis is a metabolic dependency in $FLT3^{ITD}$ acute myeloid leukemia unmasked by FLT3 tyrosine kinase inhibition. *Blood* **131:** 1639–1653. doi:10.1182/blood-2017-12-820035

Gao P, Tchernyshyov I, Chang TC, Lee YS, Kita K, Ochi T, Zeller KI, De Marzo AM, Van Eyk JE, Mendell JT, et al. 2009. c-Myc suppression of miR-23a/b enhances mitochondrial glutaminase expression and glutamine metabolism. *Nature* **458:** 762–765. doi:10.1038/nature07823

Garcia-Bermudez J, Baudrier L, La K, Zhu XG, Fidelin J, Sviderskiy VO, Papagiannakopoulos T, Molina H, Snuderl M, Lewis CA, et al. 2018. Aspartate is a limiting metabolite for cancer cell proliferation under hypoxia and in tumours. *Nat Cell Biol* **20:** 775–781. doi:10.1038/s41556-018-0118-z

Garcia-Bermudez J, Baudrier L, Bayraktar EC, Shen Y, La K, Guarecuco R, Yucel B, Fiore D, Tavora B, Freinkman E, et al. 2019. Squalene accumulation in cholesterol auxotrophic lymphomas prevents oxidative cell death. *Nature* **567:** 118–122. doi:10.1038/s41586-019-0945-5

German NJ, Yoon H, Yusuf RZ, Murphy JP, Finley LW, Laurent G, Haas W, Satterstrom FK, Guarnerio J, Zaganjor E, et al. 2016. PHD3 loss in cancer enables metabolic reliance on fatty acid oxidation via deactivation of ACC2. *Mol Cell* **63:** 1006–1020. doi:10.1016/j.molcel.2016.08.014

Goncalves MD, Lu C, Tutnauer J, Hartman TE, Hwang SK, Murphy CJ, Pauli C, Morris R, Taylor S, Bosch K, et al. 2019. High-fructose corn syrup enhances intestinal tumor growth in mice. *Science* **363:** 1345–1349. doi:10.1126/science.aat8515

Gottschalk S, Anderson N, Hainz C, Eckhardt SG, Serkova NJ. 2004. Imatinib (STI571)-mediated changes in glucose metabolism in human leukemia BCR-ABL-positive cells. *Clin Cancer Res* **10:** 6661–6668. doi:10.1158/1078-0432.CCR-04-0039

Gouw AM, Margulis K, Liu NS, Raman SJ, Mancuso A, Toal GG, Tong L, Mosley A, Hsieh AL, Sullivan DK, et al. 2019. The MYC oncogene cooperates with sterol-regulated element-binding protein to regulate lipogenesis essential for neoplastic growth. *Cell Metab* **30:** 556–572.e5. doi:10.1016/j.cmet.2019.07.012

Gregory MA, Nemkov T, Reisz JA, Zaberezhnyy V, Hansen KC, D'Alessandro A, DeGregori J. 2018. Glutaminase inhibition improves FLT3 inhibitor therapy for acute myeloid leukemia. *Exp Hematol* **58:** 52–58. doi:10.1016/j.exphem.2017.09.007

Gregory MA, Nemkov T, Park HJ, Zaberezhnyy V, Gehrke S, Adane B, Jordan CT, Hansen KC, D'Alessandro A, DeGregori J. 2019. Targeting glutamine metabolism and redox state for leukemia therapy. *Clin Cancer Res* **25:** 4079–4090. doi:10.1158/1078-0432.CCR-18-3223

Gu JJ, Singh A, Xue K, Mavis C, Barth M, Yanamadala V, Lenz P, Grau M, Lenz G, Czuczman MS, et al. 2018. Upregulation of hexokinase II contributes to rituximab-chemotherapy resistance and is a clinically relevant target for therapeutic development. *Oncotarget* **9:** 4020–4033. doi:10.18632/oncotarget.23425

Guièze R, Liu VM, Rosebrock D, Jourdain AA, Hernández-Sánchez M, Martinez Zurita A, Sun J, Ten Hacken E, Baranowski K, Thompson PA, et al. 2019. Mitochondrial reprogramming underlies resistance to BCL-2 inhibition in lymphoid malignancies. *Cancer Cell* **36:** 369–384.e13. doi:10.1016/j.ccell.2019.08.005

Hattori A, Tsunoda M, Konuma T, Kobayashi M, Nagy T, Glushka J, Tayyari F, McSkimming D, Kannan N, Tojo A, et al. 2017. Cancer progression by reprogrammed BCAA metabolism in myeloid leukaemia. *Nature* **545:** 500–504. doi:10.1038/nature22314

Hensley CT, Faubert B, Yuan Q, Lev-Cohain N, Jin E, Kim J, Jiang L, Ko B, Skelton R, Loudat L, et al. 2016. Metabolic heterogeneity in human lung tumors. *Cell* **164:** 681–694. doi:10.1016/j.cell.2015.12.034

Herranz D, Ambesi-Impiombato A, Sudderth J, Sanchez-Martin M, Belver L, Tosello V, Xu L, Wendorff AA, Castillo M, Haydu JE, et al. 2015. Metabolic reprogramming induces resistance to anti-NOTCH1 therapies in T cell acute lymphoblastic leukemia. *Nat Med* **21:** 1182–1189. doi:10.1038/nm.3955

Herst PM, Howman RA, Neeson PJ, Berridge MV, Ritchie DS. 2011. The level of glycolytic metabolism in acute myeloid leukemia blasts at diagnosis is prognostic for clinical outcome. *J Leukoc Biol* **89:** 51–55. doi:10.1189/jlb.0710417

Holleman A, Cheok MH, den Boer ML, Yang W, Veerman AJ, Kazemier KM, Pei D, Cheng C, Pui CH, Relling MV, et al. 2004. Gene-expression patterns in drug-resistant acute lymphoblastic leukemia cells and response to treatment. *N Engl J Med* **351:** 533–542. doi:10.1056/NEJMoa033513

Hopkins BD, Pauli C, Du X, Wang DG, Li X, Wu D, Amadiume SC, Goncalves MD, Hodakoski C, Lundquist MR, et al. 2018. Suppression of insulin feedback enhances the efficacy of PI3 K inhibitors. *Nature* **560:** 499–503. doi:10.1038/s41586-018-0343-4

Hosios AM, Vander Heiden MG. 2018. The redox requirements of proliferating mammalian cells. *J Biol Chem* **293:** 7490–7498. doi:10.1074/jbc.TM117.000239

Hosios AM, Hecht VC, Danai LV, Johnson MO, Rathmell JC, Steinhauser ML, Manalis SR, Vander Heiden MG. 2016. Amino acids rather than glucose account for the majority of cell mass in proliferating mammalian cells. *Dev Cell* **36:** 540–549. doi:10.1016/j.devcel.2016.02.012

Hui S, Ghergurovich JM, Morscher RJ, Jang C, Teng X, Lu W, Esparza LA, Reya T, Le Z, Yanxiang Guo J, et al. 2017.

Glucose feeds the TCA cycle via circulating lactate. *Nature* **551:** 115–118. doi:10.1038/nature24057

Huijskens MJ, Wodzig WK, Walczak M, Germeraad WT, Bos GM. 2016. Ascorbic acid serum levels are reduced in patients with hematological malignancies. *Results Immunol* **6:** 8–10. doi:10.1016/j.rinim.2016.01.001

Hulleman E, Kazemier KM, Holleman A, VanderWeele DJ, Rudin CM, Broekhuis MJ, Evans WE, Pieters R, Den Boer ML. 2009. Inhibition of glycolysis modulates prednisolone resistance in acute lymphoblastic leukemia cells. *Blood* **113:** 2014–2021. doi:10.1182/blood-2008-05-157842

Intlekofer AM, Finley LWS. 2019. Metabolic signatures of cancer cells and stem cells. *Nat Metab* **1:** 177–188. doi:10.1038/s42255-019-0032-0

Jacque N, Ronchetti AM, Larrue C, Meunier G, Birsen R, Willems L, Saland E, Decroocq J, Maciel TT, Lambert M, et al. 2015. Targeting glutaminolysis has antileukemic activity in acute myeloid leukemia and synergizes with BCL-2 inhibition. *Blood* **126:** 1346–1356. doi:10.1182/blood-2015-01-621870

Jiang P, Du W, Wang X, Mancuso A, Gao X, Wu M, Yang X. 2011. p53 regulates biosynthesis through direct inactivation of glucose-6-phosphate dehydrogenase. *Nat Cell Biol* **13:** 310–316. doi:10.1038/ncb2172

Jiang P, Du W, Mancuso A, Wellen KE, Yang X. 2013. Reciprocal regulation of p53 and malic enzymes modulates metabolism and senescence. *Nature* **493:** 689–693. doi:10.1038/nature11776

Jones CL, Stevens BM, D'Alessandro A, Reisz JA, Culp-Hill R, Nemkov T, Pei S, Khan N, Adane B, Ye H, et al. 2018. Inhibition of amino acid metabolism selectively targets human leukemia stem cells. *Cancer Cell* **34:** 724–740.e4. doi:10.1016/j.ccell.2018.10.005

Jones CL, Stevens BM, D'Alessandro A, Culp-Hill R, Reisz JA, Pei S, Gustafson A, Khan N, DeGregori J, Pollyea DA, et al. 2019. Cysteine depletion targets leukemia stem cells through inhibition of electron transport complex II. *Blood* **134:** 389–394. doi:10.1182/blood.2019898114

Ju HQ, Zhan G, Huang A, Sun Y, Wen S, Yang J, Lu WH, Xu RH, Li J, Li Y, et al. 2017. ITD mutation in FLT3 tyrosine kinase promotes Warburg effect and renders therapeutic sensitivity to glycolytic inhibition. *Leukemia* **31:** 2143–2150. doi:10.1038/leu.2017.45

Khan H, Anshu A, Prasad A, Roy S, Jeffery J, Kittipongdaja W, Yang DT, Schieke SM. 2019. Metabolic rewiring in response to biguanides is mediated by mROS/HIF-1a in malignant lymphocytes. *Cell Rep* **29:** 3009–3018.e4. doi:10.1016/j.celrep.2019.11.007

Khanim FL, Hayden RE, Birtwistle J, Lodi A, Tiziani S, Davies NJ, Ride JP, Viant MR, Gunther UL, Mountford JC, et al. 2009. Combined bezafibrate and medroxyprogesterone acetate: Potential novel therapy for acute myeloid leukaemia. *PLoS One* **4:** e8147. doi:10.1371/journal.pone.0008147

Kimmelman AC. 2015. Metabolic dependencies in RAS-driven cancers. *Clin Cancer Res* **21:** 1828–1834. doi:10.1158/1078-0432.CCR-14-2425

Kinnaird A, Zhao S, Wellen KE, Michelakis ED. 2016. Metabolic control of epigenetics in cancer. *Nat Rev Cancer* **16:** 694–707. doi:10.1038/nrc.2016.82

Koivunen P, Lee S, Duncan CG, Lopez G, Lu G, Ramkissoon S, Losman JA, Joensuu P, Bergmann U, Gross S, et al. 2012. Transformation by the (*R*)-enantiomer of 2-hydroxyglutarate linked to EGLN activation. *Nature* **483:** 484–488. doi:10.1038/nature10898

Kornblau SM, Banker DE, Stirewalt D, Shen D, Lemker E, Verstovsek S, Estrov Z, Faderl S, Cortes J, Beran M, et al. 2007. Blockade of adaptive defensive changes in cholesterol uptake and synthesis in AML by the addition of pravastatin to idarubicin + high-dose Ara-C: A phase 1 study. *Blood* **109:** 2999–3006. doi:10.1182/blood-2006-08-044446

Kuntz EM, Baquero P, Michie AM, Dunn K, Tardito S, Holyoake TL, Helgason GV, Gottlieb E. 2017. Targeting mitochondrial oxidative phosphorylation eradicates therapy-resistant chronic myeloid leukemia stem cells. *Nat Med* **23:** 1234–1240. doi:10.1038/nm.4399

Ladds M, van Leeuwen IMM, Drummond CJ, Chu S, Healy AR, Popova G, Pastor Fernández A, Mollick T, Darekar S, Sedimbi SK, et al. 2018. A DHODH inhibitor increases p53 synthesis and enhances tumor cell killing by p53 degradation blockage. *Nat Commun* **9:** 1107. doi:10.1038/s41467-018-03441-3

Lagadinou ED, Sach A, Callahan K, Rossi RM, Neering SJ, Minhajuddin M, Ashton JM, Pei S, Grose V, O'Dwyer KM, et al. 2013. BCL-2 inhibition targets oxidative phosphorylation and selectively eradicates quiescent human leukemia stem cells. *Cell Stem Cell* **12:** 329–341. doi:10.1016/j.stem.2012.12.013

Larrue C, Saland E, Vergez F, Serhan N, Delabesse E, Mansat-De Mas V, Hospital MA, Tamburini J, Manenti S, Sarry JE, et al. 2015. Antileukemic activity of 2-deoxy-*d*-glucose through inhibition of N-linked glycosylation in acute myeloid leukemia with *FLT3-ITD* or *c-KIT* mutations. *Mol Cancer Ther* **14:** 2364–2373. doi:10.1158/1535-7163.MCT-15-0163

Le A, Lane AN, Hamaker M, Bose S, Gouw A, Barbi J, Tsukamoto T, Rojas CJ, Slusher BS, Zhang H, et al. 2012. Glucose-independent glutamine metabolism via TCA cycling for proliferation and survival in B cells. *Cell Metab* **15:** 110–121. doi:10.1016/j.cmet.2011.12.009

Lee JS, Roberts A, Juarez D, Vo TT, Bhatt S, Herzog LO, Mallya S, Bellin RJ, Agarwal SK, Salem AH, et al. 2018. Statins enhance efficacy of venetoclax in blood cancers. *Sci Transl Med* **10:** eaaq1240.

Lee SC, Shestov AA, Guo L, Zhang Q, Roman JC, Liu X, Wang HY, Pickup S, Nath K, Lu P, et al. 2019. Metabolic detection of Bruton's tyrosine kinase inhibition in mantle cell lymphoma cells. *Mol Cancer Res* **17:** 1365–1377.

Lemonnier F, Cairns RA, Inoue S, Li WY, Dupuy A, Broutin S, Martin N, Fataccioli V, Pelletier R, Wakeham A, et al. 2016. The IDH2 R172 K mutation associated with angioimmunoblastic T-cell lymphoma produces 2HG in T cells and impacts lymphoid development. *Proc Natl Acad Sci* **113:** 15084–15089. doi:10.1073/pnas.1617929114

Li M, Chiang YL, Lyssiotis CA, Teater MR, Hong JY, Shen H, Wang L, Hu J, Jing H, Chen Z, et al. 2019. Non-oncogene addiction to SIRT3 plays a critical role in lymphomagenesis. *Cancer Cell* **35:** 916–931.e9. doi:10.1016/j.ccell.2019.05.002

Lin AP, Abbas S, Kim SW, Ortega M, Bouamar H, Escobedo Y, Varadarajan P, Qin Y, Sudderth J, Schulz E, et al. 2015.

D2HGDH regulates alpha-ketoglutarate levels and dioxygenase function by modulating IDH2. *Nat Commun* **6:** 7768. doi:10.1038/ncomms8768

Lin KH, Xie A, Rutter JC, Ahn YR, Lloyd-Cowden JM, Nichols AG, Soderquist RS, Koves TR, Muoio DM, MacIver NJ, et al. 2019. Systematic dissection of the metabolic-apoptotic interface in AML reveals heme biosynthesis to be a regulator of drug sensitivity. *Cell Metab* **29:** 1217–1231.e7. doi:10.1016/j.cmet.2019.01.011

Liu T, Kishton RJ, Macintyre AN, Gerriets VA, Xiang H, Liu X, Abel ED, Rizzieri D, Locasale JW, Rathmell JC. 2014. Glucose transporter 1-mediated glucose uptake is limiting for B-cell acute lymphoblastic leukemia anabolic metabolism and resistance to apoptosis. *Cell Death Dis* **5:** e1470. doi:10.1038/cddis.2014.431

Liyanage SU, Hurren R, Voisin V, Bridon G, Wang X, Xu C, MacLean N, Siriwardena TP, Gronda M, Yehudai D, et al. 2017. Leveraging increased cytoplasmic nucleoside kinase activity to target mtDNA and oxidative phosphorylation in AML. *Blood* **129:** 2657–2666. doi:10.1182/blood-2016-10-741207

Locasale JW. 2013. Serine, glycine and one-carbon units: Cancer metabolism in full circle. *Nat Rev Cancer* **13:** 572–583. doi:10.1038/nrc3557

Losman JA, Kaelin WG Jr. 2013. What a difference a hydroxyl makes: Mutant IDH, (*R*)-2-hydroxyglutarate, and cancer. *Genes Dev* **27:** 836–852. doi:10.1101/gad.217406.113

Lu C, Ward PS, Kapoor GS, Rohle D, Turcan S, Abdel-Wahab O, Edwards CR, Khanin R, Figueroa ME, Melnick A, et al. 2012. IDH mutation impairs histone demethylation and results in a block to cell differentiation. *Nature* **483:** 474–478. doi:10.1038/nature10860

Lu Z, Xie J, Wu G, Shen J, Collins R, Chen W, Kang X, Luo M, Zou Y, Huang LJ, et al. 2017. Fasting selectively blocks development of acute lymphoblastic leukemia via leptin-receptor upregulation. *Nat Med* **23:** 79–90. doi:10.1038/nm.4252

Mardis ER, Ding L, Dooling DJ, Larson DE, McLellan MD, Chen K, Koboldt DC, Fulton RS, Delehaunty KD, McGrath SD, et al. 2009. Recurring mutations found by sequencing an acute myeloid leukemia genome. *N Engl J Med* **361:** 1058–1066. doi:10.1056/NEJMoa0903840

Martín-Lorenzo A, Auer F, Chan LN, García-Ramírez I, González-Herrero I, Rodríguez-Hernández G, Bartenhagen C, Dugas M, Gombert M, Ginzel S, et al. 2018. Loss of Pax5 exploits Sca1-BCR-ABL^{p190} susceptibility to confer the metabolic shift essential for pB-ALL. *Cancer Res* **78:** 2669–2679. doi:10.1158/0008-5472.CAN-17-3262

Matre P, Velez J, Jacamo R, Qi Y, Su X, Cai T, Chan SM, Lodi A, Sweeney SR, Ma H, et al. 2016. Inhibiting glutaminase in acute myeloid leukemia: Metabolic dependency of selected AML subtypes. *Oncotarget* **7:** 79722–79735. doi:10.18632/oncotarget.12944

McBrayer SK, Mayers JR, DiNatale GJ, Shi DD, Khanal J, Chakraborty AA, Sarosiek KA, Briggs KJ, Robbins AK, Sewastianik T, et al. 2018. Transaminase inhibition by 2-hydroxyglutarate impairs glutamate biosynthesis and redox homeostasis in glioma. *Cell* **175:** 101–116.e25. doi:10.1016/j.cell.2018.08.038

McFadden K, Hafez AY, Kishton R, Messinger JE, Nikitin PA, Rathmell JC, Luftig MA. 2016. Metabolic stress is a barrier to Epstein-Barr virus-mediated B-cell immortalization. *Proc Natl Acad Sci* **113:** E782–E790. doi:10.1073/pnas.1517141113

Meyer JA, Wang J, Hogan LE, Yang JJ, Dandekar S, Patel JP, Tang Z, Zumbo P, Li S, Zavadil J, et al. 2013. Relapse-specific mutations in *NT5C2* in childhood acute lymphoblastic leukemia. *Nat Genet* **45:** 290–294. doi:10.1038/ng.2558

Michelozzi IM, Granata V, De Ponti G, Alberti G, Tomasoni C, Antolini L, Gambacorti-Passerini C, Gentner B, Dazzi F, Biondi A, et al. 2019. Acute myeloid leukaemia niche regulates response to L-asparaginase. *Br J Haematol* **186:** 420–430.

Miraki-Moud F, Ghazaly E, Ariza-McNaughton L, Hodby KA, Clear A, Anjos-Afonso F, Liapis K, Grantham M, Sohrabi F, Cavenagh J, et al. 2015. Arginine deprivation using pegylated arginine deiminase has activity against primary acute myeloid leukemia cells in vivo. *Blood* **125:** 4060–4068. doi:10.1182/blood-2014-10-608133

Mitri J, Castillo J, Pittas AG. 2008. Diabetes and risk of Non-Hodgkin's lymphoma: A meta-analysis of observational studies. *Diabetes Care* **31:** 2391–2397. doi:10.2337/dc08-1034

Moertel CG, Fleming TR, Creagan ET, Rubin J, O'Connell MJ, Ames MM. 1985. High-dose vitamin C versus placebo in the treatment of patients with advanced cancer who have had no prior chemotherapy. A randomized double-blind comparison. *N Engl J Med* **312:** 137–141. doi:10.1056/NEJM198501173120301

Molina JR, Sun Y, Protopopova M, Gera S, Bandi M, Bristow C, McAfoos T, Morlacchi P, Ackroyd J, Agip AA, et al. 2018. An inhibitor of oxidative phosphorylation exploits cancer vulnerability. *Nat Med* **24:** 1036–1046. doi:10.1038/s41591-018-0052-4

Monti S, Savage KJ, Kutok JL, Feuerhake F, Kurtin P, Mihm M, Wu B, Pasqualucci L, Neuberg D, Aguiar RC, et al. 2005. Molecular profiling of diffuse large B-cell lymphoma identifies robust subtypes including one characterized by host inflammatory response. *Blood* **105:** 1851–1861. doi:10.1182/blood-2004-07-2947

Montrose DC, Galluzzi L. 2019. Drugging cancer metabolism: Expectations vs. reality. *Int Rev Cell Mol Biol* **347:** 1–26. doi:10.1016/bs.ircmb.2019.07.007

Morrish F, Noonan J, Perez-Olsen C, Gafken PR, Fitzgibbon M, Kelleher J, VanGilst M, Hockenbery D. 2010. Myc-dependent mitochondrial generation of acetyl-CoA contributes to fatty acid biosynthesis and histone acetylation during cell cycle entry. *J Biol Chem* **285:** 36267–36274. doi:10.1074/jbc.M110.141606

Mullighan CG, Goorha S, Radtke I, Miller CB, Coustan-Smith E, Dalton JD, Girtman K, Mathew S, Ma J, Pounds SB, et al. 2007. Genome-wide analysis of genetic alterations in acute lymphoblastic leukaemia. *Nature* **446:** 758–764. doi:10.1038/nature05690

Mullighan CG, Miller CB, Radtke I, Phillips LA, Dalton J, Ma J, White D, Hughes TP, Le Beau MM, Pui CH, et al. 2008. *BCR-ABL1* lymphoblastic leukaemia is characterized by the deletion of Ikaros. *Nature* **453:** 110–114. doi:10.1038/nature06866

Murray JA, Khanim FL, Hayden RE, Craddock CF, Holyoake TL, Jackson N, Lumley M, Bunce CM, Drayson MT. 2010. Combined bezafibrate and medroxyprogesterone acetate have efficacy without haematological toxicity in elderly and relapsed acute myeloid leukaemia (AML). *Br J Haematol* **149:** 65–69. doi:10.1111/j.1365-2141.2009.08055.x

Müschen M. 2019. Metabolic gatekeepers to safeguard against autoimmunity and oncogenic B cell transformation. *Nat Rev Immunol* **19:** 337–348. doi:10.1038/s41577-019-0154-3

Mussai F, De Santo C, Abu-Dayyeh I, Booth S, Quek L, McEwen-Smith RM, Qureshi A, Dazzi F, Vyas P, Cerundolo V. 2013. Acute myeloid leukemia creates an arginase-dependent immunosuppressive microenvironment. *Blood* **122:** 749–758. doi:10.1182/blood-2013-01-480129

Mussai F, Egan S, Higginbotham-Jones J, Perry T, Beggs A, Odintsova E, Loke J, Pratt G, U KP, Lo A, et al. 2015. Arginine dependence of acute myeloid leukemia blast proliferation: A novel therapeutic target. *Blood* **125:** 2386–2396. doi:10.1182/blood-2014-09-600643

Nakajima K, Kawashima I, Koshiisi M, Kumagai T, Suzuki M, Suzuki J, Mitsumori T, Kirito K. 2019. Glycolytic enzyme hexokinase II is a putative therapeutic target in B-cell malignant lymphoma. *Exp Hematol* **78:** 46–55.e3. doi:10.1016/j.exphem.2019.09.023

Newman A, Clutterbuck RD, Powles RL, Millar JL. 1994. Selective inhibition of primary acute myeloid leukaemia cell growth by simvastatin. *Leukemia* **8:** 2023–2029.

Ni F, Yu WM, Li Z, Graham DK, Jin L, Kang S, Rossi MR, Li S, Broxmeyer HE, Qu CK. 2019. Critical role of ASCT2-mediated amino acid metabolism in promoting leukaemia development and progression. *Nat Metab* **1:** 390–403. doi:10.1038/s42255-019-0039-6

Norberg E, Lako A, Chen PH, Stanley IA, Zhou F, Ficarro SB, Chapuy B, Chen L, Rodig S, Shin D, et al. 2017. Differential contribution of the mitochondrial translation pathway to the survival of diffuse large B-cell lymphoma subsets. *Cell Death Differ* **24:** 251–262. doi:10.1038/cdd.2016.116

Noy A, Schöder H, Gönen M, Weissler M, Ertelt K, Cohler C, Portlock C, Hamlin P, Yeung HW. 2009. The majority of transformed lymphomas have high standardized uptake values (SUVs) on positron emission tomography (PET) scanning similar to diffuse large B-cell lymphoma (DLBCL). *Ann Oncol* **20:** 508–512. doi:10.1093/annonc/mdn657

Okosun J, Wolfson RL, Wang J, Araf S, Wilkins L, Castellano BM, Escudero-Ibarz L, Al Seraihi AF, Richter J, Bernhart SH, et al. 2016. Recurrent mTORC1-activating *RRAGC* mutations in follicular lymphoma. *Nat Genet* **48:** 183–188. doi:10.1038/ng.3473

Oricchio E, Katanayeva N, Donaldson MC, Sungalee S, Pasion JP, Béguelin W, Battistello E, Sanghvi VR, Jiang M, Jiang Y. 2017. Genetic and epigenetic inactivation of *SESTRIN1* controls mTORC1 and response to EZH2 inhibition in follicular lymphoma. **9:** eaak9969.

Ortega-Molina A, Deleyto-Seldas N, Carreras J, Sanz A, Lebrero-Fernández C, Menéndez C, Vandenberg A, Fernández-Ruiz B, Marín-Arraiza L, de la Calle Arregui C, et al. 2019. Oncogenic Rag GTPase signalling enhances B cell activation and drives follicular lymphoma sensitive to pharmacological inhibition of mTOR. *Nat Metab* **1:** 775–789. doi:10.1038/s42255-019-0098-8

Osthus RC, Shim H, Kim S, Li Q, Reddy R, Mukherjee M, Xu Y, Wonsey D, Lee LA, Dang CV. 2000. Deregulation of glucose transporter 1 and glycolytic gene expression by c-Myc. *J Biol Chem* **275:** 21797–21800. doi:10.1074/jbc.C000023200

Palm W, Thompson CB. 2017. Nutrient acquisition strategies of mammalian cells. *Nature* **546:** 234–242. doi:10.1038/nature22379

Pardee TS, Lee K, Luddy J, Maturo C, Rodriguez R, Isom S, Miller LD, Stadelman KM, Levitan D, Hurd D, et al. 2014. A phase I study of the first-in-class antimitochondrial metabolism agent, CPI-613, in patients with advanced hematologic malignancies. *Clin Cancer Res* **20:** 5255–5264. doi:10.1158/1078-0432.CCR-14-1019

Pardee TS, Anderson RG, Pladna KM, Isom S, Ghiraldeli LP, Miller LD, Chou JW, Jin G, Zhang W, Ellis LR, et al. 2018. A Phase I Study of CPI-613 in combination with high-dose cytarabine and mitoxantrone for relapsed or refractory acute myeloid leukemia. *Clin Cancer Res* **24:** 2060–2073. doi:10.1158/1078-0432.CCR-17-2282

Parsa S, Ortega-Molina A, Ying HY, Jiang M, Teater M, Wang J, Zhao C, Reznik E, Pasion JP, Kuo D, et al. 2020. The serine hydroxymethyltransferase-2 (SHMT2) initiates lymphoma development through epigenetic tumor suppressor silencing. *Nature Cancer* **1:** 653–664. doi:10.1038/s43018-020-0080-0

Pikman Y, Puissant A, Alexe G, Furman A, Chen LM, Frumm SM, Ross L, Fenouille N, Bassil CF, Lewis CA, et al. 2016. Targeting MTHFD2 in acute myeloid leukemia. *J Exp Med* **213:** 1285–1306. doi:10.1084/jem.20151574

Pizer ES, Wood FD, Pasternack GR, Kuhajda FP. 1996. Fatty acid synthase (FAS): A target for cytotoxic antimetabolites in HL60 promyelocytic leukemia cells. *Cancer Res* **56:** 745–751.

Pollyea DA, Stevens BM, Jones CL, Winters A, Pei S, Minhajuddin M, D'Alessandro A, Culp-Hill R, Riemondy KA, Gillen AE, et al. 2018. Venetoclax with azacitidine disrupts energy metabolism and targets leukemia stem cells in patients with acute myeloid leukemia. *Nat Med* **24:** 1859–1866. doi:10.1038/s41591-018-0233-1

Poulain L, Sujobert P, Zylbersztejn F, Barreau S, Stuani L, Lambert M, Palama TL, Chesnais V, Birsen R, Vergez F, et al. 2017. High mTORC1 activity drives glycolysis addiction and sensitivity to G6PD inhibition in acute myeloid leukemia cells. *Leukemia* **31:** 2326–2335. doi:10.1038/leu.2017.81

Qing G, Li B, Vu A, Skuli N, Walton ZE, Liu X, Mayes PA, Wise DR, Thompson CB, Maris JM, et al. 2012. ATF4 regulates *MYC*-mediated neuroblastoma cell death upon glutamine deprivation. *Cancer Cell* **22:** 631–644. doi:10.1016/j.ccr.2012.09.021

Raffel S, Falcone M, Kneisel N, Hansson J, Wang W, Lutz C, Bullinger L, Poschet G, Nonnenmacher Y, Barnert A, et al. 2017. BCAT1 restricts αKG levels in AML stem cells leading to IDH^{mut}-like DNA hypermethylation. *Nature* **551:** 384–388. doi:10.1038/nature24294

Ricciardi MR, Mirabilii S, Allegretti M, Licchetta R, Calarco A, Torrisi MR, Foà R, Nicolai R, Peluso G, Tafuri A. 2015. Targeting the leukemia cell metabolism by the CPT1a inhibition: Functional preclinical effects in leukemias. *Blood* **126:** 1925–1929. doi:10.1182/blood-2014-12-617498

Rohle D, Popovici-Muller J, Palaskas N, Turcan S, Grommes C, Campos C, Tsoi J, Clark O, Oldrini B, Komisopoulou E, et al. 2013. An inhibitor of mutant IDH1 delays growth and promotes differentiation of glioma cells. *Science* **340:** 626–630. doi:10.1126/science.1236062

Samudio I, Harmancey R, Fiegl M, Kantarjian H, Konopleva M, Korchin B, Kaluarachchi K, Bornmann W, Duvvuri S, Taegtmeyer H, et al. 2010. Pharmacologic inhibition of fatty acid oxidation sensitizes human leukemia cells to apoptosis induction. *J Clin Invest* **120:** 142–156. doi:10.1172/JCI38942

Sanchez-Martin M, Ferrando A. 2017. The NOTCH1-MYC highway toward T-cell acute lymphoblastic leukemia. *Blood* **129:** 1124–1133. doi:10.1182/blood-2016-09-692582

Saxton RA, Sabatini DM. 2017. mTOR signaling in growth, metabolism, and disease. *Cell* **168:** 960–976. doi:10.1016/j.cell.2017.02.004

Schuijers J, Manteiga JC, Weintraub AS, Day DS, Zamudio AV, Hnisz D, Lee TI, Young RA. 2018. Transcriptional dysregulation of MYC reveals common enhancer-docking mechanism. *Cell Rep* **23:** 349–360. doi:10.1016/j.celrep.2018.03.056

Scuoppo C, Miething C, Lindqvist L, Reyes J, Ruse C, Appelmann I, Yoon S, Krasnitz A, Teruya-Feldstein J, Pappin D, et al. 2012. A tumour suppressor network relying on the polyamine-hypusine axis. *Nature* **487:** 244–248. doi:10.1038/nature11126

Seam P, Juweid ME, Cheson BD. 2007. The role of FDG-PET scans in patients with lymphoma. *Blood* **110:** 3507–3516. doi:10.1182/blood-2007-06-097238

Sehn LH, Berry B, Chhanabhai M, Fitzgerald C, Gill K, Hoskins P, Klasa R, Savage KJ, Shenkier T, Sutherland J, et al. 2007. The revised International Prognostic Index (R-IPI) is a better predictor of outcome than the standard IPI for patients with diffuse large B-cell lymphoma treated with R-CHOP. *Blood* **109:** 1857–1861. doi:10.1182/blood-2006-08-038257

Shadman M, Mawad R, Dean C, Chen TL, Shannon-Dorcy K, Sandhu V, Hendrie PC, Scott BL, Walter RB, Becker PS, et al. 2015. Idarubicin, cytarabine, and pravastatin as induction therapy for untreated acute myeloid leukemia and high-risk myelodysplastic syndrome. *Am J Hematol* **90:** 483–486. doi:10.1002/ajh.23981

Sharon D, Cathelin S, Mirali S, Di Trani JM, Yanofsky DJ, Keon KA, Rubinstein JL, Schimmer AD, Ketela T, Chan SM. 2019. Inhibition of mitochondrial translation overcomes venetoclax resistance in AML through activation of the integrated stress response. *Sci Transl Med* **11:** eaax2863. doi:10.1126/scitranslmed.aax2863

Shim H, Dolde C, Lewis BC, Wu CS, Dang G, Jungmann RA, Dalla-Favera R, Dang CV. 1997. c-Myc transactivation of *LDH-A*: Implications for tumor metabolism and growth. *Proc Natl Acad Sci* **94:** 6658–6663. doi:10.1073/pnas.94.13.6658

Shojaee S, Chan LN, Buchner M, Cazzaniga V, Cosgun KN, Geng H, Qiu YH, von Minden MD, Ernst T, Hochhaus A, et al. 2016. *PTEN* opposes negative selection and enables oncogenic transformation of pre-B cells. *Nat Med* **22:** 379–387. doi:10.1038/nm.4062

Singh K, Lin J, Zhong Y, Burčul A, Mohan P, Jiang M, Sun L, Yong-Gonzalez V, Viale A, Cross JR, et al. 2019. c-MYC regulates mRNA translation efficiency and start-site selection in lymphoma. *J Exp Med.* **216:** 1509–1524.

Škrtić M, Sriskanthadevan S, Jhas B, Gebbia M, Wang X, Wang Z, Hurren R, Jitkova Y, Gronda M, Maclean N, et al. 2011. Inhibition of mitochondrial translation as a therapeutic strategy for human acute myeloid leukemia. *Cancer Cell* **20:** 674–688. doi:10.1016/j.ccr.2011.10.015

Sommermann TG, O'Neill K, Plas DR, Cahir-McFarland E. 2011. IKKβ and NF-κB transcription govern lymphoma cell survival through AKT-induced plasma membrane trafficking of GLUT1. *Cancer Res* **71:** 7291–7300. doi:10.1158/0008-5472.CAN-11-1715

Son J, Lyssiotis CA, Ying H, Wang X, Hua S, Ligorio M, Perera RM, Ferrone CR, Mullarky E, Shyh-Chang N, et al. 2013. Glutamine supports pancreatic cancer growth through a KRAS-regulated metabolic pathway. *Nature* **496:** 101–105. doi:10.1038/nature12040

Southam AD, Khanim FL, Hayden RE, Constantinou JK, Koczula KM, Michell RH, Viant MR, Drayson MT, Bunce CM. 2015. Drug redeployment to kill leukemia and lymphoma cells by disrupting SCD1-mediated synthesis of monounsaturated fatty acids. *Cancer Res* **75:** 2530–2540. doi:10.1158/0008-5472.CAN-15-0202

Sriskanthadevan S, Jeyaraju DV, Chung TE, Prabha S, Xu W, Skrtic M, Jhas B, Hurren R, Gronda M, Wang X, et al. 2015. AML cells have low spare reserve capacity in their respiratory chain that renders them susceptible to oxidative metabolic stress. *Blood* **125:** 2120–2130. doi:10.1182/blood-2014-08-594408

Stein EM, DiNardo CD, Pollyea DA, Fathi AT, Roboz GJ, Altman JK, Stone RM, DeAngelo DJ, Levine RL, Flinn IW, et al. 2017. Enasidenib in mutant *IDH2* relapsed or refractory acute myeloid leukemia. *Blood* **130:** 722–731. doi:10.1182/blood-2017-04-779405

Stine ZE, Walton ZE, Altman BJ, Hsieh AL, Dang CV. 2015. MYC, metabolism, and cancer. *Cancer Discov* **5:** 1024–1039. doi:10.1158/2159-8290.CD-15-0507

Stuart SD, Schauble A, Gupta S, Kennedy AD, Keppler BR, Bingham PM, Zachar Z. 2014. A strategically designed small molecule attacks α-ketoglutarate dehydrogenase in tumor cells through a redox process. *Cancer Metab* **2:** 4. doi:10.1186/2049-3002-2-4

Su R, Dong L, Li C, Nachtergaele S, Wunderlich M, Qing Y, Deng X, Wang Y, Weng X, Hu C, et al. 2018. R-2HG exhibits anti-tumor activity by targeting FTO/m^{6}A/MYC/CEBPA signaling. *Cell* **172:** 90–105.e23. doi:10.1016/j.cell.2017.11.031

Sulkowski PL, Corso CD, Robinson ND, Scanlon SE, Purshouse KR, Bai H, Liu Y, Sundaram RK, Hegan DC, Fons NR, et al. 2017. 2-Hydroxyglutarate produced by neomorphic IDH mutations suppresses homologous recombination and induces PARP inhibitor sensitivity. *Sci Transl Med* **9:** eaal2463. doi:10.1126/scitranslmed.aal2463

Sulkowski PL, Oeck S, Dow J, Economos NG, Mirfakhraie L, Liu Y, Noronha K, Bao X, Li J, Shuch BM, et al. 2020. Oncometabolites suppress DNA repair by disrupting local chromatin signalling. *Nature* **582:** 586–591. doi:10.1038/s41586-020-2363-0

Sullivan LB, Chandel NS. 2014. Mitochondrial reactive oxygen species and cancer. *Cancer Metab* **2:** 17. doi:10.1186/2049-3002-2-17

Sullivan LB, Gui DY, Hosios AM, Bush LN, Freinkman E, Vander Heiden MG. 2015. Supporting aspartate biosynthesis is an essential function of respiration in proliferating cells. *Cell* **162:** 552–563. doi:10.1016/j.cell.2015.07.017

Sullivan LB, Luengo A, Danai LV, Bush LN, Diehl FF, Hosios AM, Lau AN, Elmiligy S, Malstrom S, Lewis CA, et al. 2018. Aspartate is an endogenous metabolic limitation for tumour growth. *Nat Cell Biol* **20:** 782–788. doi:10.1038/s41556-018-0125-0

Sykes DB, Kfoury YS, Mercier FE, Wawer MJ, Law JM, Haynes MK, Lewis TA, Schajnovitz A, Jain E, Lee D, et al. 2016. Inhibition of dihydroorotate dehydrogenase overcomes differentiation blockade in acute myeloid leukemia. *Cell* **167:** 171–186.e15. doi:10.1016/j.cell.2016.08.057

Szlosarek PW. 2014. Arginine deprivation and autophagic cell death in cancer. *Proc Natl Acad Sci* **111:** 14015–14016. doi:10.1073/pnas.1416560111

Tiziani S, Kang Y, Harjanto R, Axelrod J, Piermarocchi C, Roberts W, Paternostro G. 2013. Metabolomics of the tumor microenvironment in pediatric acute lymphoblastic leukemia. *PLoS One* **8:** e82859. doi:10.1371/journal.pone.0082859

Trachootham D, Alexandre J, Huang P. 2009. Targeting cancer cells by ROS-mediated mechanisms: A radical therapeutic approach? *Nat Rev Drug Discov* **8:** 579–591. doi:10.1038/nrd2803

Tsai HJ, Jiang SS, Hung WC, Borthakur G, Lin SF, Pemmaraju N, Jabbour E, Bomalaski JS, Chen YP, Hsiao HH, et al. 2017. A phase II study of arginine deiminase (ADI-PEG20) in relapsed/refractory or poor-risk acute myeloid leukemia patients. *Sci Rep* **7:** 11253. doi:10.1038/s41598-017-10542-4

Turcan S, Rohle D, Goenka A, Walsh LA, Fang F, Yilmaz E, Campos C, Fabius AW, Lu C, Ward PS, et al. 2012. IDH1 mutation is sufficient to establish the glioma hypermethylator phenotype. *Nature* **483:** 479–483. doi:10.1038/nature10866

Tzoneva G, Perez-Garcia A, Carpenter Z, Khiabanian H, Tosello V, Allegretta M, Paietta E, Racevskis J, Rowe JM, Tallman MS, et al. 2013. Activating mutations in the *NT5C2* nucleotidase gene drive chemotherapy resistance in relapsed ALL. *Nat Med* **19:** 368–371. doi:10.1038/nm.3078

Tzoneva G, Dieck CL, Oshima K, Ambesi-Impiombato A, Sánchez-Martín M, Madubata CJ, Khiabanian H, Yu J, Waanders E, Iacobucci I, et al. 2018. Clonal evolution mechanisms in NT5C2 mutant-relapsed acute lymphoblastic leukaemia. *Nature* **553:** 511–514. doi:10.1038/nature25186

Vander Heiden MG, DeBerardinis RJ. 2017. Understanding the intersections between metabolism and cancer biology. *Cell* **168:** 657–669. doi:10.1016/j.cell.2016.12.039

Vander Heiden MG, Cantley LC, Thompson CB. 2009. Understanding the Warburg effect: The metabolic requirements of cell proliferation. *Science* **324:** 1029–1033. doi:10.1126/science.1160809

Wang F, Travins J, DeLaBarre B, Penard-Lacronique V, Schalm S, Hansen E, Straley K, Kernytsky A, Liu W, Gliser C, et al. 2013. Targeted inhibition of mutant IDH2 in leukemia cells induces cellular differentiation. *Science* **340:** 622–626. doi:10.1126/science.1234769

Wang YH, Israelsen WJ, Lee D, Yu VWC, Jeanson NT, Clish CB, Cantley LC, Vander Heiden MG, Scadden DT. 2014. Cell-state-specific metabolic dependency in hematopoiesis and leukemogenesis. *Cell* **158:** 1309–1323. doi:10.1016/j.cell.2014.07.048

Wang C, McKeithan TW, Gong Q, Zhang W, Bouska A, Rosenwald A, Gascoyne RD, Wu X, Wang J, Muhammad Z, et al. 2015a. *IDH2*^{R172} mutations define a unique subgroup of patients with angioimmunoblastic T-cell lymphoma. *Blood* **126:** 1741–1752. doi:10.1182/blood-2015-05-644591

Wang ES, Frankfurt O, Orford KW, Bennett M, Flinn IW, Maris M, Konopleva M. 2015b. Phase 1 study of CB-839, a first-in-class, orally administered small molecule inhibitor of glutaminase in patients with relapsed/refractory leukemia. *Blood* **126:** 2566. doi:10.1182/blood.V126.23.2566.2566

Wang P, Wu J, Ma S, Zhang L, Yao J, Hoadley KA, Wilkerson MD, Perou CM, Guan KL, Ye D, et al. 2015c. Oncometabolite D-2-hydroxyglutarate inhibits ALKBH DNA repair enzymes and sensitizes *IDH* mutant cells to alkylating agents. *Cell Rep* **13:** 2353–2361. doi:10.1016/j.celrep.2015.11.029

Wang F, Gatica D, Ying ZX, Peterson LF, Kim P, Bernard D, Saiya-Cork K, Wang S, Kaminski MS, Chang AE, et al. 2019a. Follicular lymphoma-associated mutations in vacuolar ATPase ATP6V1B2 activate autophagic flux and mTOR. *J Clin Invest* **129:** 1626–1640. doi:10.1172/JCI98288

Wang LW, Shen H, Nobre L, Ersing I, Paulo JA, Trudeau S, Wang Z, Smith NA, Ma Y, Reinstadler B, et al. 2019b. Epstein–Barr-virus-induced one-carbon metabolism drives B cell transformation. *Cell Metab* **30:** 539–555.e11. doi:10.1016/j.cmet.2019.06.003

Wang LW, Wang Z, Ersing I, Nobre L, Guo R, Jiang S, Trudeau S, Zhao B, Weekes MP, Gewurz BE. 2019c. Epstein–Barr virus subverts mevalonate and fatty acid pathways to promote infected B-cell proliferation and survival. *PLoS Pathog* **15:** e1008030. doi:10.1371/journal.ppat.1008030

Warburg O. 1924. Uber den Stoffwechsel der Karzinomezellen. *Biochem Z* **152:** 309–344.

Warburg O. 1956. On the origin of cancer cells. *Science* **123:** 309–314. doi:10.1126/science.123.3191.309

Ward PS, Patel J, Wise DR, Abdel-Wahab O, Bennett BD, Coller HA, Cross JR, Fantin VR, Hedvat CV, Perl AE, et al. 2010. The common feature of leukemia-associated IDH1 and IDH2 mutations is a neomorphic enzyme activity converting α-ketoglutarate to 2-hydroxyglutarate. *Cancer Cell* **17:** 225–234. doi:10.1016/j.ccr.2010.01.020

Weiser MA, Cabanillas ME, Konopleva M, Thomas DA, Pierce SA, Escalante CP, Kantarjian HM, O'Brien SM. 2004. Relation between the duration of remission and hyperglycemia during induction chemotherapy for acute lymphocytic leukemia with a hyperfractionated cyclophosphamide, vincristine, doxorubicin, and dexamethasone/methotrexate-cytarabine regimen. *Cancer* **100:** 1179–1185. doi:10.1002/cncr.20071

Williams RT, Guarecuco R, Gates LA, Barrows D, Passarelli MC, Carey B, Baudrier L, Jeewajee S, La K, Prizer B, et al. 2020. ZBTB1 regulates asparagine synthesis and leukemia cell response to L-asparaginase. *Cell Metab* **31:** 852–861.e6. doi:10.1016/j.cmet.2020.03.008

Wise DR, Thompson CB. 2010. Glutamine addiction: A new therapeutic target in cancer. *Trends Biochem Sci* **35:** 427–433. doi:10.1016/j.tibs.2010.05.003

Wong WW, Dimitroulakos J, Minden MD, Penn LZ. 2002. HMG-CoA reductase inhibitors and the malignant cell: The statin family of drugs as triggers of tumor-specific apoptosis. *Leukemia* **16:** 508–519. doi:10.1038/sj.leu.2402476

Wu C, Gupta N, Huang YH, Zhang HF, Alshareef A, Chow A, Lai R. 2018a. Oxidative stress enhances tumorigenicity and stem-like features via the activation of the Wnt/β-catenin/MYC/Sox2 axis in ALK-positive anaplastic large-cell lymphoma. *BMC Cancer* **18:** 361. doi:10.1186/s12885-018-4300-2

Wu D, Wang W, Chen W, Lian F, Lang L, Huang Y, Xu Y, Zhang N, Chen Y, Liu M, et al. 2018b. Pharmacological inhibition of dihydroorotate dehydrogenase induces apoptosis and differentiation in acute myeloid leukemia cells. *Haematologica* **103:** 1472–1483. doi:10.3324/haematol.2018.188185

Xia H, Wang W, Crespo J, Kryczek I, Li W, Wei S, Bian Z, Maj T, He M, Liu RJ, et al. 2017. Suppression of FIP200 and autophagy by tumor-derived lactate promotes naive T cell apoptosis and affects tumor immunity. *Sci Immunol* **2:** eaan4631.

Xiao G, Chan LN, Klemm L, Braas D, Chen Z, Geng H, Zhang QC, Aghajanirefah A, Cosgun KN, Sadras T, et al. 2018. B-cell-specific diversion of glucose carbon utilization reveals a unique vulnerability in B cell malignancies. *Cell* **173:** 470–484.e18. doi:10.1016/j.cell.2018.02.048

Xiong J, Wang L, Fei XC, Jiang XF, Zheng Z, Zhao Y, Wang CF, Li B, Chen SJ, Janin A, et al. 2017. MYC is a positive regulator of choline metabolism and impedes mitophagy-dependent necroptosis in diffuse large B-cell lymphoma. *Blood Cancer J* **7:** e0.

Xu RH, Pelicano H, Zhang H, Giles FJ, Keating MJ, Huang P. 2005. Synergistic effect of targeting mTOR by rapamycin and depleting ATP by inhibition of glycolysis in lymphoma and leukemia cells. *Leukemia* **19:** 2153–2158. doi:10.1038/sj.leu.2403968

Ye J, Kumanova M, Hart LS, Sloane K, Zhang H, De Panis DN, Bobrovnikova-Marjon E, Diehl JA, Ron D, Koumenis C. 2010. The GCN2-ATF4 pathway is critical for tumour cell survival and proliferation in response to nutrient deprivation. *EMBO J* **29:** 2082–2096. doi:10.1038/emboj.2010.81

Ye H, Adane B, Khan N, Sullivan T, Minhajuddin M, Gasparetto M, Stevens B, Pei S, Balys M, Ashton JM, et al. 2016. Leukemic stem cells evade chemotherapy by metabolic adaptation to an adipose tissue niche. *Cell Stem Cell* **19:** 23–37. doi:10.1016/j.stem.2016.06.001

Ye D, Guan KL, Xiong Y. 2018a. Metabolism, activity, and targeting of D- and L-2-hydroxyglutarates. *Trends Cancer* **4:** 151–165. doi:10.1016/j.trecan.2017.12.005

Ye H, Adane B, Khan N, Alexeev E, Nusbacher N, Minhajuddin M, Stevens BM, Winters AC, Lin X, Ashton JM, et al. 2018b. Subversion of systemic glucose metabolism as a mechanism to support the growth of leukemia cells. *Cancer Cell* **34:** 659–673.e6. doi:10.1016/j.ccell.2018.08.016

Yen K, Travins J, Wang F, David MD, Artin E, Straley K, Padyana A, Gross S, DeLaBarre B, Tobin E, et al. 2017. AG-221, a first-in-class therapy targeting acute myeloid leukemia harboring oncogenic *IDH2* mutations. *Cancer Discov* **7:** 478–493. doi:10.1158/2159-8290.CD-16-1034

Ying H, Kimmelman AC, Lyssiotis CA, Hua S, Chu GC, Fletcher-Sananikone E, Locasale JW, Son J, Zhang H, Coloff JL, et al. 2012. Oncogenic Kras maintains pancreatic tumors through regulation of anabolic glucose metabolism. *Cell* **149:** 656–670. doi:10.1016/j.cell.2012.01.058

Ying ZX, Jin M, Peterson LF, Bernard D, Saiya-Cork K, Yildiz M, Wang S, Kaminski MS, Chang AE, Klionsky DJ, et al. 2016. Recurrent mutations in the MTOR regulator RRAGC in follicular lymphoma. *Clin Cancer Res* **22:** 5383–5393. doi:10.1158/1078-0432.CCR-16-0609

Yun J, Rago C, Cheong I, Pagliarini R, Angenendt P, Rajagopalan H, Schmidt K, Willson JK, Markowitz S, Zhou S, et al. 2009. Glucose deprivation contributes to the development of *KRAS* pathway mutations in tumor cells. *Science* **325:** 1555–1559. doi:10.1126/science.1174229

Yun J, Mullarky E, Lu C, Bosch KN, Kavalier A, Rivera K, Roper J, Chio II, Giannopoulou EG, Rago C, et al. 2015. Vitamin C selectively kills *KRAS* and *BRAF* mutant colorectal cancer cells by targeting GAPDH. *Science* **350:** 1391–1396. doi:10.1126/science.aaa5004

Zhang W, Trachootham D, Liu J, Chen G, Pelicano H, Garcia-Prieto C, Lu W, Burger JA, Croce CM, Plunkett W, et al. 2012. Stromal control of cystine metabolism promotes cancer cell survival in chronic lymphocytic leukaemia. *Nat Cell Biol* **14:** 276–286. doi:10.1038/ncb2432

Zhang L, Yao Y, Zhang S, Liu Y, Guo H, Ahmed M, Bell T, Zhang H, Han G, Lorence E, et al. 2019a. Metabolic reprogramming toward oxidative phosphorylation identifies a therapeutic target for mantle cell lymphoma. *Sci Transl Med* **11:** eaau1167.

Zhang Y, Tan H, Daniels JD, Zandkarimi F, Liu H, Brown LM, Uchida K, O'Connor OA, Stockwell BR. 2019b. Imidazole ketone erastin induces ferroptosis and slows tumor growth in a mouse lymphoma model. *Cell Chem Biol* **26:** 623–633.e9.

Mouse Models of Myeloid Malignancies

Faisal Basheer[1,2,3] and George Vassiliou[1,2,3]

[1]Wellcome–MRC Cambridge Stem Cell Institute, Jeffrey Cheah Biomedical Centre, Department of Haematology, University of Cambridge, Cambridge CB2 0AW, United Kingdom

[2]Haematological Cancer Genetics, Wellcome Trust Sanger Institute, Cambridge CB10 1SA, United Kingdom

[3]Department of Haematology, Cambridge University Hospitals NHS Foundation Trust, Cambridge CB2 0QQ, United Kingdom

Correspondence: gsv20@sanger.ac.uk

Mouse models of human myeloid malignancies support the detailed and focused investigation of selected driver mutations and represent powerful tools in the study of these diseases. Carefully developed murine models can closely recapitulate human myeloid malignancies in vivo, enabling the interrogation of a number of aspects of these diseases including their preclinical course, interactions with the microenvironment, effects of pharmacological agents, and the role of non-cell-autonomous factors, as well as the synergy between co-occurring mutations. Importantly, advances in gene-editing technologies, particularly CRISPR–Cas9, have opened new avenues for the development and study of genetically modified mice and also enable the direct modification of mouse and human hematopoietic cells. In this review we provide a concise overview of some of the important mouse models that have advanced our understanding of myeloid leukemogenesis with an emphasis on models relevant to clonal hematopoiesis, myelodysplastic syndromes, and acute myeloid leukemia with a normal karyotype.

Myeloid malignancies are a spectrum of clonal disorders of hematopoietic stem cells (HSCs) variously characterized by excessive proliferation, abnormal self-renewal, defective differentiation, and ineffective hematopoiesis (Spivak 2004; Prchal 2005; Döhner et al. 2015; Kennedy and Ebert 2017). With an incidence of more than 15 cases per 100,000 per year (Visser et al. 2012), they represent a substantial health burden. At the chronic end of the spectrum, they consist of myelodysplastic syndromes (MDSs), myeloproliferative neoplasms (MPNs) that are typically preleukemic syndromes capable of transformation to secondary acute myeloid leukemia (AML) (Arber et al. 2016). Other cases of AML may result following cytotoxic therapy for unrelated malignancies, but most arise as primary or de novo AML. Studies of these disorders have markedly advanced our understanding of the clonal origins of cancer (Ben-Neriah et al. 1986; Lapidot et al. 1994; Bonnet and Dick 1997; James et al. 2005; Kralovics et al. 2005; Levine et al. 2005; Welch et al. 2012; Klampfl et al. 2013; Nangalia et al. 2013) and have established several paradigms in cancer research by paving the way with studies

Cite this article as *Cold Spring Harb Perspect Med* doi: 10.1101/cshperspect.a035535

of the molecular pathogenesis, disease classification, genetic vulnerabilities, prognostication, and monitoring/treatment (Meyer and Levine 2014; Arber et al. 2016; Tzelepis et al. 2016; Döhner et al. 2017; Montalban-Bravo and Garcia-Manero 2018).

Advances in cancer genomics have captured the set of somatic gene mutations that drive myeloid neoplasms (Table 1), revealing that many are shared between multiple different subtypes (Cancer Genome Atlas Research Network et al. 2013; Klampfl et al. 2013; Nangalia et al. 2013; Haferlach et al. 2014). Such studies have also demonstrated that some of these mutations occur early and others later in disease progression (Welch et al. 2012). More recently the discovery of the common age-related phenomenon of clonal hematopoiesis (CH) (Genovese et al. 2014; Gerstung et al. 2014; Jaiswal et al. 2014; Xie et al. 2014; McKerrell et al. 2015), the expansion of hematopoietic cell clones arising from HSCs carrying "myeloid" gene mutations, has helped put these observations into a model of myeloid cancer pathogenesis. In this model, an "early" mutation in genes such as *DNMT3A*, *TET2*, *ASXL1*, *SF3B1*, *SRSF2*, *TP53*, and *JAK2* leads to the establishment of CH clones that can stabilize in size or expand significantly during life, but only lead to a myeloid cancer in a small minority of cases. Malignant progression is usually, but not always, driven by the acquisition of "late" mutations involving proliferation genes such as *FLT3*, *NRAS*, and *KRAS*. Other genes do not fall neatly into the "early" and "late" categories, including *NPM1* and probably *RUNX1*, which almost always occur after the "early" and before the "late" mutations, and *IDH1/IDH2*, whose order varies between individual cases. Recent studies have shown that the likelihood of malignant progression is greater when particular driver genes are mutated (e.g., *U2AF1*, *SRSF2*, *IDH1/2*, and *TP53*), when clonal size is larger, and when multiple mutations are present (Abelson et al. 2018; Desai et al. 2018).

Chromosomal translocations or inversions that usually lead to the formation of fusion oncogenes are also common in myeloid cancers, found in ~20% of all cases of AML (Papaemmanuil et al. 2016) and a small proportion (~2%–3%) of the MDSs (Costa et al. 2013). Leukemia-associated chromosomal translocations were among the first cancer-associated mutations to be identified (Rowley 1973; Lindgren and Rowley 1977; Rowley et al. 1977; Knapp et al. 1985; Nowell et al. 1986) and represent "early" events. In AML, these mutations usually cause a block of differentiation of hematopoietic stem/progenitor cells (HSPCs) and, at least in some cases, can be found many years before the disease manifests itself (Greaves and Wiemels 2003). Translocations are much more common in pediatric and young adult AML, becoming uncommon in the elderly (Bolouri et al. 2018). Transformation is often driven by the acquisition of one of the "late" mutations mentioned in the previous paragraph.

Despite these advances, only 30% of patients with AML survive long term, whereas both

Table 1. Common somatic mutations noted predominantly in acute myeloid leukemia (AML) (and in some cases of clonal hematopoiesis [CH], myelodysplastic syndrome [MDS], and myeloproliferative neoplasm [MPN]) classified by functional subgroups

Biological function	Mutant gene
Activated signaling pathways	*FLT3, NRAS, KRAS, KIT, PTPN11, NF1*
Chromatin modifiers	*ASXL1, EZH2, KDM6A, MLL* fusions
Cohesin complex	*RAD21, SMC1, SMC3, STAG1, STAG2*
DNA methylation	*DNMT3A, DNMT3B, IDH1, IDH2, TET1, TET2*
Myeloid transcription factors	*CEBPA, GATA2, RUNX1*
Nucleophosmin	*NPM1*
Spliceosome complex	*SRSF2, U2AF1, SF3B1, ZRSR2*
Transcription factor fusions	*PML-RARA, RUNX1-RUNX1T1, MYH11-CBFB*
Tumor suppressors	*TP53, WT1, PHF6*

MDS and MPN remain incurable without bone marrow transplantation—an option that is open only to a fraction of patients. A change in this unsatisfactory landscape requires an improved understanding of the molecular pathogenesis of these disorders, a key step in the development of new therapeutic approaches. The characterization of the biological roles of putative cancer driver genes is critical for the development of therapeutic modalities to tackle these malignancies. Myeloid cancer cell lines harboring relevant mutations have been useful tools to validate target driver genes in vitro, but invariably have limitations that result in them not reflecting primary malignancies adequately (Sharma et al. 2010; Gillet et al. 2013). These include the acquisition of additional mutations required for in vitro growth and others that can serve to enhance subclonal fitness through multiple passages, as well as passenger mutations that can affect the way these lines behave in particular contexts. Also, in vitro culture is an artificial setting that departs significantly from the microenvironment within which myeloid cancers develop. Such factors diminish the utility of cell lines in deciphering the molecular effects of common driver mutations, an important step in developing new therapeutic approaches. The use of primary human myeloid cancer cells is an attractive alternative and does hold significant experimental utility, but these cells are often fragile ex vivo and difficult to propagate successfully in vitro. Also, the molecular heterogeneity between individual myeloid cancers makes it difficult to interrogate mutations in specific genes or gene combinations. By contrast, murine models enable the detailed and focused investigation of selected myeloid mutations, represent powerful tools in the study of these diseases, and have made a substantial contribution to the understanding of their biology. Critically, carefully developed mouse models can closely recapitulate human myeloid malignancies in vivo, enabling the interrogation of a number of aspects of these diseases including their preclinical course, their interactions with the microenvironment, the impact of aging, the effects of pharmacological agents, and the role of non-cell-autonomous factors, as well as the synergy between selected mutations. In addition, immunocompromised mice can be used to study primary human cells in xenotransplants, models that are particularly useful in the investigation of novel therapeutic intervention under controlled experimental conditions. Finally, advances in gene-editing technologies—particularly CRISPR–Cas9 (Cho et al. 2013; Koike-Yusa et al. 2014; Wang et al. 2014; Shalem et al. 2015; Shi et al. 2015)—have opened new avenues for the study of genetically modified mice, as well as mouse and human cells.

In this review we give an overview of mouse models of myeloid malignancies and their relevance to human myeloid malignancies with a particular emphasis on AML. We also discuss their relevance to the preleukemic state in the context of MDS, MPN, and the rapidly advancing area of clonal hematopoiesis and discuss future applications of these models that can help derive novel insights into cancer biology.

TYPES OF MODELS

Of the numerous organisms available in science to model disease biology, the mouse (*Mus musculus*) has become the most widely used organism for the study of human cancers and nonmalignant diseases for many reasons. These have been well-documented in recent comprehensive reviews, and the reader is directed to these for further insights (Day et al. 2015; Kohnken et al. 2017; de Ruiter et al. 2018; Landgraf et al. 2018).

Transgenic Models

Transgenic models are the simplest type of genetically engineered mouse model (GEMM), in which a DNA construct is randomly integrated into the genome after injection into the male pronucleus of fertilized eggs. Examples include cDNA constructs of mutant oncogenes expressed under the control of a ubiquitous or tissue-specific promoter (Early et al. 1996) or mutagenic transposons that can be mobilized into the genome in mutagenesis studies (Fig. 1A, left panel; Vassiliou et al. 2011).

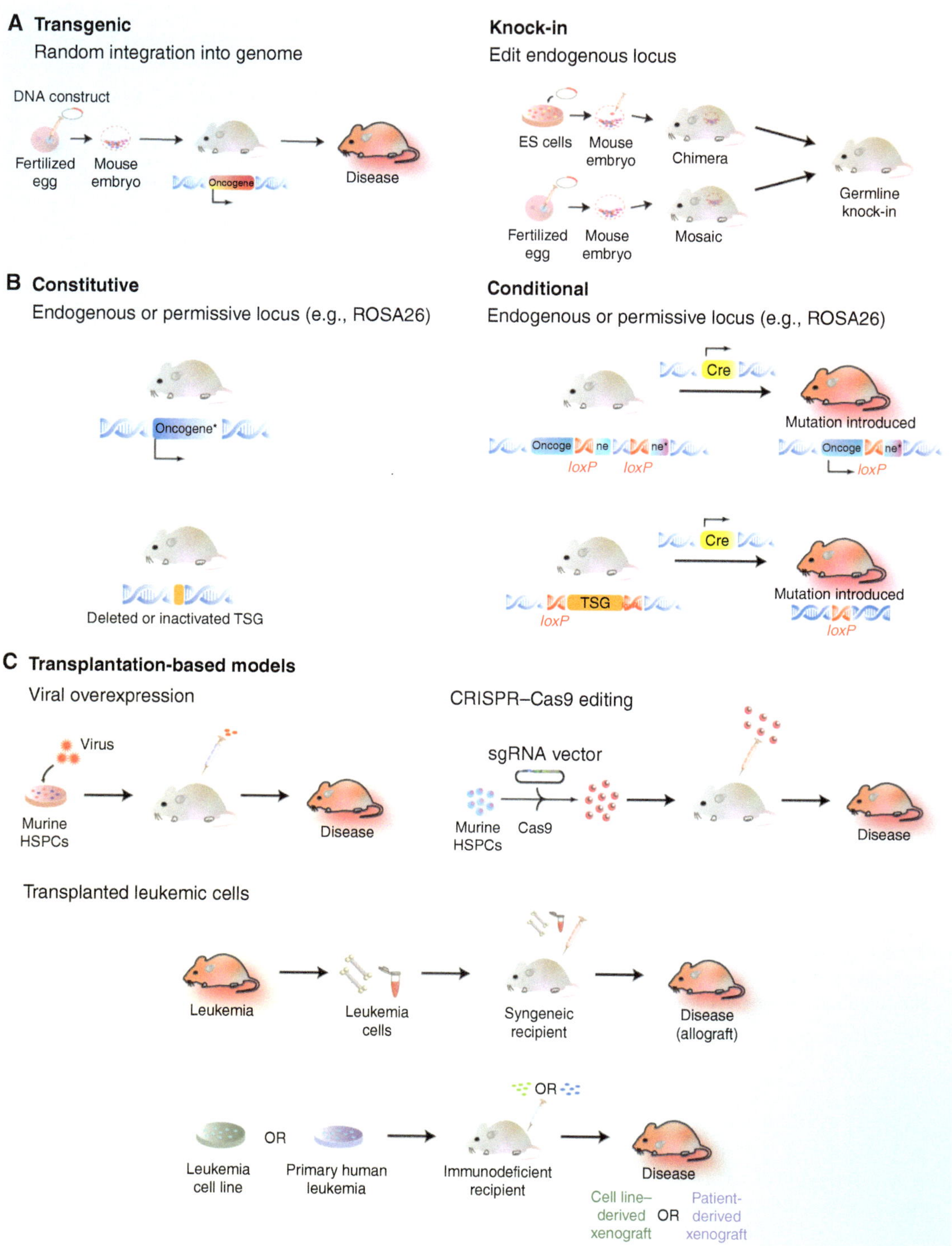

Figure 1. *(Legend on following page.)*

Knock-In Models

Knock-in models have been steadily replacing transgenic ones since the advent of embryonic stem (ES) cells (Bradley et al. 1984). Knock-in GEMMs are derived by targeted modification of the mouse genome and can involve the introduction of an activating mutation into an oncogene, a loss-of-function mutation in a tumor-suppressor gene (TSG), or the introduction of a mutant cDNA into a high-expressing location such as the *Rosa*-26 locus (Fig. 1B). Most knock-in mice have been generated by targeted modification of ES cell genomes using homologous recombination (HR) and generation of *chimeric* mice that are bred to stock mice to achieve germline transmission of the modified locus, usually through the male gametes (Fig. 1A, right panel). More recently, the advent of highly efficient genome editing tools, such as CRISPR–Cas9, is replacing or facilitating HR approaches. Importantly, CRISPR–Cas9 is enabling the direct modification of fertilized eggs at high efficiency such that the need for ES cells can be bypassed for at least some alleles. Using the latter approach can often lead to the introduction of the genetic modification only after the zygote has divided, leading to the generation of *mosaic* mice, which again have to be bred to achieve germline transmission (Fig. 1A, right panel).

Constitutive versus Conditional Models

There are broadly two types of genetically modified alleles introduced into GEMMs, constitutive and conditional (Fig. 1B). In constitutive alleles, the introduced mutation is active in all tissues/cells, whereas in conditional alleles the mutation is silent and requires activation. This is typically achieved through the Cre/*loxP* recombination system in which conditional alleles carry pairs of 34-bp-long *loxP* DNA sequences that are recognized by the Cre-recombinase enzyme, leading to recombination between the two *loxP* sites and excision of the intervening DNA as a loop (Sauer and Henderson 1988). The Cre-recombinase can be expressed under the control of a variety of promoters that (a) are tissue-specific, thereby allowing for recombination in a planned spatial manner, and (b) can be activated temporally through specific external

Figure 1. (*A*) (*Left* panel) Transgenic mouse model. A DNA construct containing gene sequence of interest is inserted into the genome through pronuclear injection into a fertilized egg, yielding transgenic offspring that develop disease (a mutant oncogene is shown as an example). (*Right* panel) Knock-in mouse model. Gene of interest is inserted into embryonic stem (ES) cell genome (*upper* half) or fertilized egg (*lower* half) to yield a chimeric or mosaic mouse knock-in mouse, respectively. Through subsequent breeding to stock mice, germline transmission of the modified locus is achieved. (*B*) Both constitutive and conditional mouse models are generated through introduction of genetically modified alleles into mice at either the endogenous locus or a highly expressive permissive locus (e.g., Rosa26 locus, as indicated). In the constitutive model (*left* panel), the introduced mutation (gain of oncogene or loss of tumor-suppressor gene [TSG]) is active in all tissues and cells. In the conditional model (*right* panel), the inserted alleles of interest are flanked by *loxP* sites, and through crossing these modified mice with a Cre-recombinase, the oncogene can be activated (*upper* half) or the TSG inactivated/removed (*lower* half) when required through activation of Cre-recombinase in a planned temporal/spatial manner. (*C*) Transplantation-based models. Lentiviral or retroviral constructs harboring oncogenes of interest are transduced into murine hematopoietic stem/progenitor cells (HSPCs) at variable transduction efficiencies to cause overexpression of the oncogene (*top left* panel). Transduced HSPCs are either selected first or transplanted in bulk through intravenous injection into irradiated syngeneic recipient mice, which later yield disease depending on factors such as nature of oncogene, transplanted cell numbers, radiation, and success of engraftment. In CRISPR–Cas9 editing, murine HSPCs can be transduced with Cas9 and sgRNA vectors designed to activate or interrupt gene of interest (*top right* panel). Alternatively, murine HSPCs derived from a native Cas9-expressing mouse can be used. Leukemic cells derived from primary murine leukemic tissues (e.g., bone marrow or spleen) can be harvested and transplanted into irradiated syngeneic recipient mice to yield disease (*bottom* panel). Alternatively, human leukemic cell lines or freshly isolated primary human leukemia cells can be isolated and injected into a native immunodeficient recipient mouse (e.g., nonobese diabetic/severe combined immunodeficiency [NOD-SCID]) yielding a cell line– or patient-derived xenograft, respectively.

mechanisms (e.g., through induction of an inflammatory response or via hormonal activation among other mechanisms) (Kuhn et al. 1995). Cre-mediated recombination can thus be used to activate oncogenes through removal of a "stop" sequence designed to block their expression or to inactivate TSG function through the deletion of important exons (Stadtfeld and Graf 2005) or entire genes or even chromosomal regions (Barlow et al. 2010). The most commonly used Cre-recombinase alleles are the transgenic alleles *Mx1*-Cre (Kuhn et al. 1995) and *Vav*-Cre (Stadtfeld and Graf 2005), both of which express in HSCs. *Vav*-Cre expresses constitutively in hematopoietic tissues, whereas the *Mx1*-Cre expresses Cre under the control of an interferon-responsive promoter. This allows inducible activation of Cre upon injection of polyinosinic polycytidilic acid (pIpC), an RNA analog that induces an antiviral interferon response.

Murine Transplantation Models

Murine transplantation models have been commonly used in understanding hematopoiesis and leukemogenesis. Whereas transgenic and conditional GEMMs are invaluable for examining the role of specific genes or gene mutations, they are expensive and time-consuming to generate. The flexibility of the hematopoietic system enables the application of genetic approaches that target mouse HSCs directly. In this setting, murine leukemia-inducing lenti-/retroviral vectors can be used to introduce and overexpress oncogenes into the cells (Rein 2011; Kohnken et al. 2017; de Ruiter et al. 2018). Cells transduced by virus are then transplanted into lethally or sublethally irradiated syngeneic recipients, which can go on to develop leukemia arising from the transformed HSPCs (Fig. 1C, top left panel). Alternatively, leukemic cells isolated can be infused into immunocompromised or irradiated recipient mice often for the study of genetic or therapeutic interventions (Fig. 1C, bottom panel). Such cells can be allografts derived from leukemic mice (primary leukemias) transplanted into syngeneic mice, which have the advantage of capturing interactions of the AML cells with their microenvironment. Alternatively, human AML cell lines or patient-derived xenografts (PDXs) can be transplanted into immunocompromised mice (Fig. 1C, bottom panel). The latter, as a more accurate representation of the original disease, is often considered the gold standard for preclinical therapeutic studies, but does not capture leukemia–niche interactions given the species barrier. Also, PDXs can be more challenging to establish because of the relative frailty of primary samples, potentially lower numbers of leukemic stem/progenitor cells being available for transplantation at sampling, and variable engraftment efficiencies. Also, subclonal selection from within the transplanted sample routinely occurs in mice, leading to a skewed representation of the patient's disease.

Transduction/transplantation models have been instrumental in deciphering the target cell for transformation for several AML-associated mutations. For example, Cozzio et al. (2003) reported that the *MLL-ENL* fusion conferred properties of self-renewal to committed myeloid progenitors and induced AML following transplantation into mice. Similarly, Huntly et al. (2004) showed that transduction of committed murine hematopoietic progenitors with *MOZ-TIF2* allowed for their propagation in vitro and subsequent ability to generate AML when transplanted into mice, in contrast to *BCR-ABL*, which did not transform these progenitors. Also, Krivtsov et al. (2006) demonstrated that in vitro–propagated murine GMP progenitors transduced with *MLL-AF9* led to AML development in recipient mice.

CRISPR–Cas9 Gene Editing

CRISPR–Cas9 gene editing enables the simultaneous targeting of one or more genes/loci within individual HSPCs to generate myeloid malignancies in mice after transplantation of edited cells (Fig. 1C, top right panel). This was highlighted in a paper by Heckl et al. (2014), in which combinations of multiple single-guide RNAs (sgRNAs) and Cas9 were delivered to mouse HSPCs with a lentiviral vector, followed by transplantation into lethally irradiated mice. The sgRNAs targeted eight genes known to be

 Cite this article as *Cold Spring Harb Perspect Med* doi: 10.1101/cshperspect.a035535

recurrently inactivated in myeloid malignancies (*Tet2, Runx1, Dnmt3a, Ezh2, Nf1, Smc3, p53,* and *Asxl1*) and led to the generation of genetically diverse AMLs harboring loss-of-function mutations in up to five genes in varying combinations (Heckl et al. 2014). Further work from the same group modeled mutations associated with CH and AML in a multiplex fashion through CRISPR–Cas9 genome editing of human cord blood and adult $CD34^+$ HSPCs (Tothova et al. 2017). Several targeted sgRNAs (including *TET2, ASXL1, DNMT3a, RUNX1, TP53, NF1, EZH2, STAG2,* and *SMC3*) were used to edit human adult $CD34^+$ cells together with lentiviral delivery of mutant *NPM1* and *FLT3*. Transplantation of these cells into immunocompromised mice led to the development of CH and MDS with morphological and genetic features similar to patients with the same genotypes. Interestingly, whereas CH and MDS were recapitulated faithfully in this system, there was no development of frank leukemia, which the authors attribute to the differences in bone marrow (BM) microenvironment and cytokine milieu between mouse and human, and the fact that many of the acquired somatic lesions, although frequently appearing in AML clones, are fundamentally associated with CH. Importantly, this study investigated therapeutic vulnerabilities of *TET2* and cohesion-mutated HSPCs and revealed in vivo sensitivity to hypomethylating agents in keeping with similar observations in human *TET2*-mutant MDS (Tothova et al. 2017).

Overall, CRISPR–Cas9 gene editing offers a powerful platform for the generation of multiple genetic lesions in a large range of cells including the primary adult stem cells required. This can facilitate the rapid generation of models with multiple mutations that are more representative of human AML, albeit as transplantation models. Also, although this can be achieved relatively easily for loss-of-function mutations, the specific mutations affecting *NPM1, IDH1, IDH2,* or *FLT3* require the co-introduction of homologous repair templates and cannot be generated with sufficient efficiency using current technologies. By contrast, although GEMMs of such mutations are laborious to create, they have now been generated for most important AML mutations and are widely available for study of mutation combinations. Nevertheless, although GEMMs remove the need to use lentiviruses or transplantation, they do rely on the specificity of *Cre* alleles for mutation activation in the desired cell/compartment. In fact, the combination of GEMMs and CRISPR-mediated models can facilitate a more detailed study of mutation combinations and also offer options for bespoke testing of therapeutic vulnerabilities of different AML subtypes.

MOUSE MODELS OF SOMATIC MUTATIONS AND PATHWAYS RELEVANT TO MYELOID MALIGNANCIES

Nucleophosmin

Nucleophosmin (NPM1) is a nucleolar protein with chaperone functions that has prominent roles in ribosomal biogenesis, chromatin remodeling, mRNA processing, maintenance of genomic stability (Okuda 2002; Swaminathan et al. 2005; Yu et al. 2006), and regulation of apoptosis (Itahana et al. 2003; Ahn et al. 2005). Importantly, NPM1 shuttles between nucleolus, nucleus, and cytoplasm using subcellular localization signals in order to carry out its normal functions (Hingorani et al. 2000). In AML, mutations disrupt its amino-terminal nucleolar localization signal and replace it with a nuclear export signal (NES), resulting in a mutant form that is predominantly located within the cytoplasm (NPM1c) (Falini et al. 2005). *NPM1c* mutations almost always affect exon 12 of the gene and are found in 27%–35% of human AML cases (Falini et al. 2005; Papaemmanuil et al. 2016), making them the most frequent genetic lesion in AML (Falini et al. 2005). Mutant NPM1 binds to and alters the distribution of several proteins including HEXIM1, p19Arf, and NF-κB (Falini et al. 2009), and some of these interactions may mediate part of its leukemogenic properties. NPM1 mutations are almost uniquely seen in AML and are frequently co-occur with mutations in signaling genes such as *FLT3, NRAS,* and *KRAS* (discussed below). Interestingly, *NPM1*-mutant AML is associated with a favorable prognosis, but this is made worse when it co-occurs with *FLT3-ITD* (Gale et al. 2008) and worse still when it co-occurs with both *DNMT3A* and *FLT3-ITD* ("triple-mutant AML") (Papaemmanuil et al. 2013).

Five years after the discovery of *NPM1c* mutations in AML, a transgenic mouse model carrying mutant *NPM1c* under the control of the *MRP8* promoter was developed by Cheng et al. (2010). When compared to control mice expressing wild-type NPM1 under the same promoter, selected lines of these transgenic mice expressed equivalent mutant mRNA and protein levels, with ~27% of mutant carrying mice displaying morphological, flow-cytometric, and pathological features of abnormal myeloproliferation at necropsy. However, the significance of this is unclear as mutant animals displayed normal peripheral blood counts, and none progressed to AML. The authors attributed this to a difference in progenitor cell types affected by the NPM1 mutant in their model compared to NPM1-mutant-positive patients and a lack of cooperating mutations. Vassiliou et al. (2011) subsequently generated a conditional knock-in mouse model of type A NPM1c mutations ($Npm1^{flox\text{-}cA}$) in which approximately one-third of all mice developed late-onset AML after activation of the $Npm1^{cA}$ mutation with *Mx1*-Cre, demonstrating the leukemogenic properties of the mutation and suggesting a need for cooperating mutations. The presence of $Npm1^{cA}$ in HSCs in these mice resulted in mRNA overexpression of homeobox genes including *HoxA*, *HoxB*, and *Nkx2.3* in HSPCs, a myeloid bias, and increased self-renewal in vitro. When aged, these mice developed AML showing morphological maturation, and these tumors were transplantable into sublethally irradiated syngeneic mice. Using insertional mutagenesis, with a Sleeping Beauty transposon capable of gene activation and disruption, they went on to identify recurrent transposon integration in genes such as signaling genes such as *Csf2, Flt3, Nf1, Kras, Ptpn1*, and *Rasgrp1*, as well as in transcriptional regulators such as *Nup98, Zfp521*, and *Bach2*. These data suggested that *Npm1c* mutations primed mutant HSPCs to leukemic transformation, which came about through activation of signaling pathways alone or in combination with altered transcriptional programs (Fig. 2).

A subsequent mouse model by Chou et al. (2012) inserted the TCTG duplication seen in human NPM1 mutations to develop a constitutive knock-in with a weaker NES. A proportion of these mice developed features of myeloproliferative disease and extramedullary hematopoiesis. Through GSEA analysis they identified down-regulation of genes in pathways related to *Cxcl12* and *Cxcr4* in this model and noted a similar pattern of gene suppression involving CXCL12 and CXCR4 pathways in a cohort of *NPM1*-mutated AML patients that was not seen in *NPM1* wild-type AML patients.

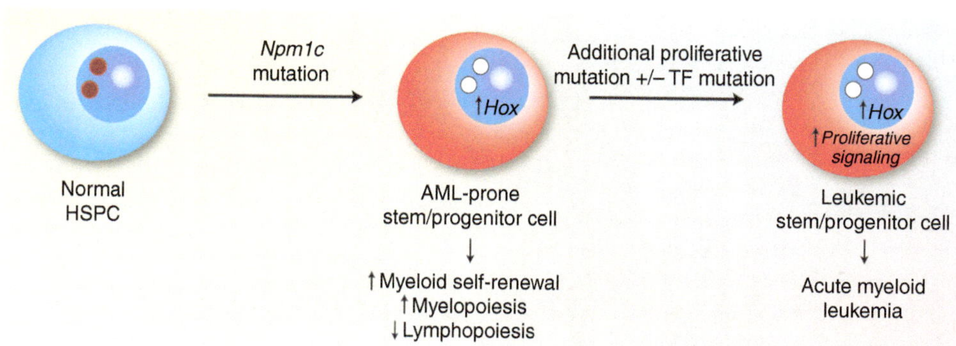

Figure 2. Normal hematopoietic stem/progenitor cells (HSPCs) acquire a somatic mutation in *NPM1c*, resulting in overexpression of the anterior homeobox genes. In turn, this facilitates increased self-renewal potential and myeloid bias and primes the cell to myeloid transformation, which occurs following the acquisition of additional proliferative mutations (e.g., *FLT3*-ITD, *NRAS*-G12D) yielding AML.

Cite this article as *Cold Spring Harb Perspect Med* doi: 10.1101/cshperspect.a035535

In addition to manipulating the constitutive genomic locus, efforts utilizing a number of permissive genomic loci to develop knock-in models have been successful in the context of *Npm1*. These permissive genomic loci include *Rosa26* (Fig. 1B, right panel) and *Hprt*. Through the insertion of human mutant *NPM1* cDNA into these loci, respectively, two separate mouse models of *NPM1* disease were generated (Mallardo et al. 2013; Sportoletti et al. 2013). Both systems contained a stop cassette flanked by *loxP* sites between promoter and cDNA allowing for conditional expression of *NPM1* through Cre-mediated recombination. In the model by Sportoletti et al. (2013), human mutant *NPM1* was conditionally expressed under the *Rosa26* promoter and demonstrated expansion within the myeloid compartment and altered megakaryocytic differentiation with thrombocytopenia similar to human AML; however, none of these mice developed AML. The conditional mouse model by Mallardo et al. (2013) utilized the *Hprt* locus to express human mutant *NPM1* conditionally in a similar fashion. In this model a small proportion of mutant *NPM1* mice developed very late AML-like disease (>400 d); however, some of these leukemias were biphenotypic (showing both myeloid and lymphoid markers).

As [50]*FLT3* internal tandem duplications (ITDs) are present in ~30%–40% of *NPM1*-mutant AMLs (Martelli et al. 2013), the combined effects of the two mutations were studied in mice, demonstrating rapid development of AML with monocytic differentiation and raised white blood cell counts, consistent with features seen in human disease (Mallardo et al. 2013; Mupo et al. 2013; Rau et al. 2014). In particular, Mupo et al. (2013) crossed the conditional $Npm1^{flox\text{-}CA}$ model (Vassiliou et al. 2011) with mice expressing *Flt3*-ITD constitutively (Lee et al. 2007) and observed short-latency AML (31–68 d) in all $Npm1^{cA/+}/Flt3^{ITD/+}$ double-mutant mice without the need to activate *Mx1-Cre* with pIpC (Mupo et al. 2013). This was thought to be due to the known "leakiness" of Mx1-Cre, highlighting the powerful synergy between the two mutations (for review, see Sportoletti et al. 2015). The majority of AMLs showed gain in copy number for the *Flt3*-ITD allele, most commonly through acquired uniparental disomy, recapitulating what happens in human AML. Another study by Dovey et al. (2017) compared double-mutant $Npm1^{cA/+}/Flt3^{ITD/+}$ to $Npm1^{cA/+}/Nras^{G12D/+}$ double-mutant mice. The latter also developed penetrant AML, albeit less rapidly than $Npm1^{cA/+}/Flt3^{ITD/+}$ mice (median 138 d vs. 52 d) and the AMLs were more differentiated. Interestingly, $Npm1^{cA/+}/Nras^{G12D/+}$ AML showed a gain in copy number for the $Nras^{G12D/+}$ allele in most cases, and in others the AMLs acquired new somatic mutations in AML driver genes (*Idh1* and *Ptpn11*), which were never seen in $Npm1^{cA/+}/Flt3^{ITD/+}$. Collectively, these findings demonstrated that molecular synergy underlies the co-occurrence patterns and phenotype of NPM1-mutant AML. More recently, triple-mutant $Dnmt3a^{R878H/+}/Npm1^{c/+}/Flt3^{ITD/+}$ mice showed that the presence in this context of the $Dnmt3a^{R878H}$ mutation (equivalent to human R882H) confers resistance to anthracycline and may in part explain the poor prognosis of triple-mutant AML (Guryanova et al. 2016). Also, a model of sequential activation of *Dnmt3a* followed by *Npm1c* using different DNA recombinase systems (Cre-*loxP*, then Flp-*FRT*) showed that the activation of the *Npm1* mutation causes malignant transformation of *Dnmt3a* mutant clonal hematopoiesis (see later) (Loberg et al. 2019).

Signaling Pathways

Somatic mutations in signal transduction pathways are frequently found in AML and most commonly involve the genes *FLT3, NRAS*, and *KRAS*. FLT3 (Fms-related tyrosine kinase 3) is a receptor tyrosine kinase expressed in immature hematopoietic cells that plays an important role in the normal myeloid and lymphoid development. FLT3 ligand (FLT3LG) binds to and activates FLT3, which then phosphorylates downstream targets to activate several signaling pathways including RAS and STAT5 (Hayakawa et al. 2000; Gilliland and Griffin 2002), to promote cell proliferation, survival, and differentiation. Approximately one-third of AMLs carry *FLT3* mutations in the form of internal tandem duplications (*FLT3*-ITD) or mutations within the tyrosine kinase domain (*FLT3*-TKD), at frequencies of ~25% and 7%–10% across all AML cases, respectively (Daver et al. 2019). ITDs are in-frame mutations of variable length affecting the juxtamembrane (JM) domain, causing disruption of its autoinhibitory activity of the kinase activity. TKD mutations typically are in the form of the D835Y or less commonly the I836 substitutions in the protein's second TKD domain (TKD2). Both *FLT3*-ITD and *FLT3*-TKD mutations result in constitutive tyrosine kinase activation and signaling (Fig. 3). Several models have provided insights into the in vivo biological effects of *Flt3*-ITD mutations. In two studies, transduction of murine BM HSPCs with retrovirus expressing a *FLT3*-ITD mutant cDNA followed by BM transplantation into recipient mice (outlined in Fig. 1C, top left panel) yielded a short-latency myeloproliferative disease characterized by splenomegaly and leukocytosis (Kelly et al. 2002a; Grundler et al. 2005). Subsequently, Lee et al. (2005) developed a transgenic mouse model (outlined in Fig. 1A) that expressed human *FLT3*-ITD in the hematopoietic system under the *vav* promoter. This also demonstrated features of a myeloproliferative disorder with splenomegaly, thrombocytosis, and megakaryocytic hyperplasia. In addition, a few mice in this study also developed clonal immature B- or T-lymphoid disease. The same group went on to generate knock-in mice through introduction of a human ITD mutation into exon 14 of the native murine *Flt3* locus using homologous recombination in ES cells (Lee et al. 2007). Homozygous $Flt3^{ITD/ITD}$ mice developed a late-onset disease similar to chronic myelomonocytic leukemia (CMML), with enhanced proliferation and survival of their hematopoietic progenitors. Of note, a small subset of patients with CMML have *FLT3*-ITD mutations. A subsequent *Flt3*-ITD conditional knock-in model, generated through the insertion of an 18-bp ITD mutation into the sequence coding the JM domain of murine *Flt3*, also generated an aggressive myeloproliferative disease with features similar to those described previously (Li et al. 2008). Collectively, these studies suggest that *Flt3*-ITD led to myeloid (and in some cases lymphoid) expansion, proliferation, and disease, but were generally insufficient to induce AML reflecting the fact that these mutations are rarely found in isolation in

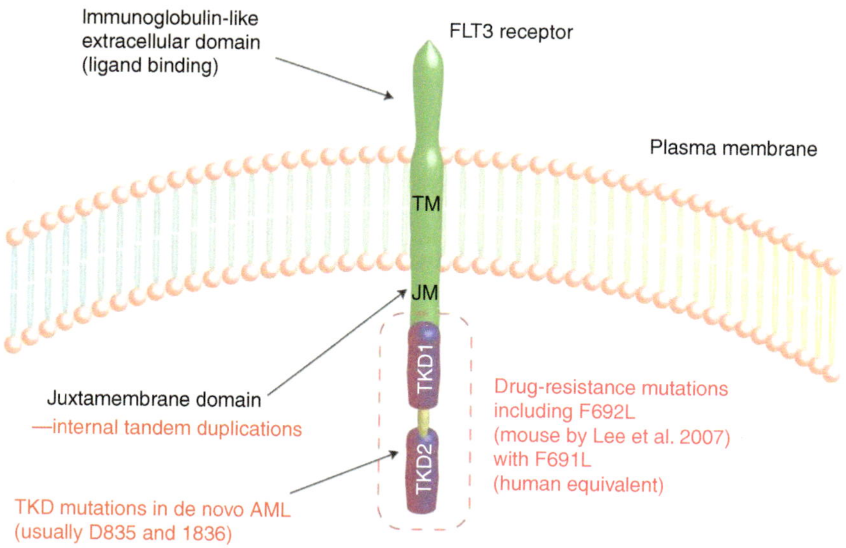

Figure 3. The FLT3 receptor consists of a transmembrane (TM), jutxamembrane (JM), and two tyrosine kinase domains (TKD1 and TKD2). Common relevant ITD/TKD and drug resistance mutations are shown.

 Cite this article as *Cold Spring Harb Perspect Med* doi: 10.1101/cshperspect.a035535

human AML. Nevertheless, as noted above for *NPM1c*, mice expressing the *Flt3*-ITD in combination with other rational AML driver mutations, including *Dnmt3a* (Meyer et al. 2016), *Tet2* (Shih et al. 2015), *PML-RARA* (Kelly et al. 2002b), *Runx1* (Mead et al. 2013), *MLL* fusion genes (Zorko et al. 2012), and *Nup98-HOXD13* (Greenblatt et al. 2012), commonly led to development of AML.

The RAS proteins signal through downstream effectors such as MAPK, PI3K, and RalGDS to drive cellular growth and proliferation upon ligand binding to different membrane receptors. Oncogenic mutations in *RAS* or RAS pathway genes are seen in diverse human cancers. *RAS* genes encode a family of guanine nucleotide binding proteins, and the RAS family consists of three GTP proteins: NRAS, KRAS, and HRAS. *RAS* mutations in myeloid malignancies were reported more than 30 years ago (Janssen et al. 1987), and mutations of *NRAS* or *KRAS* are found in ~10%–15% of AML cases (DiNardo and Cortes 2016). *RAS* mutations primarily arise at critical regulatory sites including codons G12, G13, and G61 and, in the case of KRAS, also A146, resulting in altered GTPase activity of RAS. An early mouse model expressing mutant $Kras^{G12D}$ in hematopoietic cells after conditional activation by *Mx1*-Cre resulted in a rapidly progressive myeloproliferative disorder with massive splenomegaly and marked myeloid expansion (Braun et al. 2004). In a subsequent study, *Mx1-Cre* $Nras^{G12D}$ mice were generated, and these developed an indolent myeloproliferative disorder with elevated white blood cell counts, splenomegaly, and myeloid expansion in BM and spleen (Li et al. 2011a), with mice ultimately dying of a diverse spectrum of hematologic cancers including MPD or MDS-like disorders, histiocytic sarcoma, or a lymphoproliferative disorder, but not AML. However, insertional mutagenesis with the MOL4070LTR retrovirus into these *Mx1-Cre/*$Nras^{G12D}$ mice shortly after birth induced AML in the majority of animals, but not in wild-type controls. The authors identified, in several AMLs, activating common integration sites affecting *Evi1*, a known oncogene target of chromosomal rearrangements in human AMLs (Li et al. 2011a). As discussed above, subsequent studies have shown the combination of $Nras^{G12D}$ with *Npm1c* (Dovey et al. 2017) or with other cooperative mutations such as *Cbfβ-SMMHC* (Xue et al. 2014) yielded highly penetrant AML. As with *Flt3*-ITD, these findings show that although mutations in the *Ras* family can drive myeloproliferative disease, they require other cooperative genetic events to transform and develop into AML.

Models of Mutant Epigenetic Regulators

In addition to abnormal transcription, aberrant epigenetic regulation is a common feature of myeloid malignancies, particularly AML. The study of chromatin-based events and their regulation of DNA-based processes is encompassed in the term "epigenetics," which was originally coined to describe inherited changes in gene expression independent of DNA sequence changes (Waddington 2012). Examples of this include DNA modifications such as methylation (Fig. 4), histone modifications, and RNA-associated gene silencing. Abnormal epigenetic changes and mutations are hypothesized to contribute to a preleukemic state but generally not alone enough to cause progression to AML, suggesting these lesions are present in early clones (Genovese et al. 2014; Jaiswal et al. 2014; Xie et al. 2014; McKerrell et al. 2015). Importantly, such epigenetic modifications are frequently reversible and this offers an attractive avenue for therapeutic targeting. For a systematic overview of epigenetic modifications in hematological malignancies, the reader is directed to the comprehensive reviews of Abdel-Wahab and Levine (2013), Wouters and Delwel (2016), and Gallipoli and Huntly (2018).

DNA Methylation Pathways

DNA methylation is important in embryonic development, genomic stability, and cell differentiation (Li 2002). This process involves the addition of a methyl group to the 5-carbon position of cytosines in CpG dinucleotides, resulting in 5-methylcytosine (5mC) (Fig. 4, top left). Methylated cytosine in CpG islands at promot-

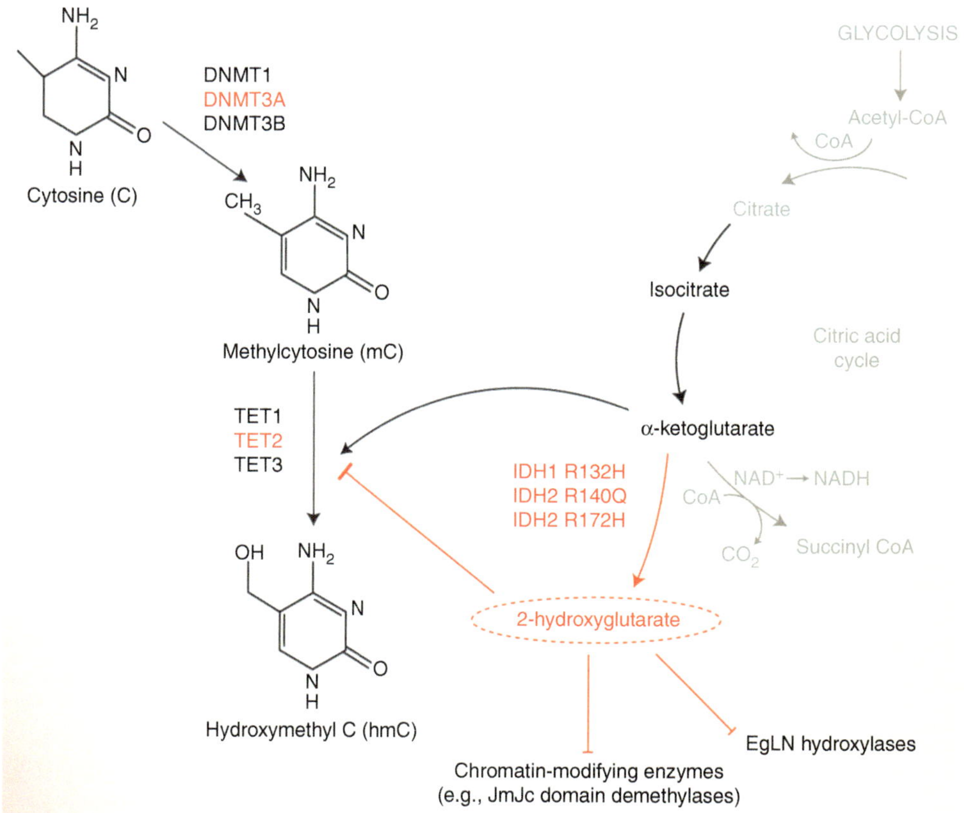

Figure 4. Conversion of cytosine to methylcytosine (mC or 5-mC) occurs through enzymatic activity of DNA methyltransferase family members DNMT1, DNMT3A, and DNMT3B, which place a methyl group at the carbon-5 position on DNA cytosine residues. In turn, 5-mC is dioxygenated to hydroxymethyl C (hmC or 5-hmC) via the TET family of enzymes (TET1/TET2/TET3) using Fe(II) and α-ketoglutarate (α-KG) as substrates. The latter is derived from the oxidative decarboxylation of isocitrate, which is catalyzed by IDH1 or IDH2 enzymes in the citric acid cycle (partially shown in black/gray). Relevant pathogenic loss of function mutations in *DNMT3A* and *TET2* (shown in red) can lead to hypermethylated states and are commonly seen in CH and MDS and are thought to represent early mutations in AML. Somatic *IDH1/IDH2* mutations (also shown in red) are typically gain of function and lead to abnormal conversion of α-KG to 2-hydroxyglutarate (2-HG), which competes with and inhibits α-KG-dependent enzyme processes and families including the JmJc histone demethylases and EgLN hydroxylases. Specifically, through inhibition of 5-mC to 5-hmC conversion, 2-HG also indirectly augments mutant TET2 activity.

ers is associated with transcriptional repression (Jones 2012), a process that can be associated with silencing of tumor-suppressor genes (Baylin and Jones 2011). DNA methylation occurs through the activity of DNA methyltransferases (DNMTs). Recurrent mutations in *DNMT3A* are early event in leukemogenesis and seen in >50% of cases of CH (Genovese et al. 2014; Jaiswal et al. 2014; Xie et al. 2014; McKerrell et al. 2015), 10%–12% of MDS and MPN (Nangalia et al. 2013; Papaemmanuil et al. 2013; Haferlach et al. 2014), and up to 36% of AML (Ley et al. 2010; Cancer Genome Atlas Research Network et al. 2013; Papaemmanuil et al. 2013). *DNMT3A* mutations can occur throughout the gene and be either missense or nonsense (including frameshift and splice site), with approximately equal numbers of each type seen in CH (Brunetti et al. 2017). Interestingly, a much greater proportion of missense mutations

(~75%) is seen in AML, with the most common mutations, affecting DNMT3A R882, seen in 50% of AML but only 17% of CH (Brunetti et al. 2017), suggesting that these mutations may impart a greater clonal fitness to the host HSC. Although we still do not know the precise manner in which *DNMT3A* mutations impart a clonal advantage to HSCs, they are thought to be associated with reduced DNMT3A function, with missense mutations (particularly R882 cases) thought to function in a dominant-negative manner over wild-type *DNMT3A* (Russler-Germain et al. 2014). *Dnmt3a*-null HSCs generated from *Dnmt3a$^{fl/fl}$* mice (Kaneda et al. 2004) crossed with *Mx1-Cre* (with the Cre recombinase then activated through pIpC injections) showed varying levels of methylation at distinct loci and down-regulation of differentiation factors leading to impaired HSC differentiation after serial transplantations into mice (Challen et al. 2011). The *Dnmt3a*-null same HSCs transplanted into mice led to a spectrum of malignancies including MDS, AML and ALL, demonstrating that loss of DNMT3A function conferred a preleukemic phenotype (Mayle et al. 2015). Another study utilizing the same conditional *Dnmt3a$^{fl/fl}$*; *Mx1-Cre* mice showed that mice transplanted with *Dnmt3a*-null BM alone developed MDS with cytopenias and myeloproliferative features. A small proportion developed AML, and these were found to have cooperating mutations in *c-Kit* (Celik et al. 2015). Furthermore, mice with an inducible deletion of *Dnmt3a* and *Flt3*-ITD mutations spontaneously developed a highly penetrant aggressive AML (Meyer et al. 2016). AML cells from these mice retained the wild-type *Dnmt3a* allele, demonstrating that Dnmt3a is haploinsufficient for AML development. Conditional expression in mice (*Mx1-Cre*) of endogenous *Dnmt3a*^{R878H} (the mouse homolog to human *DNMT3A*^{R882H}) did not lead to AML but did drive an expansion of HSPCs with features of CH (Guryanova et al. 2016). When combined with mice expressing *Flt3*-ITD and *Npm1^c* mutations, however, these *Dnmt3a*^{R878H} mice developed fully penetrant leukemia, which exhibited relative resistance to anthracycline chemotherapy (vs. AML due to *Npm1^c* and *Flt3*-ITD alone) (Guryanova et al. 2016). Another model utilizing *DNMT3A*^{R882H} overexpression through retroviral transduction of murine BM cells followed by transplantation into recipient mice demonstrated development of CMML with thrombocytosis (Xu et al. 2014). More recently, a dual recombinase inducible system was used in a murine model to independently induce *Dnmt3a*^{R878H} and *Npm1c* mutations in a stepwise fashion, so as to mimic the order in which they are acquired in humans with AML (Loberg et al. 2019). Induction of mutant *Npm1* after *Dnmt3a*^{R878H} activation resulted in progression to an MPN-like disorder. Transplantation of this MPN led to AML with an increase in myeloid progenitors and accumulation of additional detectable oncogenic mutations in signaling pathways (e.g., *Flt3*, *Ptpn11*) and epigenetic regulators including *Idh1* and *Hdac1* (Loberg et al. 2019).

After cytosine is converted to 5-mC by DNMTs, 5mC can be oxidized by the ten-eleven translocation (TET) enzymes in an α-ketoglutarate (KG)-dependent process to yield 5-hydroxymethylcytosine (5-hmC) (Fig. 4, bottom left). This can be followed by successive oxidations that eventually lead to loss of the modified methyl group and restoration of unmodified cytosine. 5-hmC is associated with more accessible chromatin and, in mouse ES cells, the transcriptional start sites (TSSs) of pluripotent genes were noted to have increased levels of 5-hmC (Ficz et al. 2011). Somatic *TET2* mutations are commonly found in 10%–20% of patients with CH (Busque et al. 2012), 10%–25% in MPN (Delhommeau et al. 2009) and MDS (Delhommeau et al. 2009; Langemeijer et al. 2009), and up to 25% of AML cases (Papaemmanuil et al. 2013). In mouse models, conditional *Tet2* deletion within the hematopoietic compartment leads to increased self-renewal and expansion of HSCs in vitro and in vivo (Li et al. 2011b; Moran-Crusio et al. 2011; Quivoron et al. 2011) and development of chronic MPN-like disorders with no progression to AML. Cimmino et al. (2017) generated a reversible RNAi transgenic *Tet2* knockdown murine model by expressing a Tet2-specific small hairpin RNA (shRNA) that could be regulated by administration of doxycycline. *Tet2* knockdown resulted in increased HSC self-renewal, expansion of myeloid compartments within the blood, spleen, and liver, and an MPN-like disease with reduced survival. Restoration of *Tet2* in BM cells derived from these mice and cultured in vitro resulted in a reversal of the aberrant self-renewal. Similarly, loss of enhanced growth and proliferation was seen in vivo when shRNA-expressing cells were transplanted into mice followed by reversal of Tet2 knockdown. In vitro, reversal of *Tet2* silencing in c-kit$^+$ HSCs from these mice resulted in decreased proliferation because of delayed cell cycle progression and increased apoptosis and promoted DNA demethylation. Interestingly, the effects of *Tet2* restoration in this model were mimicked through augmenting Tet2 activity by administration of vitamin C (L-ascorbic acid), which is known to increase 5-hmC and promote TET-driven DNA demethylation (Young et al. 2015). *Tet2*-deficient cells treated with vitamin C showed resistance to the effects of vitamin C in comparison to *Tet2*-replete cells in vitro, and mice transplanted with *Tet2*$^{-/-}$ BM treated with phosphate-buffered saline (PBS) control developed CMML-like disease, whereas those treated with vitamin C injections displayed less elevated WBC counts and delayed progression to CMML. In another study, approximately one-third of conditional *Vav-Cre+; Tet2*$^{-/-}$ mice developed MPN, and when crossed with a constitutive knock-in *Flt3*-ITD model, all animals developed aggressive AML (Shih et al. 2015).

DNA methylation can also be corrupted by mutations in the genes for the isocitrate dehydrogenase 1 and 2 (IDH1 and IDH2) enzymes. IDH1 and IDH2 are normally responsible for catalyzing the conversion of isocitrate to α-KG in the citric acid cycle in the cytosol and mitochondria, respectively. Recurrent mutations in *IDH1* were first reported in gliomas (Parsons et al. 2008; Yan et al. 2009), and mutations in both *IDH1* and *IDH2* were subsequently found in AML (Mardis et al. 2009), MPN (Green and Beer 2010), and MDS (Parsons et al. 2008). *IDH1* is mutated in up to 11% and *IDH2* in 12% of patients with cytogenetically normal AML (Thol et al. 2010; Wagner et al. 2010). *IDH1* mutations affect the R132 and *IDH2* mutations in the R140 and R172 positions (Marcucci et al. 2010). Each of these mutations impairs the conversion of isocitrate to α-KG and confers a gain-of-function activity that causes further reduction of α-KG to 2-hydroxyglutarate (2-HG). 2-HG functions as an oncometabolite by interfering with several important pathways, including the function of the TET protein family, chromatin modifiers such as the JmjC domain demethylases, and EglN hydroxylases (Fig. 4, right; Ward et al. 2010; Koivunen et al. 2012). Inhibition of these pathways leads to increased DNA and histone methylation, in association with a block in hematopoietic differentiation through interference with normal transcriptional programs (Lu et al. 2012). Conditional knock-in of the IDH1 R132H mutation into the endogenous *Idh1* locus in mice led to development of splenomegaly, anemia, and extramedullary hematopoiesis with a leukemic DNA methylation signature similar to that seen in AML patients carrying *IDH1/2* mutations (Sasaki et al. 2012). Although expansion in the myeloid compartment was observed, the lack of AML development suggested the need for secondary cooperative mutations. In a retroviral transduction/transplantation murine model, expression of mutant *IDH1* in cooperation with *HoxA9* caused an MPN-like disease and was insufficient to transform to AML (Chaturvedi et al. 2013). Chen et al. (2013) showed that transduction of HSPCs from *Nras-G12D* or *Flt3-ITD* mice with retroviral vectors expressing *IDH2*-R140Q or *IDH2*-R172K led to impaired myeloid differentiation and subsequent development of AML that was sensitive to BRD4 inhibition. A knock-in model of IDH2-R172K showed that, unlike IDH2 R140Q and *IDH1* R132H, this mutation generated high levels of 2-HG in T cells in keeping with the observation that *IDH2*-R172K is the only one of these mutations seen in human angioimmunoblastic T-cell lymphoma (Lemonnier et al. 2016).

Pathways Involved in Histone Modifications

Aberrant histone methyltransferase and demethylase functions have also been studied in murine models of myeloid malignancies to determine their effects on transcriptional networks acting in the initiation and maintenance of disease. Histone modifications, such as those affecting lysine residue H3K4, H3K9, and H3K27, are associated with changes in target gene expression, with acetylation generally associated with transcriptional activation and methylation with transcriptional repression. The mixed lineage leukemia (MLL) genes encode histone methyltransferases that methylate H3K4 and are recurrently mutated in AML, acute lymphoblastic leukemia (ALL), and lymphoma. The MLL1 gene in particular is a target of partial tandem duplications and chromosomal translocations in acute leukemias (AML, ALL, and biphenotypic) (De Braekeleer et al. 2005) with more than 135 *MLL* fusion partners recognized (Meyer et al. 2018). Mouse models driven by *MLL* fusions have been instrumental in improving our understanding of AML since the 1990s, often serving as general experimental models for acute leukemia. For a comprehensive overview of mouse models of *MLL*-driven leukemias, the reader is directed to Milne (2017) and Ottersbach et al. (2018).

Enhancer of zeste homolog 2 (EZH2) functions as a histone di- and trimethyltransferase for H3K27, resulting in transcriptional repression. It forms the core of the PRC2 Polycomb repressor complex and controls stem cell maintenance and differentiation. Although gain-of-function mutations in *EZH2* are well reported in lymphoid cancers (Morin et al. 2010; Béguelin et al. 2013; Souroullas et al. 2016), *EZH2* mutations in myeloid malignancies including MPN, MDS, and AML are generally found at low frequency, predominantly hemizygous, and predicted to cause loss of function (Ernst et al. 2010; Makishima et al. 2010; Nikoloski et al. 2010; Papaemmanuil et al. 2013). *Ezh2* loss in mouse models leads to development of multiple slowly progressing hematological malignancies including MDS and MPN (Mochizuki-Kashio et al. 2015). More recently loss of *Ezh2* in murine models has been shown to accelerate myelofibrosis (Sashida et al. 2016) and produce more aggressive JAK2V617F-driven MPNs (Shimizu et al. 2016; Yang et al. 2016). By contrast, separate mouse models have demonstrated that *Ezh2* is required for chronic myeloid leukemia (CML) (Scott et al. 2016; Xie et al. 2016) and AML (Neff et al. 2012; Tanaka et al. 2012) maintenance. Collectively, these findings suggested context-dependent oncogenic and tumor-suppressor roles for *EZH2* in hematological malignancies. Basheer et al. (2019) utilized retroviral overexpression of common AML oncogenic drivers (gene fusions *MLL-AF9* and *AML1-ETO9a*) in *Mx1-Cre* conditional $Ezh2^{fl/fl}$ mouse HSPCs at different stages followed by transplantation to recipient mice to demonstrate diametrically opposing roles of *Ezh2* during initiation and maintenance of AML. Deletion of *Ezh2* prior to transformation with oncogenic *MLL-AF9* or *AML1-ETO9a* fusion genes accelerated AML development in vivo suggesting a tumor-suppressive function in AML initiation. Conversely, deletion of *Ezh2* in secondary recipients of established *MLL-AF9*- or *AML1-ETO9a*-driven murine AMLs attenuated disease severity and prolonged survival, suggesting an oncogenic function in the same subtypes of AML. This model was the first demonstration of an epigenetic regulator possessing opposite stage-dependent oncogenic or tumor-suppressive functions in the same disease.

The H3K27 demethylase UTX (ubiquitously transcribed tetratricopeptide repeat, X-linked) is a frequent target of somatic loss-of-function mutations in solid cancers (Wang and Shilatifard 2019) and leukemias (Cancer Genome Atlas Research Network et al. 2013; Papaemmanuil et al. 2013). Previous studies had shown that loss of demethylase function is critical to the development of T-cell ALL. In a novel murine model, Gozdecka et al. (2018) showed UTX could suppress myeloid leukemogenesis through noncatalytic functions that did not significantly affect H3K27me3 status but instead resulted in changes in chromatin accessibility that altered ETS/GATA-factor binding, leading to repression of oncogenic ETS factors and up-regulation of tumor-suppressive GATA programs.

Mutations Affecting Spliceosome Genes

The spliceosome is a multiprotein complex that regulates the process of RNA splicing by catalyzing excision of intronic regions in precursor messenger RNA to yield mature mRNA. It is composed of five small nuclear ribonucleoproteins (snRNPs) and more than 80 proteins (Will and Luhrmann 2011). Mutations in splicing factor genes have been identified across several cancers and are particularly common in MDS, in which they are seen in 60%–70% of cases (Graubert et al. 2011; Papaemmanuil et al. 2011; Yoshida et al. 2011). The majority are heterozygous missense mutations in *SF3B1* (splicing factor 3b subunit 1), *SRSF2* (serine/arginine-rich splicing factor 2), and *U2AF1* (U2 small nuclear RNA auxiliary factor 1) that occur in a largely mutually exclusive manner, with loss-of-function mutations in the gene ZRSR2 also seen in a small proportion of patients (Papaemmanuil et al. 2011, 2013; Haferlach et al. 2014; Shiozawa et al. 2018). Genes whose splicing is altered by these mutations differ between mouse and human because of limited preservation of intronic sequences involved in splicing. Despite this, mice with these mutations display features reminiscent of MDS. $Srsf2^{flox\text{-}P95H/+}$ conditional knock-in mice crossed with *Mx1-Cre* mice developed several features of MDS including anemia, macrocytosis, and dysplastic changes in morphology (Kim et al. 2015). A doxycycline-inducible transgenic mouse model carrying *U2AF1-S34F*—the most abundant *U2AF1* mutation in human MDS—showed reduction in hematopoietic cell lineages and leukopenia when BM derived from these was transplanted into recipient mice (Shirai et al. 2015). Also, no functional advantage of these *U2AF1*-mutant cells was demonstrable in competitive transplantation assays, and overall survival of mutant mice was comparable to wild-type, with none developing overt features of MDS or AML. Subsequently, two conditional *Sf3b1* K700E knock-in models (Obeng et al. 2016; Mupo et al. 2017) were developed. and both showed similar phenotypic features to those seen in human MDS, including macrocytosis, anemia, and erythroid differentiation block, but lacked ringed sideroblasts. Again, both mouse models showed no growth advantage for mutant HSPCs in competitive transplantation versus wild-type HSPCs.

The impact of these mutations on the clinical consequences of cancers and potential for therapies targeting the splicing pathway has been further detailed in several comprehensive reviews (Dvinge et al. 2016; Lee and Abdel-Wahab 2016; Saez et al. 2017).

Cohesins

Mutations in the cohesin complex genes *STAG2, RAD21, SMC3,* and *SMC1A* are seen in ~13%–15% of AMLs (Cancer Genome Atlas Research Network et al. 2013; Papaemmanuil et al. 2013). The cohesin complex normally maintains polarity of sister chromatids during mitosis and facilitates their cohesion through the formation of a large ring-like structure that encircles DNA (Gligoris and Lowe 2016). They also colocalize and interact with CTCF to facilitate the formation of loop domains that stabilize interactions between two separated genomic locations in *cis*, a process thought to facilitate enhancer–promoter interactions (Fig. 5; Panigrahi and Pati 2012; Zheng and Xie 2019). Conditional $Smc3^{+/-}$ mice demonstrated increased HSPC self-renewal in vitro and in vivo and developed AML when crossed with *Flt3*-ITD (Viny et al. 2015). In another study, systematic shRNA-mediated knockdown of cohesin complex members in a mouse model led to increased proliferative capacity of mouse HSCs in vitro (Mullenders et al. 2015). When cohesin knockdown mice were aged, this resulted in development of MPN-like disorders, collectively suggesting cohesin mutations likely occur as relatively early events in leukemogenesis (Mullenders et al. 2015; Mazumdar and Majeti 2017). Other mouse models and further roles of cohesin complex members in cancer have been extensively reviewed elsewhere, and the reader is directed to Fisher et al. (2017) and Meyer et al. (2017) for further insights.

TP53

The tumor-suppressor gene *TP53* (or *P53*) encodes for a transcription factor with pleiotropic functions including control of the cell cycle, responses to DNA damage, apoptosis, cellular

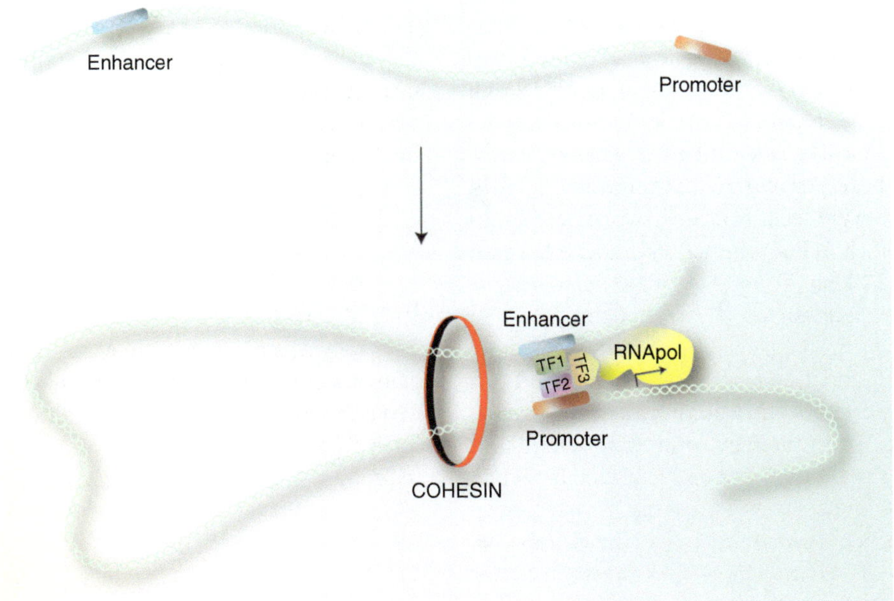

Figure 5. The cohesin complex is composed of four obligate subunits—SMC1, SMC3, RAD21, and STAG2—and forms a large ring-like structure (simplified in red) that is capable of topologically encircling DNA strands. Cohesin binding can bring enhancers and distal promoters together into close proximity via the formation of a chromatin loop leading to transcriptional activation (as shown by activity of transcription factors and RNA polymerase) and is thought to play a functional role in AML development.

senescence, and autophagy (Pant et al. 2012). *TP53* is the most frequently mutated gene in human cancers and typically associated with poor outcomes and drug resistance (Donehower et al. 2019). *TP53* mutations or deletions (often in the form of large deletions of chromosome 17p) are present in ~10% of de novo AML (Papaemmanuil et al. 2013) and up to 40% of therapy-related myeloid neoplasms (McNerney et al. 2017), conferring a very poor prognosis (Papaemmanuil et al. 2013; McNerney et al. 2017). Several mouse models of *p53* loss of function have been developed including truncation, suppression (shRNA), and dominant-negative mutation (for review, see Lozano 2010). A recent study showed that missense, frameshift, and truncating mutations impart a competitive advantage to mutant HSPCs after low-dosage irradiation in transplantation assays (Boettcher et al. 2019). Also, different mouse models of TP53 loss have been shown to develop AML, the onset of which could be significantly accelerated by *Kras-G12D* (Zhao et al. 2010) or *Nras-G12D* (Zhang et al. 2017), the latter through transformation of megakaryocyte-erythroid progenitors (MEPs). Also, a study of the gain-of-function mutant *Tp53*-R172H, representing the most common missense mutation in human AML, showed that the mutation enhanced self-renewal of myeloid progenitors, a premalignant phenotype dependent on the transcription factor *Foxh1* (Loizou et al. 2019).

With regard to the impact of TP53 on chemosensitivity, Zuber et al. (2009) reported a differential response to induction chemotherapy in mice bearing AML driven by *AML1-ETO9a/Nras-G12D* versus *MLL-ENL/Nras-G12D*, because of robust activation of p53 by induction chemotherapy in the former but not the latter. Comparison of gene expression signatures between both cohorts led to the identification of several p53 transcriptional target genes, such as *Cdkn1a*, *Mdm2*, and *Apaf1*, being up-regulated in the *AML1-ETO9a + Nras-G12D* leukemias but not in the *MLL-ENL + Nras-G12D* leukemias. In keeping with this, p53-null (vs. wild-type) *AML1-ETO9a* leukemias exhibited a more rapid onset and aggressive course with significant reduction in survival and poorer responses to induction chemotherapy, whereas MLL-ENL leukemias retained the same behavior irrespective of p53 status, suggesting they have an intrinsically disabled p53 status. This model provided a plausible explanation for the relative chemoresistance of *MLL-X-* versus *AML1-ETO*-driven human AML.

CONCLUDING REMARKS

Murine models of disease have advanced considerably with the use of novel technologies over the past few decades and have been instrumental in improving both the mechanistic understanding of human myeloid malignancies and the development of therapeutic strategies against these diseases. Although several of the models discussed above may have potential limitations and do not always fully recapitulate human disease, they collectively serve as highly informative in vivo models of the impact of leukemia-associated mutations on hematopoiesis and profoundly enhanced our understanding of disease initiation, progression, maintenance of molecular synergy, and therapeutic vulnerabilities in ways that cannot be adequately captured by in vitro studies. In addition, mouse leukemia models have enabled in vivo preclinical studies that supported the later development of clinical drugs. At present, researchers have generated sophisticated models of almost all important recurrent mutations seen in human myeloid cancers and judicious study/investigation of these models promises to deliver advances that will change the therapeutic landscape for patients, a long-awaited ambition of the leukemia scientific community.

ACKNOWLEDGMENTS

G.V. is a consultant for Kymab Ltd (Cambridge, United Kingdom) and Oxstem Ltd (Oxford, United Kingdom). The G.V. laboratory has received an educational grant from Celgene. G.V. is funded by a Cancer Research UK Senior Cancer Fellowship (C22324/A23015) and work in his laboratory is also funded by the Wellcome Trust, European Research Council, Kay Kendall Leukaemia Fund, Leukemia and Lymphoma Society (USA), Rising Tide Foundation for Clinical Cancer Research, and Bloodwise. F.B. is funded by a Clinical Lectureship from the National Institute for Health Research (United Kingdom).

REFERENCES

Abdel-Wahab O, Levine RL. 2013. Mutations in epigenetic modifiers in the pathogenesis and therapy of acute myeloid leukemia. *Blood* **121:** 3563–3572. doi:10.1182/blood-2013-01-451781

Abelson S, Collord G, Ng SWK, Weissbrod O, Mendelson Cohen N, Niemeyer E, Barda N, Zuzarte PC, Heisler L, Sundaravadanam Y, et al. 2018. Prediction of acute myeloid leukaemia risk in healthy individuals. *Nature* **559:** 400–404. doi:10.1038/s41586-018-0317-6

Ahn JY, Liu X, Cheng D, Peng J, Chan PK, Wade PA, Ye K. 2005. Nucleophosmin/B23, a nuclear PI(3,4,5)P(3) receptor, mediates the antiapoptotic actions of NGF by inhibiting CAD. *Mol Cell* **18:** 435–445. doi:10.1016/j.molcel.2005.04.010

Arber DA, Orazi A, Hasserjian R, Thiele J, Borowitz MJ, Le Beau MM, Bloomfield CD, Cazzola M, Vardiman JW. 2016. The 2016 revision to the World Health Organization classification of myeloid neoplasms and acute leukemia. *Blood* **127:** 2391–2405. doi:10.1182/blood-2016-03-643544

Barlow JL, Drynan LF, Hewett DR, Holmes LR, Lorenzo-Abalde S, Lane AL, Jolin HE, Pannell R, Middleton AJ, Wong SH, et al. 2010. A p53-dependent mechanism underlies macrocytic anemia in a mouse model of human 5q- syndrome. *Nat Med* **16:** 59–66. doi:10.1038/nm.2063

Basheer F, Giotopoulos G, Meduri E, Yun H, Mazan M, Sasca D, Gallipoli P, Marando L, Gozdecka M, Asby R, et al. 2019. Contrasting requirements during disease evolution identify EZH2 as a therapeutic target in AML. *J Exp Med* **216:** 966–981. doi:10.1084/jem.20181276

Baylin SB, Jones PA. 2011. A decade of exploring the cancer epigenome—Biological and translational implications. *Nat Rev Cancer* **11:** 726–734. doi:10.1038/nrc3130

Béguelin W, Popovic R, Teater M, Jiang Y, Bunting KL, Rosen M, Shen H, Yang SN, Wang L, Ezponda T, et al. 2013. EZH2 is required for germinal center formation and somatic EZH2 mutations promote lymphoid transformation. *Cancer Cell* **23:** 677–692. doi:10.1016/j.ccr.2013.04.011

Ben-Neriah Y, Daley GQ, Mes-Masson AM, Witte ON, Baltimore D. 1986. The chronic myelogenous leukemia-specific P210 protein is the product of the *bcr/abl* hybrid gene. *Science* **233:** 212–214. doi:10.1126/science.3460176

Boettcher S, Miller PG, Sharma R, McConkey M, Leventhal M, Krivtsov AV, Giacomelli AO, Wong W, Kim J, Chao S, et al. 2019. A dominant-negative effect drives selection of *TP53* missense mutations in myeloid malignancies. *Science* **365:** 599–604. doi:10.1126/science.aax3649

Bolouri H, Farrar JE, Triche TT Jr, Ries RE, Lim EL, Alonzo TA, Ma Y, Moore R, Mungall AJ, Marra MA, et al. 2018. The molecular landscape of pediatric acute myeloid leukemia reveals recurrent structural alterations and age-specific mutational interactions. *Nat Med* **24:** 103–112. doi:10.1038/nm.4439

Bonnet D, Dick JE. 1997. Human acute myeloid leukemia is organized as a hierarchy that originates from a primitive hematopoietic cell. *Nat Med* **3:** 730–737. doi:10.1038/nm0797-730

Bradley A, Evans M, Kaufman MH, Robertson E. 1984. Formation of germ-line chimaeras from embryo-derived teratocarcinoma cell lines. *Nature* **309:** 255–256. doi:10.1038/309255a0

Braun BS, Tuveson DA, Kong N, Le DT, Kogan SC, Rozmus J, Le Beau MM, Jacks TE, Shannon KM. 2004. Somatic activation of oncogenic *Kras* in hematopoietic cells initiates a rapidly fatal myeloproliferative disorder. *Proc Natl Acad Sci* **101:** 597–602. doi:10.1073/pnas.0307203101

Brunetti L, Gundry MC, Goodell MA. 2017. DNMT3A in leukemia. *Cold Spring Harb Perspect Med* **7:** a030320. doi:10.1101/cshperspect.a030320

Busque L, Patel JP, Figueroa ME, Vasanthakumar A, Provost S, Hamilou Z, Mollica L, Li J, Viale A, Heguy A, et al. 2012. Recurrent somatic *TET2* mutations in normal elderly individuals with clonal hematopoiesis. *Nat Genet* **44:** 1179–1181. doi:10.1038/ng.2413

Cancer Genome Atlas Research Network, Ley TJ, Miller C, Ding L, Raphael BJ, Mungall AJ, Robertson A, Hoadley K, Triche TJ Jr, Laird PW, et al. 2013. Genomic and epigenomic landscapes of adult de novo acute myeloid leukemia. *N Engl J Med* **368:** 2059–2074. doi:10.1056/NEJMoa1301689

Celik H, Mallaney C, Kothari A, Ostrander EL, Eultgen E, Martens A, Miller CA, Hundal J, Klco JM, Challen GA. 2015. Enforced differentiation of *Dnmt3a*-null bone marrow leads to failure with c-Kit mutations driving leukemic transformation. *Blood* **125:** 619–628. doi:10.1182/blood-2014-08-594564

Challen GA, Sun D, Jeong M, Luo M, Jelinek J, Berg JS, Bock C, Vasanthakumar A, Gu H, Xi Y, et al. 2011. Dnmt3a is essential for hematopoietic stem cell differentiation. *Nat Genet* **44:** 23–31. doi:10.1038/ng.1009

Chaturvedi A, Araujo Cruz MM, Jyotsana N, Sharma A, Yun H, Görlich K, Wichmann M, Schwarzer A, Preller M, Thol F, et al. 2013. Mutant IDH1 promotes leukemogenesis in vivo and can be specifically targeted in human AML. *Blood* **122:** 2877–2887. doi:10.1182/blood-2013-03-491571

Chen C, Liu Y, Lu C, Cross JR, Morris JP IV, Shroff AS, Ward PS, Bradner JE, Thompson C, Lowe SW. 2013. Cancer-associated IDH2 mutants drive an acute myeloid leukemia that is susceptible to Brd4 inhibition. *Genes Dev* **27:** 1974–1985. doi:10.1101/gad.226613.113

Cheng K, Sportoletti P, Ito K, Clohessy JG, Teruya-Feldstein J, Kutok JL, Pandolfi PP. 2010. The cytoplasmic NPM mutant induces myeloproliferation in a transgenic mouse model. *Blood* **115:** 3341–3345. doi:10.1182/blood-2009-03-208587

Cho SW, Kim S, Kim JM, Kim JS. 2013. Targeted genome engineering in human cells with the Cas9 RNA-guided endonuclease. *Nat Biotechnol* **31:** 230–232. doi:10.1038/nbt.2507

Chou SH, Ko BS, Chiou JS, Hsu YC, Tsai MH, Chiu YC, Yu IS, Lin SW, Hou HA, Kuo YY, et al. 2012. A knock-in *Npm1* mutation in mice results in myeloproliferation and implies a perturbation in hematopoietic microenvironment. *PLoS ONE* **7:** e49769. doi:10.1371/journal.pone.0049769

Cimmino L, Dolgalev I, Wang Y, Yoshimi A, Martin GH, Wang J, Ng V, Xia B, Witkowski MT, Mitchell-Flack M, et al. 2017. Restoration of TET2 function blocks aberrant self-renewal and leukemia progression. *Cell* **170:** 1079–1095 e1020. doi:10.1016/j.cell.2017.07.032

Costa D, Muñoz C, Carrió A, Nomdedeu M, Calvo X, Solé F, Luño E, Cervera J, Vallespí T, Berneaga D, et al. 2013. Reciprocal translocations in myelodysplastic syndromes and chronic myelomonocytic leukemias: Review of 5,654 patients with an evaluable karyotype. *Genes Chromosomes Cancer* **52:** 753–763. doi:10.1002/gcc.22071

Cozzio A, Passegué E, Ayton PM, Karsunky H, Cleary ML, Weissman IL. 2003. Similar MLL-associated leukemias arising from self-renewing stem cells and short-lived myeloid progenitors. *Genes Dev* **17:** 3029–3035. doi:10.1101/gad.1143403

Daver N, Schlenk RF, Russell NH, Levis MJ. 2019. Targeting *FLT3* mutations in AML: Review of current knowledge and evidence. *Leukemia* **33:** 299–312. doi:10.1038/s41375-018-0357-9

Day CP, Merlino G, Van Dyke T. 2015. Preclinical mouse cancer models: A maze of opportunities and challenges. *Cell* **163:** 39–53. doi:10.1016/j.cell.2015.08.068

De Braekeleer M, Morel F, Le Bris MJ, Herry A, Douet-Guilbert N. 2005. The *MLL* gene and translocations involving chromosomal band 11q23 in acute leukemia. *Anticancer Res* **25:** 1931–1944.

Delhommeau F, Dupont S, Della Valle V, James C, Trannoy S, Massé A, Kosmider O, Le Couedic JP, Robert F, Alberdi A, et al. 2009. Mutation in TET2 in myeloid cancers. *N Engl J Med* **360:** 2289–2301. doi:10.1056/NEJMoa0810069

de Ruiter JR, Wessels LFA, Jonkers J. 2018. Mouse models in the era of large human tumour sequencing studies. *Open Biol* **8:** 180080. doi:10.1098/rsob.180080

Desai P, Mencia-Trinchant N, Savenkov O, Simon MS, Cheang G, Lee S, Samuel M, Ritchie EK, Guzman ML, Ballman KV, et al. 2018. Somatic mutations precede acute myeloid leukemia years before diagnosis. *Nat Med* **24:** 1015–1023. doi:10.1038/s41591-018-0081-z

DiNardo CD, Cortes JE. 2016. Mutations in AML: Prognostic and therapeutic implications. *Hematology Am Soc Hematol Educ Program* **2016:** 348–355. doi:10.1182/asheducation-2016.1.348

Döhner H, Weisdorf DJ, Bloomfield CD. 2015. Acute myeloid leukemia. *N Engl J Med* **373:** 1136–1152. doi:10.1056/NEJMra1406184

Döhner H, Estey E, Grimwade D, Amadori S, Appelbaum FR, Büchner T, Dombret H, Ebert BL, Fenaux P, Larson RA, et al. 2017. Diagnosis and management of AML in adults: 2017 ELN recommendations from an international expert panel. *Blood* **129:** 424–447. doi:10.1182/blood-2016-08-733196

Donehower LA, Soussi T, Korkut A, Liu Y, Schultz A, Cardenas M, Li X, Babur O, Hsu TK, Lichtarge O, et al. 2019. Integrated analysis of TP53 gene and pathway alterations in the Cancer Genome Atlas. *Cell Rep* **28:** 3010. doi:10.1016/j.celrep.2019.08.061

Dovey OM, Cooper JL, Mupo A, Grove CS, Lynn C, Conte N, Andrews RM, Pacharne S, Tzelepis K, Vijayabaskar MS, et al. 2017. Molecular synergy underlies the co-occurrence patterns and phenotype of *NPM1*-mutant acute myeloid leukemia. *Blood* **130:** 1911–1922. doi:10.1182/blood-2017-01-760595

Dvinge H, Kim E, Abdel-Wahab O, Bradley RK. 2016. RNA splicing factors as oncoproteins and tumour suppressors. *Nat Rev Cancer* **16:** 413–430. doi:10.1038/nrc.2016.51

Early E, Moore MA, Kakizuka A, Nason-Burchenal K, Martin P, Evans RM, Dmitrovsky E. 1996. Transgenic expression of PML/RARα impairs myelopoiesis. *Proc Natl Acad Sci* **93:** 7900–7904. doi:10.1073/pnas.93.15.7900

Ernst T, Chase AJ, Score J, Hidalgo-Curtis CE, Bryant C, Jones AV, Waghorn K, Zoi K, Ross FM, Reiter A, et al. 2010. Inactivating mutations of the histone methyltransferase gene *EZH2* in myeloid disorders. *Nat Genet* **42:** 722–726. doi:10.1038/ng.621

Falini B, Mecucci C, Tiacci E, Alcalay M, Rosati R, Pasqualucci L, La Starza R, Diverio D, Colombo E, Santucci A, et al. 2005. Cytoplasmic nucleophosmin in acute myelogenous leukemia with a normal karyotype. *N Engl J Med* **352:** 254–266. doi:10.1056/NEJMoa041974

Falini B, Bolli N, Liso A, Martelli MP, Mannucci R, Pileri S, Nicoletti I. 2009. Altered nucleophosmin transport in acute myeloid leukaemia with mutated *NPM1*: Molecular basis and clinical implications. *Leukemia* **23:** 1731–1743. doi:10.1038/leu.2009.124

Ficz G, Branco MR, Seisenberger S, Santos F, Krueger F, Hore TA, Marques CJ, Andrews S, Reik W. 2011. Dynamic regulation of 5-hydroxymethylcytosine in mouse ES cells and during differentiation. *Nature* **473:** 398–402. doi:10.1038/nature10008

Fisher JB, McNulty M, Burke MJ, Crispino JD, Rao S. 2017. Cohesin mutations in myeloid malignancies. *Trends Cancer* **3:** 282–293. doi:10.1016/j.trecan.2017.02.006

Gale RE, Green C, Allen C, Mead AJ, Burnett AK, Hills RK, Linch DC; Medical Research Council Adult Leukaemia Working Party. 2008. The impact of FLT3 internal tandem duplication mutant level, number, size, and interaction with NPM1 mutations in a large cohort of young adult patients with acute myeloid leukemia. *Blood* **111:** 2776–2784. doi:10.1182/blood-2007-08-109090

Gallipoli P, Huntly BJP. 2018. Novel epigenetic therapies in hematological malignancies: Current status and beyond. *Semin Cancer Biol* **51:** 198–210. doi:10.1016/j.semcancer.2017.07.005

Genovese G, Kähler AK, Handsaker RE, Lindberg J, Rose SA, Bakhoum SF, Chambert K, Mick E, Neale BM, Fromer M, et al. 2014. Clonal hematopoiesis and blood-cancer risk inferred from blood DNA sequence. *N Engl J Med* **371:** 2477–2487. doi:10.1056/NEJMoa1409405

Gerstung M, Papaemmanuil E, Campbell PJ. 2014. Subclonal variant calling with multiple samples and prior knowledge. *Bioinformatics* **30:** 1198–1204. doi:10.1093/bioinformatics/btt750

Gillet JP, Varma S, Gottesman MM. 2013. The clinical relevance of cancer cell lines. *J Natl Cancer Inst* **105:** 452–458. doi:10.1093/jnci/djt007

Gilliland DG, Griffin JD. 2002. The roles of FLT3 in hematopoiesis and leukemia. *Blood* **100:** 1532–1542. doi:10.1182/blood-2002-02-0492

Gligoris T, Lowe J. 2016. Structural insights into ring formation of cohesin and related Smc complexes. *Trends Cell Biol* **26:** 680–693. doi:10.1016/j.tcb.2016.04.002

Gozdecka M, Meduri E, Mazan M, Tzelepis K, Dudek M, Knights AJ, Pardo M, Yu L, Choudhary JS, Metzakopian E, et al. 2018. UTX-mediated enhancer and chromatin remodeling suppresses myeloid leukemogenesis through noncatalytic inverse regulation of ETS and GATA programs. *Nat Genet* **50:** 883–894. doi:10.1038/s41588-018-0114-z

Graubert TA, Shen D, Ding L, Okeyo-Owuor T, Lunn CL, Shao J, Krysiak K, Harris CC, Koboldt DC, Larson DE, et al. 2011. Recurrent mutations in the *U2AF1* splicing factor in myelodysplastic syndromes. *Nat Genet* **44:** 53–57. doi:10.1038/ng.1031

Greaves MF, Wiemels J. 2003. Origins of chromosome translocations in childhood leukaemia. *Nat Rev Cancer* **3:** 639–649. doi:10.1038/nrc1164

Green A, Beer P. 2010. Somatic mutations of *IDH1* and IDH2 in the leukemic transformation of myeloproliferative neoplasms. *N Engl J Med* **362:** 369–370. doi:10.1056/NEJMc0910063

Greenblatt S, Li L, Slape C, Nguyen B, Novak R, Duffield A, Huso D, Desiderio S, Borowitz MJ, Aplan P, et al. 2012. Knock-in of a FLT3/ITD mutation cooperates with a NUP98-HOXD13 fusion to generate acute myeloid leukemia in a mouse model. *Blood* **119:** 2883–2894. doi:10.1182/blood-2011-10-382283

Grundler R, Miething C, Thiede C, Peschel C, Duyster J. 2005. FLT3-ITD and tyrosine kinase domain mutants induce 2 distinct phenotypes in a murine bone marrow transplantation model. *Blood* **105:** 4792–4799. doi:10.1182/blood-2004-11-4430

Guryanova OA, Shank K, Spitzer B, Luciani L, Koche RP, Garrett-Bakelman FE, Ganzel C, Durham BH, Mohanty A, Hoermann G, et al. 2016. *DNMT3A* mutations promote anthracycline resistance in acute myeloid leukemia via impaired nucleosome remodeling. *Nat Med* **22:** 1488–1495. doi:10.1038/nm.4210

Haferlach T, Nagata Y, Grossmann V, Okuno Y, Bacher U, Nagae G, Schnittger S, Sanada M, Kon A, Alpermann T, et al. 2014. Landscape of genetic lesions in 944 patients with myelodysplastic syndromes. *Leukemia* **28:** 241–247. doi: 10.1038/leu.2013.336

Hayakawa F, Towatari M, Kiyoi H, Tanimoto M, Kitamura T, Saito H, Naoe T. 2000. Tandem-duplicated Flt3 constitutively activates STAT5 and MAP kinase and introduces autonomous cell growth in IL-3-dependent cell lines. *Oncogene* **19:** 624–631. doi:10.1038/sj.onc.1203354

Heckl D, Kowalczyk MS, Yudovich D, Belizaire R, Puram RV, McConkey ME, Thielke A, Aster JC, Regev A, Ebert BL. 2014. Generation of mouse models of myeloid malignancy with combinatorial genetic lesions using CRISPR–Cas9 genome editing. *Nat Biotechnol* **32:** 941–946. doi:10.1038/nbt.2951

Hingorani K, Szebeni A, Olson MO. 2000. Mapping the functional domains of nucleolar protein B23. *J Biol Chem* **275:** 24451–24457. doi:10.1074/jbc.M003278200

Huntly BJ, Shigematsu H, Deguchi K, Lee BH, Mizuno S, Duclos N, Rowan R, Amaral S, Curley D, Williams IR, et al. 2004. *MOZ-TIF2*, but not *BCR-ABL*, confers properties of leukemic stem cells to committed murine hematopoietic progenitors. *Cancer Cell* **6:** 587–596. doi:10.1016/j.ccr.2004.10.015

Itahana K, Bhat KP, Jin A, Itahana Y, Hawke D, Kobayashi R, Zhang Y. 2003. Tumor suppressor ARF degrades B23, a nucleolar protein involved in ribosome biogenesis and cell proliferation. *Mol Cell* **12:** 1151–1164. doi:10.1016/S1097-2765(03)00431-3

Jaiswal S, Fontanillas P, Flannick J, Manning A, Grauman PV, Mar BG, Lindsley RC, Mermel CH, Burtt N, Chavez A, et al. 2014. Age-related clonal hematopoiesis associated with adverse outcomes. *N Engl J Med* **371:** 2488–2498. doi:10.1056/NEJMoa1408617

James C, Ugo V, Le Couédic JP, Staerk J, Delhommeau F, Lacout C, Garçon L, Raslova H, Berger R, Bennaceur-Griscelli A, et al. 2005. A unique clonal *JAK2* mutation leading to constitutive signalling causes polycythaemia vera. *Nature* **434:** 1144–1148. doi:10.1038/nature03546

Janssen JW, Steenvoorden AC, Lyons J, Anger B, Böhlke JU, Bos JL, Seliger H, Bartram CR. 1987. *RAS* gene mutations in acute and chronic myelocytic leukemias, chronic myeloproliferative disorders, and myelodysplastic syndromes. *Proc Natl Acad Sci* **84:** 9228–9232. doi:10.1073/pnas.84.24.9228

Jones PA. 2012. Functions of DNA methylation: Islands, start sites, gene bodies and beyond. *Nat Rev Genet* **13:** 484–492. doi:10.1038/nrg3230

Kaneda M, Okano M, Hata K, Sado T, Tsujimoto N, Li E, Sasaki H. 2004. Essential role for de novo DNA methyltransferase Dnmt3a in paternal and maternal imprinting. *Nature* **429:** 900–903. doi:10.1038/nature02633

Kelly LM, Liu Q, Kutok JL, Williams IR, Boulton CL, Gilliland DG. 2002a. FLT3 internal tandem duplication mutations associated with human acute myeloid leukemias induce myeloproliferative disease in a murine bone marrow transplant model. *Blood* **99:** 310–318. doi:10.1182/blood.V99.1.310

Kelly LM, Kutok JL, Williams IR, Boulton CL, Amaral SM, Curley DP, Ley TJ, Gilliland DG. 2002b. PML/RARα and FLT3-ITD induce an APL-like disease in a mouse model. *Proc Natl Acad Sci* **99:** 8283–8288. doi:10.1073/pnas.122233699

Kennedy JA, Ebert BL. 2017. Clinical implications of genetic mutations in myelodysplastic syndrome. *J Clin Oncol* **35:** 968–974. doi:10.1200/JCO.2016.71.0806

Kim E, Ilagan JO, Liang Y, Daubner GM, Lee SC, Ramakrishnan A, Li Y, Chung YR, Micol JB, Murphy ME, et al. 2015. *SRSF2* mutations contribute to myelodysplasia by mutant-specific effects on exon recognition. *Cancer Cell* **27:** 617–630. doi:10.1016/j.ccell.2015.04.006

Klampfl T, Gisslinger H, Harutyunyan AS, Nivarthi H, Rumi E, Milosevic JD, Them NC, Berg T, Gisslinger B, Pietra D, et al. 2013. Somatic mutations of calreticulin in myeloproliferative neoplasms. *N Engl J Med* **369:** 2379–2390. doi:10.1056/NEJMoa1311347

Knapp RH, Dewald GW, Pierre RV. 1985. Cytogenetic studies in 174 consecutive patients with preleukemic or myelodysplastic syndromes. *Mayo Clin Proc* **60:** 507–516. doi:10.1016/S0025-6196(12)60566-7

Kohnken R, Porcu P, Mishra A. 2017. Overview of the use of murine models in leukemia and lymphoma research. *Front Oncol* **7:** 22. doi:10.3389/fonc.2017.00022

Koike-Yusa H, Li Y, Tan EP, Velasco-Herrera Mdel C, Yusa K. 2014. Genome-wide recessive genetic screening in mammalian cells with a lentiviral CRISPR-guide RNA library. *Nat Biotechnol* **32:** 267–273. doi:10.1038/nbt.2800

Koivunen P, Lee S, Duncan CG, Lopez G, Lu G, Ramkissoon S, Losman JA, Joensuu P, Bergmann U, Gross S, et al. 2012. Transformation by the (R)-enantiomer of 2-hydroxyglutarate linked to EGLN activation. *Nature* **483:** 484–488. doi:10.1038/nature10898

Kralovics R, Passamonti F, Buser AS, Teo SS, Tiedt R, Passweg JR, Tichelli A, Cazzola M, Skoda RC. 2005. A gain-of-function mutation of JAK2 in myeloproliferative disorders. *N Engl J Med* **352:** 1779–1790. doi:10.1056/NEJMoa051113

Krivtsov AV, Twomey D, Feng Z, Stubbs MC, Wang Y, Faber J, Levine JE, Wang J, Hahn WC, Gilliland DG, et al. 2006. Transformation from committed progenitor to leukaemia stem cell initiated by MLL-AF9. *Nature* **442:** 818–822. doi:10.1038/nature04980

Kuhn R, Schwenk F, Aguet M, Rajewsky K. 1995. Inducible gene targeting in mice. *Science* **269:** 1427–1429. doi:10.1126/science.7660125

Landgraf M, McGovern JA, Friedl P, Hutmacher DW. 2018. Rational design of mouse models for cancer research. *Trends Biotechnol* **36:** 242–251. doi:10.1016/j.tibtech.2017.12.001

Langemeijer SM, Kuiper RP, Berends M, Knops R, Aslanyan MG, Massop M, Stevens-Linders E, van Hoogen P, van Kessel AG, Raymakers RA, et al. 2009. Acquired mutations in *TET2* are common in myelodysplastic syndromes. *Nat Genet* **41:** 838–842. doi:10.1038/ng.391

Lapidot T, Sirard C, Vormoor J, Murdoch B, Hoang T, Caceres-Cortes J, Minden M, Paterson B, Caligiuri MA, Dick JE. 1994. A cell initiating human acute myeloid leukaemia after transplantation into SCID mice. *Nature* **367:** 645–648. doi:10.1038/367645a0

Lee SC, Abdel-Wahab O. 2016. Therapeutic targeting of splicing in cancer. *Nat Med* **22:** 976–986. doi:10.1038/nm.4165

Lee BH, Williams IR, Anastasiadou E, Boulton CL, Joseph SW, Amaral SM, Curley DP, Duclos N, Huntly BJ, Fabbro D, et al. 2005. FLT3 internal tandem duplication mutations induce myeloproliferative or lymphoid disease in a transgenic mouse model. *Oncogene* **24:** 7882–7892. doi:10.1038/sj.onc.1208933

Lee BH, Tothova Z, Levine RL, Anderson K, Buza-Vidas N, Cullen DE, McDowell EP, Adelsperger J, Fröhling S, Huntly BJ, et al. 2007. FLT3 mutations confer enhanced proliferation and survival properties to multipotent progenitors in a murine model of chronic myelomonocytic leukemia. *Cancer Cell* **12:** 367–380. doi:10.1016/j.ccr.2007.08.031

Lemonnier F, Cairns RA, Inoue S, Li WY, Dupuy A, Broutin S, Martin N, Fataccioli V, Pelletier R, Wakeham A, et al.

2016. The IDH2 R172K mutation associated with angioimmunoblastic T-cell lymphoma produces 2HG in T cells and impacts lymphoid development. *Proc Natl Acad Sci* **113:** 15084–15089. doi:10.1073/pnas.1617929114

Levine RL, Wadleigh M, Cools J, Ebert BL, Wernig G, Huntly BJ, Boggon TJ, Wlodarska I, Clark JJ, Moore S, et al. 2005. Activating mutation in the tyrosine kinase JAK2 in polycythemia vera, essential thrombocythemia, and myeloid metaplasia with myelofibrosis. *Cancer Cell* **7:** 387–397. doi:10.1016/j.ccr.2005.03.023

Ley TJ, Ding L, Walter MJ, McLellan MD, Lamprecht T, Larson DE, Kandoth C, Payton JE, Baty J, Welch J, et al. 2010. *DNMT3A* mutations in acute myeloid leukemia. *N Engl J Med* **363:** 2424–2433. doi:10.1056/NEJMoa1005143

Li E. 2002. Chromatin modification and epigenetic reprogramming in mammalian development. *Nat Rev Genet* **3:** 662–673. doi:10.1038/nrg887

Li L, Piloto O, Nguyen HB, Greenberg K, Takamiya K, Racke F, Huso D, Small D. 2008. Knock-in of an internal tandem duplication mutation into murine FLT3 confers myeloproliferative disease in a mouse model. *Blood* **111:** 3849–3858. doi:10.1182/blood-2007-08-109942

Li Q, Haigis KM, McDaniel A, Harding-Theobald E, Kogan SC, Akagi K, Wong JC, Braun BS, Wolff L, Jacks T, et al. 2011a. Hematopoiesis and leukemogenesis in mice expressing oncogenic $Nras^{G12D}$ from the endogenous locus. *Blood* **117:** 2022–2032. doi:10.1182/blood-2010-04-280750

Li Z, Cai X, Cai CL, Wang J, Zhang W, Petersen BE, Yang FC, Xu M. 2011b. Deletion of Tet2 in mice leads to dysregulated hematopoietic stem cells and subsequent development of myeloid malignancies. *Blood* **118:** 4509–4518. doi:10.1182/blood-2010-12-325241

Lindgren V, Rowley JD. 1977. Comparable complex rearrangements involving 8;21 and 9;22 translocations in leukaemia. *Nature* **266:** 744–745. doi:10.1038/266744a0

Loberg MA, Bell RK, Goodwin LO, Eudy E, Miles LA, SanMiguel JM, Young K, Bergstrom DE, Levine RL, Schneider RK, et al. 2019. Sequentially inducible mouse models reveal that *Npm1* mutation causes malignant transformation of *Dnmt3a*-mutant clonal hematopoiesis. *Leukemia* **33:** 1635–1649. doi:10.1038/s41375-018-0368-6

Loizou E, Banito A, Livshits G, Ho YJ, Koche RP, Sánchez-Rivera FJ, Mayle A, Chen CC, Kinalis S, Bagger FO, et al. 2019. A gain-of-function p53-mutant oncogene promotes cell fate plasticity and myeloid leukemia through the pluripotency factor FOXH1. *Cancer Discov* **9:** 962–979. doi:10.1158/2159-8290.CD-18-1391

Lozano G. 2010. Mouse models of p53 functions. *Cold Spring Harb Perspect Biol* **2:** a001115. doi:10.1101/cshperspect.a001115

Lu C, Ward PS, Kapoor GS, Rohle D, Turcan S, Abdel-Wahab O, Edwards CR, Khanin R, Figueroa ME, Melnick A, et al. 2012. IDH mutation impairs histone demethylation and results in a block to cell differentiation. *Nature* **483:** 474–478. doi:10.1038/nature10860

Makishima H, Jankowska AM, Tiu RV, Szpurka H, Sugimoto Y, Hu Z, Saunthararajah Y, Guinta K, Keddache MA, Putnam P, et al. 2010. Novel homo- and hemizygous mutations in *EZH2* in myeloid malignancies. *Leukemia* **24:** 1799–1804. doi:10.1038/leu.2010.167

Mallardo M, Caronno A, Pruneri G, Raviele PR, Viale A, Pelicci PG, Colombo E. 2013. NPMc+ and FLT3_ITD mutations cooperate in inducing acute leukaemia in a novel mouse model. *Leukemia* **27:** 2248–2251. doi:10.1038/leu.2013.114

Marcucci G, Maharry K, Wu YZ, Radmacher MD, Mrózek K, Margeson D, Holland KB, Whitman SP, Becker H, Schwind S, et al. 2010. *IDH1* and *IDH2* gene mutations identify novel molecular subsets within de novo cytogenetically normal acute myeloid leukemia: A Cancer and Leukemia Group B study. *J Clin Oncol* **28:** 2348–2355. doi:10.1200/JCO.2009.27.3730

Mardis ER, Ding L, Dooling DJ, Larson DE, McLellan MD, Chen K, Koboldt DC, Fulton RS, Delehaunty KD, McGrath SD, et al. 2009. Recurring mutations found by sequencing an acute myeloid leukemia genome. *N Engl J Med* **361:** 1058–1066. doi:10.1056/NEJMoa0903840

Martelli MP, Sportoletti P, Tiacci E, Martelli MF, Falini B. 2013. Mutational landscape of AML with normal cytogenetics: Biological and clinical implications. *Blood Rev* **27:** 13–22. doi:10.1016/j.blre.2012.11.001

Mayle A, Yang L, Rodriguez B, Zhou T, Chang E, Curry CV, Challen GA, Li W, Wheeler D, Rebel VI, et al. 2015. *Dnmt3a* loss predisposes murine hematopoietic stem cells to malignant transformation. *Blood* **125:** 629–638. doi:10.1182/blood-2014-08-594648

Mazumdar C, Majeti R. 2017. The role of mutations in the cohesin complex in acute myeloid leukemia. *Int J Hematol* **105:** 31–36. doi:10.1007/s12185-016-2119-7

McKerrell T, Park N, Moreno T, Grove CS, Ponstingl H, Stephens J; Understanding Society Scientific Group, Crawley C, Craig J, Scott MA, et al. 2015. Leukemia-associated somatic mutations drive distinct patterns of age-related clonal hemopoiesis. *Cell Rep* **10:** 1239–1245. doi:10.1016/j.celrep.2015.02.005

McNerney ME, Godley LA, Le Beau MM. 2017. Therapy-related myeloid neoplasms: When genetics and environment collide. *Nat Rev Cancer* **17:** 513–527. doi:10.1038/nrc.2017.60

Mead AJ, Kharazi S, Atkinson D, Macaulay I, Pecquet C, Loughran S, Lutteropp M, Woll P, Chowdhury O, Luc S, et al. 2013. FLT3-ITDs instruct a myeloid differentiation and transformation bias in lymphomyeloid multipotent progenitors. *Cell Rep* **3:** 1766–1776. doi:10.1016/j.celrep.2013.04.031

Meyer SC, Levine RL. 2014. Translational implications of somatic genomics in acute myeloid leukaemia. *Lancet Oncol* **15:** e382–e394. doi:10.1016/S1470-2045(14)70008-7

Meyer SE, Qin T, Muench DE, Masuda K, Venkatasubramanian M, Orr E, Suarez L, Gore SD, Delwel R, Paietta E, et al. 2016. DNMT3A haploinsufficiency transforms $FLT3^{ITD}$ myeloproliferative disease into a rapid, spontaneous, and fully penetrant acute myeloid leukemia. *Cancer Discov* **6:** 501–515. doi:10.1158/2159-8290.CD-16-0008

Meyer AE, Rao S, Fisher JB. 2017. Cohesin mutations: Contributors to myeloid malignancies. *Oncotarget* **8:** 80107–80108. doi:10.18632/oncotarget.21050

Meyer C, Burmeister T, Gröger D, Tsaur G, Fechina L, Renneville A, Sutton R, Venn NC, Emerenciano M, Pombo-de-Oliveira MS, et al. 2018. The *MLL* recombinome of acute leukemias in 2017. *Leukemia* **32:** 273–284. doi:10.1038/leu.2017.213

Milne TA. 2017. Mouse models of MLL leukemia: Recapitulating the human disease. *Blood* **129:** 2217–2223. doi:10.1182/blood-2016-10-691428

Mochizuki-Kashio M, Aoyama K, Sashida G, Oshima M, Tomioka T, Muto T, Wang C, Iwama A. 2015. Ezh2 loss in hematopoietic stem cells predisposes mice to develop heterogeneous malignancies in an Ezh1-dependent manner. *Blood* **126:** 1172–1183. doi:10.1182/blood-2015-03-634428

Montalban-Bravo G, Garcia-Manero G. 2018. Myelodysplastic syndromes: 2018 update on diagnosis, risk-stratification and management. *Am J Hematol* **93:** 129–147. doi:10.1002/ajh.24930

Moran-Crusio K, Reavie L, Shih A, Abdel-Wahab O, Ndiaye-Lobry D, Lobry C, Figueroa ME, Vasanthakumar A, Patel J, Zhao X, et al. 2011. *Tet2* loss leads to increased hematopoietic stem cell self-renewal and myeloid transformation. *Cancer Cell* **20:** 11–24. doi:10.1016/j.ccr.2011.06.001

Morin RD, Johnson NA, Severson TM, Mungall AJ, An J, Goya R, Paul JE, Boyle M, Woolcock BW, Kuchenbauer F, et al. 2010. Somatic mutations altering EZH2 (Tyr641) in follicular and diffuse large B-cell lymphomas of germinal-center origin. *Nat Genet* **42:** 181–185. doi:10.1038/ng.518

Mullenders J, Aranda-Orgilles B, Lhoumaud P, Keller M, Pae J, Wang K, Kayembe C, Rocha PP, Raviram R, Gong Y, et al. 2015. Cohesin loss alters adult hematopoietic stem cell homeostasis, leading to myeloproliferative neoplasms. *J Exp Med* **212:** 1833–1850. doi:10.1084/jem.20151323

Mupo A, Celani L, Dovey O, Cooper JL, Grove C, Rad R, Sportoletti P, Falini B, Bradley A, Vassiliou GS. 2013. A powerful molecular synergy between mutant nucleophosmin and Flt3-ITD drives acute myeloid leukemia in mice. *Leukemia* **27:** 1917–1920. doi:10.1038/leu.2013.77

Mupo A, Seiler M, Sathiaseelan V, Pance A, Yang Y, Agrawal AA, Iorio F, Bautista R, Pacharne S, Tzelepis K, et al. 2017. Hemopoietic-specific *Sf3b1*-K700E knock-in mice display the splicing defect seen in human MDS but develop anemia without ring sideroblasts. *Leukemia* **31:** 720–727. doi:10.1038/leu.2016.251

Nangalia J, Massie CE, Baxter EJ, Nice FL, Gundem G, Wedge DC, Avezov E, Li J, Kollmann K, Kent DG, et al. 2013. Somatic *CALR* mutations in myeloproliferative neoplasms with nonmutated *JAK2*. *N Engl J Med* **369:** 2391–2405. doi:10.1056/NEJMoa1312542

Neff T, Sinha AU, Kluk MJ, Zhu N, Khattab MH, Stein L, Xie H, Orkin SH, Armstrong SA. 2012. Polycomb repressive complex 2 is required for MLL-AF9 leukemia. *Proc Natl Acad Sci* **109:** 5028–5033. doi:10.1073/pnas.1202258109

Nikoloski G, Langemeijer SM, Kuiper RP, Knops R, Massop M, Tönnissen ER, van der Heijden A, Scheele TN, Vandenberghe P, de Witte T, et al. 2010. Somatic mutations of the histone methyltransferase gene *EZH2* in myelodysplastic syndromes. *Nat Genet* **42:** 665–667. doi:10.1038/ng.620

Nowell PC, Besa EC, Stelmach T, Finan JB. 1986. Chromosome studies in preleukemic states. V. Prognostic significance of single versus multiple abnormalities. *Cancer* **58:** 2571–2575. doi:10.1002/1097-0142(19861215)58:12<2571::AID-CNCR2820581202>3.0.CO;2-O

Obeng EA, Chappell RJ, Seiler M, Chen MC, Campagna DR, Schmidt PJ, Schneider RK, Lord AM, Wang L, Gambe RG, et al. 2016. Physiologic expression of $Sf3b1^{K700E}$ causes impaired erythropoiesis, aberrant splicing, and sensitivity to therapeutic spliceosome modulation. *Cancer Cell* **30:** 404–417. doi:10.1016/j.ccell.2016.08.006

Okuda M. 2002. The role of nucleophosmin in centrosome duplication. *Oncogene* **21:** 6170–6174. doi:10.1038/sj.onc.1205708

Ottersbach K, Sanjuan-Pla A, Torres-Ruíz R, Bueno C, Velasco-Hernández T, Menendez P. 2018. The "never-ending" mouse models for MLL-rearranged acute leukemia are still teaching us. *HemaSphere* **2:** e57. doi:10.1097/HS9.0000000000000057

Panigrahi AK, Pati D. 2012. Higher-order orchestration of hematopoiesis: Is cohesin a new player? *Exp Hematol* **40:** 967–973. doi:10.1016/j.exphem.2012.09.010

Pant V, Quintas-Cardama A, Lozano G. 2012. The p53 pathway in hematopoiesis: Lessons from mouse models, implications for humans. *Blood* **120:** 5118–5127. doi:10.1182/blood-2012-05-356014

Papaemmanuil E, Cazzola M, Boultwood J, Malcovati L, Vyas P, Bowen D, Pellagatti A, Wainscoat JS, Hellstrom-Lindberg E, Gambacorti-Passerini C, et al. 2011. Somatic *SF3B1* mutation in myelodysplasia with ring sideroblasts. *N Engl J Med* **365:** 1384–1395. doi:10.1056/NEJMoa1103283

Papaemmanuil E, Gerstung M, Malcovati L, Tauro S, Gundem G, Van Loo P, Yoon CJ, Ellis P, Wedge DC, Pellagatti A, et al. 2013. Clinical and biological implications of driver mutations in myelodysplastic syndromes. *Blood* **122:** 3616–3627. quiz 3699. doi:10.1182/blood-2013-08-518886

Papaemmanuil E, Gerstung M, Bullinger L, Gaidzik VI, Paschka P, Roberts ND, Potter NE, Heuser M, Thol F, Bolli N, et al. 2016. Genomic classification and prognosis in acute myeloid leukemia. *N Engl J Med* **374:** 2209–2221. doi:10.1056/NEJMoa1516192

Parsons DW, Jones S, Zhang X, Lin JC, Leary RJ, Angenendt P, Mankoo P, Carter H, Siu IM, Gallia GL, et al. 2008. An integrated genomic analysis of human glioblastoma multiforme. *Science* **321:** 1807–1812. doi:10.1126/science.1164382

Prchal JT. 2005. Polycythemia vera and other primary polycythemias. *Curr Opin Hematol* **12:** 112–116. doi:10.1097/01.moh.0000154029.05396.d2

Quivoron C, Couronné L, Della Valle V, Lopez CK, Plo I, Wagner-Ballon O, Do Cruzeiro M, Delhommeau F, Arnulf B, Stern MH, et al. 2011. TET2 inactivation results in pleiotropic hematopoietic abnormalities in mouse and is a recurrent event during human lymphomagenesis. *Cancer Cell* **20:** 25–38. doi:10.1016/j.ccr.2011.06.003

Rau R, Magoon D, Greenblatt S, Li L, Annesley C, Duffield AS, Huso D, McIntyre E, Clohessy JG, Reschke M, et al. 2014. $NPMc^{+}$ cooperates with Flt3/ITD mutations to cause acute leukemia recapitulating human disease. *Exp*

Hematol **42:** 101–113 e105. doi:10.1016/j.exphem.2013.10.005

Rein A. 2011. Murine leukemia viruses: Objects and organisms. *Adv Virol* **2011:** 403419. doi:10.1155/2011/403419

Rowley JD. 1973. Identification of a translocation with quinacrine fluorescence in a patient with acute leukemia. *Ann Genet* **16:** 109–112.

Rowley JD, Golomb HM, Dougherty C. 1977. 15/17 translocation, a consistent chromosomal change in acute promyelocytic leukaemia. *Lancet* **1:** 549–550. doi:10.1016/S0140-6736(77)91415-5

Russler-Germain DA, Spencer DH, Young MA, Lamprecht TL, Miller CA, Fulton R, Meyer MR, Erdmann-Gilmore P, Townsend RR, Wilson RK, et al. 2014. The R882H DNMT3A mutation associated with AML dominantly inhibits wild-type DNMT3A by blocking its ability to form active tetramers. *Cancer Cell* **25:** 442–454. doi:10.1016/j.ccr.2014.02.010

Saez B, Walter MJ, Graubert TA. 2017. Splicing factor gene mutations in hematologic malignancies. *Blood* **129:** 1260–1269. doi:10.1182/blood-2016-10-692400

Sasaki M, Knobbe CB, Munger JC, Lind EF, Brenner D, Brüstle A, Harris IS, Holmes R, Wakeham A, Haight J, et al. 2012. IDH1(R132H) mutation increases murine haematopoietic progenitors and alters epigenetics. *Nature* **488:** 656–659. doi:10.1038/nature11323

Sashida G, Wang C, Tomioka T, Oshima M, Aoyama K, Kanai A, Mochizuki-Kashio M, Harada H, Shimoda K, Iwama A. 2016. The loss of Ezh2 drives the pathogenesis of myelofibrosis and sensitizes tumor-initiating cells to bromodomain inhibition. *J Exp Med* **213:** 1459–1477. doi:10.1084/jem.20151121

Sauer B, Henderson N. 1988. Site-specific DNA recombination in mammalian cells by the Cre recombinase of bacteriophage P1. *Proc Natl Acad Sci* **85:** 5166–5170. doi:10.1073/pnas.85.14.5166

Scott MT, Korfi K, Saffrey P, Hopcroft LE, Kinstrie R, Pellicano F, Guenther C, Gallipoli P, Cruz M, Dunn K, et al. 2016. Epigenetic reprogramming sensitizes CML stem cells to combined EZH2 and tyrosine kinase inhibition. *Cancer Discov* **6:** 1248–1257. doi:10.1158/2159-8290.CD-16-0263

Shalem O, Sanjana NE, Zhang F. 2015. High-throughput functional genomics using CRISPR–Cas9. *Nat Rev Genet* **16:** 299–311. doi:10.1038/nrg3899

Sharma SV, Haber DA, Settleman J. 2010. Cell line-based platforms to evaluate the therapeutic efficacy of candidate anticancer agents. *Nat Rev Cancer* **10:** 241–225. doi:10.1038/nrc2820

Shi J, Wang E, Milazzo JP, Wang Z, Kinney JB, Vakoc CR. 2015. Discovery of cancer drug targets by CRISPR–Cas9 screening of protein domains. *Nat Biotechnol* **33:** 661–667. doi:10.1038/nbt.3235

Shih AH, Jiang Y, Meydan C, Shank K, Pandey S, Barreyro L, Antony-Debre I, Viale A, Socci N, Sun Y, et al. 2015. Mutational cooperativity linked to combinatorial epigenetic gain of function in acute myeloid leukemia. *Cancer Cell* **27:** 502–515. doi:10.1016/j.ccell.2015.03.009

Shimizu T, Kubovcakova L, Nienhold R, Zmajkovic J, Meyer SC, Hao-Shen H, Geier F, Dirnhofer S, Guglielmelli P, Vannucchi AM, et al. 2016. Loss of *Ezh2* synergizes with *JAK2*-V617F in initiating myeloproliferative neoplasms and promoting myelofibrosis. *J Exp Med* **213:** 1479–1496. doi:10.1084/jem.20151136

Shiozawa Y, Malcovati L, Gallì A, Sato-Otsubo A, Kataoka K, Sato Y, Watatani Y, Suzuki H, Yoshizato T, Yoshida K, et al. 2018. Aberrant splicing and defective mRNA production induced by somatic spliceosome mutations in myelodysplasia. *Nat Commun* **9:** 3649. doi:10.1038/s41467-018-06063-x

Shirai CL, Ley JN, White BS, Kim S, Tibbitts J, Shao J, Ndonwi M, Wadugu B, Duncavage EJ, Okeyo-Owuor T, et al. 2015. Mutant U2AF1 expression alters hematopoiesis and pre-mRNA splicing in vivo. *Cancer Cell* **27:** 631–643. doi:10.1016/j.ccell.2015.04.008

Souroullas GP, Jeck WR, Parker JS, Simon JM, Liu JY, Paulk J, Xiong J, Clark KS, Fedoriw Y, Qi J, et al. 2016. An oncogenic *Ezh2* mutation induces tumors through global redistribution of histone 3 lysine 27 trimethylation. *Nat Med* **22:** 632–640. doi:10.1038/nm.4092

Spivak JL. 2004. The chronic myeloproliferative disorders: Clonality and clinical heterogeneity. *Semin Hematol* **41:** 1–5. doi:10.1053/j.seminhematol.2004.02.011

Sportoletti P, Varasano E, Rossi R, Bereshchenko O, Cecchini D, Gionfriddo I, Bolli N, Tiacci E, Intermesoli T, Zanghì P, et al. 2013. The human *NPM1* mutation A perturbs megakaryopoiesis in a conditional mouse model. *Blood* **121:** 3447–3458. doi:10.1182/blood-2012-08-449553

Sportoletti P, Varasano E, Rossi R, Mupo A, Tiacci E, Vassiliou G, Martelli MP, Falini B. 2015. Mouse models of *NPM1*-mutated acute myeloid leukemia: Biological and clinical implications. *Leukemia* **29:** 269–278. doi:10.1038/leu.2014.257

Stadtfeld M, Graf T. 2005. Assessing the role of hematopoietic plasticity for endothelial and hepatocyte development by non-invasive lineage tracing. *Development* **132:** 203–213. doi:10.1242/dev.01558

Swaminathan V, Kishore AH, Febitha KK, Kundu TK. 2005. Human histone chaperone nucleophosmin enhances acetylation-dependent chromatin transcription. *Mol Cell Biol* **25:** 7534–7545. doi:10.1128/MCB.25.17.7534-7545.2005

Tanaka S, Miyagi S, Sashida G, Chiba T, Yuan J, Mochizuki-Kashio M, Suzuki Y, Sugano S, Nakaseko C, Yokote K, et al. 2012. Ezh2 augments leukemogenicity by reinforcing differentiation blockage in acute myeloid leukemia. *Blood* **120:** 1107–1117. doi:10.1182/blood-2011-11-394932

Thol F, Damm F, Wagner K, Göhring G, Schlegelberger B, Hoelzer D, Lübbert M, Heit W, Kanz L, Schlimok G, et al. 2010. Prognostic impact of *IDH2* mutations in cytogenetically normal acute myeloid leukemia. *Blood* **116:** 614–616. doi:10.1182/blood-2010-03-272146

Tothova Z, Krill-Burger JM, Popova KD, Landers CC, Sievers QL, Yudovich D, Belizaire R, Aster JC, Morgan EA, Tsherniak A, et al. 2017. Multiplex CRISPR/Cas9-based genome editing in human hematopoietic stem cells models clonal hematopoiesis and myeloid neoplasia. *Cell Stem Cell* **21:** 547–555 e548. doi:10.1016/j.stem.2017.07.015

Tzelepis K, Koike-Yusa H, De Braekeleer E, Li Y, Metzakopian E, Dovey OM, Mupo A, Grinkevich V, Li M, Mazan M, et al. 2016. A CRISPR dropout screen identifies genetic vulnerabilities and therapeutic targets in acute myeloid leukemia. *Cell Rep* **17:** 1193–1205. doi:10.1016/j.celrep.2016.09.079

Vassiliou GS, Cooper JL, Rad R, Li J, Rice S, Uren A, Rad L, Ellis P, Andrews R, Banerjee R, et al. 2011. Mutant nucleophosmin and cooperating pathways drive leukemia initiation and progression in mice. *Nat Genet* **43:** 470–475. doi:10.1038/ng.796

Viny AD, Ott CJ, Spitzer B, Rivas M, Meydan C, Papalexi E, Yelin D, Shank K, Reyes J, Chiu A, et al. 2015. Dose-dependent role of the cohesin complex in normal and malignant hematopoiesis. *J Exp Med* **212:** 1819–1832. doi:10.1084/jem.20151317

Visser O, Trama A, Maynadié M, Stiller C, Marcos-Gragera R, De Angelis R, Mallone S, Tereanu C, Allemani C, Ricardi U, et al. 2012. Incidence, survival and prevalence of myeloid malignancies in Europe. *Eur J Cancer* **48:** 3257–3266. doi:10.1016/j.ejca.2012.05.024

Waddington CH. 2012. The epigenotype. 1942. *Int J Epidemiol* **41:** 10–13. doi:10.1093/ije/dyr184

Wagner K, Damm F, Göhring G, Görlich K, Heuser M, Schäfer I, Ottmann O, Lübbert M, Heit W, Kanz L, et al. 2010. Impact of *IDH1* R132 mutations and an *IDH1* single nucleotide polymorphism in cytogenetically normal acute myeloid leukemia: SNP rs11554137 is an adverse prognostic factor. *J Clin Oncol* **28:** 2356–2364. doi:10.1200/JCO.2009.27.6899

Wang L, Shilatifard A. 2019. UTX mutations in human cancer. *Cancer Cell* **35:** 168–176. doi:10.1016/j.ccell.2019.01.001

Wang T, Wei JJ, Sabatini DM, Lander ES. 2014. Genetic screens in human cells using the CRISPR–Cas9 system. *Science* **343:** 80–84. doi:10.1126/science.1246981

Ward PS, Patel J, Wise DR, Abdel-Wahab O, Bennett BD, Coller HA, Cross JR, Fantin VR, Hedvat CV, Perl AE, et al. 2010. The common feature of leukemia-associated IDH1 and IDH2 mutations is a neomorphic enzyme activity converting α-ketoglutarate to 2-hydroxyglutarate. *Cancer Cell* **17:** 225–234. doi:10.1016/j.ccr.2010.01.020

Welch JS, Ley TJ, Link DC, Miller CA, Larson DE, Koboldt DC, Wartman LD, Lamprecht TL, Liu F, Xia J, et al. 2012. The origin and evolution of mutations in acute myeloid leukemia. *Cell* **150:** 264–278. doi:10.1016/j.cell.2012.06.023

Will CL, Luhrmann R. 2011. Spliceosome structure and function. *Cold Spring Harb Perspect Biol* **3:** a003707. doi:10.1101/cshperspect.a003707

Wouters BJ, Delwel R. 2016. Epigenetics and approaches to targeted epigenetic therapy in acute myeloid leukemia. *Blood* **127:** 42–52. doi:10.1182/blood-2015-07-604512

Xie M, Lu C, Wang J, McLellan MD, Johnson KJ, Wendl MC, McMichael JF, Schmidt HK, Yellapantula V, Miller CA, et al. 2014. Age-related mutations associated with clonal hematopoietic expansion and malignancies. *Nat Med* **20:** 1472–1478. doi:10.1038/nm.3733

Xie H, Peng C, Huang J, Li BE, Kim W, Smith EC, Fujiwara Y, Qi J, Cheloni G, Das PP, et al. 2016. Chronic myelogenous leukemia-initiating cells require Polycomb group protein EZH2. *Cancer Discov* **6:** 1237–1247. doi:10.1158/2159-8290.CD-15-1439

Xu J, Wang YY, Dai YJ, Zhang W, Zhang WN, Xiong SM, Gu ZH, Wang KK, Zeng R, Chen Z, et al. 2014. DNMT3A Arg882 mutation drives chronic myelomonocytic leukemia through disturbing gene expression/DNA methylation in hematopoietic cells. *Proc Natl Acad Sci* **111:** 2620–2625. doi:10.1073/pnas.1400150111

Xue L, Pulikkan JA, Valk PJ, Castilla LH. 2014. NrasG12D oncoprotein inhibits apoptosis of preleukemic cells expressing Cbfβ-SMMHC via activation of MEK/ERK axis. *Blood* **124:** 426–436. doi:10.1182/blood-2013-12-541730

Yan H, Parsons DW, Jin G, McLendon R, Rasheed BA, Yuan W, Kos I, Batinic-Haberle I, Jones S, Riggins GJ, et al. 2009. *IDH1* and *IDH2* mutations in gliomas. *N Engl J Med* **360:** 765–773. doi:10.1056/NEJMoa0808710

Yang Y, Akada H, Nath D, Hutchison RE, Mohi G. 2016. Loss of Ezh2 cooperates with Jak2V617F in the development of myelofibrosis in a mouse model of myeloproliferative neoplasm. *Blood* **127:** 3410–3423. doi:10.1182/blood-2015-11-679431

Yoshida K, Sanada M, Shiraishi Y, Nowak D, Nagata Y, Yamamoto R, Sato Y, Sato-Otsubo A, Kon A, Nagasaki M, et al. 2011. Frequent pathway mutations of splicing machinery in myelodysplasia. *Nature* **478:** 64–69. doi:10.1038/nature10496

Young JI, Zuchner S, Wang G. 2015. Regulation of the epigenome by vitamin C. *Annu Rev Nutr* **35:** 545–564. doi:10.1146/annurev-nutr-071714-034228

Yu Y, Maggi LB Jr, Brady SN, Apicelli AJ, Dai MS, Lu H, Weber JD. 2006. Nucleophosmin is essential for ribosomal protein L5 nuclear export. *Mol Cell Biol* **26:** 3798–3809. doi:10.1128/MCB.26.10.3798-3809.2006

Zhang J, Kong G, Rajagopalan A, Lu L, Song J, Hussaini M, Zhang X, Ranheim EA, Liu Y, Wang J, et al. 2017. $p53^{-/-}$ synergizes with enhanced *Nras*^{G12D} signaling to transform megakaryocyte-erythroid progenitors in acute myeloid leukemia. *Blood* **129:** 358–370. doi:10.1182/blood-2016-06-719237

Zhao Z, Zuber J, Diaz-Flores E, Lintault L, Kogan SC, Shannon K, Lowe SW. 2010. p53 loss promotes acute myeloid leukemia by enabling aberrant self-renewal. *Genes Dev* **24:** 1389–1402. doi:10.1101/gad.1940710

Zheng H, Xie W. 2019. The role of 3D genome organization in development and cell differentiation. *Nat Rev Mol Cell Biol* **20:** 535–550. doi:10.1038/s41580-019-0132-4

Zorko NA, Bernot KM, Whitman SP, Siebenaler RF, Ahmed EH, Marcucci GG, Yanes DA, McConnell KK, Mao C, Kalu C, et al. 2012. *Mll* partial tandem duplication and *Flt3* internal tandem duplication in a double knock-in mouse recapitulates features of counterpart human acute myeloid leukemias. *Blood* **120:** 1130–1136. doi:10.1182/blood-2012-03-415067

Zuber J, Radtke I, Pardee TS, Zhao Z, Rappaport AR, Luo W, McCurrach ME, Yang MM, Dolan ME, Kogan SC, et al. 2009. Mouse models of human AML accurately predict chemotherapy response. *Genes Dev* **23:** 877–889. doi:10.1101/gad.1771409

Mouse Models in the Study of Mature B-Cell Malignancies

Laura Pasqualucci[1] **and Ulf Klein**[2]

[1]Department of Pathology & Cell Biology, Institute for Cancer Genetics, and the Herbert Irving Comprehensive Cancer Center, Columbia University, New York, New York 10032, USA

[2]Division of Haematology & Immunology, Leeds Institute of Medical Research at St. James's, University of Leeds, Leeds LS9 7TF, United Kingdom

Correspondence: lp171@cumc.columbia.edu

Over the past two decades, genomic analyses of several B-cell lymphoma entities have identified a large number of genes that are recurrently mutated, suggesting that their aberrant function promotes lymphomagenesis. For many of those genes, the specific role in normal B-cell development is unknown; moreover, whether and how their deregulated activity contributes to lymphoma initiation and/or maintenance is often difficult to determine. Genetically engineered mouse models that faithfully mimic lymphoma-associated genetic alterations represent valuable tools for elucidating the pathogenic roles of candidate oncogenes and tumor suppressors in vivo, as well as for the preclinical testing of novel therapeutic principles in an intact microenvironment. Here we summarize what has been learned about the mechanisms of oncogenic transformation from accurately modeling the most common and well-characterized genetic alterations identified in mature B-cell malignancies. This information is expected to guide the design of improved molecular diagnostics and mechanism-based therapeutic approaches for these diseases.

B-cell lymphomas comprise a heterogeneous group of neoplasms that originate from the oncogenic transformation of cells at various stages of mature B-cell development and, in the vast majority of cases, from germinal center (GC) B cells (Stevenson et al. 1998; Küppers et al. 1999; Swerdlow et al. 2016). A common theme that emerged from decades of studies aimed at the identification of lymphoma-associated genetic alterations is the recurrent involvement of genes that play critical regulatory roles at specific B-cell developmental stages, resulting in their aberrant expression or function and strongly implicating a mechanistic role for these proteins in lymphoma pathogenesis (Shaffer et al. 2012; Pasqualucci 2019). However, the molecular mechanisms by which these alterations contribute to lymphoma initiation and progression are often difficult to investigate, because suitable in vitro model systems that mimic the biological complexity of antigen-dependent B-cell development, and in particular the GC reaction, are lacking. The mouse is a versatile model organism for studying

Cite this article as *Cold Spring Harb Perspect Med* doi: 10.1101/cshperspect.a034827

higher vertebrates, because its immune system has the sophistication of the human counterpart and mouse embryonic stem cells are amenable to directed genetic manipulation, allowing to mimic the structural aberrations identified in cancer. As such, genetically engineered mouse models (GEMMs) have been a mainstay of cancer biology in the effort to determine the pathogenic roles of candidate oncogenes and tumor suppressors in vivo. Additionally, the availability of accurate animal models provides a valuable opportunity for preclinical studies aimed at evaluating the expanding armamentarium of molecularly targeted drugs. Of course, a number of caveats must be considered when approaching these studies, such as potential species-specific biological differences in the target cell of the oncogenic transformation process. Nevertheless, modeling lymphoma-associated genetic lesions in mice has offered critical insights into the mechanisms underlying the tumorigenic process and will continue to be a powerful filter for the nomination of potential cancer drivers among the numerous novel candidates uncovered by recent genome-sequencing studies. This review provides an examination of the advances obtained from the faithful modeling of lymphoma-associated genetic lesions in transgenic mice, as related to the molecular pathogenesis of the most common B lymphoid neoplasms: mantle cell lymphoma (MCL), Burkitt lymphoma (BL), follicular lymphoma (FL), diffuse large B-cell lymphoma (DLBCL), and chronic lymphocytic leukemia/small lymphocytic lymphoma (CLL/SLL). Emphasis will be placed on GEMMs that were proven to accurately recapitulate the human disease both genetically and phenotypically. We refer to other reviews for an in-depth discussion of alternative in vivo experimental systems that could serve as a more rapid approach to enable gain- and loss-of-function studies or the preclinical testing of novel therapeutic concepts, including the adoptive transfer of genetically modified hematopoietic progenitor cells (HPCs) (Oricchio et al. 2010) and patient-derived tumor xenograft mouse models (Townsend et al. 2016; Pizzi and Inghirami 2017).

MATURE B-CELL DEVELOPMENT

During normal B-cell development, three B-cell lineages with specific biological functions can be distinguished in higher vertebrates: $CD5^+$ B cells, marginal zone B cells, and follicular (naive) B cells. B cells expressing the CD5 antigen predominate early in life, although they continue to be generated throughout ontogeny (Baumgarth 2017). They produce polyreactive antibodies against common bacterial pathogens and provide a first line of defense against invading microorganisms. Marginal zone B cells are located at the entry site of blood-borne pathogens in the spleen, where they quickly respond to antigenic challenge by secreting antibodies that clear the pathogen (Lopes-Carvalho and Kearney 2004). Finally, in T-cell-dependent, adaptive immune responses, naive B cells undergo antibody maturation to exogenous antigens, which ultimately results in the generation of plasma cells capable of secreting high-affinity antibodies against the invading pathogen, as well as of memory B cells that quickly respond in recall responses against the same antigen (Rajewsky 1996). A key step in this process is the recruitment of naive B cells into the GC reaction following antigen encounter and guidance provided by antigen-specific T cells (Fig. 1; Victora and Nussenzweig 2012; De Silva and Klein 2015; Mesin et al. 2016; Bannard and Cyster 2017). Within the GC microenvironment, B cells first differentiate into centroblasts or dark zone (DZ) B cells. These cells proliferate at a high rate and modify their rearranged immunoglobulin variable (*IgV*) region genes through the process of activation-induced cytidine deaminase (AID)-mediated somatic hypermutation (SHM) to generate antibody specificities with improved affinity to the pathogen. Centroblasts then move to a different area within the GC, known as the light zone (LZ), where they cease proliferating and differentiate into centrocytes or LZ B cells before being selected for improved antigen binding with the help of T-follicular helper (Tfh) cells. GC B cells that are not rescued by Tfh cells because the newly introduced somatic mutations led to a decrease in affinity or disrupted the antibody structure are destined to undergo

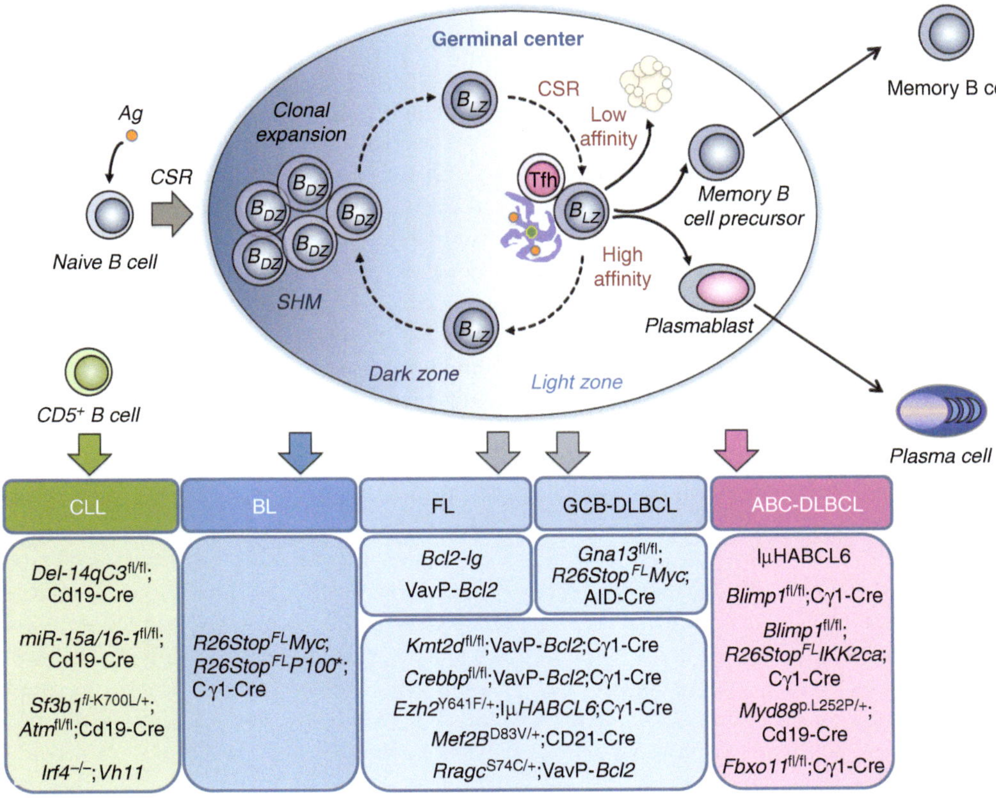

Figure 1. Presumed cellular origin of common mature B-cell malignancies for which bona fide genetically engineered mouse models (GEMMs) are available. Relationship between distinct types of B-cell neoplasms and their presumed normal counterpart, as determined based on phenotypic and genetic similarities. The major B-cell developmental steps following antigen encounter are indicated, along with $CD5^+$ mature B cells. Only GEMMs are shown that were obtained by recapitulating genetic changes observed in the human disease and that develop tumors featuring key characteristics of the corresponding human lymphoma entity. See text for details. B_{DZ}, dark zone B cells; B_{LZ}, light zone B cells; Tfh, T-follicular helper cell; CLL, chronic lymphocytic leukemia; BL, Burkitt lymphoma; FL, follicular lymphoma; GCB-DLBCL, germinal center B-cell-like diffuse large B-cell lymphoma; ABC-DLBCL, activated B-cell-like diffuse large B-cell lymphoma.

apoptosis. Positively selected LZ B cells can recycle to the DZ to undergo further rounds of SHM and selection and eventually differentiate into plasma cells or memory B cells, which constitute the immunological memory in the antibody system (Fig. 1). The GC LZ was also thought to represent the site where B cells undergo class switch recombination (CSR), a second AID-dependent B-cell-specific DNA-modification process that leads to the generation of antibodies with different effector functions but identical specificities; however, recent work provided compelling evidence that this reaction takes place predominantly prior to the GC reaction and to SHM (Roco et al. 2019). Of note, single-cell analysis of gene expression and somatically mutated *IgV* region genes in human GC B cells revealed a continuum of transcriptional changes as cells bidirectionally recirculate between the DZ and LZ compartment (Milpied et al. 2018).

CELLULAR COUNTERPARTS OF B-CELL LYMPHOMAS

A correct understanding of the putative normal counterpart of distinct lymphoid neoplasms is critical for the construction of faithful mouse models of the disease, because the genetic lesion of interest should be targeted to the proper cellular context both temporally and spatially (Fig. 1).

As an irreversible marker of transit through the GC, the determination of the *IgV* region gene SHM status, in combination with morphological and immunophenotypic analysis of normal and malignant B cells, has long provided information on the putative normal cellular counterparts of various lymphoma types (Stevenson et al. 1998; Küppers et al. 1999). The advent of genome-wide gene expression profiling technologies furthered these notions, allowing a more refined assignment of diverse lymphoma entities to their presumptive normal counterpart, as well as the identification of functionally relevant disease subtypes (Shaffer et al. 2006; Klein and Dalla-Favera 2008).

Early studies established that, with the exception of most MCL cases, the majority of B-cell lymphoid malignancies, including BL, FL, DLBCL, Hodgkin lymphoma, and possibly marginal zone lymphoma (not covered here), derive from a GC-experienced B cell, as evidenced by the expression of somatically hypermutated *IgV* region genes (Stevenson et al. 1998; Küppers et al. 1999). The cellular origin of CLL/SLL, where two major subtypes can be recognized based on the presence or absence of mutations in the *IgV* region genes, has long remained elusive and is in part still being debated (Chiorazzi and Ferrarini 2011). Nonetheless, multiple lines of evidence, including a shared gene expression profile, suggest that both CLL subtypes derive from antigen-experienced B cells (Klein et al. 2001; Rosenwald et al. 2001; Kipps et al. 2017). Of note, transcriptomic analysis has drawn a possible relationship with a mature CD5-expressing B-cell subpopulation in adults that comprises ~1% of peripheral blood B cells, expresses the CD27 memory B cell marker, and displays both mutated and unmutated *IgV* region genes (Seifert et al. 2012).

MCL cases can be distinguished by a gene and epigenetic signature that identifies conventional and leukemic nonnodal MCL, with the latter showing a more favorable outcome (Puente et al. 2018). The cellular counterpart of conventional MCL, the most common form, appears to be a naive B cell with no or few somatic mutations in its *IgV* region genes, whereas the nonnodal MCL type shows memory B-cell-like features (Clot et al. 2018).

In the case of DLBCL, at least two distinct phenotypic subtypes have been recognized based on their similarity to GC B cells (the so-called GCB-DLBCL) or in vitro activated B cells (ABC-DLBCL), with ~20% of cases remaining unclassified (Alizadeh et al. 2000). Although further subdivision within this heterogeneous disease has been revealed by genetic profiling (Chapuy et al. 2018; Schmitz et al. 2018), the historic classification into GCB-DLBCL and ABC-DLBCL has proved fundamental in the recognition of distinct normal cellular counterparts for these two tumor types. More recently, the identification of cell surface markers that distinguish DZ and LZ GC B cells —namely, CXCR4 on DZ B cells and CD86 on LZ B cells—allowed the definition of comprehensive gene expression signatures for these subpopulations (Victora et al. 2010) and a more precise assignment of BL, FL, and DLBCL to putative normal cellular counterparts (Victora et al. 2012). Perhaps surprisingly, whereas BL shows a gene expression profile that is closely related to DZ B cells, FL and GCB-DLBCL are transcriptionally more similar to LZ B cells, possibly representing an intermediate GC B-cell stage (Victora et al. 2012). The ABC-DLBCL, on the other hand, may correspond in vivo to a small subset of LZ B cells poised to undergo differentiation into plasma cells and could also include, as recently suggested, cases with similarities to memory B cells (unpublished observations) or to extrafollicular marginal zone B cells (Chapuy et al. 2018; Schmitz et al. 2018).

Although many models have been generated for the overexpression or deletion of oncogenes and tumor-suppressor genes (Ramezani-Rad and Rickert 2017), some of the strategies would not recapitulate genetic alterations found in the human disease or the exact timing of the genetic lesion, which may impact on the interpretation of the results. A major advance in this regard came from the use of Cre transgenes that can be expressed at various B-cell differentiation stages through developmentally controlled promoters, allowing them to specifically and inducibly activate or inactivate the gene of interest in the desired cell type. Thus, the crossing of floxed alleles to mb1-Cre (Hobeika et al. 2006), CD19-Cre (Rickert et al. 1997), and CD21-Cre mice (Kraus et al. 2004) allows gene recombination in B cells at a particular early B-cell developmental phase, throughout their development, or specifically in mature B cells, respectively. Cγ1-Cre and AID-Cre mouse strains are used to induce gene recombination specifically in antigen-activated B cells, including GC B cells (Casola et al. 2006; Crouch et al. 2007). Figure 2 illustrates the strategies utilized for the generation of mouse models discussed in this review.

MANTLE CELL LYMPHOMA

MCL represents 5% of all lymphoma diagnoses and comprises two recognized biological entities: an aggressive subtype characterized by unmutated or minimally mutated *IgV* region genes (conventional MCL) and a more indolent subtype that carries *IgV* mutations and is frequently leukemic (nonnodal MCL) (Jares et al. 2012; Swerdlow et al. 2016; Puente et al. 2018). The genetic hallmark of both diseases is the t(11;14) translocation that juxtaposes the *CCND1* gene (formerly known as *BCL1*), encoding for the cell-cycle regulatory protein cyclin D1 and normally not detected in resting B cells, to enhancer sequences in the *Ig* locus, leading to its constitutive expression and to loss of cell-cycle control (Jares et al. 2012).

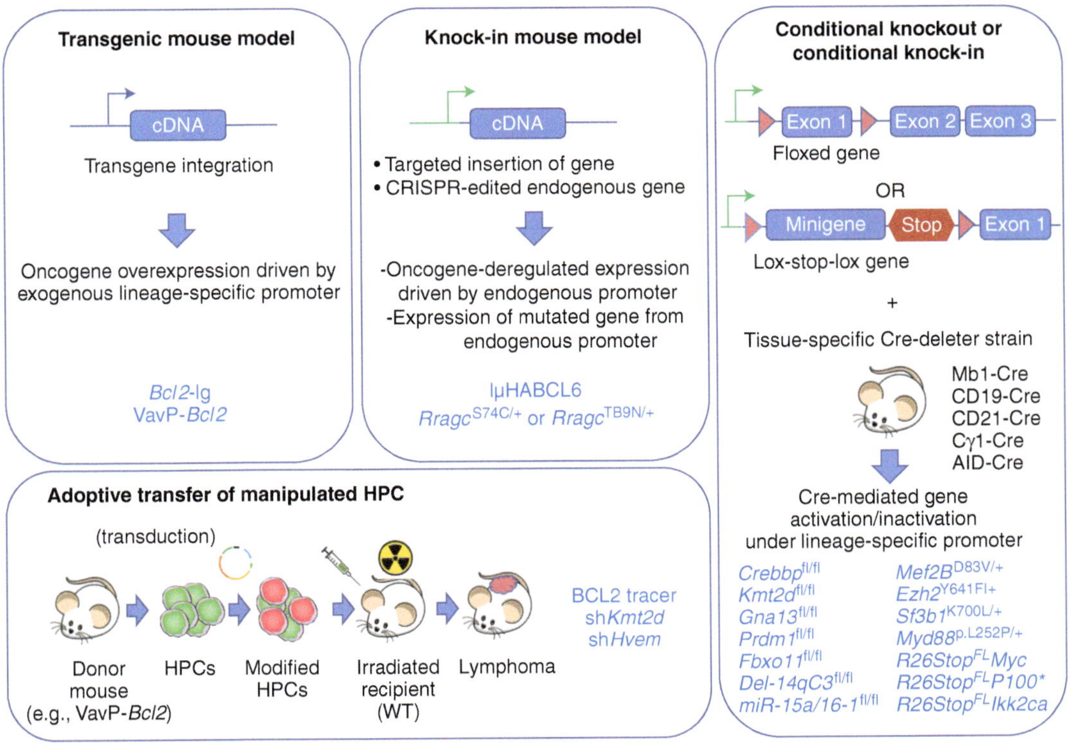

Figure 2. Strategies used for the generation of genetically engineered mouse models (GEMMs) of B-cell malignancies. Simplified schematic representation of the targeting alleles and experimental strategies used to reconstruct genetic alterations associated with human B-cell lymphomas in GEMMs (alone or in combination with additional oncogenes). The adoptive transfer approach is also illustrated as a tool to introduce conditional or inducible genetically manipulated alleles. See text for details. Only representative mouse models are listed (see Table 1 for a full list).

Table 1. Genetically engineered mouse models (GEMMs) of mature B-cell malignancies

Gene	Disease	Mutation type	Mouse model	Approach	Target cell	Phenotype	Reference(s)
Myc/PI3K	BL	Deregulated expression + gain-of-function mutation	*R26Stop*^{FL}*Myc;R26Stop*^{FL}*P100**; Cγ1- Cre	Conditional KI	GC B cells	BL	Sander et al. 2012
Bcl2	FL, GCB-DLBCL	Deregulated expression	VavP-*Bcl2*	Transgene insertion	HPC	FL	Egle et al. 2004
			Bcl2-Ig	Transgene insertion	B cells	FL	McDonnell et al. 1989
			BCL2^{trac}	TI/adoptive transfer	B cells	FL	Sungalee et al. 2014
Kmt2d[c]	FL, DLBCL	Genetic deletion	*Kmt2d*$^{fl/fl}$;VavP-*Bcl2*;Cγ1-Cre	Conditional KO	GC B cells	FL, DLBCL	Zhang et al. 2015
			Kmt2d$^{fl/fl}$;VavP-*Bcl2*;Cd19-Cre	Conditional KO	B cells	FL, DLBCL	Zhang et al. 2015
Crebbp[c]	FL, DLBCL	Genetic deletion	*Crebbp*$^{fl/+}$;VavP-*Bcl2*;Cγ1-Cre	Conditional KO	GC B cells	FL	Zhang et al. 2017
			Crebbp$^{fl/fl}$;VavP-*Bcl2*;Cd19-Cre	Conditional KO	B cells	FL	Zhang et al. 2017
			Crebbp$^{fl/fl}$;Eμ-*Bcl2*; Mb1-Cre	Conditional KO	Early B cells	FL, DLBCL	García Ramírez et al. 2017
Ezh2[c]	FL, GCB-DLBCL	Gain-of-function mutation	*Ezh2*$^{Y641F/+}$;*IμHABCL6*;Cγ1-Cre	cKI/adoptive transfer	GC B cells	DLBCL	Béguelin et al. 2016
			Ezh2$^{Y641F/N}$;VavP-Bcl2	Adoptive transfer	GC B cells	FL, DLBCL	Béguelin et al. 2013; Ennishi et al. 2019b
Mef2b	FL, DLBCL	Gain-of-function mutation	*Mef2b*$^{D83V/+}$;CD21-Cre	Conditional KI	GC B cells[a]	FL, DLBCL	Brescia et al. 2018
			Mef2b$^{D83V/+}$;*BCL2*-Ig;CD21-Cre	Conditional KI	GC B cells[a]	FL, DLBCL	Brescia et al. 2018
Rragc	FL	Gain-of-function mutation	*Rragc*$^{S74C/+}$ or *Rragc*$^{T89N/+}$; VavP-*Bcl2*	TI/adoptive transfer	All cells	FL	Ortega-Molina et al. 2019
Gna13	GCB-DLBCL, BL	Genetic deletion	*Gna13*$^{fl/fl}$;Mb1-Cre	cKO/adoptive transfer	GC B cells[b]	GC BCL	Muppidi et al. 2014
			Gna13$^{fl/fl}$;*R26Stop*^{FL}Myc;AID-Cre	Conditional KO	GC B cells	GC BCL	Healy et al. 2016
Bcl6	DLBCL	Deregulated expression	IμHABCL6	KI	GC B cells	DLBCL	Cattoretti et al. 2009

Prdm1	ABC-DLBCL	Genetic deletion	*Blimp1*$^{fl/fl}$;Cγ1-Cre	Conditional KO	GC B cells	DLBCL	Mandelbaum et al. 2010
			Blimp1$^{fl/fl}$;*R26Stop*^{FL}*Ikk2ca*; Cγ1-Cre	Conditional KO	GC B cells	DLBCL	Calado et al. 2010
Myd88	ABC-DLBCL	Gain-of-function mutation	*Myd88*$^{p.L252P/+}$;Cd19-Cre	Conditional KI	B cells	LPD, DLBCL	Knittel et al. 2016
Tet2	FL, GCB-DLBCL	Genetic deletion	*Tet2*$^{fl/fl}$;Vav-Cre	Conditional KO	HPC	BCL	Dominguez et al. 2018
			Tet2$^{fl/fl}$;IμHABCL6;Cγ1-Cre	cKO/adoptive transfer	GC B cells	BCL	Dominguez et al. 2018
miR-15a/16-1	CLL	Genetic deletion	*mir-15a/16-1*$^{fl/fl}$;Cd19-Cre	Conditional KO	B cells	CLL (DLBCL)	Klein et al. 2010
			mir-15a/16-1$^{-/-}$	KO	All cells	CLL (DLBCL)	Klein et al. 2010
13q14-MDR	CLL	Genetic deletion	*13q14-MDR*$^{fl/fl}$;Cd19-Cre	Conditional KO	B cells	CLL (DLBCL)	Klein et al. 2010
			13q14-MDR$^{-/-}$	KO	All cells	CLL (DLBCL)	Klein et al. 2010
13q14-CDR	CLL	Genetic deletion	*13q14-CDR*$^{fl/fl}$;Cd19-Cre	Conditional KO	B cells	CLL (DLBCL)	Lia et al. 2012
			13q14-CDR$^{+/-}$	KO	All cells	CLL (DLBCL)	Lia et al. 2012
Sf3b1[d]	CLL	Gain-of-function mutation	*Sf3b1K700L/+;Atm*$^{fl/fl}$;Cd19-Cre	Conditional KI	B cells	CLL	Yin et al. 2019
Irf4[d]	CLL	Genetic deletion	*Irf4*$^{-/-}$;*Vh11*	KO	All cells	CLL	Shukla et al. 2013

Listed are only GEMMs obtained by reconstructing genetic lesions associated with human B-cell malignancies and recapitulating key characteristics of the disease. See text for mouse models generated by adoptive transfer of transduced HPCs.

BL, Burkitt lymphoma; FL, follicular lymphoma; BCL, B-cell lymphoma; GCB-DLBCL, germinal center B-cell-like diffuse large B-cell lymphoma; ABC-DLBCL, BCL, B cell lymphoma activated B-cell-like diffuse large B-cell lymphoma; CLL, chronic lymphocytic lymphoma; KI, knock-in; KO, knockout; cKI, conditional knock-in; cKO, conditional knockout; TI, targeted insertion; GC, germinal center; HPC, hematopoietic progenitor cell.

[a]Cre-mediated recombination in mature B cells, but the endogenous promoter is activated in GC B cells.

[b]Cre-mediated recombination in all B cells, but the endogenous promoter is activated or up-regulated in GC B cells.

[c]GC-derived lymphomas observed only in cooperation with *Bcl2* deregulated expression.

[d]Lymphomagenesis observed only in cooperation with *Atm* deletion (*Sf3b1*) or *Vh11* (*Irf4*).

The pathogenic role of cyclin D1 deregulation in human neoplasia is supported by the ability of the overexpressed protein to accelerate B-cell lymphomagenesis in transgenic mice, when combined with other oncogenic events such as *MYC* deregulation (Bodrug et al. 1994; Lovec et al. 1994). However, the type of lymphomas produced in Eμ^{CycD1}/Eμ-*Myc* double transgenic mice resembles that found in Eμ-*Myc* mice (i.e., mainly pre-B-cell lymphomas; see next section). Moreover, MYC overexpression and/or rearrangement is rare in MCL, occurring only in the blastoid variant. Lymphomas with the classic morphologic and phenotypic (CD5^{+}CD23^{-}) appearance of the human conventional MCL were obtained by combining cyclin D1 overexpression with homozygous loss of the pro-apoptotic gene *Bim1* in Eμ^{CycD1}/CD19^{Cre}/*Bim1*$^{fl/fl}$ mice, although at very low frequencies unless challenged with serial antigenic stimulation (Katz et al. 2014). Finally, transgenic mice with a nuclear export-deficient CCND1 (D1/T286A mice) developed lymphomas by 18 mo of age with 50% penetrance, but these tumors were derived from early mature B cells, according to their IgM^{hi}IgD^{lo} immunophenotype (Gladden et al. 2006). Thus, an animal model for bona fide MCL is still lacking.

A blastoid variant of MCL has been described that frequently harbors deletions of p16^{INK4a}, an inhibitor of the cyclin-dependent kinase CDK4, and displays overexpression of both CDK4 and MYC (Beà et al. 1999). Crossing a knock-in strain that carries a mutant CDK4 protein resistant to inhibition by p16^{INK4a} with *Myc* transgenic mice (*Cdk4*^{R24C}/*Myc-3′RR* mice) leads to lymphomas that phenotypically resemble human blastoid MCL (Truffinet et al. 2007; Vincent-Fabert et al. 2012). Interestingly, a distinctive feature of these tumors is the accumulation of high amounts of CCND1/CDK4 complexes, even though this mouse model does not carry a *Ccnd1* transgene. Thus, although not recapitulating the precise genetic aberrations observed in human MCL, this system was useful in ascertaining the tumor-promoting role of genes known to be involved in MCL pathogenesis.

Recent exome-sequencing studies have provided a comprehensive picture of the coding mutations found in this lymphoma type, identifying additional candidate genes with potential roles in MCL pathogenesis (Beà et al. 2013). It is expected that such improved knowledge will lead to the development of murine MCL models more closely resembling the human disease.

BURKITT LYMPHOMA

BL, an aggressive B-cell lymphoma, is invariably associated with chromosomal translocations that bring the *MYC* gene under the control of one of the *Ig* enhancers, causing its ectopic expression in the bulk GC population in which this protein is otherwise not present (Calado et al. 2012; Dominguez-Sola et al. 2012). *MYC* translocations are found in all three clinical variants recognized within this entity by the WHO classification: (1) endemic BL (eBL), which occurs in equatorial areas (sub-Saharan Africa and South America) and is frequently associated with endemic malaria; (2) sporadic BL (sBL), which occurs elsewhere; and (3) immunodeficiency-associated BL, which most commonly occurs in HIV-positive individuals developing acquired immune deficiency syndrome (AIDS-BL). Another characteristic of BL is the frequent association with Epstein–Barr virus (EBV). The morphological features and the expression of somatically mutated *IgV* region genes in all BL cases have long identified a GC B cell as the normal cellular counterpart of this disease (Stevenson et al. 1998; Küppers et al. 1999). Moreover, the evidence of ongoing SHM in at least a fraction of cases indicated a cellular origin from DZ B cells/centroblasts that are actively undergoing SHM; this notion found support in the observation that the transcriptional profile of BL is closely related to the GC DZ signature (Victora et al. 2012). Recent whole-exome sequencing (WES) studies identified additional recurrently targeted genes in this lymphoma, including *TCF3*, which encodes the transcription factor E2A and harbors gain-of-function mutations in 10%–25% of cases, and *ID3*, a negative regulator of E2F that is typically affected by inactivating mutations in 35%–58% of all BL subtypes (Love et al. 2012; Richter et al. 2012; Schmitz et al. 2012). The TCF3-ID3 axis is predicted to promote tonic

 Cite this article as *Cold Spring Harb Perspect Med* doi: 10.1101/cshperspect.a034827

B-cell receptor (BCR) signaling, leading to the aberrant activation of the phosphoinositide-3-kinase (PI3K) signaling pathway, which is normally not active in DZ B cells. Moreover, a subset of eBL cases shows gain-of-function mutations of *CCND3*, a D-type cyclin required for GC formation and the proliferation of DZ B cells (Peled et al. 2010; Cato et al. 2011; Richter et al. 2012; Schmitz et al. 2012). Finally, the FOXO1 transcription factor is a frequent target of missense mutations, many of which cluster around the known T24 phosphorylation site (12% of cases) (Schmitz et al. 2012). Studies in transfected cell lines have shown that mutations in *FOXO1* prevent its cytoplasmic translocation and functional inactivation, which is the physiological consequence of PI3K signaling (Trinh et al. 2013). However, a mechanistic basis for the aberrant nuclear localization of FOXO1, observed in virtually all BL cases independent of genetic alterations, is presently lacking.

Because of the identification of *MYC* as the first translocated proto-oncogene in B-cell lymphomas, several transgenic mouse models were generated in the 1980s to 2000s (Adams et al. 1985; Bützler et al. 1997; Kovalchuk et al. 2000). In these mice, the expression of *MYC* transgenes was controlled by intronic heavy chain and light chain enhancers, which are active from the early stages of B-cell development but are not linked to the translocated *MYC* allele in most sporadic BLs. These mouse models all develop clonal B-cell proliferations at high penetrance, with some differences in their spectrum among the various strains, but generally unrelated to the normal counterpart of the human tumors and devoid of its pathognomonic phenotypic characteristics. For example, Eμ-*Myc* transgenic mice develop predominantly pre-B-cell lymphomas/leukemias that lack surface *Ig* expression (Adams et al. 1985; Harris et al. 1988). Lymphomas arising in λ*MYC* transgenic mice are of mature B-cell origin (IgM^+), but retain the CD43 marker and do not express somatically mutated *IgV* region genes (Kovalchuk et al. 2000), indicating that the target cell of transformation in these tumors is a transitional/pre-GC B cell rather than a GC DZ B cell. Analogous phenotypes were reported when different *Ig* enhancers were utilized to drive MYC overexpression throughout B-cell development (Park et al. 2005; Wang and Boxer 2005). As such, these mouse models have been fundamental for mechanistic studies aimed at investigating the pathogenic role of MYC in the transformation process or the cooperativity among oncogenes and the sensitivity to drugs (Hemann et al. 2003; Pasqualucci et al. 2008; Varano et al. 2017; Ravà et al. 2018). However, these models do not faithfully recapitulate key phenotypic and genetic features of human BL—or DLBCL, in which *MYC* can also be deregulated by chromosomal translocations (Chong et al. 2018)—and are not considered informative toward the dissection of the MYC oncogenic function in the pathogenesis of these cancers nor in the understanding of the cellular networks that are perturbed within the unique GC environment to license lymphomagenesis when MYC is ectopically expressed.

The generation of a BL-like lymphoma in mice was achieved by crossing two separate inducible transgenes that lead to MYC overexpression specifically in GC B cells, along with a mutant *P110** allele mimicking a constitutively active form of PI3K (Sander et al. 2012). Tumors developing in these mice closely resemble the human BL in its typical morphologic and histologic features, gene expression profile (including the expression of BCL6), and the acquisition of tertiary transforming events, such as mutations in *CCND3*. Together, the shared phenotypic and genetic features between human BLs and the BL-like tumors modeled in these mice identify the *Myc/P110** animal model as a valuable system for both mechanistic and preclinical studies. Moreover, tumors developing in this strain were instrumental in identifying a pro-proliferative and anti-apoptotic function of FOXO1 in the transformation of GC B cells toward BL (Kabrani et al. 2018).

FOLLICULAR LYMPHOMA

FL, the second most common type of B-cell lymphoma and the most frequent indolent lymphoma, is an incurable malignancy characterized by a continuous pattern of remissions and relapses that are accompanied by progressively reduced response to therapy and, in as many as 40% of cases, histologic transformation to a more aggressive disease (typically a DLBCL, or transformed FL [tFL]) (Lossos and Gascoyne 2011; Casulo et al. 2015). The genetic hallmark of FL is the t(14;18) translocation, a by-product of the VDJ recombination process that places the *BCL2* coding domain under the control of the *Ig* heavy chain enhancer, leading to ectopic and constitutive expression of the antiapoptotic protein BCL2 (Kridel et al. 2012). More recently, WES efforts have uncovered highly recurrent somatic mutations in several genes encoding for histone-modifying enzymes, such as the KMT2D methyltransferase (70% of cases), the CREBBP acetyltransferase (65% of cases), and the EZH2 methyltransferase (22% of cases), as well as multiple linker-histone family members (>44% of cases), pointing to altered epigenetic regulation as a central driving force of this malignancy (Morin et al. 2010, 2011; Pasqualucci et al. 2011; Li et al. 2014; Okosun et al. 2014). Other prevalent alterations that have been successfully modeled in the mouse include gain-of-function mutations of *MEF2B* (15% of cases) (Ying et al. 2013), loss-of-function biallelic mutations and deletions of the *TNFRSF14* gene (up to 40% of cases) (Cheung et al. 2010; Okosun et al. 2014), and point mutations of the *RRAGC* gene that, along with other genes involved in the activation of the mammalian target of rapamycin complex 1 (mTORC1) signaling, accounts for 17% of cases (Okosun et al. 2016). Of note, mutations in histone/chromatin modification genes, *MEF2B*, and *TNFRSF14* are highly frequent in both FL and DLBCL and should thus be considered reflective of both diseases. However, we discuss them in this section because of their higher prevalence in FL compared to DLBCL and the preferential development of FL-like diseases in these models.

Mouse Models Recapitulating the *BCL2* Translocation

Although several GEMMs have been generated to study the consequences of deregulated *BCL2* expression dictated by the t(14;18) translocation, only two of them were shown to develop FL-like tumors within their lifespan, indicating that the translocation alone is insufficient to drive full malignant transformation, and that additional events are required: the VavP-*Bcl2* and the *BCL2*-Ig mouse model (McDonnell et al. 1989; McDonnell and Korsmeyer 1991; Egle et al. 2004). Eμ-*BCL2* mice exhibit an expanded small B-lymphocyte population with no spontaneous tumor formation (Strasser et al. 1991); however, they have been useful to document the cooperativity between candidate oncogenic events (García-Ramírez et al. 2017). An additional mouse model (the mosaic *BCL2* tracer) is limited to the development of in situ FL, but it is worth mentioning here because it elegantly recapitulates the initial events underpinning the accumulation and expansion of *BCL2*-translocated B cells (Sungalee et al. 2014), which can be found in >50% of healthy subjects, even though most of these individuals will never develop the disease (Roulland et al. 2006).

In the VavP-*Bcl2* mouse model, the *Vav* promoter drives expression of the *BCL2* oncogene specifically in the hematopoietic compartment, hence at a stage prior to the occurrence of the *BCL2* translocation (Ogilvy et al. 1999); nonetheless, these mice develop B-cell lymphomas that accurately recapitulate critical aspects of the genetics, pathology, and GC origin of human FLs, including a follicular pattern, the expression of peanut agglutinin and BCL6 in the absence of post-GC markers, and the presence of clonally rearranged *IgV* region genes that are somatically mutated (Egle et al. 2004). These tumors require the presence of T cells, which also overexpress the *BCL2* transgene, because the GC hyperplasia could be abolished by antibodies directed against CD4 in vivo. Owing to its close resemblance to the human disease, the VavP-*Bcl2* model has been extensively used as an experimental system to assess the cooperative activity of genetic alterations that are concomitantly mutated with *BCL2* translocations, either by crossing this line with other GEMMs (e.g., $Crebbp^{fl/fl}$, $Kmt2d^{fl/fl}$, $Ezh2^{Y641N}$) or as a source of HPCs that can be transplanted into irradiated mice after retroviral transduction with constructs for gain- and loss-of-function mutants (Oricchio et al. 2014).

Different from VavP-*Bcl2* mice, expression of a *BCL2* minigene in the *BCL2*-Ig mouse model is controlled by *Ig* regulatory elements and is thus restricted to B cells (McDonnell et al. 1989). Similar to Eμ-*BCL2* mice, this strain displays an excess of B-lineage cells (both small B cells and plasma cells) exhibiting prolonged survival in vitro and, although no tumors were detected upon 12-mo follow-up in the original studies, was later shown to accumulate GC B cells and to develop PAX5$^+$BCL6$^+$ FLs in as many as 40% of cases when challenged by chronic antigenic stimulation, with a smaller fraction of mice presenting PAX5$^-$BCL6$^-$IRF4$^+$ plasmacytoid tumors (Brescia et al. 2018).

In the *BCL2* tracer mouse model, expression of a functional human *BCL2* transgene is contingent on its inversion by the V(D)J recombination process after adoptive transfer of progenitor cells into irradiated recipient wild-type mice (Fig. 2; Sungalee et al. 2014). This model mimics several aspects of FL pathogenesis as currently understood, including the sporadic nature of the t(14;18) and its induction at the appropriate developmental stage—that is, a BM pro-/pre-B cell, as a by-product of VDJ recombination (Küppers and Dalla-Favera 2001). Moreover, tracking of the BCL2-overexpressing B cells is possible in these mice by means of the unique coding joint generated by the recombination, together with the presence of an EYFP reporter and the use of specific antibodies against the human BCL2 protein. Investigation of the T-cell-dependent immune response in this model revealed that BCL2-overexpressing B cells require multiple GC reentries before disseminating and progressing to advanced preneoplastic stages of FL, analogous to the human FL in situ. In particular, although the fraction of BCL2$^+$ cells in the naive, GC, and memory B-cell compartment was not significantly different upon a single immunization, these cells were markedly enriched in the GC and memory B-cell subset following chronic antigenic recall and were able to repopulate the GCs of immunized wild-type mice in adoptive transfer experiments (Sungalee et al. 2014). Combined with the observation that t(14;18)-positive cells in healthy individuals harbor somatically mutated *IgV* region genes, these data formed the basis for the current model of FL ontogenesis, which infers an origin from a recirculating memory B cell requiring multiple transits through the GC before the acquisition of additional genetic or epigenetic disturbances would ultimately drive the development of clonal tumors.

Mouse Models Recapitulating Alterations in Histone Modification Genes

Mutations in epigenetic modification genes emerged as the most common genetic event in both FL and DLBCL, collectively accounting for almost all FL cases and >50% of DLBCL cases, and revealing a significant role for epigenetic remodeling in B-cell malignancies. One important observation made from the analysis of sequential FL and tFL biopsies was that inactivating mutations of *CREBBP* and *KMT2D* represent early events in the tumor evolutionary history, which are acquired by a common mutated precursor cell (CPC) before its divergent evolution and ultimate clonal expansion to FL or tFL in the GC (Okosun et al. 2014; Pasqualucci et al. 2014; Green et al. 2015). The precise cell differentiation stage at which *KMT2D* and *CREBBP* mutations are gained is not known and could be anywhere between a hematopoietic stem cell (HSC) and the GC B cell. Therefore, attempts to reproduce the hemizygous or homozygous genetic loss of these two enzymes were made in HSCs (Horton et al. 2017), early B cells (via a CD19-Cre recombinase) (Ortega-Molina et al. 2015; Zhang et al. 2015b, 2017), and GC B cells (via the Cγ1-Cre recombinase) (Zhang et al. 2015b, 2017).

KMT2D is a catalytic component of the mammalian COMPASS (complex of proteins associated with Set1) complex that facilitates transcription through mono- and dimethylation of histone 3 lysine 4 (H3K4) at enhancer/super-enhancer regions (Sze and Shilatifard 2016). Based on its mutational spectrum that comprises mostly truncating events, KMT2D is postulated to play a central role in suppressing the lymphomagenesis process. Interestingly, conditional deletion of *Kmt2d* in pre-B cells, that is, much earlier than the final malignant transformation step, led to a significant expansion of the GC B-cell subpopulation compared to wild-type littermates, whereas the phenotype was less pronounced when *Kmt2d* was disrupted after the initiation of the GC reaction (Zhang et al. 2015b). Analogously, GC B cells from CD19-Cre compound mice showed more robust changes in their transcriptional profile compared to cells in which deletion of *Kmt2d* was induced in the GC (Zhang et al. 2015b). These data suggest that the timing and thus the number of cell divisions completed by the cell following KMT2D inactivation may be important in allowing the epigenetic reprogramming of the CPC. This in turn may contribute to tumor formation by creating a favorable environment for the acquisition of additional genetic or epigenetic oncogenic events, including the impaired expression of terminal differentiation programs. In line with this model, loss of *Kmt2d* alone in the GC was not sufficient to drive lymphomagenesis, but when combined with deregulated expression of *BCL2* (as commonly seen in human FL and DLBCL) led to a significant increase in the percentage of bona fide FL and DLBCL carrying clonally rearranged, mutated *IgV* region genes and expressing GC-specific markers (Zhang et al. 2015b). The synergistic effect of *Kmt2d* loss and BCL2 deregulation in vivo was independently confirmed in a mouse model of adoptive transfer in which Kmt2d was silenced in VavP-*Bcl2* HPCs prior to the reconstitution of lethally irradiated, syngeneic mice (Ortega-Molina et al. 2015).

Intriguingly, the *Kmt2d*-KO mouse model shares several similarities with conditional *Crebbp*-deficient mice, as exemplified by (i) an expanded GC population with an altered DZ:LZ ratio and partially overlapping transcriptional changes; (ii) a more prominent GC phenotype in CD19-Cre compared to Cγ1-Cre mice; and (iii) the inability to induce tumor formation as a single event, but a strong synergism with BCL2 deregulation in driving FL or, at lower frequencies, DLBCL (Zhang et al. 2017). CREBBP is a histone and non-histone acetyltransferase that modulates transcription by depositing the active H3K27 acetylation mark at promoter and enhancer domains of numerous genes, and was found to occupy virtually all GC-specific super-enhancers. However, not all CREBBP-bound genes are transcriptionally affected by its loss in purified murine GC B cells, as well as DLBCL cell lines (Jiang et al. 2017; Zhang et al. 2017), in part because of the compensatory activity of its paralog EP300 (Meyer et al. 2019). Instead, *Crebbp* deletion causes focal enhancer loss of H3K27Ac and reduced expression of genes that are involved in the exit from the GC reaction (Jiang et al. 2017; Zhang et al. 2017). These include downstream effectors of the BCR and NF-κB signaling pathways, several cytokines, and a number of antigen presentation molecules, the most notable being MHC class II genes (Jiang et al. 2017; Zhang et al. 2017). Indeed, decreased MHC-II expression with reduced frequency of tumor-infiltrating T-cell subsets is a distinctive feature of *CREBBP*-mutated human FL (Green et al. 2015). Notably, the chromatin domains occupied by CREBBP are direct targets of the BCL6 oncorepressor in a complex with SMRT and HDAC3 (Jiang et al. 2017; Zhang et al. 2017); furthermore, CREBBP can directly acetylate the BCL6 protein to inactivate its function by preventing the interaction with co-repressor complexes (Bereshchenko et al. 2002; Pasqualucci et al. 2011). Thus, a major purpose of CREBBP in the GC is to oppose the oncogenic activity of BCL6 and prime the activation of terminal differentiation/antigen presentation programs as LZ B cells engage Tfh cells and prepare to exit the GC. In line with these data, *CREBBP*-mutant lymphomas show reduced expression of genes that are antagonistically regulated by the BCL6-SMRT-HDAC3 complex and become dependent on HDAC3, inhibition of which restored histone acetylation at these enhancers and suppressed lymphoma growth both in vitro and in vivo (Jiang et al. 2017; Mondello et al. 2020). The identification of HDAC3 and EP300 as vulnerabilities of *CREBBP*-mutant cells suggests potential therapeutic avenues for these lymphomas.

EZH2 is a histone methyltransferase that is highly expressed in GC B cells and is required for GC formation (Béguelin et al. 2013; Caganova et al. 2013). EZH2 sustains the GC reaction in part by catalyzing the addition of the repressive H3K27me3 mark at genes that control proliferation (e.g., *CDKN1A*, *CDKN1B*) and plasma cell differentiation (e.g., *IRF4*, *PRDM1*) to create bivalent promoters that can then be rapidly reactivated when cells exit the GC (Béguelin et al. 2013). To study the biological consequences of the hotspot gain-of-function mutations Y641F and Y641N, two mouse models have been generated in which activation of the mutant allele can be directed to the GC following the excision of a lox-stop-lox cassette by the Cγ1-Cre recombinase: a conditional *Ezh2*^{Y641F} knock-in driven by the endogenous *Ezh2* promoter (Béguelin et al. 2016) and a transgenic *Ezh2*^{Y641N} allele controlled by the *ColA1* promoter (Béguelin et al. 2013). In both, expression of mutant *Ezh2* caused massive GC hyperplasia after immunization, which was sustained by enhanced proliferation and blockade of terminal differentiation, and required the functional cooperation between EZH2 and the BCL6/BCOR repressor complex (Béguelin et al. 2013). This phenotype is also consistent with the detection of abundant H3K27me3 levels at the promoter of EZH2 target genes in the GC B cells from these animals, analogous to *EZH2*-mutant DLBCL cell lines and human tumors. Although *Ezh2* mutant mice do not develop B-cell lymphomas, the adoptive transfer of VavP-*Bcl2* bone marrow cells transduced with *Ezh2*^{Y641F} vectors were associated with accelerated lymphomagenesis (Béguelin et al. 2013; Ennishi et al. 2019a). Additionally, *EZH2* mutation cooperates with deregulated BCL6 expression to yield a transplantable GC-derived DLBCL-like disease that can be used for syngeneic immune studies (Béguelin et al. 2016; Mondello et al. 2020). Of therapeutic interest, tumors developing in the above models display significantly lower cell surface levels of both MHC-I and MHC-II, which are accompanied by an immune-"cold" environment with reduced T-cell infiltrate and could be rescued by treatment with EZH2 inhibitors (Ennishi et al. 2019a).

Truncating mutations of *TET2*, the most common event in age-associated clonal hematopoiesis (Busque et al. 2012) and a genetic hallmark of myeloid neoplasms (Moran-Crusio et al. 2011), are also detected in 3%–10% of FL/tFL (Pasqualucci et al. 2014) and 6%–12% of DLBCL (Reddy et al. 2017; Chapuy et al. 2018; Schmitz et al. 2018). To study the in vivo role of these alterations in lymphomagenesis, murine strains were engineered to model the loss of *Tet2* in HSCs or at later stages of B-cell development (Dominguez et al. 2018). Interestingly, *Tet2* deficiency facilitated the expansion of GC B cells in Vav-Cre and CD19-Cre conditional KO mice, but not when *Tet2* was deleted in the GC. These abnormal cells do not evolve into clonal DLBCL; however, effacement of the splenic architecture due to enlarged follicles or diffuse lymphoid infiltrates was observed when GC-specific *Tet2* deletion was combined with *BCL6* deregulation, even though the molecular features of these tumors, which are negative for several mature B-cell markers (CD23, CD21, IgM, IgD), require further characterization. This work also revealed a link between TET2 and CREBBP in orchestrating the GC exit transcriptional program through the activation of enhancer domains.

Collectively, the above studies illustrate a partially overlapping mechanism by which mutations in epigenetic modifiers can reprogram the epigenome of the precursor cancer cell at specific gene sets to enable malignant transformation, in cooperation with *BCL2* deregulation, and establish a link between epigenetic dysregulation and immune escape that could be exploited for therapeutic intervention.

Modeling *TNFRSF14* Loss

The GC microenvironment provides essential signals for the survival and differentiation of normal B cells and is postulated to play a particularly important role during FL development, as immune and stromal cells create a permissive niche to support the malignant B-cell population (Scott and Gascoyne 2014; Lamaison and Tarte 2019). The *TNFRSF14* gene, encoding the HVEM receptor, is one of the most frequently mutated genes in FL and GCB-DLBCL. The contribution of its genetic loss to lymphomagenesis was studied by using an shRNA-knockdown strategy in the VavP-*Bcl2* HPC adoptive transfer system (Boice et al. 2016). Although the developmental stage of the Hvem knockdown may not recapitulate the sequence of transforming events occurring in the human tumors, only a minority of CD4$^+$ and CD8$^+$ T cells were found to express the *shHvem* hairpin, whereas *shHvem*-expressing B-lymphoma cells were significantly enriched. Hvem knockdown caused marked B-cell expansion and accelerated the development of BCL2-driven FL. Mechanistically, this model was critical in demonstrating a dual role for HVEM loss during malignant transformation, which depends on its ability to (1) directly stimulate BCR signaling and B-cell proliferation, a cell-autonomous and BTLA-dependent effect exemplified by the activation of several molecules related to the BCR pathway such as SYK, BTK, BLNK, and their downstream targets ERK and IκB; and (2) induce a tumor-supportive microenvironment through the increased production of TNF-family cytokines that act as stroma-activating factors. The latter is consistent with the observation of an aberrant lymphoid stroma activation in FL that is more prominent in both murine and human *TNFRSF14*-deficient tumors. Moreover, this study offered new therapeutic perspectives for this group of tumors by showing that the administration of the soluble HVEM ectodomain protein could restore tumor suppression.

Modeling Missense *RRAGC* Mutations

The *RRAGC* gene encodes the RagC GTPase, an activator of a nutrient-sensing pathway that drives cellular anabolism (Efeyan et al. 2015). RagC forms a heterodimeric complex together with RagA that activates mTORC1 upon ample nutrient availability, leading to cell growth. To mimic the most common FL-associated *RRAGC* mutations in the mouse germline, the CRISPR–Cas9 genome engineering technology was employed. This study revealed that *Rragc*-mutant B cells show a partial insensitivity to nutrient withdrawal, which led to accelerated FL tumorigenesis on a VavP-*Bcl2*-transgenic background (Ortega-Molina et al. 2019). Mechanistically, RagC-mutant cells were found to exhibit suppression of apoptosis and a decreased requirement on microenvironmental signals provided by Tfh cells, which control the GC reaction. These data are consistent with a model in which *RRAGC* mutations increase GC B-cell fitness by inducing activation of the mTORC1 pathway; because of their competitive advantage over unmutated GC B cells, these mutant premalignant GC B cells continue to undergo cycles of selection and proliferation in the GC, which in turn could facilitate the acquisition of additional genetic alterations, ultimately transforming into a bone fide FL.

Modeling MEF2B-Activating Mutations

The MEF2B transcription factor is specifically expressed at high levels in GC B cells, where it controls the activity of a broad transcriptional network of relevance to the physiology of the GC reaction and also including the GC master regulator BCL6 (Ying et al. 2013). This function is perturbed in ~15% of FL and DLBCL because of gain-of-function mutations that can be broadly categorized into two groups: (1) amino acid substitutions in the protein amino-terminal portion, encoding for the DNA-binding domain—these mutations prevent its physical interaction to components of the HUCA complex as well as to several class IIa HDACs, all of which normally serve as negative modulators of MEF2B activity; and (2) truncating mutations in the carboxy-terminal portion of the MEF2B protein, which are postulated to interfere with negative regulatory mechanisms of its activity mediated by post-translational modifications (e.g., sumoylation), although a comprehensive characterization of this second group of alterations is still lacking (Morin et al. 2011; Ying et al. 2013). Because MEF2B transcription is specifically induced in the initial stages of GC B-cell commitment, and thus slightly earlier than Cγ1-promoter activation, a conditional knock-in mouse model for the most common D83V missense mutation was engineered using the CD21-Cre deleter strain (Brescia et al. 2018). Compared to control littermates, *Mef2b*$^{+/D83V}$; CD21-Cre mice responded to polyclonal antigenic stimulation with a significant increase in GC B cells (a phenotype also observed upon Cγ1-Cre-mediated activation of the mutant allele), which evolved over time toward clonal FL or DLBCL in ~20% of cases. This phenotype becomes fully penetrant when combined with *BCL2* deregulation in the *BCL2*-Ig mice, thus establishing MEF2B as a fundamental player in the physiologic GC reaction and a driver oncogene in lymphomagenesis.

DIFFUSE LARGE B-CELL LYMPHOMA

The most common B-cell lymphoma in the Western world, DLBCL represents a heterogeneous disease comprising phenotypically and molecularly distinct entities that are associated with distinct clinical outcome and up to five genetic subsets defined based on co-occurring mutational events (Chapuy et al. 2018; Schmitz et al. 2018). Many of the genetic alterations that segregate with GCB-DLBCL, and particularly with its genetic subtype EZB (for EZH2-BCL2) or Cluster 3, are shared with FL. Indeed, as summarized in the previous section, GEMMs for these alterations develop a spectrum of lymphoproliferative disorders ranging from in situ FL to overt DLBCL. Additional DLBCL-associated genetic lesions that have been successfully and faithfully reconstructed in the mouse include those targeting *BCL6, GNA13,* and several genes implicated in the pathogenesis of ABC-DLBCL such as *MYD88*, *PRDM1*, and components of the NF-κB pathway.

Deregulation of BCL6 Expression

As the master regulator of the GC reaction, BCL6 is expressed at high levels in GC-derived lymphoid malignancies, including FL and GCB-DLBCL, and also represents a biological dependency in these tumors, which require its activity for their proliferation and survival (Basso and Dalla-Favera 2010; Valls et al. 2017). The first in vivo model recapitulating the genetics and therefore the biology of DLBCL was obtained by engineering a knock-in allele in which expression of an HA-tagged BCL6 cassette is driven by the endogenous immunoglobulin Iμ promoter, thus mimicking a common chromosomal translocation in human DLBCL and FL (Cattoretti et al. 2009). The broader activity of the juxtaposed *Ig* promoter/enhancer sequences, which extends beyond the GC stage, disrupts the normally restricted pattern of BCL6 expression, allowing the escape from multiple negative modulatory signals that normally induce its down-regulation at the GC exit (Cattoretti et al. 2009; Basso and Dalla-Favera 2010). The translocation may also provide marginal zone B cells, which normally lack BCL6 expression, with ectopic access to its proto-oncogenic activity. This scenario is supported by the observation that BCL6 translocations are particularly enriched in a subset of ABC-DLBCL that belongs to the BN2(BCL6-Notch2) or Cluster 1 genetic subgroup, for which a marginal zone B-cell origin has been postulated (Chapuy et al. 2018; Schmitz et al. 2018).

Independent of whether caused by chromosomal translocations or simply reflecting the origin from a GC B cell, the net effect of BCL6 continuous expression is the aberrant maintenance of multiple biological programs that are normally orchestrated by BCL6 to sustain the specialized function of the GC, including the negative regulation of anti-apoptotic and DNA damage responses, plasma cell differentiation, and a variety of receptor signaling pathways (Ci et al. 2009; Basso et al. 2010). Blocked in this environment, B cells continue to be exposed to potentially deleterious events, exemplified by the high proliferative rate, replication stress, and the DNA breaks associated with SHM and CSR. Consistently, IμHABCL6 mice display massive GC hyperplasia with an increased DZ:LZ ratio, even in the absence of antigenic stimulation (Cattoretti et al. 2005). The oncogenic link between *BCL6*-deregulated expression and lymphomagenesis was conclusively proven by the evidence that Iμ*HABCL6* mice develop an array of lymphoproliferative diseases (LPDs) culminating in overt DLBCL in 40%–60% of cases and displaying evidence of AID-dependent aberrant SHM as well as Myc-IgH translocations (Cattoretti et al. 2005; Pasqualucci et al. 2008). Moreover, deregulated BCL6 expression led to a shift in the phenotype of λMYC-driven lymphomas reflecting their origin from GC-experienced cells and the requirement of AID (Pasqualucci et al. 2008).

Disruption of the Gα13 Signaling Pathway

Unlike most lymphocytes, GC B cells are strictly confined to the GC microenvironment. What prevents the exit of GC B cells into circulation is an inhibitory circuit that entails the engagement of G-protein-coupled receptors S1PR2 and P2RY8 by S1P ligands (Green and Cyster 2012). Inhibitory signals emanating from these receptors are transmitted via two G-proteins abundantly transcribed in GC B cells—namely, Gα12 and Gα13—to the effector molecule ARHGEF1, which ultimately acts by suppressing both AKT and cell migration (Green and Cyster 2012). In almost one-quarter of DLBCL, as well as in BL, the Gα13 pathway is disrupted by deleterious mutations affecting the genes *GNA13* and more rarely *S1P2R* and *ARHGEF1* (Muppidi et al. 2014). The *GNA13*-deficient state of GC B cells was modeled in the mouse by either crossing a *Gna13* conditional knockout allele with an AID-Cre transgenic strain (Healy et al. 2016) or utilizing a mixed bone marrow chimera approach (*Gna13*$^{fl/fl}$;Mb1-Cre) (Muppidi et al. 2014). In both systems, Gα13-deficient mice manifested increased numbers of GC B cells in the context of a disordered GC architecture with altered DZ/LZ distribution, increased *IgV* SHM activity, and abnormal B-cell migration behavior. The persistence of GC B cells that display impaired caspase-mediated cell death led to an increased risk of lymphoma development, as documented by the insurgence in a subset of cases of massive mesenteric lymphoadenopathies of GC origin. Clonal B-cell lymphomas reproducing morphologic, phenotypic, and genetic characteristics of the human DLBCL were also detected in 50% of mice deficient for *S1PR2*, supporting the critical role of this pathway as a lymphoma tumor suppressor (Cattoretti et al. 2009). Interestingly, deficiency of Gα13 but not of S1PR2 led to systemic dissemination in the lymph and blood, suggesting the existence of additional G-protein-coupled receptors associated with the regulation of GC confinement and prompting the discovery of P2RY8, which is also mutated in some DLBCL (Muppidi et al. 2014). These studies were instrumental in elucidating the mechanism by which *GNA13*-deficient GC B cells can exit the GC niche to spread systemically and demonstrated a tumor-suppressor function for the Gα13 signaling pathway through its dual effect in the control of B-cell positioning and AKT activation.

Deletion of *FBXO11*

F-box protein 11 (FBXO11) is a member of the F-box protein family that functions as the substrate-recognition subunit of SKP1-cullin-1-F-box-protein (SCF) E3 ligase complexes, leading to ubiquitylation and degradation of target proteins (Skaar et al. 2013). Of direct relevance to lymphoma, the BCL6 master regulator and the BLIMP1 protein were both identified as FBXO11 substrates. Indeed, monoallelic mutations and/or deletions of the *FBXO11* gene, detected in 6% of human DLBCLs, were shown to result in increased BCL6 levels, suggesting a contributing role during DLBCL pathogenesis (Duan et al. 2012). A conditional, GC-specific knockout mouse model was constructed by flanking the gene exon 4 with *loxP* sites, recombination of which results in a translational reading frameshift with production of a truncated FBXO11 protein (Schneider et al. 2016). *Fbxo11*$^{fl/fl}$;Cγ1-Cre mice display enlarged GCs with significantly increased BCL6 protein levels and reduced ability to enter the plasmablastic differentiation pathway, resembling the phenotype observed in mice with constitutive BCL6 expression or *Prdm1* deletion. Aged, chronically immunized mice develop various B-cell lymphoproliferative phenotypes ranging from expanded lymphoid follicles through LPDs disrupting the lymphoid architecture to overt DLBCL, although at very low frequency. Such low tumor penetrance implies that additional alterations are required to drive full transformation, together with *FBXO11* inactivation. Nonetheless, this model confirmed a tumor-suppressor role for *FBXO11* in lymphomagenesis, which is linked at least in part to altered BCL6 protein stability, even though multiple proteins are likely to be recognized as substrates of FBXO11-mediated degradation, in addition to BCL6 and BLIMP1.

 Cite this article as *Cold Spring Harb Perspect Med* doi: 10.1101/cshperspect.a034827

Biallelic Loss of *PRDM1/BLIMP1*

A distinctive feature of ABC-DLBCL is the presence of structural alterations that lead to genetic or epigenetic inactivation of the master plasma cell regulator BLIMP1 (also known as PRDM1), with 20% of cases carrying biallelic disruptive mutations and/or focal deletions of the *BLIMP1* locus, and an additional subset of tumors showing mutually exclusive transcriptional silencing by deregulated *BCL6* (Pasqualucci et al. 2006; Tam et al. 2006). When engineered in the mouse, conditional B-cell-specific deletion of *Blimp1* (*Blimp1*$^{fl/fl}$;CD19-Cre and *Blimp1*$^{fl/fl}$;Cγ1-Cre) induced a block in plasma cell differentiation and the development of DLBCLs recapitulating the molecular footprint of the human ABC-DLBCL (Mandelbaum et al. 2010). As in other lymphoma models, the long latency and the clonality of DLBCLs in *Blimp1* conditional KO animals indicate that oncogenic events affecting other pathways collaborate with inactivation of this transcription factor to foster a full neoplastic phenotype. One important contributor to this process is the NF-κB transcriptional complex, which is constitutively active in virtually all ABC-DLBCLs and is targeted at multiple levels by genetic alterations in more than one-half of these cases (Compagno et al. 2009), frequently together with *BLIMP1* mutations (Shaffer et al. 2012). Accordingly, the DLBCLs that develop in *Blimp1* conditional KO mice display nuclear active NF-κB (Mandelbaum et al. 2010); moreover, a mouse model with combined disruption of *Blimp1* and enforced canonical NF-κB activation, obtained via a constitutively active IKK2 protein (*R26Stop*^{FL}*Ikk2ca*;Cγ1-Cre) that can be induced in GC B cells, showed enhanced GC responses and succumbed to clonal lymphoid tumors reminiscent of human ABC-DLBCL (Calado et al. 2010).

Constitutive Activation of the NF-κB Signaling Pathway

During normal GC responses, the canonical (RELA/p50 and c-REL/p50) and noncanonical (RELB/p52) NF-κB signaling pathways have been shown to play distinct roles (Heise et al. 2014; De Silva et al. 2016), which are hijacked by lymphoma cells for their own growth advantage. In most ABC-DLBCL cases, the activity of the canonical NF-κB transcription complex is sustained by the presence of genetic alterations affecting multiple genes that encode for positive or negative regulators of the BCR, CD40 receptor, and TLR signaling cascades (Lenz et al. 2008; Compagno et al. 2009; Davis et al. 2010; Ngo et al. 2011). Among these, the TLR adaptor protein MYD88 is mutated in >30% of patient samples (Ngo et al. 2011). Consistently, AID-Cre-, CD21-Cre-, or CD19-Cre-driven expression of a *Myd88*^{L252P} allele corresponding to the most common human activating mutation (L265P) promotes the occurrence of indolent LPDs and occasional tumors that share several traits with human ABC-DLBCL (Knittel et al. 2016). Of note, a synergistic cross talk was observed between this mutation and *CD79B* mutations in a murine adoptive transfer experiment, exemplified by the accumulation of autoreactive cells (Wang et al. 2017); this finding is interesting in view of the frequent co-occurrence of *CD79B* mutations and *MYD88*-L265P alleles in ABC-DLBCL cases and the reported role for self-antigens in the survival of ABC-DLBCL cells via chronic activation of their BCR-signaling pathway (Young et al. 2015).

In a smaller subset of DLBCL, the alternative (noncanonical) NF-κB signaling cascade is also activated, as documented by the nuclear translocation of p52 (Compagno et al. 2009). This can be explained in part by the presence of truncating mutations/deletions of the *TRAF3* gene, often coexisting with *BCL6* translocations. *TRAF3* encodes for a negative regulator of the pathway, involved in the degradation of the NF-κB inducing kinase NIK. Accordingly, enforced expression of NIK and BCL6 in the GC, as obtained by conditional mutagenesis in the IμHABcl6; *Nik*^{stopFL};Cγ1-Cre mouse model, caused GC hyperplasia with blockade of terminal differentiation and ultimately premature death in 100% of the animals, because of IRF4-positive DLBCL (Zhang et al. 2015a). Notably, *Nik*^{stopFL};Cγ1-Cre mice display overt plasma cell hyperplasia but do not succumb to tumors; thus, the oncogenic function of the alternative NF-κB pathway may require the concomitant disruption of terminal B-cell differentiation, which in this case was achieved by deregulated *BCL6* expression, and thus appears to be analogous to the synergistic phenotype observed in the compound *Blimp1*$^{fl/fl}$;*R26Stop*^{FL}*Ikk2ca*;Cγ1-Cre model (Calado et al. 2010).

CHRONIC LYMPHOCYTIC LYMPHOMA/ SMALL LYMPHOCYTIC LYMPHOMA

CLL/SLL is an indolent B-cell malignancy with the tumor cells characteristically expressing the CD5 and CD23 antigens (Kipps et al. 2017). Compared to other non-Hodgkin lymphomas, CLL shows a different spectrum of genetic alterations, which mostly comprise chromosomal deletions (*13q14*, *ATM*, and *TP53*) or amplifications (trisomy of chromosome 12). Next-generation sequencing analyses could identify additional recurrent mutations in CLL/SLL, most notably those that target the *NOTCH1*, *MYD88*, and the *SF3B1* genes (Fabbri and Dalla-Favera 2016). Additionally, genome-wide association studies identified a single-nucleotide polymorphism (SNP) in a noncoding region of *IRF4*, a major transcription factor involved in B-cell development (De Silva et al. 2012), as a susceptibility locus for CLL (Di Bernardo et al. 2008).

To date, several mouse models of CLL have been obtained by reconstructing the above mentioned somatic genetic aberrations or germline SNPs. Additionally, numerous strains exist that develop CLL-like diseases but have been produced by introducing genetic changes that are not observed in the human tumors or are activated at different developmental stages compared to the putative normal counterpart of CLL. Although we refer the reader to other reviews for a detailed description of these models (Pekarsky et al. 2007; Chen and Chiorazzi 2014; Simonetti et al. 2014), we mention here the Eμ-*TCL1* transgenic mice (Bichi et al. 2002) as they are widely used in the field to study the role of the microenvironment in the disease process as well as for preclinical studies, either alone or in combination with other alterations (Johnson et al. 2006; Simonetti et al. 2014). The Eμ-*TCL1* model, however, does not recapitulate the genetics and, thus, possibly the biology of this common cancer. This circumstance needs to be considered when interpreting the findings for the human disease, although the resemblance of the lymphoproliferations developing in these mice to the more aggressive form of CLL makes them an amenable model for *IgV* unmutated CLL with unfavorable outcome.

Deletion of chromosomal region *13q14* occurs in >50% of CLL cases and at a lower frequency also in other lymphoma subtypes (Liu et al. 1995). The *13q14* region is highly conserved in the mouse genome at chromosomal region *14qC3* and has been further mapped into two characteristically deleted regions. The so-called minimal deleted region (*MDR*) encompasses two microRNAs—namely, mir-15a/16-1—located within an intron of the *deleted in leukemia 2* (*DLEU2*) gene that encodes a long noncoding RNA; the mouse *13q14* region also includes the protein-coding *Dleu5* gene. The commonly deleted region (*CDR*), present in a sizable number of CLL/SLL cases, is larger and, besides the *MDR*, includes the protein-coding *DLEU7* and *RNASEH2B* genes in both humans and mice. Three transgenic mouse lines have been generated in which only *mir-15a/16-1*, the *MDR*, or the *CDR* were deleted in B cells (Klein et al. 2010; Lia et al. 2012). Deletion of the microRNAs alone caused the development of a CLL-like disease at low penetrance (~25%), demonstrating the tumor-suppressor role of mir-15a/16-1 in vivo, as proposed in part following the observation that (i) germline mutations interfering with their normal expression occurred in some CLL patients (Calin et al. 2002, 2005), and (ii) an NZB mouse strain with a germline mutation in the 3′ flanking region of pre-miR-16-1 results in decreased expression of the mature microRNA (Raveche et al. 2007). The additional deletions of *Dleu2* and *Dleu5* in *MDR* mice increased the disease penetrance and exacerbated the disease course. Of note, besides CD5$^+$ lymphoproliferations, also CD5$^-$ lymphomas were observed. *CDR*-deleted mice showed a different spectrum of lymphoproliferations compared with the other two lines, as they predominantly developed

CLL-like lymphoid neoplasms and a more aggressive disease course. It is not clear whether the target cell of malignant transformation is the same for CLL developing in mice and humans. One clear difference is that all $CD5^+$ lymphoproliferations developing in the transgenic lines express unmutated *IgV* region genes, whereas, in humans, *IgV* mutated cases comprise a considerable fraction of all CLL diagnoses. However, all three *14qC3* mouse models expressed stereotypic antigen receptors, a characteristic feature of human CLL (Kipps et al. 2017), which indicates a critical role of antigen in the expansion of the CLL clone. One may therefore conclude that, at least with regard to the *IgV* unmutated cases, a B-cell subset with similar biological functions is targeted in both humans and mice.

The SNP identified in human CLL has been associated with a down-regulation of IRF4 expression, suggesting an atypical tumor-suppressor role for *IRF4* in CLL development (Di Bernardo et al. 2008). This hypothesis has been investigated in a mouse model in which an antibody expressing a rearranged IgV region gene of the Vh11 family that is frequently expressed in $CD5^+$ B cells was knocked into the *Ig* locus and crossed onto an *IRF4*-deficient background. *Irf4*$^{-/-}$*Vh11* knock-in mice developed a CLL-like disease with complete penetrance (Shukla et al. 2013); a follow-up study reported elevated NOTCH2 expression and hyperactivation of NOTCH signaling as the underlying mechanism (Shukla et al. 2016). Because *Irf4*$^{-/-}$ mice have multiple immune deficiencies as a result of the critical roles of IRFs in a number of immune cell types, the determination of the extent to which IRF4 deficiency affects CLL development in a B-cell-intrinsic fashion would require B-cell-specific deletion of *Irf4* on the *Vh11* background. Such a model would allow us to investigate the proposed role of reduced IRF4 expression in promoting CLL development by altering the migration properties of B cells (Simonetti et al. 2013), as a direct consequence of elevated NOTCH2 activity (Shukla et al. 2016). A B-cell-intrinsic role of IRF4-deficiency in CLL development has recently been demonstrated via conditional *Irf4* knockout on the Eμ-*TCL1* background (Asslaber et al. 2019).

Mutations in the splicing factor *SF3B1* are found in 10% of CLL cases (Wang et al. 2011). To determine the functional consequences of the most commonly occurring *SF3B1* point mutation, K700E, a conditional *Sf3b1*-K700E knock-in allele, was created that allowed to express the mutated allele in a B-cell-specific fashion using CD19-Cre mice (Yin et al. 2019). Expression of the mutated SF3B1 protein led to an enlargement of the marginal zone, although the total number of B cells was reduced, possibly in relationship to the induction of cellular senescence. Indeed, these animals did not develop B-lymphoproliferations unless bred on a conditional *ataxia telangiectasia mutated* (*ATM*)-deficient background, to reproduce the frequent co-occurrence of *SF3B1* mutations with deletion of chromosomal region *11q*, encompassing the gene, in CLL (Wang et al. 2011; Yin et al. 2019). *Atm* deletion could overcome the SF3B1-K700E-induced cellular senescence and led to the development of a clonal CLL-like disease in about one-half of the animals by 24 mo of age. Phenotypically, the tumor cells resembled human CLL cells with regard to genome instability and the dysregulation of CLL-associated cellular processes. This included down-regulation of BCR signaling, which is also observed in human CLL cells with *SF3B1* mutations. Consistent with these observations, CLL cells were more susceptible to the BTK inhibitor ibrutinib, which acts downstream of the BCR. Together, this model demonstrates the practicability of modeling specific tumor-associated genetic alterations to gain insights into the disease-underlying pathogenic mechanisms and to uncover potential Achilles' heels for therapy.

CONCLUSIONS

The advantages and versatility offered by GEMMs have revolutionized the study of cancer biology and will continue to be an invaluable resource to obtain critical insights into the multifaceted pathogenic mechanisms that underlie B-cell malignancies. However, no single model is likely to reproduce the complexity of human cancer. Moreover, the accelerated discovery of new cancer genes and the multitude of genetic interactions that are implicated in the malignant transformation process, as emerged from large-scale genome sequencing studies, pose a significant challenge to the capacity of traditional GEMMs for providing rapid advances. Finally, the plethora of novel therapeutic agents and concepts that are being considered for preclinical testing, alone or in combination, warrants the need for more effective, high-throughput approaches to modeling cancer in a faithful manner. Tumor organoids, PDXs, and the advent of increasingly sophisticated technologies such as the CRISPR–Cas9 gene editing technique may help overcome some of these limits —for example, by improving the speed at which multiple genetic changes can be simultaneously studied and by reproducing the complex interactions between the microenvironment of the patient and the malignant cells. Further efforts will also be needed by the mouse-modeling community to reduce the costs of these studies and provide more uniform systems for translational interrogation. Understanding the strength and limitations of each model remains instrumental to maximally leverage these resources.

ACKNOWLEDGMENTS

We thank the many postdocs, technicians, and students whose work contributed to form the basis of this review in the Klein, Pasqualucci, and Dalla-Favera laboratories. We apologize to those colleagues whose studies could not be cited because of space constraints. This work was supported in part by National Institutes of Health (NIH)/National Cancer Institute (NCI) grants R01-CA172492 (to L.P.), R01-CA157660 and R21-CA175461 (to U.K.), a CLL Global Research Foundation award (U.K), and a Leukemia & Lymphoma Society Translational Research Project award (L.P.).

REFERENCES

Adams JM, Harris AW, Pinkert CA, Corcoran LM, Alexander WS, Cory S, Palmiter RD, Brinster RL. 1985. The c-*myc* oncogene driven by immunoglobulin enhancers induces lymphoid malignancy in transgenic mice. *Nature* **318:** 533–538. doi:10.1038/318533a0

Alizadeh AA, Eisen MB, Davis RE, Ma C, Lossos IS, Rosenwald A, Boldrick JC, Sabet H, Tran T, Yu X, et al. 2000. Distinct types of diffuse large B-cell lymphoma identified by gene expression profiling. *Nature* **403:** 503–511. doi:10.1038/35000501

Asslaber D, Qi Y, Maeding N, Steiner M, Denk U, Höpner JP, Hartmann TN, Zaborsky N, Greil R, Egle A. 2019. B-cell–specific IRF4 deletion accelerates chronic lymphocytic leukemia development by enhanced tumor immune evasion. *Blood* **134:** 1717–1729. doi:10.1182/blood.2019000973

Bannard O, Cyster JG. 2017. Germinal centers: Programmed for affinity maturation and antibody diversification. *Curr Opin Immunol* **45:** 21–30. doi:10.1016/j.coi.2016.12.004

Basso K, Dalla-Favera R. 2010. BCL6: Master regulator of the germinal center reaction and key oncogene in B cell lymphomagenesis. *Adv Immunol* **105:** 193–210. doi:10.1016/S0065-2776(10)05007-8

Basso K, Saito M, Sumazin P, Margolin AA, Wang K, Lim WK, Kitagawa Y, Schneider C, Alvarez MJ, Califano A, et al. 2010. Integrated biochemical and computational approach identifies BCL6 direct target genes controlling multiple pathways in normal germinal center B cells. *Blood* **115:** 975–984. doi:10.1182/blood-2009-06-227017

Baumgarth N. 2017. A hard(y) look at B-1 cell development and function. *J Immunol* **199:** 3387–3394. doi:10.4049/jimmunol.1700943

Beà S, Ribas M, Hernández JM, Bosch F, Pinyol M, Hernández L, García JL, Flores T, González M, López-Guillermo A, et al. 1999. Increased number of chromosomal imbalances and high-level DNA amplifications in mantle cell lymphoma are associated with blastoid variants. *Blood* **93:** 4365–4374.

Beà S, Valdés-Mas R, Navarro A, Salaverria I, Martín-Garcia D, Jares P, Giné E, Pinyol M, Royo C, Nadeu F, et al. 2013. Landscape of somatic mutations and clonal evolution in mantle cell lymphoma. *Proc Natl Acad Sci* **110:** 18250–18255. doi:10.1073/pnas.1314608110

Béguelin W, Popovic R, Teater M, Jiang Y, Bunting KL, Rosen M, Shen H, Yang SN, Wang L, Ezponda T, et al. 2013. EZH2 is required for germinal center formation and somatic EZH2 mutations promote lymphoid transformation. *Cancer Cell* **23:** 677–692. doi:10.1016/j.ccr.2013.04.011

Béguelin W, Teater M, Gearhart MD, Calvo Fernández MT, Goldstein RL, Cárdenas MG, Hatzi K, Rosen M, Shen H, Corcoran CM, et al. 2016. EZH2 and BCL6 cooperate to assemble CBX8-BCOR complex to repress bivalent promoters, mediate germinal center formation and lymphomagenesis. *Cancer Cell* **30:** 197–213. doi:10.1016/j.ccell.2016.07.006

Bereshchenko OR, Gu W, Dalla-Favera R. 2002. Acetylation inactivates the transcriptional repressor BCL6. *Nat Genet* **32:** 606–613. doi:10.1038/ng1018

Bichi R, Shinton SA, Martin ES, Koval A, Calin GA, Cesari R, Russo G, Hardy RR, Croce CM. 2002. Human chronic lymphocytic leukemia modeled in mouse by targeted TCL1 expression. *Proc Natl Acad Sci* **99:** 6955–6960. doi:10.1073/pnas.102181599

Bodrug SE, Warner BJ, Bath ML, Lindeman GJ, Harris AW, Adams JM. 1994. Cyclin D1 transgene impedes lymphocyte maturation and collaborates in lymphomagenesis with the *myc* gene. *EMBO J* **13:** 2124–2130. doi:10.1002/j.1460-2075.1994.tb06488.x

Boice M, Salloum D, Mourcin F, Sanghvi V, Amin R, Oricchio E, Jiang M, Mottok A, Denis-Lagache N, Ciriello G, et al. 2016. Loss of the HVEM tumor suppressor in lymphoma and restoration by modified CAR-T cells. *Cell* **167:** 405–418.e13. doi:10.1016/j.cell.2016.08.032

Brescia P, Schneider C, Holmes AB, Shen Q, Hussein S, Pasqualucci L, Basso K, Dalla-Favera R. 2018. MEF2B instructs germinal center development and acts as an oncogene in B cell lymphomagenesis. *Cancer Cell* **34:** 453–465.e9. doi:10.1016/j.ccell.2018.08.006

Busque L, Patel JP, Figueroa ME, Vasanthakumar A, Provost S, Hamilou Z, Mollica L, Li J, Viale A, Heguy A, et al. 2012. Recurrent somatic *TET2* mutations in normal elderly individuals with clonal hematopoiesis. *Nat Genet* **44:** 1179–1181. doi:10.1038/ng.2413

Bützler C, Zou X, Popov AV, Brüggemann M. 1997. Rapid induction of B-cell lymphomas in mice carrying a human IgH/c-*myc*YAC. *Oncogene* **14:** 1383–1388. doi:10.1038/sj.onc.1200968

Caganova M, Carrisi C, Varano G, Mainoldi F, Zanardi F, Germain PL, George L, Alberghini F, Ferrarini L, Talukder AK, et al. 2013. Germinal center dysregulation by histone methyltransferase EZH2 promotes lymphomagenesis. *J Clin Invest* **123:** 5009–5022. doi:10.1172/JCI70626

Calado DP, Zhang B, Srinivasan L, Sasaki Y, Seagal J, Unitt C, Rodig S, Kutok J, Tarakhovsky A, Schmidt-Supprian M, et al. 2010. Constitutive canonical NF-κB activation cooperates with disruption of *BLIMP1* in the pathogenesis of activated B cell-like diffuse large cell lymphoma. *Cancer Cell* **18:** 580–589. doi:10.1016/j.ccr.2010.11.024

Calado DP, Sasaki Y, Godinho SA, Pellerin A, Kochert K, Sleckman BP, de Alboran IM, Janz M, Rodig S, Rajewsky K. 2012. The cell-cycle regulator c-Myc is essential for the formation and maintenance of germinal centers. *Nat Immunol* **13:** 1092–1100. doi:10.1038/ni.2418

Calin GA, Dumitru CD, Shimizu M, Bichi R, Zupo S, Noch E, Aldler H, Rattan S, Keating M, Rai K, et al. 2002. Frequent deletions and down-regulation of micro- RNA genes *miR15* and *miR16* at 13q14 in chronic lymphocytic leukemia. *Proc Natl Acad Sci* **99:** 15524–15529. doi:10.1073/pnas.242606799

Calin GA, Ferracin M, Cimmino A, Di Leva G, Shimizu M, Wojcik SE, Iorio MV, Visone R, Sever NI, Fabbri M, et al. 2005. A microRNA signature associated with prognosis and progression in chronic lymphocytic leukemia. *N Engl J Med* **353:** 1793–1801. doi:10.1056/NEJMoa050995

Casola S, Cattoretti G, Uyttersprot N, Koralov SB, Seagal J, Hao Z, Waisman A, Egert A, Ghitza D, Rajewsky K. 2006. Tracking germinal center B cells expressing germ-line immunoglobulin gamma1 transcripts by conditional gene targeting. *Proc Natl Acad Sci* **103:** 7396–7401. doi:10.1073/pnas.0602353103

Casulo C, Burack WR, Friedberg JW. 2015. Transformed follicular non-Hodgkin lymphoma. *Blood* **125:** 40–47. doi:10.1182/blood-2014-04-516815

Cato MH, Chintalapati SK, Yau IW, Omori SA, Rickert RC. 2011. Cyclin D3 is selectively required for proliferative expansion of germinal center B cells. *Mol Cell Biol* **31:** 127–137. doi:10.1128/MCB.00650-10

Cattoretti G, Pasqualucci L, Ballon G, Tam W, Nandula SV, Shen Q, Mo T, Murty VV, Dalla-Favera R. 2005. Deregulated BCL6 expression recapitulates the pathogenesis of human diffuse large B cell lymphomas in mice. *Cancer Cell* **7:** 445–455. doi:10.1016/j.ccr.2005.03.037

Cattoretti G, Mandelbaum J, Lee N, Chaves AH, Mahler AM, Chadburn A, Dalla-Favera R, Pasqualucci L, MacLennan AJ. 2009. Targeted disruption of the $S1P_2$ sphingosine 1-phosphate receptor gene leads to diffuse large B-cell lymphoma formation. *Cancer Res* **69:** 8686–8692. doi:10.1158/0008-5472.CAN-09-1110

Chapuy B, Stewart C, Dunford AJ, Kim J, Kamburov A, Redd RA, Lawrence MS, Roemer MGM, Li AJ, Ziepert M, et al. 2018. Molecular subtypes of diffuse large B cell lymphoma are associated with distinct pathogenic mechanisms and outcomes. *Nat Med* **24:** 679–690. doi:10.1038/s41591-018-0016-8

Chen SS, Chiorazzi N. 2014. Murine genetically engineered and human xenograft models of chronic lymphocytic leukemia. *Semin Hematol* **51:** 188–205. doi:10.1053/j.seminhematol.2014.05.001

Cheung KJ, Johnson NA, Affleck JG, Severson T, Steidl C, Ben-Neriah S, Schein J, Morin RD, Moore R, Shah SP, et al. 2010. Acquired *TNFRSF14* mutations in follicular lymphoma are associated with worse prognosis. *Cancer Res* **70:** 9166–9174. doi:10.1158/0008-5472.CAN-10-2460

Chiorazzi N, Ferrarini M. 2011. Cellular origin(s) of chronic lymphocytic leukemia: Cautionary notes and additional considerations and possibilities. *Blood* **117:** 1781–1791. doi:10.1182/blood-2010-07-155663

Chong LC, Ben-Neriah S, Slack GW, Freeman C, Ennishi D, Mottok A, Collinge B, Abrisqueta P, Farinha P, Boyle M, et al. 2018. High-resolution architecture and partner genes of MYC rearrangements in lymphoma with DLBCL morphology. *Blood Adv* **2:** 2755–2765. doi:10.1182/bloodadvances.2018023572

Ci W, Polo JM, Cerchietti L, Shaknovich R, Wang L, Yang SN, Ye K, Farinha P, Horsman DE, Gascoyne RD, et al. 2009. The BCL6 transcriptional program features repression of multiple oncogenes in primary B cells and is deregulated in DLBCL. *Blood* **113:** 5536–5548. doi:10.1182/blood-2008-12-193037

Clot G, Jares P, Giné E, Navarro A, Royo C, Pinyol M, Martín-Garcia D, Demajo S, Espinet B, Salar A, et al. 2018. A gene signature that distinguishes conventional and leukemic nonnodal mantle cell lymphoma helps predict outcome. *Blood* **132:** 413–422. doi:10.1182/blood-2018-03-838136

Compagno M, Lim WK, Grunn A, Nandula SV, Brahmachary M, Shen Q, Bertoni F, Ponzoni M, Scandurra M, Califano A, et al. 2009. Mutations of multiple genes cause deregulation of NF-κB in diffuse large B-cell lymphoma. *Nature* **459:** 717–721. doi:10.1038/nature07968

Crouch EE, Li Z, Takizawa M, Fichtner-Feigl S, Gourzi P, Montaño C, Feigenbaum L, Wilson P, Janz S, Papavasiliou FN, et al. 2007. Regulation of AID expression in the immune response. *J Exp Med* **204:** 1145–1156. doi:10.1084/jem.20061952

Davis RE, Ngo VN, Lenz G, Tolar P, Young RM, Romesser PB, Kohlhammer H, Lamy L, Zhao H, Yang Y, et al. 2010. Chronic active B-cell-receptor signalling in diffuse large

B-cell lymphoma. *Nature* **463:** 88–92. doi:10.1038/nature08638

De Silva NS, Klein U. 2015. Dynamics of B cells in germinal centres. *Nat Rev Immunol* **15:** 137–148. doi:10.1038/nri3804

De Silva NS, Simonetti G, Heise N, Klein U. 2012. The diverse roles of IRF4 in late germinal center B-cell differentiation. *Immunol Rev* **247:** 73–92. doi:10.1111/j.1600-065X.2012.01113.x

De Silva NS, Anderson MM, Carette A, Silva K, Heise N, Bhagat G, Klein U. 2016. Transcription factors of the alternative NF-κB pathway are required for germinal center B-cell development. *Proc Natl Acad Sci* **113:** 9063–9068. doi:10.1073/pnas.1602728113

Di Bernardo MC, Crowther-Swanepoel D, Broderick P, Webb E, Sellick G, Wild R, Sullivan K, Vijayakrishnan J, Wang Y, Pittman AM, et al. 2008. A genome-wide association study identifies six susceptibility loci for chronic lymphocytic leukemia. *Nat Genet* **40:** 1204–1210. doi:10.1038/ng.219

Dominguez-Sola D, Victora GD, Ying CY, Phan RT, Saito M, Nussenzweig MC, Dalla-Favera R. 2012. The proto-oncogene MYC is required for selection in the germinal center and cyclic reentry. *Nat Immunol* **13:** 1083–1091. doi:10.1038/ni.2428

Dominguez PM, Ghamlouch H, Rosikiewicz W, Kumar P, Beguelin W, Fontan L, Rivas MA, Pawlikowska P, Armand M, Mouly E, et al. 2018. TET2 deficiency causes germinal center hyperplasia, impairs plasma cell differentiation, and promotes B-cell lymphomagenesis. *Cancer Discov* **8:** 1632–1653.

Duan S, Cermak L, Pagan JK, Rossi M, Martinengo C, di Celle PF, Chapuy B, Shipp M, Chiarle R, Pagano M. 2012. FBXO11 targets BCL6 for degradation and is inactivated in diffuse large B-cell lymphomas. *Nature* **481:** 90–93. doi:10.1038/nature10688

Efeyan A, Comb WC, Sabatini DM. 2015. Nutrient-sensing mechanisms and pathways. *Nature* **517:** 302–310. doi:10.1038/nature14190

Egle A, Harris AW, Bath ML, O'Reilly L, Cory S. 2004. VavP-Bcl2 transgenic mice develop follicular lymphoma preceded by germinal center hyperplasia. *Blood* **103:** 2276–2283. doi:10.1182/blood-2003-07-2469

Ennishi D, Jiang A, Boyle M, Collinge B, Grande BM, Ben-Neriah S, Rushton C, Tang J, Thomas N, Slack GW, et al. 2019a. Double-hit gene expression signature defines a distinct subgroup of germinal center B-cell-like diffuse large B-cell lymphoma. *J Clin Oncol* **37:** 190–201. doi:10.1200/JCO.18.01583

Ennishi D, Takata K, Béguelin W, Duns G, Mottok A, Farinha P, Bashashati A, Saberi S, Boyle M, Meissner B, et al. 2019b. Molecular and genetic characterization of MHC deficiency identifies EZH2 as therapeutic target for enhancing immune recognition. *Cancer Discov* **9:** 546–563. doi:10.1159/2159–8290

Fabbri G, Dalla-Favera R. 2016. The molecular pathogenesis of chronic lymphocytic leukaemia. *Nat Rev Cancer* **16:** 145–162. doi:10.1038/nrc.2016.8

García-Ramírez I, Tadros S, González-Herrero I, Martín-Lorenzo A, Rodríguez-Hernández G, Moore D, Ruiz-Roca L, Blanco O, Alonso-López D, Rivas JL, et al. 2017. *Crebbp* loss cooperates with *Bcl2* overexpression to promote lymphoma in mice. *Blood* **129:** 2645–2656. doi:10.1182/blood-2016-08-733469

Gladden AB, Woolery R, Aggarwal P, Wasik MA, Diehl JA. 2006. Expression of constitutively nuclear cyclin D1 in murine lymphocytes induces B-cell lymphoma. *Oncogene* **25:** 998–1007. doi:10.1038/sj.onc.1209147

Green JA, Cyster JG. 2012. S1PR2 links germinal center confinement and growth regulation. *Immunol Rev* **247:** 36–51. doi:10.1111/j.1600-065X.2012.01114.x

Green MR, Kihira S, Liu CL, Nair RV, Salari R, Gentles AJ, Irish J, Stehr H, Vicente-Duenas C, Romero-Camarero I, et al. 2015. Mutations in early follicular lymphoma progenitors are associated with suppressed antigen presentation. *Proc Natl Acad Sci* **112:** E1116–E1125. doi:10.1073/pnas.1501199112

Harris AW, Pinkert CA, Crawford M, Langdon WY, Brinster RL, Adams JM. 1988. The E μ-*myc* transgenic mouse. A model for high-incidence spontaneous lymphoma and leukemia of early B cells. *J Exp Med* **167:** 353–371. doi:10.1084/jem.167.2.353

Healy JA, Nugent A, Rempel RE, Moffitt AB, Davis NS, Jiang X, Shingleton JR, Zhang J, Love C, Datta J, et al. 2016. GNA13 loss in germinal center B cells leads to impaired apoptosis and promotes lymphoma in vivo. *Blood* **127:** 2723–2731. doi:10.1182/blood-2015-07-659938

Heise N, De Silva NS, Silva K, Carette A, Simonetti G, Pasparakis M, Klein U. 2014. Germinal center B cell maintenance and differentiation are controlled by distinct NF-κB transcription factor subunits. *J Exp Med* **211:** 2103–2118. doi:10.1084/jem.20132613

Hemann MT, Fridman JS, Zilfou JT, Hernando E, Paddison PJ, Cordon-Cardo C, Hannon GJ, Lowe SW. 2003. An epi-allelic series of p53 hypomorphs created by stable RNAi produces distinct tumor phenotypes in vivo. *Nat Genet* **33:** 396–400.

Hobeika E, Thiemann S, Storch B, Jumaa H, Nielsen PJ, Pelanda R, Reth M. 2006. Testing gene function early in the B cell lineage in mb1-cre mice. *Proc Natl Acad Sci* **103:** 13789–13794. doi:10.1073/pnas.0605944103

Horton SJ, Giotopoulos G, Yun H, Vohra S, Sheppard O, Bashford-Rogers R, Rashid M, Clipson A, Chan WI, Sasca D, et al. 2017. Early loss of *Crebbp* confers malignant stem cell properties on lymphoid progenitors. *Nat Cell Biol* **19:** 1093–1104. doi:10.1038/ncb3597

Jares P, Colomer D, Campo E. 2012. Molecular pathogenesis of mantle cell lymphoma. *J Clin Invest* **122:** 3416–3423. doi:10.1172/JCI61272

Jiang Y, Ortega-Molina A, Geng H, Ying HY, Hatzi K, Parsa S, McNally D, Wang L, Doane AS, Agirre X, et al. 2017. *CREBBP* inactivation promotes the development of HDAC3-dependent lymphomas. *Cancer Discov* **7:** 38–53. doi:10.1158/2159-8290.CD-16-0975

Johnson AJ, Lucas DM, Muthusamy N, Smith LL, Edwards RB, De Lay MD, Croce CM, Grever MR, Byrd JC. 2006. Characterization of the TCL-1 transgenic mouse as a preclinical drug development tool for human chronic lymphocytic leukemia. *Blood* **108:** 1334–1338. doi:10.1182/blood-2005-12-011213

Kabrani E, Chu VT, Tasouri E, Sommermann T, Baßler K, Ulas T, Zenz T, Bullinger L, Schultze JL, Rajewsky K, et al. 2018. Nuclear FOXO1 promotes lymphomagenesis in germinal center B cells. *Blood* **132:** 2670–2683. doi:10.1182/blood-2018-06-856203

Katz SG, Labelle JL, Meng H, Valeriano RP, Fisher JK, Sun H, Rodig SJ, Kleinstein SH, Walensky LD. 2014. Mantle cell lymphoma in cyclin D1 transgenic mice with Bim-deficient B cells. *Blood* **123:** 884–893. doi:10.1182/blood-2013-04-499079

Kipps TJ, Stevenson FK, Wu CJ, Croce CM, Packham G, Wierda WG, O'Brien S, Gribben J, Rai K. 2017. Chronic lymphocytic leukaemia. *Nat Rev Dis Primers* **3:** 17008. doi:10.1038/nrdp.2017.8

Klein U, Dalla-Favera R. 2008. Germinal centres: Role in B-cell physiology and malignancy. *Nat Rev Immunol* **8:** 22–33. doi:10.1038/nri2217

Klein U, Tu Y, Stolovitzky GA, Mattioli M, Cattoretti G, Husson H, Freedman A, Inghirami G, Cro L, Baldini L, et al. 2001. Gene expression profiling of B cell chronic lymphocytic leukemia reveals a homogeneous phenotype related to memory B cells. *J Exp Med* **194:** 1625–1638. doi:10.1084/jem.194.11.1625

Klein U, Lia M, Crespo M, Siegel R, Shen Q, Mo T, Ambesi-Impiombato A, Califano A, Migliazza A, Bhagat G, et al. 2010. The *DLEU2/miR-15a/16-1* cluster controls B cell proliferation and its deletion leads to chronic lymphocytic leukemia. *Cancer Cell* **17:** 28–40. doi:10.1016/j.ccr.2009.11.019

Knittel G, Liedgens P, Korovkina D, Seeger JM, Al-Baldawi Y, Al-Maarri M, Fritz C, Vlantis K, Bezhanova S, Scheel AH, et al. 2016. B-cell–specific conditional expression of Myd88p.L252P leads to the development of diffuse large B-cell lymphoma in mice. *Blood* **127:** 2732–2741. doi:10.1182/blood-2015-11-684183

Kovalchuk AL, Qi CF, Torrey TA, Taddesse-Heath L, Feigenbaum L, Park SS, Gerbitz A, Klobeck G, Hoertnagel K, Polack A, et al. 2000. Burkitt lymphoma in the mouse. *J Exp Med* **192:** 1183–1190. doi:10.1084/jem.192.8.1183

Kraus M, Alimzhanov MB, Rajewsky N, Rajewsky K. 2004. Survival of resting mature B lymphocytes depends on BCR signaling via the Igα/β heterodimer. *Cell* **117:** 787–800. doi:10.1016/j.cell.2004.05.014

Kridel R, Sehn LH, Gascoyne RD. 2012. Pathogenesis of follicular lymphoma. *J Clin Invest* **122:** 3424–3431. doi:10.1172/JCI63186

Küppers R, Dalla-Favera R. 2001. Mechanisms of chromosomal translocations in B cell lymphomas. *Oncogene* **20:** 5580–5594. doi:10.1038/sj.onc.1204640

Küppers R, Klein U, Hansmann ML, Rajewsky K. 1999. Cellular origin of human B-cell lymphomas. *N Engl J Med* **341:** 1520–1529. doi:10.1056/NEJM199911113412007

Lamaison C, Tarte K. 2019. Impact of B cell/lymphoid stromal cell crosstalk in B-cell physiology and malignancy. *Immunol Lett* **215:** 12–18. doi:10.1016/j.imlet.2019.02.005

Lenz G, Davis RE, Ngo VN, Lam L, George TC, Wright GW, Dave SS, Zhao H, Xu W, Rosenwald A, et al. 2008. Oncogenic *CARD11* mutations in human diffuse large B cell lymphoma. *Science* **319:** 1676–1679. doi:10.1126/science.1153629

Li H, Kaminski MS, Li Y, Yildiz M, Ouillette P, Jones S, Fox H, Jacobi K, Saiya-Cork K, Bixby D, et al. 2014. Mutations in linker histone genes *HIST1H1 B, C, D,* and *E*; *OCT2* (*POU2F2*); *IRF8*; and *ARID1A* underlying the pathogenesis of follicular lymphoma. *Blood* **123:** 1487–1498. doi:10.1182/blood-2013-05-500264

Lia M, Carette A, Tang H, Shen Q, Mo T, Bhagat G, Dalla-Favera R, Klein U. 2012. Functional dissection of the Chromosome *13q14* tumor-suppressor locus using transgenic mouse lines. *Blood* **119:** 2981–2990. doi:10.1182/blood-2011-09-381814

Liu Y, Hermanson M, Grander D, Merup M, Wu X, Heyman M, Rasool O, Juliusson G, Gahrton G, Detlofsson R, et al. 1995. 13q deletions in lymphoid malignancies. *Blood* **86:** 1911–1915. doi:10.1182/blood.V86.5.1911.bloodjournal8651911

Lopes-Carvalho T, Kearney JF. 2004. Development and selection of marginal zone B cells. *Immunol Rev* **197:** 192–205. doi:10.1111/j.0105-2896.2004.0112.x

Lossos IS, Gascoyne RD. 2011. Transformation of follicular lymphoma. *Best Pract Res Clin Haematol* **24:** 147–163. doi:10.1016/j.beha.2011.02.006

Love C, Sun Z, Jima D, Li G, Zhang J, Miles R, Richards KL, Dunphy CH, Choi WW, Srivastava G, et al. 2012. The genetic landscape of mutations in Burkitt lymphoma. *Nat Genet* **44:** 1321–1325. doi:10.1038/ng.2468

Lovec H, Grzeschiczek A, Kowalski MB, Möröy T. 1994. Cyclin D1/*bcl-1* cooperates with *myc* genes in the generation of B-cell lymphoma in transgenic mice. *EMBO J* **13:** 3487–3495. doi:10.1002/j.1460-2075.1994.tb06655.x

Mandelbaum J, Bhagat G, Tang H, Mo T, Brahmachary M, Shen Q, Chadburn A, Rajewsky K, Tarakhovsky A, Pasqualucci L, et al. 2010. *BLIMP1* is a tumor suppressor gene frequently disrupted in activated B cell-like diffuse large B cell lymphoma. *Cancer Cell* **18:** 568–579. doi:10.1016/j.ccr.2010.10.030

McDonnell TJ, Korsmeyer SJ. 1991. Progression from lymphoid hyperplasia to high-grade malignant lymphoma in mice transgenic for the t(14; 18). *Nature* **349:** 254–256. doi:10.1038/349254a0

McDonnell TJ, Deane N, Platt FM, Nunez G, Jaeger U, McKearn JP, Korsmeyer SJ. 1989. *bcl-2*-immunoglobulin transgenic mice demonstrate extended B cell survival and follicular lymphoproliferation. *Cell* **57:** 79–88. doi:10.1016/0092-8674(89)90174-8

Mesin L, Ersching J, Victora GD. 2016. Germinal center B cell dynamics. *Immunity* **45:** 471–482. doi:10.1016/j.immuni.2016.09.001

Meyer SN, Scuoppo C, Vlasevska S, Bal E, Holmes AB, Holloman M, Garcia-Ibanez L, Nataraj S, Duval R, Vantrimpont T, et al. 2019. Unique and shared epigenetic programs of the CREBBP and EP300 acetyltransferases in germinal center B cells reveal targetable dependencies in lymphoma. *Immunity* **51:** 535–547.e9. doi:10.1016/j.immuni.2019.08.006

Milpied P, Cervera-Marzal I, Mollichella ML, Tesson B, Brisou G, Traverse-Glehen A, Salles G, Spinelli L, Nadel B. 2018. Human germinal center transcriptional programs are de-synchronized in B cell lymphoma. *Nat Immunol* **19:** 1013–1024. doi:10.1038/s41590-018-0181-4

Mondello P, Tadros S, Teater M, Fontan L, Chang AY, Jain N, Yang H, Singh S, Ying HY, Chu CS, et al. 2020. Selective inhibition of HDAC3 targets synthetic vulnerabilities and activates immune surveillance in lymphoma. *Cancer Discov* **10:** 440–459. doi:10.1158/2159-8290

Moran-Crusio K, Reavie L, Shih A, Abdel-Wahab O, Ndiaye-Lobry D, Lobry C, Figueroa ME, Vasanthakumar A, Patel J, Zhao X, et al. 2011. *Tet2* loss leads to increased hematopoietic stem cell self-renewal and myeloid transformation. *Cancer Cell* **20:** 11–24. doi:10.1016/j.ccr.2011.06.001

Morin RD, Johnson NA, Severson TM, Mungall AJ, An J, Goya R, Paul JE, Boyle M, Woolcock BW, Kuchenbauer F, et al. 2010. Somatic mutations altering EZH2 (Tyr641) in follicular and diffuse large B-cell lymphomas of germinal-center origin. *Nat Genet* **42:** 181–185. doi:10.1038/ng.518

Morin RD, Mendez-Lago M, Mungall AJ, Goya R, Mungall KL, Corbett RD, Johnson NA, Severson TM, Chiu R, Field M, et al. 2011. Frequent mutation of histone-modifying genes in non-Hodgkin lymphoma. *Nature* **476:** 298–303. doi:10.1038/nature10351

Muppidi JR, Schmitz R, Green JA, Xiao W, Larsen AB, Braun SE, An J, Xu Y, Rosenwald A, Ott G, et al. 2014. Loss of signalling via Gα13 in germinal centre B-cell-derived lymphoma. *Nature* **516:** 254–258. doi:10.1038/nature13765

Ngo VN, Young RM, Schmitz R, Jhavar S, Xiao W, Lim KH, Kohlhammer H, Xu W, Yang Y, Zhao H, et al. 2011. Oncogenically active *MYD88* mutations in human lymphoma. *Nature* **470:** 115–119. doi:10.1038/nature09671

Ogilvy S, Metcalf D, Print CG, Bath ML, Harris AW, Adams JM. 1999. Constitutive Bcl-2 expression throughout the hematopoietic compartment affects multiple lineages and enhances progenitor cell survival. *Proc Natl Acad Sci* **96:** 14943–14948. doi:10.1073/pnas.96.26.14943

Okosun J, Bödör C, Wang J, Araf S, Yang CY, Pan C, Boller S, Cittaro D, Bozek M, Iqbal S, et al. 2014. Integrated genomic analysis identifies recurrent mutations and evolution patterns driving the initiation and progression of follicular lymphoma. *Nat Genet* **46:** 176–181. doi:10.1038/ng.2856

Okosun J, Wolfson RL, Wang J, Araf S, Wilkins L, Castellano BM, Escudero-Ibarz L, Al Seraihi AF, Richter J, Bernhart SH, et al. 2016. Recurrent mTORC1-activating *RRAGC* mutations in follicular lymphoma. *Nat Genet* **48:** 183–188. doi:10.1038/ng.3473

Oricchio E, Wolfe AL, Schatz JH, Mavrakis KJ, Wendel HG. 2010. Mouse models of cancer as biological filters for complex genomic data. *Dis Model Mech* **3:** 701–704. doi:10.1242/dmm.006296

Oricchio E, Papapetrou EP, Lafaille F, Ganat YM, Kriks S, Ortega-Molina A, Mark WH, Teruya-Feldstein J, Huse JT, Reuter V, et al. 2014. A cell engineering strategy to enhance the safety of stem cell therapies. *Cell Rep* **8:** 1677–1685. doi:10.1016/j.celrep.2014.08.039

Ortega-Molina A, Boss IW, Canela A, Pan H, Jiang Y, Zhao C, Jiang M, Hu D, Agirre X, Niesvizky I, et al. 2015. The histone lysine methyltransferase KMT2D sustains a gene expression program that represses B cell lymphoma development. *Nat Med* **21:** 1199–1208. doi:10.1038/nm.3943

Ortega-Molina A, Deleyto-Seldas N, Carreras J, Sanz A, Lebrero-Fernández C, Menéndez C, Vandenberg A, Fernández-Ruiz B, Marín-Arraiza L, de la Calle Arregui C, et al. 2019. Oncogenic Rag GTPase signaling enhances B cell activation and drives follicular lymphoma sensitive to pharmacological inhibition of mTOR. *Nat Metab* **1:** 775–789. doi:10.1038/s42255-019-0098-8

Park SS, Kim JS, Tessarollo L, Owens JD, Peng L, Han SS, Tae Chung S, Torrey TA, Cheung WC, Polakiewicz RD, et al. 2005. Insertion of c-*Myc* into *Igh* induces B-cell and plasma-cell neoplasms in mice. *Cancer Res* **65:** 1306–1315. doi:10.1158/0008-5472.CAN-04-0268

Pasqualucci L. 2019. Molecular pathogenesis of germinal center-derived B cell lymphomas. *Immunol Rev* **288:** 240–261. doi:10.1111/imr.12745

Pasqualucci L, Compagno M, Houldsworth J, Monti S, Grunn A, Nandula SV, Aster JC, Murty VV, Shipp MA, Dalla-Favera R. 2006. Inactivation of the PRDM1/BLIMP1 gene in diffuse large B cell lymphoma. *J Exp Med* **203:** 311–317. doi:10.1084/jem.20052204

Pasqualucci L, Bhagat G, Jankovic M, Compagno M, Smith P, Muramatsu M, Honjo T, Morse HC 3rd, Nussenzweig MC, Dalla-Favera R. 2008. AID is required for germinal center-derived lymphomagenesis. *Nat Genet* **40:** 108–112. doi:10.1038/ng.2007.35

Pasqualucci L, Dominguez-Sola D, Chiarenza A, Fabbri G, Grunn A, Trifonov V, Kasper LH, Lerach S, Tang H, Ma J, et al. 2011. Inactivating mutations of acetyltransferase genes in B-cell lymphoma. *Nature* **471:** 189–195. doi:10.1038/nature09730

Pasqualucci L, Khiabanian H, Fangazio M, Vasishtha M, Messina M, Holmes AB, Ouillette P, Trifonov V, Rossi D, Tabbò F, et al. 2014. Genetics of follicular lymphoma transformation. *Cell Rep* **6:** 130–140. doi:10.1016/j.celrep.2013.12.027

Pekarsky Y, Zanesi N, Aqeilan RI, Croce CM. 2007. Animal models for chronic lymphocytic leukemia. *J Cell Biochem* **100:** 1109–1118. doi:10.1002/jcb.21147

Peled JU, Yu JJ, Venkatesh J, Bi E, Ding BB, Krupski-Downs M, Shaknovich R, Sicinski P, Diamond B, Scharff MD, et al. 2010. Requirement for cyclin D3 in germinal center formation and function. *Cell Res* **20:** 631–646. doi:10.1038/cr.2010.55

Pizzi M, Inghirami G. 2017. Patient-derived tumor xenografts of lymphoproliferative disorders: Are they surrogates for the human disease? *Curr Opin Hematol* **24:** 384–392. doi:10.1097/MOH.0000000000000349

Puente XS, Jares P, Campo E. 2018. Chronic lymphocytic leukemia and mantle cell lymphoma: Crossroads of genetic and microenvironment interactions. *Blood* **131:** 2283–2296. doi:10.1182/blood-2017-10-764373

Rajewsky K. 1996. Clonal selection and learning in the antibody system. *Nature* **381:** 751–758. doi:10.1038/381751a0

Ramezani-Rad P, Rickert RC. 2017. Murine models of germinal center derived-lymphomas. *Curr Opin Immunol* **45:** 31–36. doi:10.1016/j.coi.2016.12.002

Ravà M, D'Andrea A, Nicoli P, Gritti I, Donati G, Doni M, Giorgio M, Olivero D, Amati B. 2018. Therapeutic synergy between tigecycline and venetoclax in a preclinical model of *MYC*/*BCL2* double-hit B cell lymphoma. *Sci Transl Med* **10:** eaan8723. doi:10.1126/scitranslmed.aan8723

Raveche ES, Salerno E, Scaglione BJ, Manohar V, Abbasi F, Lin YC, Fredrickson T, Landgraf P, Ramachandra S, Huppi K, et al. 2007. Abnormal microRNA-16 locus with synteny to human 13q14 linked to CLL in NZB mice. *Blood* **109:** 5079–5086. doi:10.1182/blood-2007-02-071225

Reddy A, Zhang J, Davis NS, Moffitt AB, Love CL, Waldrop A, Leppa S, Pasanen A, Meriranta L, Karjalainen-Lindsberg ML, et al. 2017. Genetic and functional drivers of diffuse large B cell lymphoma. *Cell* **171:** 481–494.e15. doi:10.1016/j.cell.2017.09.027

Richter J, Schlesner M, Hoffmann S, Kreuz M, Leich E, Burkhardt B, Rosolowski M, Ammerpohl O, Wagener R, Bernhart SH, et al. 2012. Recurrent mutation of the *ID3* gene in Burkitt lymphoma identified by integrated genome, exome and transcriptome sequencing. *Nat Genet* **44:** 1316–1320. doi:10.1038/ng.2469

Rickert RC, Roes J, Rajewsky K. 1997. B lymphocyte-specific, Cre-mediated mutagenesis in mice. *Nucleic Acids Res* **25:** 1317–1318. doi:10.1093/nar/25.6.1317

Roco JA, Mesin L, Binder SC, Nefzger C, Gonzalez-Figueroa P, Canete PF, Ellyard J, Shen Q, Robert PA, Cappello J, et al. 2019. Class-switch recombination occurs infrequently in germinal centers. *Immunity* **51:** 337–350.e7. doi:10.1016/j.immuni.2019.07.001

Rosenwald A, Alizadeh AA, Widhopf G, Simon R, Davis RE, Yu X, Yang L, Pickeral OK, Rassenti LZ, Powell J, et al. 2001. Relation of gene expression phenotype to immunoglobulin mutation genotype in B cell chronic lymphocytic leukemia. *J Exp Med* **194:** 1639–1648. doi:10.1084/jem.194.11.1639

Roulland S, Navarro JM, Grenot P, Milili M, Agopian J, Montpellier B, Gauduchon P, Lebailly P, Schiff C, Nadel B. 2006. Follicular lymphoma-like B cells in healthy individuals: a novel intermediate step in early lymphomagenesis. *J Exp Med* **203:** 2425–2431. doi:10.1084/jem.20061292

Sander S, Calado DP, Srinivasan L, Köchert K, Zhang B, Rosolowski M, Rodig SJ, Holzmann K, Stilgenbauer S, Siebert R, et al. 2012. Synergy between PI3 K signaling and MYC in Burkitt lymphomagenesis. *Cancer Cell* **22:** 167–179. doi:10.1016/j.ccr.2012.06.012

Schmitz R, Young RM, Ceribelli M, Jhavar S, Xiao W, Zhang M, Wright G, Shaffer AL, Hodson DJ, Buras E, et al. 2012. Burkitt lymphoma pathogenesis and therapeutic targets from structural and functional genomics. *Nature* **490:** 116–120. doi:10.1038/nature11378

Schmitz R, Wright GW, Huang DW, Johnson CA, Phelan JD, Wang JQ, Roulland S, Kasbekar M, Young RM, Shaffer AL, et al. 2018. Genetics and pathogenesis of diffuse large B-cell lymphoma. *N Engl J Med* **378:** 1396–1407. doi:10.1056/NEJMoa1801445

Schneider C, Kon N, Amadori L, Shen Q, Schwartz FH, Tischler B, Bossennec M, Dominguez-Sola D, Bhagat G, Gu W, et al. 2016. FBXO11 inactivation leads to abnormal germinal-center formation and lymphoproliferative disease. *Blood* **128:** 660–666. doi:10.1182/blood-2015-11-684357

Scott DW, Gascoyne RD. 2014. The tumour microenvironment in B cell lymphomas. *Nat Rev Cancer* **14:** 517–534. doi:10.1038/nrc3774

Seifert M, Sellmann L, Bloehdorn J, Wein F, Stilgenbauer S, Dürig J, Küppers R. 2012. Cellular origin and pathophysiology of chronic lymphocytic leukemia. *J Exp Med* **209:** 2183–2198. doi:10.1084/jem.20120833

Shaffer AL III, Young RM, Staudt LM. 2012. Pathogenesis of human B cell lymphomas. *Annu Rev Immunol* **30:** 565–610. doi:10.1146/annurev-immunol-020711-075027

Shaffer AL, Wright G, Yang L, Powell J, Ngo V, Lamy L, Lam LT, Davis RE, Staudt LM. 2006. A library of gene expression signatures to illuminate normal and pathological lymphoid biology. *Immunol Rev* **210:** 67–85. doi:10.1111/j.0105-2896.2006.00373.x

Shukla V, Ma S, Hardy RR, Joshi SS, Lu R. 2013. A role for IRF4 in the development of CLL. *Blood* **122:** 2848–2855. doi:10.1182/blood-2013-03-492769

Shukla V, Shukla A, Joshi SS, Lu R. 2016. Interferon regulatory factor 4 attenuates Notch signaling to suppress the development of chronic lymphocytic leukemia. *Oncotarget* **7:** 41081–41094.

Simonetti G, Carette A, Silva K, Wang H, De Silva NS, Heise N, Siebel CW, Shlomchik MJ, Klein U. 2013. IRF4 controls the positioning of mature B cells in the lymphoid microenvironments by regulating NOTCH2 expression and activity. *J Exp Med* **210:** 2887–2902. doi:10.1084/jem.20131026

Simonetti G, Bertilaccio MT, Ghia P, Klein U. 2014. Mouse models in the study of chronic lymphocytic leukemia pathogenesis and therapy. *Blood* **124:** 1010–1019. doi:10.1182/blood-2014-05-577122

Skaar JR, Pagan JK, Pagano M. 2013. Mechanisms and function of substrate recruitment by F-box proteins. *Nat Rev Mol Cell Biol* **14:** 369–381. doi:10.1038/nrm3582

Stevenson F, Sahota S, Zhu D, Ottensmeier C, Chapman C, Oscier D, Hamblin T. 1998. Insight into the origin and clonal history of B-cell tumors as revealed by analysis of immunoglobulin variable region genes. *Immunol Rev* **162:** 247–259. doi:10.1111/j.1600-065X.1998.tb01446.x

Strasser A, Whittingham S, Vaux DL, Bath ML, Adams JM, Cory S, Harris AW. 1991. Enforced *BCL2* expression in B-lymphoid cells prolongs antibody responses and elicits autoimmune disease. *Proc Natl Acad Sci* **88:** 8661–8665. doi:10.1073/pnas.88.19.8661

Sungalee S, Mamessier E, Morgado E, Grégoire E, Brohawn PZ, Morehouse CA, Jouve N, Monvoisin C, Menard C, Debroas G, et al. 2014. Germinal center reentries of BCL2-overexpressing B cells drive follicular lymphoma progression. *J Clin Invest* **124:** 5337–5351. doi:10.1172/JCI72415

Swerdlow SH, Campo E, Harris NL, Jaffe ES, Pileri SA, Stein H, Thiele J. 2016. *WHO classification of tumours of haematopoietic and lymphoid tissues.* International Agency for Research on Cancer (IARC), Lyon.

Sze CC, Shilatifard A. 2016. MLL3/MLL4/COMPASS family on epigenetic regulation of enhancer function and cancer. *Cold Spring Harb Perspect Med* **6:** a026427.

Tam W, Gomez M, Chadburn A, Lee JW, Chan WC, Knowles DM. 2006. Mutational analysis of PRDM1 indicates a tumor-suppressor role in diffuse large B-cell lymphomas. *Blood* **107:** 4090–4100. doi:10.1182/blood-2005-09-3778

Townsend EC, Murakami MA, Christodoulou A, Christie AL, Köster J, DeSouza TA, Morgan EA, Kallgren SP, Liu H, Wu SC, et al. 2016. The public repository of xenografts enables discovery and randomized phase II-like trials in mice. *Cancer Cell* **29:** 574–586. doi:10.1016/j.ccell.2016.03.008

Trinh DL, Scott DW, Morin RD, Mendez-Lago M, An J, Jones SJ, Mungall AJ, Zhao Y, Schein J, Steidl C, et al. 2013. Analysis of *FOXO1* mutations in diffuse large B-cell lymphoma. *Blood* **121:** 3666–3674. doi:10.1182/blood-2013-01-479865

Truffinet V, Pinaud E, Cogné N, Petit B, Guglielmi L, Cogné M, Denizot Y. 2007. The 3′ *IgH* locus control region is sufficient to deregulate a c-*myc* transgene and promote mature B cell malignancies with a predominant Burkitt-like phenotype. *J Immunol* **179:** 6033–6042. doi:10.4049/jimmunol.179.9.6033

Valls E, Lobry C, Geng H, Wang L, Cardenas M, Rivas M, Cerchietti L, Oh P, Yang SN, Oswald E, et al. 2017. BCL6 antagonizes NOTCH2 to maintain survival of human follicular lymphoma cells. *Cancer Discov* **7:** 506–521. doi:10.1158/2159-8290.CD-16-1189

Varano G, Raffel S, Sormani M, Zanardi F, Lonardi S, Zasada C, Perucho L, Petrocelli V, Haake A, Lee AK, et al. 2017. The B-cell receptor controls fitness of MYC-driven lymphoma cells via GSK3β inhibition. *Nature* **546:** 302–306. doi:10.1038/nature22353

Victora GD, Nussenzweig MC. 2012. Germinal centers. *Annu Rev Immunol* **30:** 429–457. doi:10.1146/annurev-immunol-020711-075032

Victora GD, Schwickert TA, Fooksman DR, Kamphorst AO, Meyer-Hermann M, Dustin ML, Nussenzweig MC. 2010. Germinal center dynamics revealed by multiphoton microscopy with a photoactivatable fluorescent reporter. *Cell* **143:** 592–605. doi:10.1016/j.cell.2010.10.032

Victora GD, Dominguez-Sola D, Holmes AB, Deroubaix S, Dalla-Favera R, Nussenzweig MC. 2012. Identification of human germinal center light and dark zone cells and their relationship to human B-cell lymphomas. *Blood* **120:** 2240–2248. doi:10.1182/blood-2012-03-415380

Vincent-Fabert C, Fiancette R, Rouaud P, Baudet C, Truffinet V, Magnone V, Guillaudeau A, Cogné M, Dubus P, Denizot Y. 2012. A defect of the INK4-Cdk4 checkpoint and *Myc* collaborate in blastoid mantle cell lymphoma-like lymphoma formation in mice. *Am J Pathol* **180:** 1688–1701. doi:10.1016/j.ajpath.2012.01.004

Wang J, Boxer LM. 2005. Regulatory elements in the immunoglobulin heavy chain gene 3′-enhancers induce c-*myc* deregulation and lymphomagenesis in murine B cells. *J Biol Chem* **280:** 12766–12773. doi:10.1074/jbc.M412446200

Wang L, Lawrence MS, Wan Y, Stojanov P, Sougnez C, Stevenson K, Werner L, Sivachenko A, DeLuca DS, Zhang L, et al. 2011. *SF3B1* and other novel cancer genes in chronic lymphocytic leukemia. *N Engl J Med* **365:** 2497–2506. doi:10.1056/NEJMoa1109016

Wang JQ, Jeelall YS, Humburg P, Batchelor EL, Kaya SM, Yoo HM, Goodnow CC, Horikawa K. 2017. Synergistic cooperation and crosstalk between *MYD88*^{L265P} and mutations that dysregulate CD79B and surface IgM. *J Exp Med* **214:** 2759–2776. doi:10.1084/jem.20161454

Yin S, Gambe RG, Sun J, Martinez AZ, Cartun ZJ, Regis FFD, Wan Y, Fan J, Brooks AN, Herman SEM, et al. 2019. A murine model of chronic lymphocytic leukemia based on B cell-restricted expression of *Sf3b1* mutation and *Atm* deletion. *Cancer Cell* **35:** 283–296.e5. doi:10.1016/j.ccell.2018.12.013

Ying CY, Dominguez-Sola D, Fabi M, Lorenz IC, Hussein S, Bansal M, Califano A, Pasqualucci L, Basso K, Dalla-Favera R. 2013. *MEF2B* mutations lead to deregulated expression of the oncogene *BCL6* in diffuse large B cell lymphoma. *Nat Immunol* **14:** 1084–1092. doi:10.1038/ni.2688

Young RM, Wu T, Schmitz R, Dawood M, Xiao W, Phelan JD, Xu W, Menard L, Meffre E, Chan WC, et al. 2015. Survival of human lymphoma cells requires B-cell receptor engagement by self-antigens. *Proc Natl Acad Sci* **112:** 13447–13454. doi:10.1073/pnas.1514944112

Zhang B, Calado DP, Wang Z, Frohler S, Kochert K, Qian Y, Koralov SB, Schmidt-Supprian M, Sasaki Y, Unitt C, et al. 2015a. An oncogenic role for alternative NF-κB signaling in DLBCL revealed upon deregulated BCL6 expression. *Cell Rep* **11:** 715–726. doi:10.1016/j.celrep.2015.03.059

Zhang J, Dominguez-Sola D, Hussein S, Lee JE, Holmes AB, Bansal M, Vlasevska S, Mo T, Tang H, Basso K, et al. 2015b. Disruption of *KMT2D* perturbs germinal center B cell development and promotes lymphomagenesis. *Nat Med* **21:** 1190–1198. doi:10.1038/nm.3940

Zhang J, Vlasevska S, Wells VA, Nataraj S, Holmes AB, Duval R, Meyer SN, Mo T, Basso K, Brindle PK, et al. 2017. The CREBBP acetyltransferase is a haploinsufficient tumor suppressor in B-cell lymphoma. *Cancer Discov* **7:** 322–337. doi:10.1158/2159-8290.CD-16-1417

Modeling Leukemia with Human Induced Pluripotent Stem Cells

Eirini P. Papapetrou[1,2,3,4]

[1]Department of Oncological Sciences, Icahn School of Medicine at Mount Sinai, New York, New York 10029, USA

[2]Tisch Cancer Institute, Icahn School of Medicine at Mount Sinai, New York, New York 10029, USA

[3]Black Family Stem Cell Institute, Icahn School of Medicine at Mount Sinai, New York, New York 10029, USA

[4]Department of Medicine, Icahn School of Medicine at Mount Sinai, New York, New York 10029, USA

Correspondence: eirini.papapetrou@mssm.edu

The reprogramming of human somatic cells into induced pluripotent stem cells (iPSCs) a little over a decade ago raised exciting prospects to transform the study and potentially also the therapy of human diseases. iPSC models have now been created for a multitude of hematologic diseases, including malignancies. Here we discuss practical aspects of iPSC modeling of malignant diseases, review recent studies, and discuss the new opportunities that iPSC models offer, as well as their current limitations and prospects for future development.

The successful demonstration that human pluripotent stem cells (hPSCs) identical to human embryonic stem cells (hESCs), termed induced pluripotent stem cells (iPSCs), can be generated from somatic cells through the ectopic expression of a defined set of genes in 2007 was quickly succeeded by several proof-of-principle studies highlighting the potential of using iPSCs derived from patients to study and potentially cure inherited genetic diseases via gene and cell therapy and to test drugs (Hanna et al. 2007; Takahashi et al. 2007; Yu et al. 2007; Park et al. 2008; Lee et al. 2009). Modeling more complex diseases and high-throughput screening of small molecule libraries to identify lead compounds with iPSCs was demonstrated within the next few years (Brennand et al. 2011; Lee et al. 2012; Yang et al. 2013). In 2013, the development of the CRISPR/Cas9 system as a versatile and user-friendly genome editing tool took biomedical research by storm and paired with iPSC technology in a perfect marriage. More recent studies exploring the opportunities that iPSCs offer to study malignancies, with blood cancers featuring most prominently among them, are breaking new ground in cancer research (Chao et al. 2017; Kotini et al. 2017).

TECHNICAL ASPECTS OF iPSC MODELING OF BLOOD MALIGNANCIES

Reprogramming Malignant Cells

In contrast to the generation of iPSC models of inherited genetic diseases—for which the choice of starting cell type is solely based on availability

Cite this article as *Cold Spring Harb Perspect Med* doi: 10.1101/cshperspect.a034868

and convenience and encompasses any cell type of the human body—in the case of malignant diseases the composition of the starting cell population is of utmost importance. The malignant cells that iPSC models seek to capture are contained within the bone marrow (BM) and peripheral blood (PB) of patients with leukemias. These samples typically contain an admixture of normal and malignant cells with varying degrees of clonal heterogeneity of the latter. These characteristics necessitate careful genetic characterization of the derivative iPSCs to establish their provenance in relation to the different clones present in the starting cell population.

Reprogramming effectively resets the epigenome and erases any leukemia-related epigenetic abnormalities. Thus, genetic tracking is the only guide to ascertain provenance of iPSC lines from malignant cells as opposed to residual normal cells in the sample and to assign them to specific clones and subclones. Thus, although routine reprogramming of nonmalignant cells entails random picking of a small number of iPSC colonies (4–6) and, after further characterization, establishment of three or more iPSC lines, reprogramming malignant cells requires more stringent procedures to be successful. Our group has devised a reprogramming strategy tailored to the specific considerations of leukemic samples—namely, their genetic complexity and clonal heterogeneity. First, we perform comprehensive genetic characterization of the starting sample, which includes karyotype, mutational analysis with comprehensive gene panels, fluorescence in situ hybridization (FISH) for common chromosomal translocations, and potentially comparative genomic hybridization (CGH) to characterize chromosomal deletions. Second, we develop patient-specific polymerase chain reaction (PCR) (classic or quantitative)-based assays for genotyping, which enables us to easily genotype iPSC colonies in real time, as they emerge, in relatively high throughput. This, in turn, and in combination with efficient reprogramming methods—namely, Sendai virus or lentiviral vectors—enables "deep reprogramming" (i.e., the generation and screening of large numbers [which can reach the hundreds] of iPSC colonies in a single reprogramming experiment). This allows us to derive iPSC lines representing as many clones as possible, as well as normal cells. The latter typically have a reprogramming advantage over malignant cells and can most often be captured in iPSCs even if they are very rare in the starting cell sample. For the same reasons, premalignant clones can often be captured even if their representation in the starting cell sample is small or undetectable by bulk genetic analyses. This is, however, not a universal rule, as we have encountered instances in which leukemia cells reprogram with very high efficiency, surpassing that of normal cells (Kotini et al. 2017). TP53 inactivation has been documented to enhance reprogramming efficiency, and, thus, this higher reprogramming propensity may be related to TP53 activation status (Banito et al. 2009; Hong et al. 2009; Kawamura et al. 2009; Li et al. 2009; Marión et al. 2009; Utikal et al. 2009). Although oftentimes more than one clone and additionally normal cells can be captured in iPSCs, the clonal representation captured by reprogramming is often skewed (Chao et al. 2017; Kotini et al. 2017). This strongly implies that reprogramming efficiency is affected by the genetics of leukemia, including mutations, chromosomal abnormalities, and the presence or absence of genetic instability, but the underlying rules are not currently well understood.

The reprogramming efficiency of leukemic cells can be controlled by several mechanisms. Epigenetic alterations, such as DNA methylation, may very well impact the reprogramming efficiency, as aberrant DNA methylation patterns have been well documented in acute myeloid leukemia (AML) and profound methylation changes need to occur during reprogramming to pluripotency, including demethylation of promoters of key pluripotency genes (Figueroa et al. 2010; Apostolou and Stadtfeld 2018). Moreover, the capacity of leukemic cells for ex vivo growth also impacts greatly their ability to reprogram. Cell division is critically required both for efficient transduction with reprogramming vectors to initiate reprogramming, as well as for the epigenome remodeling required to complete reprogramming to pluripotency. Thus, inability to enter a proliferative state severely hampers a cell's reprogramming ability (Hanna et al. 2009; Ruiz et al. 2011; Guo et al. 2014). For example, the ability for ex vivo proliferation of myelodysplastic syndrome (MDS) and AML cells varies considerably across samples, but is generally poor. In contrast, cells from patients with myeloproliferative neoplasms (MPNs) typically grow robustly in culture, at least for a limited time period, and can be reprogrammed into iPSCs with high efficiencies (Hu et al. 2011; Kumano et al. 2012; Gandre-Babbe et al. 2013; Hosoi et al. 2014; Ye et al. 2014; Mulero-Navarro et al. 2015; Miyauchi et al. 2018). The cellular pathways underlying the capacity of leukemic cells to grow ex vivo and their putative correlation with specific genetic groups remain unknown. It is possible that an inverse correlation exists with a proapoptotic phenotype (Potter and Letai 2016). Because of all the reprogramming barriers mentioned above, several investigators have reported very low success rates of reprogramming leukemia samples, excluding MPNs (Muñoz-López et al. 2016; Lee et al. 2017). It is likely that these low success rates can be significantly increased with tailored, more efficient, and genetically informed reprogramming strategies. In our hands, approximately half of MDS and AML samples that can be induced to enter cell division by cytokine stimulation yield at least one or a few malignant iPSC lines. As more leukemias of diverse genetic groups and specific mutations are reprogrammed, principles of how reprogramming efficiency is affected by different factors discussed above will likely begin to emerge and may even provide some insights into the pathogenesis and signaling dependences of different leukemias.

The process of reprogramming per se can also be informative in elucidating the clonal architecture and evolution of a leukemia sample, in a way akin to what has been previously done using colony forming assays in methylcellulose (Fig. 1; Jan et al. 2012; Ortmann et al. 2015). First, reprogramming can determine the order of mutation acquisition (Fig. 1A). The order by which driver mutations are acquired may affect clinical features and response to therapy (Kent and Green 2017; Levine et al. 2019). Genetic analyses of the bulk tumor cannot always determine the mutational order through inference based on variant allele fractions (VAFs). Such instances may include cases in which two mutations arose close together in time and their VAFs are very similar to each other or cases of advanced disease in which the earlier clones have been almost entirely replaced by the most evolved ones. In the latter case, rare cells of a parental clone may be captured in iPSCs if they have a reprogramming advantage, which they often do, over the fully leukemic clone. Second, reprogramming can help clonal deconvolution in cases with low mutational burden, in which bulk sequencing cannot discriminate whether two mutations are present in the same or in separate clones (Fig. 1B). Capturing these clones by reprogramming can unambiguously determine the clonal composition of the starting sample. For reprogramming to inform on the clonal parameters of the starting leukemia, however, it is critical that iPSC derivation is performed in conditions ensuring and preserving clonality. These include line establishment and passaging techniques (e.g., manual picking of a single colony under a microscope, single-cell subcloning in case of mixed clonality) and mutational analyses. If integrating vectors were used for reprogramming, integration site analysis can provide an additional means to ascertain clonality (Kotini et al. 2017).

Hematopoietic Specification of iPSCs

Virtually all phenotypic and molecular assays are performed and all readouts are obtained following the in vitro directed differentiation of iPSCs into hematopoietic cells. The efficiency and robustness of this process weighs heavily on the quality of all iPSC-based studies. Most evidence to date suggests that in vitro hPSC-derived hematopoiesis consists of cells corresponding to different developmental stages, without a clear temporal separation of their emergence (Choi et al. 2012; Pearson et al. 2015). Thus, hematopoietic lineages of all three waves that are successively generated during normal development of the hematopoietic system may be present in in vitro differentiation cultures. These include a first wave, referred to as "primitive," giving rise only to erythroid, megakaryocyte,

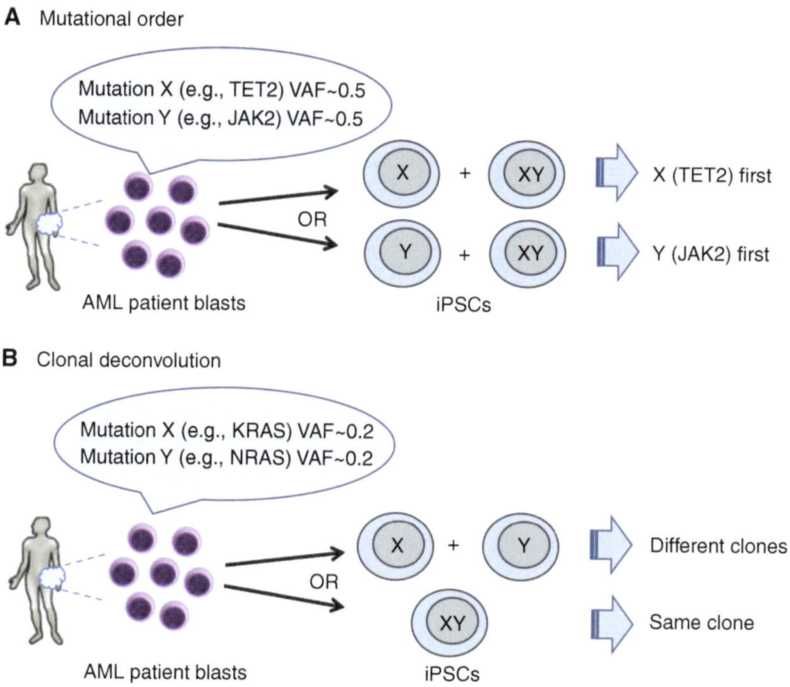

Figure 1. Mutational order reconstruction and clonal deconvolution by reprogramming. (*A*) Reprogramming into induced pluripotent stem cells (iPSCs) can decipher the order of mutation acquisition and thus illuminate the clonal history of the disease. In the example shown, two mutations (X and Y, e.g., TET2 and JAK2) have similar allele burden at presentation precluding bulk genetic analyses from determining the order by which they were acquired. iPSCs can capture the precursor single-mutant clone and thus determine which mutation occurred first. (*B*) Generation of iPSCs can deconvolute the clonal composition of a sample in the case of mutations with low variant allele fractions (VAFs) from the bulk analysis, which cannot determine whether they are present in the same or different clones. In this case, KRAS and NRAS mutations can frequently arise in divergent clonal evolution (example on *top*) or, alternatively, coexist in the same clone (example in the *bottom*).

and macrophage lineages; a second wave that consists primarily of erythro-myeloid progenitors (EMPs) and some lymphoid progenitors; and a third wave that—unlike the first two, which are extraembryonic—arises in the embryo proper and gives rise to hematopoietic stem cells (HSCs) (Ivanovs et al. 2017; Lacaud and Kouskoff 2017). The terms "primitive" and "definitive" hematopoiesis were originally coined based on pronounced differences of the erythroid products of the first and last wave (size, enucleation, and globin gene expression). With better characterization of the EMPs, the term "definitive" was extended to include the second wave (Frame et al. 2013). However, inconsistency in the use of the term remains in the literature, as some investigators save the term "definitive" exclusively for adult-type HSC-generating hematopoiesis. Notably, this confusion extends to the description of the developmental stage of hPSC-derived hematopoietic products. Earlier protocols for the in vitro hematopoietic differentiation of hPSCs yielded mostly primitive hematopoiesis. More recently, however, the findings that definitive lineages could be generated through activin inhibition or WNT stimulation, acting at the level of early mesoderm patterning, has enabled contemporary protocols to derive primarily definitive- and not primitive-type cells (Kennedy et al. 2012; Sturgeon et al. 2014). However, it is still not clear if these newer protocols better capture the second or third wave of hematopoiesis or a mixture of the two. As mentioned earlier, HSCs are only generated in the third

Cite this article as *Cold Spring Harb Perspect Med* doi: 10.1101/cshperspect.a034868

developmental wave, but it is now believed that all hematopoietic lineages can be generated by more restricted progenitors of the second wave. The fact that hPSC-derived hematopoietic cells can produce all mature lineages, but do not engraft in immunocompromised recipients (as further discussed below), has prompted the speculation that they may more closely represent EMP-type hematopoiesis.

An important limitation of hematopoietic differentiation protocols is the current inability to derive true HSCs with long-term multilineage engraftment capability, potentially related to the developmental immaturity of hPSC-derived hematopoiesis, discussed above (Vo and Daley 2015). This is a technical and not biological limitation, as multilineage engraftable hematopoiesis can be derived from human iPSCs via teratoma formation (Amabile et al. 2015; Suzuki et al. 2015). Whereas this method is impractical and not clinically translatable, it shows that HSCs can, in principle, be derived from hPSCs once the appropriate conditions are worked out, which may also include in vivo niche-derived signals. The unavailability of robust cell culture conditions to maintain and expand primary HSCs in vitro despite years of effort by several investigators is a related problem and attests to the challenge of this endeavor. Although bona-fide HSCs cannot be derived through hPSC-directed differentiation in vitro, mature cells of all hematopoietic lineages, and thus hematopoietic progenitor cells (HPCs) of all lineages, can be derived from them. However, the timing of their emergence, lineage potential, and developmental stage have not been well characterized and likely differ among differentiation protocols. Mapping the HPC populations in terms of uni- or multilineage potential and developmental origin with relation to timing of emergence and surface marker expression would greatly help boost the efficiency and reproducibility and harmonize findings across studies using diverse differentiation methods.

Genome Editing of iPSCs

Whereas for some time hPSCs were thought to be rather refractory to genetic modifications, particularly those involving homologous recombination, advances in their culture—crucially the enhancement of survival and clonal growth of hPSCs by Rho kinase (Rock) inhibition—together with the advent of more efficient gene delivery and gene editing methods, like the CRISPR/Cas9 system, has now turned the genetic engineering of hPSCs into an almost routine practice (Watanabe et al. 2007; Kim and Kim 2014; Hockemeyer and Jaenisch 2016). The genetic engineering of iPSCs uses techniques and principles from the field of genetically engineered mouse models and can, similarly, be used to create reporter, knockout, and knock-in lines. Most crucially, gene editing of iPSCs offers the unique opportunity to derive isogenic lines (i.e., lines differing in only one gene that are otherwise genetically identical) either by introducing specific mutations found in hematologic malignancies in normal iPSCs, by correcting them in patient-derived iPSCs, or, ideally, by both strategies (Chang et al. 2018). Isogenic pairs of lines are more superior controls than unrelated or even patient-matched normal lines, as the latter will still have multiple genetic differences from the disease lines, both pathogenic and nonpathogenic (Fig. 2). The CRISPR/Cas9 system can be used both to inactivate genes to model common loss-of-function mutations in leukemias (e.g., *TET2*, *RUNX1*, *EZH2*, *TP53*, cohesin) through nonhomologous end joining repair of Cas9-mediated double strand DNA breaks and to introduce hotspot mutations in oncogenic driver genes (e.g., splicing factors, *JAK2 V617F*, *DNMT3A R882H*, *NRAS G12D*, *NPM1c*, *FLT3-ITD*) through homology-directed repair from a donor DNA template.

STUDIES USING iPSC MODELS OF HEMATOLOGIC MALIGNANCIES

MPNs, including chronic myeloid leukemia (CML), essential thrombocytopenia (ET), polycythemia vera (PV), and primary myelofibrosis (PMF), were the first malignant blood diseases that were modeled with patient-derived iPSCs (Ye et al. 2009, 2014; Carette et al. 2010; Hu et al. 2011; Kumano et al. 2012; Bedel et al. 2013; Gandre-Babbe et al. 2013; Saliba et al. 2013;

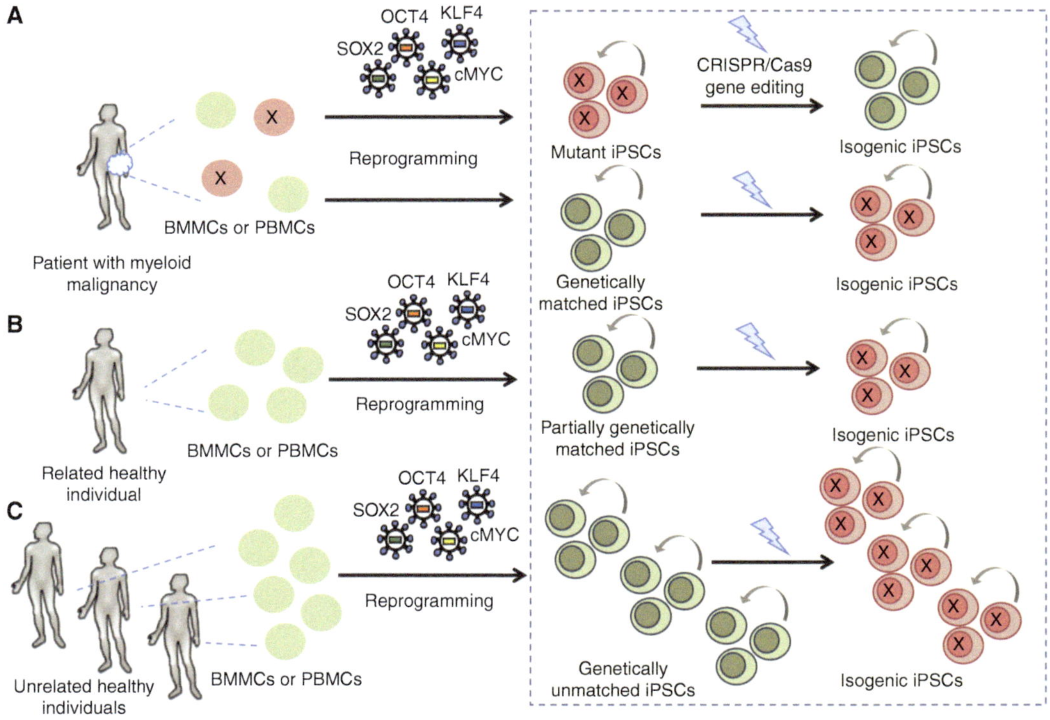

Figure 2. Control induced pluripotent stem cell (iPSC) lines. Normal iPSCs derived from the same patient (from either hematopoietic or other types of somatic cells) can be used as genetically matched controls (*A*). If these are derived from hematopoietic cells, careful genetic analyses should clarify whether they represent completely normal cells or a precursor premalignant or clonal hematopoiesis (CH) clone, by ascertaining that they harbor none of the pathogenic mutations of the patient's malignant clone. These controls share the same genetic background with the disease iPSCs derived from the same patient, but are not technically isogenic, as they almost certainly differ from the malignant iPSCs in more than one gene. Alternatively, normal lines can be derived from healthy family members of the patient, if such material is available (*B*). Finally, existing lines derived from unrelated healthy donors can be used as normal controls (*C*). In the latter case, multiple lines should be used to control for variation because of differences in the genetic background. In all cases, gene editing can be used to develop isogenic matched lines by either correcting a given mutation in patient iPSCs or introducing it in normal iPSCs. Isogenic lines are far superior controls and should always be preferred over nonisogenic controls.

Hosoi et al. 2014; Amabile et al. 2015; Mulero-Navarro et al. 2015; Suknuntha et al. 2015; Gomez Limia et al. 2017; Liu et al. 2017; Sloma et al. 2017; Miyauchi et al. 2018; Takei et al. 2018). In one study, CML-iPSCs could produce mature erythroid and myeloid cells and could not engraft leukemia in mice upon in vitro differentiation, suggesting that reprogramming and/or directed differentiation impaired their oncogenic potential. This phenotype might be related to the finding of decreased DNA methylation levels in the CML-iPSCs and the hematopoietic cells differentiated from them, compared to the primary CML cells (Amabile et al. 2015). In contrast, the dependency of CML cells on BCR-ABL could be recapitulated in patient-derived iPSCs (Carette et al. 2010; Kumano et al. 2012; Bedel et al. 2013; Suknuntha et al. 2015; Miyauchi et al. 2018). CML-iPSCs were not responsive to imatinib at the pluripotent state, but sensitivity was reestablished in hematopoietic cells in vitro differentiated from them. The finding that BCR-ABL, while expressed, does not confer dependency at the pluripotent state, highlights the requirement of cooperation between an oncogenic genetic lesion and the appropriate cellular context for malignant features to manifest. MPN patient-derived iPSCs with heterozygous and homozygous *JAK2 V617F*, *MPL*, and *CALR* mutations have been generated, reflecting the ease of reprogramming of MPN cells, but these studies have not gone beyond reproducing known cellular phenotypes from ex vivo cultured MPN cells, mainly their disease-defining ability for cytokine-independent colony formation in methylcellulose (Saliba et al. 2013; Ye et al. 2014; Gomez Limia et al. 2017; Liu et al. 2017; Takei et al. 2018). The possibility of modeling responses of JAK2 V617F MPN to JAK inhibitors was demonstrated in one study (Ye et al. 2014).

Juvenile myelomonocytic leukemia (JMML), a pediatric MDS/MPN overlap syndrome caused by various signaling mutations, has also been modeled in iPSCs (Gandre-Babbe et al. 2013; Mulero-Navarro et al. 2015; Gagne et al. 2018; Tasian et al. 2019). Specifically, patient-derived iPSCs with *PTPN11* and *CBL* mutations were generated and shown to recapitulate disease phenotypes, such as hypersensitivity to growth factors and increased proliferation. JMML-iPSC-derived myeloid cells were also shown to model differential signaling pathway activation and sensitivity to kinase inhibitors: *PTPN11*-mutant JMML-iPSC-derived hematopoietic cells exhibited constitutive activation of RAS/MAPK signaling and were sensitive to MEK inhibition, whereas *CBL*-mutant JMML-iPSC-derived hematopoietic cells showed JAK/STAT signaling activation and sensitivity to JAK inhibitors (Tasian et al. 2019).

In contrast to MPN cells, MDS and AML cells are relatively refractory to reprogramming. Our group derived the first MDS-iPSCs from two patients with chromosome 7q deletion (del7q) (Kotini et al. 2015). We found that all del7q lines had a markedly diminished potential for generation of $CD34^+/CD45^+$ HPCs upon in vitro differentiation and almost absent ability to generate all types of hematopoietic colonies in methylcellulose assays. By studying the hematopoietic potential of a series of iPSC lines with corrected chr7q dosage, as well as lines with engineered deletions spanning various chr7q regions, we were able to pinpoint a critical region whose hemizygosity was sufficient to confer this loss of differentiation potential. We then selected candidate haploinsufficient genes by means of reduced expression in the hemizygous compared to normal lines and further prioritized hits of a pooled rescue screen of 75 candidate cDNAs. Four genes, *EZH2*, *LUC7L2*, *HIPK2*, and *ATP6V0E2*, were validated to partially rescue the del7q phenotype. Interestingly, the first three genes have also been found to harbor monoallelic loss-of-function mutations in MDS, in further support of a function as haploinsufficient tumor suppressor genes in MDS. This work highlights how iPSCs combined with sophisticated genetic engineering strategies can be used to functionally map critically lost regions within recurrent chromosomal deletions, which cannot easily be modeled in the mouse or other organisms because of lack of conservation of synteny. A subsequent study focused on modeling a hotspot mutation in a splicing factor gene, *SRSF2 P95L*, in MDS-patient-derived iPSCs together with del7q and showed proof of principle of the usefulness of iPSC modeling to connect specific driver genetic lesions with cellular phenotypes and drug responses, such as sensitivity of SRSF2-mutant iPSC-derived hematopoietic cells to splicing inhibitors (Chang et al. 2018). Studies like this can inform precision medicine approaches, whereas the knowledge of which cellular phenotypes are conferred by a specific mutation (and which are not) can guide assay development for drug testing and drug discovery.

More recently, our group reported a larger collection of iPSC lines derived from patients with low-risk MDS, high-risk MDS, and secondary AML (sAML), one of which also harbored a germline *GATA2* mutation, conferring predisposition to MDS/AML (Kotini et al. 2017). Guided by comprehensive mutational analyses of the starting patient cells and the derived iPSC lines, we assembled a panel of lines capturing the different stages of disease, from familial predisposition to low-risk MDS, high-risk MDS, and sAML. By characterizing their hematopoiesis with a battery of assays, we constructed a framework of cellular phenotypes characterizing the distinct stages of myeloid malignancy from preleukemia to AML through an MDS stage. Using this system and phenotypic map we showed that we can model transitions between stages, including disease progression and reversal, by introducing and correcting, respectively, progression-associated mutations by CRISPR/Cas9. We also uncovered potential disease stage-specific effects of 5-azacytidine, a drug used as frontline therapy for MDS. Furthermore, transcriptome analyses of iPSC-derived CD34$^+$ hematopoietic progenitors of all stages revealed gene expression signatures associated with disease progression and enrichment for gene sets derived from primary AML patient cells. Surprisingly, given the inability of iPSC-derived hematopoiesis to engraft in immunodeficient mice, we found that AML-iPSC-derived hematopoietic cells robustly engrafted into NSG mice via intravenous injection, giving rise to a serially transplantable lethal myeloid leukemia. Similar findings were reported at the same time by the group of Ravi Majeti, who derived iPSCs from patients with MLL-translocated AML (Chao et al. 2017). This study also reported serial engraftment of AML-iPSC-derived hematopoietic cells administered intravenously, as well as orthotopically into NSG mice harboring human ossicles that mimic a humanized hematopoietic niche (Reinisch et al. 2016). This study additionally demonstrated, through detailed transcriptome and DNA methylation analyses, that AML-associated epigenetic changes were erased upon reprogramming, as AML-iPSCs were very similar to normal control iPSCs and clearly distinct from primary AML cells. Consistent with this, AML-iPSCs were able to differentiate into tissues of all germ layers without overt signs of malignancy in vitro and in teratomas. However, in stark contrast, their hematopoietic progeny were similar to primary AML blasts in their gene expression and DNA methylation patterns, consistent with reacquisition of phenotypic leukemic features in vitro and in vivo. No evidence of "epigenetic memory" of leukemia was found in the undifferentiated AML-iPSCs, suggesting that the reestablishment of leukemia was exclusively driven by the AML genetic lesion (MLL rearrangement) in conjunction with the acquisition of the correct cellular identity. The aforementioned studies thus uniquely highlight the sufficiency of genetic lesions for leukemia establishment on one hand and the importance of the appropriate cellular context for leukemic properties to manifest on the other (Fig. 3). In both studies, iPSCs could be derived both from major AML clones and subclones with KRAS mutations. These iPSCs shared all other leukemia-associated genetic lesions except for the KRAS mutation, highlighting the opportunities that iPSC modeling presents to isolate clones and study their properties and differential drug susceptibilities.

In contrast to myeloid malignancies, no studies of iPSC modeling of lymphoid leukemias or lymphomas have been reported to date. Although it is possible that lymphoid blasts are even harder to reprogram than myeloid blasts, the scarcity of such studies likely also reflects the challenges in the derivation of lymphoid lineages through directed in vitro differentiation of hPSCs (Muñoz-López et al. 2016; Montel-Hagen and Crooks 2019a). Of note, a recent study used gene targeting of normal human iPSCs to model childhood acute B-lymphoblastic leukemia har-

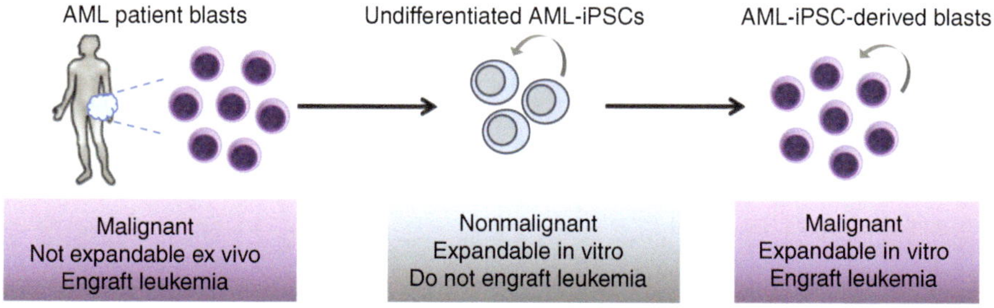

Figure 3. Induced pluripotent stem cells (iPSCs) derived from acute myeloid leukemia (AML) patients. AML-iPSCs do not exhibit malignant features at the undifferentiated pluripotent state, but only once they are differentiated along the hematopoietic lineage. Unlike primary AML blasts that have limited growth potential in vitro, iPSC-derived blasts can be extensively, potentially indefinitely, expanded in culture.

boring the ETV6-RUNX1 translocation (Böiers et al. 2018). The authors first characterized B lymphoid development in first-trimester human embryos and provided evidence of an IL-7R$^+$ progenitor cell population. They next showed that hPSCs recapitulate this developmental transition and that ETV6-RUNX1 expression specifically affects it, causing expansion of the IL-7R$^+$ progenitor compartment, block of B lineage commitment, and aberrant myeloid gene expression signatures in pro-B cells. These findings support the idea that ETV6-RUNX1 targets a specific susceptible progenitor cell type that is uniquely present in embryonic and fetal life for preleukemic initiation, which can explain why ETV6-RUNX1 translocations are rarely found in adult acute lymphoblastic leukemia (ALL).

Familial forms of predisposition to MDS/AML caused by inherited mutations have also been modeled in iPSCs. Our group described subtle phenotypic changes consistent with a preleukemic state in iPSC-derived hematopoietic cells from a patient with a germline *GATA2* mutation and modeled progression to low-risk or high-risk MDS by engineering additional genetic lesions that frequently occur in AML arising on the grounds of inherited *GATA2* deficiency—namely, mutational inactivation of the second *GATA2* allele and del7q (Kotini et al. 2017). Familial platelet disorder (FPD), caused by germline mutations of *RUNX1* and characterized by thrombocytopenia, platelet dysfunction, and predisposition to MDS/AML, has been modeled with iPSCs by several groups (Connelly et al. 2014; Sakurai et al. 2014; Antony-Debre et al. 2015; Iizuka et al. 2015). A study using iPSCs from different FPD pedigrees showed that RUNX1 haploinsufficiency causes only megakaryocytic defects, whereas dominant negative mutations confer additional phenotypic changes, supporting the idea that only the latter confer risk of leukemia progression (Antony-Debre et al. 2015). iPSC models of several inherited BM failure syndromes, which are often accompanied by predisposition to leukemia development, have been created, including Fanconi anemia, Shwachman–Diamond syndrome, Diamond–Blackfan anemia, dyskeratosis congenita, and severe congenital neutropenia. These studies mostly focused on modeling gene correction strategies and providing proof of principle of rescue of disease-relevant phenotypes by gene therapy rather than on the propensity to malignancy and have been reviewed elsewhere (Georgomanoli and Papapetrou 2019).

NEW OPPORTUNITIES AFFORDED BY iPSCs FOR THE STUDY OF LEUKEMIA BIOLOGY AND PRECLINICAL RESEARCH

Arguably the most appealing property of iPSC modeling for hematologic malignancies is the possibility to create precise genetic models. The capturing of intact human leukemic genomes enables modeling of disease-driving mutations and other genetic lesions in their native genomic context, in the appropriate cellular setting, following differentiation to the desired cell type, and in isogenic conditions. This can be particularly valuable in instances of mutations in genes whose functions are not well conserved among species or for the modeling of large-scale structural abnormalities, such as translocations, large chromosomal deletions, trisomies, or complex karyotypes that cannot be easily engineered or modeled in the mouse because of synteny issues (Kotini et al. 2015). A wealth of information on recurrent gene mutations in MDS and AML has become available in recent years, and currently no good models exist for several of them. Conventional immortalized cell lines (ICLs) with mutations such as *IDH1* and *IDH2* are lacking. Similarly, there are no hematopoietic cell lines with splicing factor mutations. Although ectopic expression of mutant genes or in situ introduction of mutations in the endogenous locus through CRISPR is often used, these approaches still suffer from uncontrolled levels of expression and stoichiometry imbalances, as most ICLs are aneuploid and contain variable numbers of copies of most endogenous genes. Altered stoichiometry and levels of expression of splicing factors can artificially affect their RNA-binding properties. Furthermore, alternative splicing and intronic sequences are not well conserved between mouse and human. Thus, the modeling of splicing factor mutations and other heterozygous hotspot mutations in iPSCs, through reprogramming or gene editing, can provide a physiological genomic context to study their downstream effects (Chang et al. 2018). Finally, the reprogramming of entire leukemic genomes offers the opportunity to capture the patient's genetic background including any inherited variation and other unknown mutations or polymorphisms that may modify the phenotype or disease risk (Kilpivaara et al. 2009).

Reprogramming technology also presents exciting opportunities to study the relative contribution of genetic and epigenetic factors in leukemogenesis. The studies of AML-iPSCs, discussed above, clearly established the requirement for an interplay between the leukemia genome and an appropriate cellular milieu (Chao et al. 2017; Kotini et al. 2017). They also showed that a leukemia genome is sufficient to establish leukemia in the correct cell type, as reprogramming erases all preexisting leukemic epigenetic alterations (Chao et al. 2017). Furthermore, these studies showed that AML-iPSC-derived blasts can model at least to some extent the transcriptome and epigenome of primary cells, as signatures shared with primary AML were found. However, more detailed comparisons between equivalent populations of iPSC-derived and primary AML blasts are required to understand how faithfully the former recapitulate the chromatin and gene expression landscape of the latter. Also, although current evidence suggests that epigenetic changes that are genetically determined by mutations in epigenetic modifiers (e.g., *TET2*, *DNMT3A*, *ASXL1*, *EZH2*, and others) should be reestablished in iPSCs upon differentiation, formal demonstration is still missing. The finding that, in contrast to AML-iPSCs, CML-iPSCs do not exhibit overt leukemic features upon differentiation is puzzling and may reflect a requirement for a specific cell type (e.g., HSCs) that was not produced in the differentiation cultures (Amabile et al. 2015). This may provide an example of how reprogramming could be used to determine the cell of origin of specific leukemias and to investigate the cell type requirements of cancers more broadly. iPSC models of familial cancer forms with different tissue preponderance may prove particularly useful for this (Lee et al. 2015).

iPSCs offer unique opportunities to model disease progression and clonal evolution of malignancy. Reprogramming can be performed in clonal conditions and often favors normal or premalignant over malignant cells (Kotini et al. 2017). Thus, unlike ICLs that can only be derived from malignant cells, iPSCs can be derived from normal and preleukemic cells harboring initiating mutations without the full set of late mutations. Additionally, the ease of stepwise addition of targeted mutations by CRISPR and the recent wealth of information on patterns of mutational cooperation open the possibility of modeling clonal evolution through synthetic biology approaches (Papaemmanuil et al. 2016).

One of the most highly advertised uses of iPSC technology from the outset was its use in drug testing and screening. Responses to DOT1L inhibitors in MLL-rearranged AML, to rigosertib and MEK inhibitors in the context of AML with KRAS mutations, and to splicing modulators in SRSF2-mutant MDS have been modeled in iPSC-derived cells, with cytotoxicity as the main readout (Chao et al. 2017; Kotini et al. 2017; Chang et al. 2018). Efforts to model drug resistance to imatinib in CML and to cytarabine-based chemotherapy in AML have also been reported (Chao et al. 2017; Miyauchi et al. 2018). Because they provide a theoretically unlimited source of cells, iPSC models can be used to develop platforms for high-throughput small-molecule screens. Additionally, they offer the possibility to perform phenotype-driven screens in cases in which there are no known targets, empowered by the availability of isogenic normal controls (Chang et al. 2018). Current work on drug screening in iPSC hematopoietic derivatives has not yet moved past proof-of-principle studies and is limited by scalability, as will be further discussed below.

COMPARISON TO OTHER PATIENT-DERIVED MODELS (IMMORTALIZED CELL LINES, PATIENT-DERIVED XENOGRAFTS)

Once established, iPSC lines can be expanded indefinitely at the pluripotent state, cryopreserved, and shared with other investigators. Thus, iPSC modeling enables experimentation with patient-derived material that, in contrast to primary cells, is unlimited, allowing for robust and well-controlled experiments that were hitherto only possible with ICLs. However, iPSCs are fundamentally different than ICLs. iPSCs are maintained in a self-renewing state by a pluripotency gene network that is self-sustaining and that, although some of its components may be shared with cancer, is clearly distinct from oncogenic signaling that maintains ICLs, which are dependent on strong viral or cellular oncogenes. iPSCs maintain normal diploid karyotypes and are genetically more stable than ICLs, which are typically aneuploid. As mentioned above, unlike ICLs that can only be derived from fully transformed cells and typically aggressive cancers, iPSCs can be derived from normal and premalignant cells. Although acquisition of genetic lesions over time is a problem with all cultured cells, measures for its mitigation are much more readily applied in iPSC research. The stem cell community is more aware of the risks of genetic diversification of cultured lines and their monitoring is a routine practice, whereas passage number is almost never tracked or reported in studies using ICLs. Aneuploid status and copy-number variation, present even among individual cells within the same ICL, can pose problems with modeling leukemia-associated mutations. Furthermore, copy-number aberrations may confound the results of CRISPR screens, as multiple Cas9-mediated DNA breaks can impair cell proliferation in a gene-independent manner, a phenomenon referred to as the CRISPR copy-number effect. While the argument can be made that iPSCs could replace ICLs in many applications, the latter are still popular because of low cost and ease of use. Generation of iPSC-derived expandable progenitor cell lines, further discussed later, may overcome most of the practical obstacles to the broader use of iPSCs.

iPSCs can be derived from leukemia cells passaged through xenotransplantation and, conversely, hematopoietic cells derived from AML-iPSCs can generate xenografts. Such "secondary" patient-derived xenografts (PDXs) can offer opportunities not afforded by primary PDXs—namely, the generation of clonal PDX models devoid of genetic drifts and amenable to extensive genetic manipulations prior to transplantation. For other applications (e.g., use as patient-specific models or avatars) in which capturing the genetic and epigenetic heterogeneity of the primary AML is desirable, primary PDXs may be preferable. Finally, how epigenetically similar iPSC xenografts are to primary PDXs and to primary AML cells is yet unknown. iPSC xenografts should thus be more valuable for genotype-to-phenotype studies, for which similarity to primary tumor is less relevant than the faithful representation of genotypes in the correct genomic environment.

MISCONCEPTIONS AND TRUE LIMITATIONS OF iPSC MODELS

As experience with iPSC modeling is building, some misconceptions are still plaguing the field, whereas important current limitations of the approach provide opportunities for future improvements.

Genetic Stability of iPSC Lines

Early studies reported a high degree of chromosome aberrations, copy-number variation, and point mutations in iPSCs and stirred serious concerns that reprogrammed cells accumulate multiple abnormalities at the chromosomal, subchromosomal, and single-base level (Mayshar et al. 2010; Gore et al. 2011; Hussein et al. 2011; Laurent et al. 2011). Subsequent studies revealed that the majority of these genetic variants are preexistent in the starting somatic cells (Abyzov et al. 2012; Cheng et al. 2012; Young et al. 2012). Numerous other studies have now established that reprogramming in itself is not mutagenic and that iPSCs are not inherently genetically unstable, as they acquire mutations during expansion in culture or during differentiation at a rate similar to that of normal adult somatic cells and consistent with spontaneous mutation acquisition rates during cell division (Cheng et al. 2012; Liang and Zhang 2013; Peterson and Loring 2014; Tapia and Schöler 2016). However, several real issues remain and need to be considered in iPSC experiments. First, reprogramming can cause "founder effects," akin to those in ICLs and other patient-derived models, by selecting for rare cells of the starting population. This can skew the representation of the primary tumor and may even select for "ultrafit" clones—for example, cells with epigenetic inactivation of *TP53*. Second, mutations will always accumulate with increased passage. Importantly, the selection forces driving genetic evolution in culture, as well as in PDX models, seem to be different than those acting in patients, leading to increased genomic divergence between the models and the primary leukemia over time (Hussein et al. 2011; Ben-David et al. 2017, 2018). In particular, aneuploidies and copy-number alterations tend to disappear in iPSCs and other models over time. In our study, we observed a growth disadvantage and strong selection pressure for correction of chr7q dosage in del7q MDS-iPSC lines over increasing passage, whereas del7q cells presumably have a selection advantage in the in vivo patient setting (Kotini et al. 2015). Third, while normal iPSCs are not more unstable than any other cell type, cancer driving mutations may involve genes regulating genome integrity and may impact genomic stability. Importantly, as further discussed below, with awareness and adherence to good laboratory practices most of these issues can be resolved.

Developmental Stage of hPSC-Derived Hematopoiesis and Its Impact on Disease Modeling

iPSC differentiation to desired cell types mimics development, and this has severe implications for disease modeling. First, developmental phenotypes may confound disease-relevant phenotypes. For example, some recurrent MDS and AML mutations, such as *GATA2*, *RUNX1*, and others, affect genes with important roles in the development of the hematopoietic system and may block the differentiation of iPSCs at early stages. For example, *RUNX1* mutations may impair or abolish the generation of HPCs from hemogenic endothelium (HE). This problem is analogous to the problem of embryonic lethality in knockout mouse models and, similarly, it could be overcome by engineering conditional alleles. Second, as discussed above, current protocols yield developmentally immature and mixed cells. Despite this, it is encouraging that several studies have shown that disease-relevant phenotypes—such as low clonogenicity, reduced proliferation, and increased apoptosis in MDS; cytokine independency in MPN; and differentiation block and increased self-renewal in AML—can be recapitulated in iPSC models (Ye et al. 2014; Kotini et al. 2015, 2017; Chao et al. 2017; Chang et al. 2018). Developmental immaturity may pose more of a problem for modeling disease features critically dependent on aging. Artificial induction of aging in iPSCs through expression of progerin could be used to reveal age-related disease manifestations (Miller et al. 2013). Most crucially, better protocols that can specify adult-type hematopoiesis exclusively or at least temporally separated from earlier waves and/or markers for purification of the former are needed. To this end, protocols that early on induce the right type of mesoderm and HE with potential for adult-type hematopoiesis will need to be devised (Kennedy et al. 2012; Sturgeon et al. 2014; Ditadi et al. 2015; Guibentif et al. 2017).

Line-to-Line Variation

Reports of large variability in differentiation propensity and phenotypes among diverse normal iPSC lines have spurred concerns over the robustness of iPSC modeling in general. Given that humans are genetically very diverse, it is hardly a surprise that most of the variation in phenotypes, differentiation propensity, gene expression, DNA methylation, and epigenetic marks has now been attributed to differences in genetic background (Kyttälä et al. 2016; DeBoever et al. 2017; Kilpinen et al. 2017; Pashos et al. 2017). Variation among genetically matched iPSC lines can also be present because of epigenetic differences established and fixed upon reprogramming (Liang and Zhang 2013). These can be further exacerbated if differentiation protocols and assays for readouts allow for a high degree of noise. Because such noise may be mistaken as disease-specific phenotypes, it is imperative that the variation of the differentiation procedure or phenotypic assay used

 Cite this article as *Cold Spring Harb Perspect Med* doi: 10.1101/cshperspect.a034868

does not exceed the effect size of the reported disease-relevant phenotype. The former can be measured by estimating the variance in the phenotypic measures among independent differentiations of the same iPSC line and among different lines of the same genotype and comparing it to the phenotypic difference between normal and disease lines (Kotini et al. 2015).

AREAS FOR IMPROVEMENT

Good Practices

Important in all areas of research, good practices are particularly critical in hPSC research and, consequently, stem cell researchers are typically alert to factors that can compromise their results and ways to mitigate the risks. Genetic diversification caused by selection imposed by culture conditions or genetic drifts can be detected by frequent karyotyping and periodic authentication of iPSC lines by DNA fingerprinting and mutational status of known mutations and prevented by routine tracking and reporting of passage number, cryopreservation, and storage of large stocks of early passage lines. Also, maintaining cultured lines at a low passage number, performing experiments of one entire study with cells at similar passage number, and avoiding unnecessary passaging and introduction of bottlenecks, such as multiple freeze–thaw cycles, extreme cell number reductions during passaging, and unnecessary subcloning, are advisable. Bottlenecks cannot be altogether avoided—for example, those imposed during initial line establishment or during genetic engineering (antibiotic selection, single-cell cloning)—and are a feature of all cancer models, including ICLs, PDXs, and organoid cultures (Ben-David et al. 2019). iPSCs offer the advantage of indefinite expansion, allowing for any inadvertent genetic changes to be traced back in time and "corrected" by retrieval of earlier passage stocks. Additional good practices include maintaining standardized cell culture conditions to decrease selection pressure, regular testing for mycoplasma contamination status, and alertness to any abrupt phenotypic changes in division time, morphological features, or any phenotype. Any such changes should be readily investigated as they often indicate underlying genetic changes. For example, our discovery of spontaneously corrected del7q MDS-iPSC clones was prompted by the observation of phenotypic rescue of hematopoiesis in the corrected clones (Kotini et al. 2015). Finally, the opportunity to have tailored control lines presents an important asset of iPSC modeling that should be harnessed (Fig. 2). Using multiple genetically identical and independently propagated lines, which can be relatively easily generated in one round of reprogramming or gene editing, can solve most issues of reproducibility arising from genetic divergence.

Future Advances

Three significant current barriers to iPSC modeling of blood cancers present opportunities for future advances.

Generation of Expandable HPCs (eHPCs)

Currently, iPSC models remain inaccessible to most of the hematology community because of a lack of hPSC culture and differentiation expertise, which are both quite laborious and costly processes. One way by which this could be sidestepped is the generation of iPSC-derived eHPCs (i.e., HPCs that can be maintained in a self-renewing state), thus bypassing the hPSC culture and differentiation steps. These eHPCs could be passaged as simple suspension cultures in media and conditions akin to those used for conventional ICLs, expanded extensively or even indefinitely, cryopreserved, and terminally differentiated on demand, while preserving all or most of their mutation-specific characteristics.

Doulatov et al. discovered five factors (HOXA9, ERG, RORA, SOX4, and MYB) that could maintain eHPCs. Discontinuation of factor expression through doxycycline withdrawal enabled differentiation along the myeloid and erythroid lineage (Doulatov et al. 2013). Furthermore, these progenitors could give rise to short-term myeloerythroid engraftment in immunocompromised mice. More recently, our group showed that a combination of 13 factors can maintain $CD34^{+}/CD45^{+}$ eHPCs long-term in vitro (Chang et al. 2018). Apart from opening up iPSC modeling to the broader community, eHPC approaches can also, very importantly, overcome limits of scale of hematopoietic differentiation and dramatically increase the throughput of assays made possible. The latter can include biochemical assays requiring large cell numbers, proteomics, and high-throughput small-molecule or genetic (e.g., CRISPR-based) synthetic lethality screens to identify therapeutic targets. For example, five-factor eHPCs derived from iPSC models of DBA enabled an unbiased chemical screen, which would not have been possible otherwise, and led to the discovery of a new small molecule stimulating erythropoiesis through induction of autophagy (Doulatov et al. 2017).

Generation of Transplantable HSCs

Although hematopoietic cells from AML-iPSCs from two different AML genotypes (MLL-rearranged and del7q) were shown to engraft in immunodeficient mice, it is currently unclear if this is a generalizable property of all AML-iPSCs. Furthermore, hematopoietic cells from CML, MDS, and normal iPSCs clearly do not engraft (Amabile et al. 2015; Chao et al. 2017; Kotini et al. 2017). This limitation, which might be at least in part a result of the developmental immaturity of hPSC-derived hematopoiesis, discussed earlier, restricts experimentation in the in vivo setting. The limited success in establishing differentiation conditions to generate engraftable hematopoiesis by many investigators over two decades has been reviewed elsewhere (Vo and Daley 2015; Rowe et al. 2016; Wahlster and Daley 2016). More recently, the Daley laboratory accomplished long-term multilineage engraftment of iPSC-derived cells, albeit at relatively modest efficiency, by forced expression of seven transcription factors (ERG, HOXA5, HOXA9, HOXA10, LCOR, RUNX1, and SPI1) (Sugimura et al. 2017).

Incorporation of Microenvironment Components and Three-Dimensional Cultures

iPSCs mainly read cellular phenotypes and do not capture nongenetic and non-cell-autonomous features of disease. Thus, future enhancements to the capabilities of the system could include cocultures with other cell types of the BM niche, such as stromal and endothelial cells. The latter could be sourced from primary cultures, autologous or allogeneic, or differentiated from iPSCs. Such cultures could be valuable to, for example, model clonal advantage conferred by specific CH- and MDS- associated mutations, which is currently not captured in vitro. For example, cells with isolated del7q or splicing factor mutations, in the absence of mutations driving overt AML, exhibit a growth disadvantage in vitro, although they clonally expand in vivo (Kotini et al. 2015, 2017; Chang et al. 2018). This discrepancy is likely a result of the in vitro conditions, as primary MDS cells also grow poorly ex vivo and ICLs with splicing factor mutations have slower division rates than wild-type cells. Culture conditions better mimicking an in vivo environment with presumably different selection pressures could enable better modeling of clonal dynamics and other disease phenotypes that are dependent on interaction with other cell types and extracellular components. 3D cultures could further enhance the capabilities of iPSC models, for example, by promoting developmental maturation and more faithful establishment of epigenetic disease components. Although the importance of 3D organoid-type cultures may be lesser for liquid tumors than solid tumors, they may enable modeling of lymphoid malignancies in the future—for example, by tissue engineering approaches recapitulating germinal center-like structures and thymic organoids to allow positive selection and maturation of T cells (Parent et al. 2013; Sun et al. 2013; Montel-Hagen et al. 2019b; Rowe and Daley 2019).

CONCLUDING REMARKS

Recent studies indicate that leukemia research can benefit tremendously from iPSC technology. Cultural aspects of hematology, like a long tradition of banking and making good use of patient material and, consequently, the size and breadth of tissue banks already in place, render iPSC modeling all the more appealing for this discipline. iPSC modeling is still a young field, and although experience is building, misconceptions are also lingering. Like all models, iPSCs have limitations, but also unique strengths. Being human models, the findings made with them can be anticipated to better translate to the clinic. As patient-derived models, iPSCs can engage in a back and forth with primary cells (i.e., hypotheses generated from clinical observations can be tested in iPSCs and findings in iPSCs can be validated in primary cells from the same patient). Because iPSCs can faithfully model human genomes, large biobanks representative of all major genetic groups and specific genotypes of blood cancers can be envisioned. These can uniquely support genotype-to-phenotype studies, target identification and validation, drug testing, screening and repurposing, and toxicity testing. Moving on from 2D single-lineage cultures to 3D and in vivo systems, capturing tissue and organ level phenotypes, in the future, can bring on the best of both worlds. In a balancing act amid doomsday scenarios and extreme hype, today iPSC technology is moving steadily toward fulfilling its promise to revolutionize the study of human physiology and disease pathogenesis.

ACKNOWLEDGMENTS

This work was supported by the National Institutes of Health (NIH) Grants Nos. R01HL121570, R01HL137219, R01HL132071, and R01CA225231, by grants from the Edward P. Evans Foundation, the New York State Stem Cell Board, the Henry and Marilyn Taub Foundation, the Alex's Lemonade Stand Foundation, and the RUNX1 research program; by a Pershing Square Sohn Prize from the Pershing Square Sohn Cancer Research Alliance; and by a Leukemia and Lymphoma Society Scholar award.

REFERENCES

Abyzov A, Mariani J, Palejev D, Zhang Y, Haney MS, Tomasini L, Ferrandino AF, Rosenberg Belmaker LA, Szekely A, Wilson M, et al. 2012. Somatic copy number mosaicism in human skin revealed by induced pluripotent stem cells. *Nature* **492:** 438–442. doi:10.1038/nature11629

Amabile G, Di Ruscio A, Müller F, Welner RS, Yang H, Ebralidze AK, Zhang H, Levantini E, Qi L, Martinelli G, et al. 2015. Dissecting the role of aberrant DNA methylation in human leukaemia. *Nat Commun* **6:** 7091. doi:10.1038/ncomms8091

Antony-Debre I, Manchev VT, Balayn N, Bluteau D, Tomowiak C, Legrand C, Langlois T, Bawa O, Tosca L, Tachdjian G, et al. 2015. Level of RUNX1 activity is critical for leukemic predisposition but not for thrombocytopenia. *Blood* **125:** 930–940. doi:10.1182/blood-2014-06-585513

Apostolou E, Stadtfeld M. 2018. Cellular trajectories and molecular mechanisms of iPSC reprogramming. *Curr Opin Genet Dev* **52:** 77–85. doi:10.1016/j.gde.2018.06.002

Banito A, Rashid ST, Acosta JC, Li S, Pereira CF, Geti I, Pinho S, Silva JC, Azuara V, Walsh M, et al. 2009. Senescence impairs successful reprogramming to pluripotent stem cells. *Genes Dev* **23:** 2134–2139. doi:10.1101/gad.1811609

Bedel A, Pasquet JM, Lippert E, Taillepierre M, Lagarde V, Dabernat S, Dubus P, Charaf L, Beliveau F, de Verneuil H, et al. 2013. Variable behavior of iPSCs derived from CML patients for response to TKI and hematopoietic differentiation. *PLoS ONE* **8:** e71596. doi:10.1371/journal.pone.0071596

Ben-David U, Ha G, Tseng YY, Greenwald NF, Oh C, Shih J, McFarland JM, Wong B, Boehm JS, Beroukhim R, et al. 2017. Patient-derived xenografts undergo mouse-specific tumor evolution. *Nat Genet* **49:** 1567–1575. doi:10.1038/ng.3967

Ben-David U, Siranosian B, Ha G, Tang H, Oren Y, Hinohara K, Strathdee CA, Dempster J, Lyons NJ, Burns R, et al. 2018. Genetic and transcriptional evolution alters cancer cell line drug response. *Nature* **560:** 325–330. doi:10.1038/s41586-018-0409-3

Ben-David U, Beroukhim R, Golub TR. 2019. Genomic evolution of cancer models: Perils and opportunities. *Nat Rev Cancer* **19:** 97–109. doi:10.1038/s41568-018-0095-3

Böiers C, Richardson SE, Laycock E, Zriwil A, Turati VA, Brown J, Wray JP, Wang D, James C, Herrero J, et al. 2018. A human IPS model implicates embryonic B-myeloid fate restriction as developmental susceptibility to B acute lymphoblastic leukemia-associated ETV6-RUNX1. *Dev Cell* **44:** 362–377.e7. doi:10.1016/j.devcel.2017.12.005

Brennand KJ, Simone A, Jou J, Gelboin-Burkhart C, Tran N, Sangar S, Li Y, Mu Y, Chen G, Yu D, et al. 2011. Modelling schizophrenia using human induced pluripotent stem cells. *Nature* **473:** 221–225. doi:10.1038/nature09915

Carette JE, Pruszak J, Varadarajan M, Blomen VA, Gokhale S, Camargo FD, Wernig M, Jaenisch R, Brummelkamp TR. 2010. Generation of iPSCs from cultured human malignant cells. *Blood* **115:** 4039–4042. doi:10.1182/blood-2009-07-231845

Chang CJ, Kotini AG, Olszewska M, Georgomanoli M, Teruya-Feldstein J, Sperber H, Sanchez R, DeVita R, Martins TJ, Abdel-Wahab O, et al. 2018. Dissecting the contributions of cooperating gene mutations to cancer phenotypes and drug responses with patient-derived iPSCs. *Stem Cell Reports* **10:** 1610–1624. doi:10.1016/j.stemcr.2018.03.020

Chao MP, Gentles AJ, Chatterjee S, Lan F, Reinisch A, Corces MR, Xavy S, Shen J, Haag D, Chanda S, et al. 2017. Human AML-iPSCs reacquire leukemic properties after differentiation and model clonal variation of disease. *Cell Stem Cell* **20:** 329–344.e7. doi:10.1016/j.stem.2016.11.018

Cheng L, Hansen NF, Zhao L, Du Y, Zou C, Donovan FX, Chou BK, Zhou G, Li S, Dowey SN, et al. 2012. Low incidence of DNA sequence variation in human induced pluripotent stem cells generated by nonintegrating plasmid expression. *Cell Stem Cell* **10:** 337–344. doi:10.1016/j.stem.2012.01.005

Choi KD, Vodyanik MA, Togarrati PP, Suknuntha K, Kumar A, Samarjeet F, Probasco MD, Tian S, Stewart R, Thomson JA, et al. 2012. Identification of the hemogenic endothelial progenitor and its direct precursor in human pluripotent stem cell differentiation cultures. *Cell Rep* **2:** 553–567. doi:10.1016/j.celrep.2012.08.002

Connelly JP, Kwon EM, Gao Y, Trivedi NS, Elkahloun AG, Horwitz MS, Cheng L, Liu PP. 2014. Targeted correction of RUNX1 mutation in FPD patient-specific induced pluripotent stem cells rescues megakaryopoietic defects. *Blood* **124:** 1926–1930. doi:10.1182/blood-2014-01-550525

DeBoever C, Li H, Jakubosky D, Benaglio P, Reyna J, Olson KM, Huang H, Biggs W, Sandoval E, D'Antonio M, et al. 2017. Large-scale profiling reveals the influence of genetic variation on gene expression in human induced pluripotent stem cells. *Cell Stem Cell* **20:** 533–546e7. doi:10.1016/j.stem.2017.03.009

Ditadi A, Sturgeon CM, Tober J, Awong G, Kennedy M, Yzaguirre AD, Azzola L, Ng ES, Stanley EG, French DL, et al. 2015. Human definitive haemogenic endothelium and arterial vascular endothelium represent distinct lineages. *Nat Cell Biol* **17:** 580–591. doi:10.1038/ncb3161

Doulatov S, Vo LT, Chou SS, Kim PG, Arora N, Li H, Hadland BK, Bernstein ID, Collins JJ, Zon LI, et al. 2013. Induction of multipotential hematopoietic progenitors from human pluripotent stem cells via respecification of lineage-restricted precursors. *Cell Stem Cell* **13:** 459–470. doi:10.1016/j.stem.2013.09.002

Doulatov S, Vo LT, Macari ER, Wahlster L, Kinney MA, Taylor AM, Barragan J, Gupta M, McGrath K, Lee HY, et al. 2017. Drug discovery for Diamond-Blackfan anemia using reprogrammed hematopoietic progenitors. *Sci Transl Med* **9:** aah5645. doi:10.1126/scitranslmed.aah5645

Figueroa ME, Lugthart S, Li Y, Erpelinck-Verschueren C, Deng X, Christos PJ, Schifano E, Booth J, van Putten W, Skrabanek L, et al. 2010. DNA methylation signatures identify biologically distinct subtypes in acute myeloid leukemia. *Cancer Cell* **17:** 13–27. doi:10.1016/j.ccr.2009.11.020

Frame JM, McGrath KE, Palis J. 2013. Erythro-myeloid progenitors: "Definitive" hematopoiesis in the conceptus prior to the emergence of hematopoietic stem cells. *Blood Cells Mol Dis* **51:** 220–225. doi:10.1016/j.bcmd.2013.09.006

Gagne AL, Maguire JA, Gandre-Babbe S, Chou ST, Tasian SK, Loh ML, Weiss MJ, Gadue P, French DL. 2018. Generation of a human Juvenile myelomonocytic leukemia iPSC line, CHOPi001-A, with a mutation in CBL. *Stem Cell Res* **31:** 157–160. doi:10.1016/j.scr.2018.07.001

Gandre-Babbe S, Paluru P, Aribeana C, Chou ST, Bresolin S, Lu L, Sullivan SK, Tasian SK, Weng J, Favre H, et al. 2013. Patient-derived induced pluripotent stem cells recapitulate hematopoietic abnormalities of juvenile myelomonocytic leukemia. *Blood* **121:** 4925–4929. doi:10.1182/blood-2013-01-478412

Georgomanoli M, Papapetrou EP. 2019. Modeling blood diseases with human induced pluripotent stem cells. *Dis Model Mech* **12:** dmm039321. doi:10.1242/dmm.039321

Gomez Limia CE, Devalle S, Reis M, Sochacki J, Carneiro M, Madeiro da Costa R, D'Andrea M, Padilha T, Zalcberg IR, Solza C, et al. 2017. Generation and characterization of a human induced pluripotent stem (iPS) cell line derived from an acute myeloid leukemia patient evolving from primary myelofibrosis carrying the CALR 52 bp deletion and the ASXL1 p.R693X mutation. *Stem Cell Res* **24:** 16–20. doi:10.1016/j.scr.2017.08.006

Gore A, Li Z, Fung HL, Young JE, Agarwal S, Antosiewicz-Bourget J, Canto I, Giorgetti A, Israel MA, Kiskinis E, et al. 2011. Somatic coding mutations in human induced pluripotent stem cells. *Nature* **471:** 63–67. doi:10.1038/nature09805

Guibentif C, Rönn RE, Böiers C, Lang S, Saxena S, Soneji S, Enver T, Karlsson G, Woods NB. 2017. Single-cell analysis identifies distinct stages of human endothelial-to-hematopoietic transition. *Cell Rep* **19:** 10–19. doi:10.1016/j.celrep.2017.03.023

Guo S, Zi X, Schulz VP, Cheng J, Zhong M, Koochaki SH, Megyola CM, Pan X, Heydari K, Weissman SM, et al. 2014. Nonstochastic reprogramming from a privileged somatic cell state. *Cell* **156:** 649–662. doi:10.1016/j.cell.2014.01.020

Hanna J, Wernig M, Markoulaki S, Sun CW, Meissner A, Cassady JP, Beard C, Brambrink T, Wu LC, Townes TM, et al. 2007. Treatment of sickle cell anemia mouse model with iPS cells generated from autologous skin. *Science* **318:** 1920–1923. doi:10.1126/science.1152092

Hanna J, Saha K, Pando B, van Zon J, Lengner CJ, Creyghton MP, van Oudenaarden A, Jaenisch R. 2009. Direct cell reprogramming is a stochastic process amenable to acceleration. *Nature* **462:** 595–601. doi:10.1038/nature08592

Hockemeyer D, Jaenisch R. 2016. Induced pluripotent stem cells meet genome editing. *Cell Stem Cell* **18:** 573–586. doi:10.1016/j.stem.2016.04.013

Hong H, Takahashi K, Ichisaka T, Aoi T, Kanagawa O, Nakagawa M, Okita K, Yamanaka S. 2009. Suppression of induced pluripotent stem cell generation by the p53-p21 pathway. *Nature* **460:** 1132–1135. doi:10.1038/nature08235

Hosoi M, Kumano K, Taoka K, Arai S, Kataoka K, Ueda K, Kamikubo Y, Takayama N, Otsu M, Eto K, et al. 2014. Generation of induced pluripotent stem cells derived from primary and secondary myelofibrosis patient samples. *Exp Hematol* **42:** 816–825. doi:10.1016/j.exphem.2014.03.010

Hu K, Yu J, Suknuntha K, Tian S, Montgomery K, Choi KD, Stewart R, Thomson JA, Slukvin II. 2011. Efficient generation of transgene-free induced pluripotent stem cells from normal and neoplastic bone marrow and cord blood mononuclear cells. *Blood* **117:** e109–119. doi:10.1182/blood-2010-07-298331

Hussein SM, Batada NN, Vuoristo S, Ching RW, Autio R, Närvä E, Ng S, Sourour M, Hämäläinen R, Olsson C, et al. 2011. Copy number variation and selection during reprogramming to pluripotency. *Nature* **471:** 58–62. doi:10.1038/nature09871

Iizuka H, Kagoya Y, Kataoka K, Yoshimi A, Miyauchi M, Taoka K, Kumano K, Yamamoto T, Hotta A, Arai S, et al. 2015. Targeted gene correction of RUNX1 in induced pluripotent stem cells derived from familial platelet disorder with propensity to myeloid malignancy restores normal megakaryopoiesis. *Exp Hematol* **43:** 849–857. doi:10.1016/j.exphem.2015.05.004

Ivanovs A, Rybtsov S, Ng ES, Stanley EG, Elefanty AG, Medvinsky A. 2017. Human haematopoietic stem cell development: From the embryo to the dish. *Development* **144:** 2323–2337. doi:10.1242/dev.134866

Jan M, Snyder TM, Corces-Zimmerman MR, Vyas P, Weissman IL, Quake SR, Majeti R. 2012. Clonal evolution of preleukemic hematopoietic stem cells precedes human acute myeloid leukemia. *Sci Transl Med* **4:** 149ra118. doi:10.1126/scitranslmed.3004315

Kawamura T, Suzuki J, Wang YV, Menendez S, Morera LB, Raya A, Wahl GM, Izpisua Belmonte JC. 2009. Linking the p53 tumour suppressor pathway to somatic cell reprogramming. *Nature* **460:** 1140–1144. doi:10.1038/nature08311

Kennedy M, Awong G, Sturgeon CM, Ditadi A, LaMotte-Mohs R, Zúñiga-Pflücker JC, Keller G. 2012. T lymphocyte potential marks the emergence of definitive hematopoietic progenitors in human pluripotent stem cell differentiation cultures. *Cell Rep* **2:** 1722–1735. doi:10.1016/j.celrep.2012.11.003

Kent DG, Green AR. 2017. Order matters: The order of somatic mutations influences cancer evolution. *Cold Spring Harb Perspect Med* **7:** a027060. doi:10.1101/cshperspect.a027060

Kilpinen H, Goncalves A, Leha A, Afzal V, Alasoo K, Ashford S, Bala S, Bensaddek D, Casale FP, Culley OJ, et al. 2017. Common genetic variation drives molecular heterogeneity in human iPSCs. *Nature* **546:** 370–375. doi:10.1038/nature22403

Kilpivaara O, Mukherjee S, Schram AM, Wadleigh M, Mullally A, Ebert BL, Bass A, Marubayashi S, Heguy A, Garcia-Manero G, et al. 2009. A germline JAK2 SNP is associated with predisposition to the development of $JAK2^{V617F}$-positive myeloproliferative neoplasms. *Nat Genet* **41:** 455–459. doi:10.1038/ng.342

Kim H, Kim JS. 2014. A guide to genome engineering with programmable nucleases. *Nat Rev Genet* **15:** 321–334. doi:10.1038/nrg3686

Kotini AG, Chang CJ, Boussaad I, Delrow JJ, Dolezal EK, Nagulapally AB, Perna F, Fishbein GA, Klimek VM, Hawkins RD, et al. 2015. Functional analysis of a chromosomal deletion associated with myelodysplastic syndromes using isogenic human induced pluripotent stem cells. *Nat Biotechnol* **33:** 646–655. doi:10.1038/nbt.3178

Kotini AG, Chang CJ, Chow A, Yuan H, Ho TC, Wang T, Vora S, Solovyov A, Husser C, Olszewska M, et al. 2017. Stage-specific human induced pluripotent stem cells map the progression of myeloid transformation to transplantable leukemia. *Cell Stem Cell* **20:** 315–328.e7. doi:10.1016/j.stem.2017.01.009

Kumano K, Arai S, Hosoi M, Taoka K, Takayama N, Otsu M, Nagae G, Ueda K, Nakazaki K, Kamikubo Y, et al. 2012. Generation of induced pluripotent stem cells from primary chronic myelogenous leukemia patient samples. *Blood* **119:** 6234–6242. doi:10.1182/blood-2011-07-367441

Kyttälä A, Moraghebi R, Valensisi C, Kettunen J, Andrus C, Pasumarthy KK, Nakanishi M, Nishimura K, Ohtaka M, Weltner J, et al. 2016. Genetic variability overrides the impact of parental cell type and determines iPSC differentiation potential. *Stem Cell Reports* **6:** 200–212. doi:10.1016/j.stemcr.2015.12.009

Lacaud G, Kouskoff V. 2017. Hemangioblast, hemogenic endothelium, and primitive versus definitive hematopoiesis. *Exp Hematol* **49:** 19–24. doi:10.1016/j.exphem.2016.12.009

Laurent LC, Ulitsky I, Slavin I, Tran H, Schork A, Morey R, Lynch C, Harness JV, Lee S, Barrero MJ, et al. 2011. Dynamic changes in the copy number of pluripotency and cell proliferation genes in human ESCs and iPSCs during reprogramming and time in culture. *Cell Stem Cell* **8:** 106–118. doi:10.1016/j.stem.2010.12.003

Lee G, Papapetrou EP, Kim H, Chambers SM, Tomishima MJ, Fasano CA, Ganat YM, Menon J, Shimizu F, Viale A, et al. 2009. Modelling pathogenesis and treatment of familial dysautonomia using patient-specific iPSCs. *Nature* **461:** 402–406. doi:10.1038/nature08320

Lee G, Ramirez CN, Kim H, Zeltner N, Liu B, Radu C, Bhinder B, Kim YJ, Choi IY, Mukherjee-Clavin B, et al. 2012. Large-scale screening using familial dysautonomia induced pluripotent stem cells identifies compounds that rescue IKBKAP expression. *Nat Biotechnol* **30:** 1244–1248. doi:10.1038/nbt.2435

Lee DF, Su J, Kim HS, Chang B, Papatsenko D, Zhao R, Yuan Y, Gingold J, Xia W, Darr H, et al. 2015. Modeling familial cancer with induced pluripotent stem cells. *Cell* **161:** 240–254. doi:10.1016/j.cell.2015.02.045

Lee JH, Salci KR, Reid JC, Orlando L, Tanasijevic B, Shapovalova Z, Bhatia M. 2017. Brief report: Human acute myeloid leukemia reprogramming to pluripotency is a rare event and selects for patient hematopoietic cells devoid of leukemic mutations. *Stem Cells* **35:** 2095–2102. doi:10.1002/stem.2655

Levine AJ, Jenkins NA, Copeland NG. 2019. The roles of initiating truncal mutations in human cancers: The order of mutations and tumor cell type matters. *Cancer Cell* **35:** 10–15. doi:10.1016/j.ccell.2018.11.009

Li H, Collado M, Villasante A, Strati K, Ortega S, Cañamero M, Blasco MA, Serrano M. 2009. The Ink4/Arf locus is a barrier for iPS cell reprogramming. *Nature* **460:** 1136–1139. doi:10.1038/nature08290

Liang G, Zhang Y. 2013. Genetic and epigenetic variations in iPSCs: Potential causes and implications for application. *Cell Stem Cell* **13:** 149–159. doi:10.1016/j.stem.2013.07.001

Liu S, Ye Z, Gao Y, He C, Williams DW, Moliterno A, Spivak J, Huang H, Cheng L. 2017. Generation of human iPSCs from an essential thrombocythemia patient carrying a V501L mutation in the MPL gene. *Stem Cell Res* **18:** 57–59. doi:10.1016/j.scr.2016.12.012

Marión RM, Strati K, Li H, Murga M, Blanco R, Ortega S, Fernandez-Capetillo O, Serrano M, Blasco MA. 2009. A p53-mediated DNA damage response limits reprogramming to ensure iPS cell genomic integrity. *Nature* **460:** 1149–1153. doi:10.1038/nature08287

Mayshar Y, Ben-David U, Lavon N, Biancotti JC, Yakir B, Clark AT, Plath K, Lowry WE, Benvenisty N. 2010. Identification and classification of chromosomal aberrations in human induced pluripotent stem cells. *Cell Stem Cell* **7:** 521–531. doi:10.1016/j.stem.2010.07.017

Miller JD, Ganat YM, Kishinevsky S, Bowman RL, Liu B, Tu EY, Mandal PK, Vera E, Shim JW, Kriks S, et al. 2013. Human iPSC-based modeling of late-onset disease via progerin-induced aging. *Cell Stem Cell* **13:** 691–705. doi:10.1016/j.stem.2013.11.006

Miyauchi M, Koya J, Arai S, Yamazaki S, Honda A, Kataoka K, Yoshimi A, Taoka K, Kumano K, Kurokawa M. 2018. ADAM8 is an antigen of tyrosine kinase inhibitor-resistant chronic myeloid leukemia cells identified by patient-derived induced pluripotent stem cells. *Stem Cell Reports* **10:** 1115–1130. doi:10.1016/j.stemcr.2018.01.015

Montel-Hagen A, Crooks GM. 2019a. From pluripotent stem cells to T cells. *Exp Hematol* **71:** 24–31. doi:10.1016/j.exphem.2018.12.001

Montel-Hagen A, Seet CS, Li S, Chick B, Zhu Y, Chang P, Tsai S, Sun V, Lopez S, Chen HC, et al. 2019b. Organoid-induced differentiation of conventional T cells from human pluripotent stem cells. *Cell Stem Cell* **24:** 376–389.e8. doi:10.1016/j.stem.2018.12.011

Mulero-Navarro S, Sevilla A, Roman AC, Lee DF, D'Souza SL, Pardo S, Riess I, Su J, Cohen N, Schaniel C, et al. 2015. Myeloid dysregulation in a human induced pluripotent stem cell model of PTPN11-associated juvenile myelomonocytic leukemia. *Cell Rep* **13:** 504–515. doi:10.1016/j.celrep.2015.09.019

Muñoz-López A, Romero-Moya D, Prieto C, Ramos-Mejía V, Agraz-Doblas A, Varela I, Buschbeck M, Palau A, Carvajal-Vergara X, Giorgetti A, et al. 2016. Development refractoriness of MLL-rearranged human B cell acute leukemias to reprogramming into pluripotency. *Stem Cell Reports* **7:** 602–618. doi:10.1016/j.stemcr.2016.08.013

Ortmann CA, Kent DG, Nangalia J, Silber Y, Wedge DC, Grinfeld J, Baxter EJ, Massie CE, Papaemmanuil E, Menon S, et al. 2015. Effect of mutation order on myeloproliferative neoplasms. *N Engl J Med* **372:** 601–612. doi:10.1056/NEJMoa1412098

Papaemmanuil E, Gerstung M, Bullinger L, Gaidzik VI, Paschka P, Roberts ND, Potter NE, Heuser M, Thol F, Bolli N, et al. 2016. Genomic classification and prognosis in acute myeloid leukemia. *N Engl J Med* **374:** 2209–2221. doi:10.1056/NEJMoa1516192

Parent AV, Russ HA, Khan IS, LaFlam TN, Metzger TC, Anderson MS, Hebrok M. 2013. Generation of functional thymic epithelium from human embryonic stem cells that supports host T cell development. *Cell Stem Cell* **13:** 219–229. doi:10.1016/j.stem.2013.04.004

Park IH, Zhao R, West JA, Yabuuchi A, Huo H, Ince TA, Lerou PH, Lensch MW, Daley GQ. 2008. Reprogramming of human somatic cells to pluripotency with defined factors. *Nature* **451:** 141–146. doi:10.1038/nature06534

Pashos EE, Park Y, Wang X, Raghavan A, Yang W, Abbey D, Peters DT, Arbelaez J, Hernandez M, Kuperwasser N, et al. 2017. Large, diverse population cohorts of hiPSCs and derived hepatocyte-like cells reveal functional genetic variation at blood lipid-associated loci. *Cell Stem Cell* **20:** 558–570.e10. doi:10.1016/j.stem.2017.03.017

Pearson S, Cuvertino S, Fleury M, Lacaud G, Kouskoff V. 2015. In vivo repopulating activity emerges at the onset of hematopoietic specification during embryonic stem cell differentiation. *Stem Cell Reports* **4:** 431–444. doi:10.1016/j.stemcr.2015.01.003

Peterson SE, Loring JF. 2014. Genomic instability in pluripotent stem cells: implications for clinical applications. *J Biol Chem* **289:** 4578–4584. doi:10.1074/jbc.R113.516419

Potter DS, Letai A. 2016. To prime, or not to prime: That is the question. *Cold Spring Harb Symp Quant Biol* **81:** 131–140. doi:10.1101/sqb.2016.81.030841

Reinisch A, Thomas D, Corces MR, Zhang X, Gratzinger D, Hong WJ, Schallmoser K, Strunk D, Majeti R. 2016. A humanized bone marrow ossicle xenotransplantation model enables improved engraftment of healthy and leukemic human hematopoietic cells. *Nat Med* **22:** 812–821. doi:10.1038/nm.4103

Rowe RG, Daley GQ. 2019. Induced pluripotent stem cells in disease modelling and drug discovery. *Nat Rev Genet* **20:** 377–388. doi:10.1038/s41576-019-0100-z

Rowe RG, Mandelbaum J, Zon LI, Daley GQ. 2016. Engineering hematopoietic stem cells: Lessons from development. *Cell Stem Cell* **18:** 707–720. doi:10.1016/j.stem.2016.05.016

Ruiz S, Panopoulos AD, Herrerías A, Bissig KD, Lutz M, Berggren WT, Verma IM, Izpisua Belmonte JC. 2011. A high proliferation rate is required for cell reprogramming and maintenance of human embryonic stem cell identity. *Curr Biol* **21:** 45–52. doi:10.1016/j.cub.2010.11.049

Sakurai M, Kunimoto H, Watanabe N, Fukuchi Y, Yuasa S, Yamazaki S, Nishimura T, Sadahira K, Fukuda K, Okano H, et al. 2014. Impaired hematopoietic differentiation of RUNX1-mutated induced pluripotent stem cells derived from FPD/AML patients. *Leukemia* **28:** 2344–2354. doi:10.1038/leu.2014.136

Saliba J, Hamidi S, Lenglet G, Langlois T, Yin J, Cabagnols X, Secardin L, Legrand C, Galy A, Opolon P, et al. 2013. Heterozygous and homozygous $JAK2^{V617F}$ states modeled by induced pluripotent stem cells from myeloproliferative neoplasm patients. *PLoS ONE* **8:** e74257. doi:10.1371/journal.pone.0074257

Sloma I, Mitjavila-Garcia MT, Feraud O, Griscelli F, Oudrhiri N, El Marsafy S, Gobbo E, Divers D, Proust A, Smadja DM, et al. 2017. Whole-genome analysis reveals unexpected dynamics of mutant subclone development in a patient with JAK2-V617F-positive chronic myeloid leukemia. *Exp Hematol* **53:** 48–58. doi:10.1016/j.exphem.2017.05.007

Sturgeon CM, Ditadi A, Awong G, Kennedy M, Keller G. 2014. Wnt signaling controls the specification of definitive and primitive hematopoiesis from human pluripotent stem cells. *Nat Biotechnol* **32:** 554–561. doi:10.1038/nbt.2915

Sugimura R, Jha DK, Han A, Soria-Valles C, da Rocha EL, Lu YF, Goettel JA, Serrao E, Rowe RG, Malleshaiah M, et al. 2017. Haematopoietic stem and progenitor cells from human pluripotent stem cells. *Nature* **545:** 432–438. doi:10.1038/nature22370

Suknuntha K, Ishii Y, Tao L, Hu K, McIntosh BE, Yang D, Swanson S, Stewart R, Wang JYJ, Thomson J, et al. 2015. Discovery of survival factor for primitive chronic myeloid leukemia cells using induced pluripotent stem cells. *Stem Cell Res* **15:** 678–693. doi:10.1016/j.scr.2015.10.015

Sun X, Xu J, Lu H, Liu W, Miao Z, Sui X, Liu H, Su L, Du W, He Q, et al. 2013. Directed differentiation of human embryonic stem cells into thymic epithelial progenitor-like cells reconstitutes the thymic microenvironment in vivo. *Cell Stem Cell* **13:** 230–236. doi:10.1016/j.stem.2013.06.014

Suzuki NM, Niwa A, Yabe M, Hira A, Okada C, Amano N, Watanabe A, Watanabe K, Heike T, Takata M, et al. 2015. Pluripotent cell models of Fanconi anemia identify the early pathological defect in human hemoangiogenic progenitors. *Stem Cells Transl Med* **4:** 333–338. doi:10.5966/sctm.2013-0172

Takahashi K, Tanabe K, Ohnuki M, Narita M, Ichisaka T, Tomoda K, Yamanaka S. 2007. Induction of pluripotent stem cells from adult human fibroblasts by defined factors. *Cell* **131:** 861–872. doi:10.1016/j.cell.2007.11.019

Takei H, Edahiro Y, Mano S, Masubuchi N, Mizukami Y, Imai M, Morishita S, Misawa K, Ochiai T, Tsuneda S, et al. 2018. Skewed megakaryopoiesis in human induced pluripotent stem cell-derived haematopoietic progenitor cells harbouring calreticulin mutations. *Br J Haematol* **181:** 791–802. doi:10.1111/bjh.15266

Tapia N, Schöler HR. 2016. Molecular obstacles to clinical translation of iPSCs. *Cell Stem Cell* **19:** 298–309. doi:10.1016/j.stem.2016.06.017

Tasian SK, Casas JA, Posocco D, Gandre-Babbe S, Gagne AL, Liang G, Loh ML, Weiss MJ, French DL, Chou ST. 2019. Mutation-specific signaling profiles and kinase inhibitor sensitivities of juvenile myelomonocytic leukemia revealed by induced pluripotent stem cells. *Leukemia* **33:** 181–190. doi:10.1038/s41375-018-0169-y

Utikal J, Polo JM, Stadtfeld M, Maherali N, Kulalert W, Walsh RM, Khalil A, Rheinwald JG, Hochedlinger K. 2009. Immortalization eliminates a roadblock during cellular reprogramming into iPS cells. *Nature* **460:** 1145–1148. doi:10.1038/nature08285

Vo LT, Daley GQ. 2015. De novo generation of HSCs from somatic and pluripotent stem cell sources. *Blood* **125:** 2641–2648. doi:10.1182/blood-2014-10-570234

Wahlster L, Daley GQ. 2016. Progress towards generation of human haematopoietic stem cells. *Nat Cell Biol* **18:** 1111–1117. doi:10.1038/ncb3419

Watanabe K, Ueno M, Kamiya D, Nishiyama A, Matsumura M, Wataya T, Takahashi JB, Nishikawa S, Nishikawa S, Muguruma K, et al. 2007. A ROCK inhibitor permits survival of dissociated human embryonic stem cells. *Nat Biotechnol* **25:** 681–686. doi:10.1038/nbt1310

Yang YM, Gupta SK, Kim KJ, Powers BE, Cerqueira A, Wainger BJ, Ngo HD, Rosowski KA, Schein PA, Ackeifi CA, et al. 2013. A small molecule screen in stem-cell-derived motor neurons identifies a kinase inhibitor as a candidate therapeutic for ALS. *Cell Stem Cell* **12:** 713–726. doi:10.1016/j.stem.2013.04.003

Ye Z, Zhan H, Mali P, Dowey S, Williams DM, Jang YY, Dang CV, Spivak JL, Moliterno AR, Cheng L. 2009. Human-induced pluripotent stem cells from blood cells of healthy donors and patients with acquired blood disorders. *Blood* **114:** 5473–5480. doi:10.1182/blood-2009-04-217406

Ye Z, Liu CF, Lanikova L, Dowey SN, He C, Huang X, Brodsky RA, Spivak JL, Prchal JT, Cheng L. 2014. Differential sensitivity to JAK inhibitory drugs by isogenic human erythroblasts and hematopoietic progenitors generated from patient-specific induced pluripotent stem cells. *Stem Cells* **32:** 269–278. doi:10.1002/stem.1545

Young MA, Larson DE, Sun CW, George DR, Ding L, Miller CA, Lin L, Pawlik KM, Chen K, Fan X, et al. 2012. Background mutations in parental cells account for most of the genetic heterogeneity of induced pluripotent stem cells. *Cell Stem Cell* **10:** 570–582. doi:10.1016/j.stem.2012.03.002

Yu J, Vodyanik MA, Smuga-Otto K, Antosiewicz-Bourget J, Frane JL, Tian S, Nie J, Jonsdottir GA, Ruotti V, Stewart R, et al. 2007. Induced pluripotent stem cell lines derived from human somatic cells. *Science* **318:** 1917–1920. doi:10.1126/science.1151526

The Molecular Genetics of Myeloproliferative Neoplasms

Anna E. Marneth[1] **and Ann Mullally**[1,2,3]

[1]Division of Hematology, Department of Medicine, Brigham and Women's Hospital, Harvard Medical School, Boston, Massachusetts 02115, USA

[2]Broad Institute, Cambridge, Massachusetts 02142, USA

[3]Dana-Farber Cancer Institute, Harvard Medical School, Boston, Massachusetts 02115, USA

Correspondence: amullally@partners.org

Activated JAK-STAT signaling is central to the pathogenesis of *BCR-ABL*-negative myeloproliferative neoplasms (MPNs) and occurs as a result of MPN phenotypic driver mutations in *JAK2*, *CALR*, or *MPL*. The spectrum of concomitant somatic mutations in other genes has now largely been defined in MPNs. With the integration of targeted next-generation sequencing (NGS) panels into clinical practice, the clinical significance of concomitant mutations in MPNs has become clearer. In this review, we describe the consequences of concomitant mutations in the most frequently mutated classes of genes in MPNs: (1) DNA methylation pathways, (2) chromatin modification, (3) RNA splicing, (4) signaling pathways, (5) transcription factors, and (6) DNA damage response/stress signaling. The increased use of molecular genetics for early risk stratification of patients brings the possibility of earlier intervention to prevent disease progression in MPNs. However, additional studies are required to decipher underlying molecular mechanisms and effectively target them.

Myeloproliferative neoplasms (MPNs) are a collection of hematopoietic disorders characterized by excessive proliferation of hematopoietic cells of the myeloid lineage. MPNs are classified based on the presence (chronic myeloid leukemia [CML]) or absence of the *BCR-ABL* translocation. In the majority of cases, *BCR-ABL*-negative MPN is caused by somatic mutations that arise in the hematopoietic stem cell (HSC) compartment and activate the JAK-STAT signaling pathway (Mead and Mullally 2017). *BCR-ABL*-negative MPN is the focus of this review and will be referred to as MPN for the remainder of the review. The JAK2-STAT signaling cascade is activated on binding of ligands to type I cytokine receptors including MPL (thrombopoietin [TPO] receptor), the erythropoietin (EPO) receptor, and the granulocyte colony-stimulating factor receptor (G-CSF) receptor. Mutations that activate the JAK-STAT signaling pathway render hematopoietic stem and progenitor cells (HSPCs) hypersensitive to cytokines. Different subtypes of MPN are classified descriptively based on the predominant lineages involved: elevated platelet count in essential thrombocythemia (ET); elevated red

Cite this article as *Cold Spring Harb Perspect Med* doi: 10.1101/cshperspect.a034876

blood cell count in polycythemia vera (PV); megakaryocytic hyperplasia and bone marrow fibrosis in myelofibrosis (MF). ET and PV can evolve into MF (termed secondary MF) or patients may present with de novo MF (termed primary MF or PMF). All subtypes of MPN can transform into secondary acute myeloid leukemia (sAML), which is typically refractory to chemotherapy and generally carries a poor prognosis.

MUTATIONS IN THE JAK-STAT SIGNALING PATHWAY

Mutations that activate the JAK-STAT signaling pathway (Fig. 1) are disease-initiating in MPNs and consequently are termed MPN phenotypic driver mutations. The most frequent MPN phenotypic driver mutation occurs in *JAK2*, a gene encoding a nonreceptor tyrosine kinase. The mutation results in a valine to phenylalanine substitution at position 617 (V617F) in the JH2 domain of the protein, negating the otherwise repressive function of this domain on kinase activity (Chen and Mullally 2014). JAK2 acts as an intermediate signaling molecule for several growth factor receptors including myeloproliferative leukemia (MPL), the EPO receptor, and G-CSF receptor. As a consequence, patients with *JAK2* mutations may have thrombocytosis (ET, 50%–60% of patients have a *JAK2*^{V617F} mutation; see Table 1), erythrocytosis (PV, 95% of patients have a *JAK2*^{V617F} mutation), and leukocytosis (observed in PV). *JAK2* exon 12 mutations, occurring in 2%–3% of PV patients, also result in constitutive activation of JAK2 signaling and typically present with isolated erythrocytosis (Scott et al. 2007). The second most frequent MPN phenotypic driver mutation is found in the endoplasmic reticulum chaperone,

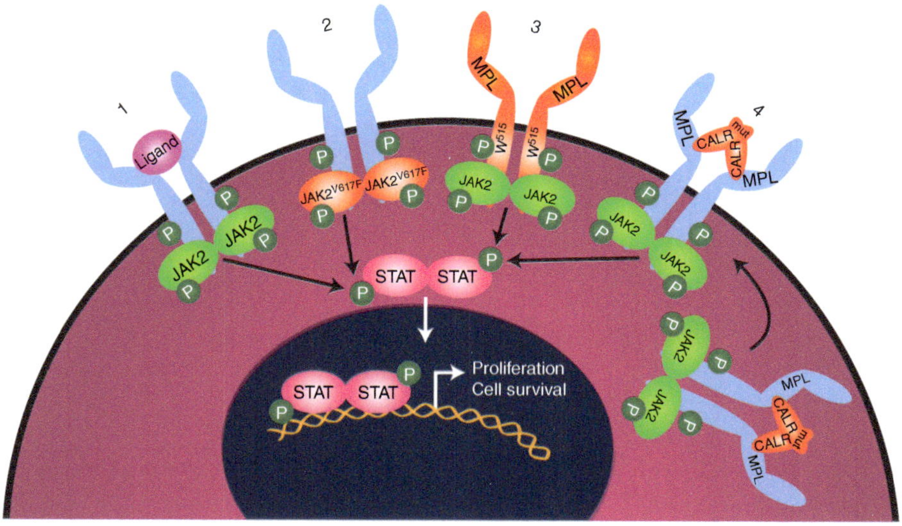

Figure 1. Mutations activating the JAK-STAT signaling pathway are sufficient to cause myeloproliferative neoplasm. In the normal situation (1), the JAK-STAT signaling pathway is activated on binding of a ligand to type I cytokine receptors including MPL (thrombopoietin [TPO] receptor), the erythropoietin (EPO) receptor, and granulocyte colony-stimulating factor (G-CSF) receptor. Activation of the JAK-STAT signaling pathway causes cell proliferation and survival of the relevant myeloid lineage cells. When JAK2 is constitutively active owing to mutations such as V617F (2), downstream signaling from type I cytokine receptors is increased, leading to clonal expansion of hematopoietic stem cells (HSCs), increased erythropoiesis (EPOR), thrombopoiesis (MPL), and granulopoiesis (G-CSFR). Situation (3) shows that MPL mutations at position W515 activate JAK-STAT signaling. In situation (4), mutant CALR develops a pathogenic binding interaction with MPL (but not with EPO or G-CSF receptor) that activates JAK-STAT signaling. In situations (3) and (4), because only the MPL receptor is involved, JAK-STAT pathway activation is restricted to MPL-expressing hematopoietic stem cell (HSC) and megakaryocyte lineage cells resulting in thrombocytosis. Mutated proteins are depicted in orange. P, Phosphorylation.

Table 1. Overview of the most frequent mutations found in MPNs and post-MPN AML

Gene	Most frequent mutation (types)	Mutation frequency				References
		ET	PV	(P)MF	Post-MPN AML	
MPN phenotypic driver mutations						
JAK2	Heterozygous and homozygous (acquired uniparental disomy) exon 12 and exon 14 mutations. V617F, located in the repressive JH2 domain, is the most frequent mutation. Also, gene/chromosomal duplications are found.	50%–60%	95%	50%–60%	37%–60%	Scott et al. 2007; Abdel-Wahab et al. 2010; Zhang et al. 2012; Vannucchi et al. 2013; Guglielmelli et al. 2014; Lundberg et al. 2014; Tefferi et al. 2016a,b; Lasho et al. 2018
CALR	Heterozygous insertion and/or deletions in exon 9, resulting in a +1 base pair frameshift and a novel carboxyl terminus.	26%	<1%	18%–32%	21%–25%	Guglielmelli et al. 2014; Lundberg et al. 2014; Rampal et al. 2014; Tefferi et al. 2016a,b: Lasho et al. 2018
MPL	Heterozygous missense mutations, W515L/K most frequent, resulting in constitutive activation of the receptor.	4%	<1%	6%–9%	8%–13%	Zhang et al. 2012; Vannucchi et al. 2013; Lundberg et al. 2014; Guglielmelli et al. 2014; Tefferi et al. 2016a,b; Lasho et al. 2018
DNA methylation						
TET2	Heterozygous or homozygous loss-of-function mutations in its catalytic domain, causing reduced conversion of methylated to hydroxymethylated cytosines.	7%–16%	19%–22%	10%–18%	19%–28%	Abdel-Wahab et al. 2010; Zhang et al. 2012; Vannucchi et al. 2013; Lundberg et al. 2014; Tefferi et al. 2016a,b; Lasho et al. 2018; Venton et al. 2018
IDH1[a]/ *IDH2*[a]	Heterozygous missense mutations in the active catalytic site, IDH1: R132, IDH2: R140 and R172, causing acquisition of the ability to convert αKG into 2-hydroxyglutatate.	1%	2%	0%–6%	19%–31%	Abdel-Wahab et al. 2010; Pardanani et al. 2010; Tefferi et al. 2010, 2016a,b; Zhang et al. 2012; Vannucchi et al. 2013; Guglielmelli et al. 2014; Lundberg et al. 2014; Rampal et al. 2014; Lasho et al. 2018; Venton et al. 2018
DNMT3A	Mutations in *DNMT3A* in MPN occur as nonsense/ frameshift mutations in addition to missense mutations (including at R882, which is located in the methyltransferase domain), resulting in reduced methyltransferase activity.	0%–9%	0%–7%	3%–15%	2%–14%	Abdel-Wahab et al. 2011; Lin et al. 2011; Stegelmann et al. 2011; Zhang et al. 2012; Vannucchi et al. 2013; Lundberg et al. 2014; Wang et al. 2014; Tefferi et al. 2016a,b: Lasho et al. 2018; Venton et al. 2018

Continued

Table 1. *Continued*

Gene	Most frequent mutation (types)	Mutation frequency				References
		ET	PV	(P)MF	Post-MPN AML	
Chromatin modification						
ASXL1[a]	Heterozygous nonsense and frameshift mutations in exon 12 leading to loss of its PHD domain.	1%–11%	3%–12%	18%–37%	17%–47%	Tefferi et al. 2016a,b, 2018d; Lasho et al. 2018; Vannucchi et al. 2013; Abdel-Wahab et al. 2010; Zhang et al. 2012; Lundberg et al. 2014; Guglielmelli et al. 2014; Rampal et al. 2014; Venton et al. 2018
EZH2[a]	Heterozygous/homozygous/hemizygous loss-of-function mutations that disrupt or delete the catalytic SET2 domain.	1%–3%	0%–3%	0%–9%	13%–15%	Vannucchi et al. 2013; Guglielmelli et al. 2014; Lundberg et al. 2014; Tefferi et al. 2016a,b; Lasho et al. 2018; Venton et al. 2018
RNA splicing						
SRSF2[a]	Heterozygous missense mutations and small in-frame deletions around hotspot P95, affecting the preferred RNA recognition sequence (wild-type GGNG and CCNG, mutant GGNG) in RNA exon splicing enhancers.	2%	3%	8%–18%	13%–22%	Zhang et al. 2012; Vannucchi et al. 2013; Guglielmelli et al. 2014; Rampal et al. 2014; Tefferi et al. 2016a,b, 2018d; Lasho et al. 2018; Venton et al. 2018
U2AF1[a]	Heterozygous missense mutations around hotspots S34 and Q157, which alter the preferred −3 (C/A >> T, S34F/Y) or +1 (G >> A, Q157P) nucleotides flanking the AG of the 3′ splice site.	1%	<1%	16%	5%–6%	Zhang et al. 2012; Tefferi et al. 2016a,b, 2018; Lasho et al. 2018d
ZRSR2	Hemizygous frameshift and nonsense mutations. Loss-of-function mutations.	3%	5%	10%	2%	Zhang et al. 2012; Tefferi et al. 2016a,b
SF3B1	Heterozygous missense mutations in exons 14–16, hotspot K700E most frequent mutation. Most commonly mutated in MDS/MPN-RS-T 80%.	5%	3%	9%–10%	4%–7%	Dunbar et al. 2008; Makishima et al. 2009; Muramatsu et al. 2010; Malcovati et al. 2011; Papaemmanuil et al. 2011; Yoshida et al. 2011; Zhang et al. 2012; Tefferi et al. 2016a,b, 2018d; Lasho et al. 2018

Cite this article as *Cold Spring Harb Perspect Med* doi: 10.1101/cshperspect.a034876

Signaling						
LNK	Mostly heterozygous missense substitutions targeting the pleckstrin homology domain in 50% of cases.	1%–3%	0%–9%	0%–6%	11%	Lundberg et al. 2014; Tefferi et al. 2016a,b; Lasho et al. 2018
CBL	Homozygous missense substitutions located in the RING and linker domain reducing E3 ligase activity.	0%–1%	0%–2%	0%–6%	4%	Grand et al. 2009; Vannucchi et al. 2013; Lundberg et al. 2014; Tefferi et al. 2016a,b; Lasho et al. 2018
NRAS/ KRAS	Heterozygous missense substitutions at codons 12, 13, and 61 causing reduced intrinsic GTP hydrolysis and resistance to GAPs.	<1%	0%–1%	3%–4%	7%–15%	Zhang et al. 2012; Lundberg et al. 2014; Tefferi et al. 2016a,b; Lasho et al. 2018; Venton et al. 2018
PTPN11	Heterozygous missense mutations in the Src-homology 2 (N-SH2) and phosphotyrosine phosphatase (PTP) domains causing increased phosphatase activity.	0%–2%	<1%	0%–2%	6%–8%	Ding et al. 2009; Lundberg et al. 2014; Rampal et al. 2014; Tefferi et al. 2016a,b; Lasho et al. 2018
Transcription factors						
RUNX1	Missense, frameshift, and nonsense mutations causing loss of function, and may act in a dominant-negative fashion over wild-type RUNX1. Both homozygous and heterozygous mutations are found.	0%–2%	0%–2%	3%–4%	4%–13%	Ding et al. 2009; Zhang et al. 2012; Lundberg et al. 2014; Tefferi et al. 2016a,b: Lasho et al. 2018; Venton et al. 2018
NFE2	Mostly heterozygous frameshift mutations causing increased expression and protein levels of wild-type NFE2.	<1%	2%–3%	0%–3%	<1%	Jutzi et al. 2013; Lundberg et al. 2014
DNA repair response/stress signaling						
TP53	Mostly missense mutations, both alleles affected. Possibly loss-of-function, gain-of-function, and/or dominant-negative.	2%–6%	1%	1%–3%	11%–36%	Harutyunyan et al. 2011; Zhang et al. 2012; Lundberg et al. 2014; Rampal et al. 2014; Tefferi et al. 2016a,b; Lasho et al. 2018; Venton et al. 2018
PPM1D	Heterozygous exon 6 mutations causing loss of carboxy-terminal degradation domain.	2%	1%	1%	NA	Grinfeld et al. 2018

MPN, Myeloproliferative neoplasm; AML, acute myeloid leukemia; ET, essential thrombocythemia; PV, polycythemis vera; (P)MF, (primary) myelofibrosis; ASXL1, EZH2, SRSF2, IDH1/2, U2AF^{Q157}, GTPase-activating proteins; αKG, α-ketgoglutarate; MDS/MPN-RS-T, myelodysplastic/myeloproliferative neoplasm with ring sideroblasts and thrombocytosis; NA, not assessed; PHD, plant homeodomain.

[a]High molecular risk mutations in (primary) myelofibrosis (Vannucchi et al. 2013; Guglielmelli et al. 2018).

CALR. *CALR* mutations occur as heterozygous insertion and/or deletions in exon 9, resulting in a +1 base pair frameshift (Klampfl et al. 2013; Nangalia et al. 2013). This frameshift changes the reading frame and results in the generation of a novel mutant-specific carboxyl terminus. CALR induces MPN by binding to and activating MPL signaling in a TPO-independent manner (Elf et al. 2016). Consistent with the observation that MPL is mostly expressed in HSCs and the megakaryocytic lineage, mutations in *CALR* occur in ET (26%) and MF but not typically in PV. The third most frequent MPN phenotypic driver mutation occurs in *MPL*, with the majority of mutations located at tryptophan 515 (W515L/K) (Pikman et al. 2006). *MPL* mutations primarily affect the megakaryocytic lineage and are present in ET (4%) and MF, but not in PV. Mutational frequencies in PMF are 50%–60% for *JAK2* mutations, 18%–32% for *CALR*, and 6%–9% for *MPL* (Table 1). Additionally, ~10% of ET and PMF patients are "triple negative"—they do not harbor *JAK2*, *CALR*, nor *MPL* mutations (Angona et al. 2016; Milosevic Feenstra et al. 2016).

It is important to note that mutations in *JAK2*, *CALR*, or *MPL* are sufficient "alone" to engender MPNs in people and in mice (Pikman et al. 2006; Mullally et al. 2013; Li et al. 2018). In 45%–50% of MPN cases, an MPN phenotypic driver mutation is the sole mutation identified based on our current knowledge of genes known to be somatically mutated in myeloid malignances (Lundberg et al. 2014; Grinfeld et al. 2018), and in a recent study all MPN patients of <39 years old had *JAK2*, *CALR*, or *MPL* as the sole mutation identified (Grinfeld et al. 2018). Furthermore, *JAK2*^{V617F} is a common mutational driver of clonal hematopoiesis of indeterminate potential (CHIP), an entity in which clonally restricted somatic mutations in genes associated with hematological malignancies are found in normal individuals (Gibson and Steensma 2018). In virtually all cases of JAK2^{V617F} CHIP, the *JAK2* mutation occurs as an isolated event indicating that JAK2^{V617F} *alone* is sufficient to cause clonal hematopoiesis (Jaiswal et al. 2014). The prevalence of JAK2^{V617F} MPN is significantly lower than that of JAK2^{V617F} CHIP (Hinds et al. 2016), suggesting there are factors that constrain and promote the transition from JAK2^{V617F} clonal hematopoiesis to MPN. Recent studies indicate that JAK2^{V617F} CHIP is itself a clinically relevant entity, being associated with an increased risk of both atherosclerotic heart disease (Jaiswal et al. 2017) and venous thrombosis (Wolach et al. 2018). These data suggest that JAK2 mutations can cause a continuum of clinically relevant disease entities, from premalignant clonal expansion to all three classical MPNs.

OTHER SOMATIC GENE MUTATIONS

Besides the three JAK-STAT activating MPN phenotypic driver mutations, >50% of MPN patients harbor additional somatic mutations (Table 1) (Grinfeld et al. 2018). Figure 2 shows an illustrative example of the acquisition of somatic mutations in different hematopoietic states (e.g., polyclonal hematopoiesis, CHIP, MPN, and post-MPN AML). The most common classes of concomitant somatic mutations found in MPN patients are (1) DNA methylation (*TET2*, *IDH1*, *IDH2*, *DNMT3A*), (2) chromatin modification (*ASXL1*, *EZH2*), (3) RNA splicing (*SRSF2*, *U2AF1*, *SF3B1*, and *ZRSR2*), (4) signaling pathways (*LNK/SH2B3*, *CBL*, *NRAS*, *KRAS*, *PTPN1*), (5) transcription factors (*RUNX1* and *NFE2*), and (6) DNA damage response/stress signaling (*TP53*, *PPM1D*) (Fig. 3). Below, we describe in which MPN subtypes these mutations are found and how specific mutations affect gene function and contribute to MPNs.

DNA METHYLATION

TET2

Consequences of Mutations on Gene Function

During DNA replication, methylated cytosines are either replaced passively by unmethylated cytosines or actively after a process of chemical modifications initiated by ten eleven translocation (TET) proteins. The TET2 enzyme catalyzes oxidation of 5-methylcytosine to 5-hy-

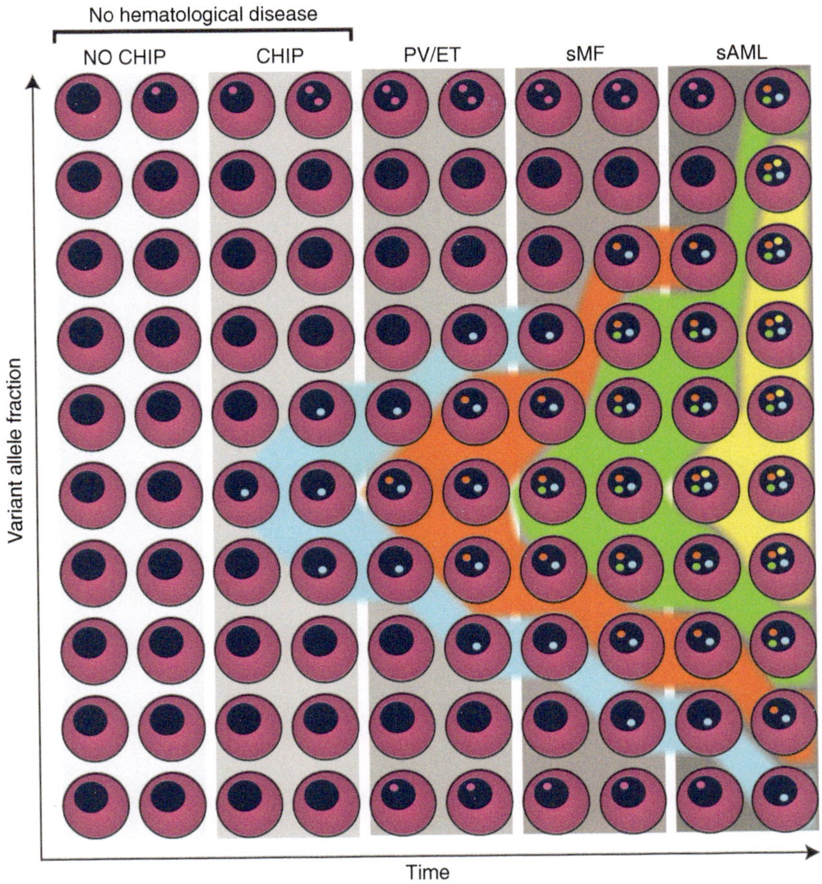

Figure 2. Illustrative example of an individual case with clonal hematopoiesis and myeloproliferative neoplasm (MPN) disease progression. Individuals without hematological diseases may have somatic mutations in genes that do not impact hematopoiesis (i.e., passenger mutations, indicated with pink dots). At some point, the individual case represented in this figure acquires a mutation (e.g., in *DNMT3A*) that causes clonal expansion of the hematopoietic stem cell (HSC) without necessarily causing an overt hematological disease (i.e., clonal hematopoiesis of indeterminate potential [CHIP]), indicated with blue dots and expansion of the blue clone from 10% to 30%. Subsequently, this individual acquires one of the MPN phenotypic "driver" mutations (e.g., $JAK2^{V617F}$, indicated with orange dots), that results in the development of an MPN (e.g., polycythemia vera [PV] or essential thrombocythemia [ET]). Chronic phase MPN (i.e., PV or ET) may then progress to secondary myelofibrosis (sMF) on acquisition of additional mutations (e.g., a mutation in EZH2 [indicated with green dots]). This clone expands over time and, finally, overt secondary acute myeloid leukemia (sAML) may arise on acquisition of a TP53 mutation (yellow dots).

droxymethylcytosine (5-hmc). TET proteins depend on α-ketoglutarate (αKG), Fe^{2+}, and ascorbate for their dioxygenase activity (Tahiliani et al. 2009; Minor et al. 2013). Mutations in *TET2* are loss-of-function causing impaired catalytic function, resulting in reduced levels of 5-hmc and resultant DNA hypermethylation (Fig. 3).

Clinical Data

All types of mutations and deletions are found throughout the *TET2* gene, with the majority of somatic missense mutations found in its catalytic domain. *TET2* mutations occur in 7%–22% of MPNs and 19%–28% of post-MPN AML patients (Table 1). Although some studies

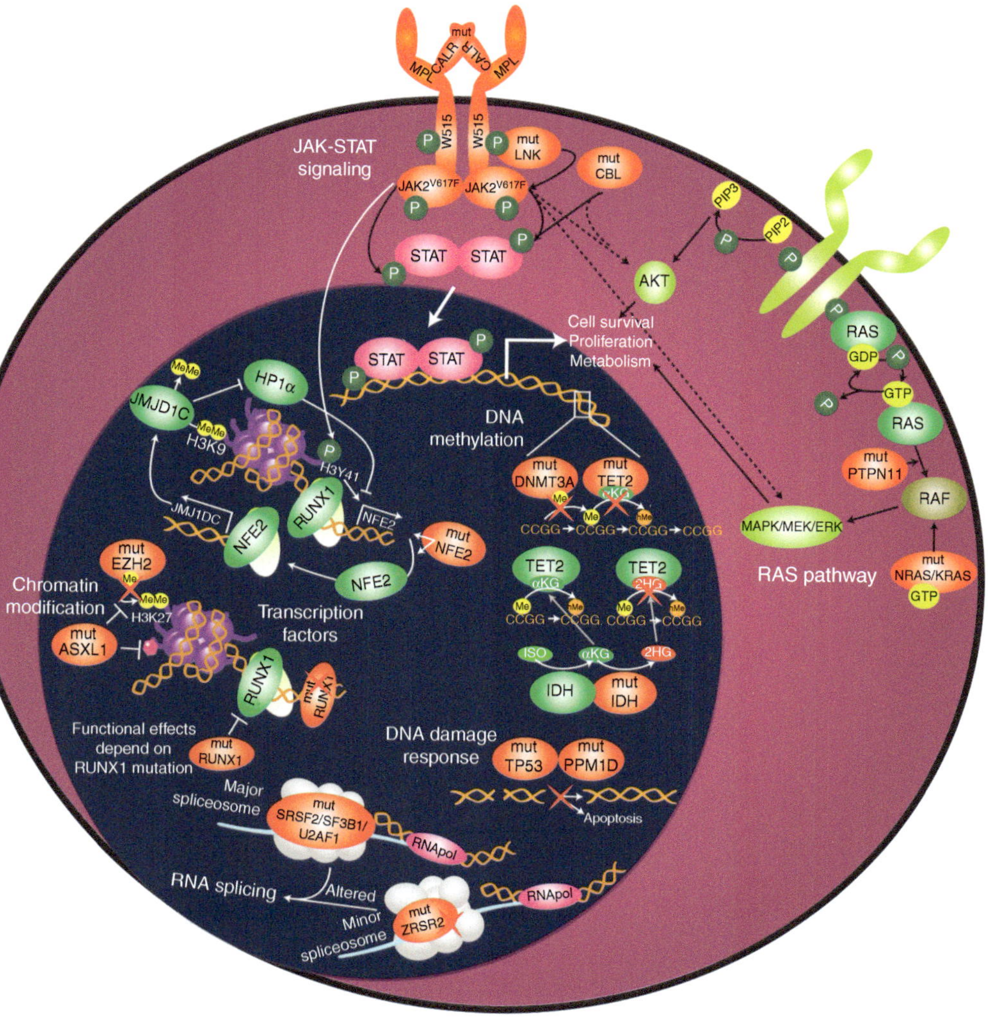

Figure 3. Overview of classes of genes found mutated in myeloproliferative neoplasms (MPNs). This includes (1) DNA methylation (*TET2*, *IDH1*, *IDH2*, and *DNMT3A*), (2) chromatin modification (*ASXL1* and *EZH2*), (3) RNA splicing (*SRSF2*, *U2AF1*, *SF3B1*, and *ZRSR2*), (4) JAK-STAT and RAS signaling pathways (*JAK2*, *CALR*, *MPL*, *LNK*/*SH2B3*, *CBL*, *NRAS*, *KRAS*, and *PTPN1*), (5) transcription factors (*RUNX1* and *NFE2*), and (6) DNA damage response/stress signaling (*TP53* and *PPM1D*). Wild-type proteins are depicted in green and mutated (mut) proteins are depicted in orange. For illustration, all genes/proteins described in this review are depicted, although some mutations may actually lead to loss of protein expression. (Refer to the main text for detailed explanations of the depicted processes.) αKG, α-ketoglutarate; GDP, guanosine diphosphate; GTP, guanosine triphosphate; 2HG, 2-hydroxyglutarate; hMe, hydroxymethyl; ISO, isocitrate; Me, methyl; P, phosphorylation; PIP2, phosphatidylinositol(4,5)-biphospate; PIP3, phosphatidylinositol(3,4,5)-triphosphate; RNApol, RNA polymerase.

have suggested that *TET2* mutations increase the risk of leukemic transformation (Abdel-Wahab et al. 2010; Beer et al. 2010; Zhang et al. 2012; Lundberg et al. 2014), more recent studies have not consistently seen this association (Tefferi et al. 2016b; Lasho et al. 2018). *TET2* mutations are the most common co-occurring mutation with the JAK2^{V617F} mutation. The order of acquisition of *JAK2* and *TET2* mutations impacts the MPN phenotype, with JAK2-first patients having a higher probability of presenting with PV than ET and a higher risk of thrombosis (Ortmann et al. 2015).

Mouse Models and Affected Cellular Pathways

In murine and xenograft HSC repopulation studies, *Tet2* knockout/knockdown/mutated HSCs have superior HSC repopulation as compared with *Tet2* wild-type cells and JAK2^{V617F+}/TET2 knockout/knockdown/mutated cells have superior HSC repopulation as compared with JAK2^{V617F+}-only HSCs (Delhommeau et al. 2009; Chen et al. 2015; Kameda et al. 2015b). When comparing JAK2^{V617F}-induced MPN with JAK2^{V617+}*Tet2* knockout/knockdown MPN, the later mice developed a more severe form of MPN and had reduced survival (Chen et al. 2015; Kameda et al. 2015b). Proposed mechanisms by which *TET2* mutations lead to more severe forms of MPN include epigenetic repression of tumor suppressor genes and increased expression of HSC self-renewal genes possibly due to enhancer hypermethylation (Kameda et al. 2015a; Rasmussen et al. 2015).

IDH1/IDH2

Consequences of Mutations on Gene Function

Wild-type isocitrate dehydrogenase (NADP$^+$) 1 and 2 (IDH1/IDH2) are metabolic enzymes that catalyze the oxidative decarboxylation of isocitrate to αKG, the cosubstrate for TET proteins. Because of missense mutations in the active catalytic site of IDH (IDH1: R132, IDH2: R140 or R172), IDH proteins acquire the ability to further convert αKG into 2-hydroxyglutatate (Fig. 3). Besides αKG, 2-hydroxyglutatate can also bind TET proteins and the Jumonji family of H3K9 and H3K36 demethylases (Xu et al. 2011). However, because 2-hydroxyglutatate cannot function as a cosubstrate, it inhibits the function of these enzymes.

Clinical Data

Missense mutations in *IDH1* and *IDH2* occur at low frequencies in MPNs and in 19%–31% of post-MPN AML (Table 1). *IDH1/2* mutations have been associated with worse prognosis in ET, and in PMF with a high risk for subsequent transformation to post-MPN sAML (Tefferi et al. 2010, 2016b; Guglielmelli et al. 2014; Yonal-Hindilerden et al. 2016).

Mouse Models and Affected Cellular Pathways

Like *Tet2* loss, expression of mutant IDH1 causes an expansion of myeloid progenitors in mouse models (Sasaki et al. 2012). Both Jak2^{V617F}-only and Jak2^{V617F}/Idh2^{R140Q} mice develop a PV phenotype with splenomegaly, but Jak2^{V617F}/Idh2^{R140Q} mice show blast-like cells in the spleen and disruption of splenic architecture that is not observed in Jak2^{V617F}-only mice (McKenney et al. 2018a). Overt leukemia was not seen in Jak2^{V617F}/Idh2^{R140Q} mice, suggesting that additional factors are required to induce leukemic transformation in Jak2^{V617F}-expressing mice.

DNMT3A

Consequences of Mutations on Gene Function

DNA methyl transferase (DNMT)3A and DNMT3B are de novo methyltransferases as opposed to DNMT1, a maintenance methyltransferase that ensures that DNA methylation is inherited by the daughter cell after cell division. Mutations in *DNMT3A* in MPN occur as nonsense/frameshift mutations, in addition to missense mutations (including at R882), resulting in reduced methyltransferase activity (Fig. 3) (Ley et al. 2010; Yamashita et al. 2010; Abdel-Wahab et al. 2011; Emperle et al. 2018). It was suggested that DNMT3A^{R882mut} acts in a dominant-negative fashion by inhibiting the function and/or oligomerization of wild-type DNMT3A, but recent evidence contradicts this finding (Emperle et al. 2018).

Clinical Data

DNMT3A mutations are found in 7% of MPNs, with lower frequency in ET and PV compared with (P)MF and post-MPN AML (Table 1). Patients are more likely to present with ET compared with PV or MF when *DNMT3A* mutations are acquired before JAK2^{V617F} compared with patients who first acquired JAK2^{V617F} (Nangalia et al. 2015).

Mouse Models and Affected Cellular Pathways

Human *DNMT3A/JAK2* and *DNMT3A/MPL* double-mutant subclones have a growth advantage compared with *JAK2* and *MPL* single-mutant subclones (Rao et al. 2012; Nangalia et al. 2015). This is consistent with in vitro serial replating assays and in vivo CRISPR knockout of *Dnmt3a* in Jak2^{V617F}-expressing mice (Jacquelin et al. 2018). When followed for 32 weeks, mice transplanted with Jak2^{V617F} control HSPCs showed a PV phenotype, whereas recipients receiving Jak2^{V617F} Cas9 Dnmt3a sgRNA HSPCs first developed a PV-like disease, but had progressed into MF by 32 weeks of age (Jacquelin et al. 2018). Mice transplanted with Jak2^{V617F}/Dnmt3a KO HSPCs showed a marked reduction in long-term and short-term HSCs and a relative accumulation of multipotent progenitors compared with Jak2^{V617F} control recipients (Jacquelin et al. 2018). Mechanistic studies in this model indicate that *DNMT3A* mutations contribute to MPN progression by deregulating Polycomb repressive complex 2 (PRC2)-mediated gene expression, through enhanced chromatin accessibility at active enhancer sites (Jacquelin et al. 2018).

CHROMATIN MODIFICATION

ASXL1

Consequences of Mutations on Gene Function

Additional sex combs like 1, transcriptional regulator (ASXL1) interacts with several chromatin-modifying proteins, including PRC2. Mutations in *ASXL1* are almost exclusively heterozygous nonsense and frameshift mutations in exon 12. There is some controversy regarding the consequences of these mutations on ASXL1 function, which could be loss- or gain-of-function and/or a dominant-negative effect. *ASXL1* exon 12 mutants lead to a detectable carboxy-terminally truncated protein lacking the plant homology domain (PHD) (Inoue et al. 2016).

Clinical Data

ASXL1 mutations are more common in PMF (18%–37%) and post-MPN AML (17%–47%) compared with early-stage MPNs (Table 1) and are associated with poor prognosis in PV and PMF patients (Vannucchi et al. 2013; Guglielmelli et al. 2014; Tefferi et al. 2014, 2016b, 2018b; Lasho et al. 2018). A worse prognosis for *ASXL1* mutated patients was also described for PMF patients undergoing allogeneic HSC transplantation (Kröger et al. 2017). Monitoring for acquisition of *ASXL1* mutations may be relevant in MPN management, because *ASXL1* mutations are the most frequent mutation acquired during ruxolitinib treatment and are associated with the development of leukocytosis and thrombocytopenia (Newberry et al. 2017).

Mouse Models and Affected Cellular Pathways

ASXL1 mutants missing the PHD domain may not interact with EZH2 (Bera et al. 2012), a member of the PRC2 complex. Consistent with this, ASXL1 mutations modeled by Asxl1 knockdown/knockout contribute to leukemogenesis through derepression of PRC2 targets, such as the Hoxa locus (Fig. 3) (Abdel-Wahab et al. 2012). In an MPN mouse model, *Asxl1* heterozygous knockout cooperated with JAK2^{V617F} to accelerate myelofibrosis and caused leukemia in several mice (Guo et al. 2019). These data show that loss of *ASXL1* promotes MPN progression.

To gain insight into mutant *Asxl1* as opposed to loss of *Asxl1*, multiple groups have generated *Asxl1* knock-in mice (Hsu et al. 2017; Nagase et al. 2018; Yang et al. 2018; Uni et al. 2019). Several mechanisms have been proposed regarding the effects of mutant ASXL1 on PRC1 and on H2AK119ub (the repressive histone mark that PRC1 deposits) (Asada et al. 2018; Nagase et al. 2018; Uni et al. 2019). In contrast to wild-type ASXL1, mutant ASXL1 binds to the

 Cite this article as *Cold Spring Harb Perspect Med* doi: 10.1101/cshperspect.a034876

PRC1 member, BMI1 (Uni et al. 2019). A well-known target of BMI1/PRC1 is the p16Ink4a locus, and Ink4a expression is increased in *Asxl1*-mutant knock-in mice, as a result of inhibition of PRC1 by mutant Asxl1 (Uni et al. 2019). Knockout of p16Ink4a in *Asxl1*-mutant knock-in mice rescued the decrease in HSC number and increased apoptosis observed in *Asxl1*-mutant mice, indicating that p16Ink4a plays a key role in *Asxl1*-mutant-driven leukemogenesis (Uni et al. 2019). Another mechanism by which mutant ASXL1 affects H2AK119ub is through the de-ubiquitinase (DUB), BAP1. Although mutant ASXL1 interacts less strongly with BAP1 than wild-type ASXL1 (Abdel-Wahab et al. 2012), it has been shown that mutant ASXL1, but not wild-type ASXL1, enhances the catalytic function of the de-ubiquitinase BAP1. This causes a reduction in global H2AK119ub and locally at HOXA and IRF8 loci in HSCs (Scheuermann et al. 2010; Asada et al. 2018). Depletion of *BAP1* abrogated mutant ASXL1-induced leukemogenesis, showing that also BAP1 plays a crucial role in *Asxl1*-mutant driven leukemia (Asada et al. 2018).

Mutant ASXL1 has been shown to interact with the acetyl lysine reader bromodomain-containing protein 4 (BRD4) (Yang et al. 2018), which plays an important role in gene transcription and regulation through its interaction with pTEFb and superenhancers. Moreover, HSPCs from transgenic *Asxl1*-mutant mice are hypersensitive to bromodomain inhibitors (Yang et al. 2018). Amongst others, one important target gene of mutant ASXL1-BRD4 is *Prdm16* (Yang et al. 2018), which is critical for the maintenance of HSCs. Finally, another mechanism by which mutant ASXL1 has been reported to contribute to leukemogenesis is through H3K and H4K deacetylation mediated repression of TGF-β (Saika et al. 2018).

EZH2

Consequences of Mutations on Gene Function

Enhancer of zeste homolog 2 (EZH2) is a component of PRC2, which harbors the histone lysine *N*-methyltransferase activity of the complex. The most well-studied function of PRC2 is methylation of H3K27 and indeed, H3K27 levels are reduced in *EZH2*-mutant cells (Fig. 3). EZH2 can act as tumor suppressor or oncogene depending on the context. Nonsense, frameshift, and missense mutations have been found in MPNs and are thought to be loss-of-function mutations, suggesting that EZH2 acts as a tumor suppressor in MPNs.

Clinical Data

EZH2 mutations are found in 0%–9% of ET, PV, and PMF patients, and in 13%–15% of post-MPN AML (Table 1). *EZH2* mutations correlate with a worse clinical phenotype with higher leukocyte counts, blast-cell counts, and larger spleens at diagnosis (Guglielmelli et al. 2011). They were shown to be an independent poor prognostic factor (overall survival 31.6 mo vs. wild-type 137 mo) (Guglielmelli et al. 2011).

Mouse Models and Affected Cellular Pathways

Similar to *ASXL1*, *EZH2*-inactivating mutations cause derepression of *HOXA9*, which supports myeloid progenitor cell self-renewal and leukemia development (Khan et al. 2013). In mouse models, concomitant loss of *Ezh2* with expression of $JAK2^{V617F}$ leads to enhanced myelofibrosis compared with $JAK2^{V617F}$ mice, impaired erythroid differentiation, expansion of HSPCs and megakaryocyte progenitors, increased thrombocytosis, and leukocytosis (Shimizu et al. 2016; Yang et al. 2016). However, $JAK2^{V617F}$/*Ezh2* *N*-methyltransferase$^{-/-}$ comutant mice did not develop leukemia, suggesting that additional hits are required for leukemic transformation of $JAK2^{V617F}$ mice.

RNA SPLICING

The third class of mutations comprises mutations in genes involved in RNA splicing (Fig. 3). Two types of spliceosomes exist: the major (U2) and minor (U12) spliceosome. The minor spliceosome splices <1% of all introns, but these are present (alongside U2-type introns) in 700–800 genes, and are evolutionarily conserved (Verma et al. 2018). Mutations in RNA splicing factors SF3B1, U2AF1, SRSF2, ZRSR2, SF3A1, PRPF40B, U2AF2, and SF1 have been reported in myeloid malignancies; the first four are most common and will be discussed below. Spliceosomal mutations are typically mutually exclusive with each other, are relatively rare in PV and ET, and occur at higher frequency in PMF (Grinfeld et al. 2018).

SRSF2

Consequences of Mutations on Gene Function

The most frequent splicing factor mutations in MPNs are found in serine and arginine rich splicing factor 2 (SRSF2), almost all affecting the hotspot proline at position 95. SRSF2 is involved in recognition of exon splicing enhancers. Whereas wild-type SRSF2 binds the RNA sequences GGNG and CCNG in exon splicing enhancers equally well, P95-mutated SRSF2 preferentially splices exons containing the CCNG sequence (Kim et al. 2015).

Clinical Data

SRSF2 mutations are infrequent in ET and PV, whereas they occur in 8%–22% of PMF and post-MPN AML (Table 1). Mutations in *SRSF2* have consistently been associated with poor prognosis in myeloid malignancies including several types of MPN and post-MPN AML, and have been associated with leukemic transformation (Lasho et al. 2012; Zhang et al. 2012; Vannucchi et al. 2013; Tefferi et al. 2018c,d; Venton et al. 2018).

Mouse Models and Affected Cellular Pathways

Mutations in *SRSF2* cause differential splicing of all classes of splicing events (Kim et al. 2015). Examples include missplicing and nonsense-mediated RNA decay-associated down-regulation of EZH2 (Kim et al. 2015) and missplicing of CASP8 causing expression of a truncated CASP8 protein that activates NF-κB signaling (Lee et al. 2018). Expression of mutant SRSF2 causes accumulation of R loops, replication stress, and activation of the ATR-Chk1 pathway (Chen et al. 2018; Nguyen et al. 2018). Wild-type SRSF2 is able to extract RNA polymerase II carboxy-terminal domain (CTD) kinase from the 7SK complex, which causes transcription pause release (Ji et al. 2013). Mutant SRSF2 loses this ability (Chen et al. 2018), which could explain the accumulation of R loops. Mutant SRSF2 also affects transcriptional regulation through predominant splicing of RUNX1 to form the short RUNX1a transcript over the longer RUNX1b transcript (Sakurai et al. 2017). Besides splicing and transcription, SRSF2 plays a role in regulating DNA stability (Xiao et al. 2007). Consistent with this, whole-exome sequencing of patient samples from different myeloid malignancies showed that *SRSF2*-mutant samples have more mutations than samples harboring other spliceosome mutations (Yoshida et al. 2011). Data on the role of *SRSF2* mutations in MPN pathogenesis and on cooperativity with JAK-STAT activating mutations are needed to better delineate their role in MPNs.

U2AF1

Consequences of Mutations on Gene Function

U2 small nuclear RNA auxiliary factor 1 (U2AF1) recognizes the 3′ splice site. U2AF1 contains two mutational hotspot regions (S34 and Q157) located in its two CCCH zinc fingers that are required for RNA binding (Webb and Wise 2004). These mutations alter the preferred −3 (C/A >> T, S34F/Y) or +1 (G >> A, Q157P) nucleotides flanking the AG of the 3′ splice site (Ilagan et al. 2015).

Clinical Data

U2AF1 mutations occur in 16% of PMF and 5%–6% of post-MPN AML patients (Table 1). As for *SF3B1*, PV and ET patients harboring *U2AF1* mutations have an inferior myelofibrosis-free survival compared with *U2AF1* wild-type patients (Tefferi et al. 2016b). Roughly

35% of U2AF1 mutations affect S34 and 65% affect Q157 or its vicinities (Tefferi et al. 2018a). Only Q157 (and near vicinity) mutations are associated with significantly shorter overall survival in MPNs (Tefferi et al. 2018a).

Mouse Models and Affected Cellular Pathways

The prognostic difference between S34 and Q157 mutations could be caused by distinct downstream effects. Indeed, besides very few common targets, U2AF1 S34- and Q157-mutant-expressing blood/MDS cells have mostly distinct expression and splicing patterns, with Q157 mutants causing missplicing of, for example, ARID2 and EZH2 (Przychodzen et al. 2013; Ilagan et al. 2015; Park et al. 2016). Like *SRSF2* mutations, $U2AF1^{S34}$ mutations cause accumulation of R loops (Q157 mutations not investigated) (Nguyen et al. 2018). Besides this canonical function, U2AF1 has been reported to bind mRNA in the cytoplasm and repress mRNA translation (Palangat et al. 2018). The S34F mutation was suggested to affect translation of hundreds of mRNAs. Whether Q157 mutations affect mRNA translation is currently unknown.

ZRSR2

Consequences of Mutations on Gene Function

Zinc finger CCCH-type, RNA binding motif, and serine/arginine-rich 2 (ZRSR2) forms a heterodimer with U2AF2 and is involved in recognizing the 3′ splice site in minor (U12-type) introns, similar to U2AF1 in the major (U2-type) spliceosome. Besides the minor spliceosome, ZRSR2 interacts with major spliceosome components SRSF1/SRSF2 and affects splicing of major introns in vitro, suggesting it also influences the major spliceosome (Shen et al. 2010) and/or other functions of these interaction partners. *ZRSR2* is located on the X chromosome; mutations predominantly occur in males and are frameshift and nonsense mutations in the majority of cases. These data indicate that *ZRSR2* mutations are loss-of-function mutations.

Clinical Data

MPN patients harboring *ZRSR2* mutations are more likely to be diagnosed with PMF (Tefferi et al. 2016a) versus ET or PV (Tefferi et al. 2016b; Grinfeld et al. 2018), suggesting that *ZRSR2* mutations promote myelofibrotic transformation.

Mouse Models and Affected Cellular Pathways

In line with a loss-of-function hypothesis and an important role for *ZRSR2* in the minor spliceosome, mutations in *ZRSR2* predominantly affect splicing of the majority of minor introns, causing intron retention (Madan et al. 2015). Pathways enriched for altered splicing in *ZRSR2*-mutant MDS cells are enriched for MAPK, ErbB signaling, and genes associated with CML and AML (Madan et al. 2015).

SF3B1

Consequences of Mutations on Gene Function

Splicing factor 3b subunit 1 (SF3B1) is part of both the major and minor spliceosome in which it recognizes the BPS as part of the U2 or U11/U12 snRNPs, respectively. Most mutations are found in exons 14–16, position 700 in particular (K700E). SF3B1 mutations cause alternative 3′ splice site selection.

Clinical Data

SF3B1 mutations occur in ~9%–10% of PMF and 4%–7% post-MPN AML patients (Table 1). In the context of MPN, *SF3B1* mutations most commonly occur in the entity MDS/MPN with ring sideroblasts and thrombocytosis (MDS/MPN-RS-T). This MDS/MPN overlap syndrome is typically characterized by the presence of both a *JAK2* and *SF3B1* mutation (Jeromin et al. 2013).

Mouse Models and Affected Cellular Pathways

As in other cancers (Darman et al. 2015; DeBoever et al. 2015; Alsafadi et al. 2016), *SF3B1*-

mutated MDS samples mainly had alternative 3′ splice site selection, in many cases leading to nonsense-mediated RNA decay (Lee et al. 2018). Differentially expressed genes included genes involved in RNA processing and metabolism, cell cycle, heme metabolism, and nonsense-mediated decay.

SIGNALING

LNK

Consequences of Mutations on Gene Function

The lymphocyte adaptor protein (LNK) or SH2B adapter protein 3 (SH2B3) is an adaptor protein. It interacts with and inhibits signaling through cytokine and tyrosine kinase receptors such as the EPO receptor and the stem cell factor receptor, c-Kit, or kinases like JAK2 (Fig. 3) (Tong et al. 2005; Bersenev et al. 2008; Simon et al. 2008). LNK inhibits the proliferation of HSCs, B-lymphoid cells, and myeloid cells mainly from the erythroid and megakaryocytic lineage (Takaki et al. 2000, 2002; Velazquez et al. 2002). Negative-feedback loops on growth stimulation are perturbed owing to mutations in *LNK* (and CBL, see below) (Takaki et al. 2002). Many mutations are missense substitutions and target the pleckstrin homology (PH) domain in the majority (~50%) of cases.

Clinical Data

LNK mutations are harbored in 0%–9% of MPN patients and 11% post-AML patients (Table 1). A reduced overall survival has been reported for ET patients harboring *LNK* mutations (Tefferi et al. 2016b).

Mouse Models and Affected Cellular Pathways

Mice lacking *Lnk* developed several characteristics of MPNs, including extramedullary hematopoiesis and splenomegaly, and an increase in HSCs and myeloid progenitor cells, predominantly of the megakaryocytic lineage (Velazquez et al. 2002; Ema et al. 2005; Buza-Vidas et al. 2006; Seita et al. 2007; Bersenev et al. 2008; Takizawa et al. 2008). The SH2 domain of LNK binds nonphosphorylated and JH2 domain-phosphorylated JAK2, thereby inhibiting JAK2 activation (Kurzer et al. 2006; Bersenev et al. 2008; Gery et al. 2009; Baran-Marszak et al. 2010). Additionally, LNK blocks binding of activators with c-Kit and activation of downstream signaling (Takaki et al. 2002; Simon et al. 2008). In addition, LNK can recruit the E3 ubiquitin ligase CBL for degradation of receptors/signaling molecules. These negative-feedback loops on growth stimulation are perturbed owing to mutations in *LNK* (Takaki et al. 2002). *LNK* mutations have been shown to enhance growth of $JAK2^{V617F}$ cells in clonogenic assays and in mice (Bersenev et al. 2008; Gery et al. 2009).

CBL

Consequences of Mutations on Gene Function

Casitas B-cell lymphoma (CBL) is a RING E3 ubiquitin ligase that promotes K63- and K48-linked ubiquitination (Thien and Langdon 2005; Mohapatra et al. 2013). It recognizes activated (receptor) tyrosine kinases such as epidermal growth factor receptor (EGFR), c-Kit, FLT3, and JAK2 by their phosphorylation and ubiquitinates them, which leads to proteasomal degradation (Thien and Langdon 2005; Mohapatra et al. 2013; Lv et al. 2017). Mutations are mostly homozygous missense substitutions located in the RING and linker domain, significantly reducing the E3 ligase activity, and thus decreasing the degradation of its substrates.

Clinical Data

Mutations in CBL are rare in ET and PV, but occur in up to 6% of MF and 4% of post-MPN AML patients (Table 1).

Mouse Models and Affected Cellular Pathways

CBL mutations lead to increased STAT5 and Akt phosphorylation, cytokine hypersensitivity, and cell proliferation (Sanada et al. 2009). *CBL* mu-

 Cite this article as *Cold Spring Harb Perspect Med* doi: 10.1101/cshperspect.a034876

tations are not merely loss-of-function mutations, because they further augmented cytokine sensitivity found in CBL knockout cells (Sanada et al. 2009).

NRAS/KRAS

Consequences of Mutations on Gene Function

Heterozygous missense substitutions at NRAS/KRAS codons 12, 13, and 61 are most common and favor the GTP-bound state of RAS because of reduced intrinsic GTP hydrolysis and resistance to GAPs (Schubbert et al. 2007). These mutations cause constitutive activation of growth signaling.

Clinical Data

Mutations in NRAS and KRAS in MPNs are associated with leukemic transformation and have been found in 7%–15% of post-MPN AML patients (Table 1), mutations in NRAS being more frequent than in KRAS.

Mouse Models and Affected Cellular Pathways

Conditional expression of $Kras^{G12D}$ in mouse models causes a myeloproliferative disease, whereas the same mutation in Nras causes a much more indolent disease (MacKenzie et al. 1999; Chan and Gilliland 2004).

PTPN11

Consequences of Mutations on Gene Function

Protein tyrosine phosphatase, nonreceptor type 11 (PTPN11) is a protein tyrosine phosphatase that acts downstream from several transmembrane receptors and dephosphorylates RAS (Bunda et al. 2015). Mutations in AML target the amino-terminal Src-homology 2 (N-SH2) and phosphotyrosine phosphatase (PTP) domains, which are important for switching between inactive and active forms of PTPN11.

Clinical Data

Heterozygous missense mutations in *PTPN11* are found in 6%–8% of post-MPN AML cases (Table 1) and are associated with shortened survival (Lasho et al. 2018).

Mouse Models and Affected Cellular Pathways

PTPN11 mutations cause a very high phosphatase activity (Tartaglia et al. 2003, 2006; Keilhack et al. 2005; Niihori et al. 2005). Dephosphorylation of RAS increases RAF–RAS association and activation of the RAS–RAF–MEK–ERK pathway (Shi et al. 2000).

TRANSCRIPTION FACTORS

RUNX1

Consequences of Mutations on Gene Function

Runt-related transcription factor 1 (RUNX1) heterodimerizes with core binding factor β (CBFβ) and regulates key hematopoietic transcriptional programs. It contains a DNA-binding and nuclear localizing Runt homology domain (RHD). Missense, frameshift, and nonsense mutations inactivate the affected RUNX1 protein, and, in addition, mutant RUNX1 may act in a dominant-negative way over the remaining wild-type RUNX1 protein.

Clinical Data

RUNX1 mutations occur in 4%–13% of post-MPN AML patients (Table 1). Multivariate analysis showed significantly shortened survival for *RUNX1* mutated versus *RUNX1* wild-type post-MPN AML patients (Lasho et al. 2018; McNamara et al. 2018).

Mouse Models and Affected Cellular Pathways

RUNX1 inactivation contributes to AML development through reduced myeloid differentiation and increased HSC self-renewal. The most frequent dominant-negative mutation, D171N, is located in its DNA-binding RHD. Mice transplanted with bone marrow cells overexpressing RUNX1^{D171N} developed MDS and MDS/AML within 4–13 mo after transplantation (Watanabe-Okochi et al. 2008). Ectopic expression of RUNX1^{D171N} in CD34^{+} HSPCs from chronic phase MPN patients seemed to keep the cells in a HSPC state and increase proliferation (Ding et al. 2009). Besides mutations in RUNX1, the short RUNX1a isoform has been shown to be overexpressed in MPN (Sakurai et al. 2017). As is the case for many leukemia-associated RUNX1 mutations, RUNX1a has been proposed to act in a dominant-negative way over the other two isoforms RUXN1b and RUNX1c. RUNX1a expression causes expansion of murine HSCs and up-regulates *Hoxa9*, *Meis1*, and *Stat1* (Tsuzuki and Seto 2012; Ran et al. 2013).

NFE2

Consequences of Mutations on Gene Function

A 4-amino acid in-frame deletion and frameshift mutations leading to expression of a carboxy-terminally truncated protein have been found in the transcription factor nuclear factor, erythroid 2 (NFE2) in MPNs. The mutations caused increased mRNA and protein expression of wild-type NFE2 (Jutzi et al. 2013).

Clinical Data

Mutations in NFE2 are carried by 0%–3% of PV and MF patients (Table 1).

Mouse Models and Affected Cellular Pathways

Mice transplanted with ectopically expressing mutant NF-E2 bone marrow cells had elevated myeloid progenitor cells as well as platelet numbers, erythrocyte numbers, and absolute neutrophil counts compared with control mice (Jutzi et al. 2013). When combined with JAK2^{V617F}, JAK2^{V617F}/NFE2 comutant mice had elevated hemoglobin and white blood cell count compared with JAK2^{V617F} mice (Jutzi et al. 2013). These data show that mutant NFE2 promotes myelopoiesis and augments the JAK2^{V617F}-induced MPN phenotype. Besides mutated NFE2, increased expression of NFE2 has been found in MPN patient samples. One of the proposed mechanisms for elevated NFE2 expression includes JAK2-dependent phosphorylation of H3Y41 in the *NFE2* promoter, leading to decreased binding of the repressive HP1α protein (Peeken et al. 2018). Increased NFE2 expression causes elevated transcription of the histone demethylase JMJD1C. In turn, JMJD1C causes positive feedback through decreasing H3K9me2 on the NFE2 promoter, also reducing HP1α binding and increasing NFE2 expression (Fig. 3) (Peeken et al. 2018).

DNA DAMAGE RESPONSE/STRESS SIGNALING

TP53

Consequences of Mutations on Gene Function

The last class of genes found mutated in MPNs includes genes involved in the DNA damage response and cellular stress. Tumor protein P53 (TP53) is a transcription factor frequently mutated in cancer. It is essential for a proper cellular response to stress and DNA damage. Many *TP53* mutations are missense mutations, which cause an abundance of mutant TP53 protein compared with wild-type TP53 (Rotter 1983). TP53 is a tumor suppressor, and *TP53* mutations can have several (nonmutually exclusive) effects: (1) loss of tumor suppressor function, (2) dominant-negative effect on wild-type TP53 protein, and (3) gain of functions that the wild-type protein does not possess.

Clinical Data

Mutations in *TP53* are uncommon in chronic phase MPNs, but exist in 11%–36% of post-MPN AML patients (Table 1). In addition to higher mutational frequency, the variant allele fraction of mutant *TP53* is higher in patient samples from transformed patients compared with chronic phase samples (Rampal et al. 2014). These data suggest that *TP53* mutations contribute to leukemic transformation in MPN.

Post-MPN AML patients harboring *TP53* mutations have an inferior overall survival compared with wild-type patients (mutant 4.4 mo vs. wild-type 6.5 mo) (Lundberg et al. 2014; Venton et al. 2018).

Mouse Models and Affected Cellular Pathways

In line with patient data, the concomitant knockout of *Tp53* and expression of $JAK2^{V617F}$ leads to leukemic transformation in mouse models (Rampal et al. 2014). Several progenitor populations from these mice were able to induce leukemia in (secondary) recipients. It has been shown that *TP53* mutations contribute to AML by increasing HSC self-renewal and resistance to cellular stress (Liu et al. 2009).

PPM1D

Consequences of Mutations on Gene Function

The serine-threonine *Protein Phosphatase* $Mg2^{+}$/$Mn2^{+}$ *1D* (*PPM1D*) gene is transcriptionally upregulated on *TP53* induction in response to DNA damage (Fiscella et al. 1997) and in turn negatively regulates TP53 and other proteins involved in the DNA damage response. Truncating and frameshift *PPM1D* mutations in exon 6 have been found in clonal hematopoiesis, MDS, and MPNs (Genovese et al. 2014; Xie et al. 2014; Coombs et al. 2017; Lindsley et al. 2017).

Clinical Data

PPM1D was recently described to be mutated in MPNs, with 1.9% of patients affected (Table 1; Grinfeld et al. 2018). Interestingly, *PPM1D* mutations are more frequent in patients who have been exposed to chemotherapy and who were diagnosed with therapy-related myeloid neoplasms (Ruark et al. 2013; Zhang et al. 2014; Kahn et al. 2018).

Mouse Models and Affected Cellular Pathways

PPM1D exon 6 mutations cause expression of a truncated PPM1D protein that lacks a carboxy-terminal degradation domain (Kahn et al. 2018). Consistent with patient data, *PPM1D*-mutant cells are selected for when treated with chemotherapy (Hsu et al. 2018; Kahn et al. 2018). This is explained by an abrogated DNA damage response, causing altered cell cycle progression, decreased apoptosis, and reduced mitochondrial priming in *PPM1D*-mutant compared with control cells (Kahn et al. 2018).

THERAPEUTIC IMPLICATIONS

Although the molecular pathogenesis of MPNs has been comprehensively defined, there are currently no curative pharmacological treatment options. The MPN phenotypic driver mutations represent attractive therapeutic targets because they are disease-initiating, activating, and can occur as the sole mutation, particularly in PV and ET. The main deficiency of JAK2 inhibitors is an absence of clonal selectivity, and efforts are ongoing to develop JAK2V617F-mutant-specific inhibitors. Mutant CALR also represents an enticing therapeutic target in MPNs, particularly from an immunological perspective, given its shared mutant-specific carboxy-terminal peptide.

Almost all of the concomitant mutations seen in MPNs do not currently have rationally designed approaches to target them, with IDH1/2 being the rare exception. Two drugs that inhibit mutant IDH1 or mutant IDH2 have been approved for the treatment of adult refractory or relapsed AML in the past 2 years: ivosidemib and enasidenib, respectively. Because mutations in IDH proteins are associated with a high risk of leukemic transformation in MPN, this is an important clinical development. Spliceosomal mutations, in particular *SRSF2* mutations, are another class of mutations associated with disease progression in MPNs, and there has been great enthusiasm around the development of spliceosomal inhibitors in myeloid malignancies more broadly. However, early clinical trial data in myelodysplastic syndrome (MDS) indicates an absence of clonal selectivity for spliceosomal inhibitors, although further studies are needed.

Another challenge posed by the genomic complexity of MPNs is that even drugs with potent, on-target, mutant-specific activity may have limited clinical efficacy depending on the clonal architecture of the MPNs (e.g., targeting a subclonal mutation as compared with a truncal lesion). Treatment paradigms that invoke early intervention to target disease-initiating genetic events and therapeutic approaches with broad efficacy regardless of molecular genetics (e.g., immunotherapy) are attractive for this reason.

CONCLUDING REMARKS

MPN phenotypic driver mutations that activate JAK-STAT signaling are central to MPN pathogenesis. However, concomitant somatic mutations are common and are often associated with disease progression. With the integration of NGS panels into MPN clinical care, molecular genetics is increasingly being used to predict prognosis and estimate the risk of disease progression (e.g., to AML) (Grinfeld et al. 2018). In myelofibrosis, clinical prognostic models that include molecular genetic parameters have already been developed (Ciboddo and Mullally 2018). The prognostic significance of concomitant somatic mutations in ET and PV is starting to be explored (Tefferi et al. 2016b; Grinfeld et al. 2018). With these advances, we have seen the development of novel mouse models to study the effects of concomitant mutations on MPN stem cells (Jacquelin et al. 2018; McKenney et al. 2018b) and identify the mechanisms by which these mutations drive disease progression. The next step is to use this knowledge to develop novel treatment approaches that exploit molecular vulnerabilities and preferentially target MPN stem cells in patients.

COMPETING INTEREST STATEMENT

The authors have declared that no conflict of interest exists.

ACKNOWLEDGMENTS

This work was supported by the National Institutes of Health (NIH) (R01HL131835 to A.M.), the MPN Research Foundation (A.M.), and the Gabrielle's Angel Foundation for Cancer Research (A.M.). A.M. is a Scholar of The Leukemia & Lymphoma Society. A.E.M. is supported by the European Molecular Biology Organization (EMBO) Long-Term Fellowship 2017-268.

REFERENCES

Abdel-Wahab O, Manshouri T, Patel J, Harris K, Yao J, Hedvat C, Heguy A, Bueso-Ramos C, Kantarjian H, Levine RL, et al. 2010. Genetic analysis of transforming events that convert chronic myeloproliferative neoplasms to leukemias. *Cancer Res* **70:** 447–452. doi:10.1158/0008-5472.CAN-09-3783

Abdel-Wahab O, Pardanani A, Rampal R, Lasho TL, Levine RL, Tefferi A. 2011. *DNMT3A* mutational analysis in primary myelofibrosis, chronic myelomonocytic leukemia and advanced phases of myeloproliferative neoplasms. *Leukemia* **25:** 1219–1220. doi:10.1038/leu.2011.82

Abdel-Wahab O, Adli M, LaFave LM, Gao J, Hricik T, Shih AH, Pandey S, Patel JP, Chung YR, Koche R, et al. 2012. *ASXL1* mutations promote myeloid transformation through loss of PRC2-mediated gene repression. *Cancer Cell* **22:** 180–193. doi:10.1016/j.ccr.2012.06.032

Alsafadi S, Houy A, Battistella A, Popova T, Wassef M, Henry E, Tirode F, Constantinou A, Piperno-Neumann S, Roman-Roman S, et al. 2016. Cancer-associated *SF3B1* mutations affect alternative splicing by promoting alternative branchpoint usage. *Nat Commun* **7:** 10615. doi:10.1038/ncomms10615

Angona A, Fernández-Rodríguez C, Alvarez-Larrán A, Camacho L, Longarón R, Torres E, Pairet S, Besses C, Bellosillo B. 2016. Molecular characterisation of triple negative essential thrombocythaemia patients by platelet analysis and targeted sequencing. *Blood Cancer J* **6:** e463. doi:10.1038/bcj.2016.75

Asada S, Goyama S, Inoue D, Shikata S, Takeda R, Fukushima T, Yonezawa T, Fujino T, Hayashi Y, Kawabata KC, et al. 2018. Mutant ASXL1 cooperates with BAP1 to promote myeloid leukaemogenesis. *Nat Commun* **9:** 2733. doi:10.1038/s41467-018-05085-9

Baran-Marszak F, Magdoud H, Desterke C, Alvarado A, Roger C, Harel S, Mazoyer E, Cassinat B, Chevret S, Tonetti C, et al. 2010. Expression level and differential JAK2-V617F-binding of the adaptor protein Lnk regulates JAK2-mediated signals in myeloproliferative neoplasms. *Blood* **116:** 5961–5971. doi:10.1182/blood-2009-12-256768

Beer PA, Delhommeau F, LeCouedic JP, Dawson MA, Chen E, Bareford D, Kusec R, McMullin MF, Harrison CN, Vannucchi AM, et al. 2010. Two routes to leukemic transformation after a *JAK2* mutation-positive myeloproliferative neoplasm. *Blood* **115:** 2891–2900. doi:10.1182/blood-2009-08-236596

Bera R, Liang D, Chiu M, Huang Y, Liang S, Shih L. 2012. PHD domain deletion mutations of ASXL1 promote myeloid leukemia transformation through epigenetic dysregulation and inhibit megakaryocytic differentiation through the inactivation of FOSB in K562 cells. Presented at the American Society of Hematology Conference. Atlanta, 8–11 December 2012.

Bersenev A, Wu C, Balcerek J, Tong W. 2008. Lnk controls mouse hematopoietic stem cell self-renewal and quiescence through direct interactions with JAK2. *J Clin Invest* **118:** 2832–2844.

Bunda S, Burrell K, Heir P, Zeng L, Alamsahebpour A, Kano Y, Raught B, Zhang ZY, Zadeh G, Ohh M. 2015. Inhibition of SHP2-mediated dephosphorylation of Ras suppresses oncogenesis. *Nat Commun* **6:** 8859. doi:10.1038/ncomms9859

Buza-Vidas N, Antonchuk J, Qian H, Mansson R, Luc S, Zandi S, Anderson K, Takaki S, Nygren JM, Jensen CT, et al. 2006. Cytokines regulate postnatal hematopoietic stem cell expansion: Opposing roles of thrombopoietin and LNK. *Genes Dev* **20:** 2018–2023. doi:10.1101/gad.385606

Chan IT, Gilliland DG. 2004. Oncogenic K-ras in mouse models of myeloproliferative disease and acute myeloid leukemia. *Cell Cycle* **3:** 536–537. doi:10.4161/cc.3.5.828

Chen E, Mullally A. 2014. How does JAK2V617F contribute to the pathogenesis of myeloproliferative neoplasms? *Hematology* **2014:** 268–276. doi:10.1182/asheducation-2014.1.268

Chen E, Schneider RK, Breyfogle LJ, Rosen EA, Poveromo L, Elf S, Ko A, Brumme K, Levine R, Ebert BL, et al. 2015. Distinct effects of concomitant Jak2V617F expression and Tet2 loss in mice promote disease progression in myeloproliferative neoplasms. *Blood* **125:** 327–335. doi:10.1182/blood-2014-04-567024

Chen L, Chen JY, Huang YJ, Gu Y, Qiu J, Qian H, Shao C, Zhang X, Hu J, Li H, et al. 2018. The augmented R-loop is a unifying mechanism for myelodysplastic syndromes induced by high-risk splicing factor mutations. *Mol Cell* **69:** 412–425.e6. doi:10.1016/j.molcel.2017.12.029

Ciboddo M, Mullally A. 2018. *JAK2* (and other genes) be nimble with MPN diagnosis, prognosis, and therapy. *Hematology* **2018:** 110–117. doi:10.1182/asheducation-2018.1.110

Coombs CC, Zehir A, Devlin SM, Kishtagari A, Syed A, Jonsson P, Hyman DM, Solit DB, Robson ME, Baselga J, et al. 2017. Therapy-related clonal hematopoiesis in patients with non-hematologic cancers is common and associated with adverse clinical outcomes. *Cell Stem Cell* **21:** 374–382.e4. doi:10.1016/j.stem.2017.07.010

Darman RB, Seiler M, Agrawal AA, Lim KH, Peng S, Aird D, Bailey SL, Bhavsar EB, Chan B, Colla S, et al. 2015. Cancer-associated SF3B1 hotspot mutations induce cryptic 3′ splice site selection through use of a different branch point. *Cell Rep* **13:** 1033–1045. doi:10.1016/j.celrep.2015.09.053

DeBoever C, Ghia EM, Shepard PJ, Rassenti L, Barrett CL, Jepsen K, Jamieson CH, Carson D, Kipps TJ, Frazer KA. 2015. Transcriptome sequencing reveals potential mechanism of cryptic 3′ splice site selection in *SF3B1*-mutated cancers. *PLoS Comput Biol* **11:** e1004105. doi:10.1371/journal.pcbi.1004105

Delhommeau F, Dupont S, Della Valle V, James C, Trannoy S, Massé A, Kosmider O, Le Couedic JP, Robert F, Alberdi A, et al. 2009. Mutation in *TET2* in myeloid cancers. *N Engl J Med* **360:** 2289–2301. doi:10.1056/NEJMoa0810069

Ding Y, Harada Y, Imagawa J, Kimura A, Harada H. 2009. *AML1/RUNX1* point mutation possibly promotes leukemic transformation in myeloproliferative neoplasms. *Blood* **114:** 5201–5205. doi:10.1182/blood-2009-06-223982

Dunbar AJ, Gondek LP, O'Keefe CL, Makishima H, Rataul MS, Szpurka H, Sekeres MA, Wang XF, McDevitt MA, Maciejewski JP. 2008. 250K single nucleotide polymorphism array karyotyping identifies acquired uniparental disomy and homozygous mutations, including novel missense substitutions of c-Cbl, in myeloid malignancies. *Cancer Res* **15:** 10349–10357. doi:10.1158/0008-5472.CAN-08-2754

Elf S, Abdelfattah NS, Chen E, Perales-Paton J, Rosen EA, Ko A, Peisker F, Florescu N, Giannini S, Wolach O, et al. 2016. Mutant calreticulin requires both its mutant C-terminus and the thrombopoietin receptor for oncogenic transformation. *Cancer Discov* **6:** 368–381. doi:10.1158/2159-8290.CD-15-1434

Ema H, Sudo K, Seita J, Matsubara A, Morita Y, Osawa M, Takatsu K, Takaki S, Nakauchi H. 2005. Quantification of self-renewal capacity in single hematopoietic stem cells from normal and *Lnk*-deficient mice. *Dev Cell* **8:** 907–914. doi:10.1016/j.devcel.2005.03.019

Emperle M, Dukatz M, Kunert S, Holzer K, Rajavelu A, Jurkowska RZ, Jeltsch A. 2018. The DNMT3A R882H mutation does not cause dominant negative effects in purified mixed DNMT3A/R882H complexes. *Sci Rep* **8:** 13242. doi:10.1038/s41598-018-31635-8

Fiscella M, Zhang H, Fan S, Sakaguchi K, Shen S, Mercer WE, Vande Woude GF, O'Connor PM, Appella E. 1997. Wip1, a novel human protein phosphatase that is induced in response to ionizing radiation in a p53-dependent manner. *Proc Natl Acad Sci* **94:** 6048–6053. doi:10.1073/pnas.94.12.6048

Genovese G, Kähler AK, Handsaker RE, Lindberg J, Rose SA, Bakhoum SF, Chambert K, Mick E, Neale BM, Fromer M, et al. 2014. Clonal hematopoiesis and blood-cancer risk inferred from blood DNA sequence. *N Engl J Med* **371:** 2477–2487. doi:10.1056/NEJMoa1409405

Gery S, Cao Q, Gueller S, Xing H, Tefferi A, Koeffler HP. 2009. Lnk inhibits myeloproliferative disorder-associated JAK2 mutant, JAK2V617F. *J Leukoc Biol* **85:** 957–965. doi:10.1189/jlb.0908575

Gibson CJ, Steensma DP. 2018. New Insights from studies of clonal hematopoiesis. *Clin Cancer Res* **24:** 4633–4642. doi:10.1158/1078-0432.CCR-17-3044

Grand FH, Hidalgo-Curtis CE, Ernst T, Zoi K, Zoi C, McGuire C, Kreil S, Jones A, Score J, Metzgeroth G, et al. 2009. Frequent CBL mutations associated with 11q acquired uniparental disomy in myeloproliferative neoplasms. *Blood* **113:** 6182–6192. doi:10.1182/blood-2008-12-194548

Grinfeld J, Nangalia J, Baxter EJ, Wedge DC, Angelopoulos N, Cantrill R, Godfrey AL, Papaemmanuil E, Gundem G, MacLean C, et al. 2018. Classification and personalized prognosis in myeloproliferative neoplasms. *N Engl J Med* **379:** 1416–1430. doi:10.1056/NEJMoa1716614

Guglielmelli P, Biamonte F, Score J, Hidalgo-Curtis C, Cervantes F, Maffioli M, Fanelli T, Ernst T, Winkelman N, Jones AV, et al. 2011. *EZH2* mutational status predicts poor survival in myelofibrosis. *Blood* **118:** 5227–5234. doi:10.1182/blood-2011-06-363424

Guglielmelli P, Lasho TL, Rotunno G, Score J, Mannarelli C, Pancrazzi A, Biamonte F, Pardanani A, Zoi K, Reiter A, et al. 2014. The number of prognostically detrimental mutations and prognosis in primary myelofibrosis: An international study of 797 patients. *Leukemia* **28:** 1804–1810. doi:10.1038/leu.2014.76

Guglielmelli P, Lasho TL, Rotunno G, Mudireddy M, Mannarelli C, Nicolosi M, Pacilli A, Pardanani A, Rumi E, Rosti V, et al. 2018. MIPSS70: Mutation-enhanced international prognostic score system for transplantation-age patients with primary myelofibrosis. *J Clin Oncol* **36:** 310–318. doi:10.1200/JCO.2017.76.4886

Guo Y, Zhou Y, Yamatomo S, Yang H, Zhang P, Chen S, Nimer SD, Zhao ZJ, Xu M, Bai J, et al. 2019. *ASXL1* alteration cooperates with *JAK2V617F* to accelerate myelofibrosis. *Leukemia* **33:** 1287–1291. doi:10.1038/s41375-018-0347-y

Harutyunyan A, Klampfl T, Cazzola M, Kralovics R. 2011. p53 lesions in leukemic transformation. *N Eng J Med* **364:** 488–490. doi:10.1056/NEJMc1012718

Hinds DA, Barnholt KE, Mesa RA, Kiefer AK, Do CB, Eriksson N, Mountain JL, Francke U, Tung JY, Nguyen HM, et al. 2016. Germ line variants predispose to both *JAK2* V617F clonal hematopoiesis and myeloproliferative neoplasms. *Blood* **128:** 1121–1128. doi:10.1182/blood-2015-06-652941

Hsu YC, Chiu YC, Lin CC, Kuo YY, Hou HA, Tzeng YS, Kao CJ, Chuang PH, Tseng MH, Hsiao TH, et al. 2017. The distinct biological implications of *Asxl1* mutation and its roles in leukemogenesis revealed by a knock-in mouse model. *J Hematol Oncol* **10:** 139. doi:10.1186/s13045-017-0508-x

Hsu JI, Dayaram T, Tovy A, De Braekeleer E, Jeong M, Wang F, Zhang J, Heffernan TP, Gera S, Kovacs JJ, et al. 2018. *PPM1D* mutations drive clonal hematopoiesis in response to cytotoxic chemotherapy. *Cell Stem Cell* **23:** 700–713.e6. doi:10.1016/j.stem.2018.10.004

Ilagan JO, Ramakrishnan A, Hayes B, Murphy ME, Zebari AS, Bradley P, Bradley RK. 2015. *U2AF1* mutations alter splice site recognition in hematological malignancies. *Genome Res* **25:** 14–26. doi:10.1101/gr.181016.114

Inoue D, Matsumoto M, Nagase R, Saika M, Fujino T, Nakayama KI, Kitamura T. 2016. Truncation mutants of *ASXL1* observed in myeloid malignancies are expressed at detectable protein levels. *Exp Hematol* **44:** 172–176.e1. doi:10.1016/j.exphem.2015.11.011

Jacquelin S, Straube J, Cooper L, Vu T, Song A, Bywater M, Baxter E, Heidecker M, Wackrow B, Porter A, et al. 2018. Jak2V617F and Dnmt3a loss cooperate to induce myelofibrosis through activated enhancer-driven inflammation. *Blood* **132:** 2707–2721. doi:10.1182/blood-2018-04-846220

Jaiswal S, Fontanillas P, Flannick J, Manning A, Grauman PV, Mar BG, Lindsley RC, Mermel CH, Burtt N, Chavez A, et al. 2014. Age-related clonal hematopoiesis associated with adverse outcomes. *N Engl J Med* **371:** 2488–2498. doi:10.1056/NEJMoa1408617

Jaiswal S, Natarajan P, Silver AJ, Gibson CJ, Bick AG, Shvartz E, McConkey M, Gupta N, Gabriel S, Ardissino D, et al. 2017. Clonal hematopoiesis and risk of atherosclerotic cardiovascular disease. *N Engl J Med* **377:** 111–121. doi:10.1056/NEJMoa1701719

Jeromin S, Haferlach T, Grossmann V, Alpermann T, Kowarsch A, Haferlach C, Kern W, Schnittger S. 2013. High frequencies of *SF3B1* and *JAK2* mutations in refractory anemia with ring sideroblasts associated with marked thrombocytosis strengthen the assignment to the category of myelodysplastic/myeloproliferative neoplasms. *Haematologica* **98:** e15–e17. doi:10.3324/haematol.2012.072538

Ji X, Zhou Y, Pandit S, Huang J, Li H, Lin CY, Xiao R, Burge CB, Fu XD. 2013. SR proteins collaborate with 7SK and promoter-associated nascent RNA to release paused polymerase. *Cell* **153:** 855–868. doi:10.1016/j.cell.2013.04.028

Jutzi JS, Bogeska R, Nikoloski G, Schmid CA, Seeger TS, Stegelmann F, Schwemmers S, Gründer A, Peeken JC, Gothwal M, et al. 2013. MPN patients harbor recurrent truncating mutations in transcription factor NF-E2. *J Exp Med* **210:** 1003–1019. doi:10.1084/jem.20120521

Kahn JD, Miller PG, Silver AJ, Sellar RS, Bhatt S, Gibson C, McConkey M, Adams D, Mar B, Mertins P, et al. 2018. *PPM1D*-truncating mutations confer resistance to chemotherapy and sensitivity to PPM1D inhibition in hematopoietic cells. *Blood* **132:** 1095–1105. doi:10.1182/blood-2018-05-850339

Kameda T, Shide K, Yamaji T, Kamiunten A, Sekine M, Hidaka T, Kubuki Y, Sashida G, Aoyama K, Yoshimitsu M, et al. 2015a. Gene expression profiling of loss of TET2 and/or *JAK2*V617F mutant hematopoietic stem cells from mouse models of myeloproliferative neoplasms. *Genom Data* **4:** 102–108. doi:10.1016/j.gdata.2015.04.002

Kameda T, Shide K, Yamaji T, Kamiunten A, Sekine M, Taniguchi Y, Hidaka T, Kubuki Y, Shimoda H, Marutsuka K, et al. 2015b. Loss of TET2 has dual roles in murine myeloproliferative neoplasms: Disease sustainer and disease accelerator. *Blood* **125:** 304–315. doi:10.1182/blood-2014-04-555508

Keilhack H, David FS, McGregor M, Cantley LC, Neel BG. 2005. Diverse biochemical properties of Shp2 mutants. Implications for disease phenotypes. *J Biol Chem* **280:** 30984–30993. doi:10.1074/jbc.M504699200

Khan SN, Jankowska AM, Mahfouz R, Dunbar AJ, Sugimoto Y, Hosono N, Hu Z, Cheriyath V, Vatolin S, Przychodzen B, et al. 2013. Multiple mechanisms deregulate EZH2 and histone H3 lysine 27 epigenetic changes in myeloid malignancies. *Leukemia* **27:** 1301–1309. doi:10.1038/leu.2013.80

Kim E, Ilagan JO, Liang Y, Daubner GM, Lee SC, Ramakrishnan A, Li Y, Chung YR, Micol JB, Murphy ME, et al. 2015. *SRSF2* mutations contribute to myelodysplasia by mutant-specific effects on exon recognition. *Cancer Cell* **27:** 617–630. doi:10.1016/j.ccell.2015.04.006

Klampfl T, Gisslinger H, Harutyunyan AS, Nivarthi H, Rumi E, Milosevic JD, Them NC, Berg T, Gisslinger B, Pietra D, et al. 2013. Somatic mutations of calreticulin in myeloproliferative neoplasms. *N Engl J Med* **369:** 2379–2390. doi:10.1056/NEJMoa1311347

Kröger N, Panagiota V, Badbaran A, Zabelina T, Triviai I, Araujo Cruz MM, Shahswar R, Ayuk F, Gehlhaar M, Wolschke C, et al. 2017. Impact of molecular genetics on outcome in myelofibrosis patients after allogeneic stem cell transplantation. *Biol Blood Marrow Transplant* **23:** 1095–1101. doi:10.1016/j.bbmt.2017.03.034

Kurzer JH, Saharinen P, Silvennoinen O, Carter-Su C. 2006. Binding of SH2-B family members within a potential negative regulatory region maintains JAK2 in an active state. *Mol Cell Biol* **26:** 6381–6394. doi:10.1128/MCB.00570-06

Lasho TL, Jimma T, Finke CM, Patnaik M, Hanson CA, Ketterling RP, Pardanani A, Tefferi A. 2012. *SRSF2* mutations in primary myelofibrosis: Significant clustering with *IDH* mutations and independent association with inferior overall and leukemia-free survival. *Blood* **120:** 4168–4171. doi:10.1182/blood-2012-05-429696

Lasho TL, Mudireddy M, Finke CM, Hanson CA, Ketterling RP, Szuber N, Begna KH, Patnaik MM, Gangat N, Pardanani A, et al. 2018. Targeted next-generation sequencing in blast phase myeloproliferative neoplasms. *Blood Adv* **2:** 370–380. doi:10.1182/bloodadvances.2018015875

Lee SC, North K, Kim E, Jang E, Obeng E, Lu SX, Liu B, Inoue D, Yoshimi A, Ki M, et al. 2018. Synthetic lethal and convergent biological effects of cancer-associated spliceosomal gene mutations. *Cancer Cell* **34:** 225–241.e8. doi:10.1016/j.ccell.2018.07.003

Ley TJ, Ding L, Walter MJ, McLellan MD, Lamprecht T, Larson DE, Kandoth C, Payton JE, Baty J, Welch J, et al. 2010. *DNMT3A* mutations in acute myeloid leukemia. *N Engl J Med* **363:** 2424–2433. doi:10.1056/NEJMoa1005143

Li J, Prins D, Park HJ, Grinfeld J, Gonzalez-Arias C, Loughran S, Dovey OM, Klampfl T, Bennett C, Hamilton TL, et al. 2018. Mutant calreticulin knockin mice develop thrombocytosis and myelofibrosis without a stem cell self-renewal advantage. *Blood* **131:** 649–661. doi:10.1182/blood-2017-09-806356

Lin J, Yao DM, Qian J, Chen Q, Qian W, Li Y, Yang J, Wang CZ, Chai HY, Qian Z, Xiao GF, Xu WR. 2011. Recurrent *DNMT3A* R882 mutations in Chinese patients with acute myeloid leukemia and myelodysplastic syndrome. *PLoS ONE* **6:** e26906. doi:10.1371/journal.pone.0026906

Lindsley RC, Saber W, Mar BG, Redd R, Wang T, Haagenson MD, Grauman PV, Hu ZH, Spellman SR, Lee SJ, et al. 2017. Prognostic mutations in myelodysplastic syndrome after stem-cell transplantation. *N Engl J Med* **376:** 536–547. doi:10.1056/NEJMoa1611604

Liu Y, Elf SE, Miyata Y, Sashida G, Liu Y, Huang G, Di Giandomenico S, Lee JM, Deblasio A, Menendez S, et al. 2009. p53 regulates hematopoietic stem cell quiescence. *Cell Stem Cell* **4:** 37–48. doi:10.1016/j.stem.2008.11.006

Lundberg P, Karow A, Nienhold R, Looser R, Hao-Shen H, Nissen I, Girsberger S, Lehmann T, Passweg J, Stern M, et al. 2014. Clonal evolution and clinical correlates of somatic mutations in myeloproliferative neoplasms. *Blood* **123:** 2220–2228. doi:10.1182/blood-2013-11-537167

Lv K, Jiang J, Donaghy R, Riling CR, Cheng Y, Chandra V, Rozenova K, An W, Mohapatra BC, Goetz BT, et al. 2017. CBL family E3 ubiquitin ligases control JAK2 ubiquitination and stability in hematopoietic stem cells and myeloid malignancies. *Genes Dev* **31:** 1007–1023. doi:10.1101/gad.297135.117

MacKenzie KL, Dolnikov A, Millington M, Shounan Y, Symonds G. 1999. Mutant N-*ras* induces myeloproliferative disorders and apoptosis in bone marrow repopulated mice. *Blood* **93:** 2043–2056.

Madan V, Kanojia D, Li J, Okamoto R, Sato-Otsubo A, Kohlmann A, Sanada M, Grossmann V, Sundaresan J, Shiraishi Y, et al. 2015. Aberrant splicing of U12-type introns is the hallmark of ZRSR2 mutant myelodysplastic syndrome. *Nat Commun* **6:** 6042. doi:10.1038/ncomms7042

Makishima H, Cazzolli H, Szpurka H, Dunbar A, Tiu R, Huh J, Muramatsu H, O'Keefe C, Hsi E, Paquette RL, et al. 2009. Mutations of e3 ubiquitin ligase cbl family members constitute a novel common pathogenic lesion in myeloid malignancies. *J Clin Oncol* **27:** 6109–6116. doi:10.1200/JCO.2009.23.7503

Malcovati L, Papaemmanuil E, Bowen DT, Boultwood J, Della Porta MG, Pascutto C, Travaglino E, Groves MJ, Godfrey AL, Ambaglio I, et al. 2011. Clinical significance of *SF3B1* mutations in myelodysplastic syndromes and myelodysplastic/myeloproliferative neoplasms. *Blood* **118:** 6239–6246. doi:10.1182/blood-2011-09-377275

McKenney AS, Lau AN, Somasundara AVH, Spitzer B, Intlekofer AM, Ahn J, Shank K, Rapaport FT, Patel MA, Papalexi E, et al. 2018a. JAK2/IDH-mutant-driven myeloproliferative neoplasm is sensitive to combined targeted inhibition. *J Clin Invest* **128:** 789–804. doi:10.1172/JCI94516

McKenney AS, Lau AN, Somasundara AVH, Spitzer B, Intlekofer AM, Ahn J, Shank K, Rapaport FT, Patel MA, Papalexi E, et al. 2018b. JAK2/IDH-mutant-driven myeloproliferative neoplasm is sensitive to combined targeted inhibition. *J Clin Invest* **128:** 4743. doi:10.1172/JCI124920

McNamara CJ, Panzarella T, Kennedy JA, Arruda A, Claudio JO, Daher-Reyes G, Ho J, Siddiq N, Devlin R, Tsui H, et al. 2018. The mutational landscape of accelerated- and blast-phase myeloproliferative neoplasms impacts patient outcomes. *Blood Adv* **2:** 2658–2671. doi:10.1182/bloodadvances.2018021469

Mead AJ, Mullally A. 2017. Myeloproliferative neoplasm stem cells. *Blood* **129:** 1607–1616. doi:10.1182/blood-2016-10-696005

Milosevic Feenstra JD, Nivarthi H, Gisslinger H, Leroy E, Rumi E, Chachoua I, Bagienski K, Kubesova B, Pietra D, Gisslinger B, et al. 2016. Whole-exome sequencing identifies novel *MPL* and *JAK2* mutations in triple-negative myeloproliferative neoplasms. *Blood* **127:** 325–332. doi:10.1182/blood-2015-07-661835

Minor EA, Court BL, Young JI, Wang G. 2013. Ascorbate induces ten-eleven translocation (Tet) methylcytosine dioxygenase-mediated generation of 5-hydroxymethylcytosine. *J Biol Chem* **288:** 13669–13674. doi:10.1074/jbc.C113.464800

Mohapatra B, Ahmad G, Nadeau S, Zutshi N, An W, Scheffe S, Dong L, Feng D, Goetz B, Arya P, et al. 2013. Protein tyrosine kinase regulation by ubiquitination: Critical roles of Cbl-family ubiquitin ligases. *Biochim Biophys Acta* **1833:** 122–139. doi:10.1016/j.bbamcr.2012.10.010

Mullally A, Bruedigam C, Poveromo L, Heidel FH, Purdon A, Vu T, Austin R, Heckl D, Breyfogle LJ, Kuhn CP, et al. 2013. Depletion of Jak2V617F myeloproliferative neoplasm-propagating stem cells by interferon-α in a murine model of polycythemia vera. *Blood* **121:** 3692–3702. doi:10.1182/blood-2012-05-432989

Muramatsu H, Makishima H, Jankowska AM, Cazzolli H, O'Keefe C, Yoshida N, Xu Y, Nishio N, Hama A, Yagasaki H, et al. 2010. Mutations of an E3 ubiquitin ligase c-Cbl but not TET2 mutations are pathogenic in juvenile myelomonocytic leukemia. *Blood* **115:** 1969–1975. doi:10.1182/blood-2009-06-226340

Nagase R, Inoue D, Pastore A, Fujino T, Hou HA, Yamasaki N, Goyama S, Saika M, Kanai A, Sera Y, et al. 2018. Expression of mutant Asxl1 perturbs hematopoiesis and promotes susceptibility to leukemic transformation. *J Exp Med* **215:** 1729–1747. doi:10.1084/jem.20171151

Nangalia J, Massie CE, Baxter EJ, Nice FL, Gundem G, Wedge DC, Avezov E, Li J, Kollmann K, Kent DG, et al. 2013. Somatic *CALR* mutations in myeloproliferative neoplasms with nonmutated *JAK2*. *N Engl J Med* **369:** 2391–2405. doi:10.1056/NEJMoa1312542

Nangalia J, Nice FL, Wedge DC, Godfrey AL, Grinfeld J, Thakker C, Massie CE, Baxter J, Sewell D, Silber Y, et al. 2015. *DNMT3A* mutations occur early or late in patients with myeloproliferative neoplasms and mutation order influences phenotype. *Haematologica* **100:** e438–e442. doi:10.3324/haematol.2015.129510

Newberry KJ, Patel K, Masarova L, Luthra R, Manshouri T, Jabbour E, Bose P, Daver N, Cortes J, Kantarjian H, et al. 2017. Clonal evolution and outcomes in myelofibrosis after ruxolitinib discontinuation. *Blood* **130:** 1125–1131. doi:10.1182/blood-2017-05-783225

Nguyen HD, Leong WY, Li W, Reddy PNG, Sullivan JD, Walter MJ, Zou L, Graubert TA. 2018. Spliceosome mutations induce R loop-associated sensitivity to ATR inhibition in myelodysplastic syndromes. *Cancer Res* **78:** 5363–5374. doi:10.1158/0008-5472.CAN-17-3970

Niihori T, Aoki Y, Ohashi H, Kurosawa K, Kondoh T, Ishikiriyama S, Kawame H, Kamasaki H, Yamanaka T, Takada F, et al. 2005. Functional analysis of PTPN11/SHP-2 mutants identified in Noonan syndrome and childhood leukemia. *J Hum Genet* **50:** 192–202. doi:10.1007/s10038-005-0239-7

Ortmann CA, Kent DG, Nangalia J, Silber Y, Wedge DC, Grinfeld J, Baxter EJ, Massie CE, Papaemmanuil E, Menon S, et al. 2015. Effect of mutation order on myeloproliferative neoplasms. *N Engl J Med* **372:** 601–612. doi:10.1056/NEJMoa1412098

Palangat M, Anastsakis D, Liang F, Lindblad K, Bradley R, Hourigan C, Hafner M, Larson D. 2018. The splicing factor U2AF1 contributes to cancer progression through a non-canonical role in translation regulation. *Genes Dev* **33:** 482–497. doi:10.1101/gad.319590.118

Papaemmanuil E, Cazzola M, Boultwood J, Malcovati L, Vyas P, Bowen D, Pellagatti A, Wainscoat JS, Hellstrom-Lindberg E, Gambacorti-Passerini C, et al. 2011. Somatic *SF3B1* mutation in myelodysplasia with ring sideroblasts. *N Eng J Med* **365:** 1384–1395. doi:10.1056/NEJMoa1103283

Pardanani A, Lasho TL, Finke CM, Mai M, McClure RF, Tefferi A. 2010. *IDH1* and *IDH2* mutation analysis in chronic- and blast-phase myeloproliferative neoplasms. *Leukemia* **24:** 1146–1151. doi:10.1038/leu.2010.77

Park SM, Ou J, Chamberlain L, Simone TM, Yang H, Virbasius CM, Ali AM, Zhu LJ, Mukherjee S, Raza A, et al. 2016. U2AF35(S34F) promotes transformation by directing aberrant ATG7 pre-mRNA 3′ end formation. *Mol Cell* **62:** 479–490. doi:10.1016/j.molcel.2016.04.011

Peeken JC, Jutzi JS, Wehrle J, Koellerer C, Staehle HF, Becker H, Schoenwandt E, Seeger TS, Schanne DH, Gothwal M, et al. 2018. Epigenetic regulation of NFE2 overexpression in myeloproliferative neoplasms. *Blood* **131:** 2065–2073. doi:10.1182/blood-2017-10-810622

Pikman Y, Lee BH, Mercher T, McDowell E, Ebert BL, Gozo M, Cuker A, Wernig G, Moore S, Galinsky I, et al. 2006. *MPLW515L* is a novel somatic activating mutation in myelofibrosis with myeloid metaplasia. *PLoS Med* **3:** e270. doi:10.1371/journal.pmed.0030270

Przychodzen B, Jerez A, Guinta K, Sekeres MA, Padgett R, Maciejewski JP, Makishima H. 2013. Patterns of missplicing due to somatic U2AF1 mutations in myeloid neoplasms. *Blood* **122:** 999–1006. doi:10.1182/blood-2013-01-480970

Rampal R, Ahn J, Abdel-Wahab O, Nahas M, Wang K, Lipson D, Otto GA, Yelensky R, Hricik T, McKenney AS, et al. 2014. Genomic and functional analysis of leukemic transformation of myeloproliferative neoplasms. *Proc Natl Acad Sci* **111:** E5401–E5410. doi:10.1073/pnas.1407792111

Ran D, Shia WJ, Lo MC, Fan JB, Knorr DA, Ferrell PI, Ye Z, Yan M, Cheng L, Kaufman DS, et al. 2013. RUNX1a enhances hematopoietic lineage commitment from human embryonic stem cells and inducible pluripotent stem cells. *Blood* **121:** 2882–2890. doi:10.1182/blood-2012-08-451641

Rao N, Butcher CM, Lewis ID, Ross DM, Melo JV, Scott HS, Bardy PG, D'Andrea RJ. 2012. Clonal and lineage analysis of somatic *DNMT3A* and *JAK2* mutations in a chronic phase polycythemia vera patient. *Br J Haematol* **156:** 268–270. doi:10.1111/j.1365-2141.2011.08837.x

Rasmussen KD, Jia G, Johansen JV, Pedersen MT, Rapin N, Bagger FO, Porse BT, Bernard OA, Christensen J, Helin K. 2015. Loss of *TET2* in hematopoietic cells leads to DNA hypermethylation of active enhancers and induction of leukemogenesis. *Genes Dev* **29:** 910–922. doi:10.1101/gad.260174.115

Rotter V. 1983. p53, a transformation-related cellular-encoded protein, can be used as a biochemical marker for the detection of primary mouse tumor cells. *Proc Natl Acad Sci* **80:** 2613–2617. doi:10.1073/pnas.80.9.2613

Ruark E, Snape K, Humburg P, Loveday C, Bajrami I, Brough R, Rodrigues DN, Renwick A, Seal S, Ramsay E, et al. 2013. Mosaic *PPM1D* mutations are associated with predisposition to breast and ovarian cancer. *Nature* **493:** 406–410. doi:10.1038/nature11725

Saika M, Inoue D, Nagase R, Sato N, Tsuchiya A, Yabushita T, Kitamura T, Goyama S. 2018. *ASXL1* and *SETBP1* mutations promote leukaemogenesis by repressing TGFβ pathway genes through histone deacetylation. *Sci Rep* **8:** 15873. doi:10.1038/s41598-018-33881-2

Sakurai H, Harada Y, Ogata Y, Kagiyama Y, Shingai N, Doki N, Ohashi K, Kitamura T, Komatsu N, Harada H. 2017. Overexpression of *RUNX1* short isoform has an important role in the development of myelodysplastic/myeloproliferative neoplasms. *Blood Adv* **1:** 1382–1386. doi:10.1182/bloodadvances.2016002725

Sanada M, Suzuki T, Shih LY, Otsu M, Kato M, Yamazaki S, Tamura A, Honda H, Sakata-Yanagimoto M, Kumano K, et al. 2009. Gain-of-function of mutated *C-CBL* tumour suppressor in myeloid neoplasms. *Nature* **460:** 904–908. doi:10.1038/nature08240

Sasaki M, Knobbe CB, Munger JC, Lind EF, Brenner D, Brustle A, Harris IS, Holmes R, Wakeham A, Haight J, et al. 2012. IDH1(R132H) mutation increases murine haematopoietic progenitors and alters epigenetics. *Nature* **488:** 656–659. doi:10.1038/nature11323

Scheuermann JC, de Ayala Alonso AG, Oktaba K, Ly-Hartig N, McGinty RK, Fraterman S, Wilm M, Muir TW, Müller J. 2010. Histone H2A deubiquitinase activity of the Polycomb repressive complex PR-DUB. *Nature* **465:** 243–247. doi:10.1038/nature08966

Schubbert S, Shannon K, Bollag G. 2007. Hyperactive Ras in developmental disorders and cancer. *Nat Rev Cancer* **7:** 295–308. doi:10.1038/nrc2109

Scott LM, Tong W, Levine RL, Scott MA, Beer PA, Stratton MR, Futreal PA, Erber WN, McMullin MF, Harrison CN, et al. 2007. *JAK2* exon 12 mutations in polycythemia vera and idiopathic erythrocytosis. *N Engl J Med* **356:** 459–468. doi:10.1056/NEJMoa065202

Seita J, Ema H, Ooehara J, Yamazaki S, Tadokoro Y, Yamasaki A, Eto K, Takaki S, Takatsu K, Nakauchi H. 2007. Lnk negatively regulates self-renewal of hematopoietic stem cells by modifying thrombopoietin-mediated signal transduction. *Proc Natl Acad Sci* **104:** 2349–2354. doi:10.1073/pnas.0606238104

Shen H, Zheng X, Luecke S, Green MR. 2010. The U2AF35-related protein Urp contacts the 3′ splice site to promote U12-type intron splicing and the second step of U2-type intron splicing. *Genes Dev* **24:** 2389–2394. doi:10.1101/gad.1974810

Shi ZQ, Yu DH, Park M, Marshall M, Feng GS. 2000. Molecular mechanism for the Shp-2 tyrosine phosphatase function in promoting growth factor stimulation of Erk activity. *Mol Cell Biol* **20:** 1526–1536. doi:10.1128/MCB.20.5.1526-1536.2000

Shimizu T, Kubovcakova L, Nienhold R, Zmajkovic J, Meyer SC, Hao-Shen H, Geier F, Dirnhofer S, Guglielmelli P, Vannucchi AM, et al. 2016. Loss of *Ezh2* synergizes with *JAK2*-V617F in initiating myeloproliferative neoplasms and promoting myelofibrosis. *J Exp Med* **213:** 1479–1496. doi:10.1084/jem.20151136

Simon C, Dondi E, Chaix A, de Sepulveda P, Kubiseski TJ, Varin-Blank N, Velazquez L. 2008. Lnk adaptor protein down-regulates specific Kit-induced signaling pathways in primary mast cells. *Blood* **112:** 4039–4047. doi:10.1182/blood-2008-05-154849

Stegelmann F, Bullinger L, Schlenk RF, Paschka P, Griesshammer M, Blersch C, Kuhn S, Schauer S, Döhner H, Döhner K. 2011. *DNMT3A* mutations in myeloproliferative neoplasms. *Leukemia* **25:** 1217–1219. doi:10.1038/leu.2011.77

Tahiliani M, Koh KP, Shen Y, Pastor WA, Bandukwala H, Brudno Y, Agarwal S, Iyer LM, Liu DR, Aravind L, et al. 2009. Conversion of 5-methylcytosine to 5-hydroxymethylcytosine in mammalian DNA by MLL partner TET1. *Science* **324:** 930–935. doi:10.1126/science.1170116

Takaki S, Sauer K, Iritani BM, Chien S, Ebihara Y, Tsuji K, Takatsu K, Perlmutter RM. 2000. Control of B cell production by the adaptor protein lnk. Definition of a conserved family of signal-modulating proteins. *Immunity* **13:** 599–609. doi:10.1016/S1074-7613(00)00060-1

Takaki S, Morita H, Tezuka Y, Takatsu K. 2002. Enhanced hematopoiesis by hematopoietic progenitor cells lacking intracellular adaptor protein, Lnk. *J Exp Med* **195:** 151–160. doi:10.1084/jem.20011170

Takizawa H, Eto K, Yoshikawa A, Nakauchi H, Takatsu K, Takaki S. 2008. Growth and maturation of megakaryocytes is regulated by Lnk/Sh2b3 adaptor protein through crosstalk between cytokine- and integrin-mediated signals. *Exp Hematol* **36:** 897–906. doi:10.1016/j.exphem.2008.02.004

Tartaglia M, Niemeyer CM, Fragale A, Song X, Buechner J, Jung A, Hählen K, Hasle H, Licht JD, Gelb BD. 2003. Somatic mutations in *PTPN11* in juvenile myelomonocytic leukemia, myelodysplastic syndromes and acute myeloid leukemia. *Nat Genet* **34:** 148–150. doi:10.1038/ng1156

Tartaglia M, Martinelli S, Stella L, Bocchinfuso G, Flex E, Cordeddu V, Zampino G, Burgt I, Palleschi A, Petrucci TC, et al. 2006. Diversity and functional consequences of germline and somatic *PTPN11* mutations in human disease. *Am J Hum Genet* **78:** 279–290. doi:10.1086/499925

Tefferi A, Lasho TL, Abdel-Wahab O, Guglielmelli P, Patel J, Caramazza D, Pieri L, Finke CM, Kilpivaara O, Wadleigh M, et al. 2010. *IDH1* and *IDH2* mutation studies in 1473 patients with chronic-, fibrotic- or blast-phase essential thrombocythemia, polycythemia vera or myelofibrosis. *Leukemia* **24:** 1302–1309. doi:10.1038/leu.2010.113

Tefferi A, Guglielmelli P, Lasho TL, Rotunno G, Finke C, Mannarelli C, Belachew AA, Pancrazzi A, Wassie EA, Ketterling RP, et al. 2014. *CALR* and *ASXL1* mutations-based molecular prognostication in primary myelofibrosis: An international study of 570 patients. *Leukemia* **28:** 1494–1500. doi:10.1038/leu.2014.57

Tefferi A, Lasho TL, Finke CM, Elala Y, Hanson CA, Ketterling RP, Gangat N, Pardanani A. 2016a. Targeted deep sequencing in primary myelofibrosis. *Blood Adv* **1:** 105–111. doi:10.1182/bloodadvances.2016000208

Tefferi A, Lasho TL, Guglielmelli P, Finke CM, Rotunno G, Elala Y, Pacilli A, Hanson CA, Pancrazzi A, Ketterling RP, et al. 2016b. Targeted deep sequencing in polycythemia vera and essential thrombocythemia. *Blood Adv* **1:** 21–30. doi:10.1182/bloodadvances.2016000216

Tefferi A, Finke CM, Lasho TL, Hanson CA, Ketterling RP, Gangat N, Pardanani A. 2018a. *U2AF1* mutation types in primary myelofibrosis: Phenotypic and prognostic distinctions. *Leukemia* **32:** 2274–2278. doi:10.1038/s41375-018-0078-0

Tefferi A, Lasho TL, Finke C, Gangat N, Hanson CA, Ketterling RP, Pardanani A. 2018b. Prognostic significance of *ASXL1* mutation types and allele burden in myelofibrosis. *Leukemia* **32:** 837–839. doi:10.1038/leu.2017.318

Tefferi A, Lasho TL, Hanson CA, Ketterling RP, Gangat N, Pardanani A. 2018c. Screening for *ASXL1* and *SRSF2* mutations is imperative for treatment decision-making in otherwise low or intermediate-1 risk patients with myelofibrosis. *Br J Haematol* **183:** 678–681. doi:10.1111/bjh.15010

Tefferi A, Nicolosi M, Mudireddy M, Szuber N, Finke CM, Lasho TL, Hanson CA, Ketterling RP, Pardanani A, Gangat N, et al. 2018d. Driver mutations and prognosis in primary myelofibrosis: Mayo-Careggi MPN alliance study of 1,095 patients. *Am J Hematol* **93:** 348–355. doi:10.1002/ajh.24978

Thien CB, Langdon WY. 2005. Negative regulation of PTK signalling by Cbl proteins. *Growth Factors* **23:** 161–167. doi:10.1080/08977190500153763

Tong W, Zhang J, Lodish HF. 2005. Lnk inhibits erythropoiesis and Epo-dependent JAK2 activation and downstream signaling pathways. *Blood* **105:** 4604–4612. doi:10.1182/blood-2004-10-4093

Tsuzuki S, Seto M. 2012. Expansion of functionally defined mouse hematopoietic stem and progenitor cells by a short isoform of RUNX1/AML1. *Blood* **119:** 727–735. doi:10.1182/blood-2011-06-362277

Uni M, Masamoto Y, Sato T, Kamikubo Y, Arai S, Hara E, Kurokawa M. 2019. Modeling *ASXL1* mutation revealed impaired hematopoiesis caused by derepression of p16Ink4a through aberrant PRC1-mediated histone modification. *Leukemia* **33:** 191–204. doi:10.1038/s41375-018-0198-6

Vannucchi AM, Lasho TL, Guglielmelli P, Biamonte F, Pardanani A, Pereira A, Finke C, Score J, Gangat N, Mannarelli C, et al. 2013. Mutations and prognosis in primary myelofibrosis. *Leukemia* **27:** 1861–1869. doi:10.1038/leu.2013.119

Velazquez L, Cheng AM, Fleming HE, Furlonger C, Vesely S, Bernstein A, Paige CJ, Pawson T. 2002. Cytokine signaling and hematopoietic homeostasis are disrupted in *Lnk*-deficient mice. *J Exp Med* **195:** 1599–1611. doi:10.1084/jem.20011883

Venton G, Courtier F, Charbonnier A, D'Incan E, Saillard C, Mohty B, Mozziconacci MJ, Birnbaum D, Murati A, Vey N, et al. 2018. Impact of gene mutations on treatment response and prognosis of acute myeloid leukemia secondary to myeloproliferative neoplasms. *Am J Hematol* **93:** 330–338. doi:10.1002/ajh.24973

Verma B, Akinyi MV, Norppa AJ, Frilander MJ. 2018. Minor spliceosome and disease. *Semin Cell Dev Biol* **79:** 103–112. doi:10.1016/j.semcdb.2017.09.036

Wang M, He N, Tian T, Liu L, Yu S, Ma D. 2014. Mutation analysis of JAK2V617F, FLT3-ITD, NPM1, and DNMT3A in Chinese patients with myeloproliferative neoplasms. *Biomed Res Int* **2014:** 485645. doi:10.1155/2014/485645

Watanabe-Okochi N, Kitaura J, Ono R, Harada H, Harada Y, Komeno Y, Nakajima H, Nosaka T, Inaba T, Kitamura T. 2008. *AML1* mutations induced MDS and MDS/AML in a mouse BMT model. *Blood* **111:** 4297–4308. doi:10.1182/blood-2007-01-068346

Webb CJ, Wise JA. 2004. The splicing factor U2AF small subunit is functionally conserved between fission yeast and humans. *Mol Cell Biol* **24:** 4229–4240. doi:10.1128/MCB.24.10.4229-4240.2004

Wolach O, Sellar RS, Martinod K, Cherpokova D, McConkey M, Chappell RJ, Silver AJ, Adams D, Castellano CA, Schneider RK, et al. 2018. Increased neutrophil extracellular trap formation promotes thrombosis in myeloproliferative neoplasms. *Sci Transl Med* **10:** eaan8292. doi:10.1126/scitranslmed.aan8292

Xiao R, Sun Y, Ding JH, Lin S, Rose DW, Rosenfeld MG, Fu XD, Li X. 2007. Splicing regulator SC35 is essential for genomic stability and cell proliferation during mammalian organogenesis. *Mol Cell Biol* **27:** 5393–5402. doi:10.1128/MCB.00288-07

Xie M, Lu C, Wang J, McLellan MD, Johnson KJ, Wendl MC, McMichael JF, Schmidt HK, Yellapantula V, Miller CA, et al. 2014. Age-related mutations associated with clonal hematopoietic expansion and malignancies. *Nat Med* **20:** 1472–1478. doi:10.1038/nm.3733

Xu W, Yang H, Liu Y, Yang Y, Wang P, Kim SH, Ito S, Yang C, Wang P, Xiao MT, et al. 2011. Oncometabolite 2-hydroxyglutarate is a competitive inhibitor of α-ketoglutarate-dependent dioxygenases. *Cancer Cell* **19:** 17–30. doi:10.1016/j.ccr.2010.12.014

Yamashita Y, Yuan J, Suetake I, Suzuki H, Ishikawa Y, Choi YL, Ueno T, Soda M, Hamada T, Haruta H, et al. 2010. Array-based genomic resequencing of human leukemia. *Oncogene* **29:** 3723–3731. doi:10.1038/onc.2010.117

Yang Y, Akada H, Nath D, Hutchison RE, Mohi G. 2016. Loss of Ezh2 cooperates with Jak2V617F in the development of myelofibrosis in a mouse model of myeloproliferative neoplasm. *Blood* **127:** 3410–3423. doi:10.1182/blood-2015-11-679431

Yang H, Kurtenbach S, Guo Y, Lohse I, Durante MA, Li J, Li Z, Al-Ali H, Li L, Chen Z, et al. 2018. Gain of function of *ASXL1* truncating protein in the pathogenesis of myeloid malignancies. *Blood* **131:** 328–341. doi:10.1182/blood-2017-06-789669

Yonal-Hindilerden I, Daglar-Aday A, Hindilerden F, Akadam-Teker B, Yilmaz C, Nalcaci M, Yavuz AS, Sargin D. 2016. The clinical significance of IDH mutations in essential thrombocythemia and primary myelofibrosis. *J Clin Med Res* **8:** 29–39. doi:10.14740/jocmr2405w

Yoshida K, Sanada M, Shiraishi Y, Nowak D, Nagata Y, Yamamoto R, Sato Y, Sato-Otsubo A, Kon A, Nagasaki M, et al. 2011. Frequent pathway mutations of splicing machinery in myelodysplasia. *Nature* **478:** 64–69. doi:10.1038/nature10496

Zhang SJ, Rampal R, Manshouri T, Patel J, Mensah N, Kayserian A, Hricik T, Heguy A, Hedvat C, Gonen M, et al. 2012. Genetic analysis of patients with leukemic transformation of myeloproliferative neoplasms shows recurrent *SRSF2* mutations that are associated with adverse outcome. *Blood* **119:** 4480–4485. doi:10.1182/blood-2011-11-390252

Zhang L, Chen LH, Wan H, Yang R, Wang Z, Feng J, Yang S, Jones S, Wang S, Zhou W, et al. 2014. Exome sequencing identifies somatic gain-of-function *PPM1D* mutations in brainstem gliomas. *Nat Genet* **46:** 726–730. doi:10.1038/ng.2995

The Role of Somatic Mutations in Acute Myeloid Leukemia Pathogenesis

Ashwin Kishtagari[1,2] **and Ross L. Levine**[3,4,5,6,7]

[1]Department of Translational Hematology and Oncology Research, [2]Department of Hematology and Oncology, Taussig Cancer Institute, Cleveland Clinic, Cleveland, Ohio 44195, USA

[3]Human Oncology and Pathogenesis Program, [4]Department of Medicine, Leukemia Service,

[5]Center for Epigenetics Research, [6]Center for Hematologic Malignancies, [7]Molecular Cancer Medicine Service, Memorial Sloan Kettering Cancer Center, New York, New York 10065, USA

Correspondence: leviner@mskcc.org

Acute myeloid leukemia (AML) is characterized by attenuation of lineage differentiation trajectories that results in impaired hematopoiesis and enhanced self-renewal. To date, sequencing studies have provided a rich landscape of information on the somatic mutations that contribute to AML pathogenesis. These studies show that most AML genomes harbor relatively fewer mutations, which are acquired in a stepwise manner. Our understanding of the genetic basis of leukemogenesis informs a broader understanding of what initiates and maintains the AML clone and informs the development of prognostic models and mechanism-based therapeutic strategies. Here, we explore the current knowledge of genetic and epigenetic aberrations in AML pathogenesis and how recent studies are expanding our knowledge of leukemogenesis and using this to accelerate therapeutic development for AML patients.

Acute myeloid leukemia (AML) is a clonal disorder initiated in hematopoietic stem and progenitor cells (HSPCs) that is characterized by impaired myeloid differentiation and abnormal proliferation at the expense of the normal hematopoietic system. AML is the most common form of acute leukemia in adults; an estimated 19,940 people will be diagnosed in 2020, and 11,180 patients will die of the disease (Siegel et al. 2020). AML is the 10th leading cause of cancer deaths in the United States. AML is most common in older adults, with a median age at diagnosis of 68 yr. Treatment of AML remains a significant challenge owing to the diverse molecular mechanisms contributing to different AML subtypes, and limited therapeutic options. Even though two-thirds of fit patients with newly diagnosed AML achieve morphological remission with intensive chemotherapy consisting of cytarabine and an anthra-

Cite this article as *Cold Spring Harb Perspect Med* doi: 10.1101/cshperspect.a034975

cycline, the majority of these patients eventually relapse (Döhner et al. 2017; Kishtagari et al. 2020).

The first whole-genome sequencing of a cancer patient was of a patient with cytogenetically normal AML, reported more than a decade ago (Ley et al. 2008). Since then, gene discovery studies have identified an extensive catalog of recurrent somatic mutations in different AML subtypes (Mardis et al. 2009; Patel et al. 2012; Cancer Genome Atlas Research et al. 2013; Papaemmanuil et al. 2016; Tyner et al. 2018). These discovery studies have led to a greater understanding of AML biology, including stepwise accumulation of genetic alterations and recurrent mutations in epigenetic modifiers in AML. The types of mutations found in AML include chromosomal rearrangements (such as translocations or inversion), gain or loss of chromosomes (aneuploidy), total or partial gene deletion, point mutation, insertion, or gene duplication/amplification. AML can develop after an antecedent myeloid malignancy (secondary AML [s-AML]), after leukemogenic therapy (therapy-related AML [t-AML]), or without an identifiable prodrome or known exposure (de novo AML). The therapeutic strategy in "fit" patients with AML (primarily influenced by patient-related factors such as advanced age, performance status, and pretreatment comorbidities) is divided into induction and postremission therapy. Induction refers to the use of cytotoxic therapy (combination of cytarabine and an anthracycline) to induce remission, preferably without measurable residual disease (MRD). Standard postremission strategies include lower-intensity cytotoxic therapy and hematopoietic stem cell transplantation (HSCT). The use of different therapies in the postremission treatment is largely determined by prognostic risk stratification (Table 1). The treatment of AML patients who are "unfit" for intensive therapy include low-dose cytarabine, hypomethylating agents, and combination treatment strategies with novel agents (e.g., venetoclax, glasdegib). Recent data suggests remarkable efficacy for venetoclax/azacytidine in older adults with AML who are not candidates for intensive therapy, such that this regimen is quickly emerging as a new alternative for first-line therapy for older adults with AML (Pollyea et al. 2018).

In this review, we provide an overview of AML pathophysiology through the prism of genomic and epigenomic alterations and discuss how these mechanisms are perturbed in leukemogenesis. Acute promyelocytic leukemia (APL), a distinct subtype of AML, will not be addressed in this review, as we would posit it is a unique malignancy with distinct mechanisms of transformation and therapeutic options. In essence, we will discuss the pathogenesis of AML by addressing the role of recurrent cytogenetic abnormalities in AML pathogenesis, the underlying molecular events that contribute to AML, how our evolving understanding of the molecular basis of AML is refining prognostic schema, and how these insights are leading to new therapeutic approaches.

CHROMSOMAL ABNORMALITIES

In AML, detection of chromosomal abnormalities by cytogenetic analysis is critically important for diagnosis, risk stratification, and therapeutic decision-making (Fig. 1). Chromosomal abnormalities are detected in ~50% of patients with AML at the time of diagnosis. Chromosomal abnormalities most commonly contribute to leukemogenesis through the production of a fusion oncoprotein and/or by altering *cis*-regulatory elements. These large-scale copy-number alterations can serve as founding events and drive disease evolution in AML. Detection of t(8:21)(q22;q22.1), inv(16)(p13.1q22), t(16;16)(p13.1;q22), or translocations generating *PML-RARA* fusion transcripts (APL) allow the diagnosis of AML, regardless of the percentage of myeloblasts in the bone marrow or peripheral blood.

Core Binding Factor Rearrangements

The inv(16)(p13;q22) or t(16;16)(p13.1;q22) and t(8;21)(q22;q22.1) translocations lead to the expression of the *CBFB-MYH11* and *RUNX1-RUNX1T1* fusion oncogenes, respectively. In steady state hematopoiesis, core bind-

Table 1. The European LeukemiaNET (ELN) 2017 risk stratification of acute myeloid leukemia (AML)

Risk category	Genetic abnormality
Favorable	t(8;21)(q22;q22.1); *RUNX1-RUNX1T1*
	inv(16)(p13.1q22) or t(16;16)(p13.1;q22); *CBFB-MYH11*
	Mutated *NPM1* without *FLT3-ITD* or with *FLT3-ITD*$^{\text{low = allelic ratio < 0.5}}$
	Biallelic mutated *CEBPA*
Intermediate	Mutated *NPM1* and *FLT3-ITD*$^{\text{high = allelic ratio > 0.5}}$
	Wild-type *NPM1* without *FLT3-ITD* or with *FLT3-ITD*^{low} (without adverse-risk genetic lesions)
	t(9;11)(p21.3;q23.3); *MLLT3-KMT2A*
	Cytogenetic abnormalities not classified as favorable or adverse
Adverse	t(6;9)(p23;q34.1); *DEK-NUP214*
	t(v;11q23.3); *KMT2A* rearranged
	t(9;22)(q34.1;q11.2); *BCR-ABL1*
	inv(3)(q21.3q26.2) or t(3;3)(q21.3;q26.2); *GATA2,MECOM(EVI1)*
	−5 or del(5q); −7; −17/abn(17p)
	Complex karyotype, monosomal karyotype
	Wild-type *NPM1* and *FLT3-ITD*^{high}
	Mutated *RUNX1*
	Mutated *ASXL1*
	Mutated *TP53*

Data reprinted from Döhner et al. (2017), with permission from The American Society of Hematology, © 2017.

ing factor beta (CBFβ) and RUNX1 heterodimerize to bind DNA and recruit lineage-defining transcription factors to regulate hematopoietic differentiation (Tahirov et al. 2001). In CBF-AML, chromosomal rearrangements alter this transcriptional complex, thus dysregulating normal hematopoiesis. These rearrangements are present in ~15% of AML cases. They are the most responsive AML subtypes to intensive chemotherapy, including postremission therapy with high-dose cytarabine (HiDAC) such that patients with these fusion oncoproteins are treated with induction chemotherapy followed by HiDAC consolidation as standard of care (Bloomfield et al. 1998; Byrd et al. 2004). Patients with CBF-AML usually have a relatively good outcome with overall survival rates of 60%–70% in adults. However, the expression of CD56 and the activating mutations in *KIT* have been correlated to greater risk of recurrence and shorter survival. The *KIT* mutations are found in 20%–25% of t(8;21)(q22;q22) and in ~30% of inv(16) (p13; q22) patients (Paschka et al. 2006). However, the role of *KIT* mutations in prognostication and in molecularly targeted therapies for AML requires further prognostic and therapeutic studies. Both *CBFB-MYH11* and *RUNX1-RUNX1T1* fusion transcripts are well-established markers for MRD monitoring by real-time quantitative polymerase chain reaction (qRT-PCR) to guide postremission therapy (Schuurhuis et al. 2018).

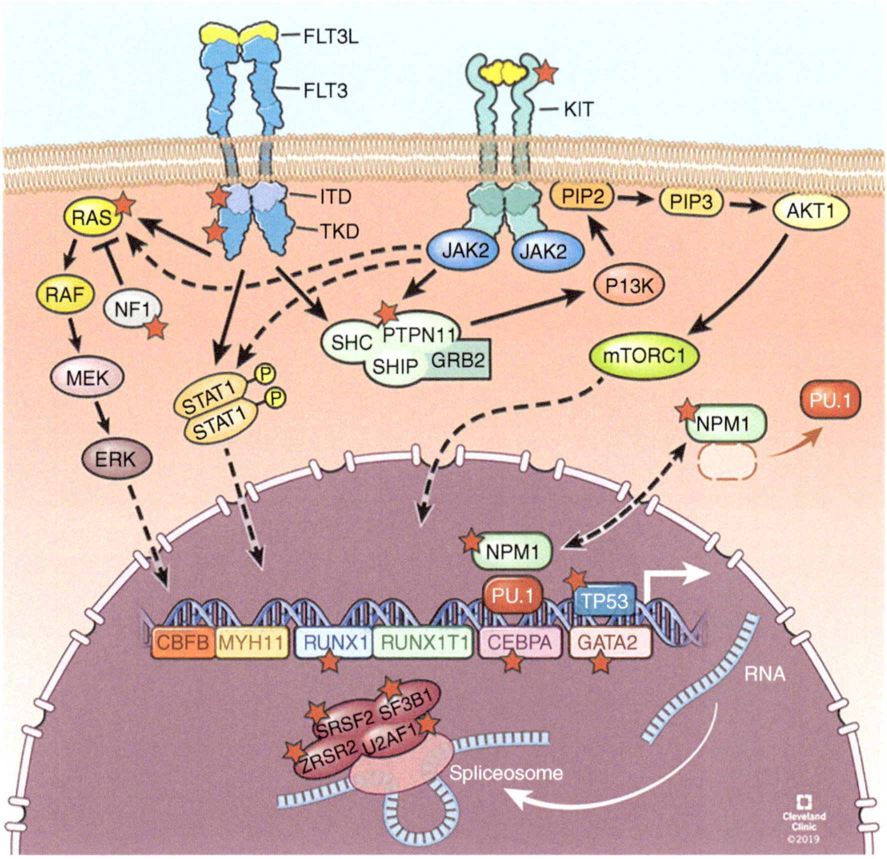

Figure 1. Overview of frequently mutated cellular pathways in acute myeloid leukemia (AML). These include (1) *CBFB-MYH11* and *RUNX1-RUNX1T1* fusion oncogenes; (2) nucleophosmin 1 (*NPM1*); (3) transcription factors *RUNX1, CEBPA,* and *GATA2*; (4) tumor suppressors *TP53*; (5) signal transduction, including *FLT3-ITD, FLT3-TKD, KIT, CBL, NRAS, KRAS, PTPN11,* and *NF1*; and (6) RNA splicing: *SF3B1, SRSF2, U2AF1,* and *ZRSR2.* Mutated genes are highlighted with a red star. (Refer to the main text for detailed explanations of the depicted processes.) (Figure reprinted with permission, Cleveland Clinic Center for Medical Art & Photography © 2019–2020. All rights reserved.)

KMT2A (*MLL1*) Rearrangements

The mixed-lineage leukemia gene (*KMT2A*, also known as *MLL1*) encodes a histone H3 lysine 4 (H3K4) methyltransferase that regulates the expression of target genes, including homoeobox (*Hox*) genes. In *MLL1* fusions, *MLL1* retains the DNA-binding amino-terminal domain, and the catalytic methyltransferase activity carboxy-terminal SET domain is replaced by a fusion partner of one of more than 70 partner genes, most commonly *AF4* t(4;11), *AF9* t(9;11), *ENL* t(11;19), *AF10* t(10;11), and *ELL* t(11;19) (Krivtsov and Armstrong 2007). The most common fusion partners of *MLL1* are members of the DOT1L complex and/or the super elongation complex (SEC), which are both involved in transcriptional control. *MLL1*-fusion leukemias are characterized by increased expression of *HOXA9*, *MEIS1*, and *MEF2C*, which encode for leukemogenic transcription factors (Armstrong et al. 2002). *MLL1* fusions occur in as many as 10% of patients with AML and are common in t-AML following exposure to topoisomerase II inhibitors (Strissel et al. 1998). *MLL1*-fusion AML carries a poor prognosis because of refractoriness to chemotherapy and shorter period to relapse (Meyer et al. 2018). Aberrant recruitment of the DOT1L by *MLL1*-fusion leukemias provided a rationale for development of small-molecule inhibitors (e.g., pinometostat) targeting DOT1L with modest results (Stein et al. 2018). Moreover, recent data showing that *MLL1* fusions, but not wild-type *MLL1*, requiring menin as a co-factor to activate downstream target gene expression has led to the development of small-molecule inhibitors of the MLL1/menin interaction, which are now entering clinical trials (Yokoyama et al. 2005; Grembecka et al. 2012; Borkin et al. 2015; Krivtsov et al. 2019; Klossowski et al. 2020). Another mechanism by which *MLL1* plays a role in leukemogenesis is through an in-frame partial tandem duplication (*MLL1-PTD*) spanning exons 3 to 9, exons 3 to 10, or exons 3 to 11 (Steudel et al. 2003). *MLL1-PTD*s occur in 3.2%–11% of adult AML and more frequently present in AML with normal karyotype and trisomy 11 (Basecke et al. 2006). They confer a worse prognosis with shortened overall survival. *MLL1-PTD* AML has a distinct gene expression signature, and concomitant *DNMT3A* and *NRAS* mutations were associated with adverse clinical outcomes (Hinai et al. 2019).

Rare Translocations and Chromosomal Alterations

inv(3)(q21.3q26.2) or t(3;3)(q21.3;q26.2); GATA2, MECOM(EVI1)

These rearrangements result in overexpression of the proto-oncogene *MECOM (EVI1)* at 3q26.2, through juxtaposition of the *EVI1* gene with a distal *GATA2* enhancer, and simultaneously confers *GATA2* haploinsufficiency (Gröschel et al. 2014). It is a distinct entity, which is present in de novo AML or AML arising from prior myelodysplastic syndromes (MDS), and is associated with aggressive disease with minimal response to standard therapies and short survival (Lugthart et al. 2010; Rogers et al. 2014). These rearrangements occur in 1%–2% of all AML cases. Mutations in genes activating RAS/receptor tyrosine kinase signaling pathways are reported in a significant proportion of the cases with these rearrangements; this may provide a target for a rational treatment strategy in this adverse-risk patient group (Gröschel et al. 2015).

t(6:9)(p23;q34.1); DEK-NUP214

This rearrangement results in a fusion of oncogene *DEK* on chromosome 6 with the nucleoporin gene *NUP214* on chromosome 9. The resulting nucleoporin chimeric fusion protein interacts with exportin-1 (XPO1)/CRM1 and may affect the export of nuclear proteins (Saito et al. 2016). It is a distinct entity reported in ~2% of AML cases and is associated with a very poor prognosis. The majority of the patients with these rearrangements have a concomitant mutation in *FLT3-ITD.* Outcomes are dismal with standard chemotherapy with the only chance of long-term remission achieved for patients who can undergo allogeneic hematopoietic stem cell transplantation in first complete remission (Díaz-Beyá et al. 2020; Kayser et al. 2020). Given the fusion chimeric protein interaction with XPO1/CRM1, it will be interesting to see whether this fusion imparts sensitivity to XPO1 inhibitors (e.g., selinexor).

Complex Karyotype, -5/5q, -7/7q, -17/17p, +8/8q

Somatically acquired chromosome copy or segment gains, chromosomal monosomies, as well as the accumulation of karyotypic abnormalities, classified as complex karyotype, defined as three or more chromosomal abnormalities, are reported in ~5%–10% of patients with AML. These alterations carry an adverse prognosis and are associated with a poor response to cytotoxic chemotherapy. Common abnormalities include those involving chromosomes 5 and 7, particularly in AML arising out of the background of MDS, and in t-AML arising in patients treated with alkylating agents and/or radiation therapy for a previous cancer. About 50% of patients with complex karyotype abnormalities have mutations in *TP53,* and it is hypothesized that *TP53* inactivation allows cells to tolerate and persist in a setting of ongoing chromosomal instability. Moreover, it remains unclear whether the poor prognosis of complex karyotype AML is due to chromosomal alterations, inactivation of the p53 pathway, or both molecular events acting in concert. Haploinsufficiency of the following genes have been implicated in myeloid malignancies with monosomy 5 or large deletions of 5q [-5/del(5q)], including *RPS14, APC, CTNNA1, HSPA9, EGR1,* and *CSNK1A1* (Joslin et al. 2007; Liu et al. 2007; Ebert et al. 2008; Wang et al. 2010; Chen et al. 2011). Haploinsufficiency or loss of heterozygosity of candidate genes involved in -7/del(7q) include *SAMD9/9L, DOCK4, EZH2, CUX1, MLL3,* and *LUC7L2*, each of which has been suggested to contribute to myeloid transformation (Zhou et al. 2011; McNerney et al. 2013; Nagamachi et al. 2013; Chen et al. 2014; Hosono et al. 2014). Loss of chromosome 17p, including the *TP53* locus at 17p13.1, is associated with complex karyotype as well as abnormalities in chromosomes 5 and 7. In contrast to AML with balanced translocations, leukemias that develop in the context of 17p alterations are characterized by greater genomic instability (Liu et al. 2016). It is important to note that *NF1* is also on chromosome 17 and that some of the events involving 17q result in haploinsufficiency/loss of *NF1* and augmented MAPK signaling (Parkin et al. 2010). Other rare rearrangements, such as t(3;17)(q26;q22), involving fusion of the *EVI1* gene located on chromosome 3q26.2 and *MSI2* (MUSASHI [MSI] family of RNA binding protein) located on 17q are found in AML (De Weer et al. 2008). Somatic acquisition of trisomy 8 is seen in ~10% of patients with AML. They contribute to leukemogenesis, at least in part, via amplification of *MYC*, which is located at chromosome 8p24 and is implicated in a spectrum of malignancies including AML (Sloand et al. 2007).

RECURRENT MUTATIONS IN AML

NPM1

More than 50% of patients with normal karyotype AML harbor mutations in nucleophosmin 1 (*NPM1*) (Fig. 1). NPM1 is a multifunctional nucleus and nucleolar phosphoprotein involved in pleiotropic cellular functions (Falini et al. 2005). *NPM1* gene mutations typically occur as insertions in exon 12, causing a frameshift mutation with an added nuclear export signal (NES) motif at the carboxy-terminus; NPM1c protein product thus accumulates aberrantly in the cytoplasm (Falini et al. 2005; Sportoletti et al. 2015). Multiple recent publications have demonstrated that mutant NPM1 is aberrantly localized in the cytoplasm (NPM1c) and this mislocalization is essential for maintaining active chromatin marks that may help maintain expression of key target genes including *HOXA* and *HOXB* genes and *MEIS1*, thereby inhibiting differentiation of leukemic cells (Brunetti et al. 2018; Gu et al. 2018). It has been suggested that NPM1c shuttles PU.1 (SPI1) into the cytoplasm, which abrogates PU.1 mediated repression of *HOX/MEIS1* transcription (Gu et al. 2018). The World Health Organization (WHO) classification of hematopoietic tumors recognizes *NPM1*-mutant AML as a distinct entity (Table 1) (Arber et al. 2016; Döhner et al. 2017). Strikingly, the majority of *NPM1*-mutated AML have mutations in *DNMT3A* and *FLT3*. AML patients with *NPM1* mutations without mutations in *DNMT3A* and *FLT3* carry a favorable prognosis, but the co-mutations *FLT3-ITD* and *DNMT3A* confer an adverse prognosis (Döhner et al. 2017). In *NPM1*-mutant AML, prediction of relapse risk by MRD assessment by qRT-PCR demonstrated that persistent *NPM1* positivity in blood was the sole predictor of relapse in multivariate analysis irrespective of the co-mutational status (Ivey et al. 2016; Dillon et al. 2020). This further supports its inclusion into daily clinical practice to better guide postremission therapy (Schuurhuis et al. 2018). *NPM1* mutation is considered to be a leukemia-initiating event and thus represents an ideal therapeutic target. In a recent study, using *Npm1c/Dnmt3a* mutant knock-in mice and cell lines, a model of AML development, showed *NPM1*-mutant induced self-renewal properties in myeloid progenitor cells, which act as leukemia-initiating cells. In mice, oral administration of the small molecule inhibitor, which targets the interaction between the histone methyltransferase MLL1 and adaptor protein menin, eradicated preleukemic *Npm1c*-mutant myeloid progenitor cells, prevented AML development, and extended survival. This study demonstrates that the elimination of at-risk preleukemic cells using targeted inhibitors may be a promising strategy (Uckelmann et al. 2020).

Mutations Disrupting Transcription Factor Function in AML (Fig. 1)

Transcription factors tightly regulate normal hematopoiesis. Abrogation of specific transcription factor activity results in block in differentiation of hematopoietic progenitor cells and the development of hematologic malignancies, including AML.

RUNX1

RUNX1 encodes the sequence-specific master hematopoietic transcription factor Runt-related transcription factor 1 (RUNX1), which is an essential regulator of hematopoiesis by maintaining the balance between cell lineage specification, self-renewal, and proliferation (Ito et al. 2015). RUNX1 has a highly conserved "Runt" homology domain (RHD), the motif responsible for heterodimerization with CBFβ, which facilitates the specificity and affinity of RUNX1 binding to target genes (Crute et al. 1996). More than 50 mutations in *RUNX1*, both point mutations and chromosomal rearrangements, have been reported in various hematologic malignancies, including AML. Loss-of-function somatic mutations in *RUNX1*, which are mechanistically distinct from rearrangements, occur in ~5%–15% of all patients with AML and confer a poor prognosis (Gaidzik et al. 2016). Mutations in *RUNX1* are enriched in patients with intermediate-risk (including normal karyotype AML) disease (Patel et al. 2012; Papaemmanuil et al. 2016). *RUNX1* mutations are usually secondary events that drive disease progression, and they are mutually exclusive with *NPM1* and *CEBPA* mutations (Hirsch et al. 2016; Papaemmanuil et al. 2016). They are associated with older age and lower complete response (CR) rates and inferior overall survival (OS) (Mendler et al. 2012). Germline mutations in *RUNX1* are associated with familial platelet disorder with propensity to myeloid malignancy (FPDMM), characterized by thrombocytopenia, platelet functional/ultrastructural defects, and a 20%–60% rate of transformation to overt myeloid malignancies (Song et al. 1999).

CEBPA

The transcription factor CCAAT/enhancer-binding protein α (CEBPA) is a master regulator involved in cell fate decisions, including myeloid-lineage commitment (Avellino and Delwel 2017). CEBPA is expressed as two isoforms: the full-length (p42) and the amino-terminally truncated isoform (p30) that lacks the full *trans*-activation potential of p42. *CEBPA* mutations in AML harbor *CEBPA* amino-terminal nonsense or frameshift mutations, resulting in the increased expression of the dominant-negative p30 isoform, diminishing p42 availability to promote myeloid differentiation. Carboxy-terminal in-frame mutations interrupt DNA binding and homodimerization properties of the proteins and often co-occur on a separate allele from amino-terminal mutations. This pattern of mutations produces p30/p30 homodimers as the functional CEBPA transcription factor entity in *CEBPA*-mutant AML (Pabst et al. 2001; Kirstetter et al. 2008). These loss-of-function *CEBPA* mutations are reported in 5%–15% of AML patients and occur mostly in younger patients with normal karyotype AML (Fröhling et al. 2004; Cancer Genome Atlas Research et al. 2013). AML patients with biallelic *CEBPA* mutations, with one allele harboring an amino-terminus mutation and the other allele having a mutation in the carboxyl terminus, exhibit a distinct gene expression signature and a favorable prognosis with the majority of younger patients achieving a cure with standard chemotherapy alone (Table 1) (Wouters et al. 2009; Fasan et al. 2014). Biallelic *CEBPA* mutations have a JAK-STAT pathway activation signature, and a high percentage of these patients also harbor gain-of-function mutations in *CSF3R* and increased sensitivity to JAK kinase inhibitors (such as ruxolitinib) ex vivo (Lavallée et al. 2016; Maxson et al. 2016). Germline mutations in *CEBPA* are associated with autosomal dominant familial AML with 100% penetrance (Smith et al. 2004).

GATA2

GATA2, a member of the zinc finger transcription factor family, is a critical transcriptional regulator of hematopoietic stem and progenitor cell differentiation and self-renewal (Crispino and Horwitz 2017). Homozygous *Gata2* knockout in mice are embryonically lethal because of the failure of definitive hematopoiesis (Tsai et al. 1994). Somatic mutations in *GATA2* are infrequent in AML, occurring in <5% of AML overall, and are clustered in normal karyotype AML with concurrent biallelic *CEBPA* mutations (Greif et al. 2012). These mutations include frameshifts, amino acid substitutions, insertions, and deletions scattered throughout the gene but most often clustered in the region encoding the zinc finger domains, leading to impaired DNA binding and affecting transcriptional activity. In its capacity as a tumor suppressor, heterozygous germline mutations in *GATA2* in coding or regulatory element regions cause a spectrum of hematopoietic disorders and a predisposition to MDS/AML, often with subsequent acquisition of somatic *ASXL1* mutations (Hahn et al. 2011; Ostergaard et al. 2011; West et al. 2014).

Mutations Altering Signal Transduction (Fig. 1)

Deregulation of signaling pathway components is frequently reported in AML. This is associated with pro-proliferative states by constitutive activation.

FLT3-ITD and FLT3-TKD

Mutations in FMS-like tyrosine kinase 3 (FLT3) occur in approximately one-third of all patients with newly diagnosed AML. These mutations can occur either as an in-frame internal tandem duplication within the juxtamembrane domain of the receptor (*FLT3-ITD*), seen in ∼20%–25% of AML, or as point mutations most commonly in the activation loop of the catalytic domain (*FLT3-TKD*). Both mutations lead to autoactivation of FLT3-kinase activity and activation of downstream signaling pathways, which lead to proliferation and block in differentiation (Meshinchi and Appelbaum 2009). AML patients with mutations in *FLT3-ITD* have an adverse prognosis compared to patients with *FLT3-TKD* or wild-type *FLT3*, and the majority of these patients relapse after chemotherapy and allogeneic HSCT (Thiede et al. 2002; Sengsayadeth et al. 2012). The poor prognosis is particularly influenced by co-mutation status (*DNMT3A* mutations, absence of *NPM1* mutations) and the allelic ratio of mutant *FLT3-ITD* to wild-type (Table 1) (Patel et al. 2012; Papaemmanuil et al. 2016). The advent of *FLT3* inhibitors (midostaurin, gilteritinib, quizartinib, and crenolinib) in various stages of clinical development represents a paradigm of targeted therapy in AML and has changed practice. These agents act through the competitive inhibition of the ATP-binding site in the FLT3 receptor; however, they vary substantially in their inhibitory properties, pharmacokinetics, and toxicity profiles. There are currently two FDA-approved small-molecule inhibitors (midostaurin and gilteritinib) of FLT3-kinase activity. In randomized clinical trial, comparing midostaurin in combination with chemotherapy or placebo with chemotherapy has been shown to significantly improve survival of untreated *FLT3*-mutant AML patients (age 18–60 yr; 74.7 vs. 25.6 mo) (Stone et al. 2017). Gilteritinib, a next-generation tyrosine kinase inhibitor, is approved for the treatment of adults who have relapsed and/or have refractory AML with *FLT3-ITD* and *FLT3-TKD* mutations (Perl et al. 2019). Of note, therapy has substantive-agent activity, whereas midostaurin has not shown significant activity when given as monotherapy.

KIT

The *KIT* gene encodes a 145-kDa transmembrane glycoprotein that is a member of the type III receptor tyrosine kinase (RTK) family (Yarden et al. 1987). Upon binding of stem cell factor (KIT ligand), the monomeric KIT receptor dimerizes and becomes autophosphorylated at key tyrosine sites and activates diverse signal transduction cascades essential for cell proliferation/survival, self-renewal, and differentiation (Malaise et al. 2009). Somatic gain-of-function *KIT* mutations occur in 10% of AML patients, but they are clustered in patients with CBF-AML rearrangements (t(8;21)/*RUNX1-RUNX1T1*, inv(16)/*CBFB-MYH11*) and may confer a more adverse prognosis in this otherwise favorable AML subtype (Paschka et al. 2006).

CBL

Casitas B cell lymphoma (CBL) protein functions as E3 ligases that ubiquitinate and negatively regulate receptor tyrosine kinases, including FLT3 and KIT (Mohapatra et al. 2013). Mutations in the E3 ubiquitin ligase *CBL* have been reported in ~1%–3% of AML patients. Mutations in *CBL* result in the loss of ubiquitin E3 ligase activity and resultant increased tyrosine kinase signaling by decreased proteasome-mediated degradation. In preclinical models, there is evidence that *FLT3-ITD* mutations cooperate with *CBL* to promote the rapid induction of AML (Taylor et al. 2015). Although, mutations in *CBL* cause biochemical loss of function, their functional consequences resemble canonical gain-of-function mutations (Sanada et al. 2009). The prognostic significance of these mutations in AML is unclear given the lack of robust data.

NRAS and KRAS

The Ras family of small GTPases, NRAS and KRAS, function as binary molecular switches by cycling between an active GTP-bound (RAS-GTP) and an inactive GDP-bound (RAS-GDP) confirmation that regulate downstream signaling effectors, such as Raf and PI3K (Schubbert et al. 2007). Somatic gain-of-function mutations in *RAS* are among the most common oncogenic drivers in cancers leading to constitutive activation of receptor tyrosine kinases (Li et al. 2018). *NRAS* (~12%) and *KRAS* (~5%) mutations are seen in a subset of AML patients at the time of diagnosis (Bacher et al. 2006). They are frequently acquired at the time of progression from MDS to AML and are associated with poor survival. In a recent study, the presence of *NRAS* and *KRAS* mutations in patients with AML receiving standard cytotoxic therapy was associated with decreased OS and event-free survival (EFS) (Ball et al. 2019). Mutations in epigenetic modifiers (*TET2*/*IDH*/*WT1*) often co-occur and cooperate with *NRAS* mutations to promote leukemogenesis (Papaemmanuil et al. 2016). Preclinical studies suggest this cooperativity and dependence on activated Ras signaling may be therapeutically exploited as they are preferentially sensitive to MAPK kinase (MEK) inhibition in mouse models and patient samples (Kunimoto et al. 2018). The emergence or co-occurrence of *NRAS* and *KRAS* mutant clones is a common and clinically relevant mechanism of resistance to *FLT3* inhibitors, *IDH* inhibitors, and BCL-2 inhibitors (Amatangelo et al. 2017; McMahon et al. 2019; DiNardo et al. 2020).

PTPN11

The non–receptor protein tyrosine phosphatase PTPN11 (also known as SRC homology 2 domain–containing phosphatase 2 or SHP2) is implicated in several signaling pathways including RAS, JAK-STAT, PI3K, and others (Tartaglia et al. 2003). Mutations in *PTPN11* are present in ~5%–10% of AML cases and enriched in patients older than 60 yr with secondary AML (Makishima et al. 2017). These mutations co-occur and cooperate with *AML1-ETO* (Hatlen et al. 2016) and *MLL-AF9* (Chen et al. 2015) rearrangements.

NF1

The neurofibromin 1 gene (*NF1*), encodes neurofibromin, a GTPase-activating protein and negative regulator of Ras. Inactivating mutations in *NF1* leading to loss of neurofibromin and resulting in prolonged activation of the RAS/RAF/MAPK signaling pathway and ultimately an increased cellular proliferation (Cichowski and Jacks 2001). Recurrent somatic inactivating mutations in *NF1* have been recently reported in ~5% patients with AML (Eisfeld et al. 2018). In the same study, *NF1*-mutant AML patients had poor outcomes with lower complete remission rates and shorter overall survival when treated with standard chemotherapy.

Mutations in Epigenetic Modifiers: *DNMT3A, TET2, IDH1/2,* and Polycomb-Group Genes (Fig. 2)

One of the hallmarks of AML pathogenesis is disruption of epigenetic regulation. The mutations in genes encoding epigenetic modifiers are commonly acquired early and are present in the initiating clone. This has led to an increasing interest in the development of epigenetic therapies for AML.

DNMT3A

DNA methyltransferase 3A (DNMT3A) is a member of the DNA methyltransferase family, which includes DNMT1, DNMT3A, DNMT3B, and DNMT3L (Okano et al. 1998). It catalyzes de novo DNA methylation at the C-5 position of cytosine bases of unmethylated CpG dinucleotides. DNA methylation is a critical epigenetic modification and plays an essential role in maintaining hematopoietic homeostasis. Consistent with its function, *Dnmt3a*-null HSCs up-regulate genes implicated in HSC self-renewal and multipotency, while down-regulating expression of genes associated with HSC differentiation (Challen et al. 2011). Mutations in *DNMT3A* are observed in ∼30% of AML cases.

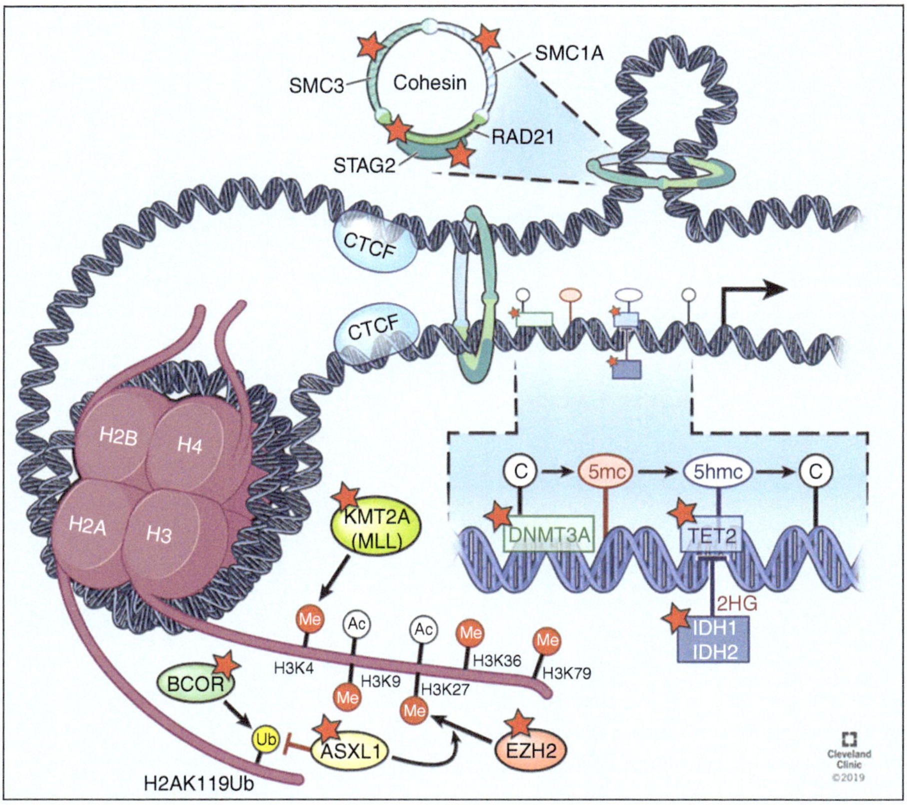

Figure 2. Overview of frequently mutated epigenetic modifiers. This includes (1) DNA cytosine modifications *DNMT3A, TET2,* and *IDH1/2*; (2) histone post-translational modifications *ASXL1, BCOR/L1,* and *MLL1 (KMT2A)*; and (3) Cohesin complex *SMC1A, SMC3,* and *RAD21*, bound to *STAG1/2*. Mutated genes are highlighted with a red star. (Refer to the main text for detailed explanations of the depicted processes.) (Figure reprinted with permission, Cleveland Clinic Center for Medical Art & Photography © 2019–2020. All rights reserved.)

DNMT3A-mutant AML patients are older and most commonly present with a normal karyotype (Ley et al. 2010; Cancer Genome Atlas Research et al. 2013). The mutations in *DNMT3A* include nonsense, frameshift, and missense alterations that are enriched within the methyltransferase domain. The recurrent mutation at codon R882 is the most frequent *DNMT3A* mutation in AML patients, the resultant protein exerts a dominant-negative effect on wild-type *DNMT3A* methyltransferase activity (Holz-Schietinger et al. 2012; Cancer Genome Atlas Research et al. 2013; Russler-Germain et al. 2014). Mutations in *DNMT3A* frequently co-occur with mutations in *NPM1* and *FLT3-ITD*, which collectively confer adverse risk (Marcucci et al. 2012; Bezerra et al. 2020). *DNMT3A* mutations at codon R882 have been shown to promote anthracycline resistance through a proximal defect in nucleosome remodeling and resultant impaired DNA damaging sensing (Guryanova et al. 2016). Clonal hierarchy studies show that mutations in *DNMT3A* are one of the founder mutations shaping the course of leukemia evolution and progression (Welch et al. 2012), making this an attractive target for the development of novel therapeutic approaches. This is further underscored by studies showing that the *DNMT3A* is the most frequently mutated gene in clonal hematopoiesis (CH) (Genovese et al. 2014; Jaiswal et al. 2014; Shlush et al. 2014; Xie et al. 2014). Although essential insights into the role of *DNMT3A* mutations in leukemogenesis have emerged from human and preclinical studies, the fundamental mechanism(s) by which mutant *DNMT3A* leads to increased self-renewal in HSCs has not been delineated.

TET2

The mammalian ten-eleven-translocation (TET) family proteins TET1, TET2, and TET3, are α-ketoglutarate-dependent dioxygenases. The TET enzymes, in the presence of oxygen, reduced Fe^{2+}, and ascorbic acid, catalyze the stepwise oxidation of 5-methylcytosine (5mC) to 5-hydroxymethylcytosine (5hmC), 5-formylcytosine (5fC), and 5-carboxylcytosine (5caC), with resultant loss of DNA methylation (Tahiliani et al. 2009; Ko et al. 2010; He et al. 2011; Ito et al. 2011). *TET2*, but not *TET1* or *TET3*, loss-of-function mutations are common across a spectrum of hematologic malignancies (Delhommeau et al. 2009; Jankowska et al. 2009). Somatic mutations in *TET2* are seen in ~20% of patients with AML, especially in patients with a prior history of MDS or myeloproliferative neoplasm (MPN) (Abdel-Wahab et al. 2009). In AML, *TET2* mutations co-occur with *NPM1*, *FLT3-ITD*, *NRAS*, and *DNMT3A* and are largely mutually exclusive with *IDH1/2* neomorphic mutations (Papaemmanuil et al. 2016; Desai et al. 2018). *TET2* mutations are among the most common mutations seen in clonal hematopoiesis (CH) (Busque et al. 2012).

Tet2$^{-/-}$ mice develop myeloid and lymphoid neoplasms, after long latencies, through the accumulation of numerous mutations, including *Apc*, *Nf1*, *Flt3*, *Cbl*, *Notch1*, and *Mll2* (Pan et al. 2017). Increased production of inflammatory mediators (IL-6) and bacterial translocation across gut mucosa may enhance leukemogenesis in *Tet2*$^{-/-}$ mice (Zhang et al. 2015; Meisel et al. 2018). Recent studies also indicate aberrant expression of diverse metabolic pathways, such as BCAT1, can decrease TET function by inhibiting α-ketoglutarate (Raffel et al. 2017). Supplementation of vitamin C (ascorbate), a co-factor of α-ketoglutarate-dependent dioxygenases like TET enzymes, has recently been shown to enhance residual *TET2* function in the heterozygous mutant state (Agathocleous et al. 2017; Cimmino et al. 2017). A clinical trial evaluating the safety and efficacy of high-dose vitamin C for *TET2*-mutated myeloid neoplasms is ongoing. Despite our mechanistic understanding of the function of TET proteins, how loss-of-function mutations in *TET2* initiates and maintains leukemogenesis is largely unknown.

IDH1 and *IDH2* Mutations

High-throughput sequencing of AML patient samples identified neomorphic mutations in cytosolic (*IDH1* at R132) or mitochondrial (*IDH2* at R140Q or R172) isoforms of isocitrate dehydrogenase, which are critical for the oxidative carboxylation of isocitrate to α-ketoglutarate. These mutations contribute to leukemogenesis through the production of the oncometabolite R enantiomer of 2-hydroxyglutratrate (R-2-HG), which, in turn, impedes epigenetic regulation via competitive inhibition of dioxygenases, including the TET family of enzymes and histone lysine demethylases (KDM), by competing with α-ketoglutarate (Mardis et al. 2009; Figueroa et al. 2010; Xu et al. 2011). This leads to a repressive chromatin landscape via DNA and histone hypermethylation, and consequent block in cellular differentiation (Lu et al. 2012; Losman et al. 2013). Mutations in *IDH1* and *IDH2* are present in ~5%–10% and ~15%–20% of patients with newly diagnosed AML, respectively. Mutations in *IDH1* and *IDH2* mutually exclusive and occur as early clonal events (Papaemmanuil et al. 2016). *IDH1* and *IDH2* mutations are more frequently observed in patients with trisomy 8 and normal karyotype AML (Medeiros et al. 2017). First-in-class, oral, selective inhibitors of mutant *IDH1* (ivosidenib) and *IDH2* (enasidenib) are U.S. Federal Drug Administration (FDA)-approved for the management of *IDH1/2*-mutant adults with refractory or relapsed AML (Stein et al. 2017; DiNardo et al. 2018). Several mechanisms of resistance to enasidenib (*IDH2* inhibitor) leading to late relapse have already been described, including acquisition of *IDH1*-mutated subclones (Quek et al. 2018) or development of additional noncatalytic second-site mutations of *IDH2* (Intlekofer et al. 2018).

ASXL1

Additional sex combs-like 1 (*ASXL1*), located at 20q11.21, is one of the three mammalian homologs of the *Drosophila* additional sex combs (*Asx*) gene. *Asx* functions as an epigenetic regulator that was originally identified as an enhancer of Trithorax (TrxG) and Polycomb group (PcG) genes (Micol and Abdel-Wahab 2016). ASXL1 interacts with BRCA1-associated protein 1 (BAP1) to form the Polycomb repressive deubiquitinase (PR-DUB) complex, which removes monoubiquitin from histone H2A at lysine 119 (H2AK119Ub) (a repressive mark) to activate genes targeted by PRC1 (Scheuermann et al. 2010). ASXL1 also interacts with the PRC2 complex to mediate histone H3 lysine 27 (H3K27) trimethylation (Abdel-Wahab et al. 2012; Inoue et al. 2013). It is yet to be determined if the observed changes in H3K27 methylation with ASXL1 loss are caused by direct interaction between ASXL1 and PRC2 or are secondary to depletion of H2AK119Ub and subsequent failure of PRC2 recruitment (Balasubramani et al. 2015). Somatic mutations in *ASXL1* are frequently detected in clonal hematopoiesis and various myeloid malignancies, suggesting they are the initial events in the leukemic transformation. *ASXL1* mutations occur in ~10%–20% of patients with AML and are enriched in those with underlying myelodysplasia (Metzeler et al. 2011). *ASXL1* mutations coexist with those mutations in the splicing factor (*SRSF2*, *U2AF1*), signal transduction (*NRAS*, *JAK2*, *NF1*), and transcription factor (*RUNX1*) (Papaemmanuil et al. 2016). *ASXL1* mutations are more common in older patients with AML and confer a poor prognosis (Schnittger et al. 2013). A mechanistic understanding of how *ASXL1* mutations in myeloid malignancies drive leukemogenesis remains to be fully elucidated

BCOR and *BCORL1*

BCL6 corepressor (*BCOR*) and its closely related homolog, BCL6 corepressor like 1 (*BCORL1*), are located on the X-chromosome and are targeted by somatic mutations in AML, MDS, chronic myelomonocytic leukemia (CMML), and aplastic anemia (Damm et al. 2013; Yoshizato et al. 2015; Papaemmanuil et al. 2016). BCOR/BCORL1 function as components of PRC1.1, a noncanonical PRC1 complex. PRC1.1 is responsible for the deposition of monoubiquitination on lysine 119 of histone 2A (H2AK119ub1) and mediates transcriptional repression by recruitment of PRC2 and subsequent deposition of H3K27me3 mark (Blackledge et al. 2014; Di Carlo et al. 2019). In mice, loss of *Bcor* function results in enhanced self-renewal of myeloid progenitor cells and cooperates with *Kras*^{G12D} to initiate leukemia in vivo (Kelly et al. 2019).

Loss-of-function somatic mutations in *BCOR* and *BCORL1* have been reported in ~1%–4% of AML, and carry an unfavorable prognosis (Grossmann et al. 2011; Damm et al. 2013).

Splicing Factor Mutations (*SF3B1, SRSF2, U2AF1, ZRSR2, U2AF2, PRPF8,* and *LUC7L2*)

Almost all human genes are subject to alternative pre-mRNA splicing, a primary source of diversity in messenger RNA species and protein isoforms, which is orchestrated by the macromolecular spliceosome complex (Fig. 1) (Lee and Rio 2015). Recent advances in high-throughput sequencing technologies have unexpectedly identified somatic mutations in the core spliceosomal proteins and associated RNA splicing factors in MDS, CMML, and AML (Anczuków and Krainer 2016). This includes mutations in *SF3B1* (splicing factor 3b subunit 1), *SRSF2* (serine/arginine rich splicing factor 2), *U2AF1* (U2 small nuclear RNA auxiliary factor 1), and *ZRSR2* (zinc finger RNA binding motif and serine/arginine rich 2). These mutations are mutually exclusive, heterozygous point mutations, suggesting synthetic lethal interactions if they were to co-occur (Yoshida et al. 2011; Lee et al. 2018). Splicing machinery mutations are most common in AML arising out of antecedent myeloid malignancy (secondary AML) (Lindsley et al. 2015). It has been shown that mutations in *SRSF2* cooperate with *IDH2*, with resultant synergy between RNA splicing and epigenetic regulation in promoting leukemogenesis (Yoshimi et al. 2019). Several groups have developed therapeutic strategies targeting the core spliceosome (SF3B1 inhibitors), splicing regulatory factors (PRMT5 inhibitor, RBM39 degraders, and SRPKs/CLKs inhibitors), and modulating pathologic splicing events (oligonucleotide-based approaches) (Lee et al. 2016; Obeng et al. 2016; Seiler et al. 2018; Fong et al. 2019; Wang et al. 2019).

Cohesin Complex

The cohesin complex is a tripartite ring including three structural proteins, SMC1A, SMC3, and RAD21, bound to either STAG1 or STAG2 (Fig. 2). This complex has many functions, most notably an essential role in aligning and stabilizing sister chromatids during metaphase (Nasmyth and Haering 2009). Cohesin complex also plays a critical role in the regulation of gene expression by cooperating with the DNA-binding protein CTCF in maintaining topologically associated domains (TADs) and regulating three-dimensional (3D) genome organization (Wendt et al. 2008). Heterozygous loss-of-function mutations in the cohesin complex occur in 12%–20% of AML and MDS patients and are more prevalent in high-risk MDS and secondary AML (Kon et al. 2013; Thota et al. 2014). These mutations are not associated with aneuploidy. Several studies have reported that the haploinsufficiency induced by the cohesin mutations enhances HSPC self-renewal and block hematopoietic differentiation (Mazumdar et al. 2015; Mullenders et al. 2015; Viny et al. 2015). *STAG2*, which is X-linked, is the most commonly mutated cohesin gene across many hematopoietic and solid tumors. A recent study demonstrated a specific role for *STAG2* (not by *STAG1*) in balancing self-renewal and differentiation in HSPCs (Viny et al. 2019).

Mutations in Tumor-Suppressor Genes: *TP53, WT1, PHF6*

TP53

The tumor-suppressor gene *TP53* is the most frequently mutated gene in human cancer and has many cellular functions, which are discussed in detail elsewhere (Fig. 1) (Kastenhuber and Lowe 2017). Mutations in *TP53* occur in 5%–20% of patients with newly diagnosed AML. There is an increased frequency of *TP53* mutations in AML patients with therapy-related myeloid neoplasms, complex karyotype, monosomal karyotype, and relapsed disease. One possible postulation for *TP53* pathogenesis in therapy-related myeloid neoplasms is that *TP53* mutations are acquired in some HSPCs during normal aging (clonal hematopoiesis) and are then selected for upon exposure to cytotoxic chemotherapy, ultimately resulting in the expansion of HSPCs with *TP53* mutations (Wong et al. 2015). The majority of *TP53* mutations are missense mutations within the central DNA-binding domain, leading to loss of function. The resulting loss of function of p53 favors genomic instability and impaired apoptosis, which can contribute to resistance to chemotherapy. AML patients with *TP53* mutations have been associated with an inadequate response to conventional cytotoxic therapies and inferior overall survival rates (median of 5–9 mo) (Stengel et al. 2017). Historically, the efforts to target p53 therapeutically have been challenging. The landscape has been changing with the development of novel therapeutic strategies targeting the *TP53* pathway. One such promising approach is APR-246, a methylated derivative of PRIMA-1 that is converted to Michael acceptor methylene quinuclidinone (MQ), which can bind covalently to mutant p53 and restore wild-type transcriptional properties to the protein (Lambert et al. 2009). There is an ongoing multicenter phase III randomized study comparing the combination of APR-246 with azacytidine compared with azacytidine alone in *TP53*-mutant MDS and AML (NCT03745716).

WT1

Wilm's tumor 1 (*WT1*) encodes for a transcription factor that regulates cell proliferation, differentiation, apoptosis, and organ development (Call et al. 1990). Somatic loss-of-function mutations target *WT1* in 6%–15% of AML patients. Also, overexpression of wild-type WT1 protein has been observed in AML, further challenging the mechanistic understanding of how *WT1* contributes to leukemogenesis (Rampal and Figueroa 2016). Heterozygous loss of *Wt1* enhances HSCs self-renewal and cooperates with *Flt3-ITD* to induce leukemic transformation (Pronier et al. 2018). Loss-of-function mutations in *WT1* led to marked promoter hypermethylation pattern and reduction in 5hmC levels similar to AML patients with mutations in *TET2* and *IDH1/2* (Rampal et al. 2014). WT1 protein has also been shown to bind directly to TET2 and recruit TET2 to specific genomic sites to activate the gene expression of WT1-target genes (Wang et al. 2015). Mutations in *WT1* are associated with younger age, often co-occur with *FLT3-ITD*, and confer adverse prognostic significance in AML with increased risk of primary refractory disease (Hou et al. 2010).

PHF6

Somatic loss-of-function mutations in the X-chromosome-linked tumor suppressor plant homeodomain factor 6 (*PHF6*) are present in ~3% of AML patients (Van Vlierberghe et al. 2011). PHF6 is involved in chromatin-mediated transcriptional regulation by binding to the nucleosome remodeling and deacetylase (NuRD) chromatin remodeling complex (Todd and Picketts 2012; Liu et al. 2015). The presence of *PHF6* mutations in preleukemic clonal hematopoiesis supports its role in leukemia initiation and HSC self-renewal (Yoshizato et al. 2015; Abelson et al. 2018). In line with this notion, in a mouse model of T-cell acute lymphoblastic anemia (T-ALL), loss of *Phf6* enhances tumor initiation and transformation and leads to increased self-renewal in mouse HSCs (Wendorff et al. 2019). Mutations in *PHF6* are associated with *RUNX1* mutations and with reduced overall survival in AML patients (Patel et al. 2012).

CONCLUDING REMARKS

Mutational studies involving large cohorts of patients with AML have identified a complex mutational landscape, including patterns of significant co-occurrence and mutual exclusivity of mutations. The mechanistic interactions between different mutations have only begun to be elucidated, and we expect these insights can be used to better inform our understanding of molecular pathogenesis of the disease, improve risk stratification, and identify novel therapeutic vulnerabilities. In specific cases, such as co-occurring *FLT3*/*TET2* (Shih et al. 2015) and *SRSF2*/*IDH2* (Yoshimi et al. 2019) mutations, mechanisms of oncogenic synergy have been elucidated; however, the basis for cooperativity between AML disease alleles requires greater investigation. Moreover, bulk sequencing studies

 Cite this article as *Cold Spring Harb Perspect Med* doi: 10.1101/cshperspect.a034975

have given us a glimpse into the temporal and spatial sequence of somatic mutations that drive leukemogenesis, from early mutations, which induce clonal hematopoiesis (*DNMT3A*, *TET2*, *ASXL1*), to disease-defining mutations present in all cells at transformation (*NPM1*), to mutations that can occur in specific subclones and further enhance the fitness of AML cells (*FLT3*, *RAS*). However, the roles of all of the different mutations in this complex sequence of genetic events that contribute to AML are not known, and many AML patients are a complex amalgam of multiple branching clones such that the AML "ecosystem" has not been fully characterized. Moreover, the observations that relapse can come from rarer AML subclones (Ding et al. 2012; Shlush et al. 2017) suggest that a better understanding of the role of specific mutations in AML heterogeneity and drug response is urgently needed.

In addition to novel mechanistic insights, we need to ensure that this knowledge is translated into improved outcomes for our patients. Most AML patients do not present with mutations for which we have a molecularly targeted therapy, and targeted therapy has limited curative potential when given as monotherapy in AML. We need to identify additional mechanisms of leukemic transformation induced by genetic/epigenetic events in AML, such that we can uncover novel therapeutic targets that lead to genotype-based combination therapies for AML patients. It is our hope that the ever-evolving understanding of AML pathogenesis will continue to lead to novel therapies for our patients.

ACKNOWLEDGMENTS

This work was supported by National Cancer Institute R35 CA197594-01A1 (R.L.L.), National Cancer Institute R01 CA216421 (R.L. L.), National Cancer Institute PS-OC U54 CA143869-05 (R.L.L.), and Leukemia & Lymphoma Society Translational Research Foundation 6499-17 (R.L.L.). This work was supported in part by Memorial Sloan Kettering Cancer Center Core Grant P30 CA008748. A.K. is supported by the VeloSano Catalyst Award.

REFERENCES

Abdel-Wahab O, Mullally A, Hedvat C, Garcia-Manero G, Patel J, Wadleigh M, Malinge S, Yao J, Kilpivaara O, Bhat R, et al. 2009. Genetic characterization of TET1, TET2, and TET3 alterations in myeloid malignancies. *Blood* **114:** 144–147. doi:10.1182/blood-2009-03-210039

Abdel-Wahab O, Adli M, LaFave LM, Gao J, Hricik T, Shih AH, Pandey S, Patel JP, Chung YR, Koche R, et al. 2012. *ASXL1* mutations promote myeloid transformation through loss of PRC2-mediated gene repression. *Cancer Cell* **22:** 180–193. doi:10.1016/j.ccr.2012.06.032

Abelson S, Collord G, Ng SWK, Weissbrod O, Mendelson Cohen N, Niemeyer E, Barda N, Zuzarte PC, Heisler L, Sundaravadanam Y, et al. 2018. Prediction of acute myeloid leukaemia risk in healthy individuals. *Nature* **559:** 400–404. doi:10.1038/s41586-018-0317-6

Agathocleous M, Meacham CE, Burgess RJ, Piskounova E, Zhao Z, Crane GM, Cowin BL, Bruner E, Murphy MM, Chen W, et al. 2017. Ascorbate regulates haematopoietic stem cell function and leukaemogenesis. *Nature* **549:** 476–481. doi:10.1038/nature23876

Amatangelo MD, Quek L, Shih A, Stein EM, Roshal M, David MD, Marteyn B, Farnoud NR, de Botton S, Bernard OA, et al. 2017. Enasidenib induces acute myeloid leukemia cell differentiation to promote clinical response. *Blood* **130:** 732–741. doi:10.1182/blood-2017-04-779447

Anczuków O, Krainer AR. 2016. Splicing-factor alterations in cancers. *RNA* **22:** 1285–1301. doi:10.1261/rna.057919.116

Arber DA, Orazi A, Hasserjian R, Thiele J, Borowitz MJ, Le Beau MM, Bloomfield CD, Cazzola M, Vardiman JW. 2016. The 2016 revision to the World Health Organization classification of myeloid neoplasms and acute leukemia. *Blood* **127:** 2391–2405. doi:10.1182/blood-2016-03-643544

Armstrong SA, Staunton JE, Silverman LB, Pieters R, den Boer ML, Minden MD, Sallan SE, Lander ES, Golub TR, Korsmeyer SJ. 2002. MLL translocations specify a distinct gene expression profile that distinguishes a unique leukemia. *Nat Genet* **30:** 41–47. doi:10.1038/ng765

Avellino R, Delwel R. 2017. Expression and regulation of C/EBPα in normal myelopoiesis and in malignant transformation. *Blood* **129:** 2083–2091. doi:10.1182/blood-2016-09-687822

Bacher U, Haferlach T, Schoch C, Kern W, Schnittger S. 2006. Implications of *NRAS* mutations in AML: A study of 2502 patients. *Blood* **107:** 3847–3853. doi:10.1182/blood-2005-08-3522

Balasubramani A, Larjo A, Bassein JA, Chang X, Hastie RB, Togher SM, Lähdesmäki H, Rao A. 2015. Cancer-associated *ASXL1* mutations may act as gain-of-function mutations of the ASXL1-BAP1 complex. *Nat Commun* **6:** 7307. doi:10.1038/ncomms8307

Ball BJ, Hsu M, Devlin SM, Famulare C, Cai SF, Dunbar A, Epstein-Peterson ZD, Menghrajani K, Glass JL, Taylor J, et al. 2019. RAS mutations are independently associated with decreased overall survival and event-free survival in patients with AML receiving induction chemotherapy. *Blood* **134:** 18. doi:10.1182/blood-2019-125319

Basecke J, Whelan JT, Griesinger F, Bertrand FE. 2006. The MLL partial tandem duplication in acute myeloid leukaemia. *Br J Haematol* **135:** 438–449. doi:10.1111/j.1365-2141.2006.06301.x

Bezerra MF, Lima AS, Piqué-Borràs MR, Silveira DR, Coelho-Silva JL, Pereira-Martins DA, Weinhäuser I, Franca-Neto PL, Quek L, Corby A, et al. 2020. Co-occurrence of DNMT3A, NPM1, FLT3 mutations identifies a subset of acute myeloid leukemia with adverse prognosis. *Blood* **135:** 870–875. doi:10.1182/blood.2019003339

Blackledge NP, Farcas AM, Kondo T, King HW, McGouran JF, Hanssen LL, Ito S, Cooper S, Kondo K, Koseki Y, et al. 2014. Variant PRC1 complex-dependent H2A ubiquitylation drives PRC2 recruitment and polycomb domain formation. *Cell* **157:** 1445–1459. doi:10.1016/j.cell.2014.05.004

Bloomfield CD, Lawrence D, Byrd JC, Carroll A, Pettenati MJ, Tantravahi R, Patil SR, Davey FR, Berg DT, Schiffer CA, et al. 1998. Frequency of prolonged remission duration after high-dose cytarabine intensification in acute myeloid leukemia varies by cytogenetic subtype. *Cancer Res* **58:** 4173–4179.

Borkin D, He S, Miao H, Kempinska K, Pollock J, Chase J, Purohit T, Malik B, Zhao T, Wang J, et al. 2015. Pharmacologic inhibition of the menin-MLL interaction blocks progression of MLL leukemia in vivo. *Cancer Cell* **27:** 589–602. doi:10.1016/j.ccell.2015.02.016

Brunetti L, Gundry MC, Sorcini D, Guzman AG, Huang YH, Ramabadran R, Gionfriddo I, Mezzasoma F, Milano F, Nabet B, et al. 2018. Mutant NPM1 maintains the leukemic state through HOX expression. *Cancer Cell* **34:** 499–512.e9. doi:10.1016/j.ccell.2018.08.005

Busque L, Patel JP, Figueroa ME, Vasanthakumar A, Provost S, Hamilou Z, Mollica L, Li J, Viale A, Heguy A, et al. 2012. Recurrent somatic *TET2* mutations in normal elderly individuals with clonal hematopoiesis. *Nat Genet* **44:** 1179–1181. doi:10.1038/ng.2413

Byrd JC, Ruppert AS, Mrózek K, Carroll AJ, Edwards CG, Arthur DC, Pettenati MJ, Stamberg J, Koduru PR, Moore JO, et al. 2004. Repetitive cycles of high-dose cytarabine benefit patients with acute myeloid leukemia and inv(16)(p13q22) or t(16;16)(p13;q22): results from CALGB 8461. *J Clin Oncol* **22:** 1087–1094. doi:10.1200/JCO.2004.07.012

Call KM, Glaser T, Ito CY, Buckler AJ, Pelletier J, Haber DA, Rose EA, Kral A, Yeger H, Lewis WH, et al. 1990. Isolation and characterization of a zinc finger polypeptide gene at the human chromosome 11 Wilms' tumor locus. *Cell* **60:** 509–520. doi:10.1016/0092-8674(90)90601-A

Cancer Genome Atlas Research Network, Ley TJ, Miller C, Ding L, Raphael BJ, Mungall AJ, Robertson A, Hoadley K, Triche TJ, Laird PW, et al. 2013. Genomic and epigenomic landscapes of adult de novo acute myeloid leukemia. *New Engl J Med* **368:** 2059–2074. doi:10.1056/NEJMoa1301689

Challen GA, Sun D, Jeong M, Luo M, Jelinek J, Berg JS, Bock C, Vasanthakumar A, Gu H, Xi Y, et al. 2011. Dnmt3a is essential for hematopoietic stem cell differentiation. *Nat Genet* **44:** 23–31. doi:10.1038/ng.1009

Chen TH, Kambal A, Krysiak K, Walshauser MA, Raju G, Tibbitts JF, Walter MJ. 2011. Knockdown of Hspa9, a del (5q31.2) gene, results in a decrease in hematopoietic progenitors in mice. *Blood* **117:** 1530–1539. doi:10.1182/blood-2010-06-293167

Chen C, Liu Y, Rappaport AR, Kitzing T, Schultz N, Zhao Z, Shroff AS, Dickins RA, Vakoc CR, Bradner JE, et al. 2014. MLL3 is a haploinsufficient 7q tumor suppressor in acute myeloid leukemia. *Cancer Cell* **25:** 652–665. doi:10.1016/j.ccr.2014.03.016

Chen L, Chen W, Mysliwski M, Serio J, Ropa J, Abulwerdi FA, Chan RJ, Patel JP, Tallman MS, Paietta E, et al. 2015. Mutated *Ptpn11* alters leukemic stem cell frequency and reduces the sensitivity of acute myeloid leukemia cells to Mcl1 inhibition. *Leukemia* **29:** 1290–1300. doi:10.1038/leu.2015.18

Cichowski K, Jacks T. 2001. NF1 tumor suppressor gene function: Narrowing the GAP. *Cell* **104:** 593–604. doi:10.1016/S0092-8674(01)00245-8

Cimmino L, Dolgalev I, Wang Y, Yoshimi A, Martin GH, Wang J, Ng V, Xia B, Witkowski MT, Mitchell-Flack M, et al. 2017. Restoration of TET2 function blocks aberrant self-renewal and leukemia progression. *Cell* **170:** 1079–1095.e20. doi:10.1016/j.cell.2017.07.032

Crispino JD, Horwitz MS. 2017. GATA factor mutations in hematologic disease. *Blood* **129:** 2103–2110. doi:10.1182/blood-2016-09-687889

Crute BE, Lewis AF, Wu Z, Bushweller JH, Speck NA. 1996. Biochemical and biophysical properties of the core-binding factor α2 (AML1) DNA-binding domain. *J Biol Chem* **271:** 26251–26260. doi:10.1074/jbc.271.42.26251

Damm F, Chesnais V, Nagata Y, Yoshida K, Scourzic L, Okuno Y, Itzykson R, Sanada M, Shiraishi Y, Gelsi-Boyer V, et al. 2013. *BCOR* and *BCORL1* mutations in myelodysplastic syndromes and related disorders. *Blood* **122:** 3169–3177. doi:10.1182/blood-2012-11-469619

Delhommeau F, Dupont S, Della Valle V, James C, Trannoy S, Massé A, Kosmider O, Le Couedic JP, Robert F, Alberdi A, et al. 2009. Mutation in *TET2* in myeloid cancers. *New Engl J Med* **360:** 2289–2301. doi:10.1056/NEJMoa0810069

Desai P, Mencia-Trinchant N, Savenkov O, Simon MS, Cheang G, Lee S, Samuel M, Ritchie EK, Guzman ML, Ballman KV, et al. 2018. Somatic mutations precede acute myeloid leukemia years before diagnosis. *Nat Med* **24:** 1015–1023. doi:10.1038/s41591-018-0081-z

De Weer A, Speleman F, Cauwelier B, Van Roy N, Yigit N, Verhasselt B, De Moerloose B, Benoit Y, Noens L, Selleslag D, et al. 2008. EVI1 overexpression in t(3;17) positive myeloid malignancies results from juxtaposition of EVI1 to the MSI2 locus at 17q22. *Haematologica* **93:** 1903–1907. doi:10.3324/haematol.13192

Díaz-Beyá M, Labopin M, Maertens J, Alijurf M, Passweg J, Dietrich B, Schouten H, Socié G, Schaap N, Schwerdtfeger R, et al. 2020. Allogeneic stem cell transplantation in AML with t(6;9)(p23;q34);*DEK-NUP214* shows a favourable outcome when performed in first complete remission. *Br J Haematol* doi: 10.1111/bjh.16433

Di Carlo V, Mocavini I, Di Croce L. 2019. Polycomb complexes in normal and malignant hematopoiesis. *J Cell Biol* **218:** 55–69. doi:10.1083/jcb.201808028

Dillon R, Hills R, Freeman S, Potter N, Jovanovic J, Ivey A, Kanda AS, Runglall M, Foot N, Valganon M, et al. 2020. Molecular MRD status and outcome after transplantation in *NPM1*-mutated AML. *Blood* **135:** 680–688. doi:10.1182/blood.2019002959

DiNardo CD, Stein EM, de Botton S, Roboz GJ, Altman JK, Mims AS, Swords R, Collins RH, Mannis GN, Pollyea DA, et al. 2018. Durable remissions with ivosidenib in *IDH1*-mutated relapsed or refractory AML. *New Engl J Med* **378:** 2386–2398. doi:10.1056/NEJMoa1716984

DiNardo CD, Tiong IS, Quaglieri A, MacRaild S, Loghavi S, Brown FC, Thijssen R, Pomilio G, Ivey A, Salmon JM, et al. 2020. Molecular patterns of response and treatment failure after frontline venetoclax combinations in older patients with AML. *Blood* **135:** 791–803. doi:10.1182/blood.2019003988

Ding L, Ley TJ, Larson DE, Miller CA, Koboldt DC, Welch JS, Ritchey JK, Young MA, Lamprecht T, McLellan MD, et al. 2012. Clonal evolution in relapsed acute myeloid leukaemia revealed by whole-genome sequencing. *Nature* **481:** 506–510. doi:10.1038/nature10738

Döhner H, Estey E, Grimwade D, Amadori S, Appelbaum FR, Büchner T, Dombret H, Ebert BL, Fenaux P, Larson RA, et al. 2017. Diagnosis and management of AML in adults: 2017 ELN recommendations from an international expert panel. *Blood* **129:** 424–447. doi:10.1182/blood-2016-08-733196

Ebert BL, Pretz J, Bosco J, Chang CY, Tamayo P, Galili N, Raza A, Root DE, Attar E, Ellis SR, et al. 2008. Identification of RPS14 as a 5q- syndrome gene by RNA interference screen. *Nature* **451:** 335–339. doi:10.1038/nature06494

Eisfeld AK, Kohlschmidt J, Mrózek K, Mims A, Walker CJ, Blachly JS, Nicolet D, Orwick S, Maharry SE, Carroll AJ, et al. 2018. *NF1* mutations are recurrent in adult acute myeloid leukemia and confer poor outcome. *Leukemia* **32:** 2536–2545. doi:10.1038/s41375-018-0147-4

Falini B, Mecucci C, Tiacci E, Alcalay M, Rosati R, Pasqualucci L, La Starza R, Diverio D, Colombo E, Santucci A, et al. 2005. Cytoplasmic nucleophosmin in acute myelogenous leukemia with a normal karyotype. *New Engl J Med* **352:** 254–266. doi:10.1056/NEJMoa041974

Fasan A, Haferlach C, Alpermann T, Jeromin S, Grossmann V, Eder C, Weissmann S, Dicker F, Kohlmann A, Schindela S, et al. 2014. The role of different genetic subtypes of *CEBPA* mutated AML. *Leukemia* **28:** 794–803. doi:10.1038/leu.2013.273

Figueroa ME, Abdel-Wahab O, Lu C, Ward PS, Patel J, Shih A, Li Y, Bhagwat N, Vasanthakumar A, Fernandez HF, et al. 2010. Leukemic IDH1 and IDH2 mutations result in a hypermethylation phenotype, disrupt TET2 function, and impair hematopoietic differentiation. *Cancer Cell* **18:** 553–567. doi:10.1016/j.ccr.2010.11.015

Fong JY, Pignata L, Goy PA, Kawabata KC, Lee SC, Koh CM, Musiani D, Massignani E, Kotini AG, Penson A, et al. 2019. Therapeutic targeting of RNA splicing catalysis through inhibition of protein arginine methylation. *Cancer Cell* **36:** 194–209.e9. doi:10.1016/j.ccell.2019.07.003

Fröhling S, Schlenk RF, Stolze I, Bihlmayr J, Benner A, Kreitmeier S, Tobis K, Döhner H, Döhner K. 2004. *CEBPA* mutations in younger adults with acute myeloid leukemia and normal cytogenetics: Prognostic relevance and analysis of cooperating mutations. *J Clin Oncol* **22:** 624–633. doi:10.1200/JCO.2004.06.060

Gaidzik VI, Teleanu V, Papaemmanuil E, Weber D, Paschka P, Hahn J, Wallrabenstein T, Kolbinger B, Köhne CH, Horst HA, et al. 2016. *RUNX1* mutations in acute myeloid leukemia are associated with distinct clinico-pathologic and genetic features. *Leukemia* **30:** 2160–2168. doi:10.1038/leu.2016.126

Genovese G, Kähler AK, Handsaker RE, Lindberg J, Rose SA, Bakhoum SF, Chambert K, Mick E, Neale BM, Fromer M, et al. 2014. Clonal hematopoiesis and blood-cancer risk inferred from blood DNA sequence. *New Engl J Med* **371:** 2477–2487. doi:10.1056/NEJMoa1409405

Greif PA, Dufour A, Konstandin NP, Ksienzyk B, Zellmeier E, Tizazu B, Sturm J, Benthaus T, Herold T, Yaghmaie M, et al. 2012. *GATA2* zinc finger 1 mutations associated with biallelic *CEBPA* mutations define a unique genetic entity of acute myeloid leukemia. *Blood* **120:** 395–403. doi:10.1182/blood-2012-01-403220

Grembecka J, He S, Shi A, Purohit T, Muntean AG, Sorenson RJ, Showalter HD, Murai MJ, Belcher AM, Hartley T, et al. 2012. Menin-MLL inhibitors reverse oncogenic activity of MLL fusion proteins in leukemia. *Nat Chem Biol* **8:** 277–284. doi:10.1038/nchembio.773

Gröschel S, Sanders MA, Hoogenboezem R, de Wit E, Bouwman BAM, Erpelinck C, van der Velden VHJ, Havermans M, Avellino R, van Lom K, et al. 2014. A single oncogenic enhancer rearrangement causes concomitant EVI1 and *GATA2* deregulation in leukemia. *Cell* **157:** 369–381. doi:10.1016/j.cell.2014.02.019

Gröschel S, Sanders MA, Hoogenboezem R, Zeilemaker A, Havermans M, Erpelinck C, Bindels EM, Beverloo HB, Döhner H, Löwenberg B, et al. 2015. Mutational spectrum of myeloid malignancies with inv(3)/t(3;3) reveals a predominant involvement of RAS/RTK signaling pathways. *Blood* **125:** 133–139. doi:10.1182/blood-2014-07-591461

Grossmann V, Tiacci E, Holmes AB, Kohlmann A, Martelli MP, Kern W, Spanhol-Rosseto A, Klein HU, Dugas M, Schindela S, et al. 2011. Whole-exome sequencing identifies somatic mutations of *BCOR* in acute myeloid leukemia with normal karyotype. *Blood* **118:** 6153–6163. doi:10.1182/blood-2011-07-365320

Gu X, Ebrahem Q, Mahfouz RZ, Hasipek M, Enane F, Radivoyevitch T, Rapin N, Przychodzen B, Hu Z, Balusu R, et al. 2018. Leukemogenic nucleophosmin mutation disrupts the transcription factor hub that regulates granulomonocytic fates. *J Clin Invest* **128:** 4260–4279. doi:10.1172/JCI97117

Guryanova OA, Shank K, Spitzer B, Luciani L, Koche RP, Garrett-Bakelman FE, Ganzel C, Durham BH, Mohanty A, Hoermann G, et al. 2016. *DNMT3A* mutations promote anthracycline resistance in acute myeloid leukemia via impaired nucleosome remodeling. *Nat Med* **22:** 1488–1495. doi:10.1038/nm.4210

Hahn CN, Chong CE, Carmichael CL, Wilkins EJ, Brautigan PJ, Li XC, Babic M, Lin M, Carmagnac A, Lee YK, et al. 2011. Heritable *GATA2* mutations associated with familial myelodysplastic syndrome and acute myeloid leukemia. *Nat Genet* **43:** 1012–1017. doi:10.1038/ng.913

Hatlen MA, Arora K, Vacic V, Grabowska EA, Liao W, Riley-Gillis B, Oschwald DM, Wang L, Joergens JE, Shih AH, et al. 2016. Integrative genetic analysis of mouse and human AML identifies cooperating disease alleles. *J Exp Med* **213:** 25–34. doi:10.1084/jem.20150524

He YF, Li BZ, Li Z, Liu P, Wang Y, Tang Q, Ding J, Jia Y, Chen Z, Li L, et al. 2011. Tet-mediated formation of 5-carboxylcytosine and its excision by TDG in mammalian DNA. *Science* **333:** 1303–1307. doi:10.1126/science.1210944

Hinai A, Pratcorona M, Grob T, Kavelaars FG, Bussaglia E, Sanders MA, Nomdedeu J, Valk PJM. 2019. The landscape of *KMT2A*-PTD AML: Concurrent mutations, gene expression signatures, and clinical outcome. *Hemasphere* **3:** e181. doi:10.1097/HS9.0000000000000181

Hirsch P, Zhang Y, Tang R, Joulin V, Boutroux H, Pronier E, Moatti H, Flandrin P, Marzac C, Bories D, et al. 2016. Genetic hierarchy and temporal variegation in the clonal history of acute myeloid leukaemia. *Nat Commun* **7:** 12475. doi:10.1038/ncomms12475

Holz-Schietinger C, Matje DM, Reich NO. 2012. Mutations in DNA methyltransferase (DNMT3A) observed in acute myeloid leukemia patients disrupt processive methylation. *J Biol Chem* **287:** 30941–30951. doi:10.1074/jbc.M112.366625

Hosono N, Makishima H, Jerez A, Yoshida K, Przychodzen B, McMahon S, Shiraishi Y, Chiba K, Tanaka H, Miyano S, et al. 2014. Recurrent genetic defects on chromosome 7q in myeloid neoplasms. *Leukemia* **28:** 1348–1351. doi:10.1038/leu.2014.25

Hou HA, Huang TC, Lin LI, Liu CY, Chen CY, Chou WC, Tang JL, Tseng MH, Huang CF, Chiang YC, et al. 2010. *WT1* mutation in 470 adult patients with acute myeloid leukemia: Stability during disease evolution and implication of its incorporation into a survival scoring system. *Blood* **115:** 5222–5231. doi:10.1182/blood-2009-12-259390

Inoue D, Kitaura J, Togami K, Nishimura K, Enomoto Y, Uchida T, Kagiyama Y, Kawabata KC, Nakahara F, Izawa K, et al. 2013. Myelodysplastic syndromes are induced by histone methylation-altering *ASXL1* mutations. *J Clin Invest* **123:** 4627–4640. doi:10.1172/JCI70739

Intlekofer AM, Shih AH, Wang B, Nazir A, Rustenburg AS, Albanese SK, Patel M, Famulare C, Correa FM, Takemoto N, et al. 2018. Acquired resistance to IDH inhibition through *trans* or *cis* dimer-interface mutations. *Nature* **559:** 125–129. doi:10.1038/s41586-018-0251-7

Ito S, Shen L, Dai Q, Wu SC, Collins LB, Swenberg JA, He C, Zhang Y. 2011. Tet proteins can convert 5-methylcytosine to 5-formylcytosine and 5-carboxylcytosine. *Science* **333:** 1300–1303. doi:10.1126/science.1210597

Ito Y, Bae SC, Chuang LS. 2015. The RUNX family: Developmental regulators in cancer. *Nat Rev Cancer* **15:** 81–95. doi:10.1038/nrc3877

Ivey A, Hills RK, Simpson MA, Jovanovic JV, Gilkes A, Grech A, Patel Y, Bhudia N, Farah H, Mason J, et al. 2016. Assessment of minimal residual disease in standard-risk AML. *New Engl J Med* **374:** 422–433. doi:10.1056/NEJMoa1507471

Jaiswal S, Fontanillas P, Flannick J, Manning A, Grauman PV, Mar BG, Lindsley RC, Mermel CH, Burtt N, Chavez A, et al. 2014. Age-related clonal hematopoiesis associated with adverse outcomes. *New Engl J Med* **371:** 2488–2498. doi:10.1056/NEJMoa1408617

Jankowska AM, Szpurka H, Tiu RV, Makishima H, Afable M, Huh J, O'Keefe CL, Ganetzky R, McDevitt MA, Maciejewski JP. 2009. Loss of heterozygosity 4q24 and TET2 mutations associated with myelodysplastic/myeloproliferative neoplasms. *Blood* **113:** 6403–6410. doi:10.1182/blood-2009-02-205690

Joslin JM, Fernald AA, Tennant TR, Davis EM, Kogan SC, Anastasi J, Crispino JD, Le Beau MM. 2007. Haploinsufficiency of *EGR1*, a candidate gene in the del(5q), leads to the development of myeloid disorders. *Blood* **110:** 719–726. doi:10.1182/blood-2007-01-068809

Kastenhuber ER, Lowe SW. 2017. Putting p53 in context. *Cell* **170:** 1062–1078. doi:10.1016/j.cell.2017.08.028

Kayser S, Hills RK, Luskin MR, Brunner AM, Terré C, Westermann J, Menghrajani K, Shaw C, Baer MR, Elliott MA, et al. 2020. Allogeneic hematopoietic cell transplantation improves outcome of adults with t(6;9) acute myeloid leukemia: Results from an international collaborative study. *Haematologica* **105:** 161–169. doi:10.3324/haematol.2018.208678

Kelly MJ, So J, Rogers AJ, Gregory G, Li J, Zethoven M, Gearhart MD, Bardwell VJ, Johnstone RW, Vervoort SJ, et al. 2019. Bcor loss perturbs myeloid differentiation and promotes leukaemogenesis. *Nat Commun* **10:** 1347. doi:10.1038/s41467-019-09250-6

Kirstetter P, Schuster MB, Bereshchenko O, Moore S, Dvinge H, Kurz E, Theilgaard-Mönch K, Månsson R, Pedersen TA, Pabst T, et al. 2008. Modeling of C/EBPα mutant acute myeloid leukemia reveals a common expression signature of committed myeloid leukemia-initiating cells. *Cancer Cell* **13:** 299–310. doi:10.1016/j.ccr.2008.02.008

Kishtagari A, Levine RL, Viny AD. 2020. Driver mutations in acute myeloid leukemia. *Curr Opin Hematol* **27:** 49–57. doi:10.1097/MOH.0000000000000567

Klossowski S, Miao H, Kempinska K, Wu T, Purohit T, Kim E, Linhares BM, Chen D, Jih G, Perkey E, et al. 2020. Menin inhibitor MI-3454 induces remission in MLL1-rearranged and *NPM1*-mutated models of leukemia. *J Clin Invest* **130:** 981–997. doi:10.1172/JCI129126

Ko M, Huang Y, Jankowska AM, Pape UJ, Tahiliani M, Bandukwala HS, An J, Lamperti ED, Koh KP, Ganetzky R, et al. 2010. Impaired hydroxylation of 5-methylcytosine in myeloid cancers with mutant *TET2*. *Nature* **468:** 839–843. doi:10.1038/nature09586

Kon A, Shih LY, Minamino M, Sanada M, Shiraishi Y, Nagata Y, Yoshida K, Okuno Y, Bando M, Nakato R, et al. 2013. Recurrent mutations in multiple components of the cohesin complex in myeloid neoplasms. *Nat Genet* **45:** 1232–1237. doi:10.1038/ng.2731

Krivtsov AV, Armstrong SA. 2007. *MLL* translocations, histone modifications and leukaemia stem-cell development. *Nat Rev Cancer* **7:** 823–833. doi:10.1038/nrc2253

Krivtsov AV, Evans K, Gadrey JY, Eschle BK, Hatton C, Uckelmann HJ, Ross KN, Perner F, Olsen SN, Pritchard T, et al. 2019. A Menin-MLL inhibitor induces specific chromatin changes and eradicates disease in models of *MLL*-rearranged leukemia. *Cancer Cell* **36:** 660–673.e11. doi:10.1016/j.ccell.2019.11.001

Kunimoto H, Meydan C, Nazir A, Whitfield J, Shank K, Rapaport F, Maher R, Pronier E, Meyer SC, Garrett-Bakelman FE, et al. 2018. Cooperative epigenetic remodeling by *TET2* loss and *NRAS* mutation drives myeloid transformation and MEK inhibitor sensitivity. *Cancer Cell* **33:** 44–59.e8. doi:10.1016/j.ccell.2017.11.012

Lambert JM, Gorzov P, Veprintsev DB, Söderqvist M, Segerback D, Bergman J, Fersht AR, Hainaut P, Wiman KG, Bykov VJ. 2009. PRIMA-1 reactivates mutant p53 by covalent binding to the core domain. *Cancer Cell* **15:** 376–388. doi:10.1016/j.ccr.2009.03.003

Lavallée VP, Krosl J, Lemieux S, Boucher G, Gendron P, Pabst C, Boivin I, Marinier A, Guidos CJ, Meloche S, et al. 2016. Chemo-genomic interrogation of *CEBPA* mutated AML reveals recurrent *CSF3R* mutations and subgroup sensitivity to JAK inhibitors. *Blood* **127:** 3054–3061. doi:10.1182/blood-2016-03-705053

Lee Y, Rio DC. 2015. Mechanisms and regulation of alternative pre-mRNA splicing. *Annu Rev Biochem* **84:** 291–323. doi:10.1146/annurev-biochem-060614-034316

Lee SC, Dvinge H, Kim E, Cho H, Micol JB, Chung YR, Durham BH, Yoshimi A, Kim YJ, Thomas M, et al. 2016. Modulation of splicing catalysis for therapeutic targeting of leukemia with mutations in genes encoding spliceosomal proteins. *Nat Med* **22:** 672–678. doi:10.1038/nm.4097

Lee SC, North K, Kim E, Jang E, Obeng E, Lu SX, Liu B, Inoue D, Yoshimi A, Ki M, et al. 2018. Synthetic lethal and convergent biological effects of cancer-associated spliceosomal gene mutations. *Cancer Cell* **34:** 225–241.e8. doi:10.1016/j.ccell.2018.07.003

Ley TJ, Mardis ER, Ding L, Fulton B, McLellan MD, Chen K, Dooling D, Dunford-Shore BH, McGrath S, Hickenbotham M, et al. 2008. DNA sequencing of a cytogenetically normal acute myeloid leukaemia genome. *Nature* **456:** 66–72. doi:10.1038/nature07485

Ley TJ, Ding L, Walter MJ, McLellan MD, Lamprecht T, Larson DE, Kandoth C, Payton JE, Baty J, Welch J, et al. 2010. *DNMT3A* mutations in acute myeloid leukemia. *New Engl J Med* **363:** 2424–2433. doi:10.1056/NEJMoa1005143

Li S, Balmain A, Counter CM. 2018. A model for RAS mutation patterns in cancers: Finding the sweet spot. *Nat Rev Cancer* **18:** 767–777. doi:10.1038/s41568-018-0076-6

Lindsley RC, Mar BG, Mazzola E, Grauman PV, Shareef S, Allen SL, Pigneux A, Wetzler M, Stuart RK, Erba HP, et al. 2015. Acute myeloid leukemia ontogeny is defined by distinct somatic mutations. *Blood* **125:** 1367–1376. doi:10.1182/blood-2014-11-610543

Liu TX, Becker MW, Jelinek J, Wu WS, Deng M, Mikhalkevich N, Hsu K, Bloomfield CD, Stone RM, DeAngelo DJ, et al. 2007. Chromosome 5q deletion and epigenetic suppression of the gene encoding α-catenin (CTNNA1) in myeloid cell transformation. *Nat Med* **13:** 78–83. doi:10.1038/nm1512

Liu Z, Li F, Zhang B, Li S, Wu J, Shi Y. 2015. Structural basis of plant homeodomain finger 6 (PHF6) recognition by the retinoblastoma binding protein 4 (RBBP4) component of the nucleosome remodeling and deacetylase (NuRD) complex. *J Biol Chem* **290:** 6630–6638. doi:10.1074/jbc.M114.610196

Liu Y, Chen C, Xu Z, Scuoppo C, Rillahan CD, Gao J, Spitzer B, Bosbach B, Kastenhuber ER, Baslan T, et al. 2016. Deletions linked to *TP53* loss drive cancer through p53-independent mechanisms. *Nature* **531:** 471–475. doi:10.1038/nature17157

Losman JA, Looper RE, Koivunen P, Lee S, Schneider RK, McMahon C, Cowley GS, Root DE, Ebert BL, Kaelin WG Jr. 2013. (*R*)-2-hydroxyglutarate is sufficient to promote leukemogenesis and its effects are reversible. *Science* **339:** 1621–1625. doi:10.1126/science.1231677

Lu C, Ward PS, Kapoor GS, Rohle D, Turcan S, Abdel-Wahab O, Edwards CR, Khanin R, Figueroa ME, Melnick A, et al. 2012. IDH mutation impairs histone demethylation and results in a block to cell differentiation. *Nature* **483:** 474–478. doi:10.1038/nature10860

Lugthart S, Gröschel S, Beverloo HB, Kayser S, Valk PJ, van Zelderen-Bhola SL, Jan Ossenkoppele G, Vellenga E, van den Berg-de Ruiter E, Schanz U, et al. 2010. Clinical, molecular, and prognostic significance of WHO type inv(3)(q21q26.2)/t(3;3)(q21;q26.2) and various other 3q abnormalities in acute myeloid leukemia. *J Clin Oncol* **28:** 3890–3898. doi:10.1200/JCO.2010.29.2771

Makishima H, Yoshizato T, Yoshida K, Sekeres MA, Radivoyevitch T, Suzuki H, Przychodzen B, Nagata Y, Meggendorfer M, Sanada M, et al. 2017. Dynamics of clonal evolution in myelodysplastic syndromes. *Nat Genet* **49:** 204–212. doi:10.1038/ng.3742

Malaise M, Steinbach D, Corbacioglu S. 2009. Clinical implications of *c-Kit* mutations in acute myelogenous leukemia. *Curr Hematol Malig Rep* **4:** 77–82. doi:10.1007/s11899-009-0011-8

Marcucci G, Metzeler KH, Schwind S, Becker H, Maharry K, Mrózek K, Radmacher MD, Kohlschmidt J, Nicolet D, Whitman SP, et al. 2012. Age-related prognostic impact of different types of *DNMT3A* mutations in adults with primary cytogenetically normal acute myeloid leukemia. *J Clin Oncol* **30:** 742–750. doi:10.1200/JCO.2011.39.2092

Mardis ER, Ding L, Dooling DJ, Larson DE, McLellan MD, Chen K, Koboldt DC, Fulton RS, Delehaunty KD, McGrath SD, et al. 2009. Recurring mutations found by sequencing an acute myeloid leukemia genome. *New Engl J Med* **361:** 1058–1066. doi:10.1056/NEJMoa0903840

Maxson JE, Ries RE, Wang YC, Gerbing RB, Kolb EA, Thompson SL, Guidry Auvil JM, Marra MA, Ma Y, Zong Z, et al. 2016. CSF3R mutations have a high degree of overlap with CEBPA mutations in pediatric AML. *Blood* **127:** 3094–3098. doi:10.1182/blood-2016-04-709899

Mazumdar C, Shen Y, Xavy S, Zhao F, Reinisch A, Li R, Corces MR, Flynn RA, Buenrostro JD, Chan SM, et al. 2015. Leukemia-associated cohesin mutants dominantly enforce stem cell programs and impair human hematopoietic progenitor differentiation. *Cell Stem Cell* **17:** 675–688. doi:10.1016/j.stem.2015.09.017

McMahon CM, Ferng T, Canaani J, Wang ES, Morrissette JJD, Eastburn DJ, Pellegrino M, Durruthy-Durruthy R, Watt CD, Asthana S, et al. 2019. Clonal selection with RAS pathway activation mediates secondary clinical resistance to selective FLT3 inhibition in acute myeloid leukemia. *Cancer Discov* **9:** 1050–1063. doi:10.1158/2159-8290.CD-18-1453

McNerney ME, Brown CD, Wang X, Bartom ET, Karmakar S, Bandlamudi C, Yu S, Ko J, Sandall BP, Stricker T, et al. 2013. *CUX1* is a haploinsufficient tumor suppressor gene on chromosome 7 frequently inactivated in acute myeloid leukemia. *Blood* **121:** 975–983. doi:10.1182/blood-2012-04-426965

Medeiros BC, Fathi AT, DiNardo CD, Pollyea DA, Chan SM, Swords R. 2017. Isocitrate dehydrogenase mutations in myeloid malignancies. *Leukemia* **31:** 272–281. doi:10.1038/leu.2016.275

Meisel M, Hinterleitner R, Pacis A, Chen L, Earley ZM, Mayassi T, Pierre JF, Ernest JD, Galipeau HJ, Thuille N, et al. 2018. Microbial signals drive pre-leukaemic myeloproliferation in a *Tet2*-deficient host. *Nature* **557:** 580–584. doi:10.1038/s41586-018-0125-z

Mendler JH, Maharry K, Radmacher MD, Mrózek K, Becker H, Metzeler KH, Schwind S, Whitman SP, Khalife J, Kohlschmidt J, et al. 2012. *RUNX1* mutations are associated with poor outcome in younger and older patients with cytogenetically normal acute myeloid leukemia and with distinct gene and MicroRNA expression signatures. *J Clin Oncol* **30:** 3109–3118. doi:10.1200/JCO.2011.40.6652

Meshinchi S, Appelbaum FR. 2009. Structural and functional alterations of FLT3 in acute myeloid leukemia. *Clin Cancer Res* **15:** 4263–4269. doi:10.1158/1078-0432.CCR-08-1123

Metzeler KH, Becker H, Maharry K, Radmacher MD, Kohlschmidt J, Mrózek K, Nicolet D, Whitman SP, Wu YZ, Schwind S, et al. 2011. *ASXL1* mutations identify a high-risk subgroup of older patients with primary cytogenetically normal AML within the ELN Favorable genetic category. *Blood* **118:** 6920–6929. doi:10.1182/blood-2011-08-368225

Meyer C, Burmeister T, Gröger D, Tsaur G, Fechina L, Renneville A, Sutton R, Venn NC, Emerenciano M, Pombo-de-Oliveira MS, et al. 2018. The *MLL* recombinome of acute leukemias in 2017. *Leukemia* **32:** 273–284. doi:10.1038/leu.2017.213

Micol JB, Abdel-Wahab O. 2016. The role of additional sex combs-like proteins in cancer. *Cold Spring Harb Perspect Med* **6:** a026526. doi:10.1101/cshperspect.a026526

Mohapatra B, Ahmad G, Nadeau S, Zutshi N, An W, Scheffe S, Dong L, Feng D, Goetz B, Arya P, et al. 2013. Protein tyrosine kinase regulation by ubiquitination: Critical roles of Cbl-family ubiquitin ligases. *Biochim Biophys Acta* **1833:** 122–139. doi:10.1016/j.bbamcr.2012.10.010

Mullenders J, Aranda-Orgilles B, Lhoumaud P, Keller M, Pae J, Wang K, Kayembe C, Rocha PP, Raviram R, Gong Y, et al. 2015. Cohesin loss alters adult hematopoietic stem cell homeostasis, leading to myeloproliferative neoplasms. *J Exp Med* **212:** 1833–1850. doi:10.1084/jem.20151323

Nagamachi A, Matsui H, Asou H, Ozaki Y, Aki D, Kanai A, Takubo K, Suda T, Nakamura T, Wolff L, et al. 2013. Haploinsufficiency of *SAMD9L*, an endosome fusion facilitator, causes myeloid malignancies in mice mimicking human diseases with monosomy 7. *Cancer Cell* **24:** 305–317. doi:10.1016/j.ccr.2013.08.011

Nasmyth K, Haering CH. 2009. Cohesin: Its roles and mechanisms. *Annu Rev Genet* **43:** 525–558. doi:10.1146/annurev-genet-102108-134233

Obeng EA, Chappell RJ, Seiler M, Chen MC, Campagna DR, Schmidt PJ, Schneider RK, Lord AM, Wang L, Gambe RG, et al. 2016. Physiologic expression of Sf3b1^{K700E} causes impaired erythropoiesis, aberrant splicing, and sensitivity to therapeutic spliceosome modulation. *Cancer Cell* **30:** 404–417. doi:10.1016/j.ccell.2016.08.006

Okano M, Xie S, Li E. 1998. Cloning and characterization of a family of novel mammalian DNA (cytosine-5) methyltransferases. *Nat Genet* **19:** 219–220. doi:10.1038/890

Ostergaard P, Simpson MA, Connell FC, Steward CG, Brice G, Woollard WJ, Dafou D, Kilo T, Smithson S, Lunt P, et al. 2011. Mutations in *GATA2* cause primary lymphedema associated with a predisposition to acute myeloid leukemia (Emberger syndrome). *Nat Genet* **43:** 929–931. doi:10.1038/ng.923

Pabst T, Mueller BU, Zhang P, Radomska HS, Narravula S, Schnittger S, Behre G, Hiddemann W, Tenen DG. 2001. Dominant-negative mutations of *CEBPA*, encoding CCAAT/enhancer binding protein-α (C/EBPα), in acute myeloid leukemia. *Nat Genet* **27:** 263–270. doi:10.1038/85820

Pan F, Wingo TS, Zhao Z, Gao R, Makishima H, Qu G, Lin L, Yu M, Ortega JR, Wang J, et al. 2017. *Tet2* loss leads to hypermutagenicity in haematopoietic stem/progenitor cells. *Nat Commun* **8:** 15102. doi:10.1038/ncomms15102

Papaemmanuil E, Gerstung M, Bullinger L, Gaidzik VI, Paschka P, Roberts ND, Potter NE, Heuser M, Thol F, Bolli N, et al. 2016. Genomic classification and prognosis in acute myeloid leukemia. *New Engl J Med* **374:** 2209–2221. doi:10.1056/NEJMoa1516192

Parkin B, Ouillette P, Wang Y, Liu Y, Wright W, Roulston D, Purkayastha A, Dressel A, Karp J, Bockenstedt P, et al. 2010. NF1 inactivation in adult acute myelogenous leukemia. *Clinical Cancer Res* **16:** 4135–4147. doi:10.1158/1078-0432.CCR-09-2639

Paschka P, Marcucci G, Ruppert AS, Mrózek K, Chen H, Kittles RA, Vukosavljevic T, Perrotti D, Vardiman JW, Carroll AJ, et al. 2006. Adverse prognostic significance of *KIT* mutations in adult acute myeloid leukemia with inv(16) and t(8;21): A cancer and Leukemia Group B Study. *J Clin Oncol* **24:** 3904–3911. doi:10.1200/JCO.2006.06.9500

Patel JP, Gönen M, Figueroa ME, Fernandez H, Sun Z, Racevskis J, Van Vlierberghe P, Dolgalev I, Thomas S, Aminova O, et al. 2012. Prognostic relevance of integrated genetic profiling in acute myeloid leukemia. *New Engl J Med* **366:** 1079–1089. doi:10.1056/NEJMoa1112304

Perl AE, Martinelli G, Cortes JE, Neubauer A, Berman E, Paolini S, Montesinos P, Baer MR, Larson RA, Ustun C, et al. 2019. Abstract CT184: Gilteritinib significantly prolongs overall survival in patients with *FLT3*-mutated (*FLT3*$^{mut+}$) relapsed/refractory (R/R) acute myeloid leukemia (AML): Results from the Phase III ADMIRAL trial. *Cancer Res* **79:** CT184.

Pollyea DA, Stevens BM, Jones CL, Winters A, Pei S, Minhajuddin M, D'Alessandro A, Culp-Hill R, Riemondy KA, Gillen AE, et al. 2018. Venetoclax with azacitidine disrupts energy metabolism and targets leukemia stem cells in patients with acute myeloid leukemia. *Nat Med* **24:** 1859–1866. doi:10.1038/s41591-018-0233-1

Pronier E, Bowman RL, Ahn J, Glass J, Kandoth C, Merlinsky TR, Whitfield JT, Durham BH, Gruet A, Hanasoge Somasundara AV, et al. 2018. Genetic and epigenetic evolution as a contributor to WT1-mutant leukemogenesis. *Blood* **132:** 1265–1278. doi:10.1182/blood-2018-03-837468

Quek L, David MD, Kennedy A, Metzner M, Amatangelo M, Shih A, Stoilova B, Quivoron C, Heiblig M, Willekens C, et al. 2018. Clonal heterogeneity of acute myeloid leukemia treated with the IDH2 inhibitor enasidenib. *Nat Med* **24:** 1167–1177. doi:10.1038/s41591-018-0115-6

Raffel S, Falcone M, Kneisel N, Hansson J, Wang W, Lutz C, Bullinger L, Poschet G, Nonnenmacher Y, Barnert A, et al.

2017. BCAT1 restricts αKG levels in AML stem cells leading to IDH^{mut}-like DNA hypermethylation. *Nature* **551:** 384–388. doi:10.1038/nature24294

Rampal R, Figueroa ME. 2016. Wilms tumor 1 mutations in the pathogenesis of acute myeloid leukemia. *Haematologica* **101:** 672–679. doi:10.3324/haematol.2015.141796

Rampal R, Alkalin A, Madzo J, Vasanthakumar A, Pronier E, Patel J, Li Y, Ahn J, Abdel-Wahab O, Shih A, et al. 2014. DNA hydroxymethylation profiling reveals that *WT1* mutations result in loss of TET2 function in acute myeloid leukemia. *Cell Rep* **9:** 1841–1855. doi:10.1016/j.celrep.2014.11.004

Rogers HJ, Vardiman JW, Anastasi J, Raca G, Savage NM, Cherry AM, Arber D, Moore E, Morrissette JJ, Bagg A, et al. 2014. Complex or monosomal karyotype and not blast percentage is associated with poor survival in acute myeloid leukemia and myelodysplastic syndrome patients with inv(3)(q21q26.2)/t(3;3)(q21;q26.2): A Bone Marrow Pathology Group study. *Haematologica* **99:** 821–829. doi:10.3324/haematol.2013.096420

Russler-Germain DA, Spencer DH, Young MA, Lamprecht TL, Miller CA, Fulton R, Meyer MR, Erdmann-Gilmore P, Townsend RR, Wilson RK, et al. 2014. The R882H DNMT3A mutation associated with AML dominantly inhibits wild-type DNMT3A by blocking its ability to form active tetramers. *Cancer Cell* **25:** 442–454. doi:10.1016/j.ccr.2014.02.010

Saito S, Cigdem S, Okuwaki M, Nagata K. 2016. Leukemia-associated Nup214 fusion proteins disturb the XPO1-mediated nuclear-cytoplasmic transport pathway and thereby the NF-κB signaling pathway. *Mol Cell Biol* **36:** 1820–1835. doi:10.1128/MCB.00158-16

Sanada M, Suzuki T, Shih LY, Otsu M, Kato M, Yamazaki S, Tamura A, Honda H, Sakata-Yanagimoto M, Kumano K, et al. 2009. Gain-of-function of mutated *C-CBL* tumour suppressor in myeloid neoplasms. *Nature* **460:** 904–908. doi:10.1038/nature08240

Scheuermann JC, de Ayala Alonso AG, Oktaba K, Ly-Hartig N, McGinty RK, Fraterman S, Wilm M, Muir TW, Müller J. 2010. Histone H2A deubiquitinase activity of the Polycomb repressive complex PR-DUB. *Nature* **465:** 243–247. doi:10.1038/nature08966

Schnittger S, Eder C, Jeromin S, Alpermann T, Fasan A, Grossmann V, Kohlmann A, Illig T, Klopp N, Wichmann HE, et al. 2013. *ASXL1* exon 12 mutations are frequent in AML with intermediate risk karyotype and are independently associated with an adverse outcome. *Leukemia* **27:** 82–91. doi:10.1038/leu.2012.262

Schubbert S, Shannon K, Bollag G. 2007. Hyperactive Ras in developmental disorders and cancer. *Nat Rev Cancer* **7:** 295–308. doi:10.1038/nrc2109

Schuurhuis GJ, Heuser M, Freeman S, Béné MC, Buccisano F, Cloos J, Grimwade D, Haferlach T, Hills RK, Hourigan CS, et al. 2018. Minimal/measurable residual disease in AML: A consensus document from the European LeukemiaNet MRD Working Party. *Blood* **131:** 1275–1291. doi:10.1182/blood-2017-09-801498

Seiler M, Yoshimi A, Darman R, Chan B, Keaney G, Thomas M, Agrawal AA, Caleb B, Csibi A, Sean E, et al. 2018. H3B-8800, an orally available small-molecule splicing modulator, induces lethality in spliceosome-mutant cancers. *Nat Med* **24:** 497–504. doi:10.1038/nm.4493

Sengsayadeth SM, Jagasia M, Engelhardt BG, Kassim A, Strickland SA, Goodman S, Lucid C, Vnencak-Jones CL, Greer JP, Savani BN. 2012. Allo-SCT for high-risk AML-CR1 in the molecular era: Impact of FLT3/ITD outweighs the conventional markers. *Bone Marrow Transplant* **47:** 1535–1537. doi:10.1038/bmt.2012.88

Shih AH, Jiang Y, Meydan C, Shank K, Pandey S, Barreyro L, Antony-Debre I, Viale A, Socci N, Sun Y, et al. 2015. Mutational cooperativity linked to combinatorial epigenetic gain of function in acute myeloid leukemia. *Cancer Cell* **27:** 502–515. doi:10.1016/j.ccell.2015.03.009

Shlush LI, Zandi S, Mitchell A, Chen WC, Brandwein JM, Gupta V, Kennedy JA, Schimmer AD, Schuh AC, Yee KW, et al. 2014. Identification of pre-leukaemic haematopoietic stem cells in acute leukaemia. *Nature* **506:** 328–333. doi:10.1038/nature13038

Shlush LI, Mitchell A, Heisler L, Abelson S, Ng SWK, Trotman-Grant A, Medeiros JJF, Rao-Bhatia A, Jaciw-Zurakowsky I, Marke R, et al. 2017. Tracing the origins of relapse in acute myeloid leukaemia to stem cells. *Nature* **547:** 104–108. doi:10.1038/nature22993

Siegel RL, Miller KD, Jemal A. 2020. Cancer statistics, 2020. *CA Cancer J Clin* **70:** 7–30. doi:10.3322/caac.21590

Sloand EM, Pfannes L, Chen G, Shah S, Solomou EE, Barrett J, Young NS. 2007. CD34 cells from patients with trisomy 8 myelodysplastic syndrome (MDS) express early apoptotic markers but avoid programmed cell death by up-regulation of antiapoptotic proteins. *Blood* **109:** 2399–2405. doi:10.1182/blood-2006-01-030643

Smith ML, Cavenagh JD, Lister TA, Fitzgibbon J. 2004. Mutation of *CEBPA* in familial acute myeloid leukemia. *New Engl J Med* **351:** 2403–2407. doi:10.1056/NEJMoa041331

Song WJ, Sullivan MG, Legare RD, Hutchings S, Tan X, Kufrin D, Ratajczak J, Resende IC, Haworth C, Hock R, et al. 1999. Haploinsufficiency of *CBFA2* causes familial thrombocytopenia with propensity to develop acute myelogenous leukaemia. *Nat Genet* **23:** 166–175. doi:10.1038/13793

Sportoletti P, Varasano E, Rossi R, Mupo A, Tiacci E, Vassiliou G, Martelli MP, Falini B. 2015. Mouse models of *NPM1*-mutated acute myeloid leukemia: Biological and clinical implications. *Leukemia* **29:** 269–278. doi:10.1038/leu.2014.257

Stein EM, DiNardo CD, Pollyea DA, Fathi AT, Roboz GJ, Altman JK, Stone RM, DeAngelo DJ, Levine RL, Flinn IW, et al. 2017. Enasidenib in mutant *IDH2* relapsed or refractory acute myeloid leukemia. *Blood* **130:** 722–731. doi:10.1182/blood-2017-04-779405

Stein EM, Garcia-Manero G, Rizzieri DA, Tibes R, Berdeja JG, Savona MR, Jongen-Lavrenic M, Altman JK, Thomson B, Blakemore SJ, et al. 2018. The DOT1L inhibitor pinometostat reduces H3K79 methylation and has modest clinical activity in adult acute leukemia. *Blood* **131:** 2661–2669. doi:10.1182/blood-2017-12-818948

Stengel A, Kern W, Haferlach T, Meggendorfer M, Fasan A, Haferlach C. 2017. The impact of *TP53* mutations and *TP53* deletions on survival varies between AML, ALL, MDS and CLL: An analysis of 3307 cases. *Leukemia* **31:** 705–711. doi:10.1038/leu.2016.263

Steudel C, Wermke M, Schaich M, Schäkel U, Illmer T, Ehninger G, Thiede C. 2003. Comparative analysis of *MLL* partial tandem duplication and *FLT3* internal tandem duplication mutations in 956 adult patients with acute myeloid leukemia. *Genes Chromosomes Cancer* **37:** 237–251. doi:10.1002/gcc.10219

Stone RM, Mandrekar SJ, Sanford BL, Laumann K, Geyer S, Bloomfield CD, Thiede C, Prior TW, Döhner K, Marcucci G, et al. 2017. Midostaurin plus chemotherapy for acute myeloid leukemia with a *FLT3* mutation. *New Engl J Med* **377:** 454–464. doi:10.1056/NEJMoa1614359

Strissel PL, Strick R, Rowley JD, Zeleznik-Le NJ. 1998. An in vivo topoisomerase II cleavage site and a DNase I hypersensitive site colocalize near exon 9 in the MLL breakpoint cluster region. *Blood* **92:** 3793–3803. doi:10.1182/blood.V92.10.3793

Tahiliani M, Koh KP, Shen Y, Pastor WA, Bandukwala H, Brudno Y, Agarwal S, Iyer LM, Liu DR, Aravind L, et al. 2009. Conversion of 5-methylcytosine to 5-hydroxymethylcytosine in mammalian DNA by MLL partner TET1. *Science* **324:** 930–935. doi:10.1126/science.1170116

Tahirov TH, Inoue-Bungo T, Morii H, Fujikawa A, Sasaki M, Kimura K, Shiina M, Sato K, Kumasaka T, Yamamoto M, et al. 2001. Structural analyses of DNA recognition by the AML1/Runx-1 Runt domain and its allosteric control by CBFβ. *Cell* **104:** 755–767. doi:10.1016/S0092-8674(01)00271-9

Tartaglia M, Niemeyer CM, Fragale A, Song X, Buechner J, Jung A, Hählen K, Hasle H, Licht JD, Gelb BD. 2003. Somatic mutations in *PTPN11* in juvenile myelomonocytic leukemia, myelodysplastic syndromes and acute myeloid leukemia. *Nat Genet* **34:** 148–150. doi:10.1038/ng1156

Taylor SJ, Thien CB, Dagger SA, Duyvestyn JM, Grove CS, Lee BH, Gilliland DG, Langdon WY. 2015. Loss of c-Cbl E3 ubiquitin ligase activity enhances the development of myeloid leukemia in FLT3-ITD mutant mice. *Exp Hematol* **43:** 191–206.e1. doi:10.1016/j.exphem.2014.11.009

Thiede C, Steudel C, Mohr B, Schaich M, Schäkel U, Platzbecker U, Wermke M, Bornhäuser M, Ritter M, Neubauer A, et al. 2002. Analysis of FLT3-activating mutations in 979 patients with acute myelogenous leukemia: Association with FAB subtypes and identification of subgroups with poor prognosis. *Blood* **99:** 4326–4335. doi:10.1182/blood.V99.12.4326

Thota S, Viny AD, Makishima H, Spitzer B, Radivoyevitch T, Przychodzen B, Sekeres MA, Levine RL, Maciejewski JP. 2014. Genetic alterations of the cohesin complex genes in myeloid malignancies. *Blood* **124:** 1790–1798. doi:10.1182/blood-2014-04-567057

Todd MA, Picketts DJ. 2012. PHF6 interacts with the nucleosome remodeling and deacetylation (NuRD) complex. *J Proteome Res* **11:** 4326–4337. doi:10.1021/pr3004369

Tsai FY, Keller G, Kuo FC, Weiss M, Chen J, Rosenblatt M, Alt FW, Orkin SH. 1994. An early haematopoietic defect in mice lacking the transcription factor GATA-2. *Nature* **371:** 221–226. doi:10.1038/371221a0

Tyner JW, Tognon CE, Bottomly D, Wilmot B, Kurtz SE, Savage SL, Long N, Schultz AR, Traer E, Abel M, et al. 2018. Functional genomic landscape of acute myeloid leukaemia. *Nature* **562:** 526–531. doi:10.1038/s41586-018-0623-z

Uckelmann HJ, Kim SM, Wong EM, Hatton C, Giovinazzo H, Gadrey JY, Krivtsov AV, Rücker FG, Döhner K, McGeehan GM, et al. 2020. Therapeutic targeting of preleukemia cells in a mouse model of *NPM1* mutant acute myeloid leukemia. *Science* **367:** 586–590. doi:10.1126/science.aax5863

Van Vlierberghe P, Patel J, Abdel-Wahab O, Lobry C, Hedvat CV, Balbin M, Nicolas C, Payer AR, Fernandez HF, Tallman MS, et al. 2011. *PHF6* mutations in adult acute myeloid leukemia. *Leukemia* **25:** 130–134. doi:10.1038/leu.2010.247

Viny AD, Ott CJ, Spitzer B, Rivas M, Meydan C, Papalexi E, Yelin D, Shank K, Reyes J, Chiu A, et al. 2015. Dose-dependent role of the cohesin complex in normal and malignant hematopoiesis. *J Exp Med* **212:** 1819–1832. doi:10.1084/jem.20151317

Viny AD, Bowman RL, Liu Y, Lavallée VP, Eisman SE, Xiao W, Durham BH, Navitski A, Park J, Braunstein S, et al. 2019. Cohesin members Stag1 and Stag2 display distinct roles in chromatin accessibility and topological control of HSC self-renewal and differentiation. *Cell Stem Cell* **25:** 682–696.e8. doi:10.1016/j.stem.2019.08.003

Wang J, Fernald AA, Anastasi J, Le Beau MM, Qian Z. 2010. Haploinsufficiency of *Apc* leads to ineffective hematopoiesis. *Blood* **115:** 3481–3488. doi:10.1182/blood-2009-11-251835

Wang Y, Xiao M, Chen X, Chen L, Xu Y, Lv L, Wang P, Yang H, Ma S, Lin H, et al. 2015. WT1 recruits TET2 to regulate its target gene expression and suppress leukemia cell proliferation. *Mol Cell* **57:** 662–673. doi:10.1016/j.molcel.2014.12.023

Wang E, Lu SX, Pastore A, Chen X, Imig J, Chun-Wei Lee S, Hockemeyer K, Ghebrechristos YE, Yoshimi A, Inoue D, et al. 2019. Targeting an RNA-binding protein network in acute myeloid leukemia. *Cancer Cell* **35:** 369–384.e7. doi:10.1016/j.ccell.2019.01.010

Welch JS, Ley TJ, Link DC, Miller CA, Larson DE, Koboldt DC, Wartman LD, Lamprecht TL, Liu F, Xia J, et al. 2012. The origin and evolution of mutations in acute myeloid leukemia. *Cell* **150:** 264–278. doi:10.1016/j.cell.2012.06.023

Wendorff AA, Quinn SA, Rashkovan M, Madubata CJ, Ambesi-Impiombato A, Litzow MR, Tallman MS, Paietta E, Paganin M, Basso G, et al. 2019. *Phf6* loss enhances HSC self-renewal driving tumor initiation and leukemia stem cell activity in T-ALL. *Cancer Discov* **9:** 436–451. doi:10.1158/2159-8290.CD-18-1005

Wendt KS, Yoshida K, Itoh T, Bando M, Koch B, Schirghuber E, Tsutsumi S, Nagae G, Ishihara K, Mishiro T, et al. 2008. Cohesin mediates transcriptional insulation by CCCTC-binding factor. *Nature* **451:** 796–801. doi:10.1038/nature06634

West RR, Hsu AP, Holland SM, Cuellar-Rodriguez J, Hickstein DD. 2014. Acquired *ASXL1* mutations are common in patients with inherited *GATA2* mutations and correlate with myeloid transformation. *Haematologica* **99:** 276–281. doi:10.3324/haematol.2013.090217

Wong TN, Ramsingh G, Young AL, Miller CA, Touma W, Welch JS, Lamprecht TL, Shen D, Hundal J, Fulton RS, et al. 2015. Role of *TP53* mutations in the origin and evolution of therapy-related acute myeloid leukaemia. *Nature* **518:** 552–555. doi:10.1038/nature13968

Wouters BJ, Löwenberg B, Erpelinck-Verschueren CA, van Putten WL, Valk PJ, Delwel R. 2009. Double *CEBPA* mutations, but not single *CEBPA* mutations, define a subgroup of acute myeloid leukemia with a distinctive gene expression profile that is uniquely associated with a favorable outcome. *Blood* **113:** 3088–3091. doi:10.1182/blood-2008-09-179895

Xie M, Lu C, Wang J, McLellan MD, Johnson KJ, Wendl MC, McMichael JF, Schmidt HK, Yellapantula V, Miller CA, et al. 2014. Age-related mutations associated with clonal hematopoietic expansion and malignancies. *Nat Med* **20:** 1472–1478. doi:10.1038/nm.3733

Xu W, Yang H, Liu Y, Yang Y, Wang P, Kim SH, Ito S, Yang C, Wang P, Xiao MT, et al. 2011. Oncometabolite 2-hydroxyglutarate is a competitive inhibitor of α-ketoglutarate-dependent dioxygenases. *Cancer Cell* **19:** 17–30. doi:10.1016/j.ccr.2010.12.014

Yarden Y, Kuang WJ, Yang-Feng T, Coussens L, Munemitsu S, Dull TJ, Chen E, Schlessinger J, Francke U, Ullrich A. 1987. Human proto-oncogene c-*kit*: A new cell surface receptor tyrosine kinase for an unidentified ligand. *EMBO J* **6:** 3341–3351. doi:10.1002/j.1460-2075.1987.tb02655.x

Yokoyama A, Somervaille TC, Smith KS, Rozenblatt-Rosen O, Meyerson M, Cleary ML. 2005. The menin tumor suppressor protein is an essential oncogenic cofactor for MLL-associated leukemogenesis. *Cell* **123:** 207–218. doi:10.1016/j.cell.2005.09.025

Yoshida K, Sanada M, Shiraishi Y, Nowak D, Nagata Y, Yamamoto R, Sato Y, Sato-Otsubo A, Kon A, Nagasaki M, et al. 2011. Frequent pathway mutations of splicing machinery in myelodysplasia. *Nature* **478:** 64–69. doi:10.1038/nature10496

Yoshimi A, Lin KT, Wiseman DH, Rahman MA, Pastore A, Wang B, Lee SC, Micol JB, Zhang XJ, de Botton S, et al. 2019. Coordinated alterations in RNA splicing and epigenetic regulation drive leukaemogenesis. *Nature* **574:** 273–277. doi:10.1038/s41586-019-1618-0

Yoshizato T, Dumitriu B, Hosokawa K, Makishima H, Yoshida K, Townsley D, Sato-Otsubo A, Sato Y, Liu D, Suzuki H, et al. 2015. Somatic mutations and clonal hematopoiesis in aplastic anemia. *New Engl J Med* **373:** 35–47. doi:10.1056/NEJMoa1414799

Zhang Q, Zhao K, Shen Q, Han Y, Gu Y, Li X, Zhao D, Liu Y, Wang C, Zhang X, et al. 2015. Tet2 is required to resolve inflammation by recruiting Hdac2 to specifically repress IL-6. *Nature* **525:** 389–393. doi:10.1038/nature15252

Zhou L, Opalinska J, Sohal D, Yu Y, Mo Y, Bhagat T, Abdel-Wahab O, Fazzari M, Figueroa M, Alencar C, et al. 2011. Aberrant epigenetic and genetic marks are seen in myelodysplastic leukocytes and reveal *Dock4* as a candidate pathogenic gene on chromosome 7q. *J Biol Chem* **286:** 25211–25223. doi:10.1074/jbc.M111.235028

Acute Megakaryocytic Leukemia

Maureen McNulty and John D. Crispino

Northwestern University, Division of Hematology/Oncology, Chicago, Illinois 60611, USA
Correspondence: j-crispino@northwestern.edu

Acute megakaryoblastic leukemia (AMKL) is a rare malignancy affecting megakaryocytes, platelet-producing cells that reside in the bone marrow. Children with Down syndrome (DS) are particularly prone to developing the disease and have a different age of onset, distinct genetic mutations, and better prognosis as compared with individuals without DS who develop the disease. Here, we discuss the contributions of chromosome 21 genes and other genetic mutations to AMKL, the clinical features of the disease, and the differing features of DS- and non-DS-AMKL. Further studies elucidating the role of chromosome 21 genes in this disease may aid our understanding of how they function in other types of leukemia, in which they are frequently mutated or differentially expressed. Although researchers have made many insights into understanding AMKL, much more remains to be learned about its underlying molecular mechanisms.

Acute megakaryoblastic leukemia (AMKL) is a subtype of acute myeloid leukemia (AML) that affects megakaryocytes. It is generally subdivided into three groups based on the characteristics of the person who has the disease: children with Down syndrome (DS), children without DS, and adults (typically without DS). Each of these subcategories has a unique subset of disease-causing or -promoting genetic alterations and have different outcomes. DS-AMKL cells are characterized by the uniform presence of trisomy 21 (T21) and *GATA1* mutations, which are accompanied by mutations in chromatin regulators such as cohesin subunits and *EZH2* or signaling molecules such as those in the JAK/STAT and RAS pathways (Yoshida et al. 2013). In contrast, leukemia cells in pediatric non-DS-AMKL do not harbor *GATA1* mutations, but rather generally have chromosomal translocations that result in expression of disease-causing fusion proteins. The prognosis for this group of children without DS is worse than that of those with DS (Radtke et al. 2009; de Rooij et al. 2017). Adults with AMKL tend to have a much worse prognosis than the pediatric groups with overall survival of less than one year (Tallman et al. 2000; de Rooij et al. 2017). The primary disease causing alterations in adult AMKL is unclear, but there are a number of cases with mutations in cohesin and splicing factor genes as well as *TP53* and *DNMT3A* (de Rooij et al. 2017).

Children with DS have a decreased risk of developing most solid tumors, but an increased risk of acquiring hematologic malignancies including AML (Nižetić and Groet 2012; Maloney et al. 2015). In particular, young children with DS are >100 times more likely to develop

Cite this article as *Cold Spring Harb Perspect Med* doi: 10.1101/cshperspect.a034884

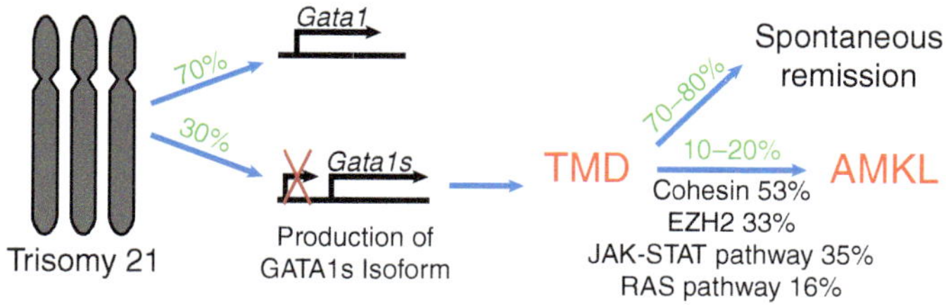

Figure 1. Genetic events in DS-AMKL. Up to 30% of neonates with Down syndrome (DS) acquire a *GATA1* mutation, which leads to exclusive expression of the short Gata1s isoform lacking the first 83 amino acids. Trisomy 21 (T21) and *GATA1* mutations are sufficient to initiate transient myeloproliferative disorder (TMD), a preleukemia, but not acute megakaryoblastic leukemia (AMKL), which is accompanied by secondary gene mutations.

AMKL (Lange 2000; Hasle et al. 2016). DS-AMKL occurs following several discrete steps, including acquisition of T21, a *GATA1* mutation, and a third genetic event which leads to malignant transformation (Fig. 1). The presence of T21 is sufficient to cause various hematologic abnormalities, such as increased numbers of megakaryocytes in utero (Chou et al. 2008; Tunstall-Pedoe et al. 2008; Malinge et al. 2012). However, T21 alone is not sufficient to promote leukemia. Patients with DS-AMKL have another critical event: mutations in the hematopoietic transcription factor *GATA1*, which result in production of the shortened GATA1s protein that lacks the first 83 amino acids (Wechsler et al. 2002). Together, T21 and a *GATA1* mutation lead to transient myeloproliferative disorder (TMD, also known as transient abnormal hematopoiesis, TAM), a self-limiting preleukemic condition seen at birth to varying degrees in up to 30% of DS neonates (Mundschau et al. 2003; Roberts et al. 2013). Although the majority of TMD cases undergo spontaneous remission, 10%–20% of clinically significant cases progress to DS-AMKL within four years (Khan et al. 2011; Maloney et al. 2015). This progression is associated with the acquisition of additional mutations in one or more genes involved in signaling or epigenetic regulatory pathways that lead to malignant transformation of residual *GATA1* mutant clones (Yoshida et al. 2013). It is not entirely clear how these additional mutations cooperate with chromosome 21 genes or GATA1s expression, or how they contribute to DS-AMKL. Although AMKL patients with DS have a favorable prognosis, these children are unusually sensitive to chemotherapy, and gaining a better understanding of the molecular mechanisms behind the disease may lead to better-tolerated targeted therapies.

TRISOMY 21

Altered Incidence of Malignancies in DS Individuals

The incidence of DS is between 1 in 319 and 1 in 1000 live births throughout the world (Asim et al. 2015). This disorder is associated with intellectual disabilities, physical characteristics such as slanted eyes, flat nasal bridges, and poor muscle tone, and an increased risk of other disorders such as Alzheimer's disease and congenital heart defects. DS is most often caused by the presence of three copies of the chromosome 21, but in ∼4% of cases it is caused by a Robertsonian translocation, in which the long arm of chromosome 21 is fused to the centromere of another chromosome or to another chromosome 21 (Mutton et al. 1996).

A 1957 mail survey first revealed that DS and leukemia occurred together more frequently than was expected by chance (Krivit and Good 1957). One percent of DS children develop a hematologic malignancy—TMD, AML, AMKL, or B-ALL—giving them a 10- to 20-fold excess risk of leukemia (Lange 2000). Children with DS are >100 times more likely than children without DS to develop AMKL (FAB AML-M7) (Lange 2000). More recent studies have indicated that

 Cite this article as *Cold Spring Harb Perspect Med* doi: 10.1101/cshperspect.a034884

blood cancers are much more common (standardized incidence ratio [SIR] 5.5, 95% confidence interval [CI] 4.2–7.1), including myeloid leukemias (SIR 11.8, 95% CI 7.11–18.5), in the DS population compared with individuals without DS (Hasle et al. 2016). In fact, leukemia represents 95% of the malignancies in the DS group, compared with 34% in children without DS (Hasle 2001). Surprisingly, individuals with DS have a decreased incidence of most solid tumors with the notable exception of testicular cancer, although the biologic basis for this remains unclear (Hasle et al. 2016).

T21 Leads to Perturbed Hematopoiesis and an Increased Propensity for Leukemia

Although multiple genetic hits are necessary in order for acute leukemia to occur, alterations in hematopoiesis occur in the presence of T21 alone. Various mouse models of DS display elevated levels of immature megakaryocytes and platelets, anemia, and extramedullary hematopoiesis (Kirsammer et al. 2008; Alford et al. 2010; Malinge et al. 2012). Similarly, fetal liver hematopoietic stem and progenitor cells (HSPCs) with T21 produce increased numbers of unusually proliferative megakaryocyte and erythroid progenitors (Chou et al. 2008; Tunstall-Pedoe et al. 2008). Highly proliferative megakaryocytes have been identified in T21 fetuses in the absence of *GATA1* mutations, and in one study, 195 of 200 neonates with DS had circulating blasts (De Vita et al. 2008; Rougemont et al. 2010; Roberts et al. 2013). It is likely that these increased numbers of early progenitors could lead to additional opportunities for acquisition of transforming mutations.

There are many factors that may contribute to the link between T21 and the amplified incidence of leukemia. Cells with T21 tend to take on several morphological characteristics associated with tumor cells, including chromosome instability, acquisition of aneuploidy on additional chromosomes, formation of telomere aggregates, and high rates of copy number alterations (Nižetić and Groet 2012). Additionally, cells from individuals with DS have increased levels of reactive oxygen species, higher rates of both genomic and mitochondrial DNA damage, and impaired single-strand break repair and base excision repair pathways (Nižetić and Groet 2012). These phenotypes may help create a permissive environment where leukemic mutations occur and persist.

Chromosome 21 Genes with Possible Roles in AMKL

There are multiple genes on chromosome 21 that are linked to hematopoiesis, megakaryopoiesis, and leukemia, and it is likely that altered dosage of these genes contributes to aberrant blood development. Acquisition of additional copies of chromosome 21 is the most common chromosomal abnormality in acute leukemia, and these trisomic clones often disappear on remission (Cavani et al. 1998; Lange 2000). Furthermore, multiple chromosome 21 genes have been linked to megakaryocyte differentiation, and individuals with monosomy 21 have thrombocytopenia and an absence of megakaryocytes (Huret and Léonard 1997).

A prominent chromosome 21 gene that is known to play a role in both megakaryopoiesis and leukemia is RUNX1 (AML1). This transcription factor is up-regulated before megakaryocyte differentiation and is essential for both hematopoietic stem cell (HSC) maintenance and megakaryocyte maturation (Elagib et al. 2003; Growney et al. 2005; Tijssen and Ghevaert 2013). Furthermore, germline *RUNX1* mutations lead to familial platelet disorder, and translocations involving this gene are frequently seen in MDS, AML, and ALL (Bellissimo and Speck 2017). In the context of DS, RUNX1 is expressed at high levels in fetal livers in which it fosters expression of early HSPC genes (De Vita et al. 2010). However, when *Runx1* was restored to disomy in a mouse model of DS, there was no effect on the megakaryocyte hyperplasia and fibrosis phenotype, suggesting that other chromosome 21 genes are responsible for the perturbed hematopoiesis of DS (Kirsammer et al. 2008).

Other candidate genes that may play a role in DS-AMKL include *ERG* and *ETS2*, transcription factors in the ETS family. ERG is induced during megakaryocyte differentiation and binds the promoters of HSC and megakaryocyte genes (Rainis et al. 2005). Furthermore, when ERG is expressed in murine fetal liver HSPCs, it is sufficient to immortalize cells and lead to leukemia when transplanted into mice (Salek-Ardakani et al. 2009). Overexpression of ERG also synergized with GATA1s to enhance megakaryopoiesis (Salek-Ardakani et al. 2009; Stankiewicz and Crispino 2009, 2013). Furthermore, restoration of *Erg* to disomy within a mouse model of DS reversed the elevated numbers of HSPCs and megakaryocytes typically seen in this model (Ng et al. 2010) and also caused a decrease in the number of immature megakaryocytes generated from T21 iPSCs (Banno et al. 2016). Likewise, ETS2 is important for megakaryocyte differentiation; its expression is elevated in T21 cells, and forced ETS2 expression is sufficient to upregulate megakaryocyte genes and induce megakaryocyte differentiation in an erythroleukemic cell line (Ge et al. 2008). These genes may each bias HSPCs in DS individuals to form megakaryocytes.

CHAF1B is a gene on chromosome 21 that delivers H3.1/H4 heterodimers to newly replicating DNA as part of the chromatin assembly factor (CAF1) complex. It was first identified as a possible disease-promoting candidate in leukemia through an shRNA screen for chromosome 21 genes in two DS-AMKL cell lines (Malinge et al. 2012). Knockdown of *CHAF1B* produced an increased population of cells carrying CD42, a marker of mature megakaryocytes, but a decrease in the degree of polyploidy (Malinge et al. 2012). It is highly expressed in multiple subtypes of blood cancers, including myeloid leukemias, in which its elevated expression is linked to worse survival. Overexpression of CHAF1B supports proliferation and blocks differentiation of HSPCs (Volk et al. 2018). It is still unclear what role this gene may play within DS-AMKL, but it is thought that increased levels of CHAF1B may contribute to the block in differentiation of AMKL blasts.

Numerous miRNAs that may play a role in cancer reside on chromosome 21. For example, mir-125b2 is overexpressed in TMD and DS-AMKL and its overexpression enhanced the proliferation and self-renewal of megakaryocyte progenitors (Klusmann et al. 2010b). Synergy with GATA1s was also observed. mir-155 is overexpressed in B-cell lymphomas and targets p53INP1, a p53 regulator (Nižetić and Groet 2012). Other microRNAs on this chromosome include let-7c, miR-99a, and miR-802 (Alexandrov et al. 2018). It is still unclear whether or how these miRNAs contribute to the myeloid disorders of DS.

Although multiple genes on chromosome 21 play a role in both normal and malignant blood development, it is still unknown which genes are specifically required for DS-AMKL. Many of these genes also cooperate with *GATA1* mutations and/or additional mutations, as described below in more detail. It is clear, however, that T21 alone is not sufficient for DS-AMKL: *GATA1* mutations are nearly always present, and across all types of hematopoietic malignancies in DS individuals, in only 0.4% of cases is T21 the only chromosomal aberration present (Mitelman et al. 1990). Other genetic events are necessary for progression to acute leukemia.

GATA1s

Role of GATA1 in Normal Blood Development

Up to 30% of newborns with DS and virtually all individuals with TMD and DS-AMKL have a detectable mutation in *GATA1*. This gene, located on the X chromosome, encodes a lineage-determining transcription factor that contains an amino-terminal transactivation domain and two DNA-binding zinc fingers. *GATA1* is expressed in megakaryocyte, erythroid, mast, basophil, and eosinophil lineages (Fujiwara et al. 1996). *GATA1* is induced in the megakaryocyte-erythroid progenitor (MEP), where its expression is necessary for differentiation down both lineages (Stachura et al. 2006). Embryonic stem cells lacking *Gata1* are able to differentiate into erythroid precursors that express several GATA1 target genes, but the cells subsequently undergo apoptosis (Weiss and Orkin 1995). When the gene was deleted in the germline, the mice died in midgestation from anemia (Fujiwara et al. 1996). In contrast, mice in which *Gata1* was deleted selectively in megakaryocytes survived but displayed thrombocytopenia with an accumulation of immature megakaryocytes and a progression to myelofibrosis (Shivdasani et al. 1997; Vannucchi et al. 2002). GATA1-deficient megakaryocytes fail to fully differentiate but rather proliferate excessively both in vitro and in vivo (Kuhl et al. 2005; Muntean and Crispino 2005) A different mouse model, in which levels of GATA1 are reduced to 5% of normal, die beginning at 5 mo of age after manifesting a disease with similarities to human myelodysplastic syndrome/myeloid leukemia (Shimizu et al. 2004). Further evidence for a critical role of GATA1 in erythroid cell and megakaryocyte development comes from human studies. Germline mutations in *GATA1* are associated with a spectrum of benign disorders including congenital thrombocytopenia and anemia (Crispino and Weiss 2014).

GATA1 Mutations in the Myeloid Malignancies of DS

GATA1 mutations have been identified in nearly all cases of TMD and DS-AMKL (Wechsler et al. 2002; Mundschau et al. 2003). These mutations generally occur within exon 2 and include nonsense, missense, insertion, and deletion mutations and result in alternative splicing of the exon or cause expression of the gene from an alternative downstream translation start site. These alterations uniformly lead to exclusive production of a short isoform termed GATA1s, which lacks the first 83 amino acids of the wild-type protein (Wechsler et al. 2002; Groet et al. 2003; Hitzler et al. 2003; Rainis et al. 2003; Xu et al. 2003). The *GATA1* mutation is an early event in DS-AMKL, occurring in utero as determined by its presence in fetuses and neonates (Mundschau et al. 2003; Taub et al. 2004; Roberts et al. 2013). Surprisingly, up to 30% of neonates with DS have *GATA1* mutations, many of which are only detectable by sensitive next-generation sequencing methods; often these infants show no clinical signs of TMD and have a disease that has been named silent TMD (or silent TAM) (Roberts et al. 2013). Notably, *GATA1* mutations have only rarely been detected in individuals with AMKL without chromosome 21 aneuploidy, other subtypes of AML, or other hematologic malignancies (Wechsler et al. 2002).

GATA1s-expressing megakaryocytes display abnormally increased levels of proliferation in vitro and in vivo (Kuhl et al. 2005; Li et al. 2005; Muntean and Crispino 2005). The mouse model that only expresses GATA1s develops a transient expansion of megakaryocyte progenitors coupled with impaired fetal erythropoiesis (Li et al. 2005). This altered proliferation and differentiation is likely caused by differential chromatin occupancy of GATA1 and GATA1s (Byrska-Bishop et al. 2015; Chlon et al. 2015; Ling et al. 2019).

GATA1s Cooperation with Genes on Chromosome 21

As discussed, the combination of T21 and a *GATA1* mutation is sufficient to cause altered hematopoiesis in both in vitro and in vivo (Yoshida et al. 2013; Maloney et al. 2015). There are multiple ways in which GATA1s could interact and cooperate with T21 genes. For example, fetal liver cells from embryos with T21 display elevated expression of both the long and short isoforms of GATA1, and studies using induced pluripotent stem cells (iPSCs), cells derived from neonates with DS, have either seen increased or variable GATA1s expression, indicating that chromosome 21 genes may play a role in regulating the GATA1 expression (Banno et al. 2016). Additionally, although mouse models of DS do not display a TMD-like disease, when bred with GATA1s mutant mice, compound mutant mice display thrombocytosis, increased fibrosis, and splenomegaly (Malinge et al. 2012).

Full-length GATA1 physically interacts with RUNX1 to activate the megakaryocyte-specific αIIb integrin promoter (Elagib et al. 2003). Of note, one study showed that a mutant GATA1 lacking the first 85 amino acids did not retain the capacity to interact with RUNX1, whereas a different study indicated that Gata1s indeed could bind RUNX1, but the ability to bind and activate the GPIbα gene was diminished (Elagib et al. 2003; Xu et al. 2006). Furthermore, GATA1 and RUNX1 share many transcriptional targets, including GPIIβ and GPIbα, JAK2, and the thrombopoietin receptor c-MPL (Goldfarb 2009).

GATA1 binding sites in megakaryocyte progenitors frequently contain ETS-like motifs, which are bound by ETS-family transcription factors such as ERG and ETS2, indicating that these proteins might cooperatively bind targets to regulate megakaryocyte differentiation (Chlon et al. 2012). Indeed, expression of ERG was sufficient to immortalize Gata1s but not GATA1 wild-type murine fetal liver HSPCs, and ERG and ETS2 overexpression each led to elevated numbers of immature megakaryocytes in a wild-type or a Gata1s context (Salek-Ardakani et al. 2009; Stankiewicz and Crispino 2009). ERG expression alone or in conjunction with Gata1s was also shown to be sufficient to cause leukemia in vivo (Salek-Ardakani et al. 2009).

Finally, DYRK1A is known to have a tumor suppressive role in the context of certain solid tumors, possibly by impairing angiogenesis, but an oncogenic role in DS-AMKL (Nižetić and Groet 2012). It is overexpressed in TMD and DS-AMKL blasts, and knockdown of DYRK1A in DS-AMKL cell lines resulted in alterations in megakaryocyte differentiation (Malinge et al. 2012). Additionally, its expression in murine bone marrow cells was sufficient to produce elevated immature megakaryocytes, and this phenotype was further enhanced in a Gata1s context.

CLINICAL AND BIOLOGICAL FEATURES OF TMD AND DS-AMKL

TMD was first defined in 1964, after several neonates with DS presented with a leukemia-like disease, including splenomegaly and leukemic blasts in the peripheral blood and marrow, which quickly and permanently resolved (Engel et al. 1964). The disease is characterized by increased numbers of small, dysplastic megakaryocytes, and blasts with megakaryocytic features in the peripheral blood and liver. It also may be accompanied by either thrombocytopenia or thrombocythemia, low WBC counts, and, rarely, anemia (Zipursky et al. 1997). Some studies have further identified the presence of elevated counts of immature eosinophils or basophils, and studies have found that TMD blasts can differentiate into eosinophils and basophils ex vivo (Maroz et al. 2014), although it should be noted that basophilic granules have been identified within the TMD blasts.

It has been estimated that ~10% of infants with DS have TMD based on visible blasts in the peripheral blood and bone marrow (Zipursky et al. 1997). A more recent study has shown that ~30% of infants with DS have detectable *GATA1* mutation (Roberts et al. 2013). The median age at diagnosis is 6.5 d (Maroz et al. 2014). As both T21 and GATA1 mutations occur in utero, it is not a surprise that signs of TMD present at the fetal or neonatal stages.

A fascinating question is why TMD spontaneously resolves in the majority of patients. It is likely that the switch from fetal liver to bone marrow hematopoiesis is involved, with the loss of the permissive environment needed to maintain the TMD clones (Gamis and Hilden 2002). Two elegant studies suggest that differences in IGF (Klusmann et al. 2010a) or interferon signaling (Woo et al. 2013) may account for the remission of TMD.

Data suggest that 10%–20% of newborns with TMD progress to AMKL within four years (Maloney et al. 2015). The median age at diagnosis is 1.7–1.8 yr (Gamis et al. 2003; Sorrell et al. 2012). Outcomes for children with AMKL who have DS are higher than those without DS, with 5-yr overall survival rates of >80% (Sorrell et al. 2012). Taub and colleagues showed that this was associated with higher rates of ara-C metabolism in T21 cells, as indicated by elevated levels of the intracellular ara-C metabolite, ara-CTP (Taub et al. 1996). A subsequent study suggested that the chromosome 21 genes involved in the altered metabolism include cystathionine-β-synthase (CBS) and superoxide dismutase 1 (SOD1) (Taub et al. 1999). When children with DS are diagnosed at 2 yr of age or older, they tend to have higher rates of relapse and worse survival (Gamis et al. 2003). In children older than 4 yr, the disease typically lacks *GATA1* mutations and is phenotypically distinct from DS-AMKL. This suggests that T21/*GATA1*

 Cite this article as *Cold Spring Harb Perspect Med* doi: 10.1101/cshperspect.a034884

mutant clones lose their propensity for transformation with time.

The cell of origin in AMKL remains unclear. Evidence suggests that other subtypes of AML originate from a population of preleukemic HSCs, which harbor early founder mutations and undergo clonal evolution to produce HSPCs that are transformed on the accumulation of further mutations (Jan et al. 2012; Corces-Zimmerman et al. 2014; Shlush et al. 2014). These leukemic stem cells (LSCs) are capable of long-term self-renewal and disease initiation and display increased resistance to many therapeutic approaches (Thomas and Majeti 2017). Leukemia blasts originating from transformed HSCs are more aggressive than those arising from myeloid lineage-committed progenitor cells such as common myeloid progenitors (CMPs) and granulocyte-monocyte progenitors (GMPs) (George et al. 2016). It is possible that AMKL stem cells may arise directly from preleukemic HSCs, as several lines of evidence suggest that megakaryocytes may be derived from HSCs rather than from an MEP or other lineage-committed progenitor (Woolthuis and Park 2016). With respect to DS-AMKL, studies by Orkin and colleagues have suggested that there may be a unique hematopoietic progenitor cell in fetal livers with T21; this cell may be highly susceptible to *GATA1* mutations, potentially explaining the strong link between the two genetic alterations (Li et al. 2005). Further studies are necessary to precisely define the cell of origin for all the subtypes of AMKL.

ACQUISITION OF TRANSFORMING MUTATIONS

Although *GATA1* mutations are seen at both the TMD and AMKL stages, progression from TMD to AMKL is associated with the acquisition of at least one additional mutation (Yoshida et al. 2013). These advanced mutations occur in multiple genes involved in multiple epigenetic or signaling pathways. In particular, more than half of DS-AMKL patients, but few if any TMD patients, harbor mutations in the cohesin complex (Yoshida et al. 2013). Cohesin, a ring-shaped complex consisting of four core subunits, is responsible for tethering sister chromatids together during mitosis, organizing chromatin within topologically active domains, and facilitating promoter–enhancer interactions within these domains to regulate gene expression (Losada 2014). Heterozygous mutations in cohesin subunit genes are also found in other subtypes of AML, albeit at lower frequencies (~10%), occur early on during leukemic development, and are mutually exclusive across subunits (Fisher et al. 2017b). Multiple in vitro and in vivo experiments have found that cohesin haploinsufficiency alone leads to a disease that resembles a myeloproliferative neoplasm but does not trigger leukemic transformation unless combined with other oncogenes (Mullenders et al. 2015; Viny et al. 2015). Furthermore, knocking down one of the core cohesin subunits or overexpressing a mutant allele imparts alterations in HSPC populations, leads to induction of stem cell genes, and causes global changes in chromatin accessibility (Mazumdar et al. 2015; Mullenders et al. 2015; Viny et al. 2015; Galeev et al. 2016). Altered cohesin complexes exert these changes in part because they fail to recruit the PRC2 complex, which deposits the repressive H3K27me3 histone mark, leading to derepression of stem cell genes *Hoxa7/9* (Fisher et al. 2017a).

Cohesin mutations likely cooperate with increased expression of chromosome 21 genes and the Gata1s leukemic isoform in the context of DS-AMKL (Fig. 2). Of note, cohesin disruption has been shown to increase expression of both RUNX1 and ERG in disomic cells, and it is possible that this effect is amplified when three copies of each gene are present cells with T21 (Mazumdar et al. 2015; Fisher et al. 2017a). Cells expressing cohesin mutants also tend to have more open, accessible chromatin surrounding the binding motifs of RUNX1 and ETS family transcription factors such as ERG, and RUNX1 displayed increased global chromatin occupancy (Mazumdar et al. 2015). Additionally, whereas expression of cohesin mutant alleles in human blood cells caused an increase in the population of $CD34^+$ HSPCs, knockdown of either RUNX1 or ERG reversed this effect, indicating that these genes play a role in the aberrant

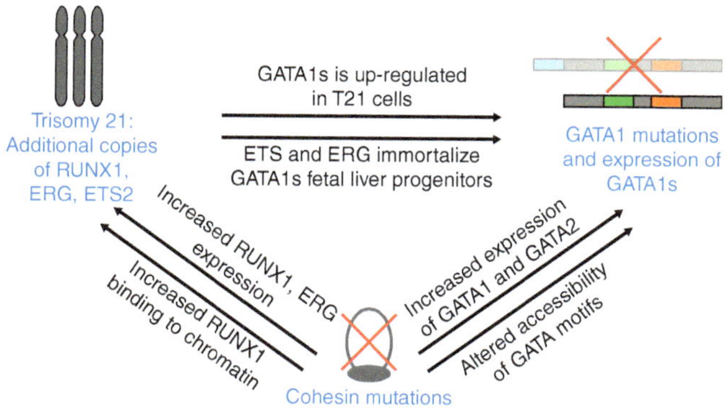

Figure 2. Model of cooperation among trisomy 21 (T21), *GATA1* mutations, and cohesin mutations. Trisomy and subsequent overexpression of chromosome 21 genes leads to enhanced self-renewal of *GATA1* mutant cells and increased expression of the Gata1s isoform. The addition of loss-of-functional mutations in cohesin complex components further increases expression of chromosome 21 genes as well as GATA1. It also is associated with increased chromatin occupancy of RUNX1 and an altered chromatin accessibility of RUNX, ETS, and GATA binding motifs.

stem cell phenotype produced by cohesin loss (Mazumdar et al. 2015). Finally, reducing the number of functional cohesin complexes may also cooperate with Gata1s, as cohesin attenuation leads to increased expression of GATA1 and GATA2 and altered accessibility of GATA motifs (Mazumdar et al. 2015; Mullenders et al. 2015; Viny et al. 2015). However, it remains unclear how alterations in cohesin would affect the activity of Gata1s, which displays altered chromatin binding compared with the full-length protein (Chlon et al. 2015) Additional studies are needed to determine how trisomy 21 genes, Gata1s, and cohesin mutations cooperate at the molecular level to lead to DS-AMKL.

Mutations in the PRC2 complex member *EZH2* were also discovered in a third of DS-AMKL patients, but no patients with TMD (Yoshida et al. 2013). EZH2 has been shown to cooperate with GATA1 to repress HSPC genes, indicating that in a Gata1s context, *EZH2* mutations might synergize with Gata1s to produce further derepression of key growth regulatory genes (Gruber and Downing 2015). Other frequently mutated genes in DS-AMKL and TMD include members of JAK-STAT, MAPK/PI3K, and WNT signaling pathways, including *JAK2*, *JAK3*, *MPL*, *FLT3*, and *APC*. Notably, *MPL* mutations in the context of TS21 and Gata1s were sufficient to induce megakaryocytic leukemia in mice (Malinge et al. 2012) Although it is unclear how these mutations may be contributing to the transformation to DS-AMKL, it is notable that these signaling pathways have been linked to up-regulation of MYC in other contexts (Malinge et al. 2008; Nikolaev et al. 2013; Yoshida et al. 2013). Furthermore, disruptions in JAK/STAT and RAS pathways have been shown to contribute to increased numbers of megakaryocyte progenitors and cytokine-independent growth (Gruber and Downing 2015). Mutations in RAS and JAK pathway genes tended to occur late in disease progression and may not exist in all AMKL clones, suggesting that these mutations are less important for disease initiation (Yoshida et al. 2013).

AMKL IN INDIVIDUALS WITHOUT DS

AMKL in children without DS is driven by different genetic pathways than is DS-AMKL. Non-DS-AMKL cells are much more likely to have copy number alterations, contain chromosomal rearrangements, and express disease-driving fusion proteins (Radtke et al. 2009). The observed translocations and the functions of their component genes are detailed in Table 1.

One of the most common chromosomal translocations seen in the disease is t(1;22)

Table 1. Common fusion events in non-DS-AMKL

Translocation	Disrupted genes	WT protein function	Fusion protein function	References
t(1;22)(p13;q13)	*RBM15* (*OTT*)	Interacts with the RBPJ transcription factor; induces RBPJ-mediated Notch signaling in myeloid progenitor cells but represses it in other cell types; conditional deletion in an in vivo model leads to increased numbers of HSPC, myeloid, and megakaryocyte cells; required for stress hematopoiesis; controls RNA splicing	Interacts with RBPJ to activate Notch signaling; human AMKL cells with the translocation have increased levels of RBPJ target genes; leads to constitutive SRF signaling; disrupts hematopoiesis and induces AMKL in vivo	Mercher et al. 2001; Miralles et al. 2003; Ma et al. 2007; Raffel et al. 2007; Descot et al. 2008; Cheng et al. 2009; Gilles et al. 2009; Mercher et al. 2009; Xiao et al. 2012; Smith et al. 2013; Zhang et al. 2015
	MKL1 (*MAL*)	Rho-actin signaling leads to its nuclear localization, where it activates serum response factor (SRF) transcriptional activity; up-regulated during megakaryocyte differentiation; its loss disrupts normal megakaryocyte differentiation and migration		
inv(16) (p13.3q24.3)	*CBFA2T3*	Acts as transcriptional corepressor; necessary for HSPC proliferation; its loss results in increased numbers of granulocyte/macrophage cells and decreased numbers of MEPs	Expression in mouse cells leads to increased self-renewal; acts as transcriptional activator and up-regulates hedgehog, BMP, and JAK-STAT signaling; cells expressing the fusion are dependent on growth factors and do not induce leukemia in vivo, indicating that additional mutations may be necessary for transformation	Chyla et al. 2008; Gruber et al. 2012; Thiollier et al. 2012; Gruber and Downing 2015
	GLIS2	Member of Hedgehog signaling pathway, not normally expressed in hematopoietic cells		
t(11;15)(p15; q35)	*NUP98*	Does not have DNA-binding domains but is able to interact with the HOXA7 and -A9 promoter; recruits CREBBP/p300 to induce histone acetylation and gene expression	May accumulate in the nucleus and result in aberrant transcription; blocks PRC2 binding and leads to derepression of PRC2 targets; up-regulates HOXA and HOXB genes, which block myeloid differentiation and maintain HSPC state; induces AML in vivo	Wang et al. 2009; Hollink et al. 2011; Thiollier et al. 2012; de Rooij et al. 2013
	JARID1A (*KDM5A*)	Demethylates H3K4, interacts with Rb and regulates expression of HOX genes		

DS, Down syndrome; AMKL, acute megakaryoblastic leukemia; WT, wild-type; HPSC, hematopoietic stem and progenitor cell; SRF, serum reponse factor; MEP, megakaryocyte-erythroid progenitor; AML, acute myeloid leukemia.

(p13;q13), which results in formation of a chimeric oncogene between RNA-binding motif protein-15 (RBM15; also known as OTT) and megakaryoblastic meukemia-1 (MKL-1; also known as MAL) (Mercher et al. 2001). This fusion protein is common in infant AMKL (Mercher et al. 2002) and found in ~12% of overall pediatric megakaryocytic leukemia cases (de Rooij et al. 2016). RBM15-MKL1 disrupts normal transcription and signaling in hematopoietic cells (Table 1). It likely cooperates with other mutations to induce leukemic transformation. In mice, expression of the fusion alone gave rise to leukemia with low penetrance and long latency (Mercher et al. 2009). However, it induced AMKL at a much higher penetrance when combined with a mutation in *MPL* (Mercher et al. 2009). Of note, mutations and altered expression levels of matrix metalloproteinase 8 (MMP8) have also been identified in AMKL patients with this translocation (Mercher et al. 2009; Kim et al. 2014). AMKL cases in children without DS who harbor this fusion have a better prognosis that those with other chromosomal alterations (de Rooij et al. 2016).

Another fusion protein often seen in pediatric non-DS-AMKL is CBFA2T3-GLIS2 (also known as ETO2-GLIS2), caused by the inv(16)(p13.3q24.3) rearrangement (Gruber et al. 2012; Thiollier et al. 2012). This translocation is observed in 12%–30% of pediatric AMKL cases (Gruber et al. 2012; Thiollier et al. 2012; de Rooij et al. 2016). The presence of this chromosomal aberration is associated with a worse overall and reduced event-free survival (de Rooij et al. 2016). CBFA2T3-GLIS2 has not been identified in adult AMKL cases, although it does occur in other pediatric AML subtypes (Gruber et al. 2012; Masetti et al. 2013). A recent study found that the fusion protein promotes self-renewal of hematopoietic progenitors by up-regulation and interaction with ERG at enhancer elements (Thirant et al. 2017). Furthermore, disruption of the transcriptional activity of the fusion by blocking its oligomerization promoted megakaryocytic differentiation.

The nuclear pore complex member NUP98 is fused to JARID1A (also known as KDM5A) in 8%–12% of pediatric AMKL cases (Gruber et al. 2012; de Rooij et al. 2016, 2017). This fusion results from the t(11;15)(p15;q35) translocation and likely promotes leukemogenesis through its aberrant up-regulation of HOX genes. It is not a statistically significant prognostic factor in AMKL, although patients with this fusion trend to show lower survival rates than other fusions (de Rooij et al. 2013, 2016, 2017).

Other recurring fusion events include rearrangements in the KMT2A gene in 9%–17% of cases, HOX gene fusions in 15% of patients, and MLL rearrangements in 10% of non-DS-AMKL cases (de Rooij et al. 2013, 2016, 2017). Other rare translocations identified include MN1-FLI1, GRB10-SDK1, C8orf76-HOXA11AS, FUS-ERG, HLXB9-ETV6, RUNX1-CBFA2T3, BCR-ABL1, MAP2K2-AF10, and THRAP-SH3BP2 (Gruber et al. 2012; Thiollier et al. 2012; de Rooij et al. 2013). It is notable that many of these genes play a role in megakaryopoiesis and leukemia. These translocations are nearly always mutually exclusive, although one case was reported to have both CBFA2T3-GLIS2 and reciprocal translocations resulting in both THRAP3-SH3BP2 and SH3BP2-THRAP3 products (Thiollier et al. 2012). The role of these rare fusion events in disease progression is largely unclear. Some are predicted to produce a functional protein and result in a gain or alteration of function of the component genes, whereas others may produce noncoding RNA and induce disease through loss of a tumor suppressive transcript (de Rooij et al. 2017). Notably, the fusion oncogenes seen in non-DS-AMKL have not been detected in AMKL patients with DS (Yoshida et al. 2013).

Several cooperating mutations have been discovered in AMKL, and these are postulated to drive disease progression. For example *JAK2*, *JAK3*, and *NRAS* mutations are also found in DS-AMKL (Gruber et al. 2012; Yoshida et al. 2013). Interestingly, some mutations seem to recur with certain fusion events. For example, nearly all NUP98-KDM5a-expressing cells also have mutated *RB1*, KMT2A rearrangements frequently co-occur with *RAS* mutations, and HOX fusion events are associated with mutations in *MPL* (de Rooij et al. 2017).

Interestingly, many cases of non-DS-AMKL that do not contain oncogenic fusions may be caused by similar genetic pathways as DS-AMKL. For example, AMKL patients without DS have sometimes been found to have acquired T21, increased copy number of Down syndrome critical region (DSCR) genes on chromosome 21, or *GATA1* mutations (Yoshida et al. 2013). In one small cohort of non-DS-AMKL patients for which copy number variation data were available, half contained amplification of the DSCR (Gruber et al. 2012). Furthermore, in pediatric non-DS-AMKL cases in which no fusion protein was found, half the patients had *GATA1* mutations (de Rooij et al. 2017). Cohesin and CTCF, which are mutated in high frequency in DS-AMKL, are altered in ~20% of all pediatric non-DS-AMKL patients; these mutations are more likely to occur in non-DS-AMKL patients with mutant *GATA1* (de Rooij et al. 2017). The cohesin pathway may also be disrupted through fusion events in these patients. For example, NIPBL, a member of the cohesin loading complex, is occasionally fused to HOXA9 or –B9. Furthermore, the core cohesin complex member *STAG2* is found in fusion events that are predicted to result in loss of function of the full-length protein in 3.5% of cases of non-DS-AMKL (Thiollier et al. 2012; de Rooij et al. 2017). Interestingly, the non-DS-AMKL patients carrying *GATA1* mutations tend to have better overall and event-free survival, mirroring the improved outcome of DS-AMKL patients (de Rooij et al. 2017).

Finally, in addition to rare cases in children, AMKL is seen in 1%–2% of adult AML; these cases have an extremely poor prognosis (Tallman et al. 2000). Although adult AMKL generally lacks chromosomal translocations, it is characterized by mutations in *TP53*, *DNMT3A*, *RB1*, and genes in the cohesin, splicing factor, and ASXL families (de Rooij et al. 2017). Additional studies on the genetics of adult AMKL are needed to better understand its basis and develop novel targeted therapies.

Given the overall poor outcomes for AMKL, new treatments are desperately needed. This also applies to DS-AMKL, as although the outcome is favorable, patients suffer from severe side effects from the therapy. Recently there has been considerable interest in leveraging differentiation therapy in cancer. With respect to AMKL, inhibition of aurora kinase A has been shown to lead to polyploidization and partial differentiation of AMKL blasts in vitro and in vivo, and to impart a significant survival advantage in animal models of the disease (Thiollier et al. 2012; Wen et al. 2012). Furthermore, a phase I study of the AURKA inhibitor alisertib revealed that the drug led to improved megakaryopoiesis in patients with myelofibrosis, a disease that is characterized by an accumulation of atypical megakaryocytes (Gangat et al. 2019). Further clinical studies are needed to assess the activity of AURKA inhibition in AMKL.

CONCLUDING REMARKS

AMKL is a rare subtype of acute myeloid leukemia in adults, but more common in pediatric patients, especially those with DS. In the recent past, a great deal has been learned about the genetic drivers of pediatric AMKL, which include *GATA1* mutations in DS-AMKL and a number of chromosome translocations in non-DS-AMKL, most notably RBM15-MKL1 and CBFA2T3-GLIS2. Nevertheless, there are many unanswered questions: Why are children with DS at such an elevated risk for development of this malignancy? How does trisomy 21 contribute to the initiation of TMD? How do mutations in genes such as *CTCF* and *RAD21* contribute to evolution of TMD to AMKL? Why are *GATA1* mutations so common in children with DS, and why are there so many different translocations in non-DS-AMKL? Answers to these questions will shed light on the initiation and progression of AMKL and may lead to the development of new, targeted therapies for this fascinating form of AML.

ACKNOWLEDGMENTS

The research work performed in this review was supported by National Institutes of Health (NIH) Grants R01 CA101774 to J.D.C. and F31 CA216976 to M.M.

REFERENCES

Alexandrov PN, Percy ME, Lukiw WJ. 2018. Chromosome 21-encoded microRNAs (mRNAs): Impact on Down's syndrome and trisomy-21 linked disease. *Cell Mol Neurobiol* **38:** 769–774. doi:10.1007/s10571-017-0514-0

Alford KA, Slender A, Vanes L, Li Z, Fisher EMC, Nizetic D, Orkin SH, Roberts I, Tybulewicz VLJ. 2010. Perturbed hematopoiesis in the Tc1 mouse model of Down syndrome. *Blood* **115:** 2928–2937. doi:10.1182/blood-2009-06-227629

Asim A, Kumar A, Muthuswamy S, Jain S, Agarwal S. 2015. Down syndrome: An insight of the disease. *J Biomed Sci* **22:** 41. doi:10.1186/s12929-015-0138-y

Banno K, Omori S, Hirata K, Nawa N, Nakagawa N, Nishimura K, Ohtaka M, Nakanishi M, Sakuma T, Yamamoto T, et al. 2016. Systematic cellular disease models reveal synergistic interaction of trisomy 21 and GATA1 mutations in hematopoietic abnormalities. *Cell Rep* **15:** 1228–1241. doi:10.1016/j.celrep.2016.04.031

Bellissimo DC, Speck NA. 2017. *RUNX1* mutations in inherited and sporadic leukemia. *Front Cell Dev Biol* **5:** 111. doi:10.3389/fcell.2017.00111

Byrska-Bishop M, VanDorn D, Campbell AE, Betensky M, Arca PR, Yao Y, Gadue P, Costa FF, Nemiroff RL, Blobel GA, et al. 2015. Pluripotent stem cells reveal erythroid-specific activities of the GATA1 N-terminus. *J Clin Invest* **125:** 993–1005. doi:10.1172/JCI75714

Cavani S, Perfumo C, Argusti A, Pierluigi M, Perroni L, Schmiegelow K, Petersen MB, Cotter FE, Strigini P, Dagna-Bricarelli F, et al. 1998. Cytogenetic and molecular study of 32 Down syndrome families: Potential leukaemia predisposing role of the most proximal segment of chromosome 21q. *Br J Haematol* **103:** 213–216. doi:10.1046/j.1365-2141.1998.00924.x

Cheng E, Luo Q, Bruscia EM, Renda MJ, Troy JA, Massaro SA, Tuck D, Schulz V, Mane SM, Berliner N, et al. 2009. Role for MKL1 in megakaryocytic maturation. *Blood* **113:** 2826–2834. doi:10.1182/blood-2008-09-180596

Chlon TM, Doré LC, Crispino JD. 2012. Cofactor-mediated restriction of GATA-1 chromatin occupancy coordinates lineage-specific gene expression. *Mol Cell* **47:** 608–621. doi:10.1016/j.molcel.2012.05.051

Chlon TM, McNulty M, Goldenson B, Rosinski A, Crispino JD. 2015. Global transcriptome and chromatin occupancy analysis reveal the short isoform of GATA1 is deficient for erythroid specification and gene expression. *Haematologica* **100:** 575–584. doi:10.3324/haematol.2014.112714

Chou ST, Opalinska JB, Yao Y, Fernandes MA, Kalota A, Brooks JSJ, Choi JK, Gewirtz AM, Danet-Desnoyers G, Nemiroff RL, et al. 2008. Trisomy 21 enhances human fetal erythro-megakaryocytic development. *Blood* **112:** 4503–4506. doi:10.1182/blood-2008-05-157859

Chyla BJ, Moreno-Miralles I, Steapleton MA, Thompson MA, Bhaskara S, Engel M, Hiebert SW. 2008. Deletion of Mtg16, a target of t(16;21), alters hematopoietic progenitor cell proliferation and lineage allocation. *Mol Cell Biol* **28:** 6234–6247. doi:10.1128/MCB.00404-08

Corces-Zimmerman MR, Hong WJ, Weissman IL, Medeiros BC, Majeti R. 2014. Preleukemic mutations in human acute myeloid leukemia affect epigenetic regulators and persist in remission. *Proc Natl Acad Sci* **111:** 2548–2553. doi:10.1073/pnas.1324297111

Crispino JD, Weiss MJ. 2014. Erythro-megakaryocytic transcription factors associated with hereditary anemia. *Blood* **123:** 3080–3088. doi:10.1182/blood-2014-01-453167

de Rooij JDE, Hollink IHIM, Arentsen-Peters STCJM, van Galen JF, Berna Beverloo H, Baruchel A, Trka J, Reinhardt D, Sonneveld E, Zimmermann M, et al. 2013. *NUP98/JARID1A* is a novel recurrent abnormality in pediatric acute megakaryoblastic leukemia with a distinct *HOX* gene expression pattern. *Leukemia* **27:** 2280–2288. doi:10.1038/leu.2013.87

de Rooij JDE, Masetti R, van den Heuvel-Eibrink MM, Cayuela J-M, Trka J, Reinhardt D, Rasche M, Sonneveld E, Alonzo TA, Fornerod M, et al. 2016. Recurrent abnormalities can be used for risk group stratification in pediatric AMKL: A retrospective intergroup study. *Blood* **127:** 3424–3430. doi:10.1182/blood-2016-01-695551

de Rooij JDE, Branstetter C, Ma J, Li Y, Walsh MP, Cheng J, Obulkasim A, Dang J, Easton J, Verboon LJ, et al. 2017. Pediatric non-Down syndrome acute megakaryoblastic leukemia is characterized by distinct genomic subsets with varying outcomes. *Nat Genet* **49:** 451–456. doi:10.1038/ng.3772

Descot A, Rex-Haffner M, Courtois G, Bluteau D, Menssen A, Mercher T, Bernard OA, Treisman R, Posern G. 2008. OTT-MAL is a deregulated activator of serum response factor-dependent gene expression. *Mol Cell Biol* **28:** 6171–6181. doi:10.1128/MCB.00303-08

De Vita S, Devoy A, Groet J, Krušlin B, Kuzmić-Prusac I, Nižetić D. 2008. Megakaryocyte hyperproliferation without *GATA1* mutation in foetal liver of a case of Down syndrome with hydrops foetalis. *Br J Haematol* **143:** 300–303. doi:10.1111/j.1365-2141.2008.07332.x

De Vita S, Canzonetta C, Mulligan C, Delom F, Groet J, Baldo C, Vanes L, Dagna-Bricarelli F, Hoischen A, Veltman J, et al. 2010. Trisomic dose of several chromosome 21 genes perturbs haematopoietic stem and progenitor cell differentiation in Down's syndrome. *Oncogene* **29:** 6102–6114. doi:10.1038/onc.2010.351

Elagib KE, Racke FK, Mogass M, Khetawat R, Delehanty LL, Goldfarb AN. 2003. RUNX1 and GATA-1 coexpression and cooperation in megakaryocytic differentiation. *Blood* **101:** 4333–4341. doi:10.1182/blood-2002-09-2708

Engel RR, Hammond D, Eitzman DV, Pearson H, Krivit W. 1964. Transient congenital leukemia in 7 infants with mongolism. *J Pediatr* **65:** 303–305. doi:10.1016/S0022-3476(64)80535-7

Fisher JB, Peterson J, Reimer M, Stelloh C, Pulakanti K, Gerbec ZJ, Abel AM, Strouse JM, Strouse C, McNulty M, et al. 2017a. The cohesin subunit Rad21 is a negative regulator of hematopoietic self-renewal through epigenetic repression of *Hoxa7* and *Hoxa9*. *Leukemia* **31:** 712–719. doi:10.1038/leu.2016.240

Fisher JB, McNulty M, Burke MJ, Crispino JD, Rao S. 2017b. Cohesin mutations in myeloid malignancies. *Trends Cancer* **3:** 282–293. doi:10.1016/j.trecan.2017.02.006

Fujiwara Y, Browne CP, Cunniff K, Goff SC, Orkin SH. 1996. Arrested development of embryonic red cell precursors in mouse embryos lacking transcription factor GATA-1. *Proc Natl Acad Sci* **93:** 12355–12358. doi:10.1073/pnas.93.22.12355

Galeev R, Baudet A, Kumar P, Rundberg Nilsson A, Nilsson B, Soneji S, Törngren T, Borg Å, Kvist A, Larsson J. 2016. Genome-wide RNAi screen identifies cohesin genes as modifiers of renewal and differentiation in human HSCs. *Cell Rep* **14:** 2988–3000. doi:10.1016/j.celrep.2016.02.082

Gamis AS, Hilden J. 2002. Transient myeloproliferative disorder, a disorder with too few data and many unanswered questions: Does it contain an important piece of the puzzle to understanding hematopoiesis and acute myelogenous leukemia? *J Pediatr Hematol Oncol* **24:** 2–5. doi:10.1097/00043426-200201000-00002

Gamis AS, Woods WG, Alonzo TA, Buxton A, Lange B, Barnard DR, Gold S, Smith FO. 2003. Increased age at diagnosis has a significantly negative effect on outcome in children with Down syndrome and acute myeloid leukemia: A report from the Children's Cancer Group Study 2891. *J Pediatr Hematol Oncol* **21:** 3415–3422. doi:10.1200/JCO.2003.08.060

Gangat N, Marinaccio C, Swords R, Watts JM, Gurbuxani S, Rademaker A, Fought AJ, Frankfurt O, Altman JK, Wen QJ, et al. 2019. Aurora kinase A inhibition provides clinical benefit, normalizes megakaryocytes, and reduces bone marrow fibrosis in patients with myelofibrosis. *Clin Cancer Res* **25:** 4898–4906. doi:10.1158/1078-0432.CCR-19-1005

Ge Y, LaFiura KM, Dombkowski AA, Chen Q, Payton SG, Buck SA, Salagrama S, Diakiw AE, Matherly LH, Taub JW. 2008. The role of the proto-oncogene ETS2 in acute megakaryocytic leukemia biology and therapy. *Leukemia* **22:** 521–529. doi:10.1038/sj.leu.2405066

George J, Uyar A, Young K, Kuffler L, Waldron-Francis K, Marquez E, Ucar D, Trowbridge JJ. 2016. Leukaemia cell of origin identified by chromatin landscape of bulk tumour cells. *Nat Commun* **7:** 12166. doi:10.1038/ncomms12166

Gilles L, Bluteau D, Boukour S, Chang Y, Zhang Y, Robert T, Dessen P, Debili N, Bernard OA, Vainchenker W, et al. 2009. MAL/SRF complex is involved in platelet formation and megakaryocyte migration by regulating MYL9 (MLC2) and MMP9. *Blood* **114:** 4221–4232. doi:10.1182/blood-2009-03-209932

Goldfarb AN. 2009. Megakaryocytic programming by a transcriptional regulatory loop: A circle connecting RUNX1, GATA-1, and P-TEFb. *J Cell Biochem* **107:** 377–382. doi:10.1002/jcb.22142

Groet J, McElwaine S, Spinelli M, Rinaldi A, Burtscher I, Mulligan C, Mensah A, Cavani S, Dagna-Bricarelli F, Basso G, et al. 2003. Acquired mutations in *GATA1* in neonates with Down's syndrome with transient myeloid disorder. *Lancet* **361:** 1617–1620. doi:10.1016/S0140-6736(03)13266-7

Growney JD, Shigematsu H, Li Z, Lee BH, Adelsperger J, Rowan R, Curley DP, Kutok JL, Akashi K, Williams IR, et al. 2005. Loss of *Runx1* perturbs adult hematopoiesis and is associated with a myeloproliferative phenotype. *Blood* **106:** 494–504. doi:10.1182/blood-2004-08-3280

Gruber TA, Downing JR. 2015. The biology of pediatric acute megakaryoblastic leukemia. *Blood* **126:** 943–949. doi:10.1182/blood-2015-05-567859

Gruber TA, Larson Gedman A, Zhang J, Koss CS, Marada S, Ta HQ, Chen S-C, Su X, Ogden SK, Dang J, et al. 2012. An Inv(16)(p13.3q24.3)-encoded *CBFA2T3-GLIS2* fusion protein defines an aggressive subtype of pediatric acute megakaryoblastic leukemia. *Cancer Cell* **22:** 683–697. doi:10.1016/j.ccr.2012.10.007

Hasle H. 2001. Pattern of malignant disorders in individuals with Down's syndrome. *Lancet Oncol* **2:** 429–436. doi:10.1016/S1470-2045(00)00435-6

Hasle H, Friedman JM, Olsen JH, Rasmussen SA. 2016. Low risk of solid tumors in persons with Down syndrome. *Genet Med* **18:** 1151–1157. doi:10.1038/gim.2016.23

Hitzler JK, Cheung J, Li Y, Scherer SW, Zipursky A. 2003. *GATA1* mutations in transient leukemia and acute megakaryoblastic leukemia of Down syndrome. *Blood* **101:** 4301–4304. doi:10.1182/blood-2003-01-0013

Hollink IHIM, van den Heuvel-Eibrink MM, Arentsen-Peters STCJM, Pratcorona M, Abbas S, Kuipers JE, van Galen JF, Beverloo HB, Sonneveld E, Kaspers GJJL, et al. 2011. *NUP98/NSD1* characterizes a novel poor prognostic group in acute myeloid leukemia with a distinct *HOX* gene expression pattern. *Blood* **118:** 3645–3656. doi:10.1182/blood-2011-04-346643

Huret JL, Léonard C. 1997. Chromosome 21 and platelets: A gene dosage effect? *Clin Genet* **51:** 140–141. doi:10.1111/j.1399-0004.1997.tb02442.x

Jan M, Snyder TM, Corces-Zimmerman MR, Vyas P, Weissman IL, Quake SR, Majeti R. 2012. Clonal evolution of preleukemic hematopoietic stem cells precedes human acute myeloid leukemia. *Sci Transl Med* **4:** 149ra118.

Khan I, Malinge S, Crispino J. 2011. Myeloid leukemia in Down syndrome. *Crit Rev Oncog* **16:** 25–36. doi:10.1615/CritRevOncog.v16.i1-2.40

Kim Y, Schulz VP, Satake N, Gruber TA, Teixeira AM, Halene S, Gallagher PG, Krause DS. 2014. Whole-exome sequencing identifies a novel somatic mutation in *MMP8* associated with a t(1;22)-acute megakaryoblastic leukemia. *Leukemia* **28:** 945–948. doi:10.1038/leu.2013.314

Kirsammer G, Jilani S, Liu H, Davis E, Gurbuxani S, Le Beau MM, Crispino JD. 2008. Highly penetrant myeloproliferative disease in the Ts65Dn mouse model of Down syndrome. *Blood* **111:** 767–775. doi:10.1182/blood-2007-04-085670

Klusmann JH, Godinho FJ, Heitmann K, Maroz A, Koch ML, Reinhardt D, Orkin SH, Li Z. 2010a. Developmental stage-specific interplay of GATA1 and IGF signaling in fetal megakaryopoiesis and leukemogenesis. *Genes Dev* **24:** 1659–1672. doi:10.1101/gad.1903410

Klusmann JH, Li Z, Böhmer K, Maroz A, Koch ML, Emmrich S, Godinho FJ, Orkin SH, Reinhardt D. 2010b. miR-125b-2 is a potential oncomiR on human chromosome 21 in megakaryoblastic leukemia. *Genes Dev* **24:** 478–490. doi:10.1101/gad.1856210

Krivit W, Good RA. 1957. Simultaneous occurrence of mongolism and leukemia: Report of a nationwide survey. *AMA Am J Dis Child* **94:** 289–293. doi:10.1001/archpedi.1957.04030040075012

Kuhl C, Atzberger A, Iborra F, Nieswandt B, Porcher C, Vyas P. 2005. GATA1-mediated megakaryocyte differentiation and growth control can be uncoupled and mapped to different domains in GATA1. *Mol Cell Biol* **25:** 8592–8606. doi:10.1128/MCB.25.19.8592-8606.2005

Lange B. 2000. The management of neoplastic disorders of haematopoiesis in children with Down's syndrome. *Br J*

Haematol **110:** 512–524. doi:10.1046/j.1365-2141.2000.02027.x

Li Z, Godinho FJ, Klusmann JH, Garriga-Canut M, Yu C, Orkin SH. 2005. Developmental stage-selective effect of somatically mutated leukemogenic transcription factor GATA1. *Nat Genet* **37:** 613–619. doi:10.1038/ng1566

Ling T, Birger Y, Stankiewicz M, Ben-Haim N, Kalisky T, Rein A, Kugler E, Chen W, Fu C, Zhang K, et al. 2019. Chromatin occupancy and epigenetic analysis reveal new insights into the function of GATA1 N terminus in erythropoiesis. *Blood* doi:10.1182/blood2019001234

Losada A. 2014. Cohesin in cancer: Chromosome segregation and beyond. *Nat Rev Cancer* **14:** 389–393. doi:10.1038/nrc3743

Ma X, Renda MJ, Wang L, Cheng EC, Niu C, Morris SW, Chi AS, Krause DS. 2007. Rbm15 modulates Notch-induced transcriptional activation and affects myeloid differentiation. *Mol Cell Biol* **27:** 3056–3064. doi:10.1128/MCB.01339-06

Malinge S, Ragu C, Della-Valle V, Pisani D, Constantinescu SN, Perez C, Villeval J-L, Reinhardt D, Landman-Parker J, Michaux L, et al. 2008. Activating mutations in human acute megakaryoblastic leukemia. *Blood* **112:** 4220–4226. doi:10.1182/blood-2008-01-136366

Malinge S, Bliss-Moreau M, Kirsammer G, Diebold L, Chlon T, Gurbuxani S, Crispino JD. 2012. Increased dosage of the chromosome 21 ortholog *Dyrk1a* promotes megakaryoblastic leukemia in a murine model of Down syndrome. *J Clin Invest* **122:** 948–962. doi:10.1172/JCI60455

Maloney KW, Taub JW, Ravindranath Y, Roberts I, Vyas P. 2015. Down syndrome preleukemia and leukemia. *Pediatr Clin North Am* **62:** 121–137. doi:10.1016/j.pcl.2014.09.009

Maroz A, Stachorski L, Emmrich S, Reinhardt K, Xu J, Shao Z, Käbler S, Dertmann T, Hitzler J, Roberts I, et al. 2014. GATA1s induces hyperproliferation of eosinophil precursors in Down syndrome transient leukemia. *Leukemia* **28:** 1259–1270. doi:10.1038/leu.2013.373

Masetti R, Pigazzi M, Togni M, Astolfi A, Indio V, Manara E, Casadio R, Pession A, Basso G, Locatelli F. 2013. *CBFA2T3-GLIS2* fusion transcript is a novel common feature in pediatric, cytogenetically normal AML, not restricted to FAB M7 subtype. *Blood* **121:** 3469–3472. doi:10.1182/blood-2012-11-469825

Mazumdar C, Shen Y, Xavy S, Zhao F, Reinisch A, Li R, Corces MR, Flynn RA, Buenrostro JD, Chan SM, et al. 2015. Leukemia-associated cohesin mutants dominantly enforce stem cell programs and impair human hematopoietic progenitor differentiation. *Cell Stem Cell* **17:** 675–688. doi:10.1016/j.stem.2015.09.017

Mercher T, Coniat MB, Monni R, Mauchauffe M, Nguyen Khac F, Gressin L, Mugneret F, Leblanc T, Dastugue N, Berger R, et al. 2001. Involvement of a human gene related to the *Drosophila spen* gene in the recurrent t(1;22) translocation of acute megakaryocytic leukemia. *Proc Natl Acad Sci* **98:** 5776–5779. doi:10.1073/pnas.101001498

Mercher T, Busson-Le Coniat M, Nguyen Khac F, Ballerini P, Mauchauffe M, Bui H, Pellegrino B, Radford I, Valensi F, Mugneret F, et al. 2002. Recurrence of OTT-MAL fusion in t(1;22) of infant AML-M7. *Genes Chromosomes Cancer* **33:** 22–28. doi:10.1002/gcc.1208

Mercher T, Raffel GD, Moore SA, Cornejo MG, Baudry-Bluteau D, Cagnard N, Jesneck JL, Pikman Y, Cullen D, Williams IR, et al. 2009. The *OTT-MAL* fusion oncogene activates RBPJ-mediated transcription and induces acute megakaryoblastic leukemia in a knockin mouse model. *J Clin Invest* **119:** 852–864.

Miralles F, Posern G, Zaromytidou AI, Treisman R. 2003. Actin dynamics control SRF activity by regulation of its coactivator MAL. *Cell* **113:** 329–342. doi:10.1016/S0092-8674(03)00278-2

Mitelman F, Heim S, Mandahl N. 1990. Trisomy 21 in neoplastic cells. *Am J Med Genet* **7:** 262–266.

Mullenders J, Aranda-Orgilles B, Lhoumaud P, Keller M, Pae J, Wang K, Kayembe C, Rocha PP, Raviram R, Gong Y, et al. 2015. Cohesin loss alters adult hematopoietic stem cell homeostasis, leading to myeloproliferative neoplasms. *J Exp Med* **212:** 1833–1850. doi:10.1084/jem.20151323

Mundschau G, Gurbuxani S, Gamis AS, Greene ME, Arceci RJ, Crispino JD. 2003. Mutagenesis of *GATA1* is an initiating event in Down syndrome leukemogenesis. *Blood* **101:** 4298–4300. doi:10.1182/blood-2002-12-3904

Muntean AG, Crispino JD. 2005. Differential requirements for the activation domain and FOG-interaction surface of GATA-1 in megakaryocyte gene expression and development. *Blood* **106:** 1223–1231. doi:10.1182/blood-2005-02-0551

Mutton D, Alberman E, Hook EB. 1996. Cytogenetic and epidemiological findings in Down syndrome, England and Wales 1989 to 1993. National Down Syndrome Cytogenetic Register and the Association of Clinical Cytogeneticists. *J Med Genet* **33:** 387–394. doi:10.1136/jmg.33.5.387

Ng AP, Hyland CD, Metcalf D, Carmichael CL, Loughran SJ, Di Rago L, Kile BT, Alexander WS. 2010. Trisomy of *Erg* is required for myeloproliferation in a mouse model of Down syndrome. *Blood* **115:** 3966–3969. doi:10.1182/blood-2009-09-242107

Nikolaev SI, Santoni F, Vannier A, Falconnet E, Giarin E, Basso G, Hoischen A, Veltman JA, Groet J, Nizetic D, et al. 2013. Exome sequencing identifies putative drivers of progression of transient myeloproliferative disorder to AMKL in infants with Down syndrome. *Blood* **122:** 554–561. doi:10.1182/blood-2013-03-491936

Nižetić D, Groet J. 2012. Tumorigenesis in Down's syndrome: Big lessons from a small chromosome. *Nat Rev Cancer* **12:** 721–732. doi:10.1038/nrc3355

Radtke I, Mullighan CG, Ishii M, Su X, Cheng J, Ma J, Ganti R, Cai Z, Goorha S, Pounds SB, et al. 2009. Genomic analysis reveals few genetic alterations in pediatric acute myeloid leukemia. *Proc Natl Acad Sci* **106:** 12944–12949. doi:10.1073/pnas.0903142106

Raffel GD, Mercher T, Shigematsu H, Williams IR, Cullen DE, Akashi K, Bernard OA, Gilliland DG. 2007. *Ott1* (*Rbm15*) has pleiotropic roles in hematopoietic development. *Proc Natl Acad Sci* **104:** 6001–6006. doi:10.1073/pnas.0609041104

Rainis L, Bercovich D, Strehl S, Teigler-Schlegel A, Stark B, Trka J, Amariglio N, Biondi A, Muler I, Rechavi G, et al. 2003. Mutations in exon 2 of *GATA1* are early events in megakaryocytic malignancies associated with trisomy 21. *Blood* **102:** 981–986. doi:10.1182/blood-2002-11-3599

Rainis L, Toki T, Pimanda JE, Rosenthal E, Machol K, Strehl S, Göttgens B, Ito E, Izraeli S. 2005. The proto-oncogene ERG in megakaryoblastic leukemias. *Cancer Res* **65:** 7596–7602. doi:10.1158/0008-5472.CAN-05-0147

Roberts I, Alford K, Hall G, Juban G, Richmond H, Norton A, Vallance G, Perkins K, Marchi E, McGowan S, et al. 2013. *GATA1*-mutant clones are frequent and often unsuspected in babies with Down syndrome: Identification of a population at risk of leukemia. *Blood* **122:** 3908–3917. doi:10.1182/blood-2013-07-515148

Rougemont A-L, Makrythanasis P, Finci V, Billieux M-H, Epiney M, McKee TA, Nizetic D, Fokstuen S. 2010. Myeloid proliferation without *GATA1* mutations in a fetus with Down syndrome presenting in utero as a pericardial effusion. *Pediatr Dev Pathol* **13:** 423–426. doi:10.2350/09-11-0743-CR.1

Salek-Ardakani S, Smooha G, de Boer J, Sebire NJ, Morrow M, Rainis L, Lee S, Williams O, Izraeli S, Brady HJM. 2009. *ERG* is a megakaryocytic oncogene. *Cancer Res* **69:** 4665–4673. doi:10.1158/0008-5472.CAN-09-0075

Shimizu R, Kuroha T, Ohneda O, Pan X, Ohneda K, Takahashi S, Philipsen S, Yamamoto M. 2004. Leukemogenesis caused by incapacitated GATA-1 function. *Mol Cell Biol* **24:** 10814–10825. doi:10.1128/MCB.24.24.10814-10825.2004

Shivdasani RA, Fujiwara Y, McDevitt MA, Orkin SH. 1997. A lineage-selective knockout establishes the critical role of transcription factor GATA-1 in megakaryocyte growth and platelet development. *EMBO J* **16:** 3965–3973. doi:10.1093/emboj/16.13.3965

Shlush LI, Zandi S, Mitchell A, Chen WC, Brandwein JM, Gupta V, Kennedy JA, Schimmer AD, Schuh AC, Yee KW, et al. 2014. Identification of pre-leukaemic haematopoietic stem cells in acute leukaemia. *Nature* **506:** 328–333. doi:10.1038/nature13038

Smith EC, Teixeira AM, Chen RC, Wang L, Gao Y, Hahn KL, Krause DS. 2013. Induction of megakaryocyte differentiation drives nuclear accumulation and transcriptional function of MKL1 via actin polymerization and RhoA activation. *Blood* **121:** 1094–1101. doi:10.1182/blood-2012-05-429993

Sorrell AD, Alonzo TA, Hilden JM, Gerbing RB, Loew TW, Hathaway L, Barnard D, Taub JW, Ravindranath Y, Smith FO, et al. 2012. Favorable survival maintained in children who have myeloid leukemia associated with Down syndrome using reduced-dose chemotherapy on Children's Oncology Group trial A2971. *Cancer* **118:** 4806–4814. doi:10.1002/cncr.27484

Stachura DL, Chou ST, Weiss MJ. 2006. Early block to erythromegakaryocytic development conferred by loss of transcription factor GATA-1. *Blood* **107:** 87–97. doi:10.1182/blood-2005-07-2740

Stankiewicz MJ, Crispino JD. 2009. ETS2 and ERG promote megakaryopoiesis and synergize with alterations in GATA-1 to immortalize hematopoietic progenitor cells. *Blood* **113:** 3337–3347. doi:10.1182/blood-2008-08-174813

Stankiewicz MJ, Crispino JD. 2013. AKT collaborates with ERG and GATA1s to dysregulate megakaryopoiesis and promote AMKL. *Leukemia* **27:** 1339–1347. doi:10.1038/leu.2013.33

Tallman MS, Neuberg D, Bennett JM, Francois CJ, Paietta E, Wiernik PH, Dewald G, Cassileth PA, Oken MM, Rowe JM. 2000. Acute megakaryocytic leukemia: The eastern cooperative oncology group experience. *Blood* **96:** 2405–2411.

Taub J, Matherly L, Stout M, Buck S, Gurney J, Ravindranath Y. 1996. Enhanced metabolism of 1-β-D-arabinofuranosylcytosine in Down syndrome cells: A contributing factor to the superior event free survival of Down syndrome children with acute myeloid leukemia. *Blood* **87:** 3395–3403.

Taub JW, Huang X, Matherly LH, Stout ML, Buck SA, Massey GV, Becton DL, Chang MN, Weinstein HJ, Ravindranath Y. 1999. Expression of chromosome 21-localized genes in acute myeloid leukemia: Differences between Down syndrome and non-Down syndrome blast cells and relationship to in vitro sensitivity to cytosine Arabinoside and Daunorubicin. *Blood* **94:** 1393–1400.

Taub JW, Mundschau G, Ge Y, Poulik JM, Qureshi F, Jensen T, James SJ, Matherly LH, Wechsler J, Crispino JD. 2004. Prenatal origin of *GATA1* mutations may be an initiating step in the development of megakaryocytic leukemia in Down syndrome. *Blood* **104:** 1588–1589. doi:10.1182/blood-2004-04-1563

Thiollier C, Lopez CK, Gerby B, Ignacimouttou C, Poglio S, Duffourd Y, Guégan J, Rivera-Munoz P, Bluteau O, Mabialah V, et al. 2012. Characterization of novel genomic alterations and therapeutic approaches using acute megakaryoblastic leukemia xenograft models. *J Exp Med* **209:** 2017–2031. doi:10.1084/jem.20121343

Thirant C, Ignacimouttou C, Lopez CK, Diop M, Le Mouël L, Thiollier C, Siret A, Dessen P, Aid Z, Rivière J, et al. 2017. ETO2-GLIS2 hijacks transcriptional complexes to drive cellular identity and self-renewal in pediatric acute megakaryoblastic leukemia. *Cancer Cell* **13:** 452–465. doi:10.1016/j.ccell.2017.02.006

Thomas D, Majeti R. 2017. Biology and relevance of human acute myeloid leukemia stem cells. *Blood* **129:** 1577–1585. doi:10.1182/blood-2016-10-696054

Tijssen MR, Ghevaert C. 2013. Transcription factors in late megakaryopoiesis and related platelet disorders. *J Thromb Haemost* **11:** 593–604. doi:10.1111/jth.12131

Tunstall-Pedoe O, Roy A, Karadimitris A, de la Fuente J, Fisk NM, Bennett P, Norton A, Vyas P, Roberts I. 2008. Abnormalities in the myeloid progenitor compartment in Down syndrome fetal liver precede acquisition of *GATA1* mutations. *Blood* **112:** 4507–4511. doi:10.1182/blood-2008-04-152967

Vannucchi AM, Bianchi L, Cellai C, Paoletti F, Rana RA, Lorenzini R, Migliaccio G, Migliaccio AR. 2002. Development of myelofibrosis in mice genetically impaired for GATA-1 expression (GATA-1^{low} mice). *Blood* **100:** 1123–1132. doi:10.1182/blood-2002-06-1913

Viny AD, Ott CJ, Spitzer B, Rivas M, Meydan C, Papalexi E, Yelin D, Shank K, Reyes J, Chiu A, et al. 2015. Dose-dependent role of the cohesin complex in normal and malignant hematopoiesis. *J Exp Med* **212:** 1819–1832. doi:10.1084/jem.20151317

Volk A, Liang K, Suraneni P, Li X, Zhao J, Bulic M, Marshall S, Pulakanti K, Malinge S, Taub J, et al. 2018. A CHAF1B-dependent molecular switch in hematopoiesis and leukemia pathogenesis. *Cancer Cell* **34:** 707–723.e7. doi:10.1016/j.ccell.2018.10.004

Wang GG, Song J, Wang Z, Dormann HL, Casadio F, Li H, Luo JL, Patel DJ, Allis CD. 2009. Haematopoietic malignancies caused by dysregulation of a chromatin-binding PHD finger. *Nature* **459:** 847–851. doi:10.1038/nature08036

Wechsler J, Greene M, McDevitt MA, Anastasi J, Karp JE, Le Beau MM, Crispino JD. 2002. Acquired mutations in *GATA1* in the megakaryoblastic leukemia of Down syndrome. *Nat Genet* **32:** 148–152. doi:10.1038/ng955

Weiss MJ, Orkin SH. 1995. Transcription factor GATA-1 permits survival and maturation of erythroid precursors by preventing apoptosis. *Proc Natl Acad Sci* **92:** 9623–9627. doi:10.1073/pnas.92.21.9623

Wen Q, Goldenson B, Silver SJ, Schenone M, Dancik V, Huang Z, Wang LZ, Lewis TA, An WF, Li X, et al. 2012. Identification of regulators of polyploidization presents therapeutic targets for treatment of AMKL. *Cell* **150:** 575–589. doi:10.1016/j.cell.2012.06.032

Woo AJ, Wieland K, Huang H, Akie TE, Piers T, Kim J, Cantor AB. 2013. Developmental differences in IFN signaling affect GATA1s-induced megakaryocyte hyperproliferation. *J Clin Invest* **123:** 3292–3304. doi:10.1172/JCI40609

Woolthuis CM, Park CY. 2016. Hematopoietic stem/progenitor cell commitment to the megakaryocyte lineage. *Blood* **127:** 1242–1248. doi:10.1182/blood-2015-07-607945

Xiao N, Jani K, Morgan K, Okabe R, Cullen DE, Jesneck JL, Raffel GD. 2012. Hematopoietic stem cells lacking *Ott1* display aspects associated with aging and are unable to maintain quiescence during proliferative stress. *Blood* **119:** 4898–4907. doi:10.1182/blood-2012-01-403089

Xu G, Nagano M, Kanezaki R, Toki T, Hayashi Y, Taketani T, Taki T, Mitui T, Koike K, Kato K, et al. 2003. Frequent mutations in the *GATA-1* gene in the transient myeloproliferative disorder of Down syndrome. *Blood* **102:** 2960–2968. doi:10.1182/blood-2003-02-0390

Xu G, Kanezaki R, Toki T, Watanabe S, Takahashi Y, Terui K, Kitabayashi I, Ito E. 2006. Physical association of the patient-specific GATA1 mutants with RUNX1 in acute megakaryoblastic leukemia accompanying Down syndrome. *Leukemia* **20:** 1002–1008. doi:10.1038/sj.leu.2404223

Yoshida K, Toki T, Okuno Y, Kanezaki R, Shiraishi Y, Sato-Otsubo A, Sanada M, Park M, Terui K, Suzuki H, et al. 2013. The landscape of somatic mutations in Down syndrome-related myeloid disorders. *Nat Genet* **45:** 1293–1299. doi:10.1038/ng.2759

Zhang L, Tran NT, Su H, Wang R, Lu Y, Tang H, Aoyagi S, Guo A, Khodadadi-Jamayran A, Zhou D, et al. 2015. Cross-talk between PRMT1-mediated methylation and ubiquitylation on RBM15 controls RNA splicing. *eLife* **4:** e07938. doi:10.7554/eLife.07938

Zipursky A, Brown E, Christensen H, Sutherland R, Doyle J. 1997. Leukemia and/or myeloproliferative syndrome in neonates with Down syndrome. *Semin Perinatol* **21:** 97–101. doi:10.1016/S0146-0005(97)80025-0

The Genetics and Mechanisms of T-Cell Acute Lymphoblastic Leukemia

Francesca Gianni,[1] Laura Belver,[1] and Adolfo Ferrando[1,2,3]

[1]Institute for Cancer Genetics, Columbia University Medical Center, New York, New York 10032, USA
[2]Department of Pathology, Columbia University Medical Center, New York, New York 10032, USA
[3]Department of Pediatrics, Columbia University Medical Center, New York, New York 10032, USA
Correspondence: af2196@columbia.edu

T-cell acute lymphoblastic leukemia (T-ALL) is an aggressive hematologic malignancy derived from early T-cell progenitors. The recognition of clinical, genetic, transcriptional, and biological heterogeneity in this disease has already translated into new prognostic biomarkers, improved leukemia animal models, and emerging targeted therapies. This work reviews our current understanding of the molecular mechanisms of T-ALL.

T-cell acute lymphoblastic leukemia (T-ALL) is an immature lymphoid tumor characterized by the diffuse infiltration of the bone marrow by malignant hematopoietic cells expressing immature T-cell markers. T-ALL represents 10%–15% of pediatric and 20%–25% of adult ALL cases and is twice more prevalent in males than in females (Dores et al. 2012; Pui et al. 2012). T-ALL patients typically present with elevated white blood cell counts and hematopoietic failure with neutropenia, anemia, and thrombocytopenia and frequently present with mediastinal thymic masses and meningeal infiltration at diagnosis (Greaves et al. 1981; Crist et al. 1988; Garand et al. 1990; Pui et al. 1990; Shuster et al. 1990; Karrman et al. 2009a).

In the early days of combination chemotherapy, T-ALL patients were recognized as a high-risk leukemia group with cure rates of ~10% (Greaves et al. 1981; Thiel 1985). Subsequently, intensified chemotherapy protocols led to a gradual improvement in outcomes with current cure rates in multicenter trials approaching 90% in children (Pui and Evans 2006; Möricke et al. 2008; Pui et al. 2008; Vrooman and Silverman 2009; Hunger et al. 2012; Conter et al. 2014) and 60% in adults (Huguet et al. 2009; Marks et al. 2009; Stock et al. 2013). However, the prognosis remains dismal for patients who fail to obtain a complete hematologic remission or whose disease relapses after initial response (Uderzo et al. 2000; Einsiedel et al. 2005; Parker et al. 2010; Tallen et al. 2010; Hof et al. 2011; Sutton et al. 2015). Although no standard-of-care savage therapy is available in the refractory setting, some drugs have been recently approved for the treatment of relapsed T-ALL. In particular, single agent nelarabine, a deoxyguanosine analog, showed efficacy in several studies conducted in children and adults (Berg et al. 2005; DeAngelo et al. 2007; Gokbuget et al. 2011). In recent years, many research efforts have been per-

Cite this article as *Cold Spring Harb Perspect Med* doi: 10.1101/cshperspect.a035246

formed to reduce the risk of relapse in T-ALL by improving induction and consolidation therapy. The inclusion of polyethylene glycol–conjugated (PEG) asparaginase and dexamethasone in frontline therapy has been reported to decrease the risk of relapse. Moreover, methotrexate intensification strategies have shown to increase event-free survival (EFS) and overall survival (OS) in T-ALL (Möricke et al. 2016; Winter et al. 2018). In addition, nelarabine is being actively explored in combination with chemotherapy as a frontline treatment in children and adult T-ALL. In the COG trial AALL0434, T-ALL patients receiving nelarabine in addition to the augmented Berlin–Frankfurt–Münster regimen showed a significant improvement in EFS (Dunsmore et al. 2018).

GENETIC AND BIOLOGIC HETEROGENEITY IN T-ALL

T-ALL is a heterogeneous disease resulting from a multistep transformation process in which accumulating genetic alterations disrupt the normal control of cell growth, proliferation, survival, and differentiation during thymocyte development. A hallmark of T-ALL is the interrelationship between key regulators of early T-cell development and T-ALL oncogenic signals. This is best illustrated by the prominent role of NOTCH1, a key factor driving T-cell fate specification and thymocyte development (Radtke et al. 2013), which is activated by oncogenic gain-of-function mutations in >60% of T-ALL cases (Weng et al. 2004). Activating mutations in *NOTCH1* in T-ALL frequently co-occur with the loss of the *CDKN2A* locus (Hebert et al. 1994) and with chromosomal translocations, resulting in the aberrant expression of a diverse group of T-ALL-specific transcription factor oncogenes including (1) basic helix-loop-helix (bHLH) factors such as *TAL1* (Begley et al. 1989; Bernard et al. 1990; Chen et al. 1990), *TAL2* (Xia et al. 1991), *LYL1* (Mellentin et al. 1989), and *BHLHB1* (Wang et al. 2000); (2) LIM-only domain (LMO) genes such as *LMO1* and *LMO2* (McGuire et al. 1989; Boehm et al. 1991; Royer-Pokora et al. 1991); (3) homeobox genes such as *TLX1* (Dube et al. 1991; Hatano et al. 1991; Kennedy et al. 1991), *TLX3* (Bernard et al. 2001; Ferrando et al. 2002; Su et al. 2006), *NKX2.1* (Homminga et al. 2011), *NKX2.2* (Homminga et al. 2011), *NKX2.5* (Nagel et al. 2003), and *HOXA* (Soulier et al. 2005); and (4) *MYC* (Erikson et al. 1986; Finger et al. 1986; Mathieu-Mahul et al. 1986), *MYB* (Clappier et al. 2007), and *SPI1* (Seki et al. 2017). In addition, somatic mutations disrupt transcription factors tumor suppressor genes (e.g., *ETV6, RUNX1, GATA3, BCL11B*) and epigenetic regulators (e.g., *EZH2, SUZ12, PHF6*), leading to the activation of oncogenic signaling pathways (Van Vlierberghe et al. 2011a, 2013; Zhang et al. 2012; Neumann et al. 2013). Numerous studies that have explored the effect of these genetic alterations on T-cell development and transformation are reviewed below.

T-ALL is classified into groups characterized by unique gene expression signatures and immunophenotypic profiles that reflect an arrest at different stages of thymocyte development (Ferrando et al. 2002; Soulier et al. 2005; Seki et al. 2017). Early T-cell precursor (ETP) leukemias show a block at the earliest stages of T-cell differentiation (CD4 CD8 double-negative), aberrant expression of myeloid and stem cell markers, and a transcriptional program related to early T-cell precursor cells, hematopoietic stem cells, and myeloid progenitors (Ferrando et al. 2002; Coustan-Smith et al. 2009; Van Vlierberghe et al. 2011a). Early-immature ETP T-ALLs have a lower prevalence of *NOTCH1* mutations, rarely have *CDKN2A* deletions, and are associated with mutations in signaling factors (e.g., *NRAS, FLT3*), epigenetic regulators (e.g., *EZH2, IDH1, IDH2, DNMT3A*), and transcription factors governing hematopoietic and T-cell development (e.g., *RUNX1, GATA3, ETV6*) (Van Vlierberghe et al. 2011a, 2013; Zhang et al. 2012; Neumann et al. 2013). Although ETP T-ALL accounts for ~10% of pediatric T-ALL cases (Coustan-Smith et al. 2009; Inukai et al. 2012; Allen et al. 2013), it comprises 40%–50% of adult T-ALLs (Van Vlierberghe et al. 2011a, 2013; Allen et al. 2013). Once described as a high-risk group with dismal outcomes and high rates of chemotherapy resistance (Gutierrez et al. 2010a; Van Vlierberghe

 Cite this article as *Cold Spring Harb Perspect Med* doi: 10.1101/cshperspect.a035246

et al. 2013), ETP T-ALL can be effectively treated using early-response-based intensification (Patrick et al. 2014; Bond et al. 2017). T-ALLs with a characteristic $CD1a^+$, $CD4^+$, and $CD8^+$ immunophenotype, corresponding to the early stages of cortical thymocyte maturation, show a favorable prognosis (Niehues et al. 1999; Wuchter et al. 2002). These leukemias are associated with activation of the *TLX1, TLX3, NKX2.1,* and *NKX2.2* homeobox genes, have the highest prevalence of *NOTCH1* mutations, and almost universally harbor deletions of the *CDKN2A* locus (Ferrando et al. 2002; Homminga et al. 2011). T-ALLs with a more mature, late-cortical-thymocyte immunophenotype with expression of CD4, CD8, and CD3 show activation of the *TAL1* transcription factor oncogene (Ferrando et al. 2002). Immunophenotypic and biological differences between ETP-ALL and T-ALL may reflect a different cell of origin for these two subsets. The close relationship of ETP-ALL with hematopoietic stem cell transcriptional signatures, the increased incidence with age, and the common presence of mutations associated with clonal hematopoiesis and myeloid leukemia support that these leukemias may originate from early hematopietic progenitors and may have a preleukemic clonal hematopoiesis phase. In the case of T-ALL tumors, the presence of TCR rearrangements to the TCR loci supports that these alterations occur during thymocyte development and point to an intrathymic progenitor as the presumed cell of origin in this case.

Non-cell-autonomous mechanisms are also relevant for the development of T-ALL. In the bone marrow, T-ALL lymphoblasts establish contacts with vascular endothelial niche cells expressing CXCL12 and are dependent on cues from the microenvironment for cell proliferation and survival (Passaro et al. 2015; Pitt et al. 2015). The disruption of leukemia–stroma cell interactions using CXCR4 antagonists suppresses leukemia-initiating cell activity in vivo and induces disease remission in both mouse models of T-ALL and primary-patient-derived T-ALL xenografts (Passaro et al. 2015; Pitt et al. 2015). Moreover, CD44 is required for the engraftment of preleukemic T cells in the bone marrow, for the bone marrow niche interactions supporting leukemia-initiating cells, and for disease progression in human T-ALL xenografts (García-Peydró et al. 2018).

ONCOGENIC NOTCH1 IN T-ALL

NOTCH1 is a class I transmembrane glycoprotein that functions as a ligand-activated transcription factor. Interaction of NOTCH with delta-like or jagged ligands expressed on the surface of a neighboring cell triggers the cleavage of NOTCH first by the ADAM10 metalloprotease and then by the γ-secretase complex, which releases the active, intracellular portion of NOTCH (ICN) from the membrane. ICN is then translocated to the nucleus where it associates with the RBPJ/CSL DNA-binding protein and activates gene expression via recruitment of mastermind-like coactivators (Bray 2016; Siebel and Lendahl 2017).

Activation of the NOTCH1 receptor in the thymus is required for early T-cell fate specification and thymocyte development (Radtke et al. 1999; Hozumi et al. 2008; Koch et al. 2008; Feyerabend et al. 2009; Germar et al. 2011; Weber et al. 2011). The pathogenic role of NOTCH1 in T-ALL was first identified in rare T-ALLs harboring the t(7;9)(q34;q34.3) chromosomal translocation, which leads to expression of a truncated and constitutively active form of NOTCH1 (Ellisen et al. 1991; Palomero et al. 2006a). An oncogenic role for NOTCH1 in T-ALL was shown by the rapid development of acute leukemia in mice transplanted with hematopoietic progenitors expressing a constitutively active intracellular form of NOTCH1 (Pear et al. 1996). Most commonly, NOTCH1 is activated as a result of somatic mutations that disrupt the negative regulatory region (NRR), an intramolecular lock protecting the extracellular portion of the receptor from cleavage by ADAM10 in the absence of ligand, or from truncation of the NOTCH1 carboxy-terminal PEST domain, which impairs the termination of NOTCH1 signaling through the proteasomal degradation of ICN (Weng et al. 2004; Sulis et al. 2008). In addition, 8%–24% of T-ALLs harbor mutations in the F-box and WD repeat domain containing

7 (*FBXW7*), which is required for the degradation of ICN (Moberg et al. 2001; Malyukova et al. 2007; O'Neil et al. 2007a; Thompson et al. 2007; Liu et al. 2017). Moreover, cyclin C likely functions in NOTCH1 degradation via phosphorylation of the NOTCH1 ICN domain and as a haploinsufficient T-ALL tumor suppressor in mouse and human leukemia (Li et al. 2014). Disruption of multiple regulatory domains of NOTCH1 provides increased signaling and transformative advantage because 20% of T-ALL patients harbor *NOTCH1* NRR mutations co-occurring with either *NOTCH1* PEST or *FBXW7* mutations (Weng et al. 2004; Mansour et al. 2006; Thompson et al. 2007). In addition, expression of the NOTCH1-ligand DLL4 in the microenvironment may provide paracrine signals for human and mouse T-ALL lymphoblasts (Minuzzo et al. 2015), and its aberrant expression in mouse T-cell precursor cells drives T-cell transformation (Xiong et al. 2013).

Oncogenic Pathways and Effector Mechanisms Controlled by NOTCH1

NOTCH1 promotes leukemic cell growth via direct transcriptional up-regulation of genes that drive anabolic pathways, such as ribosome biosynthesis, protein translation, and nucleotide and amino acid metabolism (Palomero et al. 2006b). NOTCH1 binding in super-enhancers is critical for the dynamic regulation of NOTCH1 target genes (Wang et al. 2014). The *MYC* oncogene, a direct target of NOTCH1 (Palomero et al. 2006b; Herranz et al. 2014; Yashiro-Ohtani et al. 2014), also promotes cell growth and anabolism in leukemia cells (Palomero et al. 2006b; Sharma et al. 2006; Margolin et al. 2009) and shares multiple target genes with NOTCH1 (Palomero et al. 2006b; Margolin et al. 2009). HES1, a transcriptional repressor downstream from NOTCH1 (Jarriault et al. 1995), promotes T-cell development and NOTCH1-induced leukemogenesis (Tomita et al. 1999; Wendorff et al. 2010), favoring activation of PI3K and NF-κB pathways (Palomero et al. 2008; Espinosa et al. 2010; Wong et al. 2012) via negative regulation of glucocorticoid receptor expression (Real et al. 2009) and by suppression of *BBC3* (PUMA)-mediated apoptosis (Schnell et al. 2015). In addition, NOTCH1 promotes a protective stress response in T-ALL via transcriptional up-regulation of heat shock transcription factor 1 (*HSF1*) and downstream heat shock proteins (Kourtis et al. 2018) and regulates the expression of *LUNAR1*, a potentially oncogenic T-ALL long noncoding RNA (Trimarchi et al. 2014).

The PI3K-AKT-mTOR signaling pathway is a critical mediator of cytokine-driven cell growth, proliferation, and survival (Vivanco and Sawyers 2002). NOTCH1 induces PI3K-AKT during thymocyte development to regulate cell size, glucose uptake, and glycolysis (Ciofani and Zuniga-Pflucker 2005). Moreover, PTEN, a strong negative regulator of the PI3K-AKT pathway, is transcriptionally down-regulated by HES1 in T-cell progenitors and T-ALL lymphoblasts (Palomero et al. 2007; Wong et al. 2012). NOTCH1 also induces the expression of pre-TCRα (*PTCRA*) (Reizis and Leder 2002) and other cytokine and growth factor receptors upstream of the PI3K-AKT pathway such as the interleukin 7 receptor α chain (*IL7R*) (González-García et al. 2009) and *IGF1R* (Medyouf et al. 2011). Moreover, NOTCH1 can regulate NF-κB activity in T-ALL (Shin et al. 2006; Thompson et al. 2007) and NF-κB activity is strictly required for the generation and maintenance of NOTCH1-induced tumors (Espinosa et al. 2010; D'Altri et al. 2011).

Oncogenic NOTCH1 signaling can directly promote proliferation in T-ALL inducing G_1/S cell cycle progression (Dohda et al. 2007; Joshi et al. 2009; Rao et al. 2009) via expression of the cell cycle genes *CCND3*, *CDK4*, and *CDK6* (Joshi et al. 2009) and down-regulation of the cyclin-dependent kinase inhibitors *CDKN2D* and *CDKN1B* (Rao et al. 2009). Moreover, NOTCH1 induces transcription of the S-phase kinase-associated protein 2 (*SKP2*), a negative regulator of the CDKN1A and CDKN1B cell cycle inhibitor proteins (Dohda et al. 2007).

NOTCH as a Therapeutic Target in T-ALL

The prominent role of NOTCH signaling in T-cell transformation has created major interest in the development of anti-NOTCH1 therapies for T-ALL (Weng et al. 2004). Most notably, γ-secretase inhibitors (GSIs), which block the proteolytic cleavage of NOTCH receptors by the γ-secretase complex precluding the release of intracellular NOTCH1 from the membrane, have been proposed as a potential targeted therapy in T-ALL (Milano et al. 2004; Weng et al. 2004; van Es et al. 2005; Lewis et al. 2007; Paganin and Ferrando 2011). Early on, in vitro studies showed that T-ALL cell lines treated with GSIs show a rapid clearance of intracellular activated NOTCH1 and transcriptional downregulation of NOTCH1 target genes with G_1 cell cycle arrest and a decreased cell size in T-ALL cell lines (Weng et al. 2004; Palomero et al. 2006a,b). In addition, GSI-mediated inhibition of NOTCH1 signaling abolishes the engraftment of primary T-ALL cells in mice and induces significant antitumor responses in NOTCH1-induced mouse T-ALLs (Armstrong et al. 2009; Tatarek et al. 2011) and in primary-patient-derived T-ALL xenografts (Herranz et al. 2015). Moreover, pharmacodynamic studies have documented that GSIs induce NOTCH inhibition in the clinical setting (DeAngelo et al. 2006). However, the clinical development of GSIs as anti-NOTCH1 therapy has been hampered by a paucity of therapeutic responses in early clinical trials and dose-limiting toxicities (DeAngelo et al. 2006; Wei et al. 2010; Takebe et al. 2014). The lack of therapeutic efficacy may reflect in some cases the presence of subclonal NOTCH1 mutations. However, it is also possible that even in the presence of a clonal NOTCH1 mutation T-ALL cells show weak oncogene addiction to NOTCH signaling, primary resistance, or rapid tumor adaptation via activation of parallel signaling pathways or adaptive epigenetic responses. In this regard, mutational loss of *PTEN* is associated with GSI resistance in human T-ALL cell lines (Palomero et al. 2007) and *Pten* deletion abrogates the antileukemic response to GSI therapy in mouse models of NOTCH1-induced T-ALL (Herranz et al. 2015). Mechanistically, NOTCH1 inhibition induces suppression of cellular metabolism in *Pten*-positive cells, whereas *Pten* loss and consequent activation of the PI3K-AKT pathway activates glycolysis, uncoupling NOTCH1 signaling and leukemia cell growth (Herranz et al. 2015). Similarly, aberrant expression of *MYC* can overcome the growth suppressing effects of NOTCH inhibition in some tumors (Weng et al. 2006) and mutations in *FBXW7* are highly prevalent in GSI-resistant cell lines (O'Neil et al. 2007a; Thompson et al. 2007). In addition, T-ALL cell lines seem to contain small populations of GSI-tolerant "persister" cells with distinct transcriptional programs and chromatin compaction, supporting an epigenetic mechanism of adaptation to NOTCH1 inhibition (Knoechel et al. 2014).

A second hurdle in the clinical development of GSIs is the development of dose-limiting on-target gastrointestinal toxicity as observed in a phase I clinical trials (DeAngelo et al. 2006; Papayannidis et al. 2015). GSI-induced gastrointestinal toxicity is characterized by secretory goblet cell metaplasia which results in malabsorption syndrome and diarrhea (Milano et al. 2004; van Es et al. 2005; Real et al. 2009; Wei et al. 2010). This phenotype results directly from the inhibition of NOTCH signaling in the intestinal epithelium as shown by genetic inactivation of *Rbpj* (van Es et al. 2005) or dual suppression of *Notch1* and *Notch2* in the gut (Riccio et al. 2008). Four different γ-secretase complexes contain one nicastrin and one presenilin enhancer-2 subunits that combine with a different APH-1 protein (either APH-1A or APH-1B) and a presenilin protein (PSEN, either PSEN1 or PSEN2). It has recently been shown that T-ALL specifically express PSEN1-containing-γ-secretase-complexes. Genetic deletion or pharmacological inhibition of PSEN1 impairs leukemia development and prolongs survival avoiding gut toxicities in vivo (Habets et al. 2019). Alternatively, the use of combination treatments with synergistic antileukemic effects offer the opportunity to obtain strong antitumor responses with lower toxicity. In this regard, metabolomic profiling of T-ALL cells in the context of NOTCH1 inhibition and *Pten* loss has defined a critical role for glutaminolysis in NOTCH1-induced leukemia cell growth, and small-molecule glutaminase inhibitors show strongly synergistic antitumor effects in combination with GSIs (Herranz et al. 2015). Moreover, genetic suppression of autophagy increases the antitumor effects of NOTCH inhibition in mouse models of NOTCH1-induced T-ALL (Herranz et al. 2015). In addition, GSIs show increased antitumor activity in combination with cyclin-dependent kinase inhibitors (Rao et al. 2009), histone deacetylase inhibitors (Sanda et al. 2010), proteasome inhibitors (Sanda et al. 2010), drugs targeting NF-κB signaling (Thompson et al. 2007), inhibitors of the PI3K-AKT-mTOR pathway (Chan et al. 2007; Palomero et al. 2007; Cullion et al. 2009; Sanda et al. 2010), and in the context of protein phosphatase 2A (PP2A) inhibition with perphenazine (Gutierrez et al. 2014). However, the most direct venue toward the development of a highly active and well-tolerated anti-NOTCH1 therapy in the clinic is the combination of GSIs with glucocorticoids (Real et al. 2009; Samon et al. 2012). Glucocorticoids induce apoptosis in lymphoid progenitor cells and are an essential component of ALL therapy (Inaba and Pui 2010). Early studies suggested an interaction between NOTCH1 signaling and glucocorticoid-induced apoptosis by showing that NOTCH1 activation can impair glucocorticoid-induced cell death in thymocytes (Deftos et al. 1998). Conversely, blocking NOTCH1 signaling with GSIs can reverse glucocorticoid resistance in T-ALLs (Real et al. 2009; Samon et al. 2012). The interaction between GSIs and glucocorticoids is mediated by release of the inhibitory effect of the NOTCH1-HES1 transcriptional axis on glucocorticoid receptor auto up-regulation, a critical amplification loop required for effective glucocorticoid-induced apoptosis (Real et al. 2009). Most notably, the combination of a GSI plus glucocorticoids is not only highly synergistic and active against glucocorticoid resistant leukemia models in vivo, but it also results in abrogation of GSI-induced gut toxicity (Real et al. 2009; Samon et al. 2012).

In addition to GSIs, inhibitors of sarco/endoplasmic reticulum calcium ATPase (SERCA) channels, stapled peptides targeting the NOT CH transcriptional complex, and NOTCH1-specific inhibitory antibodies have been proposed as alternative anti-NOTCH1 therapies for the treatment of T-ALL (Moellering et al. 2009; Wu et al. 2010; Roti et al. 2013; Sharma et al. 2015). SERCA inhibitors abrogate NOTCH signaling by interfering with the maturation and activity of leukemia-associated mutant forms of NOTCH1 and show on-target antileukemic effects in human T-ALL cell lines (Roti et al. 2013). SAHM1, a synthetic, cell-permeable, stabilized α-helical peptide binds to the NOTCH–RBPJ transactivation complex and prevents the recruitment of the MAML1 coactivator, thus blocking NOTCH-mediated transcription (Moellering et al. 2009). Therapeutically, SAHM1 induced strong antileukemic effects in human T-ALL cell lines and NOTCH-induced mouse leukemias without apparent gastrointestinal toxicity (Moellering et al. 2009). Finally, antibodies against the negative regulatory region of NOTCH1 (NRR1) have been shown to specifically block NOTCH1 signaling and inhibit growth in T-ALL cell lines and xenograft models with only minor changes in the intestine, suggesting that antibody-based selective inhibition of NOTCH1 could be effective and devoid of intestinal toxicity (Aste-Amezaga et al. 2010; Wu et al. 2010; Agnusdei et al. 2014; Gordon and Aster 2014; Sharma et al. 2015).

GENETIC DISRUPTION OF CELL CYCLE CONTROL

The loss of cell cycle control is a hallmark of cancer (Hanahan and Weinberg 2011). Deletions of the *CDKN2A* locus are observed in >70% of T-ALLs (Hebert et al. 1994; Ferrando et al. 2002) and cause the loss of the tumor suppressors *P16/INK4*, which inhibits G_1-S cell cycle progression, and of *P14/ARF*, which mediates cell cycle arrest and apoptosis in response to cellular stress (Kamijo et al. 1998; Zhang et al. 1998). Deletions in the cell cycle regulator *RB1*, which encodes a master regulator of cell cycle progression (Mullighan et al. 2007; Van Vlierberghe et al. 2013), and *CDKN1B*, which encodes $p27^{Kip1}$, an inhibitor of cyclin E-CDK2 and cyclin D-CDK4 complexes (Remke et al. 2009), can be found in ~15% of T-ALL cases (Liu et al. 2017). Moreover, 6% of T-ALLs harbor activating mutations in *CCND3*, which regulates the G_1/S transition (Liu et al. 2017). Finally, the t(12;14)(p13;q11) and t(7;12)(q34;p13) translocations are present in ~3% of T-ALLs and promote cell cycle progression by driving aberrantly high levels of *CCND2* expression (Clappier et al. 2006).

T-ALL TRANSCRIPTION FACTOR ONCOGENES

Oncogenic class II bHLH transcription factors, such as *TAL1*, *TAL2*, *LYL1*, and the LIM-only domain factors *LMO1* and *LMO2*, are aberrantly expressed in ~60% of T-ALLs (Ferrando et al. 2002). *TAL1* up-regulation characterizes 30%–40% of T-ALLs and can be driven by both interchromosomal and intrachromosomal rearrangements that place it under the control of T-cell-specific regulatory sequences in the *TCRA/D* locus (Begley et al. 1989; Bernard et al. 1990; Chen et al. 1990) or the SCL/TAL1 interrupting locus (*STIL*), a TAL1 neighbor gene (Aplan et al. 1990). In addition, precise heterozygous somatic mutations create de novo binding motifs for the MYB transcription factor and result in an active 5′ enhancer driving monoallelic up-regulation of *TAL1* (Mansour et al. 2014; Navarro et al. 2015). More rarely, the *TAL1*-related genes *LYL1*, *TAL2*, and *BHLHB1* are aberrantly expressed when chromosomal translocations reposition them close to TCR-loci enhancers (Mellentin et al. 1989; Xia et al. 1991; Wang et al. 2000; Homminga et al. 2012). Notably, forced expression of *TAL1* in T-cell precursors induces T-ALL in mouse models (Condorelli et al. 1996; Kelliher et al. 1996).

TAL1 transcriptional targets with T-ALL oncogenic potential include *TRIB2* (Tan et al. 2016), *NKX3.1* (Kusy et al. 2010), microRNA 223 (*MIR223*) (Mansour et al. 2013), and GTPase of immunity-associated protein (*GIMAP*) (Liau et al. 2017). Moreover, TAL1 and its binding partners GATA3 and RUNX1 form a positive autoregulatory loop involving activation of MYB that drives the initiation and maintenance of a leukemogenic transcriptional program (Sanda et al. 2012). Furthermore, the TAL1 target gene *ARID5B* encodes an epigenetic regulator that directly up-regulates *MYC*, promotes the TAL1-mediated oncogenic transcriptional program, and induces T-cell tumor formation in zebrafish (Leong et al. 2017).

The LIM-only domain factors *LMO1* and *LMO2* are overexpressed in 10% of T-ALL cases as a result of the t(11;14)(p15;q11) and t(11;14)(p13;q11) chromosomal translocations, respectively (McGuire et al. 1989; Boehm et al. 1991; Royer-Pokora et al. 1991). *LMO1* up-regulation is also driven by a promoter mutation upstream of *LMO1* that creates a new MYB binding site in 2% of T-ALLs (Li et al. 2017). *LMO2* up-regulation is found in 3%–5% of T-ALLs as a result of noncoding mutations in the *LMO2* promoter, which create putative binding sites for MYB, ETS1, or RUNX1 (Rahman et al. 2017) and in up to 5% of T-ALLs because of small chromosomal deletions in the vicinity of the *LMO2* locus (Van Vlierberghe et al. 2006; Van Vlierberghe et al. 2008a). LMO proteins do not interact directly with DNA but form transcriptional complexes with TAL1 and other bHLH factors (Larson et al. 1996), and the oncogenic activity of *Lmo1* or *Lmo2* expression in transgenic mice (Fisch et al. 1992; McGuire et al. 1992) is markedly enhanced by *Tal1* (Larson et al. 1996; Aplan et al. 1997; Tremblay et al. 2010).

Mechanistically, aberrant expression of the *LMO* genes confers properties of self-renewal to T cells. This has been observed in mouse T-cell precursors overexpressing *Lmo2*, and thymocytes from *Tal1-Lmo1* double-transgenic mice, which show up-regulation of a stem cell–like transcriptional program linked with increased self-renewal (McCormack et al. 2013; Gerby et al. 2014). Immature ETP T-ALLs, which characteristically express high levels of *LMO2* and *LYL1*, also show this stem cell–like signature (Ferrando et al. 2002; McCormack et al. 2010). Moreover, genetic suppression of *Lyl1* in *Lmo2*-expressing transgenic mice suppressed LMO2-induced stem cell–like gene expression programs, inhibited self-renewal, and precluded the development of ETP-like T-ALL (McCormack et al. 2013). Aberrant expression of LMO2 by retroviral insertion underlies the accidental development of T-ALL in X-linked severe-combined immunodeficiency patients undergoing retrovirus-based gene therapy to restore IL-2 receptor γ chain deficiency (Hacein-Bey-Abina et al. 2003, 2008; Howe et al. 2008).

Homeobox Transcription Factor Oncogenes

Homeobox genes encode for a group of strongly conserved transcription factors involved in cell lineage specification, body patterning, and embryonic organogenesis. Deregulated expression of the *HOXA9* and *HOXA10* genes can be found in ∼3% of T-ALLs harboring chromosomal translocations and inversions that relocate the *HOXA* paralog gene cluster closer to the *TCRB* and *TCRG* loci (Soulier et al. 2005; Speleman et al. 2005). Moreover, aberrant expression of *HOXA* genes is common in early-immature ETP T-ALLs (Ferrando et al. 2002, 2003; Asnafi et al. 2003; Soulier et al. 2005; Van Vlierberghe et al. 2008b) and is characteristic of T-ALLs harboring *KMT2-MLLT1* (*MLL-ENL*) (Tkachuk et al. 1992; Chervinsky et al. 1995; Rubnitz et al. 1996), *PICALM-MLLT10* (Dreyling et al. 1996; Carlson et al. 2000; Asnafi et al. 2003; Soulier et al. 2005), and *SET-NUP214* (Van Vlierberghe et al. 2008b) fusion oncogenes. In mouse models, HOXA9 expression and activating *Jak3* mutations induce accelerated development of leukemia and are linked to enhanced STAT5 transcriptional activity (de Bock et al. 2018).

Chromosomal rearrangements that drive aberrant T-cell expression of the NK-L subclass of HOX transcription factor genes, including *TLX1, TLX2, NKX2-1, NKX2-2,* and *NKX2-5,* are commonly associated with T-ALL. The t(10;14)(q24;q11) rearrangement (Dube et al. 1991; Hatano et al. 1991; Kennedy et al. 1991; Lu et al. 1991; Dear et al. 1993) places *TLX1* under the control of *TCRA/D* gene enhancers and results in *TLX1* overexpression in 5%–10% of pediatric and 30% of adult T-ALLs (Ferrando et al. 2002, 2004). The t(5;14)(q35;q32) translocation places *TLX3* under the control of T-cell regulatory elements near the *BCL11B* locus (Bernard et al. 2001) and is present in 20%–25% of pediatric and 5% of adult T-ALLs (Bernard et al. 2001; Ballerini et al. 2002; Ferrando et al. 2002, 2004; Asnafi et al. 2005). *NKX2-1-* and *NKX2-2-*rearranged leukemias are found in ∼5% of pediatric T-ALLs (Homminga et al. 2011), and chromosomal translocations involving *NKX2-5* have been reported in sporadic T-ALLs (Nagel et al. 2003; Przybylski et al. 2006). TLX1-expressing human T-ALLs are distinguished by arrest at the cortical stage of thymocyte development, which may result from disruption of VDJ recombination by TLX1 binding to *TCRA* enhancer sequences (Dadi et al. 2012). Expression of TLX1 in the mouse thymus leads to T-ALL with *Bcl11b* and *Notch1* mutations (De Keersmaecker et al. 2010; Rakowski et al. 2011). Notably, human and mouse TLX1-expressing T-cell tumors share a transcriptional program and have a defective mitotic checkpoint, and TLX1 can promote aneuploidy during T-cell transformation (Chen et al. 2010; De Keersmaecker et al. 2010).

T-ALLs harboring NK-L homeobox gene rearrangements show unique similarities. Both TLX1 and TLX3 normally down-regulate a large number of overlapping T-ALL tumor suppressor genes including *BCL11B, PHF6, RUNX1,* and *WT1* (Della Gatta et al. 2012). In addition, *TLX1-* and *TLX3-*rearranged T-ALLs frequently harbor loss-of-function mutations in the *BCL11B, WT1,* and *PHF6* tumor suppressor genes and the presence of the *NUP214-ABL1* fusion oncogene (Graux et al. 2004; Tosello et al. 2009; De Keersmaecker et al. 2010; Van Vlierberghe et al. 2010). Similarly, *NKX2-1-* and *NKX2-2-*rearranged leukemias show a TLX-1-like gene expression signature and developmental arrest (Homminga et al. 2011).

MYC

The *MYC* oncogene encodes a basic helix-loop-helix leucine zipper transcription factor that functions as a key master regulator of cell growth and proliferation and is broadly involved in the pathogenesis of human cancer (Dang 2012; Stine et al. 2015). MYC is important for thymocyte development (Dose et al. 2006) and the control of cell growth downstream from NOTCH1 and pre-TCR signaling (Dose et al. 2006). The rare (<1%) T-ALL chromosomal translocation t(8;14)(q24;q11) places the *MYC* locus under the control of *TCRA/D* enhancer elements (Erikson et al. 1986; Finger et al. 1986; Mathieu-Mahul et al. 1986) and leads to its overexpression in developing T cells. MYC oncogenic activity in T-ALL has been shown in mouse and zebrafish leukemia models in which it drives cell growth and proliferation and confers leukemia-initiating activity (Langenau et al. 2003; King et al. 2013). In addition, NOTCH1 signaling up-regulates *MYC* expression (Palomero et al. 2006b; Sharma et al. 2006), and MYC is a mediator of NOTCH1-induced transformation (Palomero et al. 2006b; Sharma et al. 2006). Mechanistically, NOTCH1 controls *MYC* via N-Me, a T-cell-specific long-range distal *MYC* enhancer (Herranz et al. 2014; Yashiro-Ohtani et al. 2014) essential for T-cell leukemogenesis and targeted by focal chromosomal duplications in ~5% of T-ALL cases (Herranz et al. 2014). Of note, and similar to NOTCH1, the MYC protein is targeted for proteasomal degradation by FBXW7 (Welcker et al. 2004; Yada et al. 2004), and T-ALL-associated *FBXW7* mutations increase both NOTCH1 and MYC protein levels (O'Neil et al. 2007a; Thompson et al. 2007). Ultimately, NOTCH1 and MYC collaborate to activate a common transcriptional program controlling leukemia cell growth and metabolism (Palomero et al. 2006b; Margolin et al. 2009).

MYB

The *MYB* oncogene encodes a leucine zipper transcription factor activated in rare cases of T-ALL harboring the t(6;7)(q23;q32) chromosomal translocation via its translocation to the vicinity of the *TCRB* locus (Clappier et al. 2007). *MYB*-translocated cases are frequently found in children under the age of 2 and show a marked increase in the expression of proliferation and mitosis genes (Clappier et al. 2007). In addition, focal duplications of the *MYB* locus driving increased MYB expression are found in ~10% of T-ALLs in both children and adults (Lahortiga et al. 2007; O'Neil et al. 2007b), and mutations leading to increased MYB activity occur in ~19% of T-ALL cases (Liu et al. 2017). *MYB* can be also up-regulated via direct transcriptional activation by TAL1 (Sanda et al. 2012) and via posttranslational up-regulation by the TAL1/miR-223/FBXW7 regulatory axis (Mansour et al. 2013) or as a result of down-regulation of MYB-targeting microRNAs (Sanghvi et al. 2014; Mets et al. 2015).

SPI1

The *SPI1* gene encodes an ETS-family transcription factor and master regulator of hematopoietic development also known as PU.1 (Burda et al. 2010). Recurrent chromosomal rearrangements involving *SPI1* are present in 4% of pediatric T-ALLs with a double-negative or CD8-single-positive immunophenotype (Seki et al. 2017). These rearrangements juxtapose *SPI1* to the *TCF7* (*TCF7-SPI1*) and the *STMN1* (*STMN1-SPI1*) loci causing increased expression of PU.1 (Seki et al. 2017). T-ALLs with SPI1 rearrangements have a distinct gene expression signature and poor prognosis (Seki et al. 2017).

TRANSCRIPTION FACTOR TUMOR SUPPRESSOR GENES

Mutations and deletions involving transcription factors tumor suppressors are frequently found in T-ALL. Mutations in *ETV6*, *RUNX1*, and *GATA3* are associated with early immature ETP T-ALLs (Van Vlierberghe et al. 2011a; Zhang et al. 2012), and mutations in *BCL11B*, *LEF1*, and *WT1* are predominantly found in early cortical T-ALLs, frequently in association with *TLX1* and *TLX3* translocations (De Keersmaecker et al. 2010; Gutierrez et al. 2010b; Della Gatta et al. 2012).

ETV6

The *ETV6* gene encodes an ETS family transcriptional repressor strictly required for the development of hematopoietic stem cells (Wang et al. 1998; Hock et al. 2004). Dominant-negative forms of ETV6 arising from amino- or carboxy-terminal truncating mutations are found in 13% of T-ALLs (Van Vlierberghe et al. 2011a).

RUNX1

The *RUNX1* tumor suppressor gene encodes a master regulator transcription factor with prominent roles in hematopoietic development (Okuda et al. 1996; Cai et al. 2000). Somatic mutations in *RUNX1* are found in ~5% of T-ALLs, typically in the immature ETP group (Della Gatta et al. 2012; Zhang et al. 2012; Grossmann et al. 2013; Van Vlierberghe et al. 2013). Germline heterozygous mutations in *RUNX1* are found in families affected with FPDMM (platelet disorder, familial, with associated myeloid malignancy; OMIM ID #601399), a leukemia predisposition syndrome characterized by a moderate decrease in platelet numbers and an increased risk of acute myeloid leukemia (Song et al. 1999) and T-ALL (Owen et al. 2008; Preudhomme et al. 2009; Nishimoto et al. 2010).

GATA3

The *GATA3* gene, which encodes an important transcriptional regulator of T-cell development and differentiation (Ting et al. 1996; Ho et al. 2009; Scripture-Adams et al. 2014) shows recurrent mutations in ETP ALL frequently involving R276, which disrupt the zinc finger DNA-binding domain (Zhang et al. 2012).

BCL11B

BCL11B encodes a zinc finger transcription factor that is mutated and deleted in mouse thymic lymphomas induced by γ-radiation (Wakabayashi et al. 2003a) and in T-ALL tumors arising in *Atm*-deficient (Ehrlich et al. 2014) and *TLX1* transgenic mice (De Keersmaecker et al. 2010). In human T-ALL, *BCL11B* mutations are present in ~10% of cases (De Keersmaecker et al. 2010; Gutierrez et al. 2011), frequently in combination with *TLX1* and *TLX3* translocations (Liu et al. 2017). *Bcl11b* inactivation in mouse T-cell progenitors results in early arrest at the DN2-DN3 stage of differentiation (Wakabayashi et al. 2003b; Ikawa et al. 2010; Li et al. 2010a) and promotes aberrant self-renewal activity (Ikawa et al. 2010) and features of natural killer T cells (Li et al. 2010a,b).

LEF1

LEF1 is a member of the lymphoid enhancer factor/T-cell factor (LEF/TCF) family of transcription factors that are critical mediators of WNT signaling (Brantjes et al. 2001). In the absence of WNT activation, LEF/TCFs block the expression of WNT target genes (Brantjes et al. 2001). However, on WNT activation, LEF/TCFs associate with active nuclear β-catenin to induce the expression of WNT target genes (van Noort and Clevers 2002). Mutations and monoallelic or biallelic deletions in the *LEF1* gene are present in ~15% of T-ALL cases (Gutierrez et al. 2010b). Notably, T-ALLs with *LEF1* inactivation show high levels of *MYC* expression and a characteristic differentiation arrest at the early cortical thymocyte stage of differentiation (Gutierrez et al. 2010b).

WT1

Deletions and mutations in the Wilms Tumor 1 (*WT1*) tumor suppressor gene are present in ~10% of T-ALLs and also in acute myeloid leukemias (Tosello et al. 2009; Heesch et al. 2010; Renneville et al. 2010; Neumann et al. 2015). T-ALL-associated *WT1* mutations are predominantly heterozygous frameshift mutations resulting in truncation of its carboxy-terminal zinc finger domains and are frequently associated with oncogenic expression of the *TLX1*, *TLX3*, or *HOXA* oncogenes (Tosello et al. 2009; Renneville et al. 2010). In T-ALL, *WT1* mutations are enriched in relapsed series and have been associated with inferior relapse-free survival (Bordin et al. 2018). Moreover, *WT1* loss confers resistance to DNA damaging agents via attenuation of TP53-induced apoptotic factors and up-regulation of the anti-apoptotic factor *XIAP* (Bordin et al. 2018).

GENETIC ALTERATIONS IN EPIGENETIC REGULATORS

Epigenetic regulators and chromatin modifiers are recurrently mutated in T-ALL. These include *PHF6* (Van Vlierberghe et al. 2010), the PRC2 complex genes *EZH2*, *EED*, and *SUZ12*

(Ntziachristos et al. 2012; Zhang et al. 2012), and the *KDM6A* histone demethylase (Ntziachristos et al. 2014; Van der Meulen et al. 2015). In addition, mutations in *IDH1*, *IDH2*, and *DNMT3A* can be specifically found in the context of ETP T-ALL (Van Vlierberghe et al. 2011a; Zhang et al. 2012).

PHF6

The plant homeodomain (PHD)-like finger 6 (*PHF6*) gene is inactivated by mutations and deletions in ~20% of T-ALL cases (Van Vlierberghe et al. 2010; Van Vlierberghe et al. 2011b), 20%–25% of mixed phenotype acute leukemia with ETP and T/myeloid characteristics (Alexander et al. 2018), and ~3% of acute myeloid leukemias (Van Vlierberghe et al. 2011b; Patel et al. 2012; Welch et al. 2012). Germline *PHF6* mutations are pathogenic in Börjeson–Forssman–Lehmann syndrome (BFLS; OMIM 301900), a rare X-linked disorder associated with intellectual disability, distinctive facial features, truncal obesity, and gynecomastia (Lower et al. 2002; Gecz et al. 2006). Interestingly, somatic mutations in the *PHF6* gene, located on Xq26, are mostly found in male T-ALL patients (Van Vlierberghe et al. 2011b). Moreover, PHF6 may function as a initiating tumor suppressor as suggested by a case of T-ALL arising in a male BFLS patient (Chao et al. 2010) and by the identification of *PHF6* mutations in clonal hemopoiesis (Yoshizato et al. 2015; Abelson et al. 2018). Consistently, in a mouse model of NOTCH1-induced T-ALL, loss of *Phf6* enhances tumor initiation, leukemia-initiating cell activity, represents an early event during T-ALL transformation and leads to increased self-renewal in mouse hematopoietic stem cells (Wendorff et al. 2018). *Phf6*-null hematopoietic stem cells are more quiescent, less prone to stress-induced activation, and confer increased hematopoietic recovery after chemotherapy (Wendorff et al. 2018). Mechanistically, PHF6 is a nucleolar protein and may function in chromatin remodeling and transcriptional regulation via interaction with the NurD nucleosome repositioning and histone deacetylation complex (Todd and Picketts 2012; Liu et al. 2015); however, it is also involved in ribosome biogenesis (Wang et al. 2013; Zhang et al. 2013) via interaction with the PAF1 transcription elongation complex (Zhang et al. 2013) and with UBF, implicated in the control of RNA polymerase I activity and ribosomal DNA (rDNA) transcription.

EZH2, EED, and *SUZ12*

The *EZH2, EED,* and *SUZ12* genes encode members of the Polycomb repressive complex 2 (PRC2), a major epigenetic regulator that mediates transcriptional repression via deposition of the H3K27me3 epigenetic mark (Cao et al. 2002; Czermin et al. 2002). Loss-of-function mutations in these genes are observed in up to 25% of T-ALLs and comprise up to 42% of ETP T-ALLs (Ntziachristos et al. 2012; Zhang et al. 2012). Conditional knockout of *Ezh2* in early hematopoietic progenitors induces γδ T-cell leukemia in mice (Simon et al. 2012), and concomitant deletion of *Runx1* and *Ezh2* induces mouse ETP T-ALL tumors in cooperation with oncogenic FLT3 (Booth et al. 2018). *PRC2* mutations have been proposed to promote T-cell transformation through increased expression and activation of FLT3 (Zhang et al. 2018) and enhanced NOTCH1 transcriptional activity (Ntziachristos et al. 2012) and may be associated with inferior response to chemotherapy (Aries et al. 2018).

KDM6A

The *KDM6A* gene (also known as *UTX*) encodes a H3K27me3 histone demethylase (Agger et al. 2007; Lan et al. 2007) that is mutated in 5%–15% of T-ALLs and functions as a tumor suppressor gene (Ntziachristos et al. 2014; Van der Meulen et al. 2015). T-ALL-associated *KMD6A* mutations are typically located in the catalytic domain, which seems to be critical for leukemia initiation and maintenance (Van der Meulen et al. 2015).

ONCOGENIC ACTIVATION OF SIGNALING PATHWAYS

In addition to genetic lesions affecting transcription factors and chromatin regulators, genes encoding critical components of signaling pathways are frequently mutated in T-ALL.

PI3K-AKT

Thymocytes are dependent on the activity of PI3Kγ and PI3Kδ for cell growth, proliferation, and survival (Webb et al. 2005; Swat et al. 2006; Ji et al. 2007), and signaling mutations in T-ALL target and activate the PI3K-AKT-mTOR signaling pathway in ~30% of cases (Liu et al. 2017). The most frequent alteration in this pathway affects the *PTEN* tumor suppressor gene through loss-of-function mutations and deletions in 10%–15% of T-ALLs (Palomero et al. 2007; Mendes et al. 2014), which could be associated with a poor prognosis (Paganin et al. 2018).

Loss of *PTEN* results in constitutive activation of the AKT-mTOR signaling axis, which directs multiple effectors to promote cell cycle progression, survival, glycolysis and protein biosynthesis (Stambolic et al. 1998; Cully et al. 2006). *Pten* heterozygous knockout mice develop lymphoid hyperplasia, T-ALL, and multiple solid tumors with loss of heterozygosity for the wild-type allele (Di Cristofano et al. 1998; Suzuki et al. 1998; Di Cristofano et al. 1999). Selective inactivation of *Pten* in hematopoietic progenitors (Yilmaz et al. 2006; Zhang et al. 2006) or in early or late thymic populations induces T-ALL (Hagenbeek et al. 2004; Hagenbeek and Spits 2008), similar to activated AKT (Mao et al. 2007). Consistently, inhibition of the PI3K/AKT/mTOR axis induces apoptosis and suppresses the growth of T-ALL in mouse models, cell lines and primary human T-ALL xenografts (Evangelisti et al. 2011; Subramaniam et al. 2012; Piovan et al. 2013; Dail et al. 2014).

In addition, activating mutations in the PI3K–AKT pathway that are detected at a lower frequency in T-ALL are found in *AKT1*, PI3K catalytic and regulatory subunit genes, PIKC3A, and PIK3CD (Gutierrez et al. 2009; Zuurbier et al. 2012; Liu et al. 2017). Moreover, the t(X;7)(q22;q34) and t(X;14)(q22;q11.2) translocations induce overexpression of IRS4 (Karrman et al. 2009b; Kang et al. 2012), a signaling factor that activates AKT (Uchida et al. 2000). Importantly, inhibition of the PI3K/AKT/mTOR axis induces apoptosis and suppresses the growth of T-ALL in mouse models, cell lines and primary human T-ALL xenografts (Evangelisti et al. 2011; Subramaniam et al. 2012; Piovan et al. 2013; Dail et al. 2014) thus representing a potential therapeutic opportunity for T-ALL patients. Notably, PTEN loss and AKT activation can also induce glucocorticoid resistance in mouse models of T-ALL (Piovan et al. 2013), and *PTEN* mutations are associated with primary glucocorticoid resistance in the clinic (Bandapalli et al. 2013). Mechanistically, AKT1 can phosphorylate the glucocorticoid receptor protein thereby blocking glucocorticoid-induced nuclear localization, and mTOR activation increases the expression of MCL1, an anti-apoptotic factor that antagonizes glucocorticoid-induced cell death (Wei et al. 2006). Consequently, PI3K–AKT–mTOR inhibition can effectively reverse glucocorticoid resistance in T-ALL (Wei et al. 2006; Subramaniam et al. 2012; Piovan et al. 2013; Burke et al. 2015).

IL7 Receptor and JAK-STAT Signaling

Activation of the JAK–STAT pathway by the interleukin-7 receptor (IL7R) supports the growth, proliferation, and survival of early T-cell progenitors (Mazzucchelli and Durum 2007). Aberrant JAK signaling was first linked to T-ALL via the t(9;12)(p24;p13) translocation, a rare rearrangement encoding the constitutively active *ETV6-JAK2* kinase fusion oncoprotein (Lacronique et al. 1997). The JAK–STAT pathway is activated in 25% of T-ALLs, because of mutations in *IL7R*, *JAK1*, *JAK3*, and *STAT5* (Liu et al. 2017), and predominantly in ETP T-ALLs, in which these mutations are found in 47% of cases (Zhang et al. 2012). T-ALL-associated *IL7R* mutations are located in the extracellular juxtamembrane-transmembrane region and lead to increased dimerization and receptor activation (Shochat et al. 2011, 2014; Zenatti et al. 2011). In addition, loss-of-function mutations in dynamin-2 (*DNM2*) impairs clathrin-mediated endocytosis of IL7R, causing increased IL7R surface density and enhanced IL-7 signaling in leukemic stem cells (Tremblay et al. 2016). Expression of mutant *IL7R* in combination with mutant *NOTCH1* accelerates leukemia development in mice (Yokoyama et al. 2013), and *IL7R* activating mutations generate ETP T-ALL when expressed in thymocytes from *p19/Arf* knockout animals (Treanor et al. 2014). *IL7R* mutations are prevalent in ETP T-ALL cases (Zhang et al. 2012,) and ETP T-ALLs show hyperactivation of STAT5 in response to interleukin-7 (Maude et al. 2015). Moreover, chromosomal rearrangements of ZEB2, which encodes a zinc finger E-box-binding transcription factor (Goossens et al. 2015) are found in ETP-ALL, and *Zeb2* overexpression in mice induces ETP-like leukemia with transcriptional activation of *IL7R* and increased JAK/STAT signaling (Goossens et al. 2015).

Activating mutations in *JAK1* and *JAK3* are found in 10% of T-ALL cases (Flex et al. 2008; Zhang et al. 2012; De Keersmaecker et al. 2013). *Jak3* mutant alleles induce T-ALL in mice albeit with long latency (Degryse et al. 2014), and treatment of these tumors with a selective JAK3 inhibitor reduces white blood cell counts and induces apoptosis in T-ALL lymphoblasts (Degryse et al. 2014). Interestingly, pharmacologic inhibition of JAK1/2 shows therapeutic activity in ETP T-ALL primary patient xenografts in vivo irrespective of JAK/STAT pathway mutations (Maude et al. 2015).

Additional mutations that affect the JAK/STAT signaling pathway are frequently found in T-ALL. Activating mutations in the *STAT5B* gene, which encodes a downstream effector of JAK1 and JAK3, have been reported in 5%–10% of T-ALLs (Bandapalli et al. 2014; Kontro et al. 2014). Genetic inactivation of *PTPN2*, encoding a tyrosine phosphatase that negatively regulates the STAT proteins, is found in ~6% of T-ALL cases (Kleppe et al. 2011). In addition, loss-of-function mutations in SH2B adaptor protein 3 (*SH2B3*), a gene that encodes a negative regulator of IL-7-mediated JAK/STAT5 signaling, are found in sporadic cases of T-ALL (Zhang et al. 2012; Perez-Garcia et al. 2013). In this context, preclinical studies have shown that JAK-STAT inhibition can induce antitumor effects in T-ALL animal models (Maude et al. 2015; Degryse et al. 2018a). Interestingly, ruxolitinib, a JAK1/2 inhibitor, showed broad antileukemic activity in xenograft models of ETP ALL, suggesting broad addiction to JAK-STAT signaling in these tumors (Maude et al. 2015). In addition, inhibition of ERK, PI3K and BCL2 in *JAK3*-mutant T-ALL cells increased the efficacy of JAK inhibitor treatment in these tumors (Degryse et al. 2018b).

ABL1-Fusion Oncogenic Kinases

About 6% of T-ALLs show rearrangements of the tyrosine kinase gene *ABL1* resulting in expression of the *NUP214-ABL1* fusion oncogene (Graux et al. 2004, 2009). T-ALL-associated *ABL1* rearrangements also generate the *EML1-ABL1* (De Keersmaecker et al. 2005) and *ETV6-ABL1* (Van Limbergen et al. 2001) fusion genes. *NUP214-ABL1* is almost exclusively found in *TLX1* and *TLX3* T-ALLs (Graux et al. 2004), and NUP214-ABL1 cooperates with TLX1 in a mouse model of T-ALL (Vanden Bempt et al. 2018). Interestingly, this group of leukemias, although not linked with a poor prognosis, shows in vitro sensitivity to different tyrosine kinase inhibitors (TKIs) (Quintas-Cardama et al. 2008). In addition, a few case reports have shown that the use of TKIs in relapsed patients harboring ABL1-fusions can induce complete or partial responses, at least temporarily (Deenik et al. 2009; Clarke et al. 2011; Chen et al. 2017), supporting the relevance of testing the activity of TKI therapy in clinical trials.

RAS–MAPK Signaling

Activating mutations in the *HRAS* and *KRAS* oncogenes have been described in 10%–15% of T-ALLs and are particularly prevalent in ETP T-ALL (Bar-Eli et al. 1989; Zhang et al. 2012; Van Vlierberghe et al. 2013; Liu et al. 2017). In addition, cryptic deletions and/or mutations in the neurofibromatosis type 1 (*NF1*) gene, which encodes a key negative regulator of Ras signaling, occur in 3% of T-ALL cases (Balgobind et al. 2008).

RIBOSOMAL PROTEIN MUTATIONS AND THE ROLE OF TRANSLATION IN T-ALL

One of the most intriguing findings of genomic profiling studies in T-ALL is the identification of recurrent mutations in ribosomal protein genes—in particular, *RPL10, RPS5*, and *RPL11* (De Keersmaecker et al. 2013; Tzoneva et al. 2013). *RPL10* mutations are present in 5%–10% of pediatric T-ALLs, with the recurrent *RPL10* R98S allele accounting for the majority (De Keersmaecker et al. 2013). This alteration up-regulates JAK-STAT signaling components thereby driving hyper-activation of the JAK–STAT pathway following cytokine stimulation (Girardi et al. 2018). *RPL10* mutations may also confer a survival advantage via a specific increase in IRES-mediated translation of the anti-apoptotic factor B-cell lymphoma 2 (*BCL-2*) (Kampen et al. 2019). The *CNOT3* gene, which encodes a component of the CCR4-NOT deadenylase complex, a master regulator of translation and mRNA stability (Bartlam and Yamamoto 2010), is mutated in ~8% of adult T-ALL cases (De Keersmaecker et al. 2013). Finally, the del(6q) chromosomal deletion, found in 30% of *TAL1*-expressing T-ALLs, leads to inactivation of two genes, *SYNCRIP* (encoding hnRNP-Q) and *SNHG5* (small nucleolar RNA host gene 5), which affect ribosomal functions, translation programs, and mitochondrial respiration (Gachet et al. 2018).

CLOSING REMARKS

The identification and mechanistic dissection of genetic alterations driving malignant transformation in T-ALL illustrates how oncogenic processes hijack the developmental programs that regulate self-renewal, lineage specification, proliferation, survival, and differentiation. Much work is yet needed to fully understand the role of autocrine and paracrine signals, tumor-microenvironment interactions, and the cross talk between different genetic and epigenetic driver alterations in the pathogenesis of T-ALL. Advanced mouse models, in vitro organoid-like culture platforms, and detailed characterization of primary patient sample–derived xenografts are called to close this gap. A thorough understanding of the genetic, transcriptional, developmental, and metabolic programs underlying the development and maintenance of T-ALL will likely offer new opportunities for the rational design of tailored therapies for this disease. Finally, it should not escape our attention that orthogonal therapeutic approaches such as emerging opportunities in immunotherapy may soon transform the treatment of this disease. Thus, chimeric antigen receptor (CAR) T cells targeting CD7 engineered via CRISPR knockout of this T-cell antigen (Cooper et al. 2018) and CAR T cells selectively directed against T-cells expressing a C1 TCRB constant chain (Maciocia et al. 2017) show remarkable activity in preclinical models of T-ALL. Moreover, CD3 activating antibodies elicit strong TCR signals in T-ALLs with surface TCR expression inducing a negative-selection-like programmed cell death mechanism (Trinquand et al. 2016).

REFERENCES

Abelson S, Collord G, Ng SWK, Weissbrod O, Mendelson Cohen N, Niemeyer E, Barda N, Zuzarte PC, Heisler L, Sundaravadanam Y, et al. 2018. Prediction of acute myeloid leukaemia risk in healthy individuals. *Nature* **559:** 400–404. doi:10.1038/s41586-018-0317-6

Agger K, Cloos PA, Christensen J, Pasini D, Rose S, Rappsilber J, Issaeva I, Canaani E, Salcini AE, Helin K. 2007. UTX and JMJD3 are histone H3K27 demethylases involved in *HOX* gene regulation and development. *Nature* **449:** 731–734. doi:10.1038/nature06145

Agnusdei V, Minuzzo S, Frasson C, Grassi A, Axelrod F, Satyal S, Gurney A, Hoey T, Seganfreddo E, Basso G, et al. 2014. Therapeutic antibody targeting of Notch1 in T-acute lymphoblastic leukemia xenografts. *Leukemia* **28:** 278–288. doi:10.1038/leu.2013.183

Alexander TB, Gu Z, Iacobucci I, Dickerson K, Choi JK, Xu B, Payne-Turner D, Yoshihara H, Loh ML, Horan J, et al. 2018. The genetic basis and cell of origin of mixed phenotype acute leukaemia. *Nature* **562:** 373–379. doi:10.1038/s41586-018-0436-0

Allen A, Sireci A, Colovai A, Pinkney K, Sulis M, Bhagat G, Alobeid B. 2013. Early T-cell precursor leukemia/lymphoma in adults and children. *Leukemia Res* **37:** 1027–1034. doi:10.1016/j.leukres.2013.06.010

Aplan PD, Lombardi DP, Ginsberg AM, Cossman J, Bertness VL, Kirsch IR. 1990. Disruption of the human SCL locus by "illegitimate" V-(D)-J recombinase activity. *Science* **250:** 1426–1429. doi:10.1126/science.2255914

Aplan PD, Jones CA, Chervinsky DS, Zhao X, Ellsworth M, Wu C, McGuire EA, Gross KW. 1997. An *scl* gene product lacking the transactivation domain induces bony abnormalities and cooperates with LMO1 to generate T-cell malignancies in transgenic mice. *EMBO J* **16:** 2408–2419. doi:10.1093/emboj/16.9.2408

Aries IM, Bodaar K, Karim SA, Chonghaile TN, Hinze L, Burns MA, Pfirrmann M, Degar J, Landrigan JT, Balbach

S, et al. 2018. PRC2 loss induces chemoresistance by repressing apoptosis in T cell acute lymphoblastic leukemia. *J Exp Med* **215:** 3094–3114. doi:10.1084/jem.20180570

Armstrong F, Brunet de la Grange P, Gerby B, Rouyez MC, Calvo J, Fontenay M, Boissel N, Dombret H, Baruchel A, Landman-Parker J, et al. 2009. NOTCH is a key regulator of human T-cell acute leukemia initiating cell activity. *Blood* **113:** 1730–1740. doi:10.1182/blood-2008-02-138172

Asnafi V, Radford-Weiss I, Dastugue N, Bayle C, Leboeuf D, Charrin C, Garand R, Lafage-Pochitaloff M, Delabesse E, Buzyn A, et al. 2003. CALM-AF10 is a common fusion transcript in T-ALL and is specific to the TCRγδ lineage. *Blood* **102:** 1000–1006. doi:10.1182/blood-2002-09-2913

Asnafi V, Buzyn A, Thomas X, Huguet F, Vey N, Boiron JM, Reman O, Cayuela JM, Lheritier V, Vernant JP, et al. 2005. Impact of TCR status and genotype on outcome in adult T-cell acute lymphoblastic leukemia: A LALA-94 study. *Blood* **105:** 3072–3078. doi:10.1182/blood-2004-09-3666

Aste-Amezaga M, Zhang N, Lineberger JE, Arnold BA, Toner TJ, Gu M, Huang L, Vitelli S, Vo KT, Haytko P, et al. 2010. Characterization of Notch1 antibodies that inhibit signaling of both normal and mutated Notch1 receptors. *PLoS ONE* **5:** e9094. doi:10.1371/journal.pone.0009094

Balgobind BV, Van Vlierberghe P, van den Ouweland AM, Beverloo HB, Terlouw-Kromosoeto JN, van Wering ER, Reinhardt D, Horstmann M, Kaspers GJ, Pieters R, et al. 2008. Leukemia-associated NF1 inactivation in patients with pediatric T-ALL and AML lacking evidence for neurofibromatosis. *Blood* **111:** 4322–4328. doi:10.1182/blood-2007-06-095075

Ballerini P, Blaise A, Busson-Le Coniat M, Su XY, Zucman-Rossi J, Adam M, van den Akker J, Perot C, Pellegrino B, Landman-Parker J, et al. 2002. *HOX11L2* expression defines a clinical subtype of pediatric T-ALL associated with poor prognosis. *Blood* **100:** 991–997. doi:10.1182/blood-2001-11-0093

Bandapalli OR, Zimmermann M, Kox C, Stanulla M, Schrappe M, Ludwig WD, Koehler R, Muckenthaler MU, Kulozik AE. 2013. NOTCH1 activation clinically antagonizes the unfavorable effect of PTEN inactivation in BFM-treated children with precursor T-cell acute lymphoblastic leukemia. *Haematologica* **98:** 928–936. doi:10.3324/haematol.2012.073585

Bandapalli OR, Schuessele S, Kunz JB, Rausch T, Stutz AM, Tal N, Geron I, Gershman N, Izraeli S, Eilers J, et al. 2014. The activating STAT5B N642H mutation is a common abnormality in pediatric T-cell acute lymphoblastic leukemia and confers a higher risk of relapse. *Haematologica* **99:** e188–e192. doi:10.3324/haematol.2014.104992

Bar-Eli M, Ahuja H, Foti A, Cline MJ. 1989. N-RAS mutations in T-cell acute lymphocytic leukaemia: Analysis by direct sequencing detects a novel mutation. *Br J Haematol* **72:** 36–39. doi:10.1111/j.1365-2141.1989.tb07648.x

Bartlam M, Yamamoto T. 2010. The structural basis for deadenylation by the CCR4-NOT complex. *Protein Cell* **1:** 443–452. doi:10.1007/s13238-010-0060-8

Begley CG, Aplan PD, Davey MP, Nakahara K, Tchorz K, Kurtzberg J, Hershfield MS, Haynes BF, Cohen DI, Waldmann TA, et al. 1989. Chromosomal translocation in a human leukemic stem-cell line disrupts the T-cell antigen receptor delta-chain diversity region and results in a previously unreported fusion transcript. *Proc Natl Acad Sci* **86:** 2031–2035. doi:10.1073/pnas.86.6.2031

Berg SL, Blaney SM, Devidas M, Lampkin TA, Murgo A, Bernstein M, Billett A, Kurtzberg J, Reaman G, Gaynon P, et al. 2005. Phase II study of nelarabine (compound 506U78) in children and young adults with refractory T-cell malignancies: A report from the Children's Oncology Group. *J Clin Oncol* **23:** 3376–3382. doi:10.1200/JCO.2005.03.426

Bernard O, Guglielmi P, Jonveaux P, Cherif D, Gisselbrecht S, Mauchauffe M, Berger R, Larsen CJ, Mathieu-Mahul D. 1990. Two distinct mechanisms for the *SCL* gene activation in the t(1;14) translocation of T-cell leukemias. *Genes Chromosomes Cancer* **1:** 194–208. doi:10.1002/gcc.2870010303

Bernard OA, Busson-LeConiat M, Ballerini P, Mauchauffe M, Della Valle V, Monni R, Nguyen Khac F, Mercher T, Penard-Lacronique V, Pasturaud P, et al. 2001. A new recurrent and specific cryptic translocation, t(5;14)(q35; q32), is associated with expression of the *Hox11L2* gene in T acute lymphoblastic leukemia. *Leukemia* **15:** 1495–1504. doi:10.1038/sj.leu.2402249

Boehm T, Foroni L, Kaneko Y, Perutz MF, Rabbitts TH. 1991. The rhombotin family of cysteine-rich LIM-domain oncogenes: Distinct members are involved in T-cell translocations to human chromosomes 11p15 and 11p13. *Proc Natl Acad Sci* **88:** 4367–4371. doi:10.1073/pnas.88.10.4367

Bond J, Graux C, Lhermitte L, Lara D, Cluzeau T, Leguay T, Cieslak A, Trinquand A, Pastoret C, Belhocine M, et al. 2017. Early response-based therapy stratification improves survival in adult early thymic precursor acute lymphoblastic leukemia: A Group for Research on Adult Acute Lymphoblastic Leukemia Study. *J Clin Oncol* **35:** 2683–2691. doi:10.1200/JCO.2016.71.8585

Booth CAG, Barkas N, Neo WH, Boukarabila H, Soilleux EJ, Giotopoulos G, Farnoud N, Giustacchini A, Ashley N, Carrelha J, et al. 2018. *Ezh2* and *Runx1* mutations collaborate to initiate lympho-myeloid leukemia in early thymic progenitors. *Cancer Cell* **33:** 274–291.e278. doi:10.1016/j.ccell.2018.01.006

Bordin F, Piovan E, Masiero E, Ambesi-Impiombato A, Minuzzo S, Bertorelle R, Sacchetto V, Pilotto G, Basso G, Zanovello P, et al. 2018. *WT1* loss attenuates the TP53-induced DNA damage response in T-cell acute lymphoblastic leukemia. *Haematologica* **103:** 266–277. doi:10.3324/haematol.2017.170431

Brantjes H, Roose J, van De Wetering M, Clevers H. 2001. All Tcf HMG box transcription factors interact with Groucho-related co-repressors. *Nucleic Acids Res* **29:** 1410–1419. doi:10.1093/nar/29.7.1410

Bray SJ. 2016. Notch signalling in context. *Nat Rev Mol Cell Biol* **17:** 722–735. doi:10.1038/nrm.2016.94

Burda P, Laslo P, Stopka T. 2010. The role of PU.1 and GATA-1 transcription factors during normal and leukemogenic hematopoiesis. *Leukemia* **24:** 1249–1257. doi:10.1038/leu.2010.104

Burke MJ, Verneris MR, Le Rademacher J, He W, Abdel-Azim H, Abraham AA, Auletta JJ, Ayas M, Brown VI, Cairo MS, et al. 2015. Transplant outcomes for children with T cell acute lymphoblastic leukemia in second remission: A report from the center for international blood and marrow transplant research. *Biol Blood Marrow Transplant* **21:** 2154–2159. doi:10.1016/j.bbmt.2015.08.023

Cai Z, de Bruijn M, Ma X, Dortland B, Luteijn T, Downing RJ, Dzierzak E. 2000. Haploinsufficiency of AML1 affects the temporal and spatial generation of hematopoietic stem cells in the mouse embryo. *Immunity* **13:** 423–431. doi:10.1016/S1074-7613(00)00042-X

Cao R, Wang L, Wang H, Xia L, Erdjument-Bromage H, Tempst P, Jones RS, Zhang Y. 2002. Role of histone H3 lysine 27 methylation in Polycomb-group silencing. *Science* **298:** 1039–1043. doi:10.1126/science.1076997

Carlson KM, Vignon C, Bohlander S, Martinez-Climent JA, Le Beau MM, Rowley JD. 2000. Identification and molecular characterization of *CALM/AF10* fusion products in T cell acute lymphoblastic leukemia and acute myeloid leukemia. *Leukemia* **14:** 100–104. doi:10.1038/sj.leu.2401629

Chan SM, Weng AP, Tibshirani R, Aster JC, Utz PJ. 2007. Notch signals positively regulate activity of the mTOR pathway in T-cell acute lymphoblastic leukemia. *Blood* **110:** 278–286. doi:10.1182/blood-2006-08-039883

Chao MM, Todd MA, Kontny U, Neas K, Sullivan MJ, Hunter AG, Picketts DJ, Kratz CP. 2010. T-cell acute lymphoblastic leukemia in association with Börjeson-Forssman-Lehmann syndrome due to a mutation in PHF6. *Pediatr Blood Cancer* **55:** 722–724. doi:10.1002/pbc.22574

Chen Q, Yang CY, Tsan JT, Xia Y, Ragab AH, Peiper SC, Carroll A, Baer R. 1990. Coding sequences of the *tal-1* gene are disrupted by chromosome translocation in human T cell leukemia. *J Exp Med* **172:** 1403–1408. doi:10.1084/jem.172.5.1403

Chen E, Huang X, Zheng Y, Li YJ, Chesney A, Ben-David Y, Yang E, Hough MR. 2010. Phosphorylation of HOX11/TLX1 on threonine-247 during mitosis modulates expression of cyclin B1. *Mol Cancer* **9:** 246. doi:10.1186/1476-4598-9-246

Chen Y, Zhang L, Huang J, Hong X, Zhao J, Wang Z, Zhang K. 2017. Dasatinib and chemotherapy in a patient with early T-cell precursor acute lymphoblastic leukemia and *NUP214-ABL1* fusion: A case report. *Exp Ther Med* **14:** 3979–3984. doi:10.3892/etm.2017.5046

Chervinsky DS, Sait SN, Nowak NJ, Shows TB, Aplan PD. 1995. Complex *MLL* rearrangement in a patient with T-cell acute lymphoblastic leukemia. *Genes Chromosomes Cancer* **14:** 76–84. doi:10.1002/gcc.2870140114

Ciofani M, Zuniga-Pflucker JC. 2005. Notch promotes survival of pre-T cells at the β-selection checkpoint by regulating cellular metabolism. *Nat Immunol* **6:** 881–888. doi:10.1038/ni1234

Clappier E, Cuccuini W, Cayuela JM, Vecchione D, Baruchel A, Dombret H, Sigaux F, Soulier J. 2006. Cyclin D2 dysregulation by chromosomal translocations to TCR loci in T-cell acute lymphoblastic leukemias. *Leukemia* **20:** 82–86. doi:10.1038/sj.leu.2404008

Clappier E, Cuccuini W, Kalota A, Crinquette A, Cayuela JM, Dik WA, Langerak AW, Montpellier B, Nadel B, Walrafen P, et al. 2007. The *C-MYB* locus is involved in chromosomal translocation and genomic duplications in human T-cell acute leukemia (T-ALL), the translocation defining a new T-ALL subtype in very young children. *Blood* **110:** 1251–1261. doi:10.1182/blood-2006-12-064683

Clarke S, O'Reilly J, Romeo G, Cooney J. 2011. *NUP214-ABL1* positive T-cell acute lymphoblastic leukemia patient shows an initial favorable response to imatinib therapy post relapse. *Leuk Res* **35:** e131–e133. doi:10.1016/j.leukres.2011.03.025

Condorelli GL, Facchiano F, Valtieri M, Proietti E, Vitelli L, Lulli V, Huebner K, Peschle C, Croce CM. 1996. T-cell-directed *TAL-1* expression induces T-cell malignancies in transgenic mice. *Cancer Res* **56:** 5113–5119.

Conter V, Valsecchi MG, Parasole R, Putti MC, Locatelli F, Barisone E, Lo Nigro L, Santoro N, Aricò M, Ziino O, et al. 2014. Childhood high-risk acute lymphoblastic leukemia in first remission: Results after chemotherapy or transplant from the AIEOP ALL 2000 study. *Blood* **123:** 1470–1478. doi:10.1182/blood-2013-10-532598

Cooper ML, Choi J, Staser K, Ritchey JK, Devenport JM, Eckardt K, Rettig MP, Wang B, Eissenberg LG, Ghobadi A, et al. 2018. An "off-the-shelf" fratricide-resistant CAR-T for the treatment of T cell hematologic malignancies. *Leukemia* **32:** 1970–1983. doi:10.1038/s41375-018-0065-5

Coustan-Smith E, Mullighan CG, Onciu M, Behm FG, Raimondi SC, Pei D, Cheng C, Su X, Rubnitz JE, Basso G, et al. 2009. Early T-cell precursor leukaemia: A subtype of very high-risk acute lymphoblastic leukaemia. *Lancet Oncol* **10:** 147–156. doi:10.1016/S1470-2045(08)70314-0

Crist WM, Shuster JJ, Falletta J, Pullen DJ, Berard CW, Vietti TJ, Alvarado CS, Roper MA, Prasthofer E, Grossi CE. 1988. Clinical features and outcome in childhood T-cell leukemia-lymphoma according to stage of thymocyte differentiation: A Pediatric Oncology Group Study. *Blood* **72:** 1891–1897.

Cullion K, Draheim KM, Hermance N, Tammam J, Sharma VM, Ware C, Nikov G, Krishnamoorthy V, Majumder PK, Kelliher MA. 2009. Targeting the Notch1 and mTOR pathways in a mouse T-ALL model. *Blood* **113:** 6172–6181. doi:10.1182/blood-2008-02-136762

Cully M, You H, Levine AJ, Mak TW. 2006. Beyond PTEN mutations: The PI3K pathway as an integrator of multiple inputs during tumorigenesis. *Nat Rev Cancer* **6:** 184–192. doi:10.1038/nrc1819

Czermin B, Melfi R, McCabe D, Seitz V, Imhof A, Pirrotta V. 2002. *Drosophila* enhancer of Zeste/ESC complexes have a histone H3 methyltransferase activity that marks chromosomal Polycomb sites. *Cell* **111:** 185–196. doi:10.1016/S0092-8674(02)00975-3

Dadi S, Le Noir S, Payet-Bornet D, Lhermitte L, Zacarias-Cabeza J, Bergeron J, Villarese P, Vachez E, Dik WA, Millien C, et al. 2012. TLX homeodomain oncogenes mediate T cell maturation arrest in T-ALL via interaction with ETS1 and suppression of TCRα gene expression. *Cancer Cell* **21:** 563–576. doi:10.1016/j.ccr.2012.02.013

D'Altri T, Gonzalez J, Aifantis I, Espinosa L, Bigas A. 2011. Hes1 expression and CYLD repression are essential events downstream of Notch1 in T-cell leukemia. *Cell Cycle* **10:** 1031–1036. doi:10.4161/cc.10.7.15067

Dail M, Wong J, Lawrence J, O'Connor D, Nakitandwe J, Chen SC, Xu J, Lee LB, Akagi K, Li Q, et al. 2014. Loss of oncogenic Notch1 with resistance to a PI3K inhibitor in

T-cell leukaemia. *Nature* **513:** 512–516. doi:10.1038/nature13495

Dang CV. 2012. MYC on the path to cancer. *Cell* **149:** 22–35. doi:10.1016/j.cell.2012.03.003

DeAngelo DJ, Stone RM, Silverman LB, Stock W, Attar EC, Fearen I, Dallob A, Matthews C, Stone J, Freedman S, et al. 2006. A phase I clinical trial of the notch inhibitor MK-0752 in patients with T-cell acute lymphoblastic leukemia/lymphoma (T-ALL) and other leukemias. *J Clin Oncol* **24:** 6585.

DeAngelo DJ, Yu D, Johnson JL, Coutre SE, Stone RM, Stopeck AT, Gockerman JP, Mitchell BS, Appelbaum FR, Larson RA. 2007. Nelarabine induces complete remissions in adults with relapsed or refractory T-lineage acute lymphoblastic leukemia or lymphoblastic lymphoma: Cancer and Leukemia Group B study 19801. *Blood* **109:** 5136–5142. doi:10.1182/blood-2006-11-056754

Dear TN, Sánchez-García I, Rabbitts TH. 1993. The *HOX11* gene encodes a DNA-binding nuclear transcription factor belonging to a distinct family of homeobox genes. *Proc Natl Acad Sci* **90:** 4431–4435. doi:10.1073/pnas.90.10.4431

de Bock CE, Demeyer S, Degryse S, Verbeke D, Sweron B, Gielen O, Vandepoel R, Vicente C, Vanden Bempt M, Dagklis A, et al. 2018. HOXA9 cooperates with activated JAK/STAT signaling to drive leukemia development. *Cancer Discov* **8:** 616–631. doi:10.1158/2159-8290.CD-17-0583

Deenik W, Beverloo HB, van der Poel-van de Luytgaarde SC, Wattel MM, van Esser JW, Valk PJ, Cornelissen JJ. 2009. Rapid complete cytogenetic remission after upfront dasatinib monotherapy in a patient with a *NUP214-ABL1*-positive T-cell acute lymphoblastic leukemia. *Leukemia* **23:** 627–629. doi:10.1038/leu.2008.318

Deftos ML, He YW, Ojala EW, Bevan MJ. 1998. Correlating notch signaling with thymocyte maturation. *Immunity* **9:** 777–786. doi:10.1016/S1074-7613(00)80643-3

Degryse S, de Bock CE, Cox L, Demeyer S, Gielen O, Mentens N, Jacobs K, Geerdens E, Gianfelici V, Hulselmans G, et al. 2014. JAK3 mutants transform hematopoietic cells through JAK1 activation, causing T-cell acute lymphoblastic leukemia in a mouse model. *Blood* **124:** 3092–3100. doi:10.1182/blood-2014-04-566687

Degryse S, Bornschein S, de Bock CE, Leroy E, Vanden Bempt M, Demeyer S, Jacobs K, Geerdens E, Gielen O, Soulier J, et al. 2018a. Mutant JAK3 signaling is increased by loss of wild-type JAK3 or by acquisition of secondary JAK3 mutations in T-ALL. *Blood* **131:** 421–425. doi:10.1182/blood-2017-07-797597

Degryse S, de Bock CE, Demeyer S, Govaerts I, Bornschein S, Verbeke D, Jacobs K, Binos S, Skerrett-Byrne DA, Murray HC, et al. 2018b. Mutant JAK3 phosphoproteomic profiling predicts synergism between JAK3 inhibitors and MEK/BCL2 inhibitors for the treatment of T-cell acute lymphoblastic leukemia. *Leukemia* **32:** 788–800. doi:10.1038/leu.2017.276

De Keersmaecker K, Graux C, Odero MD, Mentens N, Somers R, Maertens J, Wlodarska I, Vandenberghe P, Hagemeijer A, Marynen P, et al. 2005. Fusion of *EML1* to *ABL1* in T-cell acute lymphoblastic leukemia with cryptic t(9;14)(q34;q32). *Blood* **105:** 4849–4852. doi:10.1182/blood-2004-12-4897

De Keersmaecker K, Real PJ, Gatta GD, Palomero T, Sulis ML, Tosello V, Van Vlierberghe P, Barnes K, Castillo M, Sole X, et al. 2010. The *TLX1* oncogene drives aneuploidy in T cell transformation. *Nat Med* **16:** 1321–1327. doi:10.1038/nm.2246

De Keersmaecker K, Atak ZK, Li N, Vicente C, Patchett S, Girardi T, Gianfelici V, Geerdens E, Clappier E, Porcu M, et al. 2013. Exome sequencing identifies mutation in *CNOT3* and ribosomal genes *RPL5* and *RPL10* in T-cell acute lymphoblastic leukemia. *Nat Genet* **45:** 186–190. doi:10.1038/ng.2508

Della Gatta G, Palomero T, Perez-Garcia A, Ambesi-Impiombato A, Bansal M, Carpenter ZW, De Keersmaecker K, Sole X, Xu L, Paietta E, et al. 2012. Reverse engineering of *TLX* oncogenic transcriptional networks identifies *RUNX1* as tumor suppressor in T-ALL. *Nat Med* **18:** 436–440. doi:10.1038/nm.2610

Di Cristofano A, Pesce B, Cordon-Cardo C, Pandolfi PP. 1998. *Pten* is essential for embryonic development and tumour suppression. *Nat Genet* **19:** 348–355. doi:10.1038/1235

Di Cristofano A, Kotsi P, Peng YF, Cordon-Cardo C, Elkon KB, Pandolfi PP. 1999. Impaired Fas response and autoimmunity in $Pten^{+/-}$ mice. *Science* **285:** 2122–2125. doi:10.1126/science.285.5436.2122

Dohda T, Maljukova A, Liu L, Heyman M, Grandér D, Brodin D, Sangfelt O, Lendahl U. 2007. Notch signaling induces SKP2 expression and promotes reduction of p27Kip1 in T-cell acute lymphoblastic leukemia cell lines. *Exp Cell Res* **313:** 3141–3152. doi:10.1016/j.yexcr.2007.04.027

Dores GM, Devesa SS, Curtis RE, Linet MS, Morton LM. 2012. Acute leukemia incidence and patient survival among children and adults in the United States, 2001-2007. *Blood* **119:** 34–43. doi:10.1182/blood-2011-04-347872

Dose M, Khan I, Guo Z, Kovalovsky D, Krueger A, von Boehmer H, Khazaie K, Gounari F. 2006. c-Myc mediates pre-TCR-induced proliferation but not developmental progression. *Blood* **108:** 2669–2677. doi:10.1182/blood-2006-02-005900

Dreyling MH, Martinez-Climent JA, Zheng M, Mao J, Rowley JD, Bohlander SK. 1996. The t(10;11)(p13;q14) in the U937 cell line results in the fusion of the *AF10* gene and *CALM*, encoding a new member of the AP-3 clathrin assembly protein family. *Proc Natl Acad Sci* **93:** 4804–4809. doi:10.1073/pnas.93.10.4804

Dube ID, Kamel-Reid S, Yuan CC, Lu M, Wu X, Corpus G, Raimondi SC, Crist WM, Carroll AJ, Minowada J, et al. 1991. A novel human homeobox gene lies at the chromosome 10 breakpoint in lymphoid neoplasias with chromosomal translocation t(10;14). *Blood* **78:** 2996–3003.

Dunsmore KP, Winter S, Devidas M, Wood BL, Esiashvili N, Eisenberg N, Briegel N, Hayashi RJ, Gastier-Foster JM, Carroll AJ, et al. 2018. COG AALL0434: A randomized trial testing nelarabine in newly diagnosed T-cell malignancy. *J Clin Oncol* **36:** 10500. doi:10.1200/JCO.2018.36.15_suppl.10500

Ehrlich LA, Yang-Iott K, Bassing CH. 2014. *Tcrδ* translocations that delete the *Bcl11b* haploinsufficient tumor suppressor gene promote atm-deficient T cell acute lymphoblastic leukemia. *Cell Cycle* **13:** 3076–3082. doi:10.4161/15384101.2014.949144

Einsiedel HG, von Stackelberg A, Hartmann R, Fengler R, Schrappe M, Janka-Schaub G, Mann G, Hahlen K, Gobel U, Klingebiel T, et al. 2005. Long-term outcome in children with relapsed ALL by risk-stratified salvage therapy: Results of trial acute lymphoblastic leukemia-relapse study of the Berlin-Frankfurt-Munster Group 87. *J Clin Oncol* **23:** 7942–7950. doi:10.1200/JCO.2005.01.1031

Ellisen LW, Bird J, West DC, Soreng AL, Reynolds TC, Smith SD, Sklar J. 1991. *TAN-1*, the human homolog of the *Drosophila* notch gene, is broken by chromosomal translocations in T lymphoblastic neoplasms. *Cell* **66:** 649–661. doi:10.1016/0092-8674(91)90111-B

Erikson J, Finger L, Sun L, ar-Rushdi A, Nishikura K, Minowada J, Finan J, Emanuel BS, Nowell PC, Croce CM. 1986. Deregulation of c-myc by translocation of the alpha-locus of the T-cell receptor in T-cell leukemias. *Science* **232:** 884–886. doi:10.1126/science.3486470

Espinosa L, Cathelin S, D'Altri T, Trimarchi T, Statnikov A, Guiu J, Rodilla V, Ingles-Esteve J, Nomdedeu J, Bellosillo B, et al. 2010. The Notch/Hes1 pathway sustains NF-κB activation through CYLD repression in T cell leukemia. *Cancer Cell* **18:** 268–281. doi:10.1016/j.ccr.2010.08.006

Evangelisti C, Ricci F, Tazzari P, Tabellini G, Battistelli M, Falcieri E, Chiarini F, Bortul R, Melchionda F, Pagliaro P, et al. 2011. Targeted inhibition of mTORC1 and mTORC2 by active-site mTOR inhibitors has cytotoxic effects in T-cell acute lymphoblastic leukemia. *Leukemia* **25:** 781–791. doi:10.1038/leu.2011.20

Ferrando AA, Neuberg DS, Staunton J, Loh ML, Huard C, Raimondi SC, Behm FG, Pui CH, Downing JR, Gilliland DG, et al. 2002. Gene expression signatures define novel oncogenic pathways in T cell acute lymphoblastic leukemia. *Cancer Cell* **1:** 75–87. doi:10.1016/S1535-6108(02)00018-1

Ferrando AA, Armstrong SA, Neuberg DS, Sallan SE, Silverman LB, Korsmeyer SJ, Look AT. 2003. Gene expression signatures in *MLL*-rearranged T-lineage and B-precursor acute leukemias: Dominance of *HOX* dysregulation. *Blood* **102:** 262–268. doi:10.1182/blood-2002-10-3221

Ferrando AA, Neuberg DS, Dodge RK, Paietta E, Larson RA, Wiernik PH, Rowe JM, Caligiuri MA, Bloomfield CD, Look AT. 2004. Prognostic importance of *TLX1* (*HOX11*) oncogene expression in adults with T-cell acute lymphoblastic leukaemia. *Lancet* **363:** 535–536. doi:10.1016/S0140-6736(04)15542-6

Feyerabend TB, Terszowski G, Tietz A, Blum C, Luche H, Gossler A, Gale NW, Radtke F, Fehling HJ, Rodewald HR. 2009. Deletion of Notch1 converts pro-T cells to dendritic cells and promotes thymic B cells by cell-extrinsic and cell-intrinsic mechanisms. *Immunity* **30:** 67–79. doi:10.1016/j.immuni.2008.10.016

Finger LR, Harvey RC, Moore RC, Showe LC, Croce CM. 1986. A common mechanism of chromosomal translocation in T- and B-cell neoplasia. *Science* **234:** 982–985. doi:10.1126/science.3490692

Fisch P, Boehm T, Lavenir I, Larson T, Arno J, Forster A, Rabbitts TH. 1992. T-cell acute lymphoblastic lymphoma induced in transgenic mice by the *RBTN1* and *RBTN2* LIM-domain genes. *Oncogene* **7:** 2389–2397.

Flex E, Petrangeli V, Stella L, Chiaretti S, Hornakova T, Knoops L, Ariola C, Fodale V, Clappier E, Paoloni F, et al. 2008. Somatically acquired *JAK1* mutations in adult acute lymphoblastic leukemia. *J Exp Med* **205:** 751–758. doi:10.1084/jem.20072182

Gachet S, El-Chaar T, Avran D, Genesca E, Catez F, Quentin S, Delord M, Therizols G, Briot D, Meunier G, et al. 2018. Deletion 6q drives T-cell leukemia progression by ribosome modulation. *Cancer Discov* **8:** 1614–1631. doi:10.1158/2159-8290.CD-17-0831

Garand R, Vannier JP, Bene MC, Faure G, Favre M, Bernard A. 1990. Comparison of outcome, clinical, laboratory, and immunological features in 164 children and adults with T-ALL. The groupe d'etude immunologique des leucemies. *Leukemia* **4:** 739–744.

García-Peydró M, Fuentes P, Mosquera M, García-León MJ, Alcain J, Rodriguez A, García de Miguel P, Menéndez P, Weijer K, Spits H, et al. 2018. The NOTCH1/CD44 axis drives pathogenesis in a T cell acute lymphoblastic leukemia model. *J Clin Invest* **128:** 2802–2818. doi:10.1172/JCI92981

Gecz J, Turner G, Nelson J, Partington M. 2006. The Börjeson–Forssman–Lehman syndrome (BFLS, MIM #301900). *Eur J Hum Genet* **14:** 1233–1237. doi:10.1038/sj.ejhg.5201639

Gerby B, Tremblay CS, Tremblay M, Rojas-Sutterlin S, Herblot S, Hebert J, Sauvageau G, Lemieux S, Lecuyer E, Veiga DF, et al. 2014. *SCL*, *LMO1* and *Notch1* reprogram thymocytes into self-renewing cells. *PLoS Genet* **10:** e1004768. doi:10.1371/journal.pgen.1004768

Germar K, Dose M, Konstantinou T, Zhang J, Wang H, Lobry C, Arnett KL, Blacklow SC, Aifantis I, Aster JC, et al. 2011. T-cell factor 1 is a gatekeeper for T-cell specification in response to Notch signaling. *Proc Natl Acad Sci* **108:** 20060–20065. doi:10.1073/pnas.1110230108

Girardi T, Vereecke S, Sulima SO, Khan Y, Fancello L, Briggs JW, Schwab C, Op de Beeck J, Verbeeck J, Royaert J, et al. 2018. The T-cell leukemia-associated ribosomal RPL10 R98S mutation enhances JAK-STAT signaling. *Leukemia* **32:** 809–819. doi:10.1038/leu.2017.225

Gokbuget N, Basara N, Baurmann H, Beck J, Bruggemann M, Diedrich H, Guldenzoph B, Hartung G, Horst HA, Huttmann A, et al. 2011. High single-drug activity of nelarabine in relapsed T-lymphoblastic leukemia/lymphoma offers curative option with subsequent stem cell transplantation. *Blood* **118:** 3504–3511. doi:10.1182/blood-2011-01-329441

González-García S, García-Peydró M, Martin-Gayo E, Ballestar E, Esteller M, Bornstein R, de la Pompa JL, Ferrando AA, Toribio ML. 2009. CSL-MAML-dependent Notch1 signaling controls T lineage-specific IL-7Rα gene expression in early human thymopoiesis and leukemia. *J Exp Med* **206:** 779–791. doi:10.1084/jem.20081922

Goossens S, Radaelli E, Blanchet O, Durinck K, Van der Meulen J, Peirs S, Taghon T, Tremblay CS, Costa M, Farhang Ghahremani M, et al. 2015. ZEB2 drives immature T-cell lymphoblastic leukaemia development via enhanced tumour-initiating potential and IL-7 receptor signalling. *Nat Commun* **6:** 5794. doi:10.1038/ncomms6794

Gordon WR, Aster JC. 2014. Application and evaluation of anti-Notch antibodies to modulate Notch signaling.

Methods Mol Biol **1187:** 323–333. doi:10.1007/978-1-4939-1139-4_24

Graux C, Cools J, Melotte C, Quentmeier H, Ferrando A, Levine R, Vermeesch JR, Stul M, Dutta B, Boeckx N, et al. 2004. Fusion of *NUP214* to *ABL1* on amplified episomes in T-cell acute lymphoblastic leukemia. *Nat Genet* **36:** 1084–1089. doi:10.1038/ng1425

Graux C, Stevens-Kroef M, Lafage M, Dastugue N, Harrison CJ, Mugneret F, Bahloula K, Struski S, Gregoire MJ, Nadal N, et al. 2009. Heterogeneous patterns of amplification of the *NUP214-ABL1* fusion gene in T-cell acute lymphoblastic leukemia. *Leukemia* **23:** 125–133. doi:10.1038/leu.2008.278

Greaves MF, Janossy G, Peto J, Kay H. 1981. Immunologically defined subclasses of acute lymphoblastic leukaemia in children: Their relationship to presentation features and prognosis. *Br J Haematol* **48:** 179–197. doi:10.1111/j.1365-2141.1981.tb02704.x

Grossmann V, Haferlach C, Weissmann S, Roller A, Schindela S, Poetzinger F, Stadler K, Bellos F, Kern W, Haferlach T, et al. 2013. The molecular profile of adult T-cell acute lymphoblastic leukemia: Mutations in *RUNX1* and *DNMT3A* are associated with poor prognosis in T-ALL. *Genes Chromosomes Cancer* **52:** 410–422. doi:10.1002/gcc.22039

Gutierrez A, Sanda T, Grebliunaite R, Carracedo A, Salmena L, Ahn Y, Dahlberg S, Neuberg D, Moreau LA, Winter SS, et al. 2009. High frequency of *PTEN*, *PI3K*, and *AKT* abnormalities in T-cell acute lymphoblastic leukemia. *Blood* **114:** 647–650. doi:10.1182/blood-2009-02-206722

Gutierrez A, Dahlberg SE, Neuberg DS, Zhang J, Grebliunaite R, Sanda T, Protopopov A, Tosello V, Kutok J, Larson RS, et al. 2010a. Absence of biallelic *TCRγ* deletion predicts early treatment failure in pediatric T-cell acute lymphoblastic leukemia. *J Clin Oncol* **28:** 3816–3823. doi:10.1200/JCO.2010.28.3390

Gutierrez A, Sanda T, Ma W, Zhang J, Grebliunaite R, Dahlberg S, Neuberg D, Protopopov A, Winter SS, Larson RS, et al. 2010b. Inactivation of *LEF1* in T-cell acute lymphoblastic leukemia. *Blood* **115:** 2845–2851. doi:10.1182/blood-2009-07-234377

Gutierrez A, Kentsis A, Sanda T, Holmfeldt L, Chen SC, Zhang J, Protopopov A, Chin L, Dahlberg SE, Neuberg DS, et al. 2011. The *BCL11B* tumor suppressor is mutated across the major molecular subtypes of T-cell acute lymphoblastic leukemia. *Blood* **118:** 4169–4173. doi:10.1182/blood-2010-11-318873

Gutierrez A, Pan L, Groen RW, Baleydier F, Kentsis A, Marineau J, Grebliunaite R, Kozakewich E, Reed C, Pflumio F, et al. 2014. Phenothiazines induce PP2A-mediated apoptosis in T cell acute lymphoblastic leukemia. *J Clin Invest* **124:** 644–655. doi:10.1172/JCI65093

Habets RA, de Bock CE, Serneels L, Lodewijckx I, Verbeke D, Nittner D, Narlawar R, Demeyer S, Dooley J, Liston A, et al. 2019. Safe targeting of T cell acute lymphoblastic leukemia by pathology-specific NOTCH inhibition. *Sci Transl Med* **11**. doi:10.1126/scitranslmed.aau6246

Hacein-Bey-Abina S, Von Kalle C, Schmidt M, McCormack MP, Wulffraat N, Leboulch P, Lim A, Osborne CS, Pawliuk R, Morillon E, et al. 2003. *LMO2*-associated clonal T cell proliferation in two patients after gene therapy for SCID-X1. *Science* **302:** 415–419. doi:10.1126/science.1088547

Hacein-Bey-Abina S, Garrigue A, Wang GP, Soulier J, Lim A, Morillon E, Clappier E, Caccavelli L, Delabesse E, Beldjord K, et al. 2008. Insertional oncogenesis in 4 patients after retrovirus-mediated gene therapy of SCID-X1. *J Clin Invest* **118:** 3132–3142. doi:10.1172/JCI35700

Hagenbeek TJ, Spits H. 2008. T-cell lymphomas in T-cell-specific Pten-deficient mice originate in the thymus. *Leukemia* **22:** 608–619. doi:10.1038/sj.leu.2405056

Hagenbeek TJ, Naspetti M, Malergue F, Garcon F, Nunes JA, Cleutjens KB, Trapman J, Krimpenfort P, Spits H. 2004. The loss of PTEN allows TCRαβ lineage thymocytes to bypass IL-7 and pre-TCR-mediated signaling. *J Exp Med* **200:** 883–894. doi:10.1084/jem.20040495

Hanahan D, Weinberg RA. 2011. Hallmarks of cancer: The next generation. *Cell* **144:** 646–674. doi:10.1016/j.cell.2011.02.013

Hatano M, Roberts CW, Minden M, Crist WM, Korsmeyer SJ. 1991. Deregulation of a homeobox gene, *HOX11*, by the t(10;14) in T cell leukemia. *Science* **253:** 79–82. doi:10.1126/science.1676542

Hebert J, Cayuela JM, Berkeley J, Sigaux F. 1994. Candidate tumor-suppressor genes *MTS1* (p16^{INK4A}) and *MTS2* (p15^{INK4B}) display frequent homozygous deletions in primary cells from T- but not from B-cell lineage acute lymphoblastic leukemias. *Blood* **84:** 4038–4044.

Heesch S, Goekbuget N, Stroux A, Tanchez JO, Schlee C, Burmeister T, Schwartz S, Blau O, Keilholz U, Busse A, et al. 2010. Prognostic implications of mutations and expression of the Wilms tumor 1 (*WT1*) gene in adult acute T-lymphoblastic leukemia. *Haematologica* **95:** 942–949. doi:10.3324/haematol.2009.016386

Herranz D, Ambesi-Impiombato A, Palomero T, Schnell SA, Belver L, Wendorff AA, Xu L, Castillo-Martin M, Llobet-Navas D, Cordon-Cardo C, et al. 2014. A NOTCH1-driven *MYC* enhancer promotes T cell development, transformation and acute lymphoblastic leukemia. *Nat Med* **20:** 1130–1137. doi:10.1038/nm.3665

Herranz D, Ambesi-Impiombato A, Sudderth J, Sanchez-Martin M, Belver L, Tosello V, Xu L, Wendorff AA, Castillo M, Haydu JE, et al. 2015. Metabolic reprogramming induces resistance to anti-NOTCH1 therapies in T cell acute lymphoblastic leukemia. *Nat Med* **21:** 1182–1189. doi:10.1038/nm.3955

Ho IC, Tai TS, Pai SY. 2009. GATA3 and the T-cell lineage: Essential functions before and after T-helper-2-cell differentiation. *Nat Rev Immunol* **9:** 125–135. doi:10.1038/nri2476

Hock H, Meade E, Medeiros S, Schindler JW, Valk PJ, Fujiwara Y, Orkin SH. 2004. Tel/Etv6 is an essential and selective regulator of adult hematopoietic stem cell survival. *Genes Dev* **18:** 2336–2341. doi:10.1101/gad.1239604

Hof J, Krentz S, van Schewick C, Korner G, Shalapour S, Rhein P, Karawajew L, Ludwig WD, Seeger K, Henze G, et al. 2011. Mutations and deletions of the *TP53* gene predict nonresponse to treatment and poor outcome in first relapse of childhood acute lymphoblastic leukemia. *J Clin Oncol* **29:** 3185–3193. doi:10.1200/JCO.2011.34.8144

Homminga I, Pieters R, Langerak Anton W, de Rooi J, Stubbs A, Verstegen M, Vuerhard M, Buijs-Gladdines J,

Kooi C, Klous P, et al. 2011. Integrated transcript and genome analyses reveal *NKX2-1* and *MEF2C* as potential oncogenes in T cell acute lymphoblastic leukemia. *Cancer Cell* **19:** 484–497. doi:10.1016/j.ccr.2011.02.008

Homminga I, Vuerhard MJ, Langerak AW, Buijs-Gladdines J, Pieters R, Meijerink JP. 2012. Characterization of a pediatric T-cell acute lymphoblastic leukemia patient with simultaneous *LYL1* and *LMO2* rearrangements. *Haematologica* **97:** 258–261. doi:10.3324/haematol.2011.051722

Howe SJ, Mansour MR, Schwarzwaelder K, Bartholomae C, Hubank M, Kempski H, Brugman MH, Pike-Overzet K, Chatters SJ, de Ridder D, et al. 2008. Insertional mutagenesis combined with acquired somatic mutations causes leukemogenesis following gene therapy of SCID-X1 patients. *J Clin Invest* **118:** 3143–3150. doi:10.1172/JCI35798

Hozumi K, Mailhos C, Negishi N, Hirano K, Yahata T, Ando K, Zuklys S, Hollander GA, Shima DT, Habu S. 2008. Delta-like 4 is indispensable in thymic environment specific for T cell development. *J Exp Med* **205:** 2507–2513. doi:10.1084/jem.20080134

Huguet F, Leguay T, Raffoux E, Thomas X, Beldjord K, Delabesse E, Chevallier P, Buzyn A, Delannoy A, Chalandon Y, et al. 2009. Pediatric-inspired therapy in adults with Philadelphia chromosome-negative acute lymphoblastic leukemia: The GRAALL-2003 study. *J Clin Oncol* **27:** 911–918. doi:10.1200/JCO.2008.18.6916

Hunger SP, Lu X, Devidas M, Camitta BM, Gaynon PS, Winick NJ, Reaman GH, Carroll WL. 2012. Improved survival for children and adolescents with acute lymphoblastic leukemia between 1990 and 2005: A report from the children's oncology group. *J Clin Oncol* **30:** 1663–1669. doi:10.1200/JCO.2011.37.8018

Ikawa T, Hirose S, Masuda K, Kakugawa K, Satoh R, Shibano-Satoh A, Kominami R, Katsura Y, Kawamoto H. 2010. An essential developmental checkpoint for production of the T cell lineage. *Science* **329:** 93–96. doi:10.1126/science.1188995

Inaba H, Pui CH. 2010. Glucocorticoid use in acute lymphoblastic leukemia: Comparison of prednisone and dexamethasone. *Lancet Oncol* **11:** 1096–1106. doi:10.1016/S1470-2045(10)70114-5

Inukai T, Kiyokawa N, Campana D, Coustan-Smith E, Kikuchi A, Kobayashi M, Takahashi H, Koh K, Manabe A, Kumagai M, et al. 2012. Clinical significance of early T-cell precursor acute lymphoblastic leukaemia: Results of the Tokyo Children's Cancer Study Group Study L99-15. *Br J Haematol* **156:** 358–365. doi:10.1111/j.1365-2141.2011.08955.x

Jarriault S, Brou C, Logeat F, Schroeter EH, Kopan R, Israel A. 1995. Signalling downstream of activated mammalian Notch. *Nature* **377:** 355–358. doi:10.1038/377355a0

Ji H, Rintelen F, Waltzinger C, Bertschy Meier D, Bilancio A, Pearce W, Hirsch E, Wymann MP, Ruckle T, Camps M, et al. 2007. Inactivation of PI3Kγ and PI3Kδ distorts T-cell development and causes multiple organ inflammation. *Blood* **110:** 2940–2947. doi:10.1182/blood-2007-04-086751

Joshi I, Minter LM, Telfer J, Demarest RM, Capobianco AJ, Aster JC, Sicinski P, Fauq A, Golde TE, Osborne BA. 2009. Notch signaling mediates G_1/S cell-cycle progression in T cells via cyclin D3 and its dependent kinases. *Blood* **113:** 1689–1698. doi:10.1182/blood-2008-03-147967

Kamijo T, Weber JD, Zambetti G, Zindy F, Roussel MF, Sherr CJ. 1998. Functional and physical interactions of the ARF tumor suppressor with p53 and Mdm2. *Proc Natl Acad Sci* **95:** 8292–8297. doi:10.1073/pnas.95.14.8292

Kampen KR, Sulima SO, Verbelen B, Girardi T, Vereecke S, Rinaldi G, Verbeeck J, Op de Beeck J, Uyttebroeck A, Meijerink JPP, et al. 2019. The ribosomal RPL10 R98S mutation drives IRES-dependent BCL-2 translation in T-ALL. *Leukemia* **33:** 319–332. doi:10.1038/s41375-018-0176-z

Kang DH, Kim SH, Jun JW, Lee YW, Shin HB, Ahn JY, Hong DS, Lee YK, Jeon BR. 2012. Simultaneous translocation of both *TCR* loci (14q11) with rare partner loci (Xq22 and 12p13) in a case of T-lymphoblastic leukemia. *Ann Lab Med* **32:** 220–224. doi:10.3343/alm.2012.32.3.220

Karrman K, Forestier E, Heyman M, Andersen MK, Autio K, Blennow E, Borgström G, Ehrencrona H, Golovleva I, Heim S, et al. 2009a. Clinical and cytogenetic features of a population-based consecutive series of 285 pediatric T-cell acute lymphoblastic leukemias: Rare T-cell receptor gene rearrangements are associated with poor outcome. *Genes Chromosomes Cancer* **48:** 795–805. doi:10.1002/gcc.20684

Karrman K, Kjeldsen E, Lassen C, Isaksson M, Davidsson J, Andersson A, Hasle H, Fioretos T, Johansson B. 2009b. The t(X;7)(q22;q34) in paediatric T-cell acute lymphoblastic leukaemia results in overexpression of the insulin receptor substrate 4 gene through illegitimate recombination with the T-cell receptor beta locus. *Br J Haematol* **144:** 546–551. doi:10.1111/j.1365-2141.2008.07453.x

Kelliher MA, Seldin DC, Leder P. 1996. Tal-1 induces T cell acute lymphoblastic leukemia accelerated by casein kinase IIα. *EMBO J* **15:** 5160–5166. doi:10.1002/j.1460-2075.1996.tb00900.x

Kennedy MA, Gonzalez-Sarmiento R, Kees UR, Lampert F, Dear N, Boehm T, Rabbitts TH. 1991. *HOX11*, a homeobox-containing T-cell oncogene on human chromosome 10q24. *Proc Natl Acad Sci* **88:** 8900–8904. doi:10.1073/pnas.88.20.8900

King B, Trimarchi T, Reavie L, Xu L, Mullenders J, Ntziachristos P, Aranda-Orgilles B, Perez-Garcia A, Shi J, Vakoc C, et al. 2013. The ubiquitin ligase FBXW7 modulates leukemia-initiating cell activity by regulating MYC stability. *Cell* **153:** 1552–1566. doi:10.1016/j.cell.2013.05.041

Kleppe M, Soulier J, Asnafi V, Mentens N, Hornakova T, Knoops L, Constantinescu S, Sigaux F, Meijerink JP, Vandenberghe P, et al. 2011. PTPN2 negatively regulates oncogenic JAK1 in T-cell acute lymphoblastic leukemia. *Blood* **117:** 7090–7098. doi:10.1182/blood-2010-10-314286

Knoechel B, Roderick JE, Williamson KE, Zhu J, Lohr JG, Cotton MJ, Gillespie SM, Fernandez D, Ku M, Wang H, et al. 2014. An epigenetic mechanism of resistance to targeted therapy in T cell acute lymphoblastic leukemia. *Nat Genet* **46:** 364–370. doi:10.1038/ng.2913

Koch U, Fiorini E, Benedito R, Besseyrias V, Schuster-Gossler K, Pierres M, Manley NR, Duarte A, MacDonald HR, Radtke F. 2008. Delta-like 4 is the essential, nonredundant ligand for Notch1 during thymic T cell lineage commitment. *J Exp Med* **205:** 2515–2523. doi:10.1084/jem.20080829

Kontro M, Kuusanmäki H, Eldfors S, Burmeister T, Andersson EI, Bruserud Ø, Brümmendorf TH, Edgren H, Gjertsen BT, Itälä-Remes M, et al. 2014. Novel activating *STAT5B* mutations as putative drivers of T-cell acute lymphoblastic leukemia. *Leukemia* **28:** 1738–1742. doi:10.1038/leu.2014.89

Kourtis N, Lazaris C, Hockemeyer K, Balandran JC, Jimenez AR, Mullenders J, Gong Y, Trimarchi T, Bhatt K, Hu H, et al. 2018. Oncogenic hijacking of the stress response machinery in T cell acute lymphoblastic leukemia. *Nat Med* **24:** 1157–1166. doi:10.1038/s41591-018-0105-8

Kusy S, Gerby B, Goardon N, Gault N, Ferri F, Gerard D, Armstrong F, Ballerini P, Cayuela JM, Baruchel A, et al. 2010. *NKX3.1* is a direct TAL1 target gene that mediates proliferation of TAL1-expressing human T cell acute lymphoblastic leukemia. *J Exp Med* **207:** 2141–2156. doi:10.1084/jem.20100745

Lacronique V, Boureux A, Valle VD, Poirel H, Quang CT, Mauchauffe M, Berthou C, Lessard M, Berger R, Ghysdael J, et al. 1997. A TEL-JAK2 fusion protein with constitutive kinase activity in human leukemia. *Science* **278:** 1309–1312. doi:10.1126/science.278.5341.1309

Lahortiga I, De Keersmaecker K, Van Vlierberghe P, Graux C, Cauwelier B, Lambert F, Mentens N, Beverloo HB, Pieters R, Speleman F, et al. 2007. Duplication of the *MYB* oncogene in T cell acute lymphoblastic leukemia. *Nat Genet* **39:** 593–595. doi:10.1038/ng2025

Lan F, Bayliss PE, Rinn JL, Whetstine JR, Wang JK, Chen S, Iwase S, Alpatov R, Issaeva I, Canaani E, et al. 2007. A histone H3 lysine 27 demethylase regulates animal posterior development. *Nature* **449:** 689–694. doi:10.1038/nature06192

Langenau DM, Traver D, Ferrando AA, Kutok JL, Aster JC, Kanki JP, Lin S, Prochownik E, Trede NS, Zon LI, et al. 2003. Myc-induced T cell leukemia in transgenic zebrafish. *Science* **299:** 887–890. doi:10.1126/science.1080280

Larson RC, Lavenir I, Larson TA, Baer R, Warren AJ, Wadman I, Nottage K, Rabbitts TH. 1996. Protein dimerization between Lmo2 (Rbtn2) and Tal1 alters thymocyte development and potentiates T cell tumorigenesis in transgenic mice. *EMBO J* **15:** 1021–1027. doi:10.1002/j.1460-2075.1996.tb00439.x

Leong WZ, Tan SH, Ngoc PCT, Amanda S, Yam AWY, Liau WS, Gong Z, Lawton LN, Tenen DG, Sanda T. 2017. ARID5B as a critical downstream target of the TAL1 complex that activates the oncogenic transcriptional program and promotes T-cell leukemogenesis. *Genes Dev* **31:** 2343–2360. doi:10.1101/gad.302646.117

Lewis HD, Leveridge M, Strack PR, Haldon CD, O'Neil J, Kim H, Madin A, Hannam JC, Look AT, Kohl N, et al. 2007. Apoptosis in T cell acute lymphoblastic leukemia cells after cell cycle arrest induced by pharmacological inhibition of notch signaling. *Chem Biol* **14:** 209–219. doi:10.1016/j.chembiol.2006.12.010

Li L, Leid M, Rothenberg EV. 2010a. An early T cell lineage commitment checkpoint dependent on the transcription factor *Bcl11b*. *Science* **329:** 89–93. doi:10.1126/science.1188989

Li P, Burke S, Wang J, Chen X, Ortiz M, Lee SC, Lu D, Campos L, Goulding D, Ng BL, et al. 2010b. Reprogramming of T cells to natural killer-like cells upon *Bcl11b* deletion. *Science* **329:** 85–89. doi:10.1126/science.1188063

Li N, Fassl A, Chick J, Inuzuka H, Li X, Mansour MR, Liu L, Wang H, King B, Shaik S, et al. 2014. Cyclin C is a haploinsufficient tumour suppressor. *Nature cell biology* **16:** 1080–1091. doi:10.1038/ncb3046

Li Z, Abraham BJ, Berezovskaya A, Farah N, Liu Y, Leon T, Fielding A, Tan SH, Sanda T, Weintraub AS, et al. 2017. APOBEC signature mutation generates an oncogenic enhancer that drives *LMO1* expression in T-ALL. *Leukemia* **31:** 2057–2064. doi:10.1038/leu.2017.75

Liau WS, Tan SH, Ngoc PCT, Wang CQ, Tergaonkar V, Feng H, Gong Z, Osato M, Look AT, Sanda T. 2017. Aberrant activation of the *GIMAP* enhancer by oncogenic transcription factors in T-cell acute lymphoblastic leukemia. *Leukemia* **31:** 1798–1807. doi:10.1038/leu.2016.392

Liu Z, Li F, Zhang B, Li S, Wu J, Shi Y. 2015. Structural basis of plant homeodomain finger 6 (PHF6) recognition by the retinoblastoma binding protein 4 (RBBP4) component of the nucleosome remodeling and deacetylase (NuRD) complex. *J Biol Chem* **290:** 6630–6638. doi:10.1074/jbc.M114.610196

Liu Y, Easton J, Shao Y, Maciaszek J, Wang Z, Wilkinson MR, McCastlain K, Edmonson M, Pounds SB, Shi L, et al. 2017. The genomic landscape of pediatric and young adult T-lineage acute lymphoblastic leukemia. *Nat Genet* **49:** 1211–1218. doi:10.1038/ng.3909

Lower KM, Turner G, Kerr BA, Mathews KD, Shaw MA, Gedeon AK, Schelley S, Hoyme HE, White SM, Delatycki MB, et al. 2002. Mutations in *PHF6* are associated with Börjeson-Forssman-Lehmann syndrome. *Nat Genet* **32:** 661–665. doi:10.1038/ng1040

Lu M, Gong ZY, Shen WF, Ho AD. 1991. The tcl-3 protooncogene altered by chromosomal translocation in T-cell leukemia codes for a homeobox protein. *EMBO J* **10:** 2905–2910. doi:10.1002/j.1460-2075.1991.tb07840.x

Maciocia PM, Wawrzyniecka PA, Philip B, Ricciardelli I, Akarca AU, Onuoha SC, Legut M, Cole DK, Sewell AK, Gritti G, et al. 2017. Targeting the T cell receptor β-chain constant region for immunotherapy of T cell malignancies. *Nat Med* **23:** 1416–1423. doi:10.1038/nm.4444

Malyukova A, Dohda T, von der Lehr N, Akhoondi S, Corcoran M, Heyman M, Spruck C, Grander D, Lendahl U, Sangfelt O. 2007. The tumor suppressor gene *hCDC4* is frequently mutated in human T-cell acute lymphoblastic leukemia with functional consequences for Notch signaling. *Cancer Res* **67:** 5611–5616. doi:10.1158/0008-5472.CAN-06-4381

Mansour MR, Linch DC, Foroni L, Goldstone AH, Gale RE. 2006. High incidence of *Notch-1* mutations in adult patients with T-cell acute lymphoblastic leukemia. *Leukemia* **20:** 537–539. doi:10.1038/sj.leu.2404101

Mansour MR, Sanda T, Lawton LN, Li X, Kreslavsky T, Novina CD, Brand M, Gutierrez A, Kelliher MA, Jamieson CH, et al. 2013. The TAL1 complex targets the *FBXW7* tumor suppressor by activating miR-223 in human T cell acute lymphoblastic leukemia. *J Exp Med* **210:** 1545–1557. doi:10.1084/jem.20122516

Mansour MR, Abraham BJ, Anders L, Berezovskaya A, Gutierrez A, Durbin AD, Etchin J, Lawton L, Sallan SE, Silverman LB, et al. 2014. Oncogene regulation. An oncogenic super-enhancer formed through somatic mutation of a noncoding intergenic element. *Science* **346:** 1373–1377. doi:10.1126/science.1259037

Mao C, Tili EG, Dose M, Haks MC, Bear SE, Maroulakou I, Horie K, Gaitanaris GA, Fidanza V, Ludwig T, et al. 2007. Unequal contribution of Akt isoforms in the double-negative to double-positive thymocyte transition. *J Immunol* **178:** 5443–5453. doi:10.4049/jimmunol.178.9.5443

Margolin AA, Palomero T, Sumazin P, Califano A, Ferrando AA, Stolovitzky G. 2009. ChIP-on-chip significance analysis reveals large-scale binding and regulation by human transcription factor oncogenes. *Proc Natl Acad Sci* **106:** 244–249. doi:10.1073/pnas.0806445106

Marks DI, Paietta EM, Moorman AV, Richards SM, Buck G, DeWald G, Ferrando A, Fielding AK, Goldstone AH, Ketterling RP, et al. 2009. T-cell acute lymphoblastic leukemia in adults: Clinical features, immunophenotype, cytogenetics, and outcome from the large randomized prospective trial (UKALL XII/ECOG 2993). *Blood* **114:** 5136–5145. doi:10.1182/blood-2009-08-231217

Mathieu-Mahul D, Sigaux F, Zhu C, Bernheim A, Mauchauffe M, Daniel MT, Berger R, Larsen CJ. 1986. A t(8;14)(q24;q11) translocation in a T-cell leukemia (L1-ALL) with c-*myc* and TcR-α chain locus rearrangements. *Int J Cancer* **38:** 835–840. doi:10.1002/ijc.2910380609

Maude SL, Dolai S, Delgado-Martin C, Vincent T, Robbins A, Selvanathan A, Ryan T, Hall J, Wood AC, Tasian SK, et al. 2015. Efficacy of JAK/STAT pathway inhibition in murine xenograft models of early T-cell precursor (ETP) acute lymphoblastic leukemia. *Blood* **125:** 1759–1767. doi:10.1182/blood-2014-06-580480

Mazzucchelli R, Durum SK. 2007. Interleukin-7 receptor expression: Intelligent design. *Nat Rev Immunol* **7:** 144–154. doi:10.1038/nri2023

McCormack MP, Young LF, Vasudevan S, de Graaf CA, Codrington R, Rabbitts TH, Jane SM, Curtis DJ. 2010. The *Lmo2* oncogene initiates leukemia in mice by inducing thymocyte self-renewal. *Science* **327:** 879–883. doi:10.1126/science.1182378

McCormack MP, Shields BJ, Jackson JT, Nasa C, Shi W, Slater NJ, Tremblay CS, Rabbitts TH, Curtis DJ. 2013. Requirement for Lyl1 in a model of Lmo2-driven early T-cell precursor ALL. *Blood* **122:** 2093–2103. doi:10.1182/blood-2012-09-458570

McGuire EA, Hockett RD, Pollock KM, Bartholdi MF, O'Brien SJ, Korsmeyer SJ. 1989. The t(11;14)(p15;q11) in a T-cell acute lymphoblastic leukemia cell line activates multiple transcripts, including *Ttg-1*, a gene encoding a potential zinc finger protein. *Mol Cell Biol* **9:** 2124–2132. doi:10.1128/MCB.9.5.2124

McGuire EA, Rintoul CE, Sclar GM, Korsmeyer SJ. 1992. Thymic overexpression of *Ttg-1* in transgenic mice results in T-cell acute lymphoblastic leukemia/lymphoma. *Mol Cell Biol* **12:** 4186–4196. doi:10.1128/MCB.12.9.4186

Medyouf H, Gusscott S, Wang H, Tseng JC, Wai C, Nemirovsky O, Trumpp A, Pflumio F, Carboni J, Gottardis M, et al. 2011. High-level IGF1R expression is required for leukemia-initiating cell activity in T-ALL and is supported by Notch signaling. *J Exp Med* **208:** 1809–1822. doi:10.1084/jem.20110121

Mellentin JD, Smith SD, Cleary ML. 1989. *lyl*-1, a novel gene altered by chromosomal translocation in T cell leukemia, codes for a protein with a helix-loop-helix DNA binding motif. *Cell* **58:** 77–83. doi:10.1016/0092-8674(89)90404-2

Mendes RD, Sarmento LM, Canté-Barrett K, Zuurbier L, Buijs-Gladdines JG, Póvoa V, Smits WK, Abecasis M, Yunes JA, Sonneveld E, et al. 2014. *PTEN* microdeletions in T-cell acute lymphoblastic leukemia are caused by illegitimate RAG-mediated recombination events. *Blood* **124:** 567–578. doi:10.1182/blood-2014-03-562751

Mets E, Van der Meulen J, Van Peer G, Boice M, Mestdagh P, Van de Walle I, Lammens T, Goossens S, De Moerloose B, Benoit Y, et al. 2015. MicroRNA-193b-3p acts as a tumor suppressor by targeting the *MYB* oncogene in T-cell acute lymphoblastic leukemia. *Leukemia* **29:** 798–806. doi:10.1038/leu.2014.276

Milano J, McKay J, Dagenais C, Foster-Brown L, Pognan F, Gadient R, Jacobs RT, Zacco A, Greenberg B, Ciaccio PJ. 2004. Modulation of notch processing by γ-secretase inhibitors causes intestinal goblet cell metaplasia and induction of genes known to specify gut secretory lineage differentiation. *Toxicol Sci* **82:** 341–358. doi:10.1093/toxsci/kfh254

Minuzzo S, Agnusdei V, Pusceddu I, Pinazza M, Moserle L, Masiero M, Rossi E, Crescenzi M, Hoey T, Ponzoni M, et al. 2015. DLL4 regulates NOTCH signaling and growth of T acute lymphoblastic leukemia cells in NOD/SCID mice. *Carcinogenesis* **36:** 115–121. doi:10.1093/carcin/bgu223

Moberg KH, Bell DW, Wahrer DC, Haber DA, Hariharan IK. 2001. Archipelago regulates cyclin E levels in *Drosophila* and is mutated in human cancer cell lines. *Nature* **413:** 311–316. doi:10.1038/35095068

Moellering RE, Cornejo M, Davis TN, Del Bianco C, Aster JC, Blacklow SC, Kung AL, Gilliland DG, Verdine GL, Bradner JE. 2009. Direct inhibition of the NOTCH transcription factor complex. *Nature* **462:** 182–188. doi:10.1038/nature08543

Möricke A, Reiter A, Zimmermann M, Gadner H, Stanulla M, Dordelmann M, Loning L, Beier R, Ludwig WD, Ratei R, et al. 2008. Risk-adjusted therapy of acute lymphoblastic leukemia can decrease treatment burden and improve survival: Treatment results of 2169 unselected pediatric and adolescent patients enrolled in the trial ALL-BFM 95. *Blood* **111:** 4477–4489. doi:10.1182/blood-2007-09-112920

Möricke A, Zimmermann M, Valsecchi MG, Stanulla M, Biondi A, Mann G, Locatelli F, Cazzaniga G, Niggli F, Aricò M, et al. 2016. Dexamethasone vs prednisone in induction treatment of pediatric ALL: Results of the randomized trial AIEOP-BFM ALL 2000. *Blood* **127:** 2101–2112. doi:10.1182/blood-2015-09-670729

Mullighan CG, Goorha S, Radtke I, Miller CB, Coustan-Smith E, Dalton JD, Girtman K, Mathew S, Ma J, Pounds SB, et al. 2007. Genome-wide analysis of genetic alterations in acute lymphoblastic leukaemia. *Nature* **446:** 758–764. doi:10.1038/nature05690

Nagel S, Kaufmann M, Drexler HG, MacLeod RA. 2003. The cardiac homeobox gene *NKX2-5* is deregulated by juxtaposition with *BCL11B* in pediatric T-ALL cell lines via a novel t(5;14)(q35.1;q32.2). *Cancer Res* **63:** 5329–5334.

Navarro JM, Touzart A, Pradel LC, Loosveld M, Koubi M, Fenouil R, Le Noir S, Maqbool MA, Morgado E, Gregoire C, et al. 2015. Site- and allele-specific Polycomb dysregulation in T-cell leukaemia. *Nat Commun* **6:** 6094. doi:10.1038/ncomms7094

Neumann M, Heesch S, Schlee C, Schwartz S, Gokbuget N, Hoelzer D, Konstandin NP, Ksienzyk B, Vosberg S, Graf A, et al. 2013. Whole-exome sequencing in adult ETP-ALL reveals a high rate of *DNMT3A* mutations. *Blood* **121:** 4749–4752. doi:10.1182/blood-2012-11-465138

Neumann M, Vosberg S, Schlee C, Heesch S, Schwartz S, Gokbuget N, Hoelzer D, Graf A, Krebs S, Bartram I, et al. 2015. Mutational spectrum of adult T-ALL. *Oncotarget* **6:** 2754–2766. doi:10.18632/oncotarget.2218

Niehues T, Kapaun P, Harms DO, Burdach S, Kramm C, Korholz D, Janka-Schaub G, Gobel U. 1999. A classification based on T cell selection-related phenotypes identifies a subgroup of childhood T-ALL with favorable outcome in the COALL studies. *Leukemia* **13:** 614–617. doi:10.1038/sj.leu.2401382

Nishimoto N, Imai Y, Ueda K, Nakagawa M, Shinohara A, Ichikawa M, Nannya Y, Kurokawa M. 2010. T cell acute lymphoblastic leukemia arising from familial platelet disorder. *Int J Hematol* **92:** 194–197. doi:10.1007/s12185-010-0612-y

Ntziachristos P, Tsirigos A, Van Vlierberghe P, Nedjic J, Trimarchi T, Flaherty MS, Ferres-Marco D, da Ros V, Tang Z, Siegle J, et al. 2012. Genetic inactivation of the Polycomb repressive complex 2 in T cell acute lymphoblastic leukemia. *Nat Med* **18:** 298–301. doi:10.1038/nm.2651

Ntziachristos P, Tsirigos A, Welstead GG, Trimarchi T, Bakogianni S, Xu L, Loizou E, Holmfeldt L, Strikoudis A, King B, et al. 2014. Contrasting roles of histone 3 lysine 27 demethylases in acute lymphoblastic leukaemia. *Nature* **514:** 513–517. doi:10.1038/nature13605

O'Neil J, Grim J, Strack P, Rao S, Tibbitts D, Winter C, Hardwick J, Welcker M, Meijerink JP, Pieters R, et al. 2007a. *FBW7* mutations in leukemic cells mediate NOTCH pathway activation and resistance to γ-secretase inhibitors. *J Exp Med* **204:** 1813–1824. doi:10.1084/jem.20070876

O'Neil J, Tchinda J, Gutierrez A, Moreau L, Maser RS, Wong KK, Li W, McKenna K, Liu XS, Feng B, et al. 2007b. Alu elements mediate *MYB* gene tandem duplication in human T-ALL. *J Exp Med* **204:** 3059–3066. doi:10.1084/jem.20071637

Okuda T, van Deursen J, Hiebert SW, Grosveld G, Downing JR. 1996. AML1, the target of multiple chromosomal translocations in human leukemia, is essential for normal fetal liver hematopoiesis. *Cell* **84:** 321–330. doi:10.1016/S0092-8674(00)80986-1

Owen CJ, Toze CL, Koochin A, Forrest DL, Smith CA, Stevens JM, Jackson SC, Poon MC, Sinclair GD, Leber B, et al. 2008. Five new pedigrees with inherited *RUNX1* mutations causing familial platelet disorder with propensity to myeloid malignancy. *Blood* **112:** 4639–4645. doi:10.1182/blood-2008-05-156745

Paganin M, Ferrando A. 2011. Molecular pathogenesis and targeted therapies for NOTCH1-induced T-cell acute lymphoblastic leukemia. *Blood Rev* **25:** 83–90. doi:10.1016/j.blre.2010.09.004

Paganin M, Grillo MF, Silvestri D, Scapinello G, Buldini B, Cazzaniga G, Biondi A, Valsecchi MG, Conter V, te Kronnie G, et al. 2018. The presence of mutated and deleted PTEN is associated with an increased risk of relapse in childhood T cell acute lymphoblastic leukaemia treated with AIEOP-BFM ALL protocols. *Br J Haematol* **182:** 705–711. doi:10.1111/bjh.15449

Palomero T, Barnes KC, Real PJ, Glade Bender JL, Sulis ML, Murty VV, Colovai AI, Balbin M, Ferrando AA. 2006a. CUTLL1, a novel human T-cell lymphoma cell line with t(7;9) rearrangement, aberrant NOTCH1 activation and high sensitivity to γ-secretase inhibitors. *Leukemia* **20:** 1279–1287. doi:10.1038/sj.leu.2404258

Palomero T, Lim WK, Odom DT, Sulis ML, Real PJ, Margolin A, Barnes KC, O'Neil J, Neuberg D, Weng AP, et al. 2006b. NOTCH1 directly regulates c-*MYC* and activates a feed-forward-loop transcriptional network promoting leukemic cell growth. *Proc Natl Acad Sci* **103:** 18261–18266. doi:10.1073/pnas.0606108103

Palomero T, Sulis ML, Cortina M, Real PJ, Barnes K, Ciofani M, Caparros E, Buteau J, Brown K, Perkins SL, et al. 2007. Mutational loss of *PTEN* induces resistance to NOTCH1 inhibition in T-cell leukemia. *Nat Med* **13:** 1203–1210. doi:10.1038/nm1636

Palomero T, Dominguez M, Ferrando AA. 2008. The role of the PTEN/AKT Pathway in NOTCH1-induced leukemia. *Cell Cycle* **7:** 965–970. doi:10.4161/cc.7.8.5753

Papayannidis C, DeAngelo DJ, Stock W, Huang B, Shaik MN, Cesari R, Zheng X, Reynolds JM, English PA, Ozeck M, et al. 2015. A Phase 1 study of the novel γ-secretase inhibitor PF-03084014 in patients with T-cell acute lymphoblastic leukemia and T-cell lymphoblastic lymphoma. *Blood Cancer J* **5:** e350. doi:10.1038/bcj.2015.80

Parker C, Waters R, Leighton C, Hancock J, Sutton R, Moorman AV, Ancliff P, Morgan M, Masurekar A, Goulden N, et al. 2010. Effect of mitoxantrone on outcome of children with first relapse of acute lymphoblastic leukaemia (ALL R3): An open-label randomised trial. *Lancet* **376:** 2009–2017. doi:10.1016/S0140-6736(10)62002-8

Passaro D, Irigoyen M, Catherinet C, Gachet S, Da Costa De Jesus C, Lasgi C, Tran Quang C, Ghysdael J. 2015. CXCR4 is required for leukemia-initiating cell activity in T cell acute lymphoblastic leukemia. *Cancer Cell* **27:** 769–779. doi:10.1016/j.ccell.2015.05.003

Patel JL, Smith LM, Anderson J, Abromowitch M, Campana D, Jacobsen J, Lones MA, Gross TG, Cairo MS, Perkins SL. 2012. The immunophenotype of T-lymphoblastic lymphoma in children and adolescents: A Children's Oncology Group report. *Br J Haematol* **159:** 454–461. doi:10.1111/bjh.12042

Patrick K, Wade R, Goulden N, Mitchell C, Moorman AV, Rowntree C, Jenkinson S, Hough R, Vora A. 2014. Outcome for children and young people with early T-cell precursor acute lymphoblastic leukaemia treated on a contemporary protocol, UKALL 2003. *Br J Haematol* **166:** 421–424. doi:10.1111/bjh.12882

Pear WS, Aster JC, Scott ML, Hasserjian RP, Soffer B, Sklar J, Baltimore D. 1996. Exclusive development of T cell neoplasms in mice transplanted with bone marrow expressing activated Notch alleles. *J Exp Med* **183:** 2283–2291. doi:10.1084/jem.183.5.2283

Perez-Garcia A, Ambesi-Impiombato A, Hadler M, Rigo I, LeDuc CA, Kelly K, Jalas C, Paietta E, Racevskis J, Rowe JM, et al. 2013. Genetic loss of *SH2B3* in acute lymphoblastic leukemia. *Blood* **122:** 2425–2432. doi:10.1182/blood-2013-05-500850

Piovan E, Yu J, Tosello V, Herranz D, Ambesi-Impiombato A, Da Silva AC, Sanchez-Martin M, Perez-Garcia A, Rigo I, Castillo M, et al. 2013. Direct reversal of glucocorticoid resistance by AKT inhibition in acute lymphoblastic leukemia. *Cancer Cell* **24:** 766–776. doi:10.1016/j.ccr.2013.10.022

Pitt LA, Tikhonova AN, Hu H, Trimarchi T, King B, Gong Y, Sanchez-Martin M, Tsirigos A, Littman DR, Ferrando AA, et al. 2015. CXCL12-producing vascular endothelial niches control acute T cell leukemia maintenance. *Cancer Cell* **27:** 755–768. doi:10.1016/j.ccell.2015.05.002

Preudhomme C, Renneville A, Bourdon V, Philippe N, Roche-Lestienne C, Boissel N, Dhedin N, André JM, Cornillet-Lefebvre P, Baruchel A, et al. 2009. High frequency of *RUNX1* biallelic alteration in acute myeloid leukemia secondary to familial platelet disorder. *Blood* **113:** 5583–5587. doi:10.1182/blood-2008-07-168260

Przybylski GK, Dik WA, Grabarczyk P, Wanzeck J, Chudobska P, Jankowski K, von Bergh A, van Dongen JJ, Schmidt CA, Langerak AW. 2006. The effect of a novel recombination between the homeobox gene *NKX2-5* and the TRD locus in T-cell acute lymphoblastic leukemia on activation of the *NKX2-5* gene. *Haematologica* **91:** 317–321.

Pui CH, Evans WE. 2006. Treatment of acute lymphoblastic leukemia. *N Engl J Med* **354:** 166–178. doi:10.1056/NEJMra052603

Pui CH, Behm FG, Singh B, Schell MJ, Williams DL, Rivera GK, Kalwinsky DK, Sandlund JT, Crist WM, Raimondi SC. 1990. Heterogeneity of presenting features and their relation to treatment outcome in 120 children with T-cell acute lymphoblastic leukemia. *Blood* **75:** 174–179.

Pui CH, Robison LL, Look AT. 2008. Acute lymphoblastic leukaemia. *Lancet* **371:** 1030–1043. doi:10.1016/S0140-6736(08)60457-2

Pui CH, Mullighan CG, Evans WE, Relling MV. 2012. Pediatric acute lymphoblastic leukemia: Where are we going and how do we get there? *Blood* **120:** 1165–1174. doi:10.1182/blood-2012-05-378943

Quintas-Cardama A, Tong W, Manshouri T, Vega F, Lennon PA, Cools J, Gilliland DG, Lee F, Cortes J, Kantarjian H, et al. 2008. Activity of tyrosine kinase inhibitors against human *NUP214-ABL1*-positive T cell malignancies. *Leukemia* **22:** 1117–1124. doi:10.1038/leu.2008.80

Radtke F, Wilson A, Stark G, Bauer M, van Meerwijk J, MacDonald HR, Aguet M. 1999. Deficient T cell fate specification in mice with an induced inactivation of *Notch1*. *Immunity* **10:** 547–558. doi:10.1016/S1074-7613(00)80054-0

Radtke F, MacDonald HR, Tacchini-Cottier F. 2013. Regulation of innate and adaptive immunity by Notch. *Nat Rev Immunol* **13:** 427–437. doi:10.1038/nri3445

Rahman S, Magnussen M, Leon TE, Farah N, Li Z, Abraham BJ, Alapi KZ, Mitchell RJ, Naughton T, Fielding AK, et al. 2017. Activation of the *LMO2* oncogene through a somatically acquired neomorphic promoter in T-cell acute lymphoblastic leukemia. *Blood* **129:** 3221–3226. doi:10.1182/blood-2016-09-742148

Rakowski LA, Lehotzky EA, Chiang MY. 2011. Transient responses to NOTCH and TLX1/HOX11 inhibition in T-cell acute lymphoblastic leukemia/lymphoma. *PLoS One* **6:** e16761. doi:10.1371/journal.pone.0016761

Rao SS, O'Neil J, Liberator CD, Hardwick JS, Dai X, Zhang T, Tyminski E, Yuan J, Kohl NE, Richon VM, et al. 2009. Inhibition of NOTCH signaling by gamma secretase inhibitor engages the RB pathway and elicits cell cycle exit in T-cell acute lymphoblastic leukemia cells. *Cancer Res* **69:** 3060–3068. doi:10.1158/0008-5472.CAN-08-4295

Real PJ, Tosello V, Palomero T, Castillo M, Hernando E, de Stanchina E, Sulis ML, Barnes K, Sawai C, Homminga I, et al. 2009. γ-secretase inhibitors reverse glucocorticoid resistance in T cell acute lymphoblastic leukemia. *Nat Med* **15:** 50–58. doi:10.1038/nm.1900

Reizis B, Leder P. 2002. Direct induction of T lymphocyte-specific gene expression by the mammalian Notch signaling pathway. *Genes Dev* **16:** 295–300. doi:10.1101/gad.960702

Remke M, Pfister S, Kox C, Toedt G, Becker N, Benner A, Werft W, Breit S, Liu S, Engel F, et al. 2009. High-resolution genomic profiling of childhood T-ALL reveals frequent copy-number alterations affecting the TGF-β and PI3K-AKT pathways and deletions at 6q15-16.1 as a genomic marker for unfavorable early treatment response. *Blood* **114:** 1053–1062. doi:10.1182/blood-2008-10-186536

Renneville A, Kaltenbach S, Clappier E, Collette S, Micol JB, Nelken B, Lepelley P, Dastugue N, Benoit Y, Bertrand Y, et al. 2010. Wilms tumor 1 (*WT1*) gene mutations in pediatric T-cell malignancies. *Leukemia* **24:** 476–480. doi:10.1038/leu.2009.221

Riccio O, van Gijn ME, Bezdek AC, Pellegrinet L, van Es JH, Zimber-Strobl U, Strobl LJ, Honjo T, Clevers H, Radtke F. 2008. Loss of intestinal crypt progenitor cells owing to inactivation of both Notch1 and Notch2 is accompanied by derepression of CDK inhibitors $p27^{Kip1}$ and $p57^{Kip2}$. *EMBO Rep* **9:** 377–383. doi:10.1038/embor.2008.7

Roti G, Carlton A, Ross KN, Markstein M, Pajcini K, Su AH, Perrimon N, Pear WS, Kung AL, Blacklow SC, et al. 2013. Complementary genomic screens identify SERCA as a therapeutic target in *NOTCH1* mutated cancer. *Cancer Cell* **23:** 390–405. doi:10.1016/j.ccr.2013.01.015

Royer-Pokora B, Loos U, Ludwig WD. 1991. *TTG-2*, a new gene encoding a cysteine-rich protein with the LIM motif, is overexpressed in acute T-cell leukaemia with the t(11;14)(p13;q11). *Oncogene* **6:** 1887–1893.

Rubnitz JE, Behm FG, Curcio-Brint AM, Pinheiro RP, Carroll AJ, Raimondi SC, Shurtleff SA, Downing JR. 1996. Molecular analysis of t(11;19) breakpoints in childhood acute leukemias. *Blood* **87:** 4804–4808.

Samon JB, Castillo-Martin M, Hadler M, Ambesi-Impiobato A, Paietta E, Racevskis J, Wiernik PH, Rowe JM, Jakubczak J, Randolph S, et al. 2012. Preclinical analysis of the γ-secretase inhibitor PF-03084014 in combination with glucocorticoids in T-cell acute lymphoblastic leukemia. *Mol Cancer Ther* **11:** 1565–1575. doi:10.1158/1535-7163.MCT-11-0938

Sanda T, Li X, Gutierrez A, Ahn Y, Neuberg DS, O'Neil J, Strack PR, Winter CG, Winter SS, Larson RS, et al. 2010. Interconnecting molecular pathways in the pathogenesis and drug sensitivity of T-cell acute lymphoblastic leukemia. *Blood* **115:** 1735–1745. doi:10.1182/blood-2009-07-235143

Sanda T, Lawton LN, Barrasa MI, Fan ZP, Kohlhammer H, Gutierrez A, Ma W, Tatarek J, Ahn Y, Kelliher MA, et al. 2012. Core transcriptional regulatory circuit controlled by the TAL1 complex in human T cell acute lymphoblastic leukemia. *Cancer Cell* **22:** 209–221. doi:10.1016/j.ccr.2012.06.007

Sanghvi VR, Mavrakis KJ, Van der Meulen J, Boice M, Wolfe AL, Carty M, Mohan P, Rondou P, Socci ND, Benoit Y, et al. 2014. Characterization of a set of tumor suppressor microRNAs in T cell acute lymphoblastic leukemia. *Sci Signal* **7:** ra111. doi:10.1126/scisignal.2005500

Schnell SA, Ambesi-Impiombato A, Sanchez-Martin M, Belver L, Xu L, Qin Y, Kageyama R, Ferrando AA. 2015. Therapeutic targeting of HES1 transcriptional programs in T-ALL. *Blood* **125:** 2806–2814. doi:10.1182/blood-2014-10-608448

Scripture-Adams DD, Damle SS, Li L, Elihu KJ, Qin S, Arias AM, Butler RR III, Champhekar A, Zhang JA, Rothenberg EV. 2014. GATA-3 dose-dependent checkpoints in early T cell commitment. *J Immunol* **193:** 3470–3491. doi:10.4049/jimmunol.1301663

Seki M, Kimura S, Isobe T, Yoshida K, Ueno H, Nakajima-Takagi Y, Wang C, Lin L, Kon A, Suzuki H, et al. 2017. Recurrent *SPI1* (PU.1) fusions in high-risk pediatric T cell acute lymphoblastic leukemia. *Nat Genet* **49:** 1274–1281. doi:10.1038/ng.3900

Sharma VM, Calvo JA, Draheim KM, Cunningham LA, Hermance N, Beverly L, Krishnamoorthy V, Bhasin M, Capobianco AJ, Kelliher MA. 2006. Notch1 contributes to mouse T-cell leukemia by directly inducing the expression of c-*myc*. *MolCell Biol* **26:** 8022–8031. doi:10.1128/MCB.01091-06

Sharma A, Gadkari RA, Ramakanth SV, Padmanabhan K, Madhumathi DS, Devi L, Appaji L, Aster JC, Rangarajan A, Dighe RR. 2015. A novel monoclonal antibody against Notch1 targets leukemia-associated mutant Notch1 and depletes therapy resistant cancer stem cells in solid tumors. *Sci Rep* **5:** 11012. doi:10.1038/srep11012

Shin HM, Minter LM, Cho OH, Gottipati S, Fauq AH, Golde TE, Sonenshein GE, Osborne BA. 2006. Notch1 augments NF-κB activity by facilitating its nuclear retention. *EMBO J* **25:** 129–138. doi:10.1038/sj.emboj.7600902

Shochat C, Tal N, Bandapalli OR, Palmi C, Ganmore I, te Kronnie G, Cario G, Cazzaniga G, Kulozik AE, Stanulla M, et al. 2011. Gain-of-function mutations in interleukin-7 receptor-α (IL7R) in childhood acute lymphoblastic leukemias. *J Exp Med* **208:** 901–908. doi:10.1084/jem.20110580

Shochat C, Tal N, Gryshkova V, Birger Y, Bandapalli OR, Cazzaniga G, Gershman N, Kulozik AE, Biondi A, Mansour MR, et al. 2014. Novel activating mutations lacking cysteine in type I cytokine receptors in acute lymphoblastic leukemia. *Blood* **124:** 106–110. doi:10.1182/blood-2013-10-529685

Shuster JJ, Falletta JM, Pullen DJ, Crist WM, Humphrey GB, Dowell BL, Wharam MD, Borowitz M. 1990. Prognostic factors in childhood T-cell acute lymphoblastic leukemia: A Pediatric Oncology Group study. *Blood* **75:** 166–173.

Siebel C, Lendahl U. 2017. Notch signaling in development, tissue homeostasis, and disease. *Physiol Rev* **97:** 1235–1294. doi:10.1152/physrev.00005.2017

Simon C, Chagraoui J, Krosl J, Gendron P, Wilhelm B, Lemieux S, Boucher G, Chagnon P, Drouin S, Lambert R, et al. 2012. A key role for *EZH2* and associated genes in mouse and human adult T-cell acute leukemia. *Genes Dev* **26:** 651–656. doi:10.1101/gad.186411.111

Song WJ, Sullivan MG, Legare RD, Hutchings S, Tan X, Kufrin D, Ratajczak J, Resende IC, Haworth C, Hock R, et al. 1999. Haploinsufficiency of *CBFA2* causes familial thrombocytopenia with propensity to develop acute myelogenous leukaemia. *Nat Genet* **23:** 166–175. doi:10.1038/13793

Soulier J, Clappier E, Cayuela JM, Regnault A, García-Peydró M, Dombret H, Baruchel A, Toribio ML, Sigaux F. 2005. *HOXA* genes are included in genetic and biologic networks defining human acute T-cell leukemia (T-ALL). *Blood* **106:** 274–286. doi:10.1182/blood-2004-10-3900

Speleman F, Cauwelier B, Dastugue N, Cools J, Verhasselt B, Poppe B, Van Roy N, Vandesompele J, Graux C, Uyttebroeck A, et al. 2005. A new recurrent inversion, inv(7)(p15q34), leads to transcriptional activation of *HOXA10* and *HOXA11* in a subset of T-cell acute lymphoblastic leukemias. *Leukemia* **19:** 358–366. doi:10.1038/sj.leu.2403657

Stambolic V, Suzuki A, de la Pompa JL, Brothers GM, Mirtsos C, Sasaki T, Ruland J, Penninger JM, Siderovski DP, Mak TW. 1998. Negative regulation of PKB/Akt-dependent cell survival by the tumor suppressor PTEN. *Cell* **95:** 29–39. doi:10.1016/S0092-8674(00)81780-8

Stine ZE, Walton ZE, Altman BJ, Hsieh AL, Dang CV. 2015. MYC, metabolism, and cancer. *Cancer Discov* **5:** 1024–1039. doi:10.1158/2159-8290.CD-15-0507

Stock W, Johnson JL, Stone RM, Kolitz JE, Powell BL, Wetzler M, Westervelt P, Marcucci G, DeAngelo DJ, Vardiman JW, et al. 2013. Dose intensification of daunorubicin and cytarabine during treatment of adult acute lymphoblastic leukemia: Results of Cancer and Leukemia Group B Study 19802. *Cancer* **119:** 90–98. doi:10.1002/cncr.27617

Su XY, Della-Valle V, Andre-Schmutz I, Lemercier C, Radford-Weiss I, Ballerini P, Lessard M, Lafage-Pochitaloff M, Mugneret F, Berger R, et al. 2006. *HOX11L2/TLX3* is transcriptionally activated through T-cell regulatory elements downstream of *BCL11B* as a result of the t(5;14)(q35;q32). *Blood* **108:** 4198–4201. doi:10.1182/blood-2006-07-032953

Subramaniam PS, Whye DW, Efimenko E, Chen J, Tosello V, De Keersmaecker K, Kashishian A, Thompson MA, Castillo M, Cordon-Cardo C, et al. 2012. Targeting nonclassical oncogenes for therapy in T-ALL. *Cancer Cell* **21:** 459–472. doi:10.1016/j.ccr.2012.02.029

Sulis ML, Williams O, Palomero T, Tosello V, Pallikuppam S, Real PJ, Barnes K, Zuurbier L, Meijerink JP, Ferrando AA. 2008. NOTCH1 extracellular juxtamembrane expansion mutations in T-ALL. *Blood* **112:** 733–740. doi:10.1182/blood-2007-12-130096

Sutton R, Shaw PJ, Venn NC, Law T, Dissanayake A, Kilo T, Haber M, Norris MD, Fraser C, Alvaro F, et al. 2015. Persistent MRD before and after allogeneic BMT predicts relapse in children with acute lymphoblastic leukaemia. *Br J Haematol* **168:** 395–404. doi:10.1111/bjh.13142

Suzuki A, de la Pompa JL, Stambolic V, Elia AJ, Sasaki T, del Barco Barrantes I, Ho A, Wakeham A, Itie A, Khoo W, et al. 1998. High cancer susceptibility and embryonic lethality associated with mutation of the *PTEN* tumor suppressor gene in mice. *Curr Biol* **8:** 1169–1178. doi:10.1016/S0960-9822(07)00488-5

Swat W, Montgrain V, Doggett TA, Douangpanya J, Puri K, Vermi W, Diacovo TG. 2006. Essential role of PI3Kδ and PI3Kγ in thymocyte survival. *Blood* **107:** 2415–2422. doi:10.1182/blood-2005-08-3300

Takebe N, Nguyen D, Yang SX. 2014. Targeting notch signaling pathway in cancer: Clinical development advances and challenges. *Pharmacol Ther* **141:** 140–149. doi:10.1016/j.pharmthera.2013.09.005

Tallen G, Ratei R, Mann G, Kaspers G, Niggli F, Karachunsky A, Ebell W, Escherich G, Schrappe M, Klingebiel T, et al. 2010. Long-term outcome in children with relapsed acute lymphoblastic leukemia after time-point and site-of-relapse stratification and intensified short-course multidrug chemotherapy: Results of trial ALL-REZ BFM 90. *J Clin Oncol* **28:** 2339–2347. doi:10.1200/JCO.2009.25.1983

Tan SH, Yam AW, Lawton LN, Wong RW, Young RA, Look AT, Sanda T. 2016. TRIB2 reinforces the oncogenic transcriptional program controlled by the TAL1 complex in T-cell acute lymphoblastic leukemia. *Leukemia* **30:** 959–962. doi:10.1038/leu.2015.195

Tatarek J, Cullion K, Ashworth T, Gerstein R, Aster JC, Kelliher MA. 2011. Notch1 inhibition targets the leukemia-initiating cells in a *Tal1/Lmo2* mouse model of T-ALL. *Blood* **118:** 1579–1590. doi:10.1182/blood-2010-08-300343

Thiel E. 1985. Cell surface markers in leukemia: Biological and clinical correlations. *Crit Rev Oncol Hematol* **2:** 209–260. doi:10.1016/S1040-8428(85)80003-2

Thompson BJ, Buonamici S, Sulis ML, Palomero T, Vilimas T, Basso G, Ferrando A, Aifantis I. 2007. The SCF^{FBW7} ubiquitin ligase complex as a tumor suppressor in T cell leukemia. *J Exp Med* **204:** 1825–1835. doi:10.1084/jem.20070872

Ting CN, Olson MC, Barton KP, Leiden JM. 1996. Transcription factor GATA-3 is required for development of the T-cell lineage. *Nature* **384:** 474–478. doi:10.1038/384474a0

Tkachuk DC, Kohler S, Cleary ML. 1992. Involvement of a homolog of *Drosophila* trithorax by 11q23 chromosomal translocations in acute leukemias. *Cell* **71:** 691–700. doi:10.1016/0092-8674(92)90602-9

Todd MA, Picketts DJ. 2012. PHF6 interacts with the nucleosome remodeling and deacetylation (NuRD) complex. *J Proteome Res* **11:** 4326–4337. doi:10.1021/pr3004369

Tomita K, Hattori M, Nakamura E, Nakanishi S, Minato N, Kageyama R. 1999. The bHLH gene *Hes1* is essential for expansion of early T cell precursors. *Genes Dev* **13:** 1203–1210. doi:10.1101/gad.13.9.1203

Tosello V, Mansour MR, Barnes K, Paganin M, Sulis ML, Jenkinson S, Allen CG, Gale RE, Linch DC, Palomero T, et al. 2009. *WT1* mutations in T-ALL. *Blood* **114:** 1038–1045. doi:10.1182/blood-2008-12-192039

Treanor LM, Zhou S, Janke L, Churchman ML, Ma Z, Lu T, Chen SC, Mullighan CG, Sorrentino BP. 2014. Interleukin-7 receptor mutants initiate early T cell precursor leukemia in murine thymocyte progenitors with multipotent potential. *J Exp Med* **211:** 701–713. doi:10.1084/jem.20122727

Tremblay M, Tremblay CS, Herblot S, Aplan PD, Hebert J, Perreault C, Hoang T. 2010. Modeling T-cell acute lymphoblastic leukemia induced by the *SCL* and *LMO1* oncogenes. *Genes Dev* **24:** 1093–1105. doi:10.1101/gad.1897910

Tremblay CS, Brown FC, Collett M, Saw J, Chiu SK, Sonderegger SE, Lucas SE, Alserihi R, Chau N, Toribio ML, et al. 2016. Loss-of-function mutations of dynamin 2 promote T-ALL by enhancing IL-7 signalling. *Leukemia* **30:** 1993–2001. doi:10.1038/leu.2016.100

Trimarchi T, Bilal E, Ntziachristos P, Fabbri G, Dalla-Favera R, Tsirigos A, Aifantis I. 2014. Genome-wide mapping and characterization of Notch-regulated long noncoding RNAs in acute leukemia. *Cell* **158:** 593–606. doi:10.1016/j.cell.2014.05.049

Trinquand A, dos Santos NR, Tran Quang C, Rocchetti F, Zaniboni B, Belhocine M, de Costa de Jesus C, Lhermitte L, Tesio M, Dussiot M, et al. 2016. Triggering the TCR developmental checkpoint activates a therapeutically targetable tumor suppressive pathway in T-cell leukemia. *Cancer Discov* **6:** 972–985. doi:10.1158/2159-8290.CD-15-0675

Tzoneva G, Perez-Garcia A, Carpenter Z, Khiabanian H, Tosello V, Allegretta M, Paietta E, Racevskis J, Rowe JM, Tallman MS, et al. 2013. Activating mutations in the *NT5C2* nucleotidase gene drive chemotherapy resistance in relapsed ALL. *Nat Med* **19:** 368–371. doi:10.1038/nm.3078

Uchida T, Myers MJ, White MF. 2000. IRS-4 mediates protein kinase B signaling during insulin stimulation without promoting antiapoptosis. *Mol Cell Biol* **20:** 126–138. doi:10.1128/MCB.20.1.126-138.2000

Uderzo C, Dini G, Locatelli F, Miniero R, Tamaro P. 2000. Treatment of childhood acute lymphoblastic leukemia after the first relapse: Curative strategies. *Haematologica* **85:** 47–53.

Vanden Bempt M, Demeyer S, Broux M, De Bie J, Bornschein S, Mentens N, Vandepoel R, Geerdens E, Radaelli E, Bornhauser BC, et al. 2018. Cooperative enhancer activation by TLX1 and STAT5 drives development of NUP214-ABL1/TLX1-positive T cell acute lymphoblastic leukemia. *Cancer Cell* **34:** 271–285.e277. doi:10.1016/j.ccell.2018.07.007

Van der Meulen J, Sanghvi V, Mavrakis K, Durinck K, Fang F, Matthijssens F, Rondou P, Rosen M, Pieters T, Vandenberghe P, et al. 2015. The H3K27me3 demethylase UTX is a gender-specific tumor suppressor in T-cell acute lymphoblastic leukemia. *Blood* **125:** 13–21. doi:10.1182/blood-2014-05-577270

van Es JH, van Gijn ME, Riccio O, van den Born M, Vooijs M, Begthel H, Cozijnsen M, Robine S, Winton DJ, Radtke F, et al. 2005. Notch/γ-secretase inhibition turns proliferative cells in intestinal crypts and adenomas into goblet cells. *Nature* **435:** 959–963. doi:10.1038/nature03659

Van Limbergen H, Beverloo HB, van Drunen E, Janssens A, Hahlen K, Poppe B, Van Roy N, Marynen P, De Paepe A, Slater R, et al. 2001. Molecular cytogenetic and clinical findings in ETV6/ABL1-positive leukemia. *Genes Chromosomes Cancer* **30:** 274–282. doi:10.1002/1098-2264(2000)9999:9999<1::AID-GCC1089>3.0.CO;2-1 van Noort M, Clevers H. 2002. TCF transcription factors, mediators of Wnt-signaling in development and cancer. *Dev Biol* **244:** 1–8. doi:10.1006/dbio.2001.0566

Van Vlierberghe P, van Grotel M, Beverloo HB, Lee C, Helgason T, Buijs-Gladdines J, Passier M, van Wering ER, Veerman AJ, Kamps WA, et al. 2006. The cryptic chromosomal deletion del(11)(p12p13) as a new activation mechanism of *LMO2* in pediatric T-cell acute lymphoblastic leukemia. *Blood* **108:** 3520–3529. doi:10.1182/blood-2006-04-019927

Van Vlierberghe P, Beverloo HB, Buijs-Gladdines J, van Wering ER, Horstmann M, Pieters R, Meijerink JP. 2008a. Monoallelic or biallelic *LMO2* expression in relation to the *LMO2* rearrangement status in pediatric T-cell acute lymphoblastic leukemia. *Leukemia* **22:** 1434–1437. doi:10.1038/sj.leu.2405063

Van Vlierberghe P, van Grotel M, Tchinda J, Lee C, Beverloo HB, van der Spek PJ, Stubbs A, Cools J, Nagata K, Fornerod M, et al. 2008b. The recurrent *SET-NUP214* fusion as a new *HOXA* activation mechanism in pediatric T-cell acute lymphoblastic leukemia. *Blood* **111:** 4668–4680. doi:10.1182/blood-2007-09-111872

Van Vlierberghe P, Palomero T, Khiabanian H, Van der Meulen J, Castillo M, Van Roy N, De Moerloose B, Philippé J, González-García S, Toribio ML, et al. 2010. *PHF6* mutations in T-cell acute lymphoblastic leukemia. *Nat Genet* **42:** 338–342. doi:10.1038/ng.542

Van Vlierberghe P, Ambesi-Impiombato A, Perez-Garcia A, Haydu JE, Rigo I, Hadler M, Tosello V, Della Gatta G, Paietta E, Racevskis J, et al. 2011a. *ETV6* mutations in early immature human T cell leukemias. *J Exp Med* **208:** 2571–2579. doi:10.1084/jem.20112239

Van Vlierberghe P, Patel J, Abdel-Wahab O, Lobry C, Hedvat CV, Balbin M, Nicolas C, Payer AR, Fernandez HF, Tallman MS, et al. 2011b. *PHF6* mutations in adult acute myeloid leukemia. *Leukemia* **25:** 130–134. doi:10.1038/leu.2010.247

Van Vlierberghe P, Ambesi-Impiombato A, De Keersmaecker K, Hadler M, Paietta E, Tallman MS, Rowe JM, Forne C, Rue M, Ferrando AA. 2013. Prognostic relevance of integrated genetic profiling in adult T-cell acute lymphoblastic leukemia. *Blood* **122:** 74–82. doi:10.1182/blood-2013-03-491092

Vivanco I, Sawyers CL. 2002. The phosphatidylinositol 3-kinase-AKT pathway in human cancer. *Nat Rev Cancer* **2:** 489–501. doi:10.1038/nrc839

Vrooman LM, Silverman LB. 2009. Childhood acute lymphoblastic leukemia: Update on prognostic factors. *Curr Opin Pediatr* **21:** 1–8. doi:10.1097/MOP.0b013e32831f1f24

Wakabayashi Y, Inoue J, Takahashi Y, Matsuki A, Kosugi-Okano H, Shinbo T, Mishima Y, Niwa O, Kominami R. 2003a. Homozygous deletions and point mutations of the *Rit1/Bcl11b* gene in γ-ray induced mouse thymic lymphomas. *Biochem Biophys Res Commun* **301:** 598–603. doi:10.1016/S0006-291X(02)03069-3

Wakabayashi Y, Watanabe H, Inoue J, Takeda N, Sakata J, Mishima Y, Hitomi J, Yamamoto T, Utsuyama M, Niwa O, et al. 2003b. *Bcl11b* is required for differentiation and survival of αβ T lymphocytes. *Nat Immunol* **4:** 533–539. doi:10.1038/ni927

Wang LC, Swat W, Fujiwara Y, Davidson L, Visvader J, Kuo F, Alt FW, Gilliland DG, Golub TR, Orkin SH. 1998. The *TEL/ETV6* gene is required specifically for hematopoiesis in the bone marrow. *Genes Dev* **12:** 2392–2402. doi:10.1101/gad.12.15.2392

Wang J, Jani-Sait SN, Escalon EA, Carroll AJ, de Jong PJ, Kirsch IR, Aplan PD. 2000. The t(14;21)(q11.2;q22) chromosomal translocation associated with T-cell acute lymphoblastic leukemia activates the *BHLHB1* gene. *Proc Natl Acad Sci* **97:** 3497–3502. doi:10.1073/pnas.97.7.3497

Wang J, Leung JW, Gong Z, Feng L, Shi X, Chen J. 2013. PHF6 regulates cell cycle progression by suppressing ribosomal RNA synthesis. *J Biol Chem* **288:** 3174–3183. doi:10.1074/jbc.M112.414839

Wang H, Zang C, Taing L, Arnett KL, Wong YJ, Pear WS, Blacklow SC, Liu XS, Aster JC. 2014. NOTCH1-RBPJ complexes drive target gene expression through dynamic interactions with superenhancers. *Proc Natl Acad Sci* **111:** 705–710. doi:10.1073/pnas.1315023111

Webb LM, Vigorito E, Wymann MP, Hirsch E, Turner M. 2005. Cutting edge: T cell development requires the combined activities of the p110γ and p110δ catalytic isoforms of phosphatidylinositol 3-kinase. *J Immunol* **175:** 2783–2787. doi:10.4049/jimmunol.175.5.2783

Weber BN, Chi AW, Chavez A, Yashiro-Ohtani Y, Yang Q, Shestova O, Bhandoola A. 2011. A critical role for TCF-1 in T-lineage specification and differentiation. *Nature* **476:** 63–68. doi:10.1038/nature10279

Wei G, Twomey D, Lamb J, Schlis K, Agarwal J, Stam RW, Opferman JT, Sallan SE, den Boer ML, Pieters R, et al. 2006. Gene expression-based chemical genomics identifies rapamycin as a modulator of MCL1 and glucocorticoid resistance. *Cancer Cell* **10:** 331–342. doi:10.1016/j.ccr.2006.09.006

Wei P, Walls M, Qiu M, Ding R, Denlinger RH, Wong A, Tsaparikos K, Jani JP, Hosea N, Sands M, et al. 2010. Evaluation of selective gamma-secretase inhibitor PF-03084014 for its antitumor efficacy and gastrointestinal safety to guide optimal clinical trial design. *Mol Cancer Ther* **9:** 1618–1628. doi:10.1158/1535-7163.MCT-10-0034

Welch JS, Ley TJ, Link DC, Miller CA, Larson DE, Koboldt DC, Wartman LD, Lamprecht TL, Liu F, Xia J, et al. 2012. The origin and evolution of mutations in acute myeloid leukemia. *Cell* **150:** 264–278. doi:10.1016/j.cell.2012.06.023

Welcker M, Orian A, Jin J, Grim JE, Harper JW, Eisenman RN, Clurman BE. 2004. The Fbw7 tumor suppressor regulates glycogen synthase kinase 3 phosphorylation-dependent c-Myc protein degradation. *Proc Natl Acad Sci* **101:** 9085–9090. doi:10.1073/pnas.0402770101

Wendorff AA, Koch U, Wunderlich FT, Wirth S, Dubey C, Brüning JC, MacDonald HR, Radtke F. 2010. Hes1 is a critical but context-dependent mediator of canonical Notch signaling in lymphocyte development and transformation. *Immunity* **33:** 671–684. doi:10.1016/j.immuni.2010.11.014

Wendorff AA, Quinn SA, Rashkovan M, Madubata CJ, Ambesi-Impiombato A, Litzow MR, Tallman MS, Paietta E, Paganin M, Basso G, et al. 2018. *Phf6* loss enhances HSC self-renewal driving tumor initiation and leukemia stem cell activity in T-ALL. *Cancer Discov* **9:** 436–451. doi:10.1158/2159-8290.CD-18-1005

Weng AP, Ferrando AA, Lee W, Morris J, Silverman LB, Sanchez-Irizarry C, Blacklow SC, Look AT, Aster JC. 2004. Activating mutations of *NOTCH1* in human T cell acute lymphoblastic leukemia. *Science* **306:** 269–271. doi:10.1126/science.1102160

Weng AP, Millholland JM, Yashiro-Ohtani Y, Arcangeli ML, Lau A, Wai C, Del Bianco C, Rodriguez CG, Sai H, Tobias J, et al. 2006. c-*Myc* is an important direct target of Notch1 in T-cell acute lymphoblastic leukemia/lymphoma. *Genes Dev* **20:** 2096–2109. doi:10.1101/gad.1450406

Winter SS, Dunsmore KP, Devidas M, Wood BL, Esiashvili N, Chen Z, Eisenberg N, Briegel N, Hayashi RJ, Gastier-Foster JM, et al. 2018. Improved survival for children and young adults with T-lineage acute lymphoblastic leukemia: Results From the Children's Oncology Group AALL0434 Methotrexate Randomization. *J Clin Oncol* **36:** 2926–2934. doi:10.1200/JCO.2018.77.7250

Wong GW, Knowles GC, Mak TW, Ferrando AA, Zuñiga-Pflücker JC. 2012. HES1 opposes a PTEN-dependent check on survival, differentiation, and proliferation of TCRβ-selected mouse thymocytes. *Blood* **120:** 1439–1448. doi:10.1182/blood-2011-12-395319

Wu Y, Cain-Hom C, Choy L, Hagenbeek TJ, de Leon GP, Chen Y, Finkle D, Venook R, Wu X, Ridgway J, et al. 2010. Therapeutic antibody targeting of individual Notch receptors. *Nature* **464:** 1052–1057. doi:10.1038/nature08878

Wuchter C, Ruppert V, Schrappe M, Dorken B, Ludwig WD, Karawajew L. 2002. In vitro susceptibility to dexamethasone- and doxorubicin-induced apoptotic cell death in context of maturation stage, responsiveness to interleukin 7, and early cytoreduction in vivo in childhood T-cell acute lymphoblastic leukemia. *Blood* **99:** 4109–4115. doi:10.1182/blood.V99.11.4109

Xia Y, Brown L, Yang CY, Tsan JT, Siciliano MJ, Espinosa R III, Le Beau MM, Baer RJ. 1991. *TAL2*, a helix-loop-helix gene activated by the (7;9)(q34;q32) translocation in human T-cell leukemia. *Proc Natl Acad Sci* **88:** 11416–11420. doi:10.1073/pnas.88.24.11416

Xiong H, Maraver A, Latkowski JA, Henderson T, Schlessinger K, Ding Y, Shen J, Tadokoro CE, Lafaille JJ. 2013. Characterization of two distinct lymphoproliferative diseases caused by ectopic expression of the Notch ligand DLL4 on T cells. *PLoS ONE* **8:** e84841. doi:10.1371/journal.pone.0084841

Yada M, Hatakeyama S, Kamura T, Nishiyama M, Tsunematsu R, Imaki H, Ishida N, Okumura F, Nakayama K, Nakayama KI. 2004. Phosphorylation-dependent degradation of c-*Myc* is mediated by the F-box protein Fbw7. *EMBO J* **23:** 2116–2125. doi:10.1038/sj.emboj.7600217

Yashiro-Ohtani Y, Wang H, Zang C, Arnett KL, Bailis W, Ho Y, Knoechel B, Lanauze C, Louis L, Forsyth KS, et al. 2014. Long-range enhancer activity determines *Myc* sensitivity to Notch inhibitors in T cell leukemia. *Proc Natl Acad Sci* **111:** E4946–E4953. doi:10.1073/pnas.1407079111

Yilmaz OH, Valdez R, Theisen BK, Guo W, Ferguson DO, Wu H, Morrison SJ. 2006. Pten dependence distinguishes haematopoietic stem cells from leukaemia-initiating cells. *Nature* **441:** 475–482. doi:10.1038/nature04703

Yokoyama K, Yokoyama N, Izawa K, Kotani A, Harashima A, Hozumi K, Tojo A. 2013. In vivo leukemogenic potential of an interleukin 7 receptor α chain mutant in hematopoietic stem and progenitor cells. *Blood* **122:** 4259–4263. doi:10.1182/blood-2012-08-451278

Yoshizato T, Dumitriu B, Hosokawa K, Makishima H, Yoshida K, Townsley D, Sato-Otsubo A, Sato Y, Liu D, Suzuki H, et al. 2015. Somatic mutations and clonal hematopoiesis in aplastic anemia. *N Engl J Med* **373:** 35–47. doi:10.1056/NEJMoa1414799

Zenatti PP, Ribeiro D, Li W, Zuurbier L, Silva MC, Paganin M, Tritapoe J, Hixon JA, Silveira AB, Cardoso BA, et al. 2011. Oncogenic *IL7R* gain-of-function mutations in childhood T-cell acute lymphoblastic leukemia. *Nat Genet* **43:** 932–939. doi:10.1038/ng.924

Zhang Y, Xiong Y, Yarbrough WG. 1998. ARF promotes MDM2 degradation and stabilizes p53: *ARF-INK4a* locus deletion impairs both the Rb and p53 tumor suppression pathways. *Cell* **92:** 725–734. doi:10.1016/S0092-8674(00)81401-4

Zhang J, Grindley JC, Yin T, Jayasinghe S, He XC, Ross JT, Haug JS, Rupp D, Porter-Westpfahl KS, Wiedemann LM, et al. 2006. PTEN maintains haematopoietic stem cells and acts in lineage choice and leukaemia prevention. *Nature* **441:** 518–522. doi:10.1038/nature04747

Zhang J, Ding L, Holmfeldt L, Wu G, Heatley SL, Payne-Turner D, Easton J, Chen X, Wang J, Rusch M, et al. 2012. The genetic basis of early T-cell precursor acute lymphoblastic leukaemia. *Nature* **481:** 157–163. doi:10.1038/nature10725

Zhang C, Mejia LA, Huang J, Valnegri P, Bennett EJ, Anckar J, Jahani-Asl A, Gallardo G, Ikeuchi Y, Yamada T, et al. 2013. The X-linked intellectual disability protein PHF6 associates with the PAF1 complex and regulates neuronal migration in the mammalian brain. *Neuron* **78:** 986–993. doi:10.1016/j.neuron.2013.04.021

Zhang J, Zhang Y, Zhang M, Liu C, Liu X, Yin J, Wu P, Chen X, Yang W, Zhang L, et al. 2018. FLT3 pathway is a potential therapeutic target for PRC2-mutated T-cell acute lymphoblastic leukemia. *Blood* **132:** 2520–2524. doi:10.1182/blood-2018-04-845628

Zuurbier L, Petricoin EF III, Vuerhard MJ, Calvert V, Kooi C, Buijs-Gladdines JG, Smits WK, Sonneveld E, Veerman AJ, Kamps WA, et al. 2012. The significance of *PTEN* and *AKT* aberrations in pediatric T-cell acute lymphoblastic leukemia. *Haematologica* **97:** 1405–1413. doi:10.3324/haematol.2011.059030

The Biology of B-Progenitor Acute Lymphoblastic Leukemia

Kathryn G. Roberts and Charles G. Mullighan

Department of Pathology, St. Jude Children's Research Hospital, Memphis, Tennessee 38105, USA

Correspondence: charles.mullighan@stjude.org

Genomic analyses have revolutionized our understanding of the biology of B-progenitor acute lymphoblastic leukemia (ALL). Studies of thousands of cases across the age spectrum have revised the taxonomy of B-ALL by identifying multiple new subgroups with diverse sequence and structural initiating events that vary substantially by age at diagnosis and prognostic significance. There is a growing appreciation of the role of inherited genetic variation in predisposition to ALL and drug responsiveness and of the nature of genetic variegation and clonal evolution that may be targeted for improved diagnostic, risk stratification, disease monitoring, and therapeutic intervention. This review provides an overview of the current state of knowledge of the genetic basis of B-ALL, with an emphasis on recent discoveries that have changed our approach to diagnosis and monitoring.

B-progenitor acute lymphoblastic leukemia (B-ALL) is the most common childhood cancer, with cure rates exceeding 90% in most developed countries (Hunger and Mullighan 2015). However, the prognosis for ALL declines with increasing age, with historic cure rates of just 30%–40% in adults (age ≥ 40 yr) (Frey and Luger 2015). B-progenitor acute lymphoblastic leukemia (B-ALL) comprises multiple subtypes characterized by recurrent disease-initiating genetic alterations that are important for risk stratification. These include aneuploidy (gain or loss of whole chromosomes) or chromosomal translocations that deregulate genes through the formation of chimeric fusions or by juxtaposition to strong enhancers and commonly involve hematopoietic transcription factors, epigenetic modifiers, cytokine receptors, and tyrosine kinases (Iacobucci and Mullighan 2017). Cooperating genetic events that contribute to leukemogenesis include copy number alterations and sequence mutations that perturb multiple cellular pathways. In recent years, the rapid development and implementation of next-generation sequencing techniques has revolutionized our understanding of the genomic landscape of ALL by identifying genomic alterations that were previously cryptic and by enabling comprehensive characterization of both germline and somatic alterations that define each subtype across the age spectrum, as well as characterizing the nature of clonal variegation, genetic heterogeneity, and disease progression (Mullighan et al. 2008b; Ma et al. 2015; Tzoneva et al. 2018). In addition to refining risk stratification, these studies have also identified new therapeu-

Cite this article as *Cold Spring Harb Perspect Med* doi: 10.1101/cshperspect.a034835

tic targets that guide precision medicine approaches intended to improve the cure rate while reducing adverse treatment effects.

Here, we will review the genomic landscape of B-ALL with particular emphasis on new subtypes and prognosis and discuss both somatic and inherited variants that contribute to leukemogenesis. The role of the interaction between leukemic cells and the bone marrow microenvironment in disease development and response to treatment will also be discussed.

RECURRENT CHROMOSOMAL ALTERATIONS AND PROGNOSIS

The frequency of subtype-defining alterations varies with age (Table 1; Fig. 1). Secondary genetic alterations may be acquired or enriched during disease progression (Mullighan et al. 2007, 2008b; Moorman et al. 2012). Common targets include lymphoid transcription factors (*IKZF1, PAX5, EBF1, ETV6*), cell cycle regulators and tumor suppressors (*CDKN2A/B, TP53, RB1*), regulators of lymphoid signaling (*BTLA* and *CD200*), Ras pathway signaling (*NRAS, KRAS, PTPN11*), and chromatin modifiers (*CREBBP, SETD2, WHSC1*) (Kuiper et al. 2007; Mullighan et al. 2007). The prevalence, gene, and type of alteration vary between subtypes and have different prognostic relevance. Current risk stratification and treatment algorithms incorporate age, sex, presentation white blood cell count, established cytogenetic alterations, and response to initial therapy as measured by levels of minimal residual disease (MRD). Genomic alterations including composite copy number alterations have recently been proposed as important factors for determining prognosis (Hamadeh et al. 2019). Because MRD is such a central component of risk stratification, future clinical trials should aim to integrate new genomic information with response to therapy to develop a comprehensive relapse prediction model (O'Connor et al. 2018).

Gross Chromosomal Abnormalities

High hyperdiploidy (nonrandom gain of at least five chromosomes) is present in ~25% of childhood ALL patients, but accounts for <5% of adolescents and young adults (16–39 yr old; AYA) and adults, and is associated with a favorable outcome. The patterns of chromosomal gain are nonrandom, and most commonly involve chromosomes 4, 10, 14, and 21 and the X chromosome. Mutations involving the Ras pathway (*KRAS, NRAS, PTPN11*) and epigenetic modifiers are frequent genetic events in hyperdiploid patients (Paulsson et al. 2015). Hypodiploid ALL with less than 44 chromosomes comprises two principal subtypes with distinct transcriptional profiles and genetic alterations. Historically, hypodiploid ALL has been associated with an unfavorable prognosis (Harrison et al. 2004); however, the outcome is improved with contemporary studies utilizing MRD risk-stratified regimens, and transplantation provides no additional survival benefit compared to chemotherapy alone in MRD-negative patients (Mullighan et al. 2015; Pui et al. 2019). Patients with low hypodiploidy (31–39 chromosomes) commonly harbor deletion of *IKZF2* and sequence mutations of *TP53* that are frequently inherited (Holmfeldt et al. 2013). This subtype is rare in children (<1%), but increases with age, accounting for >10% of adults, and is associated with a very poor outcome (Moorman et al. 2007; Gu et al. 2019). Patients with near-haploid ALL (24–30 chromosomes) present at a younger age, accounting for ~2% of childhood ALL (Holmfeldt et al. 2013). Frequent secondary alterations in this subtype include Ras-activating mutations and deletions of *IKZF3* (Holmfeldt et al. 2013; Gu et al. 2019). Doubling of the hypodiploid clone (known as masked hypodiploidy) is common in both near-haploid and low-hypodiploid ALL and results in a modal chromosome number in the hyperdiploid range. Given the markedly differing prognoses of hypodiploid and hyperdiploid ALL, it is important to distinguish masked hypodiploidy (which typically shows four copies of multiple chromosomes in the doubled clone, and copy-neutral loss of heterozygosity of multiple chromosomes) from hyperdiploidy (which typically has multiple trisomic chromosomes).

ALL with intrachromosomal amplification of chromosome 21 (iAMP21) defines a subtype

Table 1. Prevalence and prognosis of subtypes in B-ALL

ALL subtype	Category	Median age (yr)	Prevalence	Genomic alterations	Clinical features	Reference(s)
Hyperdiploid (>50 chromosomes)	Aneuploid	4	High in children (25%)	Ras pathway Epigenetic modifiers	Excellent prognosis	Paulsson et al. 2015
Low-hypodiploid (31–39 chromosomes)	Aneuploid	47	High in adults (10%–15%)	*IKZF2* del, *TP53* mut (commonly inherited)	Poor prognosis	Holmfeldt et al. 2013
Near-haploid (24–30 chromosomes)	Aneuploid	5.4	<3% in all ages	Ras pathway, *IKZF3* del	Intermediate prognosis	Holmfeldt et al. 2013
iAMP21	Copy number gain	10	~3% in children and AYA	Complex structural alterations of chromosome 21	Good prognosis with intensive therapy, low WBC	Harrison 2015
ETV6-RUNX1 t(12;21)(p13;q22)	TF rearrangement	4	High in children (25%)	*PAX5* del, *WHSC1* mut	Excellent prognosis	Mullighan et al. 2007; Jaffe et al. 2013
ETV6-RUNX1-like	TF rearrangement	3	~3% in children	*ETV6* fusions and del, *IKZF1* fusions and del	Unknown	Lilljebjörn et al. 2016; Zaliova et al. 2017
DUX4-rearranged	TF rearrangement	14.3	Peak in AYA (~8%)	*ERG* del, *IKZF1* del, Ras pathway	Excellent prognosis	Lilljebjörn et al. 2016; Yasuda et al. 2016; Zhang et al. 2016
KMT2A-rearranged	TF rearrangement	40	High in infants (~90%) and adults (~15%)	Ras pathway (commonly subclonal)	Poor prognosis, sensitive to bortezomib or DOT1L inhibition	Andersson et al. 2015
TCF3-PBX1 t(1;19)(q23;p13)	TF rearrangement	8	~5% in children, rarely in adults		Good prognosis, CNS relapse	Barber et al. 2007; Burmeister et al. 2010
ZNF384-rearranged	TF rearrangement	15	Peak in AYA (~5%)	Epigenetic modifiers, Ras pathway	Intermediate prognosis	Liu et al. 2016; Shago et al. 2016; Yasuda et al. 2016
MEF2D-rearranged	TF rearrangement	14	Peak in AYA (~7%)	Ras pathway	Intermediate prognosis, sensitive to HDAC inhibition	Gu et al. 2016; Suzuki et al. 2016
NUTM1-rearranged	TF rearrangement	3	Exclusively in children (1%)	Unknown	Excellent prognosis	Li et al. 2018; Gu et al. 2019

Continued

Table 1. *Continued*

ALL subtype	Category	Median age (yr)	Prevalence	Genomic alterations	Clinical features	Reference(s)
TCF3-HLF t(17;19)(q22;p13)	TF rearrangement	15	Very rare in all ages (<1%)	*TCF3* mut, *PAX5* del, Ras pathway	Very poor prognosis, sensitive to Bcl2 inhibition	Fischer et al. 2015
PAX5alt	Other TF-driven	10	Highest in children (~11%)	*PAX5* fusion, mut, amp	Intermediate prognosis	Li et al. 2018; Gu et al. 2019
PAX5 P80R	Other TF-driven	22	Highest in adults (~4%)	Ras pathway	Intermediate prognosis	Li et al. 2018; Gu et al. 2019
IKZF1 N159Y	Other TF-driven		Very rare in all ages (<1%)	Unknown	Unknown	Li et al. 2018; Gu et al. 2019
BCL2/*MYC*-rearranged	Other TF-driven	48	Almost exclusively in AYA and adults (~3%)	Unknown	Poor prognosis	Gu et al. 2019
Ph-like	Kinase-driven	21	Peaks in AYA (25%–30%)	Multiple kinase alterations, *IKZF1* del and mut, *CDKN2A/B* del	Poor prognosis, amenable to TKI therapy	Roberts et al. 2014a, 2017a
BCR-ABL1 t(9;22)(q34;q11.2)	Kinase-driven	40–45	5% in children, highest in adults (40%–50%)	*IKZF1* del and mut, *CDKN2A/B* del	Historically poor prognosis, improved with TKI	Mullighan et al. 2008a; Roberts et al. 2014a, 2017a
Other		16	~5% in children, ~10% in AYA and adults	Unknown	Intermediate prognosis	

(AYA) Adolescent and young adult, (amp) amplification, (B-ALL) B-progenitor acute lymphoblastic leukemia, (CNS) central nervous system, (del) deletion, (HDAC) histone deacetylase, (mut) sequence mutation, (TF) transcription factor, (TKI) tyrosine kinase inhibitor.

Cite this article as *Cold Spring Harb Perspect Med* doi: 10.1101/cshperspect.a034835

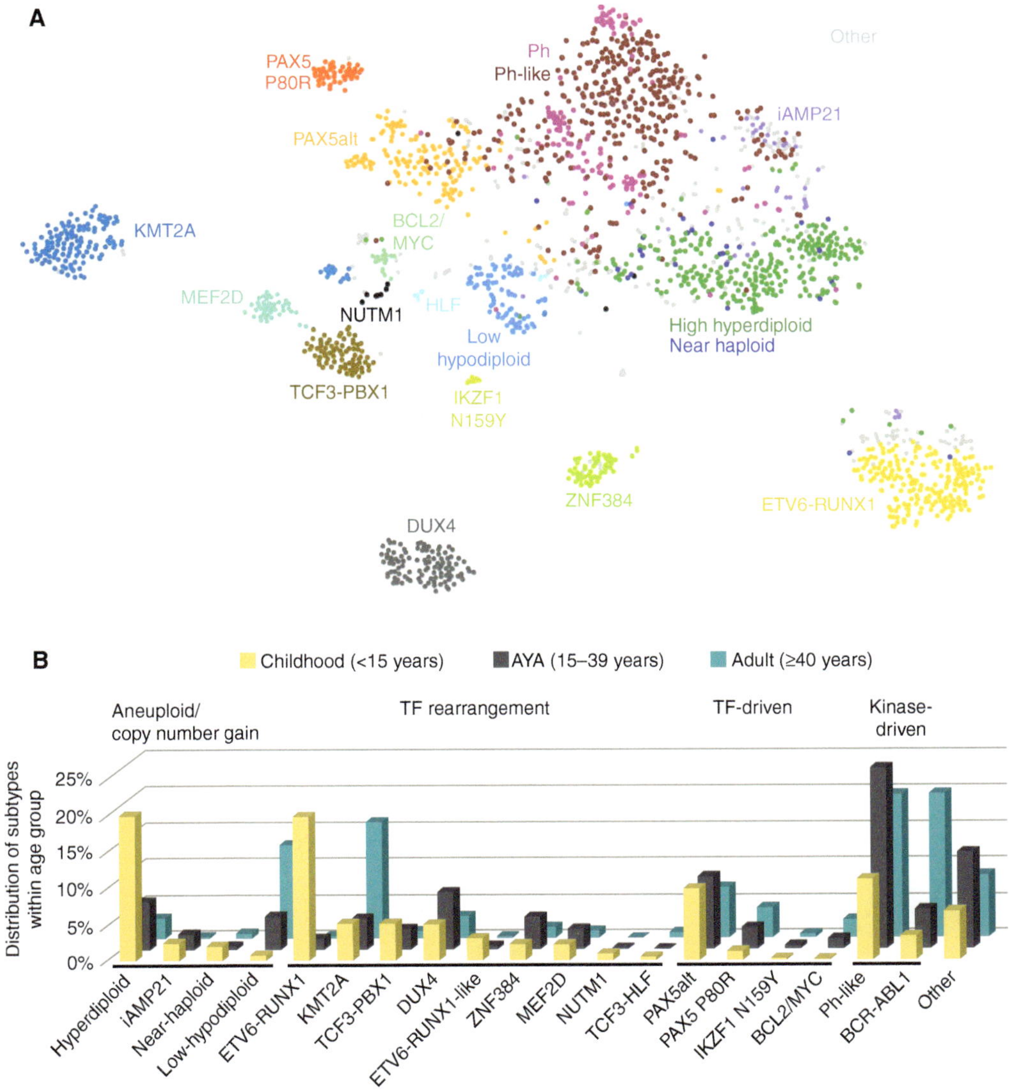

Figure 1. (*A*) tSNE plot showing B-progenitor acute lymphoblastic leukemia (B-ALL) subtypes based on RNA-seq gene expression profiling of 1988 cases. (*B*) Distribution of B-ALL subtypes within each age group. Subtypes are grouped as gross chromosomal abnormalities (aneuploidy or copy number gain), transcription factor (TF) rearrangement, other TF-driven, kinase-driven, and all others (Gu et al. 2019).

of ALL that is more common in older children (median age 10 yr), and is rarely observed in patients older than 30 yr (Harrison et al. 2014). The role of iAMP21 in leukemogenesis is unclear, but a common region of amplification includes *ERG* and *DYRK1A* with gain of at least two copies of *RUNX1* (Li et al. 2014). Secondary events include the *P2RY8-CRLF2* fusion and genetic alterations in kinase signaling, including *IL7R* and *FLT3*. Improved risk stratification and treatment with intensive therapy can rescue the poor outcome of these patients when treated as standard-risk (Moorman et al. 2013).

Translocations

ETV6-RUNX1, encoded by the t(12;21)(p13;q22) translocation, is another favorable cytogenetic alteration with a high frequency in childhood ALL (25%) and <5% in AYAs and adults. Secondary DNA copy number alterations, notably *PAX5* deletion, and mutation of *WHSC1* are frequent genetic events in patients harboring *ETV6-RUNX1* (Mullighan et al. 2007; Jaffe et al. 2013; Papaemmanuil et al. 2014). *KMT2A* (*MLL*) rearrangements are a hallmark of infant ALL (age < 1 yr). They also account for a significant proportion of adults with ALL (~15%) and are associated with a poor prognosis in all ages (Hunger and Mullighan 2015). The reasons underlying the biphasic distribution in age are not well understood. In infant cases, *KMT2A* rearrangement is frequently acquired in utero (Ford et al. 1993), and patients harbor very few cooperating lesions, suggesting the rearrangement itself is sufficient to induce leukemia (Andersson et al. 2015). The most commonly perturbed pathways include PI3K and Ras signaling, with the majority of mutations present at a low tumor burden (Driessen et al. 2013; Andersson et al. 2015; Agraz-Doblas et al. 2019). Subclonal activating mutations of *FLT3* were recently shown to accelerate disease onset in a mouse model of *KMT2A*-rearranged leukemia, suggesting these alterations can influence the rate of leukemogenesis even at low levels (Hyrenius-Wittsten et al. 2018).

TCF3-PBX1, encoded by the t(1;19)(q23;p13) translocation, is present in ~5% of children and less in AYAs and adults. Previously considered a high-risk subtype with a propensity to central nervous system relapse, it is now associated with a favorable outcome on contemporary ALL therapies (Barber et al. 2007; Burmeister et al. 2010). By contrast the t(17;19)(q22;p13) translocation, encoding the *TCF3-HLF* fusion gene, defines a rare subtype of ALL (<1% in all ages) with a distinct transcriptional profile that is typically associated with an overall survival of <2 yr from diagnosis (Inaba et al. 1992; Hunger 1996). Interestingly, primary leukemic cells harboring *TCF3-HLF* show sensitivity to the BCL2 inhibitor venetoclax (ABT-199), identifying a new therapeutic option for this fatal subtype (Fischer et al. 2015).

BCR-ABL1 ALL is uncommon in children (2%–5% of patients), but accounts for at least 25% of adults (Roberts et al. 2014a, 2017a). The addition of ABL1 tyrosine kinase inhibitors (TKIs) to chemotherapeutic regimens in both children and adults has significantly improved the survival of *BCR-ABL1*-positive patients (Ravandi et al. 2010; Schultz et al. 2014; Slayton et al. 2018). *IKZF1* alterations (deletion or mutation) are a hallmark of kinase-driven ALL (Ph+ and Ph-like) and are associated with treatment failure and relapse, even in the era of TKI therapy (Mullighan et al. 2008a; Martinelli et al. 2009; Roberts et al. 2014a; Slayton et al. 2018). The co-occurrence of *IKZF1* deletions with *CDKN2A/B*, *PAX5*, or PAR1 deletions in the absence of *ERG* deletions (termed *IKZF1*^{plus}) detected by multiplex ligation probe amplification (MLPA) in childhood ALL confers a worse prognosis compared to patients with *IKZF1* deletion who do not fulfill the criteria for *IKZF1*^{plus} (Stanulla et al. 2018). Although technically straightforward, identification of *IKZF1*^{plus} as a biomarker of poor outcome is limited by the inability of the MLPA approach to identify the full spectrum of *IKZF1* alterations, cases with high-risk ALL that do not have *IKZF1* alterations, and the lack of *ERG* deletion in approximately one-third of *DUX4* cases that commonly have *IKZF1* alterations and favorable outcome.

NEW SUBTYPES IN B-ALL

The application of comprehensive sequencing and integrative analyses continues to refine the genomic landscape of ALL, resulting in the identification of new entities with prognostic and therapeutic significance. Rearrangements in these new subtypes involve a diverse range of partners that converge on a single gene (e.g., *MEF2D* and *ZNF384*-rearranged ALL) or are cryptic by cytogenetic analysis (e.g., *DUX4*-rearranged ALL). Other subtypes may harbor alteration of a range of driver genes by diverse mechanisms (e.g., Ph-like ALL) or are initiated by sequence mutations (e.g., PAX5 P80R and IKZF1 N159Y). Additional groups have similar gene expression profiles to known subtypes with different genetic alterations (Ph-like and *ETV6-RUNX1*-like ALL).

Ph-like ALL: An Opportunity for Targeted Therapies

Philadelphia chromosome like (Ph-like or *BCR-ABL1*-like) ALL was incorporated as a provisional entity to the revision of the World Health Organization (WHO) classification of acute leukemia in 2016 (Arber et al. 2016). Leukemic cells from patients with Ph-like ALL have similar transcriptional profiles to Ph+ ALL but lack the *BCR-ABL1* fusion gene (Den Boer et al. 2009; Mullighan et al. 2009). Similar to with Ph+ ALL, the incidence of Ph-like ALL increases with age, comprising 10%–15% of childhood ALL cases, >20% of adults, and peaking at 25%–30% in AYAs (Loh et al. 2013; Roberts et al. 2014a, 2017a, 2018; Jain et al. 2017a; Reshmi et al. 2017; Tasian et al. 2017a). In all ages, Ph-like ALL is associated with elevated MRD levels and/or higher rates of treatment failure compared to non-Ph-like ALL patients (Roberts et al. 2014a, 2017a; Tasian et al. 2017b). Thus, the inferior treatment outcomes in AYA and adults may be partly explained by the high prevalence of Ph-like ALL. In Children's Oncology Group (COG) cohorts of National Cancer Institute (NCI) standard-risk (SR) ALL, Ph-like ALL is less common and confers a better prognosis compared to children with high-risk (HR) ALL (Roberts et al. 2018). Furthermore, children with Ph-like ALL treated on St. Jude Total XV studies had a favorable outcome with MRD risk-directed therapy intensification (Roberts et al. 2014b).

Ph-like ALL is genetically heterogeneous and is characterized by rearrangements, copy number alterations, and sequence mutations that activate tyrosine kinase or cytokine receptor signaling. Despite this complexity, most alterations can be divided into a limited number of distinct subgroups based on the activated kinase and signaling pathways. These include rearrangements or, less commonly, sequence mutations of *CRLF2 (IGH-CRLF2, P2RY8-CRLF2)*, fusions involving ABL-class genes (*ABL1, ABL2, CSF1R, LYN, PDGFRA, PDGFRB*), alterations activating JAK-STAT signaling (including rearrangements of *JAK2, EPOR* or *TYK2*) and mutations/deletions of *IL7R, SH2B3, JAK1, JAK3, TYK2, IL2RB*), Ras signaling pathways (*NRAS, KRAS, PTPN11*), and less common fusions (*FLT3, FGFR1, NTRK3, PTK2B*) (Fig. 2A; Roberts et al. 2014a, 2017a; Reshmi et al. 2017). The frequency of each kinase subgroup varies with age, particularly with respect to *CRLF2*-rearrangements, in which *IGH-CRLF2* accounts for almost 50% of Ph-like ALL in AYAs and adults but is less common in children. ABL-class fusions are most prevalent in children with HR ALL (Fig. 2B). Fewer kinase alterations are identified in Ph-like ALL patients with SR ALL (Roberts et al. 2018). A small subset of children harboring rearrangement of *CRLF2*—most commonly *P2RY8-CRLF2* and with Down syndrome ALL—lack the Ph-like ALL gene expression signature (Gu et al. 2019).

The majority of Ph-like alterations can be targeted effectively in preclinical models using a combinatorial approach of chemotherapy with ABL1 (e.g., dasatinib) or JAK inhibition (e.g., ruxolitinib) (Roberts et al. 2017b), and a number of case reports demonstrate efficacy of ABL1 TKI treatment in Ph-like ALL patients with refractory disease (Lengline et al. 2013; Weston et al. 2013; Kobayashi et al. 2015; Schwab et al. 2016). This approach is currently being tested in frontline studies of patients treated at St. Jude Children's Research Hospital (Total XVII, NCT03117751) (Inaba et al. 2017) and on COG protocols (AALL1131, NCT01406756; AALL1521, NCT02723994) (Tasian et al. 2017b).

ETV6-RUNX1-Like ALL

Analogous to Ph-like ALL, *ETV6-RUNX1*-like ALL is defined by having a gene expression profile and immunophenotype (CD27 positive, CD44 low to negative) similar to *ETV6-RUNX1* ALL, but lacking the *ETV6-RUNX1* fusion (Lilljebjörn et al. 2016; Zaliova et al. 2017). Unsurprisingly, like *ETV6-RUNX1* ALL, *ETV6-RUNX1*-like ALL is almost exclusively identified in children (~3%) and confers a favorable prognosis. This subtype is associated with alternate lesions (gene fusions or copy number alterations) in *ETV6*, *IKZF1*, or *TCF3*, suggesting global deregulation of lymphoid development is a hallmark of this transcriptional signature (Gu et al. 2019).

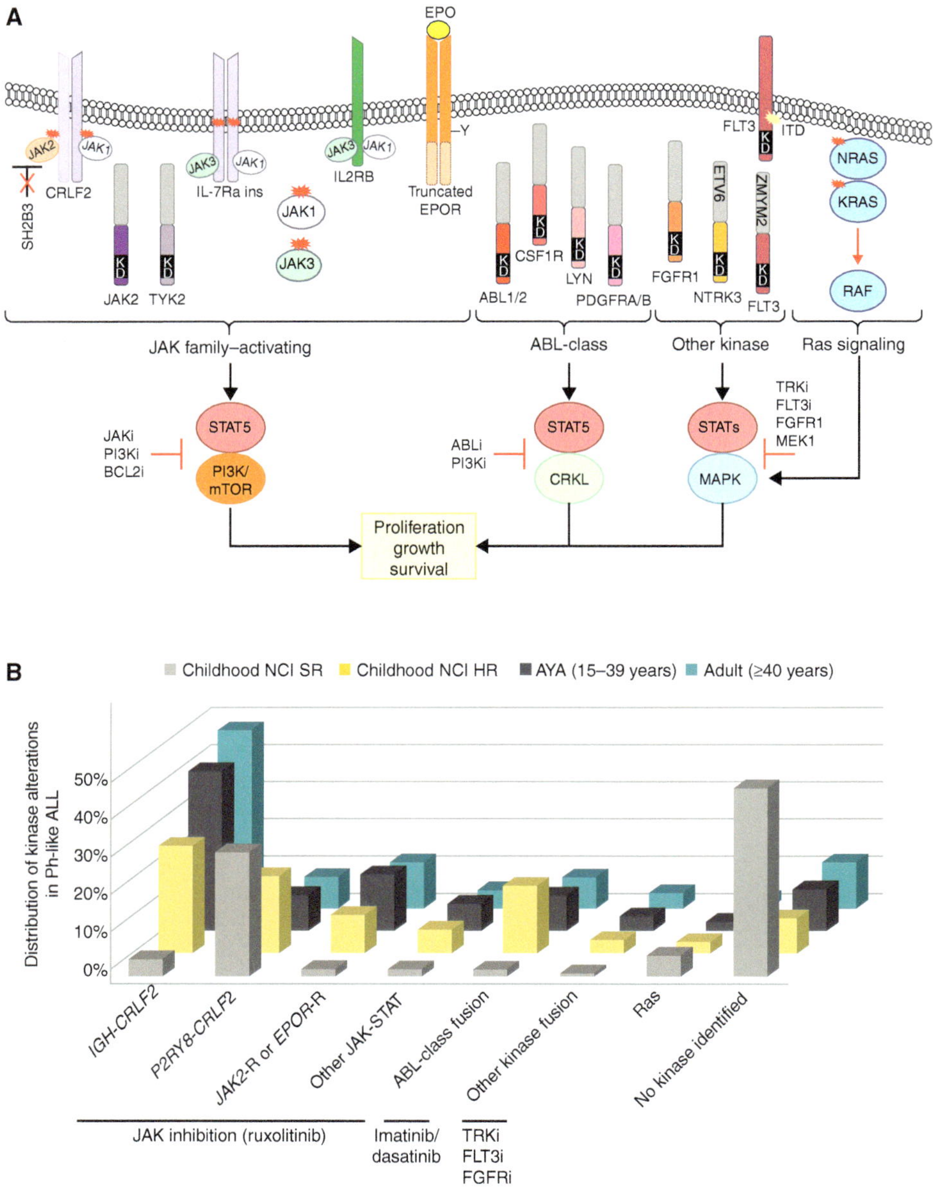

Figure 2. (*A*) Kinase alterations and signaling pathways dysregulated in Philadelphia chromosome-like (Ph-like) ALL. The majority of kinase and cytokine receptor alterations converge on two pathways that activate JAK-family member signaling or ABL signaling. Alterations that activate JAK-STAT signaling can be targeted with JAK and PI3K inhibitors. ABL-class alterations can be targeted with ABL-inhibitors such as dasatinib. Other kinase alterations and those that activate Ras signaling can be targeted with specific inhibitors including those that inactivate TRK, FLT3, FGFR1, and MEK for the MAPK pathway. (*B*) Distribution of kinase subtypes in Ph-like ALL within each age group (Roberts et al. 2014a, 2017a, 2018; Reshmi et al. 2017). Combined prevalence of Ph-like ALL subtypes in childhood National Cancer Institute (NCI) standard-risk (SR; age 1–9.99 yr and WBC < 50,000/μL), NCI high-risk (HR; age 10–15 yr or WBC ≥ 50,000/μL), adolescent and young adults (1639 yr), and adults (≥40 yr). Genomic subtypes include *IGH-CRLF2*, *P2RY8-CRLF2*, and ABL-class fusions (*ABL1*, *ABL2*, *CSF1R*, *LYN*, *PDGFRA*, and *PDGFRB*); *JAK2* and *EPOR* rearrangements and other mutations in JAK–STAT signaling (*JAK1/3*, *IL7R*, *SH2B3*, *TYK2*, and *IL2RB*); and other kinase alterations (*FLT3*, *FGFR1*, *NTRK3*), Ras mutations (*KRAS*, *NRAS*, *NF1*, *PTPN11*, *BRAF*, and *CBL*), and unknown alterations.

 Cite this article as *Cold Spring Harb Perspect Med* doi: 10.1101/cshperspect.a034835

DUX4-rearranged ALL

An interesting subtype of B-ALL with a very distinctive gene expression profile and immunophenotype (CD2 and CD371 positive) is characterized by genetic alterations and deregulation of the transcription factor genes *DUX4* (double homeobox 4) and *ERG* (ETS-related gene) (Yeoh et al. 2002; Harvey et al. 2010; Lilljebjörn et al. 2016; Yasuda et al. 2016; Zhang et al. 2016; Schinnerl et al. 2019). *DUX4* is located in microsatellite *D4Z4* repeat domains in the subtelomeric region of chromosome 4 that is duplicated on chromosome 10q and is normally exclusively expressed in germinal tissues (Gatica and Rosa 2016). In *DUX4*-rearranged ALL, translocation or insertion of *DUX4* to *IGH* is the initiating event that results in overexpression of a 3′ truncated isoform of *DUX4* not normally expressed in B cells. The aberrantly expressed *DUX4* binds to an intragenic region of *ERG*, resulting in gross transcriptional deregulation of *ERG*, and, commonly, expression of ERGalt, a transcript that utilizes a noncanonical first exon that encodes a truncated carboxy-terminal ERG protein. ERGalt retains the DNA-binding and transactivating domain of ERG, inhibits the transcriptional activity of wild-type ERG, and is transforming in mouse models of B-ALL (Zhang et al. 2016). This subtype accounts for 5%–10% of B-ALL, with a slight peak in AYAs. Of clinical relevance, *DUX4*-rearranged ALL is associated with an excellent prognosis in both children and adults (Gu et al. 2019), even despite the presence of secondary genetic alterations otherwise associated with poor outcome, such as *IKZF1* deletions, which are present in ~40% of *DUX4*-rearranged ALL (Zhang et al. 2016).

New Transcription Factors: *MEF2D* and *ZNF384*

Recurrent rearrangements of *MEF2D* and *ZNF384* account for ~4% and 5% of children and up to 7% and 10% in AYA patients, respectively. Accordingly, both subtypes are associated with older age of onset (median age 14 and 15 yr) (Gu et al. 2016; Liu et al. 2016; Suzuki et al. 2016).

Multiple 3′ partners have been identified for *MEF2D* (encoding myocyte enhancer factor 2D), including *BCL9*, *CSF1R*, *DAZAP1*, *FOXJ2*, *HNRNPUL1*, *HNRNPH1*, and *SS18* (Gu et al. 2016; Ohki et al. 2019). All fusions preserve the MEF2D MADS-box domain that mediates DNA binding, resulting in enhanced transcriptional activity and deregulation of MEF2D targets (Gu et al. 2016). An exception is *MEF2D-CFS1R*, which displays the Ph-like gene expression profile (Roberts et al. 2014a). *MEF2D*-rearranged ALL is associated with an aberrant immunophenotype (CD10 negative, CD38 positive) and an intermediate to poor outcome (Gu et al. 2016; Suzuki et al. 2016; Ohki et al. 2019). Alterations of *PHF6*, recurrently mutated in T-cell ALL, were the most frequent cooperating lesions identified by targeted sequencing (Ohki et al. 2019). Deregulation of *MEF2D* also results in the overexpression of *HDAC9* (histone deacetylase 9), which can be targeted therapeutically using HDAC inhibitors (Gu et al. 2016).

Rearrangements of *ZNF384* (encoding zinc finger 384) define a subtype of acute leukemia that transcends immunophenotypic classification and may manifest as classical pre-B ALL without lineage aberrancy, B-ALL with expression of the myeloid markers (CD13/33), or B/myeloid mixed phenotype acute leukemia (Alexander et al. 2018). To date, 11 different 5′ fusion partners, usually involving a transcriptional regulator or chromatin modifier, have been identified for *ZNF384*: *ARIDIB*, *BMP2K*, *CLTC*, *CREBBP*, *EP300*, *EWSR1*, *NIPBL*, *SMARCA2*, *SYNRG*, *TAF15*, and *TCF3* (Liu et al. 2016; Shago et al. 2016; Yasuda et al. 2016; Hirabayashi et al. 2017). An intermediate prognosis has been described in small pediatric cohorts (Liu et al. 2016). The rearrangements are also distinctive, usually involving the entire coding region of *ZNF384*, resulting in the expression of wild-type *ZNF384* in a lineage inappropriate manner, as well as the chimeric fusion protein. Studies of hematopoietic progenitor cells from primary leukemia samples, as well as xenografting of immunophenotypically multiclonal populations, has shown that *ZNF384* rearrangements are acquired in a subset of hematopoietic stem cells and prime leukemic cells for lineage plasticity (Alexander et al. 2018). More recently, cases harboring rearrangement of the zinc finger *ZNF362* to *SMARCA2* and *TAF15* were shown to cluster with *ZNF384*-rearranged ALL, indicating deregulation of similar downstream targets (Li et al. 2018).

REDEFINING "OTHER" B-ALL

Despite the advances made in refining the classification of B-ALL, until recently, almost one-quarter of cases across the age spectrum lacked a subtype defining lesion and were collectively known as "Other." These cases were excluded from risk stratification, commonly relapsed, and lacked targeted therapeutic approaches. To systematically define the frequency and prognostic significance of subtypes across the age spectrum, two groups recently performed an integrated large scale genomic analysis of 1223 and 1988 B-ALL cases, respectively, using transcriptional profiling to refine subtype classification (Li et al. 2018; Gu et al. 2019). In addition to known groups, including those defined by aneuploidy, up to five new subtypes were identified with distinct gene expression signatures, accounting for an additional 15% of B-ALL. As such, >90% of ALL cases may be classified into distinct genetic subtypes using these algorithms.

PAX5-Driven Subtypes

PAX5 is largely considered to function as a haploinsufficient tumor suppressor in ALL, with secondary heterozygous deletions and loss-of-function mutations present in one-third of all patients with B-ALL across a range of subtypes (Kuiper et al. 2007; Mullighan et al. 2007). In mouse models, *Pax5* heterozygosity cooperates with constitutive activation of the JAK-STAT pathway to promote B-ALL development, supporting its role as a tumor suppressor (Dang et al. 2015). *PAX5* translocations are reported in 2%–3% of B-ALL (Nebral et al. 2009; Coyaud et al. 2010). Recent analyses identified two *PAX5* subtypes defined by distinct transcriptional profiles and genetic alterations. The first subtype, referred to as PAX5-altered (PAX5alt), comprises cases with diverse *PAX5* rearrangements (most commonly to *ETV6* or *NOL4L*), sequence mutations or intragenic amplification (Schwab et al. 2017), with the highest prevalence observed in children and AYA (10% each vs. 7% in adults) (Gu et al. 2019). The second group of PAX5-driven ALL is defined by the presence of the PAX5 P80R mutation, which is homozygous in almost all cases because of deletion or frameshift mutation of the wild-type *PAX5* allele, suggesting that loss of both *PAX5* alleles drives the unique gene expression profile of this subtype (Fig. 3; Li et al. 2018; Gu et al. 2019; Passet et al. 2019). The prevalence of PAX5 P80R increases with age, accounting for almost 5% of adults. This subtype confers an intermediate to favorable prognosis in both children and adults (Bastian et al. 2019; Gu et al. 2019; Passet et al. 2019; Zaliova et al. 2019). Cooperating lesions identified in PAX5 P80R patients include a high frequency of signaling mutations, particularly in the Ras, JAK-STAT, and other kinase signaling pathways (*FLT3*, *PIK3CA*), highlighting the potential for targeted therapies (Gu et al. 2019; Passet et al. 2019). Notably, heterozygous $Pax5^{P80R/+}$ or homozygous $Pax5^{P80R/P80R}$ knock-in mice develop B-progenitor ALL that is transplantable, and tumors that arise in $Pax5^{P80R/+}$ mice genetically inactivate the wild-type *Pax5* allele by deletion or truncation, recapitulating the loss of wild-type *PAX5* observed in human ALL (Gu et al. 2019). In a mouse model of B-ALL, PAX5-ETV6 activated distinct transcriptional pathways including pre-B cell receptor signaling and migration/adhesion, confirming its role as an oncoprotein rather than simply acting as a competitive inhibitor of the wild-type PAX5 protein (Smeenk et al. 2017). The identification of PAX5 subtypes as distinct entities highlights the importance of this gene in regulating B-cell differentiation, and confirms *PAX5* alterations as founding lesions in B-lymphoid leukemogenesis as opposed to secondary cooperating events as previously thought.

IKZF1 N159Y

Another uncommon subtype (accounting for <1% of ALL) defined by a single mutation in a lymphoid transcription factor includes cases

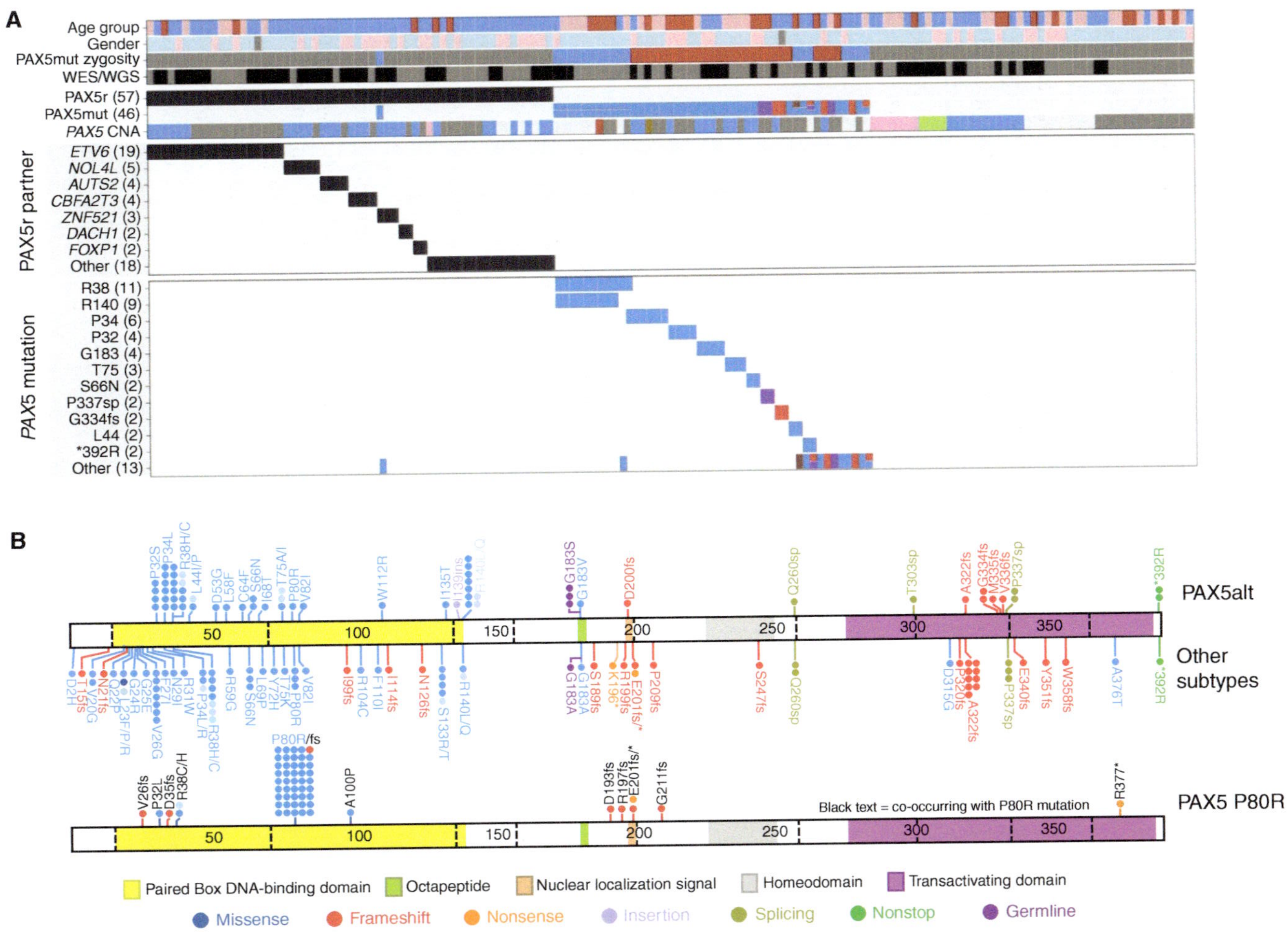

Figure 3. (*A*) Genetic alterations of PAX5, including gene rearrangements (PAX5r), sequence mutations (PAX5mut). and focal intragenic amplifications (PAX5amp, pink in PAX5 CNA) observed in the PAX5alt cohort. (*B*) Protein domain plot of PAX5 showing the mutations detected in PAX5alt and other B-ALL subtypes (*top* panel) and in the PAX5 P80R subtype (*bottom* panel). (CNA) Copy number alteration.

harboring a heterozygous N159Y missense mutation in *IKZF1* (Li et al. 2018; Gu et al. 2019). In contrast to PAX5 P80R ALL, the nonmutated wild-type allele of *IKZF1* is retained in patients with IKZF1 N159Y ALL. The N159 residue is located within the DNA-binding domain of IKZF1. Mutation of this residue results in nuclear mislocalization and enhanced intercellular adhesion that is characteristic of perturbed IKZF1 function (Churchman et al. 2015). Such cases exhibit a distinct gene expression profile compared to other *IKZF1*-altered cases, with increased expression of genes involved in oncogenesis (YAP1), chromatin remodeling (SALL1), and JAK-STAT signaling (Li et al. 2018; Gu et al. 2019).

IGH Rearrangements

Rearrangements of the *IGH* locus to a range of partners—including *CRLF2*, *CEBP* family members (CCAAT/enhancer binding protein), and *ID4*—are frequent in AYA and adult ALL (~10%) and generally confer a poor prognosis (Russell et al. 2014). In addition to these partners, we identified a subset of cases with pre-B immunophenotype and a unique transcriptional signature characterized by rearrangement of *IGH* to *BCL2*, *MYC*, and/or *BCL6* (BCL2/MYC) (Gu et al. 2019) that resemble those observed in "double-hit" lymphoma and are rarely identified in ALL (Moorman et al. 2012; Russell et al. 2014; Uchida et al. 2017; Wagener et al. 2018). This subtype is predominantly identified in adults (median age 48.5 yr) and is associated with an extremely unfavorable outcome.

NUTM1 Rearrangements

An additional subtype present exclusively in 1% of childhood ALL (median age 3 yr) involves fusion of almost all the coding region of *NUTM1* (nuclear protein in testis midline carcinoma family 1) to six different 5′ partners—*ACIN1*, *BRD9*, *CUX1*, *IKZF1*, *SLC12A6*, and *ZNF618*—resulting in increased expression of *NUTM1* (Li et al. 2018; Gu et al. 2019). *NUTM1* is normally expressed in the testis and acts as a chromatin modifier by recruiting EP300 (p300) to increase local histone acetylation (Alekseyenko et al. 2015). Fusions of *NUTM1* (commonly *BRD4-NUTM1*) are a hallmark of NUT midline carcinoma (NMC), an aggressive and fatal subtype of squamous cell carcinoma that also arises frequently in children (French 2014). *BRD4-NUTM1* acts to repress differentiation in NMC by recruiting histone acetyltransferases and other transcriptional cofactors to regions of chromatin that are actively transcribing pro-proliferative and antidifferentiation genes, including MYC (French 2014). Thus, fusions such as *BRD9-NUTM1* in ALL may have a similar mechanism of action, although experimental studies are required to elucidate the role of *NUTM1* in leukemogenesis. In contrast to NMC, ALL patients with *NUTM1* rearrangements have an excellent prognosis. Given the involvement of *BRD9*, bromodomain or HDAC inhibitors would be a logical targeted therapeutic approach for these patients.

MIXED PHENOTYPE ALL

Mixed phenotype acute leukemia (MPAL) is characterized by expression of cell surface proteins characteristic of multiple lineages, most commonly B and myeloid (B/M MPAL) or T and myeloid (T/M MPAL) markers, either in a single (biphenotypic) or multiple (bilineal) immunophenotypic subpopulations. Prior studies had identified rearrangements of *KMT2A* (MLL) or the *BCR-ABL1* fusion in a minority of cases, but until recently the genetics of MPAL had been poorly understood. However, this is of great interest given the phenotypic plasticity and poor prognosis of this form of leukemia. Genomic analyses have shown that T/M and B/M are genetically distinct, with T/M leukemia characterized by founder mutations or rearrangements in transcription factors and chromatin modifiers (*WT1*, *ETV6*, *RUNX1*, *CEBPA*) and the majority of B/M cases to harbor rearrangements of *ZNF384* (Alexander et al. 2018; Takahashi et al. 2018; Xiao et al. 2018). The phenotypic plasticity and characteristic of MPAL (that has bedeviled the selection of appropriate therapy) is largely independent of genetic variegation and, rather, is due to the acquisition of founding lesions in very early hematopoietic progenitors. Thus, MPAL forms part of a spectrum of immature/stem cell leukemias (for T/M MPAL, like early T cell precursor ALL) (Zhang et al. 2012), and future studies are integrating ALL-directed therapy and genomic analysis to further refine optimal diagnostic and classification approaches (Hrusak et al. 2018).

INHERITED VARIANTS IN ALL

Genome-wide association studies (GWASs) have identified risk loci with common genetic polymorphisms that are associated with a modest increase in ALL susceptibility, including *IKZF1* (7p12.2), *CDKN2A/CDKN2B* (9p21), *PIP4K2A* (10p12.2), *GATA3* (10p14), *ARID5B* (10q21.2), *CEBPE*, and *ERG* (14q11.2) (Moriyama et al. 2015b; Qian et al. 2019). Associations with several of these loci exhibit a degree of ALL subtype specificity—for example, *GATA3* with Ph-like ALL (Perez-Andreu et al. 2013; Jain et al. 2017b) and *ERG* with *TCF3-PBX1*—suggesting an interplay of germline and somatic alterations in leukemogenesis. More recently, studies of families with multiple individuals with ALL and complementary examinations of large cohorts of patients with presumed sporadic ALL have identified deleterious germline variants in genes that are also targets of somatic mutation in ALL, including *PAX5*, *ETV6*, *IKZF1*, *TP53*, and *ERG*.

A role for *PAX5* in autosomal dominant predisposition to B-ALL was identified by the description of three unrelated families who harbored a germline *PAX5* c547G > A mutation in the octapeptide domain (PAX5 G183S) that resulted in moderate attenuation of transcriptional activity in vitro (Shah et al. 2013; Auer et al. 2014). Notably, all affected individuals had somatic loss of the wild-type allele, suggesting that biallelic inactivation of *PAX5* is also important for B-cell leukemogenesis in this context.

Deleterious germline variants within the DNA-binding domain of *ETV6* are present in 1% of sporadic B-ALL and affect transcriptional repression either by abrogating binding to ETS-containing DNA sequences or through altered intracellular localization (Moriyama et al. 2015a; Noetzli et al. 2015; Topka et al. 2015; Zhang et al. 2015). Multiple subsequent reports suggest that *ETV6* sequence mutations may be the most common germline alterations predisposing to ALL (Feurstein and Godley 2017; Hock and Shimamura 2017; Duployez et al. 2018). Moreover, a focal germline *ETV6* splice site deletion resulting in exon skipping and protein truncation has been reported in a highly penetrant family (Rampersaud et al. 2019). Another report identified a constitutional translocation disrupting *ETV6* (Jarviaho et al. 2019). These studies indicate that careful analysis of germline structural variants is required to describe the full repertoire of deleterious germline alterations in ALL.

Churchman et al. reported inherited germline variants in *IKZF1* that impair its function in a similar manner to somatic mutations. In contrast to somatic *IKZF1* alterations that are most commonly deletions or mutations in the amino-terminal (DNA-binding) or carboxy-terminal (dimerizing) zinc fingers (Churchman et al. 2015), the germline variants are scattered throughout the gene in regions of poorly characterized function and were not predicted to be deleterious by in silico analyses, but were highly deleterious in more sophisticated cellular assays including subcellular mislocalization, cell–cell adhesion, and cell stromal adhesion in vivo (Churchman et al. 2018).

TP53 alterations are a hallmark of low-hypodiploid ALL, with almost half occurring in the germline, suggesting that low-hypodiploid ALL is another manifestation of Li–Fraumeni syndrome (Holmfeldt et al. 2013). In a large cohort of childhood ALL, 49 nonsilent rare *TP53* coding variants were identified in 77 patients, of which 22 variants were classified as pathogenic (Qian et al. 2018). Children with *TP53* pathogenic variants presented at an older age, had inferior outcomes to children with wild-type *TP53*, and were more likely to develop second malignancies. This study also confirmed the association of inherited *TP53* variants with hypodiploid ALL (Qian et al. 2018). A recent GWAS identified novel susceptibility variants at the *ERG* locus that were enriched in Hispanics (Qian et al. 2019), providing additional insight into the relationship of germline genetic variation in racial occurrence and outcomes in ALL (Yang et al. 2011; Karol et al. 2017). Together, these studies highlight the importance of these genes in both de novo and familial ALL.

RELAPSED ALL

Relapsed ALL remains a leading cause of childhood cancer death (Curtin et al. 2016) and is associated with high rates of treatment failure and death in older individuals (Fielding et al. 2007; Stock 2010; Frey and Luger 2015). The main curative approach for adults is an allogenic stem cell transplant; however, survival rates for relapsed ALL are improving with the implementation of new immunotherapeutic approaches including blinatumomab (CD19/CD3 bispecific T-cell engager), inotuzumab ozagamicin (anti-CD22 antibody conjugated to calicheamicin), and CAR T cells (chimeric antigen receptor) (Davila et al. 2014; Kantarjian et al. 2016, 2017; Maude et al. 2018; Park et al. 2018).

Genomic studies in childhood ALL show that predominant clones at diagnosis are often eradicated, and relapse arises from a minor clone that already harbors and/or acquires additional genomic alterations that drive resistance in a drug-specific or -agnostic manner (Fig. 4; Mullighan et al. 2008b, 2011; Li et al. 2015; Ma et al. 2015; Oshima et al. 2016; Tzoneva et al. 2018). Mutations in genes encoding epigenetic regulators and chromatin modifiers are recurrent events in relapsed ALL and can directly influence response to treatment (Mullighan et al. 2011; Mar et al. 2014; Ma et al. 2015). In particular, mutations in the transcriptional coactivator and acetyl transferase

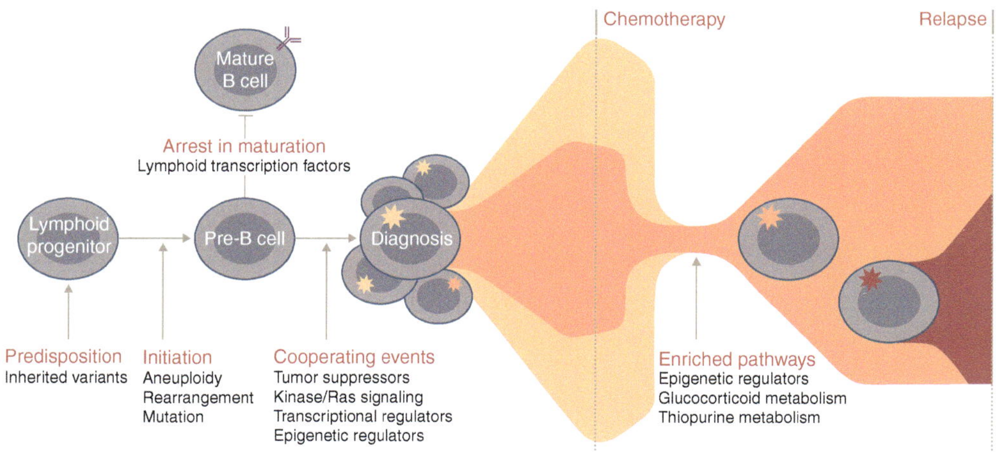

Figure 4. Commonly altered pathways and stepwise progression of B-progenitor acute lymphoblastic leukemia (B-ALL). Common genetic polymorphisms (*IKZF1*, *CDKN2A/B*, *PIP4K2A*, *GATA3*, *ARID5B*, *CEBPE*, and *ERG*) and deleterious nonsilent inherited variants (*PAX5*, *ETV6*, *IKZF1*, *TP53*, and *ERG*) increase the risk of ALL susceptibility. Driving or founding lesions of ALL define genomic subtypes: aneuploidy and other chromosomal abnormalities (hyperdiploid, low-hypodiploid, near-haploid, iAMP21), rearrangements deregulating transcription factors (*ETV6-RUNX1*, *ETV6-RUNX1*-like, *KMT2A*, *TCF3-PBX1*, *DUX4*, *ZNF384*, *MEF2D*, *NUTM1*, *TCF3-HLF*, *PAX5*, *BCL2/MYC*) or kinase genes (Ph-like, *BCR-ABL1*), and specific mutations in lymphoid transcription factors (PAX5 P80R, IKZF1, N195Y). Deletion and loss of lymphoid transcription factors (e.g., *IKZF1*, *PAX5*, *EBF1*) coupled with the alteration of tumor suppressors and cell cycle regulators (*CDKN2A/B*, *TP53*), kinase signaling pathway genes (e.g., *NRAS*, *KRAS*, *FLT3*), other transcriptional regulators (e.g., *ETV6*, *ERG*), or epigenetic regulators (e.g., *CREBBP*, *WHSC1*, *CTCF*) result in the accumulation of immature lymphoid blasts and presentation at diagnosis. During treatment, the predominant diagnosis clone is commonly eradicated and relapse arises from a minor clone that already harbors and/or acquires additional genetic alterations that drive resistance. Pathways that are enriched at relapse include those involving epigenetic regulators (e.g., *CREBBP*, *SETD2*, *KDM6A*), the glucocorticoid response (e.g., *CREBBP*, *NR3C1*), and thiopurine metabolism (e.g., *NT5C2*, *MSH6*).

 Cite this article as *Cold Spring Harb Perspect Med* doi: 10.1101/cshperspect.a034835

CREBBP occur in up to 20% of relapsed ALL and impair sensitivity to glucocorticoid therapy (Mullighan et al. 2011). Mutations in *NT5C2* (5′-nucleotidase catalytic enzyme II) confer increased resistance to purine analogs at the cost of impaired leukemia cell growth and leukemia-initiating cell activity (Meyer et al. 2013; Tzoneva et al. 2018). In addition, loss of *MSH6*, a major component of the mismatch repair (MMR) system, results in intrinsic chemoresistance to thiopurines because of an inability to recognize thioguanine nucleotide mismatching and failure to initiate MMR. Thus, cells defective for MSH6 do not undergo cell cycle arrest or apoptosis and continue to proliferate in the presence of thiopurine (Evensen et al. 2018). Other recurrent somatic alterations in relapsed ALL include deletions of the glucocorticoid receptor *NR3C1* and mutations in the H3K36 trimethyltransferase *SETD2*, the lysine-specific demethylase *KDM6A*, and the epigenetic regulator *MLL2* (Mar et al. 2014; Ma et al. 2015). Enhancing our knowledge of relapse-enriched or acquired alterations is important for initial risk stratification and has implications for molecular monitoring given the increasingly widespread application of deep sequencing approaches to identify low levels of MRD.

ROLE OF THE MICROENVIRONMENT IN ALL

Most studies of mechanisms of leukemogenesis and treatment response have focused on leukemic cell-intrinsic features, but it is increasingly apparent that tumor cell-extrinsic factors, including the nature of nonleukemic hematopoietic cells, and the interaction of leukemic cells with the bone marrow microenvironment, are important determinants of response to therapy and may also be directly influenced by genetic alterations of the leukemic cell. This is exemplified by the finding that alterations of *IKZF1* (Ikaros) in kinase-driven (Ph+ and Ph-like) ALL drive high-risk disease by derepressing expression of adhesion molecules that result in acquisition of a hematopoietic stem cell like phenotype and aberrant leukemic intercellular and cell-stromal adhesion (Joshi et al. 2014; Churchman et al. 2015). This leads to perturbed bone marrow mislocalization and resistance to therapy that may be circumvented, at least in this context, by rexinoids (that bind to retinoid X receptor α, which is also derepressed by loss of Ikaros) that result in differentiation and up-regulation of wild-type Ikaros. Another approach is focal adhesion kinase (FAK) inhibitors, which inhibit FAK signaling downstream of integrin activation (Churchman et al. 2016), an approach that is entering the clinic for the treatment of solid tumors (Lee et al. 2015) and in conjunction with immunotherapy (Jiang et al. 2016).

Although there is extensive evidence that remodeling of, and interaction with, the bone marrow hematopoietic niche has an important role in the survival of acute myeloid leukemia cells (Tabe and Konopleva 2014), the nature and importance of the ALL cell microenvironment interaction is less well studied, but is likely important in light of findings that disruption of CXCR4-CXCL12-mediated interaction can improve drug responsiveness in experimental models of B-ALL and T-cell acute lymphoblastic leukemia (T-ALL) (Pitt et al. 2015; Randhawa et al. 2016). Our recent data indicate that interaction of leukemic cells with bone marrow stromal cells results in profound deregulation of adhesion, signaling cascades, and epithelial to mesenchymal transition–like phenotype in ALL cells and accompanying drug resistance that can potentially be exploited therapeutically (Yoshihara et al. 2018).

CONCLUSIONS

Within the last decade, integrated genomic analyses of large cohorts of childhood ALL, and more recently AYA and adult ALL, has revolutionized our understanding of the genetic basis of ALL by identifying new subtypes, dysregulated pathways, and therapeutic targets that have led to improved risk stratification and treatment strategies. Despite these advances, a proportion of ALL cases cannot be categorized into any of the currently established subtypes, and ongoing discovery studies are required to fully define the genomic landscape. Recent discoveries have already had substantial impact on diagnosis and management of the disease.

For example, targeted approaches are being tested in multiple trials of Ph-like ALL, and the appreciation that accurate classification and risk stratification requires genomic approaches that detect complex structural events in addition to sequence alterations has led to the increasingly widespread adoption of RNA sequencing and, in some centers, whole-genome sequencing. It is envisaged that genomic sequencing will become the clinical standard of care, and the field will continue to explore novel and sensitive approaches to detect and monitor disease, including cell-free technology and mutation-directed measurement of measurable residual disease.

ACKNOWLEDGMENTS

The authors thank colleagues at St. Jude, the Children's Oncology Group, and the multiple centers and leukemia cooperative study groups that have contributed samples and expertise to many of the studies described in this review, including Joshua Stokes from Biomedical Communications at St. Jude. The authors are supported by a National Institutes of Health Outstanding Investigator Award, a St. Baldrick's Foundation Robert J. Arceci Innovation Award, and the Henry Schueler 41&9 Foundation (to C.G.M.).

REFERENCES

Agraz Doblas A, Bueno C, Bashford-Rogers R, Roy A, Schneider P, Bardini M, Ballerini P, Cazzaniga G, Moreno T, Revilla C, et al. 2019. Unraveling the cellular origin and clinical prognostic markers of infant B-cell acute lymphoblastic leukemia using genome-wide analysis. *Haematologica* **104:** 1176–1188. doi:10.3324/haematol.2018.206375

Alekseyenko AA, Walsh EM, Wang X, Grayson AR, Hsi PT, Kharchenko PV, Kuroda MI, French CA. 2015. The oncogenic BRD4-NUT chromatin regulator drives aberrant transcription within large topological domains. *Genes Dev* **29:** 1507–1523. doi:10.1101/gad.267583.115

Alexander TB, Gu Z, Iacobucci I, Dickerson K, Choi JK, Xu B, Payne-Turner D, Yoshihara H, Loh ML, Horan J, et al. 2018. The genetic basis and cell of origin of mixed phenotype acute leukaemia. *Nature* **562:** 373–379. doi:10.1038/s41586-018-0436-0

Andersson AK, Ma J, Wang J, Chen X, Gedman AL, Dang J, Nakitandwe J, Holmfeldt L, Parker M, Easton J, et al. 2015. The landscape of somatic mutations in infant MLL-rearranged acute lymphoblastic leukemias. *Nat Genet* **47:** 330–337. doi:10.1038/ng.3230

Arber DA, Orazi A, Hasserjian R, Thiele J, Borowitz MJ, Le Beau MM, Bloomfield CD, Cazzola M, Vardiman JW. 2016. The 2016 revision to the World Health Organization classification of myeloid neoplasms and acute leukemia. *Blood* **127:** 2391–2405. doi:10.1182/blood-2016-03-643544

Auer F, Rüschendorf F, Gombert M, Husemann P, Ginzel S, Izraeli S, Harit M, Weintraub M, Weinstein OY, Lerer I, et al. 2014. Inherited susceptibility to pre B-ALL caused by germline transmission of PAX5 c.547G>A. *Leukemia* **28:** 1136–1138. doi:10.1038/leu.2013.363

Barber KE, Harrison CJ, Broadfield ZJ, Stewart AR, Wright SL, Martineau M, Strefford JC, Moorman AV. 2007. Molecular cytogenetic characterization of *TCF3 (E2A)*/19p13.3 rearrangements in B-cell precursor acute lymphoblastic leukemia. *Genes Chromosomes Cancer* **46:** 478–486. doi:10.1002/gcc.20431

Bastian L, Schroeder MP, Eckert C, Schlee C, Tanchez JO, Kampf S, Wagner DL, Schulze V, Isaakidis K, Lazaro-Navarro J, et al. 2019. PAX5 biallelic genomic alterations define a novel subgroup of B-cell precursor acute lymphoblastic leukemia. *Leukemia* **33:** 1895–1909. doi:10.1038/s41375-019-0430-z

Burmeister T, Gokbuget N, Schwartz S, Fischer L, Hubert D, Sindram A, Hoelzer D, Thiel E. 2010. Clinical features and prognostic implications of *TCF3-PBX1* and *ETV6-RUNX1* in adult acute lymphoblastic leukemia. *Haematologica* **95:** 241–246. doi:10.3324/haematol.2009.011346

Churchman ML, Low J, Qu C, Paietta EM, Kasper LH, Chang Y, Payne-Turner D, Althoff MJ, Song G, Chen SC, et al. 2015. Efficacy of retinoids in IKZF1-mutated BCR-ABL1 acute lymphoblastic leukemia. *Cancer Cell* **28:** 343–356. doi:10.1016/j.ccell.2015.07.016

Churchman ML, Evans K, Richmond J, Robbins A, Jones L, Shapiro IM, Pachter JA, Weaver DT, Houghton PJ, Smith MA, et al. 2016. Synergism of FAK and tyrosine kinase inhibition in Ph^+ B-ALL. *JCI Insight* **1:** e86082. doi:10.1172/jci.insight.86082

Churchman ML, Qian M, Te Kronnie G, Zhang R, Yang W, Zhang H, Lana T, Tedrick P, Baskin R, Verbist K, et al. 2018. Germline genetic *IKZF1* variation and predisposition to childhood acute lymphoblastic leukemia. *Cancer Cell* **33:** 937–948.e8. doi:10.1016/j.ccell.2018.03.021

Coyaud E, Struski S, Prade N, Familiades J, Eichner R, Quelen C, Bousquet M, Mugneret F, Talmant P, Pages MP, et al. 2010. Wide diversity of PAX5 alterations in B-ALL: A groupe francophone de cytogénétique hématologique study. *Blood* **115:** 3089–3097. doi:10.1182/blood-2009-07-234229

Curtin SC, Miniño AM, Adnderson RN. 2016. *Declines in cancer death rates among children and adolescents in the United States, 1999–2014,* NCHS data brief, no 257. National Center for Health Statistics, Hyattsville, MD.

Dang J, Wei L, de Ridder J, Su X, Rust AG, Roberts KG, Payne-Turner D, Cheng J, Ma J, Qu C, et al. 2015. PAX5 is a tumor suppressor in mouse mutagenesis models of acute lymphoblastic leukemia. *Blood* **125:** 3609–3617. doi:10.1182/blood-2015-02-626127

Davila ML, Riviere I, Wang X, Bartido S, Park J, Curran K, Chung SS, Stefanski J, Borquez-Ojeda O, Olszewska M, et al. 2014. Efficacy and toxicity management of 19-28z CAR T cell therapy in B cell acute lymphoblastic leukemia. *Sci Transl Med* **6:** 224ra25. doi:10.1126/scitranslmed.3008226

Den Boer ML, van Slegtenhorst M, De Menezes RX, Cheok MH, Buijs-Gladdines JG, Peters ST, Van Zutven LJ, Beverloo HB, Van der Spek PJ, Escherich G, et al. 2009. A subtype of childhood acute lymphoblastic leukaemia with poor treatment outcome: A genome-wide classification study. *Lancet Oncol* **10:** 125–134. doi:10.1016/S1470-2045(08)70339-5

Driessen EM, van Roon EH, Spijkers-Hagelstein JA, Schneider P, de Lorenzo P, Valsecchi MG, Pieters R, Stam RW. 2013. Frequencies and prognostic impact of RAS mutations in MLL-rearranged acute lymphoblastic leukemia in infants. *Haematologica* **98:** 937–944. doi:10.3324/haematol.2012.067983

Duployez N, Abou Chahla W, Lejeune S, Marceau-Renaut A, Letizia G, Boyer T, Geffroy S, Peyrouze P, Grardel N, Nelken B, et al. 2018. Detection of a new heterozygous germline *ETV6* mutation in a case with hyperdiploid acute lymphoblastic leukemia. *Eur J Haematol* **100:** 104–107. doi:10.1111/ejh.12981

Evensen NA, Madhusoodhan PP, Meyer J, Saliba J, Chowdhury A, Araten DJ, Nersting J, Bhatla T, Vincent TL, Teachey D, et al. 2018. MSH6 haploinsufficiency at relapse contributes to the development of thiopurine resistance in pediatric B-lymphoblastic leukemia. *Haematologica* **103:** 830–839. doi:10.3324/haematol.2017.176362

Feurstein S, Godley LA. 2017. Germline ETV6 mutations and predisposition to hematological malignancies. *Int J Hematol* **106:** 189–195. doi:10.1007/s12185-017-2259-4

Fielding AK, Richards SM, Chopra R, Lazarus HM, Litzow MR, Buck G, Durrant IJ, Luger SM, Marks DI, Franklin IM, et al. 2007. Outcome of 609 adults after relapse of acute lymphoblastic leukemia (ALL); an MRC UKALL12/ECOG 2993 study. *Blood* **109:** 944–950. doi:10.1182/blood-2006-05-018192

Fischer U, Forster M, Rinaldi A, Risch T, Sungalee S, Warnatz HJ, Bornhauser B, Gombert M, Kratsch C, Stütz AM, et al. 2015. Genomics and drug profiling of fatal *TCF3-HLF*–positive acute lymphoblastic leukemia identifies recurrent mutation patterns and therapeutic options. *Nat Genet* **47:** 1020–1029. doi:10.1038/ng.3362

Ford AM, Ridge SA, Cabrera ME, Mahmoud H, Steel CM, Chan LC, Greaves M. 1993. In utero rearrangements in the trithorax-related oncogene in infant leukaemias. *Nature* **363:** 358–360. doi:10.1038/363358a0

French C. 2014. NUT midline carcinoma. *Nat Rev Cancer* **14:** 149–150. doi:10.1038/nrc3659

Frey NV, Luger SM. 2015. How I treat adults with relapsed or refractory Philadelphia chromosome-negative acute lymphoblastic leukemia. *Blood* **126:** 589–596. doi:10.1182/blood-2014-09-551937

Gatica LV, Rosa AL. 2016. A complex interplay of genetic and epigenetic events leads to abnormal expression of the *DUX4* gene in facioscapulohumeral muscular dystrophy. *Neuromuscul Disord* **26:** 844–852. doi:10.1016/j.nmd.2016.09.015

Gu Z, Churchman M, Roberts K, Li Y, Liu Y, Harvey RC, McCastlain K, Reshmi SC, Payne-Turner D, Iacobucci I, et al. 2016. Genomic analyses identify recurrent *MEF2D* fusions in acute lymphoblastic leukaemia. *Nat Commun* **7:** 13331. doi:10.1038/ncomms13331

Gu Z, Churchman ML, Roberts KG, Moore I, Zhou X, Nakitandwe J, Hagiwara K, Pelletier S, Gingras S, Berns H, et al. 2019. *PAX5*-driven subtypes of B-progenitor acute lymphoblastic leukemia. *Nat Genet* **51:** 296–307. doi:10.1038/s41588-018-0315-5

Hamadeh L, Enshaei A, Schwab C, Alonso CN, Attarbaschi A, Barbany G, den Boer ML, Boer JM, Braun M, Dalla Pozza L, et al. 2019. Validation of the United Kingdom copy-number alteration classifier in 3239 children with B-cell precursor ALL. *Blood Adv* **3:** 148–157. doi:10.1182/bloodadvances.2018025718

Harrison CJ. 2015. Blood spotlight on iAMP21 acute lymphoblastic leukemia (ALL), a high-risk pediatric disease. *Blood* **125:** 1383–1386. doi:10.1182/blood-2014-08-569228

Harrison CJ, Moorman AV, Broadfield ZJ, Cheung KL, Harris RL, Reza Jalali G, Robinson HM, Barber KE, Richards SM, Mitchell CD, et al. 2004. Three distinct subgroups of hypodiploidy in acute lymphoblastic leukemia. *Br J Haematol* **125:** 552–559. doi:10.1111/j.1365-2141.2004.04948.x

Harrison CJ, Moorman AV, Schwab C, Carroll AJ, Raetz EA, Devidas M, Strehl S, Nebral K, Harbott J, Teigler-Schlegel A, et al. 2014. An international study of intrachromosomal amplification of chromosome 21 (iAMP21): cytogenetic characterization and outcome. *Leukemia* **28:** 1015–1021. doi:10.1038/leu.2013.317

Harvey RC, Mullighan CG, Wang X, Dobbin KK, Davidson GS, Bedrick EJ, Chen IM, Atlas SR, Kang H, Ar K, et al. 2010. Identification of novel cluster groups in pediatric high-risk B-precursor acute lymphoblastic leukemia with gene expression profiling: Correlation with genome-wide DNA copy number alterations, clinical characteristics, and outcome. *Blood* **116:** 4874–4884. doi:10.1182/blood-2009-08-239681

Hirabayashi S, Ohki K, Nakabayashi K, Ichikawa H, Momozawa Y, Okamura K, Yaguchi A, Terada K, Saito Y, Yoshimi A, et al. 2017. *ZNF384*-related fusion genes define a subgroup of childhood B-cell precursor acute lymphoblastic leukemia with a characteristic immunotype. *Haematologica* **102:** 118–129. doi:10.3324/haematol.2016.151035

Hock H, Shimamura A. 2017. *ETV6* in hematopoiesis and leukemia predisposition. *Semin Hematol* **54:** 98–104. doi:10.1053/j.seminhematol.2017.04.005

Holmfeldt L, Wei L, Diaz-Flores E, Walsh M, Zhang J, Ding L, Payne-Turner D, Churchman M, Andersson A, Chen SC, et al. 2013. The genomic landscape of hypodiploid acute lymphoblastic leukemia. *Nat Genet* **45:** 242–252. doi:10.1038/ng.2532

Hrusak O, de Haas V, Stancikova J, Vakrmanova B, Janotova I, Mejstrikova E, Capek V, Trka J, Zaliova M, Luks A, et al. 2018. International cooperative study identifies treatment strategy in childhood ambiguous lineage leukemia. *Blood* **132:** 264–276. doi:10.1182/blood-2017-12-821363

Hunger SP. 1996. Chromosomal translocations involving the E2A gene in acute lymphoblastic leukemia: Clinical features and molecular pathogenesis. *Blood* **87:** 1211–1224.

Hunger SP, Mullighan CG. 2015. Acute lymphoblastic leukemia in children. *N Engl J Med* **373:** 1541–1552. doi:10.1056/NEJMra1400972

Hyrenius-Wittsten A, Pilheden M, Sturesson H, Hansson J, Walsh MP, Song G, Kazi JU, Liu J, Ramakrishan R, Garcia-Ruiz C, et al. 2018. De novo activating mutations drive clonal evolution and enhance clonal fitness in *KMT2A*-rearranged leukemia. *Nat Commun* **9:** 1770. doi:10.1038/s41467-018-04180-1

Iacobucci I, Mullighan CG. 2017. Genetic basis of acute lymphoblastic leukemia. *J Clin Oncol* **35:** 975–983. doi:10.1200/JCO.2016.70.7836

Inaba T, Roberts WM, Shapiro LH, Jolly KW, Raimondi SC, Smith SD, Look AT. 1992. Fusion of the leucine zipper gene HLF to the E2A gene in human acute B-lineage leukemia. *Science* **257:** 531–534. doi:10.1126/science.1386162

Inaba H, Azzato EM, Mullighan CG. 2017. Integration of next-generation sequencing to treat acute lymphoblastic leukemia with targetable lesions: The St. Jude Children's Research Hospital approach. *Front Pediatr* **5:** 258. doi:10.3389/fped.2017.00258

Jaffe JD, Wang Y, Chan HM, Zhang J, Huether R, Kryukov GV, Bhang HE, Taylor JE, Hu M, Englund NP, et al. 2013. Global chromatin profiling reveals *NSD2* mutations in pediatric acute lymphoblastic leukemia. *Nat Genet* **45:** 1386–1391. doi:10.1038/ng.2777

Jain N, Roberts KG, Jabbour E, Patel K, Eterovic AK, Chen K, Zweidler-McKay P, Lu X, Fawcett G, Wang SA, et al. 2017a. Ph-like acute lymphoblastic leukemia: A high-risk subtype in adults. *Blood* **129:** 572–581. doi:10.1182/blood-2016-07-726588

Jain N, Zhang H, Roberts KG, Qian MX, Yang WJ, Jabbour EJ, Kantarjian HM, Mullighan CG, Yang JJ, Konopleva M. 2017b. GATA3 rs3824662A allele is overrepresented in adult patients with Ph-like ALL, especially in patients with CRLF2 abnormalities. *Blood* **130:** 1430. doi:10.1182/blood-2017-03-771576

Jarviaho T, Bang B, Zachariadis V, Taylan F, Moilanen J, Mottonen M, Smith CIE, Harila-Saari A, Niinimaki R, Nordgren A. 2019. Predisposition to childhood acute lymphoblastic leukemia caused by a constitutional translocation disrupting *ETV6*. *Blood Adv* **24:** 2722–2731. doi:10.1182/blood advances.2018028795

Jiang H, Hegde S, Knolhoff BL, Zhu Y, Herndon JM, Meyer MA, Nywening TM, Hawkins WG, Shapiro IM, Weaver DT, et al. 2016. Targeting focal adhesion kinase renders pancreatic cancers responsive to checkpoint immunotherapy. *Nat Med* **22:** 851–860. doi:10.1038/nm.4123

Joshi I, Yoshida T, Jena N, Qi X, Zhang J, Van Etten RA, Georgopoulos K. 2014. Loss of Ikaros DNA-binding function confers integrin-dependent survival on pre-B cells and progression to acute lymphoblastic leukemia. *Nat Immunol* **15:** 294–304. doi:10.1038/ni.2821

Kantarjian HM, DeAngelo DJ, Stelljes M, Martinelli G, Liedtke M, Stock W, Gokbuget N, O'Brien S, Wang K, Wang T, et al. 2016. Inotuzumab ozogamicin versus standard therapy for acute lymphoblastic leukemia. *N Engl J Med* **375:** 740–753. doi:10.1056/NEJMoa1509277

Kantarjian H, Stein A, Gökbuget N, Fielding AK, Schuh AC, Ribera JM, Wei A, Dombret H, Foà R, Bassan R, et al. 2017. Blinatumomab versus chemotherapy for advanced acute lymphoblastic leukemia. *N Engl J Med* **376:** 836–847. doi:10.1056/NEJMoa1609783

Karol SE, Larsen E, Cheng C, Cao X, Yang W, Ramsey LB, Fernandez CA, McCorkle JR, Paugh SW, Autry RJ, et al. 2017. Genetics of ancestry-specific risk for relapse in acute lymphoblastic leukemia. *Leukemia* **31:** 1325–1332. doi:10.1038/leu.2017.24

Kobayashi K, Miyagawa N, Mitsui K, Matsuoka M, Kojima Y, Takahashi H, Ootsubo K, Nagai J, Ueno H, Ishibashi T, et al. 2015. TKI dasatinib monotherapy for a patient with Ph-like ALL bearing *ATF7IP/PDGFRB* translocation. *Pediatr Blood Cancer* **62:** 1058–1060. doi:10.1002/pbc.25327

Kuiper RP, Schoenmakers EF, van Reijmersdal SV, Hehir-Kwa JY, van Kessel AG, van Leeuwen FN, Hoogerbrugge PM. 2007. High-resolution genomic profiling of childhood ALL reveals novel recurrent genetic lesions affecting pathways involved in lymphocyte differentiation and cell cycle progression. *Leukemia* **21:** 1258–1266. doi:10.1038/sj.leu.2404691

Lee BY, Timpson P, Horvath LG, Daly RJ. 2015. FAK signaling in human cancer as a target for therapeutics. *Pharmacol Ther* **146:** 132–149. doi:10.1016/j.pharmthera.2014.10.001

Lengline E, Beldjord K, Dombret H, Soulier J, Boissel N, Clappier E. 2013. Successful tyrosine kinase inhibitor therapy in a refractory B-cell precursor acute lymphoblastic leukemia with *EBF1-PDGFRB* fusion. *Haematologica* **98:** e146–e148. doi:10.3324/haematol.2013.095372

Li Y, Schwab C, Ryan SL, Papaemmanuil E, Robinson HM, Jacobs P, Moorman AV, Dyer S, Borrow J, Griffiths M, et al. 2014. Constitutional and somatic rearrangement of chromosome 21 in acute lymphoblastic leukaemia. *Nature* **508:** 98–102. doi:10.1038/nature13115

Li B, Li H, Bai Y, Kirschner-Schwabe R, Yang JJ, Chen Y, Lu G, Tzoneva G, Ma X, Wu T, et al. 2015. Negative feedback-defective PRPS1 mutants drive thiopurine resistance in relapsed childhood ALL. *Nat Med* **21:** 563–571. doi:10.1038/nm.3840

Li JF, Dai YT, Lilljebjörn H, Shen SH, Cui BW, Bai L, Liu YF, Qian MX, Kubota Y, Kiyoi H, et al. 2018. Transcriptional landscape of B cell precursor acute lymphoblastic leukemia based on an international study of 1,223 cases. *Proc Natl Acad Sci* **115:** E11711–E11720. doi:10.1073/pnas.1814397115

Lilljebjörn H, Henningsson R, Hyrenius-Wittsten A, Olsson L, Orsmark-Pietras C, von Palffy S, Askmyr M, Rissler M, Schrappe M, Cario G, et al. 2016. Identification of *ETV6-RUNX1*-like and *DUX4*-rearranged subtypes in paediatric B-cell precursor acute lymphoblastic leukaemia. *Nat Commun* **7:** 11790. doi:10.1038/ncomms11790

Liu YF, Wang BY, Zhang WN, Huang JY, Li BS, Zhang M, Jiang L, Li JF, Wang MJ, Dai YJ, et al. 2016. Genomic profiling of adult and pediatric B-cell acute lymphoblastic leukemia. *EBioMedicine* **8:** 173–183. doi:10.1016/j.ebiom.2016.04.038

Loh ML, Zhang J, Harvey RC, Roberts K, Payne-Turner D, Kang H, Wu G, Chen X, Becksfort J, Edmonson M, et al. 2013. Tyrosine kinome sequencing of pediatric acute lymphoblastic leukemia: A report from the children's oncology group TARGET project. *Blood* **121:** 485–488. doi:10.1182/blood-2012-04-422691

Ma X, Edmonson M, Yergeau D, Muzny DM, Hampton OA, Rusch M, Song G, Easton J, Harvey RC, Wheeler DA, et al. 2015. Rise and fall of subclones from diagnosis to relapse in pediatric B-acute lymphoblastic leukaemia. *Nat Commun* **6:** 6604. doi:10.1038/ncomms7604

Mar BG, Bullinger LB, McLean KM, Grauman PV, Harris MH, Stevenson K, Neuberg DS, Sinha AU, Sallan SE, Silverman LB, et al. 2014. Mutations in epigenetic regulators including SETD2 are gained during relapse in paediatric acute lymphoblastic leukaemia. *Nat Commun* **5:** 3469. doi:10.1038/ncomms4469

Martinelli G, Iacobucci I, Storlazzi CT, Vignetti M, Paoloni F, Cilloni D, Soverini S, Vitale A, Chiaretti S, Cimino G, et al. 2009. *IKZF1* (Ikaros) deletions in *BCR-ABL1*-positive acute lymphoblastic leukemia are associated with short disease-free survival and high rate of cumulative incidence of relapse: A GIMEMA AL WP report. *J Clin Oncol* **27:** 5202–5207. doi:10.1200/JCO.2008.21.6408

Maude SL, Laetsch TW, Buechner J, Rives S, Boyer M, Bittencourt H, Bader P, Verneris MR, Stefanski HE, Myers GD, et al. 2018. Tisagenlecleucel in children and young adults with B-cell lymphoblastic leukemia. *N Engl J Med* **378:** 439–448. doi:10.1056/NEJMoa1709866

Meyer JA, Wang J, Hogan LE, Yang JJ, Dandekar S, Patel JP, Tang Z, Zumbo P, Li S, Zavadil J, et al. 2013. Relapse-specific mutations in *NT5C2* in childhood acute lymphoblastic leukemia. *Nat Genet* **45:** 290–294. doi:10.1038/ng.2558

Moorman AV, Harrison CJ, Buck GA, Richards SM, Secker-Walker LM, Martineau M, Vance GH, Cherry AM, Higgins RR, Fielding AK, et al. 2007. Karyotype is an independent prognostic factor in adult acute lymphoblastic leukemia (ALL): Analysis of cytogenetic data from patients treated on the Medical Research Council (MRC) UKALLXII/Eastern Cooperative Oncology Group (ECOG) 2993 trial. *Blood* **109:** 3189–3197. doi:10.1182/blood-2006-10-051912

Moorman AV, Schwab C, Ensor HM, Russell LJ, Morrison H, Jones L, Masic D, Patel B, Rowe JM, Tallman M, et al. 2012. *IGH@* translocations, *CRLF2* deregulation, and microdeletions in adolescents and adults with acute lymphoblastic leukemia. *J Clin Oncol* **30:** 3100–3108. doi:10.1200/JCO.2011.40.3907

Moorman AV, Robinson H, Schwab C, Richards SM, Hancock J, Mitchell CD, Goulden N, Vora A, Harrison CJ. 2013. Risk-directed treatment intensification significantly reduces the risk of relapse among children and adolescents with acute lymphoblastic leukemia and intrachromosomal amplification of chromosome 21: a comparison of the MRC ALL97/99 and UKALL2003 trials. *J Clin Oncol* **31:** 3389–3396. doi:10.1200/JCO.2013.48.9377

Moriyama T, Metzger ML, Wu G, Nishii R, Qian M, Devidas M, Yang W, Cheng C, Cao X, Quinn E, et al. 2015a. Germline genetic variation in *ETV6* and risk of childhood acute lymphoblastic leukaemia: A systematic genetic study. *Lancet Oncol* **16:** 1659–1666. doi:10.1016/S1470-2045(15)00369-1

Moriyama T, Relling MV, Yang JJ. 2015b. Inherited genetic variation in childhood acute lymphoblastic leukemia. *Blood* **125:** 3988–3995. doi:10.1182/blood-2014-12-580001

Mullighan CG, Goorha S, Radtke I, Miller CB, Coustan-Smith E, Dalton JD, Girtman K, Mathew S, Ma J, Pounds SB, et al. 2007. Genome-wide analysis of genetic alterations in acute lymphoblastic leukaemia. *Nature* **446:** 758–764. doi:10.1038/nature05690

Mullighan CG, Miller CB, Radtke I, Phillips LA, Dalton J, Ma J, White D, Hughes TP, Le Beau MM, Pui CH, et al. 2008a. BCR-ABL1 lymphoblastic leukaemia is characterized by the deletion of Ikaros. *Nature* **453:** 110–114. doi:10.1038/nature06866

Mullighan CG, Phillips LA, Su X, Ma J, Miller CB, Shurtleff SA, Downing JR. 2008b. Genomic analysis of the clonal origins of relapsed acute lymphoblastic leukemia. *Science* **322:** 1377–1380. doi:10.1126/science.1164266

Mullighan CG, Su X, Zhang J, Radtke I, Phillips LA, Miller CB, Ma J, Liu W, Cheng C, Schulman BA, et al. 2009. Deletion of *IKZF1* and prognosis in acute lymphoblastic leukemia. *N Engl J Med* **360:** 470–480. doi:10.1056/NEJMoa0808253

Mullighan CG, Zhang J, Kasper LH, Lerach S, Payne-Turner D, Phillips LA, Heatley SL, Holmfeldt L, Collins-Underwood JR, Ma J, et al. 2011. *CREBBP* mutations in relapsed acute lymphoblastic leukaemia. *Nature* **471:** 235–239. doi:10.1038/nature09727

Mullighan CG, Jeha S, Pei D, Payne-Turner D, Coustan-Smith E, Roberts KG, Waanders E, Choi JK, Ma X, Raimondi SC, et al. 2015. Outcome of children with hypodiploid ALL treated with risk-directed therapy based on MRD levels. *Blood* **126:** 2896–2899. doi:10.1182/blood-2015-09-671131

Nebral K, Denk D, Attarbaschi A, König M, Mann G, Haas OA, Strehl S. 2009. Incidence and diversity of PAX5 fusion genes in childhood acute lymphoblastic leukemia. *Leukemia* **23:** 134–143. doi:10.1038/leu.2008.306

Noetzli L, Lo RW, Lee-Sherick AB, Callaghan M, Noris P, Savoia A, Rajpurkar M, Jones K, Gowan K, Balduini CL, et al. 2015. Germline mutations in *ETV6* are associated with thrombocytopenia, red cell macrocytosis and predisposition to lymphoblastic leukemia. *Nat Genet* **47:** 535–538. doi:10.1038/ng.3253

O'Connor D, Enshaei A, Bartram J, Hancock J, Harrison CJ, Hough R, Samarasinghe S, Schwab C, Vora A, Wade R, et al. 2018. Genotype-specific minimal residual disease interpretation improves stratification in pediatric acute lymphoblastic leukemia. *J Clin Oncol* **36:** 34–43. doi:10.1200/JCO.2017.74.0449

Ohki K, Kiyokawa N, Saito Y, Hirabayashi S, Nakabayashi K, Ichikawa H, Momozawa Y, Okamura K, Yoshimi A, Ogata-Kawata H, et al. 2019. Clinical and molecular characteristics of *MEF2D* fusion-positive B-cell precursor acute lymphoblastic leukemia in childhood, including a novel translocation resulting in *MEF2D-HNRNPH1* gene fusion. *Haematologica* **104:** 128–137. doi:10.3324/haematol.2017.186320

Oshima K, Khiabanian H, da Silva-Almeida AC, Tzoneva G, Abate F, Ambesi-Impiombato A, Sanchez-Martin M, Carpenter Z, Penson A, Perez-Garcia A, et al. 2016. Mutational landscape, clonal evolution patterns, and role of RAS mutations in relapsed acute lymphoblastic leukemia. *Proc Natl Acad Sci* **113:** 11306–11311. doi:10.1073/pnas.1608420113

Papaemmanuil E, Rapado I, Li Y, Potter NE, Wedge DC, Tubio J, Alexandrov LB, Van Loo P, Cooke SL, Marshall J, et al. 2014. RAG-mediated recombination is the predominant driver of oncogenic rearrangement in *ETV6-RUNX1* acute lymphoblastic leukemia. *Nat Genet* **46:** 116–125. doi:10.1038/ng.2874

Park JH, Rivière I, Gonen M, Wang X, Sénéchal B, Curran KJ, Sauter C, Wang Y, Santomasso B, Mead E, et al. 2018. Long-term follow-up of CD19 CAR therapy in acute lymphoblastic leukemia. *N Engl J Med* **378:** 449–459. doi:10.1056/NEJMoa1709919

Passet M, Boissel N, Sigaux F, Saillard C, Bargetzi M, Ba I, Thomas X, Graux C, Chalandon Y, Leguay T, et al. 2019. *PAX5* P80R mutation identifies a novel subtype of B-cell precursor acute lymphoblastic leukemia with favorable outcome. *Blood* **133:** 280–284. doi:10.1182/blood-2018-10-882142

Paulsson K, Lilljebjörn H, Biloglav A, Olsson L, Rissler M, Castor A, Barbany G, Fogelstrand L, Nordgren A, Sjogren H, et al. 2015. The genomic landscape of high hyperdiploid childhood acute lymphoblastic leukemia. *Nat Genet* **47:** 672–676. doi:10.1038/ng.3301

Perez-Andreu V, Roberts KG, Harvey RC, Yang W, Cheng C, Pei D, Xu H, Gastier-Foster J ES, Lim JY, et al. 2013. Inherited *GATA3* variants are associated with Ph-like childhood acute lymphoblastic leukemia and risk of relapse. *Nat Genet* **45:** 1494–1498. doi:10.1038/ng.2803

Pitt LA, Tikhonova AN, Hu H, Trimarchi T, King B, Gong Y, Sanchez-Martin M, Tsirigos A, Littman DR, Ferrando AA, et al. 2015. CXCL12-producing vascular endothelial niches control acute T cell leukemia maintenance. *Cancer Cell* **27:** 755–768. doi:10.1016/j.ccell.2015.05.002

Pui CH, Rebora P, Schrappe M, Attarbaschi A, Baruchel A, Basso G, Cave H, Elitzur S, Koh K, Liu HC, et al. 2019. Outcome of children with hypodiploid acute lymphoblastic leukemia: A retrospective multinational study. *J Clin Oncol* **37:** 770–779. doi:10.1200/JCO.18.00822

Qian M, Cao X, Devidas M, Yang W, Cheng C, Dai Y, Carroll A, Heerema NA, Zhang H, Moriyama T, et al. 2018. *TP53* germline variations influence the predisposition and prognosis of B-cell acute lymphoblastic leukemia in children. *J Clin Oncol* **36:** 591–599. doi:10.1200/JCO.2017.75.5215

Qian M, Xu H, Perez-Andreu V, Roberts KG, Zhang H, Yang W, Zhang S, Zhao X, Smith C, Devidas M, et al. 2019. Novel susceptibility variants at the *ERG* locus for childhood acute lymphoblastic leukemia in Hispanics. *Blood* **133:** 724–729. doi:10.1182/blood-2018-07-862946

Rampersaud E, Ziegler DS, Iacobucci I, Payne-Turner D, Churchman ML, Schrader KA, Vijai J, Offit K, Tucker K, Sutton R, et al. 2019. Germline deletion of *ETV6* in familial acute lymphoblastic leukemia. *Blood Adv* **3:** 1039–1046. doi:10.1182/bloodadvances.2018030635

Randhawa S, Cho BS, Ghosh D, Sivina M, Koehrer S, Müschen M, Peled A, Davis RE, Konopleva M, Burger JA. 2016. Effects of pharmacological and genetic disruption of CXCR4 chemokine receptor function in B-cell acute lymphoblastic leukaemia. *Br J Haematol* **174:** 425–436. doi:10.1111/bjh.14075

Ravandi F, O'Brien S, Thomas D, Faderl S, Jones D, Garris R, Dara S, Jorgensen J, Kebriaei P, Champlin R, et al. 2010. First report of phase 2 study of dasatinib with hyper-CVAD for the frontline treatment of patients with Philadelphia chromosome-positive (Ph^+) acute lymphoblastic leukemia. *Blood* **116:** 2070–2077. doi:10.1182/blood-2009-12-261586

Reshmi SC, Harvey RC, Roberts KG, Stonerock E, Smith A, Jenkins H, Chen IM, Valentine M, Liu Y, Li Y, et al. 2017. Targetable kinase gene fusions in high-risk B-ALL: A study from the children's oncology group. *Blood* **129:** 3352–3361.

Roberts KG, Li Y, Payne-Turner D, Harvey RC, Yang YL, Pei D, McCastlain K, Ding L, Lu C, Song G, et al. 2014a. Targetable kinase-activating lesions in Ph-like acute lymphoblastic leukemia. *N Engl J Med* **371:** 1005–1015. doi:10.1056/NEJMoa1403088

Roberts KG, Pei D, Campana D, Payne-Turner D, Li Y, Cheng C, Sandlund JT, Jeha S, Easton J, Becksfort J, et al. 2014b. Outcomes of children with *BCR-ABL1*–like acute lymphoblastic leukemia treated with risk-directed therapy based on the levels of minimal residual disease. *J Clin Oncol* **32:** 3012–3020. doi:10.1200/JCO.2014.55.4105

Roberts KG, Gu Z, Payne-Turner D, McCastlain K, Harvey RC, Chen IM, Pei D, Iacobucci I, Valentine M, Pounds SB, et al. 2017a. High frequency and poor outcome of Philadelphia chromosome-like acute lymphoblastic leukemia in adults. *J Clin Oncol* **35:** 394–401. doi:10.1200/JCO.2016.69.0073

Roberts KG, Yang YL, Payne-Turner D, Lin W, Files JK, Dickerson K, Gu Z, Taunton J, Janke LJ, Chen T, et al. 2017b. Oncogenic role and therapeutic targeting of ABL-class and JAK-STAT activating kinase alterations in Ph-like ALL. *Blood Adv* **1:** 1657–1671. doi:10.1182/bloodadvances.2017000547

Roberts KG, Reshmi SC, Harvey RC, Chen IM, Patel K, Stonerock E, Jenkins H, Dai Y, Valentine M, Gu Z, et al. 2018. Genomic and outcome analyses of Ph-like ALL in NCI standard-risk patients: A report from the children's oncology group. *Blood* **132:** 815–824.

Russell LJ, Enshaei A, Jones L, Erhorn A, Masic D, Bentley H, Laczko KS, Fielding AK, Goldstone AH, Goulden N, et al. 2014. *IGH@* translocations are prevalent in teenagers and young adults with acute lymphoblastic leukemia and are associated with a poor outcome. *J Clin Oncol* **32:** 1453–1462. doi:10.1200/JCO.2013.51.3242

Schinnerl D, Mejstrikova E, Schumich A, Zaliova M, Fortschegger K, Nebral K, Attarbaschi A, Fiser K, Kauer MO, Popitsch N, et al. 2019. CD371 cell surface expression: A unique feature of *DUX4*-rearranged acute lymphoblastic leukemia. *Haematologica* **104:** e352–e355. doi:10.3324/haematol.2018.214353

Schultz KR, Carroll A, Heerema NA, Bowman WP, Aledo A, Slayton WB, Sather H, Devidas M, Zheng HW, Davies SM, et al. 2014. Long-term follow-up of imatinib in pediatric Philadelphia chromosome-positive acute lymphoblastic leukemia: Children's oncology group study AALL0031. *Leukemia* **28:** 1467–1471. doi:10.1038/leu.2014.30

Schwab C, Ryan SL, Chilton L, Elliott A, Murray J, Richardson S, Wragg C, Moppett J, Cummins M, Tunstall O, et al. 2016. *EBF1-PDGFRB* fusion in pediatric B-cell precursor acute lymphoblastic leukemia (BCP-ALL): Genetic profile and clinical implications. *Blood* **127:** 2214–2218. doi:10.1182/blood-2015-09-670166

Schwab C, Nebral K, Chilton L, Leschi C, Waanders E, Boer JM, Žaliová M, Sutton R, Öfverholm II, Ohki K, et al. 2017. Intragenic amplification of *PAX5*: A novel subgroup in B-cell precursor acute lymphoblastic leukemia? *Blood Adv* **1:** 1473–1477. doi:10.1182/bloodadvances.2017006734

Shago M, Abla O, Hitzler J, Weitzman S, Abdelhaleem M. 2016. Frequency and outcome of pediatric acute lymphoblastic leukemia with *ZNF384* gene rearrangements including a novel translocation resulting in an *ARID1B/ZNF384* gene fusion. *Pediatr Blood Cancer* **63:** 1915–1921. doi:10.1002/pbc.26116

Shah S, Schrader KA, Waanders E, Timms AE, Vijai J, Miething C, Wechsler J, Yang J, Hayes J, Klein RJ, et al. 2013. A recurrent germline *PAX5* mutation confers susceptibility to pre-B cell acute lymphoblastic leukemia. *Nat Genet* **45:** 1226–1231. doi:10.1038/ng.2754

Slayton WB, Schultz KR, Kairalla JA, Devidas M, Mi X, Pulsipher MA, Chang BH, Mullighan C, Iacobucci I, Silverman LB, et al. 2018. Dasatinib plus intensive chemotherapy in children, adolescents, and young adults with Philadelphia chromosome-positive acute lymphoblastic leukemia: Results of Children's Oncology Group trial AALL0622. *J Clin Oncol* **36:** 2306–2314. doi:10.1200/JCO.2017.76.7228

Smeenk L, Fischer M, Jurado S, Jaritz M, Azaryan A, Werner B, Roth M, Zuber J, Stanulla M, den Boer ML, et al. 2017. Molecular role of the PAX5-ETV6 oncoprotein in promoting B-cell acute lymphoblastic leukemia. *EMBO J* **36:** 718–735. doi:10.15252/embj.201695495

Stanulla M, Dagdan E, Zaliova M, Möricke A, Palmi C, Cazzaniga G, Eckert C, Te Kronnie G, Bourquin JP, Bornhauser B, et al. 2018. *IKZF1*^{plus} defines a new minimal residual disease-dependent very-poor prognostic profile in pediatric B-cell precursor acute lymphoblastic leukemia. *J Clin Oncol* **36:** 1240–1249. doi:10.1200/JCO.2017.74.3617

Stock W. 2010. Adolescents and young adults with acute lymphoblastic leukemia. *Hematology Am Soc Hematol Educ Program* **2010:** 21–29. doi:10.1182/asheducation-2010.1.21

Suzuki K, Okuno Y, Kawashima N, Muramatsu H, Okuno T, Wang X, Kataoka S, Sekiya Y, Hamada M, Murakami N, et al. 2016. *MEF2D-BCL9* fusion gene is associated with high-risk acute B-cell precursor lymphoblastic leukemia in adolescents. *J Clin Oncol* **34:** 3451–3459. doi:10.1200/JCO.2016.66.5547

Tabe Y, Konopleva M. 2014. Advances in understanding the leukaemia microenvironment. *Br J Haematol* **164:** 767–778. doi:10.1111/bjh.12725

Takahashi K, Wang F, Morita K, Yan Y, Hu P, Zhao P, Zhar AA, Wu CJ, Gumbs C, Little L, et al. 2018. Integrative genomic analysis of adult mixed phenotype acute leukemia delineates lineage associated molecular subtypes. *Nat Commun* **9:** 2670. doi:10.1038/s41467-018-04924-z

Tasian SK, Hurtz C, Wertheim GB, Bailey NG, Lim MS, Harvey RC, Chen IM, Willman CL, Astles R, Zebrowski A, et al. 2017a. High incidence of Philadelphia chromosome-like acute lymphoblastic leukemia in older adults with B-ALL. *Leukemia* **31:** 981–984. doi:10.1038/leu.2016.375

Tasian SK, Loh ML, Hunger SP. 2017b. Philadelphia chromosome-like acute lymphoblastic leukemia. *Blood* **130:** 2064–2072. doi:10.1182/blood-2017-06-743252

Topka S, Vijai J, Walsh MF, Jacobs L, Maria A, Villano D, Gaddam P, Wu G, McGee RB, Quinn E, et al. 2015. Germline *ETV6* mutations confer susceptibility to acute lymphoblastic leukemia and thrombocytopenia. *PLoS Genet* **11:** e1005262. doi:10.1371/journal.pgen.1005262

Tzoneva G, Dieck CL, Oshima K, Ambesi-Impiombato A, Sánchez-Martín M, Madubata CJ, Khiabanian H, Yu J, Waanders E, Iacobucci I, et al. 2018. Clonal evolution mechanisms in *NT5C2* mutant-relapsed acute lymphoblastic leukaemia. *Nature* **553:** 511–514. doi:10.1038/nature25186

Uchida A, Isobe Y, Uemura Y, Nishio Y, Sakai H, Kato M, Otsubo K, Hoshikawa M, Takagi M, Miura I. 2017. De novo acute lymphoblastic leukemia-like disease of high grade B-cell lymphoma with *MYC* and *BCL2* and/or *BCL6* rearrangements: A case report and literature review. *BMC Clin Pathol* **17:** 21. doi:10.1186/s12907-017-0060-1

Wagener R, López C, Kleinheinz K, Bausinger J, Aukema SM, Nagel I, Toprak UH, Seufert J, Altmüller J, Thiele H, et al. 2018. *IG-MYC*$^{+}$ neoplasms with precursor B-cell phenotype are molecularly distinct from Burkitt lymphomas. *Blood* **132:** 2280–2285. doi:10.1182/blood-2018-03-842088

Weston BW, Hayden MA, Roberts KG, Bowyer S, Hsu J, Fedoriw G, Rao KW, Mullighan CG. 2013. Tyrosine kinase inhibitor therapy induces remission in a patient with refractory *EBF1-PDGFRB*-positive acute lymphoblastic leukemia. *J Clin Oncol* **31:** e413–e416. doi:10.1200/JCO.2012.47.6770

Xiao W, Bharadwaj M, Levine M, Farnhoud N, Pastore F, Getta BM, Hultquist A, Famulare C, Medina JS, Patel MA, et al. 2018. *PHF6* and *DNMT3A* mutations are enriched in distinct subgroups of mixed phenotype acute leukemia with T-lineage differentiation. *Blood Adv* **2:** 3526–3539. doi:10.1182/bloodadvances.2018023531

Yang JJ, Cheng C, Devidas M, Cao X, Fan Y, Campana D, Yang W, Neale G, Cox NJ, Scheet P, et al. 2011. Ancestry and pharmacogenomics of relapse in acute lymphoblastic leukemia. *Nat Genet* **43:** 237–241. doi:10.1038/ng.763

Yasuda T, Tsuzuki S, Kawazu M, Hayakawa F, Kojima S, Ueno T, Imoto N, Kohsaka S, Kunita A, Doi K, et al. 2016. Recurrent *DUX4* fusions in B cell acute lymphoblastic leukemia of adolescents and young adults. *Nat Genet* **48:** 569–574. doi:10.1038/ng.3535

Yeoh EJ, Ross ME, Shurtleff SA, Williams WK, Patel D, Mahfouz R, Behm FG, Raimondi SC, Relling MV, Patel A, et al. 2002. Classification, subtype discovery, and prediction of outcome in pediatric acute lymphoblastic leukemia by gene expression profiling. *Cancer Cell* **1:** 133–143. doi:10.1016/S1535-6108(02)00032-6

Yoshihara H, Churchman ML, Peters JL, Finkelstein DB, Paietta EM, Litzow MR, Mullighan CG. 2018. Functional and genomic characterization of the interaction between acute lymphoblastic leukemia cells and the microenvironment identifies pathways for therapeutic intervention. *Blood* **132:** 1550. doi:10.1182/blood-2018-08-867010

Zaliova M, Kotrova M, Bresolin S, Stuchly J, Stary J, Hrusak O, Te Kronnie G, Trka J, Zuna J, Vaskova M. 2017. *ETV6/RUNX1*-like acute lymphoblastic leukemia: A novel B-cell precursor leukemia subtype associated with the CD27/CD44 immunophenotype. *Genes Chromosomes Cancer* **56:** 608–616. doi:10.1002/gcc.22464

Zaliova M, Stuchly J, Winkowska L, Musilova A, Fiser K, Slamova M, Starkova J, Vaskova M, Hrusak O, Sramkova L, et al. 2019. Genomic landscape of pediatric B-other acute lymphoblastic leukemia in a consecutive European cohort. *Haematolica* **104:** 1396–1406. doi:10.3324/haematol.2018.204974

Zhang J, Ding L, Holmfeldt L, Wu G, Heatley SL, Payne-Turner D, Easton J, Chen X, Wang J, Rusch M, et al. 2012. The genetic basis of early T-cell precursor acute lymphoblastic leukaemia. *Nature* **481:** 157–163. doi:10.1038/nature10725

Zhang MY, Churpek JE, Keel SB, Walsh T, Lee MK, Loeb KR, Gulsuner S, Pritchard CC, Sanchez-Bonilla M, Delrow JJ, et al. 2015. Germline *ETV6* mutations in familial thrombocytopenia and hematologic malignancy. *Nat Genet* **47:** 180–185. doi:10.1038/ng.3177

Zhang J, McCastlain K, Yoshihara H, Xu B, Chang Y, Churchman ML, Wu G, Li Y, Wei L, Iacobucci I, et al. 2016. Deregulation of DUX4 and ERG in acute lymphoblastic leukemia. *Nat Genet* **48:** 1481–1489. doi:10.1038/ng.3691

Chronic Lymphocytic Leukemia

Nicholas Chiorazzi,[1] Shih-Shih Chen,[1] and Kanti R. Rai[2]

[1]The Feinstein Institutes for Medical Research, Northwell Health, Manhasset, New York 11030, USA
[2]The Donald and Barbara Zucker School of Medicine at Hofstra/Northwell, Hempstead, New York 11549, USA
Correspondence: NChizzi@Northwell.edu

Patients with chronic lymphocytic leukemia can be divided into three categories: those who are minimally affected by the problem, often never requiring therapy; those that initially follow an indolent course but subsequently progress and require therapy; and those that from the point of diagnosis exhibit an aggressive disease necessitating treatment. Likewise, such patients pass through three phases: development of the disease, diagnosis, and need for therapy. Finally, the leukemic clones of all patients appear to require continuous input from the exterior, most often through membrane receptors, to allow them to survive and grow. This review is presented according to the temporal course that the disease follows, focusing on those external influences from the tissue microenvironment (TME) that support the time lines as well as those internal influences that are inherited or develop as genetic and epigenetic changes occurring over the time line. Regarding the former, special emphasis is placed on the input provided via the B-cell receptor for antigen and the C-X-C-motif chemokine receptor-4 and the therapeutic agents that block these inputs. Regarding the latter, prominence is laid upon inherited susceptibility genes and the genetic and epigenetic abnormalities that lead to the developmental and progression of the disease.

Chronic lymphocytic leukemia (CLL) is a disease of aging adults. Because it often begins as a relatively indolent condition with many patients having long survival, CLL has a high prevalence rate, making it the most common adult leukemia in western countries. The disease results from the overgrowth of a single $CD5^+$ B lymphocyte co-expressing low levels of surface membrane immunoglobulin (smIg) of a single IG light (L) chain type and of CD79b, CD20, and CD23. The clinical consequences of this clonal overgrowth are highly variable: Some patients die within 2–3 yr of diagnosis, whereas others survive decades beyond. This variability is due to factors intrinsic to the leukemic B cell (e.g., genetic and epigenetic changes in coding and noncoding genes) and factors extrinsic to the leukemic cell (e.g., inputs delivered by various signaling pathways in the tissue microenvironment [TME]).

This perspective is organized according to the order CLL evolves in patients. It starts with epidemiologic, genetic, and environmental factors that influence development of the disease, follows with features leading to the clinical presentation, diagnosis, and initial treatment, if necessary, and concludes with elements causing disease progression or therapy refractoriness,

Cite this article as *Cold Spring Harb Perspect Med* doi: 10.1101/cshperspect.a035220

describing current and emerging therapeutic options. Emphasis is placed on recent findings relating to these three periods.

DISEASE DEVELOPMENT

Epidemiology

According to the National Cancer Institute's Surveillance, Epidemiology, and End Results Program (SEER), the estimated number of new cases of CLL in the United States in 2018 was 20,940, representing ~1.2% of new cancer diagnoses and the number of deaths from CLL was 4510, ~0.7% of all cancer deaths (SEER Cancer Stat Facts: Chronic Lymphocytic Leukemia, National Cancer Institute, Bethesda, MD; https://seer.cancer.gov/statfacts/html/clyl.html). Median age at diagnosis was 70, with the highest numbers of cases identified in the 65–74 yr age group.

However, these statistics are not relevant worldwide as the incidence of CLL varies based on race/ethnicity: White > Black > Hispanic > Asian/Pacific Islander. Incidence also varies based on gender, being approximately two-fold more frequent in males.

Environmental Considerations

Exposure to pesticides, specifically deltamethrin (Leon et al. 2019), and herbicides (Alavanja et al. 2014; Coggon et al. 2015) has been associated with the development of CLL; the most convincing is Agent Orange used during the Vietnam War (Baumann Kreuziger et al. 2014; Mescher et al. 2018). Radon exposure has shown a similar relationship (Schwartz and Klug 2016).

The link with ionizing radiation is controversial. Because CLL incidence did not increase among Japanese exposed to atomic bomb blasts in World War II (Preston et al. 1994), ionizing radiation was not considered a risk factor. However, epidemiologic studies of people in the vicinity of the Grenoble nuclear power plant breakdown suggest an increased incidence among exposed individuals (Gluzman et al. 2006; Chumak et al. 2008; Kesminiene et al. 2008; Romanenko et al. 2008; Zablotska et al. 2013), so this conclusion needs reconsideration.

Finally, respiratory tract infections, cellulitis, and herpes zoster can presage CLL (Landgren et al. 2007a,b; Lesley et al. 2009), implying an underlying immune defect predisposing to disease development. Consistent with this, hypogammaglobulinemia is common in CLL and can precede diagnosis (Lenders et al. 1984; Tsai et al. 2009).

Genetic Considerations

Inheritance of Susceptibility Genes

CLL has the highest incidence of familial association among leukemias, with first-degree relatives having more than eight-fold higher likelihood of developing the disease (Goldin et al. 2004). Conversely, the low CLL incidence among Asians/Pacific Islanders, particularly Japanese, does not increase when living in the United States (Gale et al. 2000). Both observations strongly imply involvement of inheritable susceptibility alleles that promote or prevent disease. Genome-wide association studies (GWASs) identified several polymorphic genetic loci (Di Bernardo et al. 2008; Crowther-Swanepoel et al. 2010a; Slager et al. 2011, 2012; Berndt et al. 2013, 2016; Speedy et al. 2014). These have been refined to the nine most likely (Law et al. 2017), which are transcriptionally active in CLL cells and contain genes involved in the control of human B-cell development and signaling or of immune function (Law et al. 2017). Consistent with this, GWASs of CLL and myeloma patients uncovered shared risk loci influenced by polymorphisms in B-cell regulatory elements affecting genes involved in B-cell development (Went et al. 2019).

Normal B-lymphocyte development proceeds by an ordered process of cellular maturation occurring in the bone marrow (BM), beginning with a hematopoietic stem cell (HSC) and culminating with a mature B cell (Fig. 1A). Mature B lymphocytes evolve to memory and/or plasma cells based on the types of antigens encountered in the periphery and the maturation pathways they are guided to follow by cells of the hematopoietic and nonhematopoietic lineages. Thus, susceptibility genes can exert in-

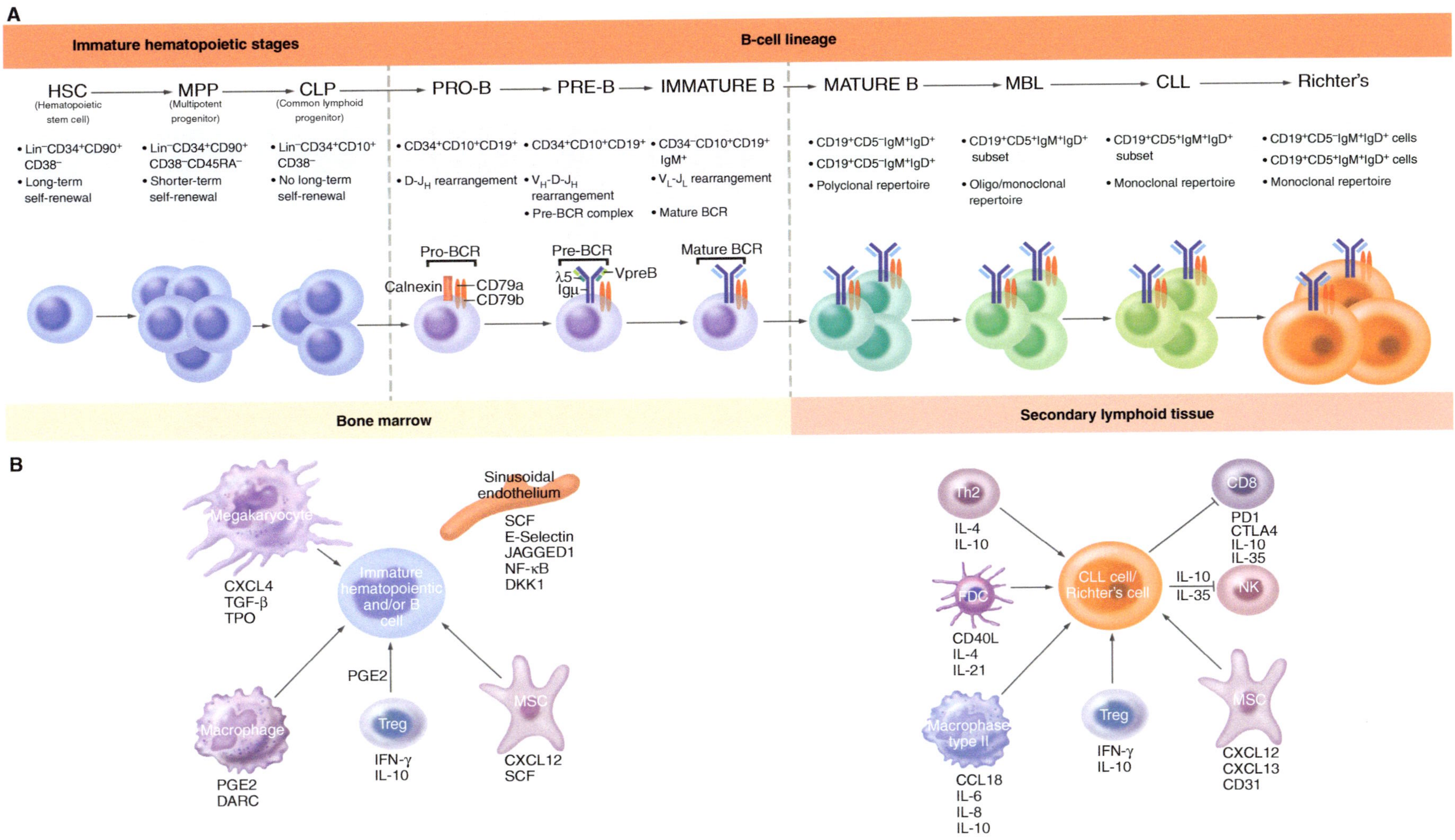

Figure 1. (*Legend on following page.*)

fluences at many points along the B-cell differentiation path.

Noninherited Recurrent Genetic Mutations in CLL Cells

The leukemic cells from the majority of patients exhibit chromosomal abnormalities at some point in the course of disease. Moreover, normal cells at early stages of hematopoiesis taken from CLL patients have mutations present in their leukemic clone (Damm et al. 2014; Marsilio et al. 2018). Transplantation of HSCs from CLL patients into immune-compromised mice leads to mature $CD5^+$ B cells resembling those in CLL patients (Kikushige et al. 2011). These early mutations, however, are not sufficient to yield the full-fledged disease (Kikushige et al. 2011) but result in a pre-leukemic state resembling monoclonal B lymphocytosis (Rawstron et al. 2002b).

The most common somatic abnormalities found in mature CLL cells are del13q, tri12, del11q, and del17p, in this order of frequency (Döhner et al. 2000; Haferlach et al. 2007; Zenz et al. 2010a; Stilgenbauer 2014). Deletions at 13q and tri12 are found at diagnosis, suggesting these are initiating events; del11q and del17p are most often found later in disease, implying they promote clonal evolution and disease progression. The incriminating genetic elements in del13q are two microRNAs, *miR15a/16b* (Calin et al. 2002). Loss of *miR15a/16b* leads to overproduction of the anti-apoptotic protein Bcl-2 (Cimmino et al. 2005) and heightened cell-cycle progression (Klein et al. 2010), both oncogene-like effects. Moreover, mice with a defective *miR15/16* spontaneously develop a CLL-like disease (Raveche et al. 2007; Hayakawa et al. 2016), and deletion of the chromosomal region corresponding to 13q in mice leads to murine CLL (Klein et al. 2010; Kasar et al. 2016).

The advent of high-throughput, next-generation deep DNA sequencing enabled the demonstration that CLL cells also exhibit specific gene aberrations. Beginning in 2011 (Fabbri et al. 2011; Puente et al. 2011; Quesada et al.

Figure 1. Microenvironment-supported B-lymphocyte development in patients with chronic lymphocytic leukemia (CLL). (*A*) Differentiation scheme assumed for CLL and Richter's transformation (RT) cells. Normal B lymphocytes progress through an ordered differentiation program that begins with hematopoietic stem cells (HSCs), proceeds through multipotent progenitor cells (MPPs), and then common lymphoid precursors (CLPs). After this point, commitment is made to the B-lymphocyte lineage. Pro-, pre-, and immature B cells differ based on the progressive rearrangements of *IGHV*, *IGHD*, and *IGHJ* genes. *IGHD-IGHJ* rearrangement is completed in pro-B cells, followed by *IGHV-IGHD-IGHJ* rearrangement in pre-B cells, and both *IGHV-IGHD-IGHJ* + *IGLV-IGLJ* rearrangements in immature B cells. Thus, antibodies that can create a complete B-cell receptor (BCR) exist from the pre-B cell–immature B cell interphase and at later stages of B-cell development (transitional, mature, etc.). Mutations in CLL HSCs and MPPs have been documented (Damm et al. 2014; Marsilio et al. 2018), and xenografting CLL HSCs/MPPs into severely immune-compromised mice (Kikushige et al. 2011) leads to a condition resembling monoclonal B-lymphocytosis (Rawstron et al. 2002a). If leukemia stem cells exist in CLL, HSCs, MPPs, CLPs, and pro-B cells carrying genetic abnormalities would be considered "pre-leukemic stem cells" and not "leukemic stem cells," because they could not give rise to a CLL cell with the same *IGHV-IGHD-IGHJ* + *IGLV-IGLJ* rearrangements. The latter is relevant because, upon disease relapse, the emerging cells express a complete B-cell receptor (*IGHV-IGHD-IGHJ* + *IGLV-IGLJ* rearrangements) that indicates it is a member of the original CLL clone. Hence, we suggest the true leukemic stem cell in CLL resides at a differentiation stage at or beyond the pre-B cell–immature B cell interphase. CLL cells proliferate in secondary lymphoid organs and can transformation to Richter's cells, often as CLL-derived diffused large B-cell lymphoma (DLBCL) that have larger cells with prominent nuclei. (*B*) Microenvironmental signals associated with clonal expansion. (*Left*) Bone marrow microenvironment that supports normal and abnormal hematopoietic development. Bone marrow niche supports the differentiation and maturation of B cells. Immature HSCs and B cells are maintained and regulated by niche factors (i.e., CXCL12 and SCF produced by MSC), endothelial cell–derived signals (i.e., SCF, E-selectin, JAGGED1), and the progeny of HSCs including macrophages and megakaryocyte and regulatory T cells. (*Right*) The secondary lymphoid microenvironment sustains CLL and RT cells. CLL and RT cells receive growth promotion (e.g., IL-4, IL-21, CD40L, CCL19) and suppression (e.g., IL-10, IL-35, and PDL1-PD1 interaction) signals, as well as cell homing and retention cues (CXCL12, CXCL13, and CD31). Th2, T helper 2 cells; FDC, follicular dendritic cell; NK, natural-killer cell; MSC, mesenchymal stromal cell; Treg, T regulatory cell.

 Cite this article as *Cold Spring Harb Perspect Med* doi: 10.1101/cshperspect.a035220

2011; Wang et al. 2011) and now involving approximately 1000 CLL exomes (Quesada et al. 2012; Landau et al. 2013, 2015; Puente et al. 2015; Ljungström et al. 2016), a series of gene mutations was identified in CLL, although not as plentiful as in solid tumors (Table 1; Pleasance et al. 2010). Most of these lead to amino acid changes, suggesting selection for pathogenicity. Pathways controlling DNA damage repair/cell cycle control, Notch signaling, IL-1R family signaling, Wnt signaling, and RNA processing and export, MYC activity, and MAPK signaling are affected (Wang et al. 2011; Landau et al. 2015).

More disease-driving aberrations are found in *IGHV*-unmutated CLL (U-CLL) than in *IGHV*-mutated CLL (M-CLL). Additionally, certain mutations occur more frequently in U-CLL (*NOTCH1*, *XPO1*, and *POT1*) and others in M-CLL (del(13q), *MyD88*, and *CHD2*), or in CLL subsets with specific genomic aberrations (e.g., *MyD88* with del13q; *SF3B1* with del11q; *NOTCH1*, *BIRC3*, *FBXW7*, and BCOR with tri12 [Table 1]). Moreover, sets of mutations associate with the use of certain stereotyped *IGHV-IGHD-IGHJ* gene rearrangements (Rossi et al. 2009b; Sutton et al. 2016). Selected mutations occur in specific regions of individual genes (e.g., PEST domain of *NOTCH1* and HEAT domain of *SF3B1*). In some instances, a relationship exists between a specific abnormality and aggressive clinical course and/or shortened survival (Rossi et al. 2012a); this might be caused by development of Richter's transformation (RT) (Richter 1928) (Table 2; Fabbri et al. 2011; Rossi et al. 2012b).

Collectively, these associations and the fact that no single mutation is found in every CLL clone strongly suggest the development of CLL differs for distinct subsets of patients. In this

Table 1. Recurrent mutations in chronic lymphocytic leukemia (CLL) B cells that associate with chromosomal aberrations, IGHV genes, and mutation status and stereotyped subsets

Mutation	Chromosomal aberrations[a]	IGHV gene[b]	Stereotyped subset[c]
SF3B1	del11q	*IGHV1-69* (unmutated)	#3, #7
	del13q	*IGHV3-21* (unmutated)	#2
		IGHV3-21 (mutated)	#2
ATM	del11q	*IGHV3-21* (unmutated)	#2
	del13q	*IGHV3-21* (mutated)	#2
NOTCH1	Trisomy 12	*IGHV1-69* (unmutated)	#6
		IGHV4-39 (unmutated)	#8
		Clan I genes (unmutated)	#1, #99, #59,
BCOR	Trisomy 12		
BIRC3	Trisomy 12		
FBXW7	Trisomy 12		
XPO1	del11q	U-CLL > M-CLL	
	del13q		
POT1	del11q	U-CLL > M-CLL	
	del13q		
CHD2	del13q	M-CLL > U-CLL	
TP53	del13q	Clan I genes (unmutated)	#1, #99
	del17p		
MYD88	del13q	M-CLL > U-CLL	
SAMHD1	del13q		

[a]Main recurrent genetic aberrations associated with chromosomal abnormalities of known prognostic significance in CLL.

[b]*IGHV* (immunoglobulin heavy variable) gene and mutation status associated with common genetic aberrations. *IGHV* gene mutations are determined based on degree of identity with the germline (≥98% identity = "unmutated," U-CLL; <98% germline identity = "mutated," M-CLL). Mutations of *XPO1*, *POT1*, *CHD2*, and *MYD88* are not associated with a specific *IGHV* gene mutation but occur more frequently in M-CLL or U-CLL.

[c]Stereotyped subset-biased acquisition of recurrent gene mutations. *MYD88* and *BIRC3* mutations are rare in all subsets.

Table 2. Biological pathways associated with common mutations

Type of pathway	Common mutations
RNA and ribosomal-processing	*SF3B1, XPO1, RPS15, DOX3X, ZNF292, MED12, NXF1*
DNA-damage and cell-cycle-control	*ATM, TP53, POT1*
Chromatin-modification	*CHD2, ZMYM3, BAZ2A, ASXL1, SETD2*
Notch-signaling	*NOTCH1, FBXW7*
Inflammatory	*BIRC3, MYD88, TRAF3, SAMHD1*
MAPK-ERK	*BRAF, KRAS, MAP2K1, NRAS*
WNT-signaling and MYC-related	*MGA, PTPN11*
BCR-signaling	*EGR2, PAX5, BCOR, IRF4, IKZF3*

MAPK, Mitogen-activated protein kinases; ERK, extracellular signal–regulated kinases; WNT, wingless/integrated; BCR, B-cell receptor.

regard, mutations in U-CLL patients are more often found in coding regions of driver genes, and mutations in M-CLL tend to target promoter and enhancer regions. Moreover, the former mutations carry signatures suggesting a mutation mechanism associated with aging, whereas the latter suggest a mechanism associated with activation-induced cytidine deaminase (AID) activity (Burns et al. 2018). These mutational mechanisms have been suggested as active in CLL, albeit not in an *IGHV*-defined subset setting (Alexandrov et al. 2013; Kasar et al. 2015).

Influences of B-Lymphocyte Surface Receptors on CLL

In addition to genetic and environmental factors, normal B lymphocytes are influenced by cell-autonomous and cell-extrinsic signals that promote clonal survival and expansion.

Signals Initiated by the B-Cell Receptor for Antigen

Normal B lymphocytes respond to insults (often microbial) from the exterior and from within. In each instance, engagement of (auto)antigens by the smIg of the B-cell receptor (BCR) transmits an activating signal leading to survival and growth or anergy or death (Fig. 2). Based on structural studies of variable domains of Igs made by the leukemic B lymphocytes, the (auto)antigens they can bind, and the consequences of initiating such signals in vitro, it appears CLL B cells respond similarly to such inputs.

Consistent with derivation from a human B-cell subpopulation analogous to the murine $CD5^+/Ly1^+/B1^+$ B-cell subset (Hayakawa et al. 1983), initial studies of the genes coding for the variable domains of CLL Igs suggested these were restricted in use (Fong et al. 1985; Kipps et al. 1988) and were minimally, if at all, different from the germline sequence (Meeker et al. 1988; Pratt et al. 1989; Küppers et al. 1991; Friedman et al. 1992; Wagner and Luzzatto 1993; Pan et al. 1996). Subsequent studies confirmed restricted gene use (Johnson et al. 1997; Fais et al. 1998; Widhopf and Kipps 2001; Kröber et al. 2002; Ghiotto et al. 2006; Hadzidimitriou et al. 2009), although a review of available CLL sequences (Schroeder and Dighiero 1994) and prospective analyses of IgG^+ (Hashimoto et al. 1995) and IgM^+ (Fais et al. 1998) clones showed that >50% of randomly chosen IgM^+ CLL cases as well as ~75% of IgG^+ and IgA^+ cases exhibited significant numbers of *IGHV* mutations (>2% differences from the most similar germline gene). Thus, CLL clones are molecularly heterogeneous and can be subgrouped based on *IGHV* gene mutations. Notably, these two CLL types, M-CLL and U-CLL, have dramatically different clinical courses and outcomes (Damle et al. 1999; Hamblin et al. 1999), and segregating CLL patients this way is a valuable prognostic indicator for patient outcome.

Furthermore, certain CLL IGs have remarkably similar amino acid *IGHV-IGHD-IGHJ* rearrangements with characteristic HCDR3 amino acid motifs (Tobin et al. 2003, 2004; Ghiotto et al. 2004; Messmer et al. 2004; Stamatopoulos

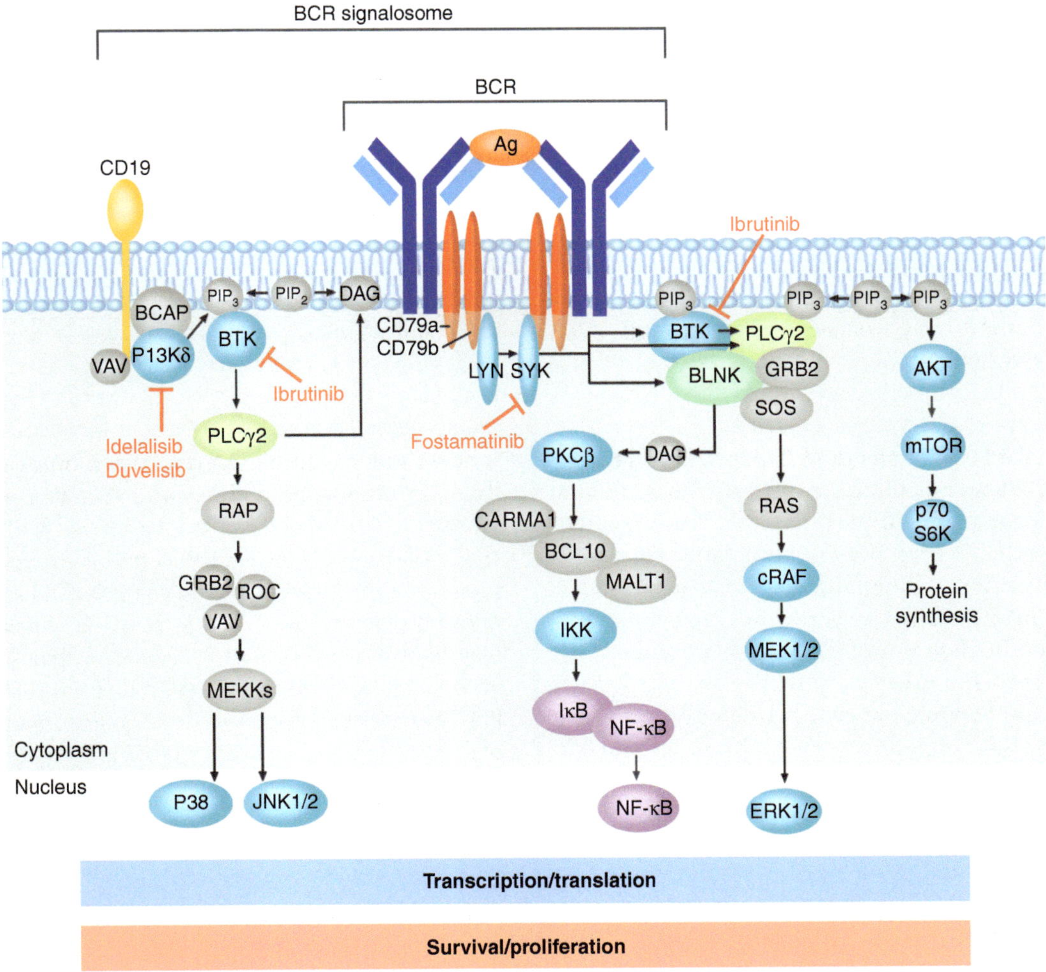

Figure 2. B-cell receptor (BCR) signaling pathway and the effects of kinase inhibition. Upon antigen interaction with the membrane IG component of the BCR, Lyn is activated and in turn phosphorylates CD79 on tyrosine residues—in particular, those in ITAM motifs. This permits binding of SYK and various adaptor molecules that initiate signaling that proceeds through key kinases including BTK, PI3Kδ, and AKT. (For a comprehensive review, see Slupsky [2014)].) The sites of action for kinase inhibitors are indicated: BTK (ibrutinib), PI3Kδ (idelalisib), PI3Kδ+γ (duvelisib), and SYK (fostamatinib).

et al. 2007, 2017; Vardi et al. 2014; Agathangelidis et al. 2019); these are referred to as "stereotyped BCRs" (Messmer et al. 2004). The likelihood such rearrangements occur by chance is infinitesimally small (10^{-12}), indicating selection of normal B lymphocytes with defined and in some cases quasi-unique BCR structures rarely found in large amounts in the normal B-cell repertoire. Stereotyped BCRs are found in ~33% of CLL cases (Stamatopoulos et al. 2007; Murray et al. 2008; Agathangelidis et al. 2012, 2019). When considering U-CLL, ~50% of cases fall into a stereotyped subset.

Foreign or autologous antigens engage smIg leading to a series of stimulatory events activating various B-cell fates: survival, expansion, anergy, or death. The state or type of B cell as well as concomitant signals delivered via membrane molecules on other cells or their secreted factors determine which fate occurs. For CLL cells, the antigens or classes of antigens involved are foreign (e.g., viral [Steininger et al. 2012], fungal

[Hoogeboom et al. 2013], and bacterial [Hatzi et al. 2016]) or autologous (e.g., self-antigens characteristic of autoimmune disorders [Bröker et al. 1988; Sthoeger et al. 1989; Borche et al. 1990; Hervé et al. 2005]) and self-antigens developing during apoptosis or normal catabolism (Catera et al. 2006; Chu et al. 2008, 2010; Lanemo Myhrinder et al. 2008). B-cell interactions with antigens that support survival and expansion most likely occur in solid tissues where most CLL cells divide (Calissano et al. 2011; Herishanu et al. 2011; Herndon et al. 2017) and hematopoietic and nonhematopoietic cells support survival and expansion.

Another important type of autoreactivity characteristic of CLL IGs is their ability to bind themselves (Binder et al. 2011, 2013; Dühren-von Minden et al. 2012), leading to self-association/homodimerization (Minici et al. 2017). This interaction results in BCR signaling without binding antigenic epitopes external to the B cell and extrinsic to the BCR, referred to as "autonomous signaling" (Dühren-von Minden et al. 2012). Although not yet studied thoroughly, the affinity of self-association, and hence the frequency of autonomous signaling, correlates with patient outcome: High affinity correlates with better outcome and low affinity with bad outcome (Minici et al. 2017). It has been suggested that this type of signaling promotes survival or anergy, whereas signaling resulting from smIg binding of non-IG antigens leads to proliferation (Chiorazzi and Efremov 2013). Self-association/autonomous signaling occurs in normal pre-B cells (Köhler et al. 2008; Eschbach et al. 2011) and B-1 cells in mice (Köhler et al. 2008), and findings from a mouse model of CLL support its importance in the human disease (Iacovelli et al. 2015).

Signals Initiated by Other Membrane-Associated Pathways

Several other signaling pathways affect the biology of CLL cells. The C-X-C-motif chemokine receptor-4 (CXCR4) is critical in allowing CLL cells to traffic to survival niches in solid tissues (Burger and Bürkle 2007) and delivers survival signals to normal B lymphocytes and CLL cells (Burger and Kipps 2002). Similarly, CD38 and CD49d, two membrane molecules whose levels of expression correlate with clinical course in CLL (Damle et al. 1999; Bulian et al. 2008; Gattei et al. 2008; Rossi et al. 2008; Shanafelt et al. 2008a), deliver trophic signals to CLL cells (Deaglio et al. 2003, 2007; Zucchetto et al. 2009, 2012; Vaisitti et al. 2010). The orphan receptor ROR-1, initially identified by gene expression analyses of CLL B cells (Klein et al. 2001; Rosenwald et al. 2001) and subsequently found on CLL cells (Baskar et al. 2008; Daneshmanesh et al. 2008; Fukuda et al. 2008), delivers signals, either constitutively (Hojjat-Farsangi et al. 2013) or after interacting with Wnt family ligands (Yu et al. 2016). Because ROR-1 signaling promotes CLL cell survival, growth, and migration (Cui et al. 2016; Hasan et al. 2017, 2019; Yu et al. 2017) and ROR-1 is expressed only on CLL cells and certain other B-cell lymphoproliferative disorders and not on immature and mature normal B lymphocytes (Broome et al. 2011), targeting the molecule is a potential therapy (Yang et al. 2011). Clinical trials with anti-ROR-1 monoclonal antibodies (mAbs) (Choi et al. 2015) and with chimeric antigen-receptor (CAR)-T cells bearing anti-ROR-1 mAbs (Hudecek et al. 2010) are under way.

Other Microenvironmental Signals Associated with Clonal Expansion

Other hematopoietic and nonhematopoietic cells foster clonal expansion, either by cell–cell contact or by elaborating cytokines and chemokines (Fig. 1B). For example, nurse-like cells, a CLL equivalent of tumor-associated macrophages (Tsukada et al. 2002), secrete the CXCR4 ligand, CXCL12; this attracts leukemic B cells to these trophic elements that secrete BAFF and APRIL (Nishio et al. 2005). Additionally, classical macrophages, particularly those of the M2 type, promote survival, and elimination of these cells prevents CLL-cell growth (Galletti et al. 2016; Hanna et al. 2016). In addition, although T lymphocytes in CLL are defective in interacting with leukemic B cells (Ramsay et al. 2008) and hence do not effectively carry out cytolysis, they do promote survival and expansion in vitro (Granziero et al. 2001; Os et al. 2013) and

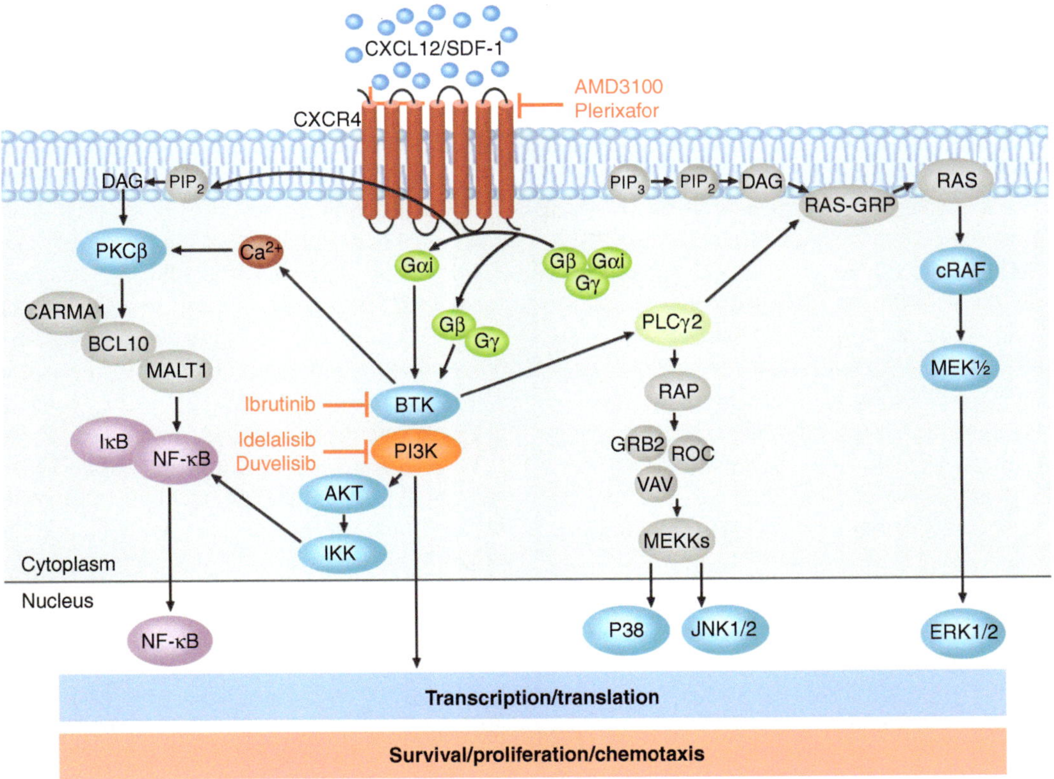

Figure 3. CXCR4 signaling pathway and the effects of kinase inhibition. CXCR4 (C-X-C-motif chemokine receptor-4) is a G protein–coupled receptor (GPCR) that binds CXCL12/stromal-derived-factor-1 (SDF-1). CXCR4 signaling in response to CXCL12/SDF-1 mediates migration of circulating CLL cells. As a GPCR, CXCR4 engagement activates G protein–mediated signaling resulting in intracellular Ca^{2+} flux and subsequent activation of downstream pathways such as Ras and PI3Kδ. Activated JNK and PI3Kδ signaling lead to cell survival and migration. CXCR4 induces downstream signaling by several pathways such as those involving BTK and PLCγ2 signaling. Blocking CXCR4 signaling can be achieved by AMD3100 and plerixafor, which prevent CXCR4/SDF-1 binding, and by BTK inhibitor by ibrutinib. Other small molecular inhibitors like idelalisib and duvelisib target PI3K to block CXCR4 downstream signaling.

in xenografts (Bagnara et al. 2011; Patten et al. 2016). CLL cells, especially from poor-outcome U-CLL patients, secrete CCL3 and CCL4 that draw T cells into their vicinity, thereby receiving trophic signals (Burger et al. 2009). IL-4 is especially relevant for survival and reprogramming smIg expression (Fig. 3; Aguilar-Hernandez et al. 2016; Guo et al. 2016). Finally, mesenchymal stromal cells support CLL-cell survival by secreting cytokines and chemokines (Trimarco et al. 2015), as do vascular endothelial cells expressing CD31, the co-receptor for CD38 on hematopoietic cells including CLL cells (Deaglio et al. 1996, 2000).

Monoclonal B-Cell Lymphocytosis

B lymphocytes bearing a CLL phenotype can be found in the blood of normal individuals, in some instances years before the diagnosis of CLL (Landgren et al. 2009; Georgiadis et al. 2017). This condition, termed monoclonal B-cell lymphocytosis (MBL), is defined by elevated numbers of $CD5^{+}CD19^{+}CD20^{low}CD79b^{low}Ig^{low}$ cells in the blood and no evidence for CLL or small lymphocytic lymphoma (SLL) (Marti et al. 2005; Shanafelt et al. 2010).

MBL is surprisingly common. Approximately 5% of the general population after the age of 40 has MBL, increasing to ∼15% after the age of 70 (Rawstron et al. 2002a; Ghia et al. 2004). Moreover, first-degree relatives in familial CLL cohorts have a ∼15% incidence of MBL after the age of 40, and first-degree relatives in families with sporadic CLL have a similar incidence after age 60 (Rawstron et al. 2002b; Marti et al. 2003; Matos et al. 2009; Goldin et al. 2010). Because annually only 1% of subjects with MBL progress to CLL requiring therapy (Rawstron et al. 2002a,b; Fung et al. 2007; Rossi 2009a; Shanafelt et al. 2009b; Molica et al. 2011), additional events, most likely genetic aberrations, are needed to usher this common condition to leukemia. Elevated serum β_2-microglobulin levels and expression of an unmutated *IGHV* by the MBL clone predict a shorter transformation time to CLL (Parikh et al. 2018).

The common genetic abnormalities (Rawstron et al. 2008; Shanafelt et al. 2009a; Molica et al. 2011) and susceptibility loci (Crowther-Swanepoel et al. 2010b) characteristic of CLL are found in MBL. Although limited, genetic studies using next-generation sequencing (NGS) reveal similarities between MBL and early-stage CLL (Rasi et al. 2012; Greco et al. 2013; Ojha et al. 2014; Agathangelidis et al. 2018; Popp et al. 2019). MBL and CLL samples have similar mutation burdens; however, when analyzed for specific driver mutations, less are found in MBL (Puente et al. 2015), consistent with the stepwise evolution from one to the other.

Finally, as in CLL, there are implications for a more global immune defect in people with MBL. Such individuals have a higher incidence of severe infections (Lesley et al. 2009; Casabonne et al. 2012; Moreira et al. 2013) and nonhematologic cancers (Solomon et al. 2016) and may have an increased incidence of hypogammaglobulinemia (Glancy and Siles 2016).

Normal Cell Equivalents of Full-Fledged CLL B Cells

CLL cells are identified by CD5 expression and hence could be derived from a normal CD5$^+$ human B lymphocyte. It is believed that this human B-cell subset is evolutionarily aligned with the murine B-1 subset (Hayakawa et al. 1983). Although murine CD5$^+$ B-1 cells have been extensively studied, it is controversial whether they derive from a one-of-a-kind hematopoietic precursor, hence embodying a distinct B-cell lineage (Montecino-Rodriguez et al. 2006; Ghosn et al. 2011), or represent sets of B lymphocytes that acquire a unique surface membrane phenotype and functional features based on the maturational path followed during development (Haughton et al. 1993). The same conundrum exists for CLL—that is, one precursor cell type that follows different maturation stages, thereby accumulating or not somatic *IGHV* mutations, or two (or more) fundamentally distinct precursors. Candidate precursors include mature CD5$^+$ B cells (Seifert et al. 2012) and a B-cell subset bearing the CD20$^+$CD27$^+$CD43$^+$CD70$^-$ surface membrane phenotype (Griffin et al. 2011).

Because CLL B cells fall into two categories based on *IGHV* gene mutations, it has been suggested U-CLL cells derive from naive B lymphocytes and M-CLL from memory B cells. However, because both CLL subtypes appear to be chronically activated cells based on membrane phenotype (Damle et al. 2002), telomere lengths (Damle et al. 2004; Strefford et al. 2015), gene expression profiling (Klein et al. 2001; Rosenwald et al. 2001), and epigenetic analyses (Oakes et al. 2016), precursors for both CLL subtypes are likely antigen-experienced. In this regard, because U-CLL clones can spontaneously (Gurrieri et al. 2002; Bagnara et al. 2006) or upon stimulation (Patten et al. 2012, 2016) acquire new *IGHV* mutations, it is possible the lack of mutations in the majority of cells in these clones is due to the developmental path the normal B cell followed prior to transformation (Chiorazzi and Ferrarini 2003).

Collectively, the above suggests CLL develops in genetically susceptible people upon exposure to still ill-defined environmental antigens possibly acting in concert with common autoantigens. This might be a stepwise process beginning early in hematopoietic and B-cell ontogeny and ending in cells downstream in the B-cell developmental pathway at a point after rearrangement of the *IGHV-IGHD-IGHJ* and *IGLV-IGLJ* segments (Fig. 1A). This selection is mediated either by classical interactions of smIg with (auto)antigens or by smIg self-association and consequent autonomous signaling. Chronic stimulation over time, probably due to ongoing stimulation through the BCR and possibly other pathways (e.g., TLR9 or TLR7), leads to repetitive rounds of DNA replication and development of genetic abnormalities that complement each other and create a leukemic clone. This occurs in normal B cells selected for transformation based on the structure of their BCRs.

DIAGNOSIS AND INITIAL TREATMENT OF CLL

Clinical and Laboratory Parameters

In most western countries in which health care is readily accessible, diagnosis of CLL is made during a routine medical visit by finding an elevated number of lymphocytes on a complete blood count. If lymphocyte expansion persists, flow cytometric analysis of the number of $CD5^+CD19^+$ B cells is carried out, searching for an increased number of cells with low levels of smIg of a single IG L chain type co-expressing CD20, CD79b, and CD23. Because most patients are asymptomatic at this time, clinical history is often not revealing, although weight loss, lethargy, night sweats, and complaints of "swollen glands" may be reported. Physical examination focuses on identifying lymphadenopathy and hepatosplenomegaly and evidence of red blood cell or platelet deficiencies. Guidelines for the diagnosis and treatment of CLL have recently been updated (Hallek et al. 2018).

Prognostic Markers

Upon diagnosis of CLL, a series of prognostic indicators may assist in defining the stage of the disease and in predicting the clinical course that an individual patient will follow. Clinical stage is assigned according to algorithms defined by Rai et al. (1975) or Binet et al. (1981), using physical findings and the results of a complete blood count. These time-honored approaches remain the mainstays of clinical care.

Predictions of clinical course and outcome can be made by analyzing a series of laboratory parameters. Perhaps the most reliable prognostic indicator is "*IGHV* mutation status": the presence or absence of significant numbers of somatic mutations in the *IGHV* gene expressed by the CLL clone. As discussed, CLL clones can be divided into two categories, based on mutations in the heavy chain variable gene, *IGHV*-unmutated ("U-CLL; $\leq$2% difference from the most similar germline gene) and *IGHV*-mutated ("M-CLL"; >2% difference from the most similar germline gene) (Schroeder and Dighiero 1994; Hashimoto et al. 1995; Fais et al. 1998), with patients bearing a U-CLL clone having a more aggressive clinical course (Damle et al. 1999; Hamblin et al. 1999).

Other cell-based indicators suggesting an inferior clinical course include increased percentages of CLL cells bearing membrane CD38 (Damle et al. 1999) or CD49d (Shanafelt et al. 2008a; Bulian et al. 2014; Baumann et al. 2016) or intracellular levels of ZAP70 (Crespo et al. 2003; Rassenti et al. 2008). Furthermore, β_2-microglobulin (Simonsson et al. 1980; Di Giovanni et al. 1989; Keating et al. 1995) and thymidine kinase (Hallek et al. 1999) serum levels provide prognostic information; the former is easier to analyze and is preferred in clinical settings.

Finally, serial absolute lymphocyte counts afford helpful information. Patients whose absolute lymphocyte counts double in <1 yr are more likely to follow an aggressive course (Montserrat et al. 1986; Molica and Alberti 1987).

Predictive Markers

Whereas prognostic markers try to presage the likelihood of disease progression and hence clinical outcome, predictive markers try to foresee the response to a given therapy (Oldenhuis et al. 2008; Mandrekar and Sargent 2010; Zenz et al. 2010b; Montserrat 2012). Because CLL is a heterogeneous disease at the clinical and molecular levels, it is difficult to define parameters that best predict outcome to a specific therapy. Moreover, because the therapies for CLL are currently under major flux, the principles defined for one approach might not apply to another. With these caveats in mind, genetic abnormalities, particularly loss or mutation of *TP53*, are predictive for certain therapies. Patients with TP53 disruption do not respond to chemoimmunotherapy and might be compromised by it (Gonzalez et al. 2011). Moreover, although patients with this genetic lesion respond to signaling inhibitors better than to chemoimmunotherapy, these patients are more likely to relapse (Byrd et al. 2015; Farooqui et al. 2015). Additionally, the presence of mutations in NOTCH1 can signal ineffectiveness of anti-CD20 mAb treatment because of diminished numbers of membrane CD20 molecules (Pozzo et al. 2016).

Possibly the most reliable predictive indicator for patients treated with chemotherapy and chemoimmunotherapy is the level of minimal residual disease (MRD) detectable after therapy. MRD is evaluated using multiparameter flow cytometry (Rawstron et al. 2013; Böttcher 2019), using polymerase chain reaction detection of the signature VH CDR3 segment of the CLL clone (van Dongen et al. 2003), and, recently, by next-generation deep sequencing of the CLL *IGHV-IGHD-IGHJ* rearrangement (Logan et al. 2011, 2013; Rawstron et al. 2015; Rodríguez-Vicente et al. 2017).

The extent of MRD independently predicts progression-free survival and overall survival in patients receiving various chemotherapy and chemoimmunotherapy regimens in the front-line, follow-up, and consolidation settings (Böttcher et al. 2012; Kwok et al. 2016; Varghese et al. 2017). Hence, MRD can be used as a surrogate for progression-free survival in therapeutic clinical trials (Dimier et al. 2018). However, a role for MRD in patients treated with the signaling pathway inhibitors or anti-BCL2 therapy is not clear, especially for the former because most patients receiving these medications continue to have detectable leukemic cells.

Combinatorial Indices

Because of the complexity and variability in clinical course and in leukemia-cell biology in individual patients, combinatorial algorithms incorporating several prognostic and predictive markers have been devised to better predict outcome and response to therapy (Wierda et al. 2007, 2011; Molica et al. 2010; Rossi et al. 2013).

The Chronic Lymphocytic Leukemia International Prognostic Index (CLL-IPI) incorporates patient age, disease stage (Rai or Binet systems), TP53 disruption, *IGHV* mutation status, and serum β2-microglobulin levels (International CLL-IPI Working Group 2016). These five parameters are weighted individually, and a composite score assigns patients to one of four risk groups. Another algorithm using only *IGHV* mutations and high-risk fluorescence in situ hybridization (FISH) cytogenetics (del17p and del11q) divides CLL patients into three groups: low-risk, comprised of M-CLL clones without high-risk cytogenetics; intermediate-risk, containing either U-CLL or high-risk cytogenetics; and high-risk, consisting of U-CLL and high-risk cytogenetics (Delgado et al. 2017). Time to first treatment and overall survival follow the order of the risk categories for both approaches. Should the same conclusions be drawn for treatments with the signaling inhibitors and the BCL-2 family blocker (Molica et al. 2018), these might eventually be useful in daily practice and to stratify patients in clinical trials.

Finally, despite the information that prognostic, predictive, and combination indicators suggest, the decision to begin therapy in clinical practice is still based on an educated synthesis of patient information and symptoms, physical examination findings, and laboratory data to define active disease (Hallek et al. 2018).

Options for the Initial Treatment of CLL

A physician treating CLL patients in 2019 has many previously unavailable options. Because most CLL patients are aging and might have compromised organ systems that reduce treatment tolerability, patient fitness and comorbidities influence therapy goals (complete remission vs. symptom alleviation/palliation). Table 3 provides therapeutic options for patients in various fitness and disease categories. At this point, the most frequently employed are chemoimmunotherapy, mAbs to B-cell surface molecules, and inhibitors of signaling and anti-apoptotic pathways.

 Cite this article as *Cold Spring Harb Perspect Med* doi: 10.1101/cshperspect.a035220

Table 3. Therapeutic options for chronic lymphocytic leukemia (CLL) patients in various fitness and disease categories for front-line and advanced disease settings

Co-morbidities	CLL cell genetic profile	*IGHV* mutation status	Suggested front-line therapy	Therapeutic goals for front-line therapy	Suggested therapy for relapsed/refractory patients	Therapeutic goals for secondary therapies
None/mild	Absence of del17p/TP53 mutation	M-CLL	FCR < 65 yr Ibrutinib Obinu + CLB	Long-term remission with prolonged survival	Ibrutinib Idelalisib + Ritux Venetoclax Obinu + CLB Duvelisib	Long-term remission
		U-CLL	Obinu + CLB Ibrutinib			
	Presence of del17p/TP53 mutation	Not relevant	Ibrutinib	Long-term remission with prolonged survival	Venetoclax + Ritux Ibrutinib HSC transplantation	Long-term remission
Significant	Absence of del17p/TP53 mutation	Not relevant	Ibrutinib Obinu + CLB BR	Disease control and improved quality of life	Ibrutinib Idelalisib + Ritux Obinu + CLB Venetoclax Duvelisib	Disease control
	Presence of del17p/TP53 mutation	Not relevant	Ibrutinib	Disease control and improved quality of life	Ibrutinib Venetoclax	Disease control
Overriding	Irrelevant	Irrelevant	Ibrutinib Obinu + CLB Ritux ± CLB Ofa ± CLB BR	Palliation	Ibrutinib Idelalisib + Ritux Venetoclax Obinu + CLB	Palliation

FCR, Fludarabine/cyclophosphamide/rituximab; Obinu, obinutuzumab; CLB, chlorambucil; Ritux, rituximab; Ofa, ofatumumab; BR, bendamustine/rituximab; M-CLL, IGHV-mutated CLL; U-CLL IGHV-unmutated CLL.

Chemoimmunotherapy

Historically, chemotherapy has been the mainstay of cancer therapy, with addition of mAbs leading to improved regimens. In CLL, fludarabine plus cyclophosphamide (FC) were synergistic (Keating et al. 1989; Yamauchi et al. 2001); adding rituximab (FCR) resulted in an even more effective regimen (Keating et al. 2005; Tam et al. 2008; Hallek et al. 2010; Fischer et al. 2016; Thompson et al. 2016). Presently, FCR is considered state-of-the-art therapy for physically fit CLL patients. Remarkably, ~50% of previously untreated M-CLL patients are alive without progression at ~13 yr, compared to only <10% of U-CLL patients (Thompson et al. 2016), suggesting this treatment may cure some M-CLL patients. Studies with shorter follow-up times (Fischer et al. 2016) and fewer cases (Rossi et al. 2015) report similar results, although high serum β_2-microglobulin levels and del17p and/or del11q herald less durable remissions (Rossi et al. 2015). Bone marrow (BM) and immune suppression following this regimen (Benjamini et al. 2015), however, raise concerns about secondary malignancies, especially in patients receiving FCR as frontline therapy (Zhou et al. 2012; Benjamini et al. 2015; Falchi et al. 2016).

Monoclonal Antibodies

Three anti-CD20 mAbs, classified as Type I or II based on binding properties (Beers et al. 2010), are approved for use in CLL. Type I mAbs (rituximab and ofatumumab) effectively promote cytotoxicity but are less effective at inducing apoptosis (Cragg et al. 2003), whereas type II (obinutuzumab) is superior at inducing apoptosis but inferior at carrying out cytotoxicity (Chan et al. 2003). In previously untreated CLL patients, type II obinutuzumab, in combination with chlorambucil, is superior to type I rituximab plus chlorambucil (Goede et al. 2014).

Specific Pathway Inhibition

Studies associating unique structural BCR features with clinical outcome and differences in signaling capacities brought small molecules blocking enzymes critical for this signaling pathway into the clinic. Orally administered inhibitors of Bruton's tyrosine kinase (Btk), ibrutinib, and of phospatidylinositol-4,5-bisphosphate 3-kinase delta (PI3Kδ), idelalisib, yielded dramatic responses in relapsed/refractory patients by blocking signaling through the BCR, chemokine receptors, and integrins (Figs. 2 and 3; Spaargaren et al. 2003; Ortolano et al. 2006; de Gorter et al. 2007; de Rooij et al. 2012; Herman et al. 2015; Maffei et al. 2015; Chen et al. 2016). Ibrutinib is efficacious in patients with del17p, del11q, and unmutated *IGHV* (Farooqui et al. 2015) and in patients refractory or unresponsive to other therapies (Byrd et al. 2013; Furman et al. 2014b). Both molecules inhibit cell replication (Herman et al. 2011, 2014a; Ponader et al. 2012), trafficking to/retention in lymphoid tissues (Niedermeier et al. 2009; Herman et al. 2011, 2014a,b; Ponader et al. 2012; Fiorcari et al. 2013; Göckeritz et al. 2015), and production of pro-inflammatory cytokines (Ponader et al. 2012; Herman et al. 2014a; Niemann et al. 2016). Upon initiating ibrutinib or idelalisib therapy, lymphadenopathy and splenomegaly rapidly regress and peripheral blood lymphocyte counts increase because of redistribution of cells from tissue compartments to the blood (Woyach et al. 2014b; Chen et al. 2016; Burger et al. 2017). In most patients, lymphocytosis diminishes over time and circulating B-cell numbers in the blood fall to or below pretreatment levels. Ibrutinib is FDA-approved for first- and second-line therapy of CLL and for patients with del17p; idelalisib in combination with rituximab is approved for relapsed CLL. Recently, an inhibitor of both PI3Kδ and PI3Kγ (duvelisib) was approved for the treatment of relapsed/refractory CLL and SLL (Flinn et al. 2018).

As single agents, these medications rarely lead to complete remissions (Burger et al. 2010). Also, occurrence of long-term side effects and development of resistance have not been fully investigated. Ibrutinib and idelalisib are generally well-tolerated, and severe side effects occur in a minority of patients (de Weerdt et al. 2017). For ibrutinib, these are bleeding (Lipsky et al. 2015), hypertension (Caldeira et al. 2019), and atrial fibrillation (McMullen et al. 2014;

Lentz et al. 2019). For idelalisib, neutropenia and inflammatory reactions (Brown 2014; Furman et al. 2014b), particularly in treatment-naive patients (Lampson et al. 2016), are major adverse events, and hence idelalisib plus rituximab is reserved for relapsed, refractory disease.

Targeting Anti-Apoptotic Proteins

CLL lymphocytes characteristically overexpress anti-apoptotic BCL-2 (Schena et al. 1992), the parent molecule in a family of proteins controlling suppression or initiation of apoptosis (Adams and Cory 2018). BCL-2 family members containing BCL-2 homology domain-3 (BH3-only proteins) promote apoptosis by blocking pro-survival members of the family (Ruefli-Brasse and Reed 2017). Venetoclax, an orally administered BH3-protein mimetic selectively targeting BCL-2 (Souers et al. 2013), is effective in refractory CLL patients with del17p, del11q, or *IGHV*-unmutated clones (Anderson et al. 2016) and is FDA-approved for previously treated CLL patients bearing del17p clones. Overall remissions and complete remissions have been achieved in 82% and 10% of patients, respectively, and in 5%, residual disease was not detectable at 15 mo (Roberts et al. 2016). Because of the propensity to cause tumor lysis syndrome, patients are started on very low drug doses initially.

DISEASE PROGRESSION AND THERAPEUTIC REFRACTORINESS TO INITIAL THERAPY

Factors Promoting Development of More Aggressive Clonal Variants

Like other cancers, progression of CLL develops from the emergence of intraclonal variants with genetic changes fostering growth, survival, and therapeutic resistance. These disrupt the balance between cellular proliferation and death (Chiorazzi 2007) and in some patients become a major component of the leukemic clone. Such variants can develop spontaneously or are generated by processes inherent to normal cells or unique to a cancer cell; certain treatments targeting replicating DNA can do the same.

CLL cells contain high levels of reactive oxygen species (Oltra et al. 2001; Zhou et al. 2003), a characteristic of cancer cells, which can act as mutagens (Cerutti 1994; Wiseman and Halliwell 1996; Nogueira and Hay 2013). Also, as B lymphocytes, CLL cells can make the mutagenic enzyme, AID (Albesiano et al. 2003; McCarthy et al. 2003; Oppezzo et al. 2003). AID carries out a normal role in the development of more effective immune responses by inducing mutations in genes coding the variable domains of Abs/IGs (*IGHV, IGHD, IGHJ* and *IGLV, IGLJ*) and in the gene segments that support switching from IgM to IgG, IgA, and IgE (Muramatsu et al. 1999, 2000). However, AID can act aberrantly, creating mutations outside IG loci (Pasqualucci et al. 1998; Yamane et al. 2011), leading to genetic changes and B-cell lymphomas (Pasqualucci et al. 2001; Lenz et al. 2007; Robbiani et al. 2009).

A small fraction (~0.01%–1%) of circulating CLL B cells express AID mRNA (Albesiano et al. 2003), and so AID protein is rarely detectable (Pasqualucci et al. 2004). However, CLL cells in tissue proliferation centers (Leuenberger et al. 2010; Patten et al. 2012) and those activated in vitro (Cerutti et al. 2002; Albesiano et al. 2003; Oppezzo et al. 2003) and growing in xenografts (Patten et al. 2016) synthesize AID protein, consistent with the link of AID production to cell division (Rush et al. 2005). The protein is functional as evidenced by detection of new, spontaneous mutations in the clonal *IGHV-IGHD-IGHJ* (Patten et al. 2012, 2016) and hence could create off-target mutations and intraclonal variants that might lead to disease progression. Although certain chemotherapeutic agents can induce DNA mutations (Tan et al. 2015), based on next-generation deep-sequencing analyses many/most mutations that emerge after cancer therapy in CLL patients are present before treatment. Mathematical modeling suggests this is likely for ibrutinib (Komarova et al. 2014). Also, because the drug prevents CLL B-cell division (Honigberg et al. 2010; Herman et al. 2011; Burger et al. 2017) and AID is produced upon cell proliferation (Rush et al. 2005), it is likely that additional clonal mutations are halted by ibrutinib.

Clonal Evolution

The common genetic abnormalities identified by FISH and the recurrent genetic mutations defined by NGS (Table 1) have been used to follow clonal evolution in patients (Finn et al. 1998; Shanafelt et al. 2008b; Landau et al. 2013, 2014a, 2015; Lawrence et al. 2013; Nadeu et al. 2018). Similarly, epigenetic diversity can identify similar events (Kulis et al. 2012; Oakes et al. 2014; Landau et al. 2014b; Guièze and Wu 2015; Queirós et al. 2015; Mansouri et al. 2018). Resulting clonal architectures can be informative (Messina et al. 2014; Wang et al. 2014; Ojha et al. 2015). Whereas linear development from a starting genetic template is seen more often, branching patterns are also found (Braggio et al. 2012), indicating distinct intraclonal variants can evolve in parallel. These chronologic genetic and epigenetic variations provide insights into disease progression and into the clinical courses for individual patients (Quesada et al. 2013; Villamor et al. 2013; Rose-Zerilli et al. 2016).

Role of CLL-Cell Growth Rate in Disease Progression

CLL progresses at a slower rate than acute leukemias and more aggressive lymphomas, as reflected by clonal birth rates and by the relatively low baseline levels of genomic mutations. Approximately 0.1%–2% of a CLL clone is added daily, based on deuterium (^{2}H)-labeling of replicating DNA provided as "heavy water" (^2H_2O) to measure CLL B-cell growth in patients (Messmer et al. 2005; Defoiche et al. 2008; van Gent et al. 2008). Clonal birth rates directly correlate with clinical course, as patients with higher birth rates require treatment sooner (Murphy et al. 2017). Also, most CLL-cell growth occurs in lymph nodes (LNs) (Herndon et al. 2017), suggesting CLL cells divide in secondary lymphoid tissues and traffic to the BM, where they reside mostly in a resting state (Fig. 4; Calissano et al. 2011). This model for growth and survival based on tissue residence has been recapitulated in murine models (Chen et al. 2013). Hence, CLL cells at different anatomic sites can behave differently, which may relate to effectiveness of certain therapeutic agents.

Relapsed/Refractory, Accelerated, and Transformed Disease

Here we assume that first-line treatments mentioned in Table 1 have failed, and the patient again requires therapy. Consistent with clonal evolution and disease progression being a function of increased cell growth in LNs, patients in this category often have nodal, splenic, or extranodal disease. A suspicion of Richter's transformation (RT) (Richter 1928), often as diffuse large B-cell lymphoma (DLBCL) that has large B cells with nuclear sizes more than twice that of a normal B lymphocyte, is raised when LN or spleen enlargement occurs rapidly and when extranodal sites are defined; elevated LDH levels are often found (Jain and Young 2014; Allan and Furman 2019). In those instances in which RT is not found, patients might have "accelerated CLL," defined by highly proliferative CLL cells in expanded, substantially more active proliferation centers that contain T cells, especially CD4$^+$ cells, and dendritic cells. Although the frequencies of accelerated CLL and RT are only ~23% and ~10% of all CLLs, they are increased for those relapsed/refractory patients with adenopathy (~25% accelerated CLL, ~50% standard refractory CLL, and ~25% RT) (Gine et al. 2010). Survival in the three categories are distinct: ~76 mo in nonaccelerated CLL, 34 mo for accelerated CLL, and only 8–12 mo for RT.

The mechanisms leading to accelerated CLL and RT are unclear, although they might involve BCR and TLR signaling to stimulate CLL-cell proliferation (Balogh et al. 2011), especially stereotyped subset #8 CLLs (Rossi et al. 2009b) that display polyreactivity to multiple antigens (Gounari et al. 2015). The lymphoma that develops in RT is usually clonally related to the CLL clone (Mao et al. 2007), and when that is the case the outcome for the patient is worse than if the lymphoma has a distinct genetic origin (Condoluci and Rossi 2017). Several genetic alterations are associated with RT: elevated AID levels in leukemic B cells (Reiniger et al. 2006), disruption of TP53 and CDKN2A, and activation of NOTCH1 and c-MYC (Fabbri et al. 2013). TP53 and CDKNA2 mutations are found in >50% of cases, whereas trisomy 12 and

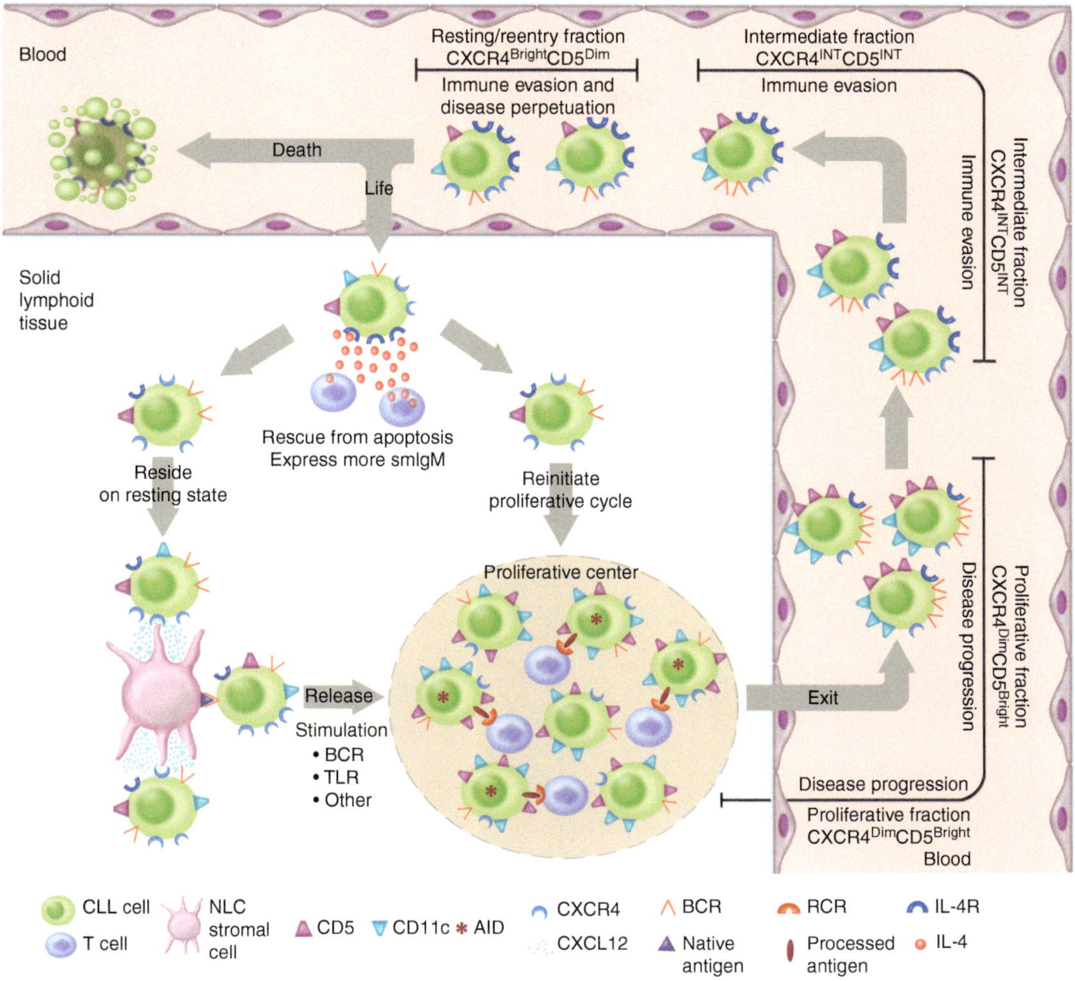

Figure 4. Life cycle of a chronic lymphocytic leukemia (CLL) B lymphocyte. In primary and secondary lymphoid tissues (*bottom left*) CLL B lymphocytes nestle, in a resting state, on survival-nurturing cells (e.g., nurse-like cells [Burger et al. 2000] or less well-defined, nonhematopoietic "stromal cells"). Docking is facilitated by several receptor–ligand interactions, including CXCL12-CXCR4. When cell division initiates, spontaneously or after stimulation via receptors (e.g., B-cell receptor [BCR] or Toll-like receptors [TLRs]), cells internalize CXCR4, detach, and migrate to structures resembling germinal centers ("proliferation centers" [Swerdlow et al. 1984; Schmid and Isaacson 1994; Bonato et al. 1998]), sites of CLL B-cell expansion. Activated/dividing cells up-regulate a number of surface proteins that promote interactions with T lymphocytes. These interactions up-regulate the DNA-mutating enzyme AID, which can cause mutations in genes genome-wide, leading to clonal evolution and possibly more aggressive disease. After expansion, some recently divided CLL cells exit the lymphoid tissue, entering the circulation bearing the $CXCR4^{Dim}CD5^{Bright}$ phenotype ("proliferative fraction" [Calissano et al. 2011]). Over time, the circulating cells express more CXCR4 and less CD5, eventually morphing into a $CXCR4^{Bright}CD5^{Dim}$ resting fraction (RF) phenotype. These cells are best suited to follow a CXCL12/SDF1 gradient because of high levels of CXCR4, returning back to nutrient-rich niches in tissues and being rescued from apoptosis by IL-4 and likely other cytokines. Cells that cannot reenter tissues or do not arrive soon enough die. Once rescued, CLL cells proceed to a proliferation center to re-initiate the proliferative process and potential further clonal evolution or dock on a stromal element, where they again reside in the resting state.

NOTCH1 mutations are found in >30% of cases (Allan and Furman 2019). A microRNA expression signature has also been identified in RT (Van Roosbroeck et al. 2018).

Therapy for Relapsed/Refractory and Accelerated Disease and for Richter's Transformation

Table 3 lists a series of therapies for patients in these categories, again based on the physical condition of the patient and the goal of treatment. For patients relapsing on ibrutinib, progression appears accelerated and less well-controlled (Jain et al. 2015; Maddocks et al. 2015). Leukemic cells of patients failing ibrutinib can contain mutations at the site in the Btk molecule where the drug binds (cysteine 481) or in downstream signaling molecules (Furman et al. 2014a; Woyach et al. 2014a; Cheng et al. 2015); such variants appear to be selected from cells bearing these mutations existing prior to treatment (Woyach et al. 2014a).

Outcomes for RT patients treated with chemoimmunotherapy remain dismal. Because of the ineffectiveness of chemoimmunotherapy and the dysfunction of T cells, NK cells, and other immune subsets, novel agents targeting RT cells and their interaction with immune subsets in LNs are being developed.

In a few reports, treatment with ibrutinib induced partial responses or retained stable disease in RT patients (Giri et al. 2015; Fischer et al. 2018); this could be caused by reduced proliferation of CLL/RS cells expressing AID (Reiniger et al. 2006). However, CLL patients that develop accelerated CLL or RT can progress on ibrutinib (Kadri et al. 2017); because ibrutinib is now used as front-line therapy, finding an effective therapy for this subset of patients is urgently needed. The BCL-2 inhibitor, venetoclax, alone (Jones et al. 2018) or in combination with ibrutinib (Flinn et al. 2019; Rogers 2019) may be beneficial for relapse/refractory patients and for RT (Roberts et al. 2016), although the effectiveness of these and resistance to venetoclax (Blombery et al. 2019) are evolving.

T-cell exhaustion and impaired T cell–B cell interactions promote disease progression in patients with RT. Improving T-cell function with anti-PD1 or anti-PDL1 mAb treatments (pembrolizumab or nivolumab) was therapeutic in a CLL mouse model (McClanahan et al. 2015), in patients with relapsed/refractory Hodgkin lymphoma (Ansell et al. 2015), and in patients with CLL-derived RT (Ding et al. 2015). The combination of pembrolizumab and ibrutinib in patients with RT is being evaluated (NCT20332980). Overall, BCR inhibitors and immune checkpoint inhibitors appear promising, although the number of patients treated is limited, and studies of larger patient cohorts are needed to define optimal therapeutic strategies.

An approach to enhancing actions of cytolytic T lymphocytes comes from work inserting, into the T-cell surface membrane, the antigen-binding portion of an antibody that binds B lymphocytes (e.g., CD19) linked to the constant and signaling regions of a T-cell receptor (Gross et al. 1989; Eshhar et al. 1993). These engineered CAR-T cells kill target cells independent of histocompatibility constraints and the requirements for antibody-dependent and complement-dependent cytotoxicty.

CAR-T therapy has had dramatic results in selected relapsed/refractory CLL patients (Brentjens et al. 2011; Porter et al. 2011), and larger studies indicate beneficial responses in ~30%–50% of patients (Frey and Porter 2016; Romero 2017; Turtle et al. 2017). Using T cells from patients who received ibrutinib (Fraietta et al. 2016; Harper 2019) or cells expanded in the presence of PI3Kδ inhibitors (Petersen et al. 2018) or the selective expansion of autologous $CD4^+$ and $CD8^+$ cells infused at defined CD4 to CD8 ratios (Sommermeyer et al. 2016; Turtle et al. 2016) have improved effectiveness.

However, CAR-T cells can result in major complications. A cytokine release syndrome (Lee et al. 2014) from liberation of pro-inflammatory cytokines (Kochenderfer et al. 2012), including IL-6 (Lee et al. 2014), can occur. Blocking the IL-6 receptor with mAbs is helpful (Lee et al. 2014). The use of CAR-T therapy will increase as effective ways of lessening complications emerge (Acharya et al. 2019). Moreover, because CAR-Ts use anti-B-cell antibodies to target CLL cells, normal B lymphocytes are also eliminated, leading to hypogammaglobulinemia (Kochenderfer et al. 2010).

Implications for More Effective Disease Interventions and Possible Cures

Several avenues could lead to new therapies and hopefully cures. Considering the major beneficial impact inhibitors of BTK and PI3K signaling have had on CLL, it is likely that combinations of these drugs with newly approved agents such as venetoclax will lead to more profound, long-lasting effects and longer overall survival; several such studies are under way. Moreover, targeting other signaling pathways supporting survival and growth of CLL cells may be valuable adjuncts to current enzyme inhibitors.

As deep DNA sequencing becomes more available, rapid, and inexpensive, therapeutic decisions might take into consideration specific gene abnormalities and clonal architecture in individual patients. Personalized therapy might involve replacing/overexpressing/removing microRNAs because they can be oncogenic or tumor-inhibitory. Similarly, targeting patient-specific driver mutations and the pathways they derange, early or during disease progression, could achieve this goal.

Because of their shared features, targeting stereotyped BCRs might be feasible for discrete groups of patients. Development of small molecules reactive with stereotypes (Liu et al. 2013; Sarkar et al. 2014, 2016) and humanized mAbs binding specific *IGHV*s (Chang et al. 2016) support this possibility.

Finally, safer and more specific and effective CAR-T cells, and the reinfusion of functionally competent autologous T cells capable of recognizing CLL-specific antigens, similar to those emerging in myeloma (Thompson et al. 2003), may advance cellular therapy.

REFERENCES

Acharya UH, Dhawale T, Yun S, Jacobson CA, Chavez JC, Ramos JD, Appelbaum J, Maloney DG. 2019. Management of cytokine release syndrome and neurotoxicity in chimeric antigen receptor (CAR) T cell therapy. *Expert Rev Hematol* **12:** 195–205. doi:10.1080/17474086.2019.1585238

Adams JM, Cory S. 2018. The BCL-2 arbiters of apoptosis and their growing role as cancer targets. *Cell Death Differ* **25:** 27–36. doi:10.1038/cdd.2017.161

Agathangelidis A, Darzentas N, Hadzidimitriou A, Brochet X, Murray F, Yan XJ, Davis Z, van Gastel-Mol EJ, Tresoldi C, Chu CC, et al. 2012. Stereotyped B-cell receptors in one-third of chronic lymphocytic leukemia: A molecular classification with implications for targeted therapies. *Blood* **119:** 4467–4475. doi:10.1182/blood-2011-11-393694

Agathangelidis A, Ljungström V, Scarfò L, Fazi C, Gounari M, Pandzic T, Sutton L-A, Stamatopoulos K, Tonon G, Rosenquist R, et al. 2018. Highly similar genomic landscapes in monoclonal B-cell lymphocytosis and ultra-stable chronic lymphocytic leukemia with low frequency of driver mutations. *Haematologica* **103:** 865–873. doi:10.3324/haematol.2017.177212

Agathangelidis A, Psomopoulos F, Stamatopoulos K. 2019. Stereotyped B cell receptor immunoglobulins in B cell lymphomas. *Methods Mol Biol* **1956:** 139–155. doi:10.1007/978-1-4939-9151-8_7

Aguilar-Hernandez MM, Blunt MD, Dobson R, Yeomans A, Thirdborough S, Larrayoz M, Smith LD, Linley A, Strefford JC, Davies A, et al. 2016. IL-4 enhances expression and function of surface IgM in CLL cells. *Blood* **127:** 3015–3025. doi:10.1182/blood-2015-11-682906

Alavanja MC, Hofmann JN, Lynch CF, Hines CJ, Barry KH, Barker J, Buckman DW, Thomas K, Sandler DP, Hoppin JA, et al. 2014. Non-Hodgkin lymphoma risk and insecticide, fungicide and fumigant use in the agricultural health study. *PLoS One* **9:** e109332. doi:10.1371/journal.pone.0109332

Albesiano E, Messmer BT, Damle RN, Allen SL, Rai KR, Chiorazzi N. 2003. Activation-induced cytidine deaminase in chronic lymphocytic leukemia B cells: Expression as multiple forms in a dynamic, variably sized fraction of the clone. *Blood* **102:** 3333–3339. doi:10.1182/blood-2003-05-1585

Alexandrov LB, Nik-Zainal S, Wedge DC, Aparicio SA, Behjati S, Biankin AV, Bignell GR, Bolli N, Borg A, Borresen-Dale AL, et al. 2013. Signatures of mutational processes in human cancer. *Nature* **500:** 415–421. doi:10.1038/nature12477

Allan JN, Furman RR. 2019. Current trends in the management of Richter's syndrome. *Int J Hematol Oncol* **7:** IJH09. doi:10.2217/ijh-2018-0010

Anderson MA, Deng J, Seymour JF, Tam C, Kim SY, Fein J, Yu L, Brown JR, Westerman D, Si EG, et al. 2016. The BCL2 selective inhibitor venetoclax induces rapid onset apoptosis of CLL cells in patients via a TP53-independent mechanism. *Blood* **127:** 3215–3224. doi:10.1182/blood-2016-01-688796

Ansell SM, Lesokhin AM, Borrello I, Halwani A, Scott EC, Gutierrez M, Schuster SJ, Millenson MM, Cattry D, Freeman GJ, et al. 2015. PD-1 blockade with nivolumab in relapsed or refractory Hodgkin's lymphoma. *New Engl J Med* **372:** 311–319. doi:10.1056/NEJMoa1411087

Bagnara D, Callea V, Stelitano C, Morabito F, Fabris S, Neri A, Zanardi S, Ghiotto F, Ciccone E, Grossi CE, et al. 2006.

IgV gene intraclonal diversification and clonal evolution in B-cell chronic lymphocytic leukaemia. *Br J Haematol* **133:** 50–58.

Bagnara D, Kaufman MS, Calissano C, Marsilio S, Patten PE, Simone R, Chum P, Yan XJ, Allen SL, Kolitz JE, et al. 2011. A novel adoptive transfer model of chronic lymphocytic leukemia suggests a key role for T lymphocytes in the disease. *Blood* **117:** 5463–5472. doi:10.1182/blood-2010-12-324210

Balogh Z, Reiniger L, Rajnai H, Csomor J, Szepesi A, Balogh A, Deak L, Gagyi E, Bodor C, Matolcsy A. 2011. High rate of neoplastic cells with genetic abnormalities in proliferation centers of chronic lymphocytic leukemia. *Leuk Lymphoma* **52:** 1080–1084. doi:10.3109/10428194.2011.555889

Baskar S, Kwong KY, Hofer T, Levy JM, Kennedy MG, Lee E, Staudt LM, Wilson WH, Wiestner A, Rader C. 2008. Unique cell surface expression of receptor tyrosine kinase ROR1 in human B-cell chronic lymphocytic leukemia. *Clin Cancer Res* **14:** 396–404. doi:10.1158/1078-0432.CCR-07-1823

Baumann Kreuziger LM, Tarchand G, Morrison VA. 2014. The impact of Agent Orange exposure on presentation and prognosis of patients with chronic lymphocytic leukemia. *Leuk Lymphoma* **55:** 63–66. doi:10.3109/10428194.2013.794267

Baumann T, Delgado J, Santacruz R, Martínez-Trillos A, Rozman M, Aymerich M, López C, Costa D, Carrió A, Villamor N, et al. 2016. CD49d (ITGA4) expression is a predictor of time to first treatment in patients with chronic lymphocytic leukaemia and mutated *IGHV* status. *Br J Haematol* **172:** 48–55. doi:10.1111/bjh.13788

Beers SA, Chan CH, French RR, Cragg MS, Glennie MJ. 2010. CD20 as a target for therapeutic type I and II monoclonal antibodies. *Semin Hematol* **47:** 107–114. doi:10.1053/j.seminhematol.2010.01.001

Benjamini O, Jain P, Trinh L, Qiao W, Strom SS, Lerner S, Wang X, Burger J, Ferrajoli A, Kantarjian H, et al. 2015. Second cancers in patients with chronic lymphocytic leukemia who received frontline fludarabine, cyclophosphamide and rituximab therapy: Distribution and clinical outcomes. *Leuk Lymphoma* **56:** 1643–1650. doi:10.3109/10428194.2014.957203

Berndt SI, Skibola CF, Joseph V, Camp NJ, Nieters A, Wang Z, Cozen W, Monnereau A, Wang SS, Kelly RS, et al. 2013. Genome-wide association study identifies multiple risk loci for chronic lymphocytic leukemia. *Nat Genet* **45:** 868–876. doi:10.1038/ng.2652

Berndt SI, Camp NJ, Skibola CF, Vijai J, Wang Z, Gu J, Nieters A, Kelly RS, Smedby KE, Monnereau A, et al. 2016. Meta-analysis of genome-wide association studies discovers multiple loci for chronic lymphocytic leukemia. *Nat Commun* **7:** 10933. doi:10.1038/ncomms10933

Binder M, Müller F, Jackst A, Léchenne B, Pantic M, Bacher U, Zu Eulenburg C, Veelken H, Mertelsmann R, Pasqualini R, et al. 2011. B-cell receptor epitope recognition correlates with the clinical course of chronic lymphocytic leukemia. *Cancer* **117:** 1891–1900. doi:10.1002/cncr.25755

Binder M, Müller F, Frick M, Wehr C, Simon F, Leistler B, Veelken H, Mertelsmann R, Trepel M. 2013. CLL B-cell receptors can recognize themselves: Alternative epitopes and structural clues for autostimulatory mechanisms in CLL. *Blood* **121:** 239–241. doi:10.1182/blood-2012-09-454439

Binet JL, Auquier A, Dighiero G, Chastang C, Piguet H, Goasguen J, Vaugier G, Potron G, Colona P, Oberling F, et al. 1981. A new prognostic classification of chronic lymphocytic leukemia derived from a multivariate survival analysis. *Cancer* **48:** 198–206.

Blombery P, Anderson MA, Gong JN, Thijssen R, Birkinshaw RW, Thompson ER, Teh CE, Nguyen T, Xu Z, Flensburg C, et al. 2019. Acquisition of the recurrent Gly101Val mutation in BCL2 confers resistance to venetoclax in patients with progressive chronic lymphocytic leukemia. *Cancer Discov* **9:** 342–353. doi:10.1158/2159-8290.CD-18-1119

Bonato M, Pittaluga S, Tierens A, Criel A, Verhoef G, Wlodarska I, Vanutysel L, Michaux L, Vandekerckhove P, Van den Berghe H, et al. 1998. Lymph node histology in typical and atypical chronic lymphocytic leukemia. *Am J Surg Pathol* **22:** 49–56. doi:10.1097/00000478-199801000-00006

Borche L, Lim A, Binet JL, Dighiero G. 1990. Evidence that chronic lymphocytic leukemia B lymphocytes are frequently committed to production of natural autoantibodies. *Blood* **76:** 562–569. doi:10.1182/blood.V76.3.562.562

Böttcher S. 2019. Flow cytometric MRD detection in selected mature B-cell malignancies. *Methods Mol Biol* **1956:** 157–197. doi:10.1007/978-1-4939-9151-8_8

Böttcher S, Ritgen M, Fischer K, Stilgenbauer S, Busch RM, Fingerle-Rowson G, Fink AM, Bühler A, Zenz T, Wenger MK, et al. 2012. Minimal residual disease quantification is an independent predictor of progression-free and overall survival in chronic lymphocytic leukemia: A multivariate analysis from the randomized GCLLSG CLL8 trial. *J Clin Oncol* **30:** 980–988. doi:10.1200/JCO.2011.36.9348

Braggio E, Kay NE, Vanwier S, Tschumper RC, Smoley S, Eckel-Passow JE, Sassoon T, Barrett M, Van Dyke DL, Byrd JC, et al. 2012. Longitudinal genome-wide analysis of patients with chronic lymphocytic leukemia reveals complex evolution of clonal architecture at disease progression and at the time of relapse. *Leukemia* **26:** 1698–1701. doi:10.1038/leu.2012.14

Brentjens RJ, Rivière I, Park JH, Davila ML, Wang X, Stefanski J, Taylor C, Yeh R, Bartido S, Borquez-Ojeda O, et al. 2011. Safety and persistence of adoptively transferred autologous CD19-targeted T cells in patients with relapsed or chemotherapy refractory B-cell leukemias. *Blood* **118:** 4817–4828. doi:10.1182/blood-2011-04-348540

Bröker BM, Klajman A, Youinou P, Jouquan J, Worman CP, Murphy J, Mackenzie L, Quartey-Papafio R, Blaschek M, Collins P, et al. 1988. Chronic lymphocytic leukemic (CLL) cells secrete multispecific autoantibodies. *J Autoimmun* **1:** 469–481. doi:10.1016/0896-8411(88)90068-6

Broome HE, Rassenti LZ, Wang HY, Meyer LM, Kipps TJ. 2011. ROR1 is expressed on hematogones (non-neoplastic human B-lymphocyte precursors) and a minority of precursor-B acute lymphoblastic leukemia. *Leuk Res* **35:** 1390–1394. doi:10.1016/j.leukres.2011.06.021

Brown J, Byrd JC, Coutre SE, Benson DM, Flinn IW, Wagner-Johnston ND, Spurgeon SE, Kahl BS, Bello C, Webb HK, et al. 2014. Idelalisib, an inhibitor of phosphatidylinositol 3-kinase p110δ, for relapsed/refractory chronic lymphocytic leukemia. *Blood* **123:** 3390–3397. doi:10.1182/blood-2013-11-535047

Bulian P, Gaidano G, Del Poeta G, Gattei V. 2008. CD49d expression in chronic lymphocytic leukemia: A prognostic parameter and a therapeutic target. *Future Oncol* **4:** 355–358. doi:10.2217/14796694.4.3.355

Bulian P, Shanafelt TD, Fegan C, Zucchetto A, Cro L, Nückel H, Baldini L, Kurtova AV, Ferrajoli A, Burger JA, et al. 2014. CD49d is the strongest flow cytometry–based predictor of overall survival in chronic lymphocytic leukemia. *J Clin Oncol* **32:** 897–904. doi:10.1200/JCO.2013.50.8515

Burger JA, Bürkle A. 2007. The CXCR4 chemokine receptor in acute and chronic leukaemia: A marrow homing receptor and potential therapeutic target. *Br J Haematol* **137:** 288–296. doi:10.1111/j.1365-2141.2007.06590.x

Burger JA, Kipps TJ. 2002. Chemokine receptors and stromal cells in the homing and homeostasis of chronic lymphocytic leukemia B cells. *Leuk Lymphoma* **43:** 461–466. doi:10.1080/10428190290011921

Burger JA, Tsukada N, Burger M, Zvaifler NJ, Dell'Aquila M, Kipps TJ. 2000. Blood-derived nurse-like cells protect chronic lymphocytic leukemia B cells from spontaneous apoptosis through stromal cell-derived factor-1. *Blood* **96:** 2655–2663. doi:10.1182/blood.V96.8.2655

Burger JA, Quiroga MP, Hartmann E, Bürkle A, Wierda WG, Keating MJ, Rosenwald A. 2009. High-level expression of the T-cell chemokines CCL3 and CCL4 by chronic lymphocytic leukemia B cells in nurselike cell cocultures and after BCR stimulation. *Blood* **113:** 3050–3058. doi:10.1182/blood-2008-07-170415

Burger J, O'Brien S, Fowler N, Advani R, Sharman JP, Furman RR, Izumi R, Buggy J, Loury D, Hamdy A, et al. 2010. The Bruton's tyrosine kinase inhibitor, PCI-32765, is well tolerated and demonstrates promising clinical activity in chronic lymphocytic leukemia (CLL) and small lymphocytic lymphoma (SLL): An update on ongoing phase 1 studies. *Blood* **116:** 57. doi:10.1182/blood.V116.21.57.57 53rd ASH meeting abstract

Burger JA, Li KW, Keating MJ, Sivina M, Amer AM, Garg N, Ferrajoli A, Huang X, Kantarjian H, Wierda WG, et al. 2017. Leukemia cell proliferation and death in chronic lymphocytic leukemia patients on therapy with the BTK inhibitor ibrutinib. *JCI Insight* **2:** e89904. doi:10.1172/jci.insight.89904

Burns A, Alsolami R, Becq J, Timbs A, Bruce D, Robbe P, Vavoulis D, Cabes M, Dreau H, Taylor J, et al. 2018. Whole-genome sequencing of chronic lymphocytic leukemia reveals distinct differences in the mutational landscape between $IgHV^{mut}$ and $IgHV^{unmut}$ subgroups. *Leukemia* **32:** 332–342. doi:10.1038/leu.2017.177

Byrd JC, Furman RR, Coutre SE, Flinn IW, Burger JA, Blum KA, Grant B, Sharman JP, Coleman M, Wierda WG, et al. 2013. Targeting BTK with Ibrutinib in relapsed chronic lymphocytic leukemia. *New Engl J Med* **369:** 32–42. doi:10.1056/NEJMoa1215637

Byrd JC, Furman RR, Coutre SE, Burger JA, Blum KA, Coleman M, Wierda WG, Jones JA, Zhao W, Heerema NA, et al. 2015. Three-year follow-up of treatment-naïve and previously treated patients with CLL and SLL receiving single-agent ibrutinib. *Blood* **125:** 2497–2506. doi:10.1182/blood-2014-10-606038

Caldeira D, Alves D, Costa J, Ferreira JJ, Pinto FJ. 2019. Ibrutinib increases the risk of hypertension and atrial fibrillation: Systematic review and meta-analysis. *PLoS One* **14:** e0211228. doi:10.1371/journal.pone.0211228

Calin GA, Dumitru CD, Shimizu M, Bichi R, Zupo S, Noch E, Aldler H, Rattan S, Keating M, Rai K, et al. 2002. Nonlinear partial differential equations and applications: Frequent deletions and down-regulation of micro-RNA genes *miR15* and *miR16* at 13q14 in chronic lymphocytic leukemia. *Proc Natl Acad Sci* **99:** 15524–15529. doi:10.1073/pnas.242606799

Calissano C, Damle RN, Marsilio S, Yan XJ, Yancopoulos S, Hayes G, Emson C, Murphy EJ, Hellerstein MK, Sison C, et al. 2011. Intraclonal complexity in chronic lymphocytic leukemia: Fractions enriched in recently born/divided and older/quiescent cells. *Mol Med* **17:** 1374–1382. doi:10.2119/molmed.2011.00360

Casabonne D, Almeida J, Nieto WG, Romero A, Fernández-Navarro P, Rodriguez-Caballero A, Muñoz-Criado S, Díaz MG, Benavente Y, de Sanjosé S, et al. 2012. Common infectious agents and monoclonal B-cell lymphocytosis: A cross-sectional epidemiological study among healthy adults. *PLoS One* **7:** e52808. doi:10.1371/journal.pone.0052808

Catera R, Hatzi K, Chu CC, Herve' M, Meffre E, Ferrarini M, Oscier D, Davis Z, Allen S, Rai K, et al. 2006. Polyreactive monoclonal antibodies synthesized by some B-CLL cells recognize specific antigens on viable and apoptotic T cells. *Blood* **108:** 2813. doi:10.1182/blood.V108.11.2813.2813

Cerutti PA. 1994. Oxy-radicals and cancer. *Lancet* **344:** 862–863. doi:10.1016/S0140-6736(94)92832-0

Cerutti A, Zan H, Kim EC, Shah S, Schattner EJ, Schaffer A, Casali P. 2002. Ongoing in vivo immunoglobulin class switch DNA recombination in chronic lymphocytic leukemia B cells. *J Immunol* **169:** 6594–6603. doi:10.4049/jimmunol.169.11.6594

Chan HT, Hughes D, French RR, Tutt AL, Walshe CA, Teeling JL, Glennie MJ, Cragg MS. 2003. CD20-induced lymphoma cell death is independent of both caspases and its redistribution into triton X-100 insoluble membrane rafts. *Cancer Res* **63:** 5480–5489.

Chang DK, Kurella VB, Biswas S, Avnir Y, Sui J, Wang X, Sun J, Wang Y, Panditrao M, Peterson E, et al. 2016. Humanized mouse G6 anti-idiotypic monoclonal antibody has therapeutic potential against *IGHV1-69* germline gene-based B-CLL. *MAbs* **8:** 787–798. doi:10.1080/19420862.2016.1159365

Chen SS, Batliwalla F, Holodick NE, Yan XJ, Yancopoulos S, Croce CM, Rothstein TL, Chiorazzi N. 2013. Autoantigen can promote progression to a more aggressive TCL1 leukemia by selecting variants with enhanced B-cell receptor signaling. *Proc Natl Acad Sci* **110:** E1500–E1507. doi:10.1073/pnas.1300616110

Chen SS, Chang BY, Chang S, Tong T, Ham S, Sherry B, Burger JA, Rai KR, Chiorazzi N. 2016. BTK inhibition results in impaired CXCR4 chemokine receptor surface expression, signaling and function in chronic lymphocytic leukemia. *Leukemia* **30:** 833–843. doi:10.1038/leu.2015.316

Cheng S, Guo A, Lu P, Ma J, Coleman M, Wang YL. 2015. Functional characterization of BTK^{C481S} mutation that confers ibrutinib resistance: Exploration of alternative kinase inhibitors. *Leukemia* **29:** 895–900. doi:10.1038/leu.2014.263

Chiorazzi N. 2007. Cell proliferation and death: Forgotten features of chronic lymphocytic leukemia B cells. *Best Pract Res Clin Haematol* **20:** 399–413. doi:10.1016/j.beha.2007.03.007

Chiorazzi N, Efremov DG. 2013. Chronic lymphocytic leukemia: A tale of one or two signals? *Cell Res* **23:** 182–185. doi:10.1038/cr.2012.152

Chiorazzi N, Ferrarini M. 2003. B cell chronic lymphocytic leukemia: Lessons learned from studies of the B cell antigen receptor. *Annu Rev Immunol* **21:** 841–894. doi:10.1146/annurev.immunol.21.120601.141018

Choi MY, Widhopf GF II, Wu CC, Cui B, Lao F, Sadarangani A, Cavagnaro J, Prussak C, Carson DA, Jamieson C, et al. 2015. Pre-clinical specificity and safety of UC-961, a first-in-class monoclonal antibody targeting ROR1. *Clin Lymphoma Myeloma Leuk* **15**(Suppl.): S167–S169. doi:10.1016/j.clml.2015.02.010

Chu CC, Catera R, Hatzi K, Yan XJ, Zhang L, Wang XB, Fales HM, Allen SL, Kolitz JE, Rai KR, et al. 2008. Chronic lymphocytic leukemia antibodies with a common stereotypic rearrangement recognize nonmuscle myosin heavy chain IIA. *Blood* **112:** 5122–5129. doi:10.1182/blood-2008-06-162024

Chu CC, Catera R, Zhang L, Didier S, Agagnina BM, Damle RN, Kaufman MS, Kolitz JE, Allen SL, Rai KR, et al. 2010. Many chronic lymphocytic leukemia antibodies recognize apoptotic cells with exposed nonmuscle myosin heavy chain IIA: Implications for patient outcome and cell of origin. *Blood* **115:** 3907–3915. doi:10.1182/blood-2009-09-244251

Chumak VV, Romanenko AY, Voillequé PG, Bakhanova EV, Gudzenko N, Hatch M, Zablotska LB, Golovanov IA, Luckyanov NK, Sholom SV, et al. 2008. The Ukrainian–American study of leukemia and related disorders among chornobyl cleanup workers from Ukraine: II. Estimation of bone marrow doses. *Radiat Res* **170:** 698–710. doi:10.1667/RR1403.1

Cimmino A, Calin GA, Fabbri M, Iorio MV, Ferracin M, Shimizu M, Wojcik SE, Aqeilan RI, Zupo S, Dono M, et al. 2005. *miR-15* and *miR-16* induce apoptosis by targeting BCL2. *Proc Natl Acad Sci* **102:** 13944–13949. doi:10.1073/pnas.0506654102

Coggon D, Ntani G, Harris EC, Jayakody N, Palmer KT. 2015. Soft tissue sarcoma, non-Hodgkin's lymphoma and chronic lymphocytic leukaemia in workers exposed to phenoxy herbicides: Extended follow-up of a UK cohort. *Occup Environ Med* **72:** 435–441. doi:10.1136/oemed-2014-102654

Condoluci A, Rossi D. 2017. Treatment of Richter's syndrome. *Curr Treat Options Oncol* **18:** 75. doi:10.1007/s11864-017-0512-y

Cragg MS, Morgan SM, Chan HT, Morgan BP, Filatov AV, Johnson PW, French RR, Glennie MJ. 2003. Complement-mediated lysis by anti-CD20 mAb correlates with segregation into lipid rafts. *Blood* **101:** 1045–1052. doi:10.1182/blood-2002-06-1761

Crespo M, Bosch F, Villamor N, Bellosillo B, Colomer D, Rozman M, Marcé S, López-Guillermo A, Campo E, Montserrat E. 2003. ZAP-70 expression as a surrogate for immunoglobulin-variable-region mutations in chronic lymphocytic leukemia. *N Engl J Med* **348:** 1764–1775. doi:10.1056/NEJMoa023143

Crowther-Swanepoel D, Broderick P, Di Bernardo MC, Dobbins SE, Torres M, Mansouri M, Ruiz-Ponte C, Enjuanes A, Rosenquist R, Carracedo A, et al. 2010a. Common variants at 2q37.3, 8q24.21, 15q21.3 and 16q24.1 influence chronic lymphocytic leukemia risk. *Nat Genet* **42:** 132–136. doi:10.1038/ng.510

Crowther-Swanepoel D, Corre T, Lloyd A, Gaidano G, Olver B, Bennett FL, Doughty C, Toniolo D, Caligaris-Cappio F, Ghia P, et al. 2010b. Inherited genetic susceptibility to monoclonal B-cell lymphocytosis. *Blood* **116:** 5957–5960. doi:10.1182/blood-2010-07-294975

Cui B, Ghia EM, Chen L, Rassenti LZ, DeBoever C, Widhopf GF, Yu J, Neuberg DS, Wierda WG, Rai KR, et al. 2016. High-level ROR1 associates with accelerated disease progression in chronic lymphocytic leukemia. *Blood* **128:** 2931–2940. doi:10.1182/blood-2016-04-712562

Damle RN, Wasil T, Fais F, Ghiotto F, Valetto A, Allen SL, Buchbinder A, Budman D, Dittmar K, Kolitz J, et al. 1999. Ig V gene mutation status and CD38 expression as novel prognostic indicators in chronic lymphocytic leukemia. *Blood* **94:** 1840–1847. doi:10.1182/blood.V94.6.1840

Damle RN, Ghiotto F, Valetto A, Albesiano E, Fais F, Yan XJ, Sison CP, Allen SL, Kolitz J, Schulman P, et al. 2002. B-cell chronic lymphocytic leukemia cells express a surface membrane phenotype of activated, antigen-experienced B lymphocytes. *Blood* **99:** 4087–4093. doi:10.1182/blood.V99.11.4087

Damle RN, Batliwalla FM, Ghiotto F, Valetto A, Albesiano E, Sison C, Allen SL, Kolitz J, Vinciguerra VP, Kudalkar P, et al. 2004. Telomere length and telomerase activity delineate distinctive replicative features of the B-CLL subgroups defined by immunoglobulin V gene mutations. *Blood* **103:** 375–382. doi:10.1182/blood-2003-04-1345

Damm F, Mylonas E, Cosson A, Yoshida K, Della Valle V, Mouly E, Diop M, Scourzic L, Shiraishi Y, Chiba K, et al. 2014. Acquired initiating mutations in early hematopoietic cells of CLL patients. *Cancer Discov* **4:** 1088–1101. doi:10.1158/2159-8290.CD-14-0104

Daneshmanesh AH, Mikaelsson E, Jeddi-Tehrani M, Bayat AA, Ghods R, Ostadkarampour M, Akhondi M, Lagercrantz S, Larsson C, Osterborg A, et al. 2008. Ror1, a cell surface receptor tyrosine kinase is expressed in chronic lymphocytic leukemia and may serve as a putative target for therapy. *Int J Cancer* **123:** 1190–1195. doi:10.1002/ijc.23587

Deaglio S, Dianzani U, Horenstein AL, Fernandez JE, van Kooten C, Bragardo M, Funaro A, Garbarino G, Di Virgilio F, Banchereau J, et al. 1996. Human CD38 ligand. A 120-KDA protein predominantly expressed on endothelial cells. *J Immunol* **156:** 727–734.

Deaglio S, Mallone R, Baj G, Arnulfo A, Surico N, Dianzani U, Mehta K, Malavasi F. 2000. CD38/CD31, a receptor/ligand system ruling adhesion and signaling in human leukocytes. *Chem Immunol* **75:** 99–120. doi:10.1159/000058765

Deaglio S, Capobianco A, Bergui L, Dürig J, Morabito F, Dührsen U, Malavasi F. 2003. CD38 is a signaling molecule in B-cell chronic lymphocytic leukemia cells. *Blood* **102:** 2146–2155. doi:10.1182/blood-2003-03-0989

Deaglio S, Vaisitti T, Aydin S, Bergui L, D'Arena G, Bonello L, Omede P, Scatolini M, Jaksic O, Chiorino G, et al. 2007. CD38 and ZAP-70 are functionally linked and mark CLL cells with high migratory potential. *Blood* **110:** 4012–4021. doi:10.1182/blood-2007-06-094029

Defoiche J, Debacq C, Asquith B, Zhang Y, Burny A, Bron D, Lagneaux L, Macallan D, Willems L. 2008. Reduction of B cell turnover in chronic lymphocytic leukaemia. *Br J Haematol* **143:** 240–247. doi:10.1111/j.1365-2141.2008.07348.x

de Gorter DJJ, Beuling EA, Kersseboom R, Middendorp S, van Gils JM, Hendriks RW, Pals ST, Spaargaren M. 2007. Bruton's tyrosine kinase and phospholipase Cγ2 mediate chemokine-controlled B cell migration and homing. *Immunity* **26:** 93–104. doi:10.1016/j.immuni.2006.11.012

Delgado J, Doubek M, Baumann T, Kotaskova J, Molica S, Mozas P, Rivas-Delgado A, Morabito F, Pospisilova S, Montserrat E. 2017. Chronic lymphocytic leukemia: A prognostic model comprising only two biomarkers (*IGHV* mutational status and FISH cytogenetics) separates patients with different outcome and simplifies the CLL-IPI. *Am J Hematol* **92:** 375–380. doi:10.1002/ajh.24660

de Rooij MF, Kuil A, Geest CR, Eldering E, Chang BY, Buggy JJ, Pals ST, Spaargaren M. 2012. The clinically active BTK inhibitor PCI-32765 targets B-cell receptor- and chemokine-controlled adhesion and migration in chronic lymphocytic leukemia. *Blood* **119:** 2590–2594. doi:10.1182/blood-2011-11-390989

de Weerdt I, Koopmans SM, Kater AP, van Gelder M. 2017. Incidence and management of toxicity associated with ibrutinib and idelalisib: A practical approach. *Haematologica* **102:** 1629–1639. doi:10.3324/haematol.2017.164103

Di Bernardo MC, Crowther-Swanepoel D, Broderick P, Webb E, Sellick G, Wild R, Sullivan K, Vijayakrishnan J, Wang Y, Pittman AM, et al. 2008. A genome-wide association study identifies six susceptibility loci for chronic lymphocytic leukemia. *Nat Genet* **40:** 1204–1210. doi:10.1038/ng.219

Di Giovanni S, Valentini G, Carducci P, Giallonardo P. 1989. β-2-microglobulin is a reliable tumor marker in chronic lymphocytic leukemia. *Acta Haematol* **81:** 181–185. doi:10.1159/000205558

Dimier N, Delmar P, Ward C, Morariu-Zamfir R, Fingerle-Rowson G, Bahlo J, Fischer K, Eichhorst B, Goede V, van Dongen JJM, et al. 2018. A model for predicting effect of treatment on progression-free survival using MRD as a surrogate end point in CLL. *Blood* **131:** 955–962. doi:10.1182/blood-2017-06-792333

Ding W, Dong H, Call TG, Shanafelt TD, Parikh SA, Leis JF, Laplant BR, He R, Witzig TE, Lin Y, et al. 2015. PD-1 blockade with pembrolizumab (MK-3475) in relapsed/refractory CLL including Richter transformation: An early efficacy report from a phase 2 trial (MC1485). *Blood* **126:** 834. doi:10.1182/blood.V126.23.834.834

Döhner H, Stilgenbauer S, Benner A, Leupolt E, Kröber A, Bullinger L, Döhner K, Bentz M, Lichter P. 2000. Genomic aberrations and survival in chronic lymphocytic leukemia. *N Engl J Med* **343:** 1910–1916. doi:10.1056/NEJM200012283432602

Dühren-von Minden M, Übelhart R, Schneider D, Wossning T, Bach MP, Buchner M, Hofmann D, Surova E, Follo M, Köhler F, et al. 2012. Chronic lymphocytic leukaemia is driven by antigen-independent cell-autonomous signalling. *Nature* **489:** 309–312. doi:10.1038/nature11309

Eschbach C, Bach MP, Fidler I, Pelanda R, Köhler F, Rajewsky K, Jumaa H. 2011. Efficient generation of B lymphocytes by recognition of self-antigens. *Eur J Immunol* **41:** 2397–2403. doi:10.1002/eji.201041344

Eshhar Z, Waks T, Gross G, Schindler DG. 1993. Specific activation and targeting of cytotoxic lymphocytes through chimeric single chains consisting of antibody-binding domains and the γ or ζ subunits of the immunoglobulin and T-cell receptors. *Proc Natl Acad Sci* **90:** 720–724. doi:10.1073/pnas.90.2.720

Fabbri G, Rasi S, Rossi D, Trifonov V, Khiabanian H, Ma J, Grunn A, Fangazio M, Capello D, Monti S, et al. 2011. Analysis of the chronic lymphocytic leukemia coding genome: Role of NOTCH1 mutational activation. *J Exp Med* **208:** 1389–1401. doi:10.1084/jem.20110921

Fabbri G, Khiabanian H, Holmes AB, Wang J, Messina M, Mullighan CG, Pasqualucci L, Rabadan R, Dalla-Favera R. 2013. Genetic lesions associated with chronic lymphocytic leukemia transformation to Richter syndrome. *J Exp Med* **210:** 2273–2288. doi:10.1084/jem.20131448

Fais F, Ghiotto F, Hashimoto S, Sellars B, Valetto A, Allen SL, Schulman P, Vinciguerra VP, Rai K, Rassenti LZ, et al. 1998. Chronic lymphocytic leukemia B cells express restricted sets of mutated and unmutated antigen receptors. *J Clin Invest* **102:** 1515–1525. doi:10.1172/JCI3009

Falchi L, Vitale C, Keating MJ, Lerner S, Wang X, Elhor Gbito KY, Strom S, Wierda WG, Ferrajoli A. 2016. Incidence and prognostic impact of other cancers in a population of long-term survivors of chronic lymphocytic leukemia. *Ann Oncol* **27:** 1100–1106. doi:10.1093/annonc/mdw072

Farooqui MZ, Valdez J, Martyr S, Aue G, Saba N, Niemann CU, Herman SE, Tian X, Marti G, Soto S, et al. 2015. Ibrutinib for previously untreated and relapsed or refractory chronic lymphocytic leukaemia with *TP53* aberrations: A phase 2, single-arm trial. *Lancet Oncol* **16:** 169–176. doi:10.1016/S1470-2045(14)71182-9

Finn WG, Kay NE, Kroft SH, Church S, Peterson LC. 1998. Secondary abnormalities of chromosome 6q in B-cell chronic lymphocytic leukemia: A sequential study of karyotypic instability in 51 patients. *Am J Hematol* **59:** 223–229. doi:10.1002/(SICI)1096-8652(199811)59:3<223::AID-AJH7>3.0.CO;2-Y

Fiorcari S, Brown WS, McIntyre BW, Estrov Z, Maffei R, O'Brien S, Sivina M, Hoellenriegel J, Wierda WG, Keating MJ, et al. 2013. The PI3-kinase δ inhibitor idelalisib (GS-1101) targets integrin-mediated adhesion of chronic lymphocytic leukemia (CLL) cell to endothelial and marrow stromal cells. *PLoS One* **8:** e83830. doi:10.1371/journal.pone.0083830

Fischer K, Bahlo J, Fink AM, Goede V, Herling CD, Cramer P, Langerbeins P, von Tresckow J, Engelke A, Maurer C, et al. 2016. Long-term remissions after FCR chemoimmunotherapy in previously untreated patients with CLL: Updated results of the CLL8 trial. *Blood* **127:** 208–215. doi:10.1182/blood-2015-06-651125

Fischer A, Bastian S, Cogliatti S, Mey U, Saub J, Schanz U, Padberg B, Hohloch K. 2018. Ibrutinib-induced rapid response in chemotherapy-refractory Richter's syndrome. *Hematol Oncol* **36:** 370–371. doi:10.1002/hon.2464

Flinn IW, Hillmen P, Montillo M, Nagy Z, Illés Á, Etienne G, Delgado J, Kuss BJ, Tam CS, Gasztonyi Z, et al. 2018. The phase 3 DUO trial: Duvelisib vs ofatumumab in relapsed and refractory CLL/SLL. *Blood* **132:** 2446–2455. doi:10.1182/blood-2018-05-850461

Flinn IW, Gribben JG, Dyer MJS, Wierda W, Maris MB, Furman RR, Hillmen P, Rogers KA, Padmanabhan Iyer S, Quillet-Mary A, et al. 2019. Phase 1b study of venetoclax-obinutuzumab in previously untreated and relapsed/refractory chronic lymphocytic leukemia. *Blood* **133:** 2765–2775. doi:10.1182/blood-2019-01-896290

Fong S, Chen PP, Gilbertson TA, Fox RI, Vaughan JH, Carson DA. 1985. Structural similarities in the κ light chains of human rheumatoid factor paraproteins and serum immunoglobulins bearing a cross-reactive idiotype. *J Immunol* **135:** 1955–1960.

Fraietta JA, Beckwith KA, Patel PR, Ruella M, Zheng Z, Barrett DM, Lacey SF, Melenhorst JJ, McGettigan SE, Cook DR, et al. 2016. Ibrutinib enhances chimeric antigen receptor T-cell engraftment and efficacy in leukemia. *Blood* **127:** 1117–1127. doi:10.1182/blood-2015-11-679134

Frey NV, Porter DL. 2016. CAR T-cells merge into the fast lane of cancer care. *Am J Hematol* **91:** 146–150. doi:10.1002/ajh.24238

Friedman DF, Moore JS, Erikson J, Manz J, Goldman J, Nowell PC, Silberstein LE. 1992. Variable region gene analysis of an isotype-switched (IgA) variant of chronic lymphocytic leukemia. *Blood* **80:** 2287–2297. doi:10.1182/blood.V80.9.2287.2287

Fukuda T, Chen L, Endo T, Tang L, Lu D, Castro JE, Widhopf GF II, Rassenti LZ, Cantwell MJ, Prussak CE, et al. 2008. Antisera induced by infusions of autologous Ad-CD154-leukemia B cells identify ROR1 as an oncofetal antigen and receptor for Wnt5a. *Proc Natl Acad Sci* **105:** 3047–3052. doi:10.1073/pnas.0712148105

Fung SS, Hillier KL, Leger CS, Sandhu I, Vickars LM, Galbraith PF, Li CH, Leitch HA. 2007. Clinical progression and outcome of patients with monoclonal B-cell lymphocytosis. *Leuk Lymphoma* **48:** 1087–1091. doi:10.1080/10428190701321277

Furman RR, Cheng S, Lu P, Setty M, Perez AR, Guo A, Racchumi J, Xu G, Wu H, Ma J, et al. 2014a. Ibrutinib resistance in chronic lymphocytic leukemia. *New Engl J Med* **370:** 2352–2354. doi:10.1056/NEJMc1402716

Furman RR, Sharman JP, Coutre SE, Cheson BD, Pagel JM, Hillmen P, Barrientos JC, Zelenetz AD, Kipps TJ, Flinn I, et al. 2014b. Idelalisib and rituximab in relapsed chronic lymphocytic leukemia. *New Engl J Med* **370:** 997–1007. doi:10.1056/NEJMoa1315226

Gale RP, Cozen W, Goodman MT, Wang FF, Bernstein L. 2000. Decreased chronic lymphocytic leukemia incidence in Asians in Los Angeles county. *Leuk Res* **24:** 665–669. doi:10.1016/S0145-2126(00)00038-2

Galletti G, Scielzo C, Barbaglio F, Rodriguez TV, Riba M, Lazarevic D, Cittaro D, Simonetti G, Ranghetti P, Scarfo L, et al. 2016. Targeting macrophages sensitizes chronic lymphocytic leukemia to apoptosis and inhibits disease progression. *Cell Rep* **14:** 1748–1760. doi:10.1016/j.celrep.2016.01.042

Gattei V, Bulian P, Del Principe MI, Zucchetto A, Maurillo L, Buccisano F, Bomben R, Dal-Bo M, Luciano F, Rossi FM, et al. 2008. Relevance of CD49d protein expression as overall survival and progressive disease prognosticator in chronic lymphocytic leukemia. *Blood* **111:** 865–873. doi:10.1182/blood-2007-05-092486

Georgiadis P, Liampa I, Hebels DG, Krauskopf J, Chatziioannou A, Valavanis I, de Kok TMCM, Kleinjans JCS, Bergdahl IA, Melin B, et al. 2017. Evolving DNA methylation and gene expression markers of B-cell chronic lymphocytic leukemia are present in pre-diagnostic blood samples more than 10 years prior to diagnosis. *BMC Genomics* **18:** 728. doi:10.1186/s12864-017-4117-4

Ghia P, Prato G, Scielzo C, Stella S, Geuna M, Guida G, Caligaris-Cappio F. 2004. Monoclonal $CD5^+$ and $CD5^-$ B-lymphocyte expansions are frequent in the peripheral blood of the elderly. *Blood* **103:** 2337–2342. doi:10.1182/blood-2003-09-3277

Ghiotto F, Fais F, Valetto A, Albesiano E, Hashimoto S, Dono M, Ikematsu H, Allen SL, Kolitz J, Rai KR, et al. 2004. Remarkably similar antigen receptors among a subset of patients with chronic lymphocytic leukemia. *J Clin Invest* **113:** 1008–1016. doi:10.1172/JCI19399

Ghiotto F, Fais F, Albesiano E, Sison C, Valetto A, Gaidano G, Reinhardt J, Kolitz JE, Rai K, Allen SL, et al. 2006. Similarities and differences between the light and heavy chain Ig variable region gene repertoires in chronic lymphocytic leukemia. *Mol Med* **12:** 300–308. doi:10.2119/2006-00080.Ghiotto

Ghosn EE, Sadate-Ngatchou P, Yang Y, Herzenberg LA. 2011. Distinct progenitors for B-1 and B-2 cells are present in adult mouse spleen. *Proc Natl Acad Sci* **108:** 2879–2884. doi:10.1073/pnas.1019764108

Gine E, Martinez A, Villamor N, Lopez-Guillermo A, Camos M, Martinez D, Esteve J, Calvo X, Muntanola A, Abrisqueta P, et al. 2010. Expanded and highly active proliferation centers identify a histological subtype of chronic lymphocytic leukemia ("accelerated" chronic lymphocytic leukemia) with aggressive clinical behavior. *Haematologica* **95:** 1526–1533. doi:10.3324/haematol.2010.022277

Giri S, Hahn A, Yaghmour G, Martin MG. 2015. Ibrutinib has some activity in Richter's syndrome. *Blood Cancer J* **5:** e277. doi:10.1038/bcj.2014.98

Glancy E, Siles R. 2016. Monoclonal B-cell lymphocytosis and hypogammaglobulinaemia. *Br J Haematol* **173:** 316–317. doi:10.1111/bjh.13585

Gluzman D, Imamura N, Sklyarenko L, Nadgornaya V, Zavelevich M, Machilo V. 2006. Patterns of hematological malignancies in Chernobyl clean-up workers (1996-2005). *Exp Oncol* **28:** 60–63.

Göckeritz E, Kerwien S, Baumann M, Wigger M, Vondey V, Neumann L, Landwehr T, Wendtner CM, Klein C, Liu N, et al. 2015. Efficacy of phosphatidylinositol-3 kinase inhibitors with diverse isoform selectivity profiles for inhibiting the survival of chronic lymphocytic leukemia cells. *Int J Cancer* **137:** 2234–2242. doi:10.1002/ijc.29579

Goede V, Fischer K, Busch R, Engelke A, Eichhorst B, Wendtner CM, Chagorova T, de la Serna J, Dilhuydy MS, Illmer T, et al. 2014. Obinutuzumab plus chlorambucil in patients with CLL and coexisting conditions. *N Engl J Med* **370:** 1101–1110. doi:10.1056/NEJMoa1313984

Goldin LR, Pfeiffer RM, Li X, Hemminki K. 2004. Familial risk of lymphoproliferative tumors in families of patients with chronic lymphocytic leukemia: Results from the Swedish family-cancer database. *Blood* **104:** 1850–1854. doi:10.1182/blood-2004-01-0341

Goldin LR, Landgren O, Marti GE, Caporaso NE. 2010. Familial aspects of chronic lymphocytic leukemia, monoclonal B-cell lymphocytosis (MBL), and related lymphomas. *European J Clin Med Oncol* **2:** 119–126.

Gonzalez D, Martinez P, Wade R, Hockley S, Oscier D, Matutes E, Dearden CE, Richards SM, Catovsky D, Morgan GJ. 2011. Mutational status of the TP53 gene as a predictor of response and survival in patients with chronic lymphocytic leukemia: Results from the LRF CLL4 trial. *J Clin Oncol* **29:** 2223–2229. doi:10.1200/JCO.2010.32.0838

Gounari M, Ntoufa S, Appolino B, Papakonstantinou N, Chu C, Rossi D, Gaidano G, Chiorazzi N, Stamatopoulos K, Ghia P. 2015. Excessive antigen reactivity may underlie the clinical aggressiveness of chronic lymphocytic leukemia stereotyped subset #8. *Blood* **125:** 3580–3587. doi:10.1182/blood-2014-09-603217

Granziero L, Ghia P, Circosta P, Gottardi D, Strola G, Geuna M, Montagna L, Piccoli P, Chilosi M, Caligaris-Cappio F. 2001. Survivin is expressed on CD40 stimulation and interfaces proliferation and apoptosis in B-cell chronic lymphocytic leukemia. *Blood* **97:** 2777–2783. doi:10.1182/blood.V97.9.2777

Greco M, Capello D, Bruscaggin A, Spina V, Rasi S, Monti S, Ciardullo C, Cresta S, Fangazio M, Gaidano G, et al. 2013. Analysis of *SF3B1* mutations in monoclonal B-cell lymphocytosis. *Hematol Oncol* **31:** 54–55. doi:10.1002/hon.2013

Griffin DO, Holodick NE, Rothstein TL. 2011. Human B1 cells in umbilical cord and adult peripheral blood express the novel phenotype $CD20^+CD27^+CD43^+CD70^-$. *J Exp Med* **208:** 67–80. doi:10.1084/jem.20101499

Gross G, Waks T, Eshhar Z. 1989. Expression of immunoglobulin-T-cell receptor chimeric molecules as functional receptors with antibody-type specificity. *Proc Natl Acad Sci* **86:** 10024–10028. doi:10.1073/pnas.86.24.10024

Guièze R, Wu CJ. 2015. Genomic and epigenomic heterogeneity in chronic lymphocytic leukemia. *Blood* **126:** 445–453. doi:10.1182/blood-2015-02-585042

Guo B, Zhang L, Chiorazzi N, Rothstein TL. 2016. IL-4 rescues surface IgM expression in chronic lymphocytic leukemia. *Blood* **128:** 553–562. doi:10.1182/blood-2015-11-682997

Gurrieri C, McGuire P, Zan H, Yan XJ, Cerutti A, Albesiano E, Allen SL, Vinciguerra V, Rai KR, Ferrarini M, et al. 2002. Chronic lymphocytic leukemia B cells can undergo somatic hypermutation and intraclonal immunoglobulin V_HDJ_H gene diversification. *J Exp Med* **196:** 629–639. doi:10.1084/jem.20011693

Hadzidimitriou A, Darzentas N, Murray F, Smilevska T, Arvaniti E, Tresoldi C, Tsaftaris A, Laoutaris N, Anagnostopoulos A, Davi F, et al. 2009. Evidence for the significant role of immunoglobulin light chains in antigen recognition and selection in chronic lymphocytic leukemia. *Blood* **113:** 403–411. doi:10.1182/blood-2008-07-166868

Haferlach C, Dicker F, Schnittger S, Kern W, Haferlach T. 2007. Comprehensive genetic characterization of CLL: A study on 506 cases analysed with chromosome banding analysis, interphase FISH, IgVH status and immunophenotyping. *Leukemia* **21:** 2442–2451. doi:10.1038/sj.leu.2404935

Hallek M, Langenmayer I, Nerl C, Knauf W, Dietzfelbinger H, Adorf D, Ostwald M, Busch R, Kuhn-Hallek I, Thiel E, et al. 1999. Elevated serum thymidine kinase levels identify a subgroup at high risk of disease progression in early, nonsmoldering chronic lymphocytic leukemia. *Blood* **93:** 1732–1737.

Hallek M, Fischer K, Fingerle-Rowson G, Fink AM, Busch R, Mayer J, Hensel M, Hopfinger G, Hess G, von Grünhagen U, et al. 2010. Addition of rituximab to fludarabine and cyclophosphamide in patients with chronic lymphocytic leukaemia: A randomised, open-label, phase 3 trial. *The Lancet* **376:** 1164–1174. doi:10.1016/S0140-6736(10)61381-5

Hallek M, Cheson BD, Catovsky D, Caligaris-Cappio F, Dighiero G, Döhner H, Hillmen P, Keating M, Montserrat E, Chiorazzi N, et al. 2018. iwCLL guidelines for diagnosis, indications for treatment, response assessment, and supportive management of CLL. *Blood* **131:** 2745–2760. doi:10.1182/blood-2017-09-806398

Hamblin TJ, Davis Z, Gardiner A, Oscier DG, Stevenson FK. 1999. Unmutated Ig V_H genes are associated with a more aggressive form of chronic lymphocytic leukemia. *Blood* **94:** 1848–1854. doi:10.1182/blood.V94.6.1848

Hanna BS, McClanahan F, Yazdanparast H, Zaborsky N, Kalter V, Rößner PM, Benner A, Durr C, Egle A, Gribben JG, et al. 2016. Depletion of CLL-associated patrolling monocytes and macrophages controls disease development and repairs immune dysfunction in vivo. *Leukemia* **30:** 570–579. doi:10.1038/leu.2015.305

Harper K. 2019. Ibrutinib may boost efficacy of CAR T cells. *Cancer Discov* **9:** OF3.

Hasan K, Yu J, Chen L, Cui B, Widhopf GF, Rassenti L, Shen Z, Briggs SP, Kipps TJ. 2017. Wnt5a induces ROR1 to complex with HS1 to enhance migration of chronic lymphocytic leukemia cells. *Leukemia* **31:** 2615–2622. doi:10.1038/leu.2017

Hasan MK, Rassenti L, Widhopf GF, Yu J, Kipps TJ. 2019. Wnt5a causes ROR1 to complex and activate cortactin to enhance migration of chronic lymphocytic leukemia cells. *Leukemia* **33:** 653–661. doi:10.1038/s41375-018-0306-7

Hashimoto S, Dono M, Wakai M, Allen SL, Lichtman SM, Schulman P, Vinciguerra VP, Ferrarini M, Silver J, Chiorazzi N. 1995. Somatic diversification and selection of immunoglobulin heavy and light chain variable region genes in IgG^+ $CD5^+$ chronic lymphocytic leukemia B cells. *J Exp Med* **181:** 1507–1517. doi:10.1084/jem.181.4.1507

Hatzi K, Catera R, Moreno Atanasio C, Fischetti VA, Allen SL, Kolitz JE, Rai KR, Chu CC, Chiorazzi N. 2016. Chronic lymphocytic leukemia immunoglobulins display bacterial reactivity that converges and diverges from auto-/poly-reactivity and IGHV mutation status. *Clin Immunol* **172:** 44–51. doi:10.1016/j.clim.2016.08.020

Haughton G, Arnold LW, Whitmore AC, Clarke SH. 1993. B-1 cells are made, not born. *Immunol Today* **14:** 84–87. discussion 87–91. doi:10.1016/0167-5699(93)90064-R

Hayakawa K, Hardy RR, Parks DR, Herzenberg LA. 1983. The "Ly-1 B" cell subpopulation in normal immunodefective, and autoimmune mice. *J Exp Med* **157:** 202–218. doi:10.1084/jem.157.1.202

Hayakawa K, Formica AM, Colombo MJ, Shinton SA, Brill-Dashoff J, Morse Iii HC, Li YS, Hardy RR. 2016. Loss of a chromosomal region with synteny to human 13q14 occurs in mouse chronic lymphocytic leukemia that originates from early-generated B-1 B cells. *Leukemia* **30:** 1510–1519. doi:10.1038/leu.2016.61

Herishanu Y, Pérez-Galán P, Liu D, Biancotto A, Pittaluga S, Vire B, Gibellini F, Njuguna N, Lee E, Stennett L, et al. 2011. The lymph node microenvironment promotes B-cell receptor signaling, NF-κB activation, and tumor proliferation in chronic lymphocytic leukemia. *Blood* **117:** 563–574. doi:10.1182/blood-2010-05-284984

Herman SE, Gordon AL, Hertlein E, Ramanunni A, Zhang X, Jaglowski S, Flynn J, Jones J, Blum KA, Buggy JJ, et al. 2011. Bruton tyrosine kinase represents a promising therapeutic target for treatment of chronic lymphocytic leukemia and is effectively targeted by PCI-32765. *Blood* **117:** 6287–6296. doi:10.1182/blood-2011-01-328484

Herman SEM, Mustafa RZ, Gyamfi JA, Pittaluga S, Chang S, Chang B, Farooqui M, Wiestner A. 2014a. Ibrutinib inhibits B-cell receptor and NF-κB signaling and reduces tumor proliferation in tissue-resident cells of patients with chronic lymphocytic leukemia. *Blood* **123:** 3286–3295. doi:10.1182/blood-2014-02-548610

Herman SEM, Niemann CU, Farooqui M, Jones J, Mustafa RZ, Lipsky A, Saba N, Martyr S, Soto S, Valdez J, et al. 2014b. Ibrutinib-induced lymphocytosis in patients with chronic lymphocytic leukemia: Correlative analyses from a phase II study. *Leukemia* **28:** 2188–2196. doi:10.1038/leu.2014.122

Herman SEM, Mustafa RZ, Jones J, Wong DH, Farooqui M, Wiestner A. 2015. Treatment with ibrutinib inhibits BTK- and VLA-4-dependent adhesion of chronic lymphocytic leukemia cells in vivo. *Clin Cancer Res* **21:** 4642–4651. doi:10.1158/1078-0432.CCR-15-0781

Herndon TM, Chen SS, Saba NS, Valdez J, Emson C, Gatmaitan M, Tian X, Hughes TE, Sun C, Arthur DC, et al. 2017. Direct in vivo evidence for increased proliferation of CLL cells in lymph nodes compared to bone marrow and peripheral blood. *Leukemia* **31:** 1340–1347. doi:10.1038/leu.2017.11

Hervé M, Xu K, Ng YS, Wardemann H, Albesiano E, Messmer BT, Chiorazzi N, Meffre E. 2005. Unmutated and mutated chronic lymphocytic leukemias derive from self-reactive B cell precursors despite expressing different antibody reactivity. *J Clin Invest* **115:** 1636–1643. doi:10.1172/JCI24387

Hojjat-Farsangi M, Khan AS, Daneshmanesh AH, Moshfegh A, Sandin A, Mansouri L, Palma M, Lundin J, Osterborg A, Mellstedt H. 2013. The tyrosine kinase receptor ROR1 is constitutively phosphorylated in chronic lymphocytic leukemia (CLL) cells. *PLoS One* **8:** e78339. doi:10.1371/journal.pone.0078339

Honigberg LA, Smith AM, Sirisawad M, Verner E, Loury D, Chang B, Li S, Pan Z, Thamm DH, Miller RA, et al. 2010. The Bruton tyrosine kinase inhibitor PCI-32765 blocks B-cell activation and is efficacious in models of autoimmune disease and B-cell malignancy. *Proc Natl Acad Sci* **107:** 13075–13080. doi:10.1073/pnas.1004594107

Hoogeboom R, van Kessel KP, Hochstenbach F, Wormhoudt TA, Reinten RJ, Wagner K, Kater AP, Guikema JE, Bende RJ, van Noesel CJ. 2013. A mutated B cell chronic lymphocytic leukemia subset that recognizes and responds to fungi. *J Exp Med* **210:** 59–70. doi:10.1084/jem.20121801

Hudecek M, Schmitt TM, Baskar S, Lupo-Stanghellini MT, Nishida T, Yamamoto TN, Bleakley M, Turtle CJ, Chang WC, Greisman HA, et al. 2010. The B-cell tumor–associated antigen ROR1 can be targeted with T cells modified to express a ROR1-specific chimeric antigen receptor. *Blood* **116:** 4532–4541. doi:10.1182/blood-2010-05-283309

Iacovelli S, Hug E, Bennardo S, Duehren-von Minden M, Gobessi S, Rinaldi A, Suljagic M, Bilbao D, Bolasco G, Eckl-Dorna J, et al. 2015. Two types of BCR interactions are positively selected during leukemia development in the Eμ-TCL1 transgenic mouse model of CLL. *Blood* **125:** 1578–1588. doi:10.1182/blood-2014-07-587790

Jain P, Young KH. 2014. Haematological cancer: Richter's transformation in CLL—A distinct lymphoma. *Nat Rev Clin Oncol* **11:** 6–8. doi:10.1038/nrclinonc.2013.229

Jain P, Keating M, Wierda W, Estrov Z, Ferrajoli A, Jain N, George B, James D, Kantarjian H, Burger J, et al. 2015. Outcomes of patients with chronic lymphocytic leukemia after discontinuing ibrutinib. *Blood* **125:** 2062–2067. doi:10.1182/blood-2014-09-603670

Johnson TA, Rassenti LZ, Kipps TJ. 1997. Ig VH1 genes expressed in B cell chronic lymphocytic leukemia exhibit distinctive molecular features. *J Immunol* **158:** 235–246.

Jones JA, Mato AR, Wierda WG, Davids MS, Choi M, Cheson BD, Furman RR, Lamanna N, Barr PM, Zhou L, et al. 2018. Venetoclax for chronic lymphocytic leukaemia progressing after ibrutinib: An interim analysis of a multicentre, open-label, phase 2 trial. *Lancet Oncol* **19:** 65–75. doi:10.1016/S1470-2045(17)30909-9

Kadri S, Lee J, Fitzpatrick C, Galanina N, Sukhanova M, Venkataraman G, Sharma S, Long B, Petras K, Theissen M, et al. 2017. Clonal evolution underlying leukemia progression and Richter transformation in patients with ibrutinib-relapsed CLL. *Blood Adv* **1:** 715–727. doi:10.1182/bloodadvances.2016003632

Kasar S, Kim J, Improgo R, Tiao G, Polak P, Haradhvala N, Lawrence MS, Kiezun A, Fernandes SM, Bahl S, et al. 2015. Whole-genome sequencing reveals activation-induced cytidine deaminase signatures during indolent chronic lymphocytic leukaemia evolution. *Nat Commun* **6:** 8866. doi:10.1038/ncomms9866

Kasar S, Underbayev C, Hassan M, Ilev I, Degheidy H, Bauer S, Marti G, Lutz C, Raveche E, Batish M. 2016. Alterations in the *mir-15a/16-1* loci impairs its processing and augments B-1 expansion in de novo mouse model of chronic lymphocytic leukemia (CLL). *PLoS One* **11:** e0149331. doi:10.1371/journal.pone.0149331

Keating MJ, Kantarjian H, Talpaz M, Redman J, Koller C, Barlogie B, Velasquez W, Plunkett W, Freireich EJ, McCredie KB. 1989. Fludarabine: A new agent with major activity against chronic lymphocytic leukemia. *Blood* **74:** 19–25. doi:10.1182/blood.V74.1.19.bloodjournal74119

Keating MJ, Lerner S, Kantarjian H, Freireich EJ, O'Brien S. 1995. The serum β2-microglobulin level is more powerful than stage in predicting response and survival in chronic lymphocytic leukemia. *Blood* **86:** 606A.

Keating MJ, O'Brien S, Albitar M, Lerner S, Plunkett W, Giles F, Andreeff M, Cortes J, Faderl S, Thomas D, et al. 2005. Early results of a chemoimmunotherapy regimen of fludarabine, cyclophosphamide, and rituximab as initial therapy for chronic lymphocytic leukemia. *J Clin Oncol* **23:** 4079–4088. doi:10.1200/JCO.2005.12.051

Kesminiene A, Evrard A-S, Ivanov VK, Malakhova IV, Kurtinaitis J, Stengrevics A, Tekkel M, Anspaugh LR, Bouville A, Chekin S, et al. 2008. Risk of hematological malignancies among Chernobyl liquidators. *Radiat Res* **170:** 721–735. doi:10.1667/RR1231.1

Kikushige Y, Ishikawa F, Miyamoto T, Shima T, Urata S, Yoshimoto G, Mori Y, Iino T, Yamauchi T, Eto T, et al. 2011. Self-renewing hematopoietic stem cell is the primary target in pathogenesis of human chronic lymphocytic leukemia. *Cancer Cell* **20:** 246–259. doi:10.1016/j.ccr.2011.06.029

Kipps TJ, Tomhave E, Chen PP, Carson DA. 1988. Autoantibody-associated κ light chain variable region gene expressed in chronic lymphocytic leukemia with little or no somatic mutation. Implications for etiology and immunotherapy. *J Exp Med* **167:** 840–852. doi:10.1084/jem.167.3.840

Klein U, Tu Y, Stolovitzky GA, Mattioli M, Cattoretti G, Husson H, Freedman A, Inghirami G, Cro L, Baldini L, et al. 2001. Gene expression profiling of B cell chronic lymphocytic leukemia reveals a homogeneous phenotype related to memory B cells. *J Exp Med* **194:** 1625–1638. doi:10.1084/jem.194.11.1625

Klein U, Lia M, Crespo M, Siegel R, Shen Q, Mo T, Ambesi-Impiombato A, Califano A, Migliazza A, Bhagat G, et al. 2010. The *DLEU2/miR-15a/16-1* cluster controls B cell proliferation and its deletion leads to chronic lymphocytic leukemia. *Cancer Cell* **17:** 28–40. doi:10.1016/j.ccr.2009.11.019

Kochenderfer JN, Wilson WH, Janik JE, Dudley ME, Stetler-Stevenson M, Feldman SA, Maric I, Raffeld M, Nathan DA, Lanier BJ, et al. 2010. Eradication of B-lineage cells and regression of lymphoma in a patient treated with autologous T cells genetically engineered to recognize CD19. *Blood* **116:** 4099–4102. doi:10.1182/blood-2010-04-281931

Kochenderfer JN, Dudley ME, Feldman SA, Wilson WH, Spaner DE, Maric I, Stetler-Stevenson M, Phan GQ, Hughes MS, Sherry RM, et al. 2012. B-cell depletion and remissions of malignancy along with cytokine-associated toxicity in a clinical trial of anti-CD19 chimeric-antigen-receptor–transduced T cells. *Blood* **119:** 2709–2720. doi:10.1182/blood-2011-10-384388

Köhler F, Hug E, Eschbach C, Meixlsperger S, Hobeika E, Kofer J, Wardemann H, Jumaa H. 2008. Autoreactive B cell receptors mimic autonomous pre-B cell receptor signaling and induce proliferation of early B cells. *Immunity* **29:** 912–921. doi:10.1016/j.immuni.2008.10.013

Komarova NL, Burger JA, Wodarz D. 2014. Evolution of ibrutinib resistance in chronic lymphocytic leukemia (CLL). *Proc Natl Acad Sci* **111:** 13906–13911. doi:10.1073/pnas.1409362111

Kröber A, Seiler T, Benner A, Bullinger L, Bruckle E, Lichter P, Döhner H, Stilgenbauer S. 2002. V_H mutation status, CD38 expression level, genomic aberrations, and survival in chronic lymphocytic leukemia. *Blood* **100:** 1410–1416. doi:10.1182/blood.V100.4.1410.h81602001410_1410_1416

Kulis M, Heath S, Bibikova M, Queirós AC, Navarro A, Clot G, Martínez-Trillos A, Castellano G., Brun-Heath I, Pinyol M, et al. 2012. Epigenomic analysis detects widespread gene-body DNA hypomethylation in chronic lymphocytic leukemia. *Nat Genet* **44:** 1236–1242. doi:10.1038/ng.2443

Küppers R, Gause A, Rajewsky K. 1991. B cells of chronic lymphatic leukemia express V genes in unmutated form. *Leuk Res* **15:** 487–496. doi:10.1016/0145-2126(91)90060-7

Kwok M, Rawstron AC, Varghese A, Evans PAS, O'Connor SJM, Doughty C, Newton DJ, Moreton P, Hillmen P. 2016. Minimal residual disease is an independent predictor for 10-year survival in CLL. *Blood* **128:** 2770–2773. doi:10.1182/blood-2016-05-714162

Lampson BL, Kasar SN, Matos TR, Morgan EA, Rassenti L, Davids MS, Fisher DC, Freedman AS, Jacobson CA, Armand P, et al. 2016. Idelalisib given front-line for treatment of chronic lymphocytic leukemia causes frequent immune-mediated hepatotoxicity. *Blood* **128:** 195–203. doi:10.1182/blood-2016-03-707133

Landau DA, Carter Scott L, Stojanov P, McKenna A, Stevenson K, Lawrence Michael S, Sougnez C, Stewart C, Sivachenko A, Wang L, et al. 2013. Evolution and impact of subclonal mutations in chronic lymphocytic leukemia. *Cell* **152:** 714–726. doi:10.1016/j.cell.2013.01.019

Landau DA, Carter SL, Getz G, Wu CJ. 2014a. Clonal evolution in hematological malignancies and therapeutic implications. *Leukemia* **28:** 34–43. doi:10.1038/leu.2013.248

Landau DA, Clement K, Ziller Michael J, Boyle P, Fan J, Gu H, Stevenson K, Sougnez C, Wang L, Li S, et al. 2014b. Locally disordered methylation forms the basis of intratumor methylome variation in chronic lymphocytic leukemia. *Cancer Cell* **26:** 813–825. doi:10.1016/j.ccell.2014.10.012

Landau DA, Tausch E, Taylor-Weiner AN, Stewart C, Reiter JG, Bahlo J, Kluth S, Bozic I, Lawrence M, Bottcher S, et al. 2015. Mutations driving CLL and their evolution in progression and relapse. *Nature* **526:** 525–530. doi:10.1038/nature15395

Landgren O, Gridley G, Check D, Caporaso NE, Morris Brown L. 2007a. Acquired immune-related and inflammatory conditions and subsequent chronic lymphocytic leukaemia. *Br J Haematol* **139:** 791–798. doi:10.1111/j.1365-2141.2007.06859.x

Landgren O, Rapkin JS, Caporaso NE, Mellemkjaer L, Gridley G, Goldin LR, Engels EA. 2007b. Respiratory tract infections and subsequent risk of chronic lymphocytic leukemia. *Blood* **109:** 2198–2201. doi:10.1182/blood-2006-08-044008

Landgren O, Albitar M, Ma W, Abbasi F, Hayes RB, Ghia P, Marti GE, Caporaso N. 2009. B-cell clones as early markers for chronic lymphocytic leukemia. *N Engl J Med* **360:** 659–667. doi:10.1056/NEJMoa0806122

Lanemo Myhrinder A, Hellqvist E, Sidorova E, Söderberg A, Baxendale H, Dahle C, Willander K, Tobin G, Bäckman E,

Söderberg O, et al. 2008. A new perspective: Molecular motifs on oxidized LDL, apoptotic cells, and bacteria are targets for chronic lymphocytic leukemia antibodies. *Blood* **111:** 3838–3848. doi:10.1182/blood-2007-11-125450

Law PJ, Berndt SI, Speedy HE, Camp NJ, Sava GP, Skibola CF, Holroyd A, Joseph V, Sunter NJ, Nieters A, et al. 2017. Genome-wide association analysis implicates dysregulation of immunity genes in chronic lymphocytic leukaemia. *Nat Commun* **8:** 14175. doi:10.1038/ncomms14175

Lawrence MS, Stojanov P, Polak P, Kryukov GV, Cibulskis K, Sivachenko A, Carter SL, Stewart C, Mermel CH, Roberts SA, et al. 2013. Mutational heterogeneity in cancer and the search for new cancer-associated genes. *Nature* **499:** 214–218. doi:10.1038/nature12213

Lee DW, Gardner R, Porter DL, Louis CU, Ahmed N, Jensen M, Grupp SA, Mackall CL. 2014. Current concepts in the diagnosis and management of cytokine release syndrome. *Blood* **124:** 188–195.

Lenders JW, de Pauw BE, Bogman MJ, Haanen C. 1984. Combined immunodeficiency preceding chronic lymphocytic leukemia. *Blut* **48:** 171–175. doi:10.1007/BF00320340

Lentz R, Feinglass J, Ma S, Akhter N. 2019. Risk factors for the development of atrial fibrillation on ibrutinib treatment. *Leuk Lymphoma* **60:** 1447–1453. doi:10.1080/10428194.2018.1533129

Lenz G, Nagel I, Siebert R, Roschke AV, Sanger W, Wright GW, Dave SS, Tan B, Zhao H, Rosenwald A, et al. 2007. Aberrant immunoglobulin class switch recombination and switch translocations in activated B cell–like diffuse large B cell lymphoma. *J Exp Med* **204:** 633–643. doi:10.1084/jem.20062041

Leon ME, Ferro G, Schüz J, Schinasi LH, Kjaerheim K, Straif K, Lebailly P, Tual S, Hofmann JN, Beane Freeman LE, et al. 2019. Pesticide use and risk of non-Hodgkin lymphoid malignancies in agricultural cohorts from France, Norway and the USA: A pooled analysis from the AGRICOH consortium. *Int J Epidemiol* **48:** 1519–1535. doi:10.1093/ije/dyz017

Lesley AA, Ola L, Eric AE. 2009. Common community acquired infections and subsequent risk of chronic lymphocytic leukaemia. *Br J Haematol* **147:** 444–449. doi:10.1111/j.1365-2141.2009.07849.x

Leuenberger M, Frigerio S, Wild PJ, Noetzli F, Korol D, Zimmermann DR, Gengler C, Probst-Hensch NM, Moch H, Tinguely M. 2010. AID protein expression in chronic lymphocytic leukemia/small lymphocytic lymphoma is associated with poor prognosis and complex genetic alterations. *Mod Pathol* **23:** 177–186. doi:10.1038/modpathol.2009.156

Lipsky AH, Farooqui MZ, Tian X, Martyr S, Cullinane AM, Nghiem K, Sun C, Valdez J, Niemann CU, Herman SE, et al. 2015. Incidence and risk factors of bleeding-related adverse events in patients with chronic lymphocytic leukemia treated with ibrutinib. *Haematologica* **100:** 1571–1578. doi:10.3324/haematol.2015.126672

Liu Y, Higgins CD, Overstreet CM, Rai KR, Chiorazzi N, Lai JR. 2013. Peptides that bind specifically to an antibody from a chronic lymphocytic leukemia clone expressing unmutated immunoglobulin variable region genes. *Mol Med* **19:** 245–252. doi:10.2119/molmed.2013.00082

Ljungström V, Cortese D, Young E, Pandzic T, Mansouri L, Plevova K, Ntoufa S, Baliakas P, Clifford R, Sutton LA, et al. 2016. Whole-exome sequencing in relapsing chronic lymphocytic leukemia: Clinical impact of recurrent *RPS15* mutations. *Blood* **127:** 1007–1016. doi:10.1182/blood-2015-10-674572

Logan AC, Gao H, Wang C, Sahaf B, Jones CD, Marshall EL, Buño I, Armstrong R, Fire AZ, Weinberg KI, et al. 2011. High-throughput VDJ sequencing for quantification of minimal residual disease in chronic lymphocytic leukemia and immune reconstitution assessment. *Proc Natl Acad Sci* **108:** 21194–21199. doi:10.1073/pnas.1118357109

Logan AC, Zhang B, Narasimhan B, Carlton V, Zheng J, Moorhead M, Krampf MR, Jones CD, Waqar AN, Faham M, et al. 2013. Minimal residual disease quantification using consensus primers and high-throughput IGH sequencing predicts post-transplant relapse in chronic lymphocytic leukemia. *Leukemia* **27:** 1659–1665. doi:10.1038/leu.2013.52

Maddocks KJ, Ruppert AS, Lozanski G, Heerema NA, Zhao W, Abruzzo L, Lozanski A, Davis M, Gordon A, Smith LL, et al. 2015. Etiology of ibrutinib therapy discontinuation and outcomes in patients with chronic lymphocytic leukemia. *JAMA Oncol* **1:** 80–87. doi:10.1001/jamaoncol.2014.218

Maffei R, Fiorcari S, Martinelli S, Potenza L, Luppi M, Marasca R. 2015. Targeting neoplastic B cells and harnessing microenvironment: The "double face" of ibrutinib and idelalisib. *J Hematol Oncol* **8:** 60. doi:10.1186/s13045-015-0157-x

Mandrekar SJ, Sargent DJ. 2010. Predictive biomarker validation in practice: Lessons from real trials. *Clin Trials* **7:** 567–573. doi:10.1177/1740774510368574

Mansouri L, Wierzbinska JA, Plass C, Rosenquist R. 2018. Epigenetic deregulation in chronic lymphocytic leukemia: Clinical and biological impact. *Semin Cancer Biol* **51:** 1–11. doi:10.1016/j.semcancer.2018.02.001

Mao Z, Quintanilla-Martinez L, Raffeld M, Richter M, Krugmann J, Burek C, Hartmann E, Rudiger T, Jaffe ES, Müller-Hermelink HK, et al. 2007. IgVH mutational status and clonality analysis of Richter's transformation: Diffuse large B-cell lymphoma and Hodgkin lymphoma in association with B-cell chronic lymphocytic leukemia (B-CLL) represent 2 different pathways of disease evolution. *Am J Surg Pathol* **31:** 1605–1614. doi:10.1097/PAS.0b013e31804bdaf8

Marsilio S, Khiabanian H, Fabbri G, Vergani S, Scuoppo C, Montserrat E, Shpall EJ, Hadigol M, Marin P, Rai KR, et al. 2018. Somatic CLL mutations occur at multiple distinct hematopoietic maturation stages: Documentation and cautionary note regarding cell fraction purity. *Leukemia* **32:** 1041–1044. doi:10.1038/leu.2017.343

Marti GE, Carter P, Abbasi F, Washington GC, Jain N, Zenger VE, Ishibe N, Goldin L, Fontaine L, Weissman N, et al. 2003. B-cell monoclonal lymphocytosis and B-cell abnormalities in the setting of familial B-cell chronic lymphocytic leukemia. *Cytometry B Clin Cytom* **52B:** 1–12. doi:10.1002/cyto.b.10013

Marti GE, Rawstron AC, Ghia P, Hillmen P, Houlston RS, Kay N, Schleinitz TA, Caporaso N. 2005. Diagnostic criteria for monoclonal B-cell lymphocytosis. *Br J Haematol* **130:** 325–332. doi:10.1111/j.1365-2141.2005.05550.x

Matos DM, Ismael SJ, Scrideli CA, de Oliveira FM, Rego EM, Falcão RP. 2009. Monoclonal B-cell lymphocytosis in first-degree relatives of patients with sporadic (non-familial) chronic lymphocytic leukaemia. *Br J Haematol* **147:** 339–346. doi:10.1111/j.1365-2141.2009.07861.x

McCarthy H, Wierda WG, Barron LL, Cromwell CC, Wang J, Coombes KR, Rangel R, Elenitoba-Johnson KS, Keating MJ, Abruzzo LV. 2003. High expression of activation-induced cytidine deaminase (AID) and splice variants is a distinctive feature of poor-prognosis chronic lymphocytic leukemia. *Blood* **101:** 4903–4908. doi:10.1182/blood-2002-09-2906

McClanahan F, Hanna B, Miller S, Clear AJ, Lichter P, Gribben JG, Seiffert M. 2015. PD-L1 checkpoint blockade prevents immune dysfunction and leukemia development in a mouse model of chronic lymphocytic leukemia. *Blood* **126:** 203–211. doi:10.1182/blood-2015-01-622936

McMullen JR, Boey EJ, Ooi JY, Seymour JF, Keating MJ, Tam CS. 2014. Ibrutinib increases the risk of atrial fibrillation, potentially through inhibition of cardiac PI3K-Akt signaling. *Blood* **124:** 3829–3830. doi:10.1182/blood-2014-10-604272

Meeker TC, Grimaldi JC, O'Rourke R, Loeb J, Juliusson G, Einhorn S. 1988. Lack of detectable somatic hypermutation in the V region of the Ig H chain gene of a human chronic B lymphocytic leukemia. *J Immunol* **141:** 3994–3998.

Mescher C, Gilbertson D, Randall NM, Tarchand G, Tomaska J, Baumann Kreuziger L, Morrison VA. 2018. The impact of Agent Orange exposure on prognosis and management in patients with chronic lymphocytic leukemia: A National Veteran Affairs Tumor Registry study. *Leuk Lymphoma* **59:** 1348–1355. doi:10.1080/10428194.2017

Messina M, Del Giudice I, Khiabanian H, Rossi D, Chiaretti S, Rasi S, Spina V, Holmes AB, Marinelli M, Fabbri G, et al. 2014. Genetic lesions associated with chronic lymphocytic leukemia chemo-refractoriness. *Blood* **123:** 2378–2388. doi:10.1182/blood-2013-10-534271

Messmer BT, Albesiano E, Efremov DG, Ghiotto F, Allen SL, Kolitz J, Foa R, Damle RN, Fais F, Messmer D, et al. 2004. Multiple distinct sets of stereotyped antigen receptors indicate a role for antigen in promoting chronic lymphocytic leukemia. *J Exp Med* **200:** 519–525. doi:10.1084/jem.20040544

Messmer BT, Messmer D, Allen SL, Kolitz JE, Kudalkar P, Cesar D, Murphy EJ, Koduru P, Ferrarini M, Zupo S, et al. 2005. In vivo measurements document the dynamic cellular kinetics of chronic lymphocytic leukemia B cells. *J Clin Invest* **115:** 755–764. doi:10.1172/JCI23409

Minici C, Gounari M, Übelhart R, Scarfò L, Dühren-von Minden M, Schneider D, Tasdogan A, Alkhatib A, Agathangelidis A, Ntoufa S, et al. 2017. Distinct homotypic B-cell receptor interactions shape the outcome of chronic lymphocytic leukaemia. *Nat Commun* **8:** 15746. doi:10.1038/ncomms15746

Molica S, Alberti A. 1987. Prognostic value of the lymphocyte doubling time in chronic lymphocytic leukemia. *Cancer* **60:** 2712–2716. doi:10.1002/1097-0142(19871201)60:11<2712::AID-CNCR2820601122>3.0.CO;2-1

Molica S, Mauro FR, Callea V, Giannarelli D, Lauria F, Rotoli B, Cortelezzi A, Liso V, Foa R. 2010. The utility of a prognostic index for predicting time to first treatment in early chronic lymphocytic leukemia: The GIMEMA experience. *Haematologica* **95:** 464–469. doi:10.3324/haematol.2009.011767

Molica S, Mauro FR, Giannarelli D, Lauria F, Cortelezzi A, Brugiatelli M, Liso V, Cuneo A, Foà R. 2011. Differentiating chronic lymphocytic leukemia from monoclonal B-lymphocytosis according to clinical outcome: On behalf of the GIMEMA chronic lymphoproliferative diseases working group. *Haematologica* **96:** 277–283. doi:10.3324/haematol.2010.030189

Molica S, Giannarelli D, Mirabelli R, Levato L, Kay NE, Shanafelt TD. 2018. Chronic lymphocytic leukemia international prognostic index: A systematic review and meta-analysis. *Blood* **131:** 365–368. doi:10.1182/blood-2017-09-806034

Montecino-Rodriguez E, Leathers H, Dorshkind K. 2006. Identification of a B-1 B cell–specified progenitor. *Nat Immunol* **7:** 293–301. doi:10.1038/ni1301

Montserrat E. 2012. CLL therapy: The increasing importance of predictive markers. *Oncology (Williston Park)* **26:** 1064–1066.

Montserrat E, Sanchez-Bisono J, Viñolas N, Rozman C. 1986. Lymphocyte doubling time in chronic lymphocytic leukaemia: Analysis of its prognostic significance. *Br J Haematol* **62:** 567–575. doi:10.1111/j.1365-2141.1986.tb02969.x

Moreira J, Rabe KG, Cerhan JR, Kay NE, Wilson JW, Call TG, Leis JF, Jelinek DF, Schwager SM, Bowen DA, et al. 2013. Infectious complications among individuals with clinical monoclonal B-cell lymphocytosis (MBL): A cohort study of newly diagnosed cases compared to controls. *Leukemia* **27:** 136–141. doi:10.1038/leu.2012.187

Muramatsu M, Sankaranand VS, Anant S, Sugai M, Kinoshita K, Davidson NO, Honjo T. 1999. Specific expression of activation-induced cytidine deaminase (AID), a novel member of the RNA-editing deaminase family in germinal center B cells. *J Biol Chem* **274:** 18470–18476. doi:10.1074/jbc.274.26.18470

Muramatsu M, Kinoshita K, Fagarasan S, Yamada S, Shinkai Y, Honjo T. 2000. Class switch recombination and hypermutation require activation-induced cytidine deaminase (AID), a potential RNA editing enzyme. *Cell* **102:** 553–563. doi:10.1016/S0092-8674(00)00078-7

Murphy EJ, Neuberg DS, Rassenti LZ, Hayes G, Redd R, Emson C, Li K, Brown JR, Wierda WG, Turner S, et al. 2017. Leukemia-cell proliferation and disease progression in patients with early stage chronic lymphocytic leukemia. *Leukemia* **31:** 1348–1354. doi:10.1038/leu.2017.34

Murray F, Darzentas N, Hadzidimitriou A, Tobin G, Boudjogra M, Scielzo C, Laoutaris N, Karlsson K, Baran-Marzsak F, Tsaftaris A, et al. 2008. Stereotyped patterns of somatic hypermutation in subsets of patients with chronic lymphocytic leukemia: Implications for the role of antigen selection in leukemogenesis. *Blood* **111:** 1524–1533. doi:10.1182/blood-2007-07-099564

Nadeu F, Clot G, Delgado J, Martín-García D, Baumann T, Salaverria I, Beà S, Pinyol M, Jares P, Navarro A, et al. 2018. Clinical impact of the subclonal architecture and mutational complexity in chronic lymphocytic leukemia. *Leukemia* **32:** 645–653. doi:10.1038/leu.2017.291

Niedermeier M, Hennessy BT, Knight ZA, Henneberg M, Hu J, Kurtova AV, Wierda WG, Keating MJ, Shokat KM, Burger JA. 2009. Isoform-selective phosphoinositide 3′-kinase inhibitors inhibit CXCR4 signaling and overcome stromal cell-mediated drug resistance in chronic lymphocytic leukemia: A novel therapeutic approach. *Blood* **113:** 5549–5557. doi:10.1182/blood-2008-06-165068

Niemann CU, Herman SE, Maric I, Gomez-Rodriguez J, Biancotto A, Chang BY, Martyr S, Stetler-Stevenson M, Yuan CM, Calvo KR, et al. 2016. Disruption of in vivo chronic lymphocytic leukemia tumor–microenvironment interactions by ibrutinib—Findings from an investigator-initiated phase II study. *Clin Cancer Res* **22:** 1572–1582. doi:10.1158/1078-0432.CCR-15-1965

Nishio M, Endo T, Tsukada N, Ohata J, Kitada S, Reed JC, Zvaifler NJ, Kipps TJ. 2005. Nurselike cells express BAFF and APRIL, which can promote survival of chronic lymphocytic leukemia cells via a paracrine pathway distinct from that of SDF-1α. *Blood* **106:** 1012–1020. doi:10.1182/blood-2004-03-0889

Nogueira V, Hay N. 2013. Molecular pathways: Reactive oxygen species homeostasis in cancer cells and implications for cancer therapy. *Clin Cancer Res* **19:** 4309–4314. doi:10.1158/1078-0432.CCR-12-1424

Oakes CC, Claus R, Gu L, Assenov Y, Hüllein J, Zucknick M, Bieg M, Brocks D, Bogatyrova O, Schmidt CR, et al. 2014. Evolution of DNA methylation is linked to genetic aberrations in chronic lymphocytic leukemia. *Cancer Discov* **4:** 348–361. doi:10.1158/2159-8290.CD-13-0349

Oakes CC, Seifert M, Assenov Y, Gu L, Przekopowitz M, Ruppert AS, Wang Q, Imbusch CD, Serva A, Koser SD, et al. 2016. DNA methylation dynamics during B cell maturation underlie a continuum of disease phenotypes in chronic lymphocytic leukemia. *Nat Genet* **48:** 253–264. doi:10.1038/ng.3488

Ojha J, Secreto C, Rabe K, Ayres-Silva J, Tschumper R, Dyke DV, Slager S, Fonseca R, Shanafelt T, Kay N, et al. 2014. Monoclonal B-cell lymphocytosis is characterized by mutations in CLL putative driver genes and clonal heterogeneity many years before disease progression. *Leukemia* **28:** 2395–2398. doi:10.1038/leu.2014.226

Ojha J, Ayres J, Secreto C, Tschumper R, Rabe K, Van Dyke D, Slager S, Shanafelt T, Fonseca R, Kay NE, et al. 2015. Deep sequencing identifies genetic heterogeneity and recurrent convergent evolution in chronic lymphocytic leukemia. *Blood* **125:** 492–498. doi:10.1182/blood-2014-06-580563

Oldenhuis CNAM, Oosting SF, Gietema JA, de Vries EGE. 2008. Prognostic versus predictive value of biomarkers in oncology. *Eur J Cancer* **44:** 946–953. doi:10.1016/j.ejca.2008.03.006

Oltra AM, Carbonell F, Tormos C, Iradi A, Sáez GT. 2001. Antioxidant enzyme activities and the production of MDA and 8-oxo-dG in chronic lymphocytic leukemia. *Free Radic Biol Med* **30:** 1286–1292. doi:10.1016/S0891-5849(01)00521-4

Oppezzo P, Vuillier F, Vasconcelos Y, Dumas G, Magnac C, Payelle-Brogard B, Pritsch O, Dighiero G. 2003. Chronic lymphocytic leukemia B cells expressing AID display dissociation between class switch recombination and somatic hypermutation. *Blood* **101:** 4029–4032. doi:10.1182/blood-2002-10-3175

Ortolano S, Hwang IY, Han SB, Kehrl JH. 2006. Roles for phosphoinositide 3-kinases, Bruton's tyrosine kinase, and Jun kinases in B lymphocyte chemotaxis and homing. *Eur J Immunol* **36:** 1285–1295. doi:10.1002/eji.200535799

Os A, Bürgler S, Ribes Anna P, Funderud A, Wang D, Thompson Keith M, Tjønnfjord Geir E, Bogen B, Munthe Ludvig A. 2013. Chronic lymphocytic leukemia cells are activated and proliferate in response to specific T helper cells. *Cell Rep* **4:** 566–577. doi:10.1016/j.celrep.2013.07.011

Pan LX, Diss TC, Peng HZ, Norton AJ, Isaacson PG. 1996. Nodular lymphocyte predominance Hodgkin's disease: A monoclonal or polyclonal B-cell disorder? *Blood* **87:** 2428–2434. doi:10.1182/blood.V87.6.2428.bloodjournal8762428

Parikh SA, Chaffee KG, Larson MC, Hampel PJ, Call TG, Ding W, Kenderian SS, Leis JF, Chanan-Khan AA, Conte MJ, et al. 2018. Outcomes of a large cohort of individuals with clinically ascertained high-count monoclonal B-cell lymphocytosis. *Haematologica* **103:** e237–e240. doi:10.3324/haematol.2017.183194

Pasqualucci L, Migliazza A, Fracchiolla N, William C, Neri A, Baldini L, Chaganti RSK, Klein U, Kuppers R, Rajewsky K, et al. 1998. BCL-6 mutations in normal germinal center B cells: Evidence of somatic hypermutation acting outside Ig loci. *Proc Natl Acad Sci* **95:** 11816–11821. doi:10.1073/pnas.95.20.11816

Pasqualucci L, Neumeister P, Goossens T, Nanjangud G, Chaganti RS, Küppers R, Dalla-Favera R. 2001. Hypermutation of multiple proto-oncogenes in B-cell diffuse large-cell lymphomas. *Nature* **412:** 341–346. doi:10.1038/35085588

Pasqualucci L, Guglielmino R, Houldsworth J, Mohr J, Aoufouchi S, Polakiewicz R, Chaganti RSK, Dalla-Favera R. 2004. Expression of the AID protein in normal and neoplastic B cells. *Blood* **104:** 3318–3325. doi:10.1182/blood-2004-04-1558

Patten PE, Chu CC, Albesiano E, Damle RN, Yan XJ, Kim D, Zhang L, Magli AR, Barrientos J, Kolitz JE, et al. 2012. IGHV-unmutated and IGHV-mutated chronic lymphocytic leukemia cells produce activation-induced deaminase protein with a full range of biologic functions. *Blood* **120:** 4802–4811. doi:10.1182/blood-2012-08-449744

Patten PE, Ferrer G, Chen SS, Simone R, Marsilio S, Yan XJ, Gitto Z, Yuan C, Kolitz JE, Barrientos J, et al. 2016. Chronic lymphocytic leukemia cells diversify and differentiate in vivo via a nonclassical Th1-dependent, Bcl-6-deficient process. *JCI Insight* **1:** e86288. doi:10.1172/jci.insight.86288

Petersen CT, Hassan M, Morris AB, Jeffery J, Lee K, Jagirdar N, Staton AD, Raikar SS, Spencer HT, Sulchek T, et al. 2018. Improving T-cell expansion and function for adoptive T-cell therapy using ex vivo treatment with PI3Kδ inhibitors and VIP antagonists. *Blood Adv* **2:** 210–223. doi:10.1182/bloodadvances.2017011254

Pleasance ED, Stephens PJ, O'Meara S, McBride DJ, Meynert A, Jones D, Lin ML, Beare D, Lau KW, Greenman C, et al. 2010. A small-cell lung cancer genome with complex signatures of tobacco exposure. *Nature* **463:** 184–190. doi:10.1038/nature08629

Ponader S, Chen S-S, Buggy JJ, Balakrishnan K, Gandhi V, Wierda WG, Keating MJ, O'Brien S, Chiorazzi N, Burger JA. 2012. The Bruton tyrosine kinase inhibitor PCI-32765 thwarts chronic lymphocytic leukemia cell survival and tissue homing in vitro and in vivo. *Blood* **119:** 1182–1189. doi:10.1182/blood-2011-10-386417

Popp HD, Flach J, Brendel S, Ruppenthal S, Kleiner H, Seifarth W, Schneider S, Schulze TJ, Weiss C, Wenz F, et al. 2019. Accumulation of DNA damage and alteration of the DNA damage response in monoclonal B-cell lymphocytosis and chronic lymphocytic leukemia. *Leuk Lymphoma* **60:** 795–804. doi:10.1080/10428194.2018.1498494

Porter DL, Levine BL, Kalos M, Bagg A, June CH. 2011. Chimeric antigen receptor-modified T cells in chronic lymphoid leukemia. *N Engl J Med* **365:** 725–733. doi:10.1056/NEJMoa1103849

Pozzo F, Bittolo T, Arruga F, Bulian P, Macor P, Tissino E, Gizdic B, Rossi FM, Bomben R, Zucchetto A, et al. 2016. NOTCH1 mutations associate with low CD20 level in chronic lymphocytic leukemia: Evidence for a NOTCH1 mutation-driven epigenetic dysregulation. *Leukemia* **30:** 182–189. doi:10.1038/leu.2015.182

Pratt LF, Rassenti L, Larrick J, Robbins B, Banks PM, Kipps TJ. 1989. Ig V region gene expression in small lymphocytic lymphoma with little or no somatic hypermutation. *J Immunol* **143:** 699–705.

Preston DL, Kusumi S, Tomonaga M, Izumi S, Ron E, Kuramoto A, Kamada N, Dohy H, Matsuo T, Matsui T, et al. 1994. Cancer incidence in atomic bomb survivors. Part III: Leukemia, lymphoma and multiple myeloma, 1950–1987. *Radiat Res* **137:** S68–S97. doi:10.2307/3578893

Puente XS, Pinyol M, Quesada V, Conde L, Ordóñez GR, Villamor N, Escaramis G, Jares P, Beà S, González-Díaz M, et al. 2011. Whole-genome sequencing identifies recurrent mutations in chronic lymphocytic leukaemia. *Nature* **475:** 101–105. doi:10.1038/nature10113

Puente XS, Beà S, Valdés-Mas R, Villamor N, Gutiérrez-Abril J, Martín-Subero JI, Munar M, Rubio-Pérez C, Jares P, Aymerich M, et al. 2015. Non-coding recurrent mutations in chronic lymphocytic leukaemia. *Nature* **526:** 519–524. doi:10.1038/nature14666

Queirós AC, Villamor N, Clot G, Martinez-Trillos A, Kulis M, Navarro A, Penas EMM, Jayne S, Majid A, Richter J, et al. 2015. A B-cell epigenetic signature defines three biological subgroups of chronic lymphocytic leukemia with clinical impact. *Leukemia* **29:** 598–605. doi:10.1038/leu.2014.252

Quesada V, Conde L, Villamor N, Ordóñez GR, Jares P, Bassaganyas L, Ramsay AJ, Beà S, Pinyol M, Martínez-Trillos A, et al. 2011. Exome sequencing identifies recurrent mutations of the splicing factor SF3B1 gene in chronic lymphocytic leukemia. *Nat Genet* **44:** 47–52. doi:10.1038/ng.1032

Quesada V, Ramsay AJ, Lopez-Otin C. 2012. Chronic lymphocytic leukemia with SF3B1 mutation. *N Engl J Med* **366:** 2530. doi:10.1056/NEJMc1204033

Quesada V, Ramsay AJ, Rodriguez D, Puente XS, Campo E, Lopez-Otin C. 2013. The genomic landscape of chronic lymphocytic leukemia: clinical implications. *BMC Med* **11:** 124. doi:10.1186/1741-7015-11-124

Rai KR, Sawitsky A, Cronkite EP, Chanana AD, Levy RN, Pasternack BS. 1975. Clinical staging of chronic lymphocytic leukemia. *Blood* **46:** 219–234. doi:10.1182/blood.V46.2.219.219

Ramsay AG, Johnson AJ, Lee AM, Gorgun G, Le Dieu R, Blum W, Byrd JC, Gribben JG. 2008. Chronic lymphocytic leukemia T cells show impaired immunological synapse formation that can be reversed with an immunomodulating drug. *J Clin Invest* **118:** 2427–2437.

Rasi S, Monti S, Spina V, Foà R, Gaidano G, Rossi D. 2012. Analysis of NOTCH1 mutations in monoclonal B-cell lymphocytosis. *Haematologica* **97:** 153–154. doi:10.3324/haematol.2011.053090

Rassenti LZ, Jain S, Keating MJ, Wierda WG, Grever MR, Byrd JC, Kay NE, Brown JR, Gribben JG, Neuberg DS, et al. 2008. Relative value of ZAP-70, CD38, and immunoglobulin mutation status in predicting aggressive disease in chronic lymphocytic leukemia. *Blood* **112:** 1923–1930. doi:10.1182/blood-2007-05-092882

Raveche ES, Salerno E, Scaglione BJ, Manohar V, Abbasi F, Lin Y-C, Fredrickson T, Landgraf P, Ramachandra S, Huppi K, et al. 2007. Abnormal microRNA-16 locus with synteny to human 13q14 linked to CLL in NZB mice. *Blood* **109:** 5079–5086. doi:10.1182/blood-2007-02-071225

Rawstron AC, Green MJ, Kuzmicki A, Kennedy B, Fenton JA, Evans PA, O'Connor SJ, Richards SJ, Morgan GJ, Jack AS, et al. 2002a. Monoclonal B lymphocytes with the characteristics of "indolent" chronic lymphocytic leukemia are present in 3.5% of adults with normal blood counts. *Blood* **100:** 635–639. doi:10.1182/blood.V100.2.635

Rawstron AC, Yuille MR, Fuller J, Cullen M, Kennedy B, Richards SJ, Jack AS, Matutes E, Catovsky D, Hillmen P, et al. 2002b. Inherited predisposition to CLL is detectable as subclinical monoclonal B-lymphocyte expansion. *Blood* **100:** 2289–2290. doi:10.1182/blood-2002-03-0892

Rawstron AC, Bennett FL, O'Connor SJM, Kwok M, Fenton JAL, Plummer M, de Tute R, Owen RG, Richards SJ, Jack AS, et al. 2008. Monoclonal B-cell lymphocytosis and chronic lymphocytic leukemia. *N Engl J Med* **359:** 575–583. doi:10.1056/NEJMoa075290

Rawstron AC, Böttcher S, Letestu R, Villamor N, Fazi C, Kartsios H, de Tute RM, Shingles J, Ritgen M, Moreno C, et al. 2013. Improving efficiency and sensitivity: European Research Initiative in CLL (ERIC) update on the international harmonised approach for flow cytometric residual disease monitoring in CLL. *Leukemia* **27:** 142–149. doi:10.1038/leu.2012.216

Rawstron AC, Fazi C, Agathangelidis A, Villamor N, Letestu R, Nomdedeu J, Palacio C, Stehlikova O, Kreuzer KA, Liptrot S, et al. 2015. A complementary role of multiparameter flow cytometry and high-throughput sequencing for minimal residual disease detection in chronic lymphocytic leukemia: An European research initiative on CLL study. *Leukemia* **30:** 929–936. doi:10.1038/leu.2015.313

Reiniger L, Bödör C, Bognár A, Balogh Z, Csomor J, Szepesi A, Kopper L, Matolcsy A. 2006. Richter's and prolymphocytic transformation of chronic lymphocytic leukemia are associated with high mRNA expression of activation-induced cytidine deaminase and aberrant somatic hypermutation. *Leukemia* **20:** 1089–1095. doi:10.1038/sj.leu.2404183

Richter MN. 1928. Generalized reticular cell sarcoma of lymph nodes associated with lymphatic leukemia. *Am J Pathol* **4:** 285–292 287.

Robbiani DF, Bunting S, Feldhahn N, Bothmer A, Camps J, Deroubaix S, McBride KM, Klein IA, Stone G, Eisenreich TR, et al. 2009. AID produces DNA double-strand breaks in non-Ig genes and mature B cell lymphomas with reciprocal chromosome translocations. *Mol Cell* **36:** 631–641. doi:10.1016/j.molcel.2009.11.007

Roberts AW, Davids MS, Pagel JM, Kahl BS, Puvvada SD, Gerecitano JF, Kipps TJ, Anderson MA, Brown JR, Gressick L, et al. 2016. Targeting BCL2 with venetoclax in relapsed chronic lymphocytic leukemia. *N Engl J Med* **374:** 311–322. doi:10.1056/NEJMoa1513257

Rodríguez-Vicente AE, Bikos V, Hernández-Sánchez M, Malcikova J, Hernández-Rivas JM, Pospisilova S. 2017. Next-generation sequencing in chronic lymphocytic leukemia: Recent findings and new horizons. *Oncotarget* **8:** 71234–71248. doi:10.18632/oncotarget.19525

Rogers KA, Huang Y, Dotson E, Lundberg J, Andritsos LA, Awan FT, Woyach JA, Byrd JC. 2019. Use of PD-1 (PDCD1) inhibitors for the treatment of Richter syndrome: Experience at a single academic centre. *B J Haematol* **185:** 363–366. doi:10.1111/bjh.15508

Romanenko A, Bebeshko V, Hatch M, Bazyka D, Finch S, Dyagil I, Reiss R, Chumak V, Bouville A, Gudzenko N, et al. 2008. The Ukrainian–American study of leukemia and related disorders among Chernobyl cleanup workers from Ukraine: I. Study methods. *Radiat Res* **170:** 691–697. doi:10.1667/RR1402.1

Romero D. 2017. After ibrutinib, CAR T cells induce responses. *Nat Rev Clin Oncol* **14:** 588. doi:10.1038/nrclinonc.2017.124

Rosenwald A, Alizadeh AA, Widhopf G, Simon R, Davis RE, Yu X, Yang L, Pickeral OK, Rassenti LZ, Powell J, et al. 2001. Relation of gene expression phenotype to immunoglobulin mutation genotype in B cell chronic lymphocytic leukemia. *J Exp Med* **194:** 1639–1648. doi:10.1084/jem.194.11.1639

Rose-Zerilli MJ, Gibson J, Wang J, Tapper W, Davis Z, Parker H, Larrayoz M, McCarthy H, Walewska R, Forster J, et al. 2016. Longitudinal copy number, whole exome and targeted deep sequencing of 'good risk' IGHV-mutated CLL patients with progressive disease. *Leukemia* **30:** 1301–1310. doi:10.1038/leu.2016.10

Rossi D, Zucchetto A, Rossi FM, Capello D, Cerri M, Deambrogi C, Cresta S, Rasi S, De Paoli L, Bodoni CL, et al. 2008. CD49d expression is an independent risk factor of progressive disease in early stage chronic lymphocytic leukemia. *Haematologica* **93:** 1575–1579. doi:10.3324/haematol.13103

Rossi D, Sozzi E, Puma A, De Paoli L, Rasi S, Spina V, Gozzetti A, Tassi M, Cencini E, Raspadori D, et al. 2009a. The prognosis of clinical monoclonal B cell lymphocytosis differs from prognosis of Rai 0 chronic lymphocytic leukaemia and is recapitulated by biological risk factors. *Br J Haematol* **146:** 64–75. doi:10.1111/j.1365-2141.2009.07711.x

Rossi D, Spina V, Cerri M, Rasi S, Deambrogi C, De Paoli L, Laurenti L, Maffei R, Forconi F, Bertoni F, et al. 2009b. Stereotyped B-cell receptor is an independent risk factor of chronic lymphocytic leukemia transformation to Richter syndrome. *Clin Cancer Res* **15:** 4415–4422. doi:10.1158/1078-0432.CCR-08-3266

Rossi D, Rasi S, Fabbri G, Spina V, Fangazio M, Forconi F, Marasca R, Laurenti L, Bruscaggin A, Cerri M, et al. 2012a. Mutations of NOTCH1 are an independent predictor of survival in chronic lymphocytic leukemia. *Blood* **119:** 521–529. doi:10.1182/blood-2011-09-379966

Rossi D, Rasi S, Spina V, Fangazio M, Monti S, Greco M, Ciardullo C, Famà R, Cresta S, Bruscaggin A, et al. 2012b. Different impact of NOTCH1 and SF3B1 mutations on the risk of chronic lymphocytic leukemia transformation to Richter syndrome. *Br J Haematol* **158:** 426–429. doi:10.1111/j.1365-2141.2012.09155.x

Rossi D, Rasi S, Spina V, Bruscaggin A, Monti S, Ciardullo C, Deambrogi C, Khiabanian H, Serra R, Bertoni F, et al. 2013. Integrated mutational and cytogenetic analysis identifies new prognostic subgroups in chronic lymphocytic leukemia. *Blood* **121:** 1403–1412. doi:10.1182/blood-2012-09-458265

Rossi D, Terzi-di-Bergamo L, De Paoli L, Cerri M, Ghilardi G, Chiarenza A, Bulian P, Visco C, Mauro FR, Morabito F, et al. 2015. Molecular prediction of durable remission after first-line fludarabine-cyclophosphamide-rituximab in chronic lymphocytic leukemia. *Blood* **126:** 1921–1924. doi:10.1182/blood-2015-05-647925

Ruefli-Brasse A, Reed JC. 2017. Therapeutics targeting Bcl-2 in hematological malignancies. *Biochem J* **474:** 3643–3657. doi:10.1042/BCJ20170080

Rush JS, Liu M, Odegard VH, Unniraman S, Schatz DG. 2005. Expression of activation-induced cytidine deaminase is regulated by cell division, providing a mechanistic basis for division-linked class switch recombination. *Proc Natl Acad Sci* **102:** 13242–13247. doi:10.1073/pnas.0502779102

Sarkar M, Liu Y, Morimoto J, Peng H, Aquino C, Rader C, Chiorazzi N, Kodadek T. 2014. Recognition of antigen-specific B-cell receptors from chronic lymphocytic leukemia patients by synthetic antigen surrogates. *Chem Biol* **21:** 1670–1679. doi:10.1016/j.chembiol.2014.10.010

Sarkar M, Liu Y, Qi J, Peng H, Morimoto J, Rader C, Chiorazzi N, Kodadek T. 2016. Targeting stereotyped B cell receptors from chronic lymphocytic leukemia patients with synthetic antigen surrogates. *J Biol Chem* **291:** 7558–7570. doi:10.1074/jbc.M115.701656

Schena M, Larsson LG, Gottardi D, Gaidano G, Carlsson M, Nilsson K, Caligaris-Cappio F. 1992. Growth- and differentiation-associated expression of bcl-2 in B-chronic lymphocytic leukemia cells. *Blood* **79:** 2981–2989. doi:10.1182/blood.V79.11.2981.2981

Schmid C, Isaacson PG. 1994. Proliferation centres in B-cell malignant lymphoma, lymphocytic (B-CLL): An immunophenotypic study. *Histopathology* **24:** 445–451. doi:10.1111/j.1365-2559.1994.tb00553.x

Schroeder HW Jr, Dighiero G. 1994. The pathogenesis of chronic lymphocytic leukemia: Analysis of the antibody repertoire. *Immunol Today* **15:** 288–294. doi:10.1016/0167-5699(94)90009-4

Schwartz GG, Klug MG. 2016. Incidence rates of chronic lymphocytic leukemia in US states are associated with residential radon levels. *Future Oncol* **12:** 165–174. doi:10.2217/fon.15.275

Seifert M, Sellmann L, Bloehdorn J, Wein F, Stilgenbauer S, Durig J, Küppers R. 2012. Cellular origin and pathophysiology of chronic lymphocytic leukemia. *J Exp Med* **209:** 2183–2198. doi:10.1084/jem.20120833

Shanafelt TD, Geyer SM, Bone ND, Tschumper RC, Witzig TE, Nowakowski GS, Zent CS, Call TG, Laplant B, Dewald GW, et al. 2008a. CD49d expression is an independent predictor of overall survival in patients with chronic lymphocytic leukaemia: A prognostic parameter with therapeutic potential. *Br J Haematol* **140:** 537–546. doi:10.1111/j.1365-2141.2007.06965.x

Shanafelt TD, Hanson C, Dewald GW, Witzig TE, LaPlant B, Abrahamzon J, Jelinek DF, Kay NE. 2008b. Karyotype evolution on fluorescent in situ hybridization analysis is associated with short survival in patients with chronic lymphocytic leukemia and is related to CD49d expression. *J Clin Oncol* **26:** e5–e6. doi:10.1200/JCO.2008.16.7874

Shanafelt TD, Kay NE, Jenkins G, Call TG, Zent CS, Jelinek DF, Morice WG, Boysen J, Zakko L, Schwager S, et al. 2009a. B-cell count and survival: Differentiating chronic lymphocytic leukemia from monoclonal B-cell lymphocytosis based on clinical outcome. *Blood* **113:** 4188–4196. doi:10.1182/blood-2008-09-176149

Shanafelt TD, Kay NE, Rabe KG, Call TG, Zent CS, Maddocks K, Jenkins G, Jelinek DF, Morice WG, Boysen J, et al. 2009b. Brief report: Natural history of individuals with clinically recognized monoclonal B-cell lymphocytosis compared with patients with Rai 0 chronic lymphocytic leukemia. *J Clin Oncol* **27:** 3959–3963. doi:10.1200/JCO.2008.21.2704

Shanafelt TD, Ghia P, Lanasa MC, Landgren O, Rawstron AC. 2010. Monoclonal B-cell lymphocytosis (MBL): Biology, natural history and clinical management. *Leukemia* **24:** 512–520. doi:10.1038/leu.2009.287

Simonsson B, Wibell L, Nilsson K. 1980. β2-microglobulin in chronic lymphocytic leukaemia. *Scand J Haematol* **24:** 174–180. doi:10.1111/j.1600-0609.1980.tb02364.x

Slager SL, Rabe KG, Achenbach SJ, Vachon CM, Goldin LR, Strom SS, Lanasa MC, Spector LG, Rassenti LZ, Leis JF, et al. 2011. Genome-wide association study identifies a novel susceptibility locus at 6p21.3 among familial CLL. *Blood* **117:** 1911–1916. doi:10.1182/blood-2010-09-308205

Slager SL, Skibola CF, Di Bernardo MC, Conde L, Broderick P, McDonnell SK, Goldin LR, Croft N, Holroyd A, Harris S, et al. 2012. Common variation at 6p21.31 (BAK1) influences the risk of chronic lymphocytic leukemia. *Blood* **120:** 843–846. doi:10.1182/blood-2012-03-413591

Slupsky JR. 2014. Does B cell receptor signaling in chronic lymphocytic leukaemia cells differ from that in other B cell types? *Scientifica (Cairo)* **2014:** 208928. doi:10.1155/2014/208928

Solomon BM, Chaffee KG, Moreira J, Schwager SM, Cerhan JR, Call TG, Kay NE, Slager SL, Shanafelt TD. 2016. Risk of non-hematologic cancer in individuals with high-count monoclonal B-cell lymphocytosis. *Leukemia* **30:** 331–336. doi:10.1038/leu.2015.235

Sommermeyer D, Hudecek M, Kosasih PL, Gogishvili T, Maloney DG, Turtle CJ, Riddell SR. 2016. Chimeric antigen receptor-modified T cells derived from defined $CD8^+$ and $CD4^+$ subsets confer superior antitumor reactivity in vivo. *Leukemia* **30:** 492–500. doi:10.1038/leu.2015.247

Souers AJ, Leverson JD, Boghaert ER, Ackler SL, Catron ND, Chen J, Dayton BD, Ding H, Enschede SH, Fairbrother WJ, et al. 2013. ABT-199, a potent and selective BCL-2 inhibitor, achieves antitumor activity while sparing platelets. *Nat Med* **19:** 202–208. doi:10.1038/nm.3048

Spaargaren M, Beuling EA, Rurup ML, Meijer HP, Klok MD, Middendorp S, Hendriks RW, Pals ST. 2003. The B cell antigen receptor controls integrin activity through Btk and PLCγ2. *J Exp Med* **198:** 1539–1550. doi:10.1084/jem.20011866

Speedy HE, Bernardo MC, Sava GP, Dyer MJS, Holroyd A, Wang Y, Sunter NJ, Mansouri L, Juliusson G, Smedby KE, et al. 2014. A genome-wide association study identifies multiple susceptibility loci for chronic lymphocytic leukemia. *Nat Genet* **46:** 56–60. doi:10.1038/ng.2843

Stamatopoulos K, Belessi C, Moreno C, Boudjograh M, Guida G, Smilevska T, Belhoul L, Stella S, Stavroyianni N, Crespo M, et al. 2007. Over 20% of patients with chronic lymphocytic leukemia carry stereotyped receptors: Pathogenetic implications and clinical correlations. *Blood* **109:** 259–270. doi:10.1182/blood-2006-03-012948

Stamatopoulos K, Agathangelidis A, Rosenquist R, Ghia P. 2017. Antigen receptor stereotypy in chronic lymphocytic leukemia. *Leukemia* **31:** 282–291. doi:10.1038/leu.2016.322

Steininger C, Widhopf GF II, Ghia EM, Morello CS, Vanura K, Sanders R, Spector D, Guiney D, Jäger U, Kipps TJ. 2012. Recombinant antibodies encoded by IGHV1-69 react with pUL32, a phosphoprotein of cytomegalovirus and B-cell superantigen. *Blood* **119:** 2293–2301. doi:10.1182/blood-2011-08-374058

Sthoeger ZM, Wakai M, Tse DB, Vinciguerra VP, Allen SL, Budman DR, Lichtman SM, Schulman P, Weiselberg LR, Chiorazzi N. 1989. Production of autoantibodies by CD5-expressing B lymphocytes from patients with chronic lymphocytic leukemia. *J Exp Med* **169:** 255–268. doi:10.1084/jem.169.1.255

Stilgenbauer S, Schnaiter A, Paschka P, Zenz T, Rossi M, Döhner K, Bühler A, Böttcher S, Ritgen M, Kneba M, et al. 2014. Gene mutations and treatment outcome in chronic lymphocytic leukemia: Results from the CLL8 trial. *Blood* **123:** 3247–3254. doi:10.1182/blood-2014-01-546150

Strefford JC, Kadalayil L, Forster J, Mjj R-Z, Parker A, Lin TT, Heppel N, Norris K, Gardiner A, Davies Z, et al. 2015. Telomere length predicts progression and overall survival in chronic lymphocytic leukemia: Data from the UK LRF CLL4 trial. *Leukemia* **29:** 2411–2414. doi:10.1038/leu.2015.217

Sutton LA, Young E, Baliakas P, Hadzidimitriou A, Moysiadis T, Plevova K, Rossi D, Kminkova J, Stalika E, Pedersen LB, et al. 2016. Different spectra of recurrent gene mutations in subsets of chronic lymphocytic leukemia harboring stereotyped B-cell receptors. *Haematologica* **101:** 959–967. doi:10.3324/haematol.2016.141812

Swerdlow SH, Murray LJ, Habeshaw JA, Stansfeld AG. 1984. Lymphocytic lymphoma/B-chronic lymphocytic leukaemia—An immunohistopathological study of peripheral B lymphocyte neoplasia. *Br J Cancer* **50:** 587–599. doi:10.1038/bjc.1984.225

Tam CS, O'Brien S, Wierda W, Kantarjian H, Wen S, Do KA, Thomas DA, Cortes J, Lerner S, Keating MJ. 2008. Long-term results of the fludarabine, cyclophosphamide, and rituximab regimen as initial therapy of chronic lymphocytic leukemia. *Blood* **112:** 975–980. doi:10.1182/blood-2008-02-140582

Tan SH, Sapari NS, Miao H, Hartman M, Loh M, Chng WJ, Iau P, Buhari SA, Soong R, Lee SC. 2015. High-throughput mutation profiling changes before and 3 weeks after chemotherapy in newly diagnosed breast cancer patients. *PLoS One* **10:** e0142466. doi:10.1371/journal.pone.0142466

Thompson JA, Figlin RA, Sifri-Steele C, Berenson RJ, Frohlich MW. 2003. A phase I trial of CD3/CD28-activated T cells (Xcellerated T cells) and interleukin-2 in patients with metastatic renal cell carcinoma. *Clin Cancer Res* **9:** 3562–3570.

Thompson PA, Tam CS, O'Brien SM, Wierda WG, Stingo F, Plunkett W, Smith SC, Kantarjian HM, Freireich EJ, Keating MJ. 2016. Fludarabine, cyclophosphamide, and rituximab treatment achieves long-term disease-free survival in IGHV-mutated chronic lymphocytic leukemia. *Blood* **127:** 303–309. doi:10.1182/blood-2015-09-667675

Tobin G, Thunberg U, Johnson A, Eriksson I, Söderberg O, Karlsson K, Merup M, Juliusson G, Vilpo J, Enblad G, et al. 2003. Chronic lymphocytic leukemias utilizing the VH3-21 gene display highly restricted Vλ2-14 gene use and homologous CDR3s: Implicating recognition of a common antigen epitope. *Blood* **101:** 4952–4957. doi:10.1182/blood-2002-11-3485

Tobin G, Thunberg U, Karlsson K, Murray F, Laurell A, Willander K, Enblad G, Merup M, Vilpo J, Juliusson G, et al. 2004. Subsets with restricted immunoglobulin gene rearrangement features indicate a role for antigen selection in the development of chronic lymphocytic leukemia. *Blood* **104:** 2879–2885. doi:10.1182/blood-2004-01-0132

Trimarco V, Ave E, Facco M, Chiodin G, Frezzato F, Martini V, Gattazzo C, Lessi F, Giorgi CA, Visentin A, et al. 2015. Cross-talk between chronic lymphocytic leukemia (CLL) tumor B cells and mesenchymal stromal cells (MSCs): Implications for neoplastic cell survival. *Oncotarget* **6:** 42130–42149. doi:10.18632/oncotarget.6239

Tsai H-T, Caporaso NE, Kyle RA, Katzmann JA, Dispenzieri A, Hayes RB, Marti GE, Albitar M, Ghia P, Rajkumar SV, et al. 2009. Evidence of serum immunoglobulin abnormalities up to 9.8 years before diagnosis of chronic lymphocytic leukemia: A prospective study. *Blood* **114:** 4928–4932. doi:10.1182/blood-2009-08-237651

Tsukada N, Burger JA, Zvaifler NJ, Kipps TJ. 2002. Distinctive features of "nurselike" cells that differentiate in the context of chronic lymphocytic leukemia. *Blood* **99:** 1030–1037. doi:10.1182/blood.V99.3.1030

Turtle CJ, Hanafi L-A, Berger C, Hudecek M, Pender B, Robinson E, Hawkins R, Chaney C, Cherian S, Chen X, et al. 2016. Immunotherapy of non-Hodgkin's lymphoma with a defined ratio of $CD8^+$ and $CD4^+$ CD19-specific chimeric antigen receptor-modified T cells. *Sci Transl Med* **8:** 355ra116. doi:10.1126/scitranslmed.aaf8621

Turtle CJ, Hay KA, Hanafi LA, Li D, Cherian S, Chen X, Wood B, Lozanski A, Byrd JC, Heimfeld S, et al. 2017. Durable molecular remissions in chronic lymphocytic leukemia treated with CD19-specific chimeric antigen receptor-modified T cells after failure of ibrutinib. *J Clin Oncol* **35:** 3010–3020. doi:10.1200/JCO.2017.72.8519

Vaisitti T, Aydin S, Rossi D, Cottino F, Bergui L, D'Arena G, Bonello L, Horenstein AL, Brennan P, Pepper C, et al. 2010. CD38 increases CXCL12-mediated signals and homing of chronic lymphocytic leukemia cells. *Leukemia* **24:** 958–969. doi:10.1038/leu.2010.36

van Dongen JJM, Langerak AW, Bruggemann M, Evans PAS, Hummel M, Lavender FL, Delabesse E, Davi F, Schuuring E, Garcia-Sanz R, et al. 2003. Design and standardization of PCR primers and protocols for detection of clonal immunoglobulin and T-cell receptor gene recombinations in suspect lymphoproliferations: Report of the BIOMED-2 Concerted Action BMH4-CT98-3936. *Leukemia* **17:** 2257–2317. doi:10.1038/sj.leu.2403202

van Gent R, Kater AP, Otto SA, Jaspers A, Borghans JA, Vrisekoop N, Ackermans MA, Ruiter AF, Wittebol S, Eldering E, et al. 2008. In vivo dynamics of stable chronic lymphocytic leukemia inversely correlate with somatic hypermutation levels and suggest no major leukemic turnover in bone marrow. *Cancer Res* **68:** 10137–10144. doi:10.1158/0008-5472.CAN-08-2325

Van Roosbroeck K, Bayraktar R, Calin S, Bloehdorn J, Dragomir MP, Okubo K, Bertilaccio MTS, Zupo S, You MJ, Gaidano G, et al. 2018. miRNAs involvement in the pathogenesis of Richter's syndrome. *Haematologica* **104:** 1004–1015.

Vardi A, Agathangelidis A, Sutton LA, Ghia P, Rosenquist R, Stamatopoulos K. 2014. Immunogenetic studies of chronic lymphocytic leukemia: Revelations and speculations about ontogeny and clinical evolution. *Cancer Res* **74:** 4211–4216. doi:10.1158/0008-5472.CAN-14-0630

Varghese AM, Howard DR, Pocock C, Rawstron AC, Follows G, McCarthy H, Dearden C, Fegan C, Milligan D, Smith AF, et al. 2017. Eradication of minimal residual disease improves overall and progression-free survival in patients with chronic lymphocytic leukaemia, evidence from NCRN CLL207: A phase II trial assessing alemtuzumab consolidation. *Br J Haematol* **176:** 573–582. doi:10.1111/bjh.14342

Villamor N, Conde L, Martinez-Trillos A, Cazorla M, Navarro A, Bea S, Lopez C, Colomer D, Pinyol M, Aymerich M, et al. 2013. *NOTCH1* mutations identify a genetic subgroup of chronic lymphocytic leukemia patients with high risk of transformation and poor outcome. *Leukemia* **27:** 1100–1106. doi:10.1038/leu.2012.357

Wagner SD, Luzzatto L. 1993. Vχ gene segments rearranged in chronic lymphocytic leukemia are distributed over a large portion of the Vχ locus and do not show somatic mutation. *Eur J Immunol* **23:** 391–397. doi:10.1002/eji.1830230214

Wang L, Lawrence MS, Wan Y, Stojanov P, Sougnez C, Stevenson K, Werner L, Sivachenko A, DeLuca DS, Zhang L, et al. 2011. *SF3B1* and other novel cancer genes in chronic lymphocytic leukemia. *N Engl J Med* **365:** 2497–2506. doi:10.1056/NEJMoa1109016

Wang J, Khiabanian H, Rossi D, Fabbri G, Gattei V, Forconi F, Laurenti L, Marasca R, Del Poeta G, Foa R, et al. 2014. Tumor evolutionary directed graphs and the history of chronic lymphocytic leukemia. *Elife* **3:** e02869. doi:10.7554/eLife.02869

Went M, Sud A, Speedy H, Sunter NJ, Försti A, Law PJ, Johnson DC, Mirabella F, Holroyd A, Li N, et al. 2019. Genetic correlation between multiple myeloma and chronic lymphocytic leukaemia provides evidence for shared aetiology. *Blood Cancer J* **9:** 1. doi:10.1038/s41408-018-0162-8

Widhopf GF II, Kipps TJ. 2001. Normal B cells express *51p1*-encoded Ig heavy chains that are distinct from those expressed by chronic lymphocytic leukemia B cells. *J Immunol* **166:** 95–102. doi:10.4049/jimmunol.166.1.95

Wierda WG, O'Brien S, Wang X, Faderl S, Ferrajoli A, Do KA, Cortes J, Thomas D, Garcia-Manero G, Koller C, et al. 2007. Prognostic nomogram and index for overall survival in previously untreated patients with chronic lymphocytic leukemia. *Blood* **109:** 4679–4685. doi:10.1182/blood-2005-12-051458

Wierda WG, O'Brien S, Wang X, Faderl S, Ferrajoli A, Do K-A, Garcia-Manero G, Cortes J, Thomas D, Koller CA, et al. 2011. Multivariable model for time to first treatment in patients with chronic lymphocytic leukemia. *J Clinl Oncol* **29:** 4088–4095. doi:10.1200/JCO.2010.33.9002

Wiseman H, Halliwell B. 1996. Damage to DNA by reactive oxygen and nitrogen species: Role in inflammatory disease and progression to cancer. *Biochem J* **313:** 17–29. doi:10.1042/bj3130017

Woyach JA, Furman RR, Liu T-M, Ozer HG, Zapatka M, Ruppert AS, Xue L, Li DH-H, Steggerda SM, Versele M, et al. 2014a. Resistance mechanisms for the Bruton's tyrosine kinase inhibitor ibrutinib. *New Engl J Med* **370:** 2286–2294. doi:10.1056/NEJMoa1400029

Woyach JA, Smucker K, Smith LL, Lozanski A, Zhong Y, Ruppert AS, Lucas D, Williams K, Zhao W, Rassenti L, et al. 2014b. Prolonged lymphocytosis during ibrutinib therapy is associated with distinct molecular characteristics and does not indicate a suboptimal response to therapy. *Blood* **123:** 1810–1817. doi:10.1182/blood-2013-09-527853

Yamane A, Resch W, Kuo N, Kuchen S, Li Z, Sun HW, Robbiani DF, McBride K, Nussenzweig MC, Casellas R. 2011. Deep-sequencing identification of the genomic targets of the cytidine deaminase AID and its cofactor RPA in B lymphocytes. *Nat Immunol* **12:** 62–69. doi:10.1038/ni.1964

Yamauchi T, Nowak BJ, Keating MJ, Plunkett W. 2001. DNA repair initiated in chronic lymphocytic leukemia lymphocytes by 4-hydroperoxycyclophosphamide is inhibited by fludarabine and clofarabine. *Clin Cancer Res* **7:** 3580–3589.

Yang J, Baskar S, Kwong KY, Kennedy MG, Wiestner A, Rader C. 2011. Therapeutic potential and challenges of targeting receptor tyrosine kinase ROR1 with monoclonal antibodies in B-cell malignancies. *PLoS One* **6:** e21018. doi:10.1371/journal.pone.0021018

Yu J, Chen L, Cui B, Widhopf GF II, Shen Z, Wu R, Zhang L, Zhang S, Briggs SP, Kipps TJ. 2016. Wnt5a induces ROR1/ROR2 heterooligomerization to enhance leukemia chemotaxis and proliferation. *J Clin Invest* **126:** 585–598. doi:10.1172/JCI83535

Yu J, Chen L, Chen Y, Hasan K, Ghia EM, Zhang L, Wu R, Rassenti LZ, Widhopf GF, Shen Z, et al. 2017. Wnt5a induces ROR1 to associate with 14-3-3ζ for enhanced chemotaxis and proliferation of chronic lymphocytic leukemia cells. *Leukemia* **31:** 2608–2614. doi:10.1038/leu.2017.132

Zablotska LB, Bazyka D, Lubin JH, Gudzenko N, Little MP, Hatch M, Finch S, Dyagil I, Reiss RF, Chumak VV, et al. 2013. Radiation and the risk of chronic lymphocytic and other leukemias among Chornobyl cleanup workers. *Environ Health Perspect* **121:** 59–65. doi:10.1289/ehp.1204996

Zenz T, Eichhorst B, Busch R, Denzel T, Habe S, Winkler D, Buhler A, Edelmann J, Bergmann M, Hopfinger G, et al. 2010a. TP53 Mutation and survival in chronic lymphocytic leukemia. *J Clin Oncol* **8:** 4473–4479. doi:10.1200/JCO.2009.2027.8762

Zenz T, Fröhling S, Mertens D, Döhner H, Stilgenbauer S. 2010b. Moving from prognostic to predictive factors in chronic lymphocytic leukaemia (CLL). *Best Pract Res Clin Haematol* **23:** 71–84. doi:10.1016/j.beha.2009.12.003

Zhou Y, Hileman EO, Plunkett W, Keating MJ, Huang P. 2003. Free radical stress in chronic lymphocytic leukemia cells and its role in cellular sensitivity to ROS-generating anticancer agents. *Blood* **101:** 4098–4104. doi:10.1182/blood-2002-08-2512

Zhou Y, Tang G, Medeiros LJ, McDonnell TJ, Keating MJ, Wierda WG, Wang SA. 2012. Therapy-related myeloid neoplasms following fludarabine, cyclophosphamide, and rituximab (FCR) treatment in patients with chronic lymphocytic leukemia/small lymphocytic lymphoma. *Mod Pathol* **25:** 237–245. doi:10.1038/modpathol.2011.158

Zucchetto A, Benedetti D, Tripodo C, Bomben R, Dal Bo M, Marconi D, Bossi F, Lorenzon D, Degan M, Rossi FM, et al. 2009. CD38/CD31, the CCL3 and CCL4 chemokines, and CD49d/vascular cell adhesion molecule-1 are interchained by sequential events sustaining chronic lymphocytic leukemia cell survival. *Cancer Res* **69:** 4001–4009. doi:10.1158/0008-5472.CAN-08-4173

Zucchetto A, Vaisitti T, Benedetti D, Tissino E, Bertagnolo V, Rossi D, Bomben R, Dal Bo M, Del Principe MI, Gorgone A, et al. 2012. The CD49d/CD29 complex is physically and functionally associated with CD38 in B-cell chronic lymphocytic leukemia cells. *Leukemia* **26:** 1301–1312. doi:10.1038/leu.2011.369

MAP-Kinase-Driven Hematopoietic Neoplasms: A Decade of Progress in the Molecular Age

Rikhia Chakraborty,[1,2] Omar Abdel-Wahab,[3,4] and Benjamin H. Durham[3,5]

[1]Texas Children's Cancer Center, Texas Children's Hospital, Houston, Texas 77030, USA

[2]Department of Pediatrics, Division of Pediatric Hematology-Oncology, Baylor College of Medicine, Houston, Texas 77030, USA

[3]Human Oncology and Pathogenesis Program, Department of Medicine, [4]Leukemia Service, Department of Medicine, [5]Department of Pathology, Memorial Sloan Kettering Cancer Center, New York, New York 10065, USA

Correspondence: abdelwao@mskcc.org, durhamb@mskcc.org

Mutations in members of the mitogen-activated protein kinase (MAPK) pathway are extensively studied in epithelial malignancies, with *BRAF* mutations being one of the most common alterations activating this pathway. However, *BRAF* mutations are overall quite rare in hematological malignancies. Studies over the past decade have identified high-frequency *BRAF*^{V600E}, *MAP2K1*, and other kinase alterations in two groups of MAPK-driven hematopoietic neoplasms: hairy cell leukemia (HCL) and the systemic histiocytoses. Despite HCL and histiocytoses sharing common molecular alterations, these are phenotypically distinct malignancies that differ in respect to clinical presentation and suspected cell of origin. The purpose of this review is to highlight the molecular advancements over the last decade in the histiocytic neoplasms and HCL and discuss the impact these insights have had on our understanding of the molecular pathophysiology, cellular origins, and therapy of these enigmatic diseases as well as perspectives for future research directions.

The mitogen-activated protein kinase (MAPK) pathway has a long association with human neoplasia. A key member in this pathway is the BRAF serine/threonine kinase belonging to the RAF family of serine/threonine kinases, which also includes ARAF and RAF1. RAF kinases transduce mitogenic signals from the cell membrane to the nucleus and regulate MEK-ERK signaling. Of the RAF kinases, BRAF is most frequently mutated in cancer with *BRAF*^{V600E} accounting for 90% of activating mutations (Wellbrock et al. 2004). Similarly, the neoplastic cells of the systemic histiocytoses (SHs) and hairy cell leukemia (HCL) have nearly universal ERK overexpression suggesting constitutive activation of MAPK signaling in these distinct hematological neoplasms (Fig. 1; Badalian-Very et al. 2010; Tiacci et al. 2011; Haroche et al. 2012).

Although quite rare in hematological disorders overall, *BRAF* mutations are strikingly enriched in two sets of diseases: classical HCL

Cite this article as *Cold Spring Harb Perspect Med* doi: 10.1101/cshperspect.a034892

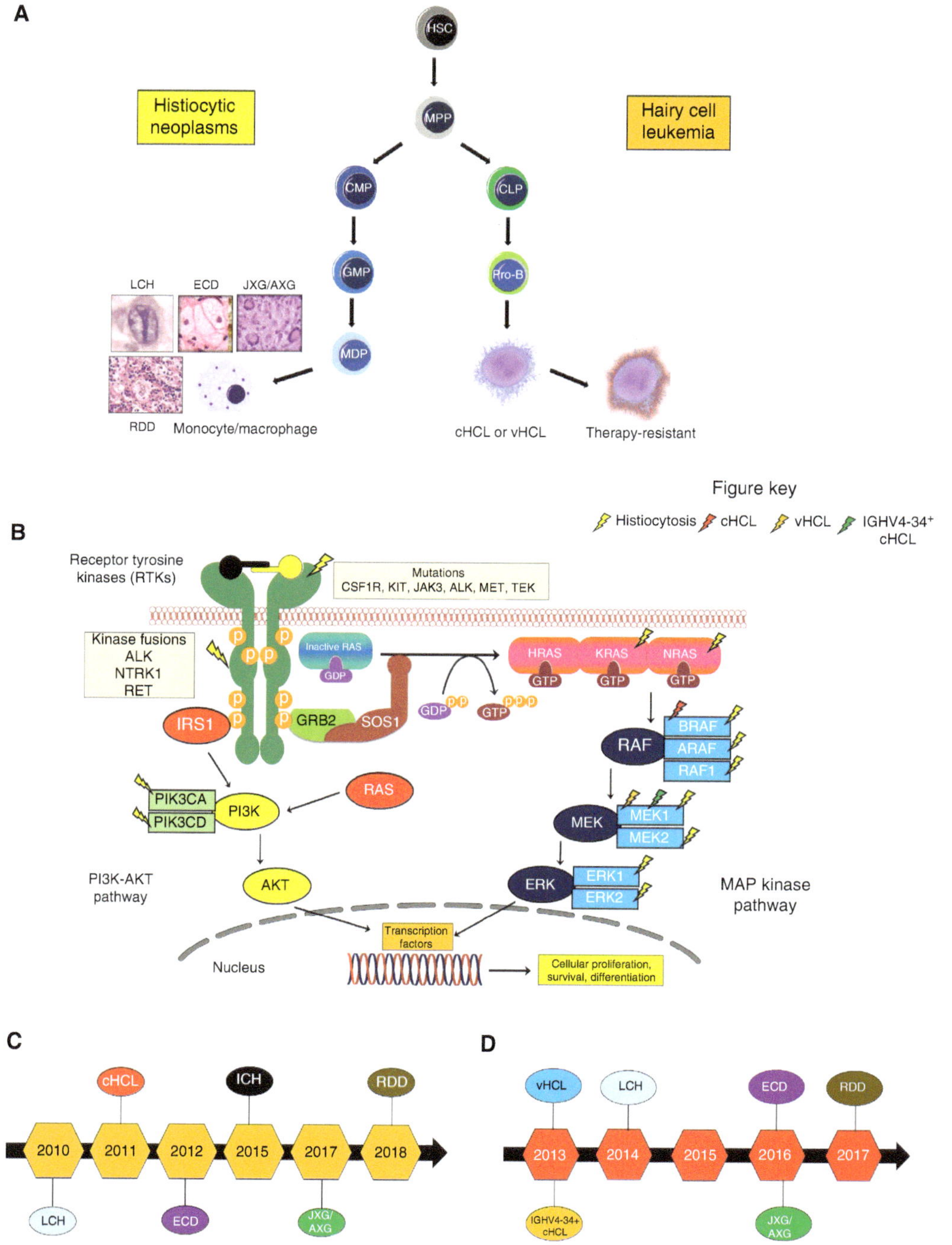

Figure 1. Overview of the mitogen-activated protein kinase (MAPK)-driven hematopoietic neoplasms with common molecular alterations but divergent phenotypes. (*A*) Diagram demonstrating the divergent hematopoietic development of histiocytic neoplasms and hairy cell leukemia. (*B*) Diagram of the MAPK and PI3K-AKT signaling pathways with description of the activation of the RAS proteins (HRAS, KRAS, and NRAS) with annotation of the signaling proteins affected by genetic alterations in the histiocytic neoplasms, classical hairy cell leukemia, IGHV4-34^{+} classical hairy cell leukemia, and hairy cell leukemia variant. (*C*) Timeline of the discovery of recurrent *BRAF*^{V600E} mutations in the MAPK-driven hematological neoplasms. (*D*) Timeline of the discovery of recurrent *MAP2K1* mutations in the MAPK-driven hematological neoplasms. LCH, Langerhans cell histiocytosis; ECD, Erdheim–Chester disease; JXG/AXG, juvenile xanthogranuloma/adult xanthogranuloma; RDD, Rosai–Dorfman–Destombes disease; ICH, indeterminate cell histiocytosis; cHCL, classical hairy cell leukemia; vHCL, hairy cell leukemia variant; *IGHV*, immunoglobulin heavy chain variable; HSC, hematopoietic stem cell; MPP, multipotent progenitor; CMP, common myeloid progenitor; GMP, granulocyte–monocyte progenitor; MDP, monocyte–dendritic cell progenitor; CLP, common lymphoid progenitor; Pro-B, pro-B-lymphocyte; RTK, receptor tyrosine kinase.

(cHCL) (Tiacci et al. 2011; Arcaini et al. 2012; Swerdlow et al. 2017) and SH—Langerhans cell histiocytosis (LCH) (Badalian-Very et al. 2010) and Erdheim–Chester disease (ECD) (Haroche et al. 2012). Furthermore, additional sequencing efforts identified recurrent mutations in *MAP2K1* (MEK1) in variant HCL (vHCL) (Waterfall et al. 2014), LCH (Brown et al. 2014; Chakraborty et al. 2014), ECD, and other non-LCH neoplasms (Diamond et al. 2016; Durham et al. 2016). Interestingly, *BRAF*^{V600E} is frequently present in cHCL (~100%) (Tiacci et al. 2011) and LCH and ECD (50%–60%) (Badalian-Very et al. 2010; Haroche et al. 2012); meanwhile, *MAP2K1* mutations are present in vHCL (~50%) (Waterfall et al. 2014; Durham et al. 2017a) and SH (~25%) (Figs. 1–5; Brown et al. 2014; Chakraborty et al. 2014; Diamond et al. 2016; Durham et al. 2016). However, despite their common molecular alterations, these are distinct malignancies with different clinical presentations and biology. Nonetheless, the discovery of recurrent *BRAF*^{V600E} and *MAP2K1* mutations in both malignancies has guided new therapeutic approaches, as well as an opportunity to explore how a common genetic event gives rise to these enigmatic diseases (Fig. 1; Haroche et al. 2013; Hyman et al. 2015; Tiacci et al. 2015; Diamond et al. 2016, 2018, 2019; Durham et al. 2019). This review discusses the amalgamation of diverse kinase alterations uncovered in SH and HCL during the last decade and underscore how new insights have refined our understanding of these disorders as clonal neoplasms with constitutive MAPK and PI3K-AKT activation. We will also highlight how our concepts of the cellular origins of the MAPK-driven hematological neoplasms and molecular therapeutics have started evolving.

OVERVIEW OF HISTIOCYTIC NEOPLASMS

Histiocytic neoplasms are a heterogeneous group of disorders broadly classified as LCH and non-LCH that share the common pathological features of infiltration and accumulation of neoplastic histiocytes in tissues with nearly universal ERK activation and an accompanying inflammatory milieu (Badalian-Very et al. 2010; Haroche et al. 2012; Swerdlow et al. 2017; Ozkaya et al. 2018). However, a revised classification recategorized LCH and non-LCH into the following: "L" Langerhans group [LCH, ECD, disseminated juvenile/adult xanthogranuloma (JXG/AXG), and indeterminate cell histiocytosis (ICH)]; "C" group (cutaneous JXG/AXG and Rosai–Dorfman–Destombes disease [RDD]); "R" group (noncutaneous RDD) (Table 1; Emile et al. 2016).

LANGERHANS CELL HISTIOCYTOSIS

Historical Perspective

The first historical descriptions of LCH patients occurred in case series. Hippocrates reported a patient with a nonfatal disease with painful skull lesions ~400 BC, a presentation that could be consistent with LCH (Donadieu and Pritchard 1999). Later, Hand–Schüller–Christian described patients with rash, lytic bone lesions, and diabetes insipidus (DI) and Letterer–Siwe discussed a fatal disseminated disease (Hand 1893; Schüller 1915; Christian 1919; Letterer 1924; Siwe 1933). Afterward, Farber characterized single lytic bone lesions as "eosinophilic granulomas" (Farber 1941). However, Lichtenstein noted a similar histology in these clinically diverse descriptions and posited they constitute a common syndrome he called "histiocytosis X," with the "X" indicating uncertain cellular origin (Lichtenstein 1953). Eventually, Nezelof utilized electron microscopy and reported Birbeck granules in both LCH lesions and epidermal Langerhans cells (LCs), leading to the hypothesis that LCH arises from pathologically activated LCs (Nezelof et al. 1973; Lampert 1998; Arceci 1999).

Clinical Presentation

LCH has diverse manifestations from self-resolving, single-organ lesions to multi-organ disease, which is associated with 10%–20% mortality (Arceci 1999; McClain et al. 2004). Bone (75%) and skin (34%) are the most commonly involved organs with lytic bone lesions frequently involving the skull (Table 1; Guyot-Goubin

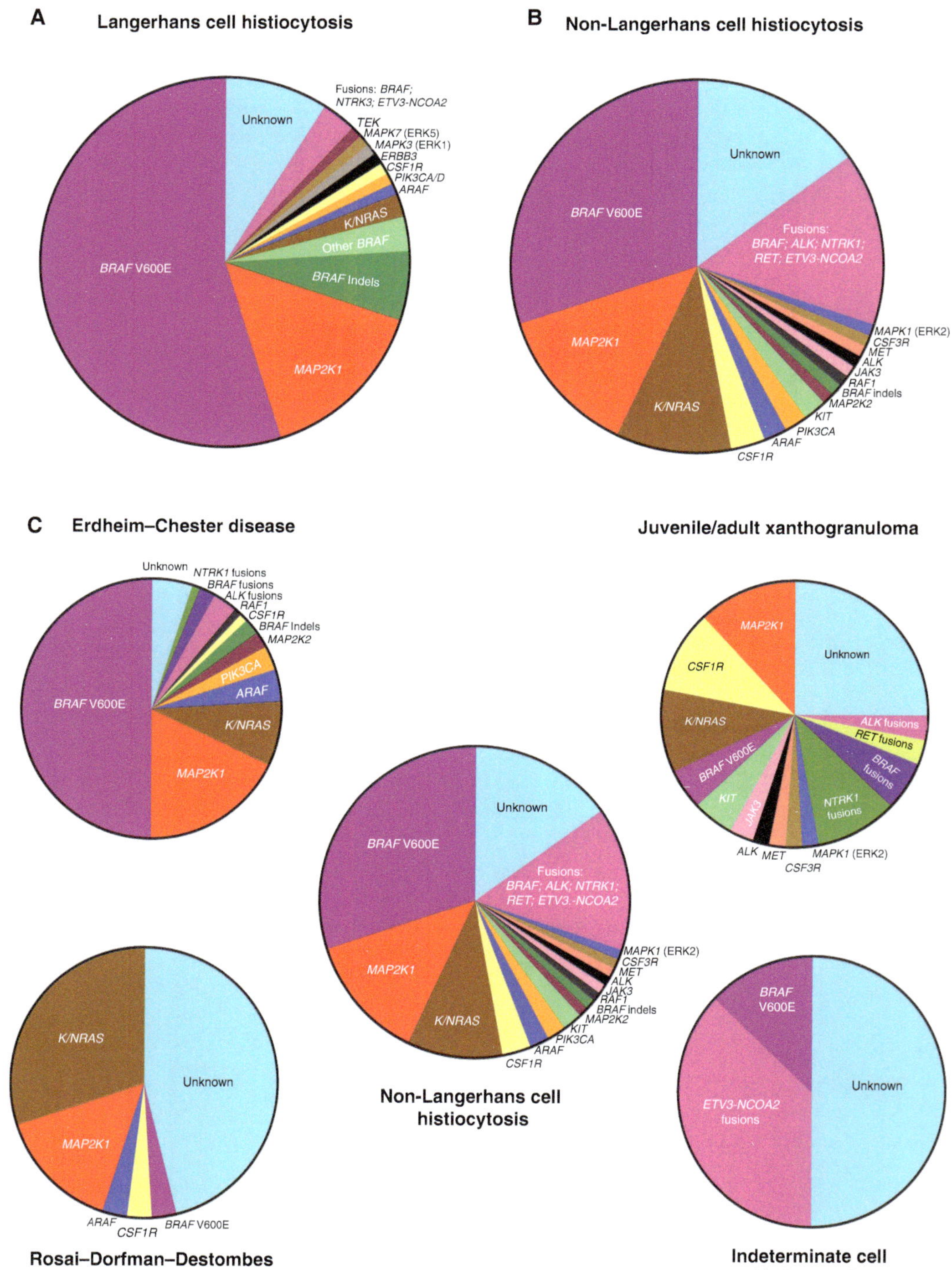

Figure 2. Summary of diverse kinase alterations discovered in the histiocytic neoplasms. (*A*) Pie chart illustrating a composite of the known kinase alterations in Langerhans cell histiocytosis. (*B*) Pie chart showing a composite of the known kinase alterations in non-Langerhans cell histiocytoses. (*C*) Pie charts demonstrating the published kinase alterations in the four discussed subcategories of the non-Langerhans cell histiocytic neoplasms.

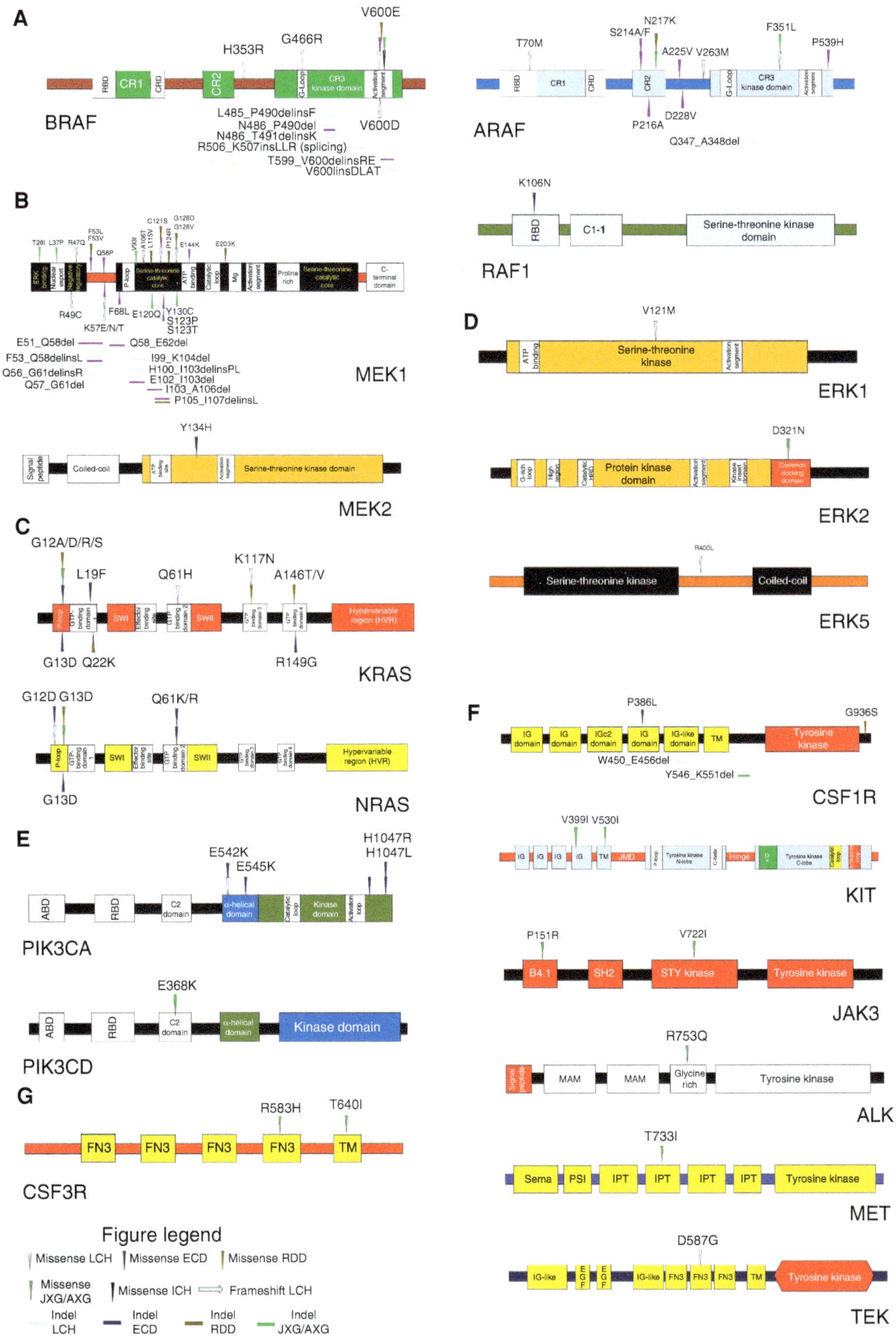

Figure 3. Summary of the diverse kinase mutations in histiocytic neoplasms. (*A*) Protein diagrams cataloging the published somatic mutations described in the RAF isoforms (BRAF, ARAF, and RAF1 [CRAF]). (*B*) Protein diagrams cataloging the somatic mutations discovered in MEK1 and MEK2. (*C*) Protein diagrams cataloging the somatic mutations uncovered in the RAS isoforms (KRAS and NRAS). (*D*) Protein diagrams cataloging somatic mutations described in ERK1, ERK2, and ERK5. (*E*) Protein diagrams cataloging somatic mutations involving the PI3K isoforms (PIK3CA and PIK3CD). (*F*) Protein diagrams documenting somatic mutations recently discovered in the receptor tyrosine kinases. (*G*) Protein diagram cataloging somatic mutations in CSF3R. LCH, Langerhans cell histiocytosis; ECD, Erdheim–Chester disease; JXG/AXG, juvenile xanthogranuloma/adult xanthogranuloma; RDD, Rosai–Dorfman–Destombes disease; ICH, indeterminate cell histiocytosis.

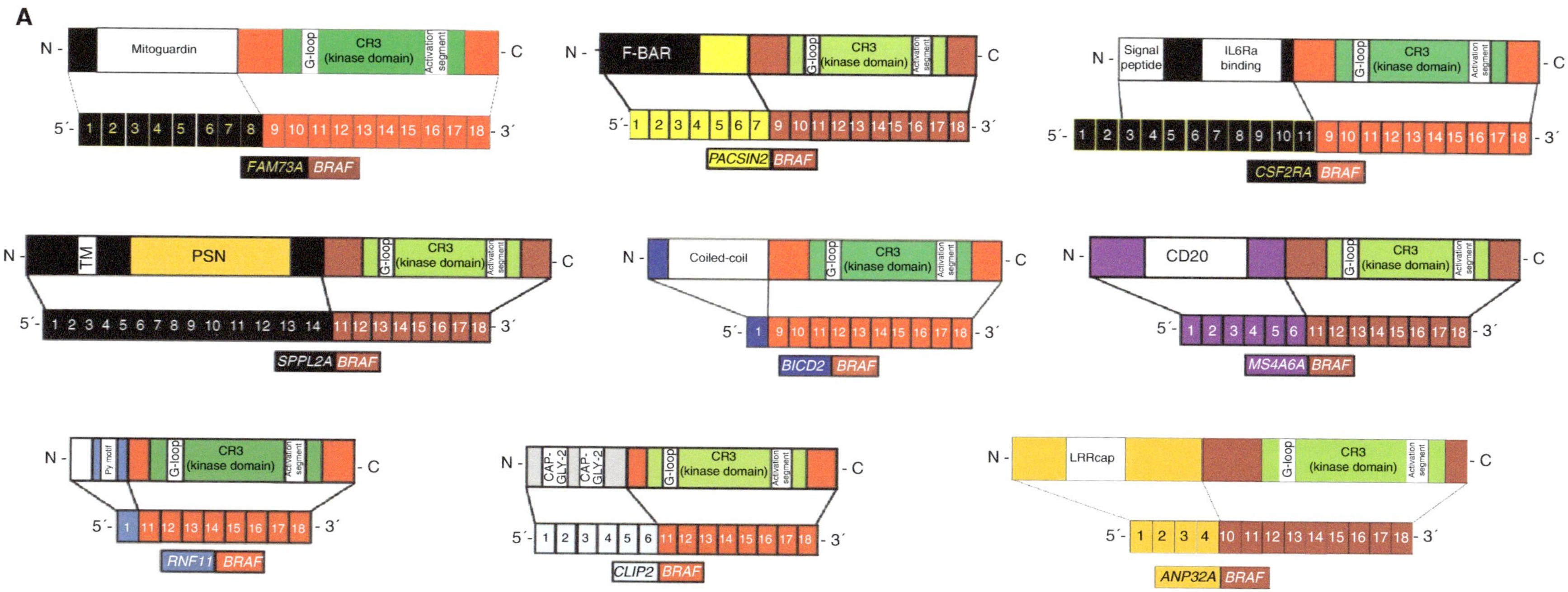

Figure 4. Summary of the diverse kinase fusions in histiocytic neoplasms. (*A*) Illustrations of recurrent *BRAF* fusions discovered in the histiocytic neoplasms. (*B*) Illustrations of the recurrent *NTRK1* fusions uncovered in non-Langerhans cell histiocytoses and an *NTRK3* fusion in Langerhans cell histiocytosis. (*C*) Illustrations of recurrent *ALK* fusions described in the non-Langerhans cell histiocytic neoplasms. (*D*) Illustration of the recurrent *ETV3-NCOA2* fusion discovered in both Langerhans cell histiocytosis and non-Langerhans cell histiocytosis. (*E*) Illustration of the recurrent *NCOA4-RET* fusion recently discovered in non-Langerhans cell histiocytosis. (*Continued on following page.*)

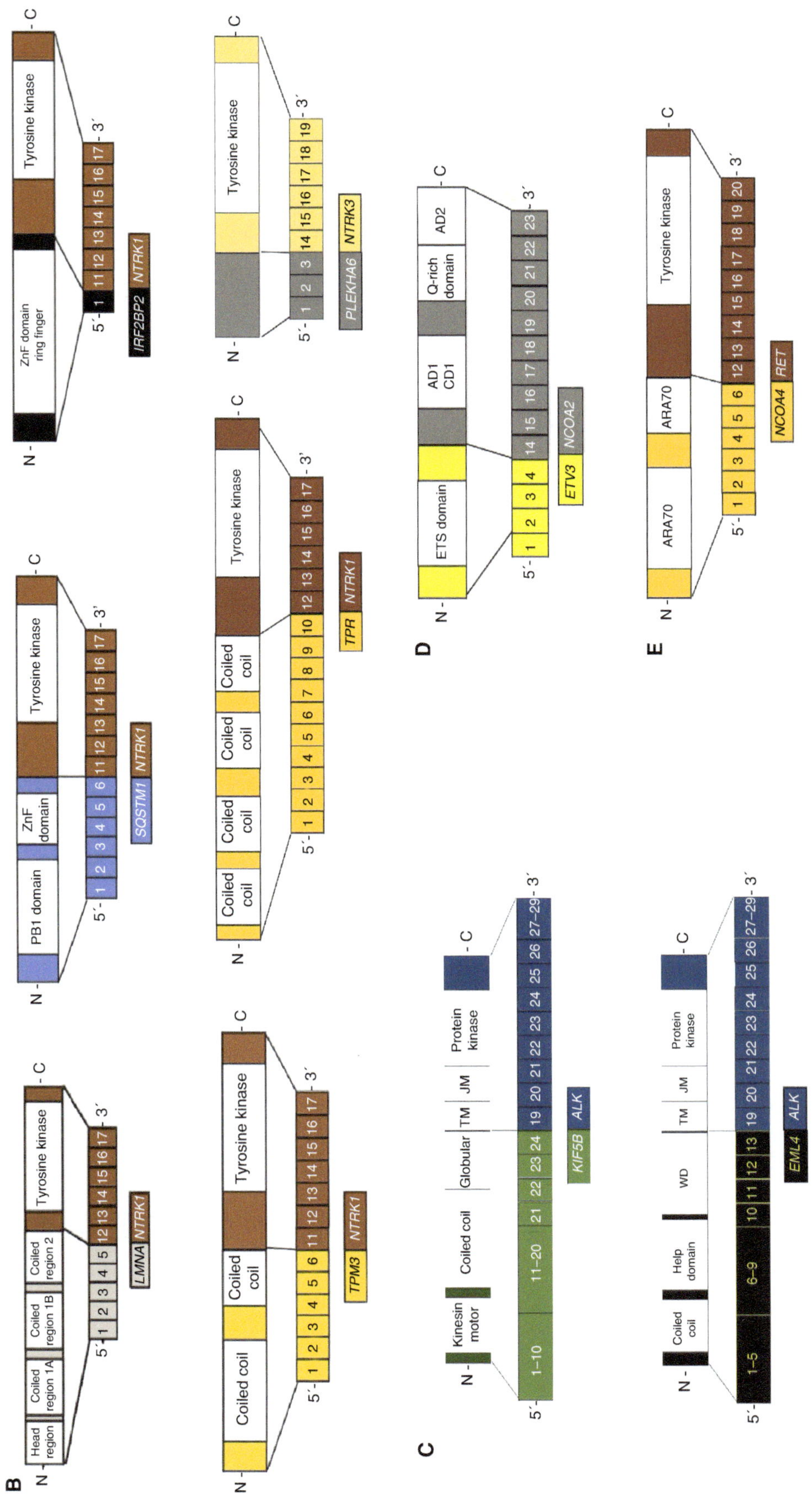

Figure 4. *(Continued from previous page.)*

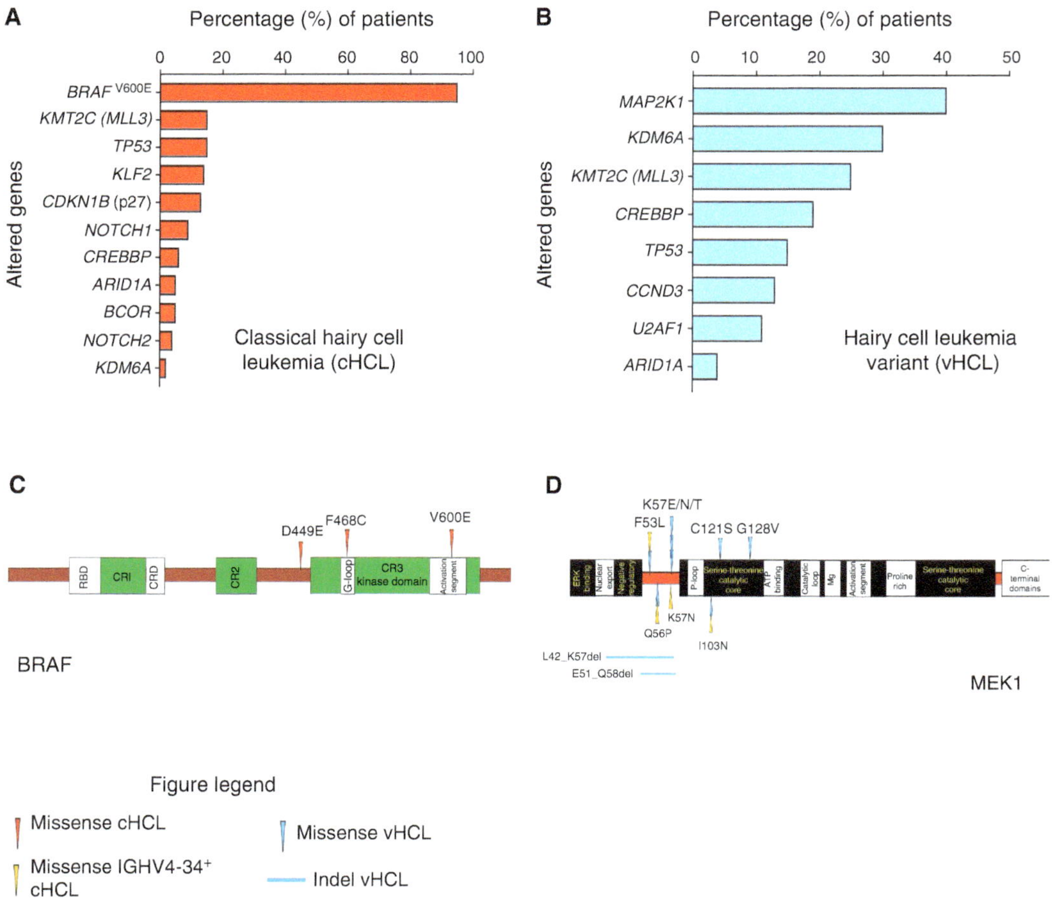

Figure 5. Summary of genetic alterations in hairy cell leukemia. (*A*) Histogram of driver and co-occurring mutations reported in classical hairy cell leukemia. (*B*) Histogram of driver and co-occurring mutations described in hairy cell leukemia variant. (*C*) Protein diagram mapping somatic mutations involving BRAF that have been uncovered in classical hairy cell leukemia. (*D*) Protein diagram mapping somatic mutations in MEK1 discovered in hairy cell leukemia variant and *IGHV4-34*$^+$ classical hairy cell leukemia. cHCL, Classical hairy cell leukemia; vHCL, hairy cell leukemia variant; *IGHV*, immunoglobulin heavy chain variable.

et al. 2008; Stålemark et al. 2008). Besides skin, LCH may arise in any mucosal tissue (gingiva, gastrointestinal tract) (Broadbent et al. 1994; Guyot-Goubin et al. 2008). "High-risk" LCH includes diffuse infiltration or focal lesions of spleen, liver, or bone marrow with a 5-yr survival rate of 84% compared to 99% in "low-risk" LCH (Gadner et al. 2013). LCH may also involve the central nervous system (LCH-CNS), presenting with mass lesions, diabetes insipidus, or progressive neurodegenerative symptoms (LCH-ND) arising decades after initial presentation (Grois et al. 1998, 2010; Héritier et al. 2018).

Pathologically, LCH is characterized by lesions composed of clonal, pathological "histiocytes" with reniform (coffee-bean-shaped) nuclei and abundant, pink cytoplasm with immunoreactivity for CD1a and langerin (CD207) and pathognomonic Birbeck granules (Table 1; Nezelof et al. 1973; Favara et al. 1997; Chikwava and Jaffe 2004; Swerdlow et al. 2017). Histology also shows a milieu of pathologic dendritic cells (DCs) and recruited inflammatory cells (lymphocytes, eosinophils, and macrophages) (Laman et al. 2003; Senechal et al. 2007; Allen et al. 2010; Berres et al. 2014).

Table 1. Summary of the classification, pathological, and radiological features of the histiocytic neoplasms.

Disease	LCH	ECD	JXG/AXG	RDD	ICH
Broad classification	LCH	Non-LCH	Non-LCH	Non-LCH	Non-LCH
Revised classification groupings	L	L	L (extracutaneous) and C (cutaneous)	C (cutaneous) and R (other RDD)	L
Immunophenotypic features					
CD68	+	++	++	++	+
CD163	–	++	++	++	–
CD14	–	++	++	++	–
CD1a	++	–	–	–	++
CD207 (Langerin)	++	–	–	–	–
S100	+	–/+	–/+	+	+
Factor XIIIa	–	+	+	+	–
CD45	+	+	+	+	+
Histological features					
Birbeck granules	Yes	No	No	No	No
Xanthomatous histiocytes	No	Yes	Yes	No	No
Touton giant cells	No	Yes	Yes	No	No
Emperipolesis (intractyoplasmic lymphocytes)	No	Occasional	Occasional	Abundant	No
Radiological features					
Bilateral, symmetric osteosclerosis involving meta-diaphysis of femur, tibia, and fibula	Rare	Frequent, pathognomonic	No	No	No
Lytic, "punched-out" lesions of skull and axial skeleton	Frequent	Rare	No	No	No
Infiltrative, perinephric soft tissue thickening ("hairy kidney")	No	Frequent	Rare	No	No

LCH, Langerhans cell histiocytosis; ECD, Erdheim–Chester disease; JXG, juvenile xanthogranuloma; AXG, adult xanthogranuloma; RDD, Rosai–Dorfman–Destombes disease; ICH, indeterminate cell histiocytosis; L group, Langerhans-related; C group, cutaneous and mucocutaneous; R group, Rosai–Dorfman–Destombes disease; +, low expression; ++, high expression; –, no expression.

JUVENILE/ADULT XANTHOGRANULOMA

Clinical Presentation

JXG/AXG was originally described in the early 1900s and was believed to be endothelium derived and was named "nevoxanthoendothelioma" (McDonagh and McDonagh 1912). JXG/AXG is usually self-limiting with dermal lesions in most patients; but 4% present with disseminated disease (Weitzman and Jaffe 2005; Allen and Parsons 2015). Histologically, JXG/AXG shows xanthomatous histiocytes with admixed multinucleated and Touton giant cells that are immunoreactive for CD68, CD163, CD14, fascin, and Factor XIIIa with variable positivity for S100 and no immunoreactivity for CD1a or CD207 (Table 1; Weitzman and Jaffe 2005; Diamond et al. 2014; Haroche and Abla 2015; Swerdlow et al. 2017).

ERDHEIM–CHESTER DISEASE

Clinical Presentation

ECD is a rare, systemic, non-LCH disease with around 800 reported cases in the literature that was first described as a "lipoid granulomatosis" in 1930 by Erdheim and Chester. ECD has diverse clinical manifestations ranging from localized presentations (bone-only disease) to multisystem disease that are extensively discussed elsewhere (Chester 1930; Weitzman and Jaffe 2005; Diamond et al. 2014; Haroche and Abla 2015; Estrada-Veras et al. 2017; Haroche et al. 2017; Cohen-Aubart et al. 2018). The diagnosis of ECD requires combining the histological criteria and the appropriate clinical and radiological setting (Weitzman and Jaffe 2005; Diamond et al. 2014; Haroche and Abla 2015; Swerdlow et al. 2017). Radiographically, bilateral and symmetric diaphyseal and metaphyseal osteosclerosis of the legs is observed in most patients. Histologically, ECD shows xanthomatous histiocytes with surrounding fibrosis, as well as admixed multinucleated giant cells with immunoreactivity for CD68, CD163, CD14, fascin, and Factor XIIIa and negativity for CD1a and CD207 (Table 1; Weitzman and Jaffe 2005; Diamond et al. 2014; Haroche and Abla 2015; Swerdlow et al. 2017).

ROSAI–DORFMAN–DESTOMBES DISEASE

Clinical Presentation

RDD is a rare, non-LCH hematological disorder known as "sinus histiocytosis with massive lymphadenopathy" that was first described by Destombes, Rosai, and Dorfman (Destombes 1965; Rosai and Dorfman 1969, 1972; Haroche and Abla 2015). RDD has heterogeneous clinical manifestations and can occur as an isolated disorder or in association with hereditary, autoimmune, or neoplastic conditions. The majority of RDD patients present with classical (nodal) RDD that primarily manifests as bilateral, massive, and painless cervical lymphadenopathy with or without fever, night sweats, and weight loss. However, 43% of patients develop extranodal RDD with 19% showing multisystem RDD, and prognosis has been correlated with the number of extranodal systems affected with a detailed clinical discussion reviewed elsewhere (Haroche and Abla 2015; Abla et al. 2018). Histologically, the abnormal, xanthomatous histiocytes of RDD demonstrate abundant emperipolesis of erythrocytes, lymphocytes, and plasma cells. The abnormal histiocytes are immunoreactive for CD14, CD68, CD163, and S100 with negativity for CD1a and CD207 (Table 1; Weitzman and Jaffe 2005; Haroche and Abla 2015; Swerdlow et al. 2017; Durham 2019).

INDETERMINANT CELL HISTIOCYTOSIS

Clinical Presentation

ICH is a rare, non-LCH neoplasm first described in 1985 that predominantly involves the skin and is characterized by the presence of dendritic cells that are morphologically and immunophenotypically like LCH. However, ICH shows a dense dermal infiltration of neoplastic histiocytes admixed with lymphocytes without significant eosinophilic infiltration and is immunoreactive for CD68, S100, and CD1a but not for CD163 and CD207. Therefore, unlike LCH, ICH lacks CD207 and Birbeck granules (Table 1; Wood et al. 1985; Rezk et al. 2008).

MOLECULAR PATHOPHYSIOLOGY OF HISTIOCYTIC NEOPLASMS

Prior to the molecular era, the determination of whether SHs were reactive or neoplastic was unclear and constituted a historical debate (Arceci et al. 1998; Degar and Rollins 2009). Furthermore, the cellular heterogeneity of histiocytoses and the limitations of molecular technology precluded classification of SHs as neoplasms (Merad et al. 2002; Senechal et al. 2007; da Costa et al. 2009). However, the dawning of the molecular era revealed a series of activating kinase alterations involved in MAPK, PI3K-AKT, and RTK signaling within the SHs (Figs. 2–4).

RAF Isoforms

The discovery of *BRAF* mutations in the histiocytoses occurred after $BRAF^{V600E}$ was reported in 57% of LCH (Badalian-Very et al. 2010) and 54% of ECD (Haroche et al. 2012). Later studies uncovered *BRAF*^{V600E} in JXG/AXG, RDD, and ICH but were not prevalent in SHs other than LCH and ECD (O'Malley et al. 2015; Techavichit et al. 2017; Fatobene et al. 2018; Durham et al. 2019). Besides *BRAF*^{V600E}, SH case reports have revealed other activation segment *BRAF* mutations (*BRAF*^{V600D}; *BRAF*^{V600insDLAT}) (Satoh et al. 2012; Kansal et al. 2013). Additionally, a *BRAF* splicing mutation (*BRAF* c.1511_1517 + 2 duplication) was reported (Héritier et al. 2017). Furthermore, activating, in-frame deletions in *BRAF* exon 12 (encodes the β3-αC loop critical for kinase activation) and numerous *BRAF* fusions have been described in SHs (Figs. 2, 3A, 4A; Chakraborty et al. 2016; Lee et al. 2017; Zarnegar et al. 2018; Durham et al. 2019). Other whole-exome sequencing (WES) studies have revealed activating *ARAF* mutations in LCH (Nelson et al. 2014) and non-LCH (ECD; JXG/AXG; RDD) along with *RAF1* mutations in ECD (Figs. 2, 3A; Diamond et al. 2016, 2019; Durham et al. 2019).

MAP2K1/MAP2K2

In *BRAF*^{V600E}-negative histiocytoses, NGS studies found *MAP2K1* to be a second recurrently mutated gene locus in LCH (Brown et al. 2014; Chakraborty et al. 2014) and non-LCH (ECD, JXG/AXG, and RDD) (Diamond et al. 2016; Garces et al. 2017). Functionally, the *MAP2K1* mutations occurred within mutational hotspots and clustered in the amino-terminal regulatory domain (exon 2) and amino-terminal kinase domain (exon 3) resulting in MAPK activation (Chakraborty et al. 2014; Nelson et al. 2015; Diamond et al. 2016; Garces et al. 2017). Additionally, ECD sequencing found recurrent *MAP2K2*^{Y134H} in the MEK2 kinase domain that activated MAPK signaling (Figs. 2, 3B; Diamond et al. 2019; Durham et al. 2019).

RAS Isoforms

The RAS isoforms encode small GTPases that regulate the MAPK and PI3K-AKT signaling pathways. First, *NRAS* mutations were found in single cases of LCH and ECD (Ozono et al. 2011; Diamond et al. 2013). Afterward, studies confirmed that *NRAS*/*KRAS* mutations are recurrent in SH and affected the GTP-binding domains leading to constitutive MAPK activation (Figs. 2, 3C; Emile et al. 2014; Diamond et al. 2016; Shanmugam et al. 2016; Garces et al. 2017; Lee et al. 2017; Durham et al. 2019).

Extracellular-Signal-Regulated Kinases (ERK) Isoforms

As the molecular age continued to interrogate *BRAF*^{V600}-negative histiocytoses, rare mutations started to emerge in the ERK isoforms. An activating *MAPK1*^{D321N} affecting the ERK2 carboxy-terminal-docking domain surfaced in JXG and showed in vitro sensitivity to ERK inhibition but not RAF or MEK inhibition (Chakraborty et al. 2017). Another WES study of LCH found *MAPK3*^{V121M} in the ERK1 kinase domain and *MAPK7*^{R400L} affecting the ERK5 carboxy-terminal domain with both mutations influencing MAPK signaling (Figs. 2, 3D; Durham et al. 2019).

PI3K Isoforms

The PI3K isoforms include phosphatidylinositol-4,5-bisphosphate-3-kinase catalytic subunit alpha (*PIK3CA*) and catalytic subunit delta (*PIK3CD*), members of the PI3K-AKT signaling pathway. Recurrent *PIK3CA* mutations were first revealed in ECD (Emile et al. 2014) and then in LCH (Héritier et al. 2015). Later studies primarily identified *PIK3CA* mutations as recurrent events in ECD with rare *PIK3CD* mutations in JXG and LCH. *PIK3CA* mutations clustered in the α-helical and kinase domains leading to PI3K-AKT activation (Figs. 2, 3E; Chakraborty et al. 2014; Diamond et al. 2016; Durham et al. 2019).

Receptor Tyrosine Kinases

Continued sequencing of histiocytoses implicated the RTKs. A WES study found a case of *ERBB3*-mutated LCH (Chakraborty et al. 2014). Later studies uncovered recurrent *ALK* and

NTRK1 fusions in ECD and JXG/AXG (Diamond et al. 2016; Lee et al. 2017). Then, a large WES/NGS study evaluated 270 histiocytoses patients and discovered recurrent, activating mutations in *CSF1R*, the RTK critical for monocyte and macrophage development, which was enriched in JXG/AXG but found across histiocytoses; and this study was really the first time that activating *CSF1R* mutations have been implicated in cancer. Additionally, other RTK alterations were uncovered in JXG/AXG (*KIT, JAK3, ALK, MET,* and *CSF3R*) and in LCH (TEK), as well as the first *RET* and *NTRK3* fusions in the histiocytoses (Figs. 2, 3F–G, 4; Cai et al. 2019; Durham et al. 2019).

ETV3-NCOA2 Fusions

ETV3-NCOA2 fusions were described in ICH and then reported in one LCH case (Brown et al. 2015; Lee et al. 2017). These fusions involve exons 1–4 of *ETV3* and exons 14–23 of *NCOA2*. This leads to the preservation and fusion of the carboxy-terminal transcriptional activation domains of NCOA2 to the amino-terminal ETS domain of ETV3 (Fig. 4D; Wang et al. 2012; Mesquita et al. 2013; Brown et al. 2015), and prior studies of *NCOA2* gene fusions have demonstrated that the AD1 and CID domains in the carboxyl terminus are required for the transformation of NCOA2 fusion proteins (Figs. 2, 4D; Carapeti et al. 1998; Deguchi et al. 2003; Strehl et al. 2008; Sumegi et al. 2010; Wang et al. 2012; Brown et al. 2015; Durham 2019). However, extensive functional characterization of the role of the *ETV3-NCOA2* fusion in SH pathogenesis is warranted.

Overall, the molecular age demonstrates most SH patients harbor diverse alterations in MAPK, PI3K-AKT, and RTK pathway genes supporting that histiocytoses are clonal, hematopoietic neoplasms with many molecularly directed therapeutic targets.

CELLULAR-ORIGIN STUDIES IN HISTIOCYTOSES

Identification of MAPK mutations has provided a molecular etiology for the SHs and a tool to trace potential precursor cells in these neoplasms. Thus, there has been an accumulation of evidence building on Nezelof's historical proposal of a pathological hematopoietic precursor for LCH ("pathological LCs") that has initiated new cellular origin studies into the SHs (Nezelof and Basset 2001). Gene expression studies in LCH and non-LCH have documented SH lesions have expression profiles of myeloid-derived precursors and not epidermal LCs (Allen et al. 2010; Diamond et al. 2016). Additionally, *BRAF*^{V600E} was traced to CD34^{+} hematopoietic stem/progenitor cells (HSPCs) in studies of high-risk pediatric and adult multisystem LCH and ECD patients but not in patients with single-system or low-risk, multifocal LCH (Berres et al. 2014; Milne et al. 2017; Durham et al. 2017b).

Furthermore, several groups have generated murine models with enforced *BRAF*^{V600E}-expression in langerin^{+} cells resulting in formation of localized LCH-like lesions and in CD11c^{+} cells resulting in a more aggressive phenotype similar to high-risk LCH (Berres et al. 2014; Mass et al. 2017). Notably, xenotransplantation studies using CD34^{+} HSPCs from histiocytosis patients gave rise to genetically and phenotypically accurate xenografts, which provided functional evidence of the self-renewal capacity of kinase-altered HSPCs in SH patients (Durham et al. 2017b). Cumulatively, current evidence led to the proposal of a revised model of histiocytosis pathogenesis, the misguided myeloid differentiation model, in which the developmental stage at which an ERK-activating alteration arises determines the clinical manifestations. Thus, the cell of origin of at least a proportion of SH patients resides in the HSPC compartment prior to committed monocyte or dendritic cell differentiation (Milne et al. 2017; Durham et al. 2017b).

Additional murine studies into alternate cells of origin demonstrated that mosaic expression of *Braf*^{V600E} in yolk sac–derived, erythromyeloid progenitors (EMPs), the cell of origin of murine tissue–resident macrophages (e.g., microglia and Kupffer cells), led to clonal expansion and the accumulation of ERK-activated microglia in the CNS of these models. These mice developed a severe, late-onset neurodegenerative disorder but lacked the systemic accumulation of histiocytes outside the CNS as was seen in models with *Braf*^{V600E} expression in HSC-derived cells. Therefore, these results illustrate yolk sac–derived EMPs can be a potential cell of origin in the histiocytoses (Gomez Perdiguero et al. 2015; Mass et al. 2017). Thus, more than one immediate cellular precursor and the potential for alternate cells-of-origin exist for SHs. However, more investigation is required.

MOLECULARLY BASED HISTIOCYTOSIS THERAPY

Over the past 5 years, SH therapy has dramatically changed with the emergence of targeted therapy and the first U.S. Food and Drug Administration (FDA)-approved SH treatment (Fig. 6A,B) resulting in an improved prognosis for ECD (5-yr survival of 43% in 1996 but 83% currently) (Veyssier-Belot et al. 1996; Cohen-Aubart et al. 2018).

Because 50%–60% of SH patients harbor *BRAF*^{V600E} (Badalian-Very et al. 2010; Haroche et al. 2012), a vemurafenib phase II clinical trial studied *BRAF*^{V600}-mutated ECD and LCH and demonstrated a nearly 100% metabolic response rate, as did several case series. As a result, the U.S. FDA–approved vemurafenib for use in *BRAF*^{V600}-mutated ECD in November 2017 (Fig. 6A; Haroche et al. 2013, 2015; Cohen-Aubart et al. 2014; Hyman et al. 2015; Borys et al. 2016; Bhatia et al. 2018; Diamond et al. 2018). Although BRAF inhibition generally achieves robust and durable responses in *BRAF*^{V600}-mutated histiocytoses, the LOVE study showed 75% of patients who discontinued vemurafenib relapsed in 6 mo but were able to recapture their prior responses when restarted on BRAF inhibitors (vemurafenib; dabrafenib) (Cohen Aubart et al. 2017; Vaglio and Diamond 2017). Additionally, BRAF inhibitor resistance in the SH is rare and has only been reported in one instance where a dabrafenib-treated *BRAF*^{V600E}-mutated ECD patient acquired a *KRAS* mutation, which responded to trametinib (Nordmann et al. 2017).

It is important to note that the extreme sensitivity and durability of response of SH to vemurafenib are quite unique across cancers. Although *BRAF*^{V600E} mutations are seen in ∼8% of all cancer types overall, very few cancers have been shown to have high response rates to BRAF inhibitors as single agents as has been seen in SHs (for review, see Holderfield et al. 2014; Crispo et al. 2019). The largest experience with BRAF inhibition has been in the setting of *BRAF*^{V600E}-mutant metastatic melanoma in which BRAF inhibition is most commonly combined with MEK inhibition to improve efficacy and durability of response and reduce side effects from single-agent BRAF inhibition. But even with this approach, although 63%–76% of all patients with advanced *BRAF*^{V600E}-mutant melanoma derive clinical benefit from combined BRAF/MEK inhibition, median progression-free survival lasts only about 9 mo and 90% of patients develop resistance within 1 yr (for review, see Crispo et al. 2019). Currently, BRAF inhibitors are FDA-approved for the therapy of *BRAF*^{V600E}-mutant metastatic melanoma, either alone or in combination with MEK inhibitors, and there are three BRAF/MEK inhibitors approved for this setting (vemurafenib/debrafinib, dabrafenib and trametinib, and encorafenib plus binimetinib). In addition, BRAF inhibitors are approved in three specific settings for thyroid cancers: (1) vemurafenib for *BRAF*^{V600E}-mutant advanced radioactive iodine-refractory thyroid cancer, (2) dabrafenib for *BRAF*^{V600E}-mutated metastatic papillary thyroid cancer, and (3) debrafenib plus trametinib for the treatment of locally advanced or metastatic anaplastic thyroid cancer with a *BRAF*^{V600E} mutation and no satisfactory locoregional treatment options.

Accumulating molecular knowledge in *BRAF*^{V600}-negative SH led to investigations into MEK inhibitors (cobimetinib; trametinib) (Diamond et al. 2016, 2019; Cohen Aubart et al. 2017, 2018) with the cobimetinib phase II clinical trial showing an 89% overall response rate (ORR) by positron emission tomography (PET)-computed tomography (CT) with fluorodeoxyglucose (FDG) tracer irrespective of disease site. As a result, the U.S. FDA granted

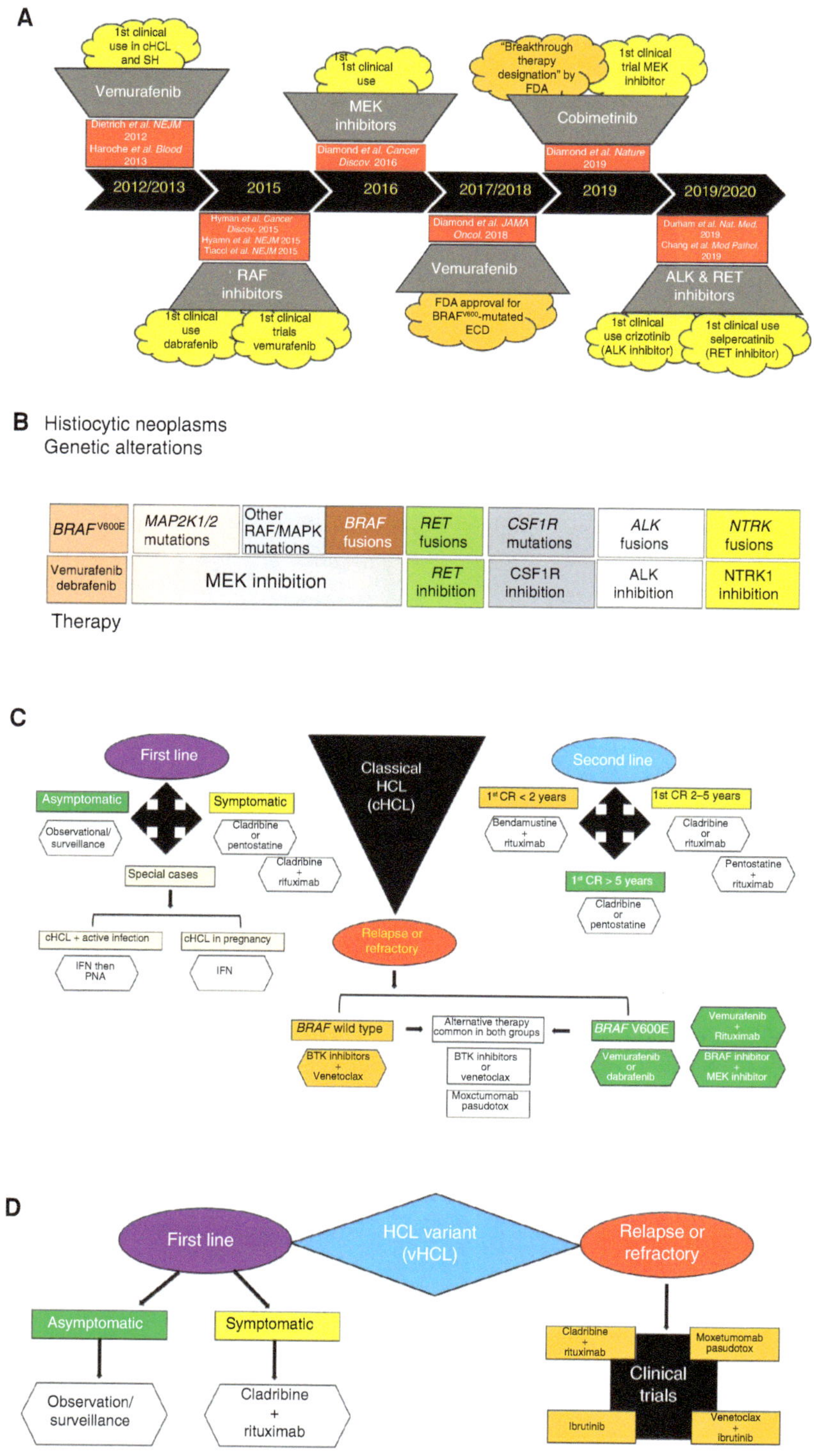

Figure 6. Therapeutic advancements achieved during a progressive molecular age for MAPK-driven hematopoietic neoplasms. (*A*) Timeline documenting the targeted therapeutic achievements in the histiocytic neoplasms and hairy cell leukemia over the past decade. (*B*) Diagram summarizing the molecular targeted therapies that have or may demonstrate clinical efficacy in the histiocytic neoplasms. (*C*) Diagram of a composite therapeutic algorithm for the first-line, second-line, and relapsed/refractory treatment of classical hairy cell leukemia based on current advancements during the molecular age. (*D*) Diagram of a composite therapeutic algorithm for the first-line and relapsed/refractory treatment of hairy cell leukemia variant founded on current molecular progress. SH, Systemic histiocytoses; ECD, Erdheim–Chester disease; cHCL, classical hairy cell leukemia; vHCL, hairy cell leukemia variant; FDA, Food and Drug Administration; PNA, purine analog; IFN, interferon; BTK, Bruton tyrosine kinase; CR, complete response.

"Breakthrough Therapy Designation" to cobimetinib in the treatment of *BRAF*^{V600}-negative histiocytoses (Fig. 6A; Diamond et al. 2019).

Moreover, molecular discovery of *ALK*, *NTRK1*, and *RET* fusions, as well as *CSF1R* mutations in diverse histioctyoses, have stimulated investigations into other targeted therapies. These studies have provided in vitro functional data or clinical reports supporting the use of ALK inhibitors (crizotinib; alectinib), the RET-specific inhibitor selpercatinib, NTRK inhibitors, and *CSF1R*-inhibitors (pexidartinib) in SHs (Fig. 6B; Diamond et al. 2016; Lee et al. 2017; Taylor et al. 2018; Chang et al. 2019; Durham et al. 2019). Therefore, the molecular age has provided many exciting therapeutic options for SH patients, but molecularly targeted therapies beyond BRAF and MEK inhibitors need to be scrutinized in future clinical trials. Also, questions about the optimal dosing, treatment duration, and therapy response assessments require further study, especially in pediatric SH patients.

HAIRY CELL LEUKEMIA

Clinical Presentation

HCL was originally named "leukemic reticuloendotheliosis" and described based on the existence of numerous "hairy" surface projections (Bouroncle et al. 1958). Classical HCL is a rare, mature B-lymphocytic neoplasm comprising 2% of lymphoid leukemias. Meanwhile, vHCL is a similar mature B-lymphocytic neoplasm with variant clinical, cytological, and immunophenotypical features and is 10% as common as cHCL (Swerdlow et al. 2017; Maitre et al. 2019).

Patients with HCL commonly present with weakness, fatigue, bleeding, and fever, and the immunophenotypical profile has emerged as the key component to distinguish cHCL and vHCL. Therefore, HCL is a group of hematological malignancies consisting of cHCL, *IGHV4-34*$^{+}$ cHCL, and vHCL that are morphologically similar with subtle pathological differences but have distinct clinical and laboratory features, immunophenotypes, and molecular characteristics that are compared in Table 2 (Tiacci et al. 2011; Waterfall et al. 2014; Dietrich et al. 2015; Falini et al. 2016; Swerdlow et al. 2017; Thompson and Ravandi 2017; Durham et al. 2017a; Maitre et al. 2019). Furthermore, newly discovered molecular features (Fig. 5; Table 2) assist in further characterization of the pathophysiology and therapeutic options for cHCL and vHCL and have been correlated with other HCL risk stratification parameters as detailed in Table 3 (Arons et al. 2009; Forconi et al. 2009; Xi et al. 2012; Poret et al. 2015; Falini et al. 2016; Swerdlow et al. 2017; Durham et al. 2017a; Maitre et al. 2019).

Pathophysiology

Genomic Profiling

In 2011, WES of cHCL uncovered *BRAF*^{V600E} as the driving genetic event in ~97% of cHCL (Tiacci et al. 2011; Waterfall et al. 2014; Dietrich et al. 2015; Durham et al. 2017a). Occasional *BRAF*^{V600E}-negative cHCL patients were shown to have *BRAF* exon 11 mutations (*BRAF*^{D449E}; *BRAF*^{F468C}) (Figs. 1C, 5) that were predicted but not proven to be activating (Tschernitz et al. 2014). Meanwhile, another WES study evaluated vHCL and *IGHV4-34*$^{+}$ cHCL and found activating *MAP2K1* mutations in ~50% of these cases (Figs. 1D, 5; Waterfall et al. 2014; Dietrich et al. 2015; Durham et al. 2017a). Therefore, through MAPK pathway activation by *BRAF* and *MAP2K1* mutations, the neoplastic hairy cells demonstrate increased proliferation and survival (Tiacci et al. 2011; Waterfall et al. 2014; Dietrich et al. 2015; Durham et al. 2017a).

Recently, the discovery of co-occurring genetic alterations that may cooperate with *BRAF*^{V600E} in cHCL and *MAP2K1* mutations in vHCL have provided further insights into their pathogenesis. Alterations in genes involved in cell cycle regulation (*CCND1*; *CDKN1B/p27*; *CCND3*), NF-κB pathway and B-lymphocyte differentiation (*KLF2*), the spliceosome (*U2AF1*), and epigenetic regulation (*KMT2C/MLL3*, *KDM6A*, *CREBBP*, *ARID1A*) are potentially key players in the pathophysiology of cHCL or vHCL but will require further study to elucidate their mechanistic roles (Fig. 5A,B;

Table 2. Summary of the characteristic features of classical hairy cell leukemia and hairy cell leukemia variant

Characteristic Features	IGHV4-34- cHCL	IGHV4-34$^+$ cHCL	vHCL
Laboratory parameters			
Pancytopenia	Present	Absent	Absent
Monocytopenia	Present	Absent	Absent
Absolute neutrophil count	Decreased	Normal	Normal
Leukocytosis	Absent	Present	Present
Soluble IL2 receptor (plasma)	Elevated	Unknown	Normal
Bone marrow aspiration	Dry tap	Easily aspirated	Easily aspirated
Immunophenotypic profile			
CD19	++	++	++
CD20	++	++	++
CD22	++	++	++
FMC7	+	+	+
CD11c	++	++	++
CD103	+	+	+
CD25	+	+	--
CD123	+	+	--
CD200	+	+	--
Annexin A1	+	+	--
Histological features			
Nucleus (Wright–Giemsa)	Oval/kidney-shaped	Oval/kidney-shaped	Round/oval
Nucleolus (Wright–Giemsa)	Absent	Absent	Prominent
Cytoplasm (Wright–Giemsa)	Abundant, pale	Abundant, pale	Abundant, pale
Cellular surface	Thin, often long circumferential projections	Thin, often long circumferential projections	Thin, often long circumferential projections
Infiltration pattern (bone marrow)	Diffuse and/or interstitial	Diffuse and/or interstitial	Diffuse, intrasinusoidal, and/or interstitial
Infiltration pattern (spleen)	Red pulp with effacement of white pulp	Red pulp with effacement of white pulp	Red pulp
TRAP immunocytochemistry	+	+	--
Annexin A1 immunohistochemistry	+	+	--
BRAF^{V600E} immunohistochemistry	+	--	--
Molecular features			
BRAF^{V600E} mutations	Present (~97%)	Absent	Absent
MAP2K1 alterations	Absent	Present	Present (~50%)
IGHV somatic hypermutation	Frequent	Absent	Rare
IGHV4-34 usage	Absent	Present	Frequent
CDKN1B (p27) co-occurring mutations	Present	Unknown	Absent
KLF2 co-occurring mutations	Present	Unknown	Absent

Continued

Table 2. *Continued*

Characteristic Features	IGHV4-34- cHCL	IGHV4-34⁺ cHCL	vHCL
NOTCH1 co-occurring mutations	Rare	Unknown	Absent
NOTCH2 co-occurring mutations	Rare	Unknown	Absent
BCOR co-occurring mutations	Rare	Unknown	Absent
KDM6A co-occurring mutations	Rare	Unknown	Frequent
CREBBP co-occurring mutations	Rare	Unknown	Frequent
CCND3 co-occurring mutations	Absent	Unknown	Present
U2AF1 co-occurring mutations	Absent	Unknown	Present

cHCL, Classical hairy cell leukemia; vHCL, hairy cell leukemia variant; IL2, interleukin 2; CD, cluster of differentiation; *IGHV*, immunoglobulin heavy chain variable; +, low expression; ++, high expression; –, not detected.

(Waterfall et al. 2014; Clipson et al. 2015; Dietrich et al. 2015; Piva et al. 2015; Falini et al. 2016; Jallades et al. 2017; Durham et al. 2017a; Maitre et al. 2018, 2019).

Gene Expression and Methylation Profiling

The molecular era has refined epigenetic advancements, which has yielded new insights into the peculiar clinical-pathological features of cHCL, whereas few notable studies have investigated *IGHV4-34*$^{+}$ cHCL or vHCL. The methylation and gene expression profiles in cHCL supported the constitutive activation of the MAPK pathway. Also, hypomethylation and overexpression of genes that inhibit matrix metalloproteinase activity and hypermethylation and underexpression of chemokine receptors critical for B-lymphocyte migration to peripheral lymphoid organ follicles result in neoplastic hairy cells homing to bone marrow, splenic red pulp, and hepatic sinusoids rather than splenic white pulp and lymph nodes. Additionally, cHCL showed hypomethylation and overexpression of genes that stimulate fibronectin production and may contribute to the bone marrow reticulin fibrosis and poor bone marrow aspiration in cHCL (Basso et al. 2004; Arribas et al. 2019). Furthermore, overexpression of *TGFB1*, which stimulates neoplastic hairy cells to produce TGF-β, has been posited as a reason for the inhibition of normal hematopoiesis in cHCL (leukopenia; monocytopenia) (Basso et al. 2004; Swerdlow et al. 2017). Meanwhile, other studies support *LST1* (leukocyte transcript 1) and *ACTB* (actin β) genes are enriched in and important for the formation of actin-containing, circumferential "hairy" membrane projections characteristic of HCL (Pettirossi et al. 2015; Falini et al. 2016).

Cellular Origins of cHCL

Through the discovery of *BRAF*^{V600E} in cHCL, a biomarker for the evaluation of the cell of origin of cHCL appeared. Although epigenetic profiling suggests cHCL is derived from transformed, postgerminal center B-lymphocytes (Basso et al. 2004; Falini et al. 2016; Arribas et al. 2019), recent cellular-origin studies reported that the HSCs in cHCL harbor the *BRAF*^{V600E} mutation. Furthermore, xenografting of purified, *BRAF*^{V600E}-mutated HSCs into immunodeficient mice resulted in stable engraftment, which functionally demonstrated the self-renewal capacity of *BRAF*^{V600E}-mutant HSCs in cHCL. However, the transplanted mice did not develop the complete cHCL phenotype, and this

Table 3. Summary of risk-stratification parameters in hairy cell leukemia that predict a poor prognosis and resistance to purine analogs

Parameters	Measurement
Clinical	
Splenomegaly	>3 cm below the costal margin
Laboratory	
Leukocytosis	>1 × 10^9 cells/L
Hairy cells in peripheral blood	>5 g/L
Beta-2 microglobulin level	>2× the upper limit of normal (High)
CD38 by immunophenotype	Present
Molecular features	
BRAF^{V600E}	Absent
IGHV mutational status	Unmutated
IGHV4-34 rearrangement	Present
Telomere length	Short

cHCL, Classical hairy cell leukemia; vHCL, hairy cell leukemia variant; CD, cluster of differentiation; *IGHV*, immunoglobulin heavy chain variable

raises the question as to whether or not a permissive epigenetic background and acquisition of cooperating genetic alterations are required for phenotypically accurate cHCL (Chung et al. 2014; Falini et al. 2016). Therefore, more functional studies and murine modeling are required to attain a faithful cHCL animal model.

TREATMENT

HCL patients should be treated when symptomatic or when presenting with one of these hematological parameters: hemoglobin <11 g/dL; platelet count <100,000/µL; or ANC <1,000 cells/µL. Meanwhile, asymptomatic cHCL patients are to be managed with observation/surveillance (Grever et al. 2017; Andrasiak et al. 2018; Maitre et al. 2019).

Chemotherapy

First-line treatment in cHCL patients involves purine analog (PNA) monotherapy (cladribine or pentostatin) because large studies have shown 76%–83% of patients achieved a complete response (CR) and 31%–33% a partial response (PR) (Dearden et al. 2011; Cornet et al. 2014; Else et al. 2015; Maitre et al. 2019). Additionally, a phase II trial of chemoimmunotherapy with cladribine followed by rituximab demonstrated a CR of 100% and has high efficacy as a first-line therapy. However, special cases do arise and include patients with symptomatic cHCL and a febrile infection requiring infection management prior to PNA treatment (INF-α before PNA). Also, pregnant cHCL patients should be treated with interferon (IFN) (Fig. 6C; Maitre et al. 2019).

Second-line chemotherapy is necessary for the 50% of cHCL patients who relapse during the first 5 yr following first-line chemotherapy, and the consensus on treatment options is stratified based on duration of the first CR (CR > 5 yr; CR = 2–5 yr; CR < 2 yr) (Fig. 6C; Else et al. 2011, 2015; Burotto et al. 2013; Cornet et al. 2014; Chihara et al. 2016; Sadeghi and Li 2018; Maitre et al. 2019).

First-line chemotherapy in symptomatic vHCL patients has no current consensus; however, a combination of cladribine/rituximab is the common treatment used when managing vHCL (Fig. 6D; Kreitman et al. 2013; Maitre et al. 2019).

Targeted Therapy

The molecular era spawned the discovery of *BRAF*^{V600E} in >97% of cHCL and the first molecular target in these neoplasms (Fig. 6A; Tiacci et al. 2011; Dietrich et al. 2012; Falini et al. 2016). The first clinical trials of vemurafenib in relapsed/refractory cHCL showed an ORR approaching 100% with 35%–40% CRs, and the median relapse-free survival was ~19 mo (CR patients) and 6 mo (PR patients) (Tiacci et al. 2015; Falini et al. 2016; Maitre et al. 2019). Thus, the most promising therapeutic options for relapsed/refractory cHCL include targeted therapeutics: BRAF inhibitors in *BRAF*^{V600E}-mutated cHCL (Hyman et al. 2015; Tiacci et al. 2015); BRAF/MEK inhibitor combinations in *BRAF*^{V600E}-mutated cHCL; recombinant immunoconjugates targeting CD22 (moxetumomab pasudotox), which has promising preliminary results in a phase I clinical trial (91% ORR, including 59% with CRs) (Kreitman et al. 2018; Maitre et al. 2019); and the first-in-class Bruton tyrosine kinase (BTK) inhibitor ibrutinib approved for treating relapsed/refractory B-cell malignancies (e.g., chronic lymphocytic leukemia [CLL]/small lymphocytic leukemia [SLL]) (Fig. 6C; Byrd et al. 2015; Sarvaria et al. 2016; Maitre et al. 2019). Furthermore, clinical trials utilizing moxetumomab pasudotox, ibrutinib, and ibrutinib/venetoclax are suggested for the treatment of relapsed/refractory vHCL (Fig. 6D; Bohn et al. 2017; Maitre et al. 2019). Future directions for molecular treatments in HCL should include trials combining BRAF/MEK inhibitors in cHCL, MEK inhibitors in vHCL and *IGHV4-34*$^{+}$ cHCL, CDK4/6 inhibitors in *CCND3*-mutated vHCL, and ibrutinib in both cHCL and vHCL (Maitre et al. 2019).

Mechanisms of Vemurafenib Resistance

As in metastatic melanoma, the dramatic clinical efficacy of vemurafenib in refractory/relapsed cHCL has now shown relapse, which suggests the development of resistance mechanisms (Tiacci et al. 2015; Falini et al. 2016). However, knowledge of the vemurafenib resistance mechanisms in cHCL has just begun to emerge. For example, resistance in two patients treated in a phase II cHCL clinical trial was secondary to acquired mutations in *KRAS/NRAS* following treatment with vemurafenib, which induce reactivation of the MAPK pathway through *RAF1* (Trunzer et al. 2013; Tiacci et al. 2015; Durham et al. 2017a). Another patient experienced complete, de novo vemurafenib resistance, and genomic analysis of his pretreatment sample revealed a gain-of-function mutation in *IRS1* (*IRS1*^{P1201S}) that functionally activated PI3K-AKT signaling. Furthermore, this patient had heterozygous deletions of *NF1* and *NF2* that functionally induced vemurafenib resistance in vitro (Whittaker et al. 2013; Shalem et al. 2014; Durham et al. 2017a). Nonetheless, more functional and sequencing studies are required to better elucidate and catalog cHCL vemurafenib-resistance mechanisms.

Frequency and Implication of BRAF Mutations in Hematologic Malignancies outside of HCL and SH

In contrast to the very high frequency of *BRAF*^{V600E} mutations in HCL and SH, BRAF mutations are far rarer in more common hematologic malignancies. Outside of HCL and SH, recurrent BRAF mutations have been reported in 4%–10% of multiple myeloma (Andrulis et al. 2013; Lohr et al. 2014), 2%–5% of patients with CLL (Jebaraj et al. 2013; Leeksma et al. 2019), and 1%–2% patients with acute myeloid leukemia (AML) (Papaemmanuil et al. 2016). To date, the only formal evaluation of the use of BRAF inhibition in BRAF-mutant hematologic malignancies outside of HCL and SH was the use of vemurafenib for nine patients with *BRAF*^{V600E}-mutant multiple myeloma as part of the VE-BASKET Study (Raje et al. 2018). The best confirmed overall response rate in this cohort was 33% with two patients achieving partial remissions. In the single published report of an AML patient treated with a BRAF inhibitor, a refractory AML patient was treated with combined dabrafenib/trametinib with only a very transient response (Wander et al. 2017). It is important to note that in CLL and myeloma, *BRAF* mutations are often subclonal. Moreover, in CLL, *BRAF* mutations frequently occur outside of the V600 residue (most commonly at the G466, D594, and K601 residues). Given the use of vemurafenib and dabrafenib for *BRAF*^{V600E}/K-mutant diseases specifically, the therapeutic implications of BRAF inhibition with approved

BRAF inhibitors has an unclear role in CLL and has never been evaluated.

CONCLUDING REMARKS

Molecular advancements over the past decade helped unravel the molecular pathophysiology, cellular origins, and therapeutic targets in the MAPK-driven hematological neoplasms. Since the description of *BRAF*^{V600E} in SH and cHCL (Badalian-Very et al. 2010; Tiacci et al. 2011; Haroche et al. 2012), there has been an onslaught of molecular progress linking diverse kinase alterations activating MAPK, PI3K-AKT, and RTK signaling to the histiocytic neoplasms, as well as *MAP2K1* mutations in *IGHV4-34*$^{+}$ cHCL and vHCL (Figs. 1–5). These recent discoveries have refined the current pathological understanding of the histiocytoses as clonal, myeloid neoplasms with constitutive activation of MAPK and PI3K-AKT signaling and confirm HCL belongs to the MAPK-driven, hematological neoplasms. Furthermore, molecular progress has re-imagined therapeutic options for patients with these disorders (Fig. 6). Additionally, many biomarkers are now available that have enhanced our biological understanding of the cellular pathogenesis and ontogeny of the SH and HCL. However, our functional genomic conceptualization of the molecular pathogenesis and histogenesis of SH and HCL are just emerging with many aspects still enshrouded in mystery requiring systematic dissection with studies employing single-cell molecular and epigenetic analyses, as well as preclinical models. Finally, as the molecular era continues to unfold, future studies to elucidate why HCL and SH share common MAPK alterations but are phenotypically distinct neoplasms with differing clinical presentations, pathophysiology, and suspected cellular origins are a desperately needed dimension of investigation.

ACKNOWLEDGMENTS

O.A.-W. is supported by 1 R01 CA201247-01A1 from the National Cancer Institute (NCI) of the National Institutes of Health (NIH). B.H.D. is supported by the Fellow Scholar Award in Basic/Translational Research from the American Society of Hematology (ASH), a grant from the Erdheim–Chester Disease Global Alliance Foundation, and K08 CA218901 from the NCI/NIH. R.C. is supported by U.S. Department of Defense Peer Reviewed Cancer Research Program Career Development Award W81XWH1910167.

REFERENCES

Abla O, Jacobsen E, Picarsic J, Krenova Z, Jaffe R, Emile JF, Durham BH, Braier J, Charlotte F, Donadieu J, et al. 2018. Consensus recommendations for the diagnosis and clinical management of Rosai–Dorfman–Destombes disease. *Blood* **131:** 2877–2890. doi:10.1182/blood-2018-03-839753

Allen CE, Parsons DW. 2015. Biological and clinical significance of somatic mutations in Langerhans cell histiocytosis and related histiocytic neoplastic disorders. *Hematology Am Soc Hematol Educ Program* **2015:** 559–564. doi:10.1182/asheducation-2015.1.559

Allen CE, Li L, Peters TL, Leung HC, Yu A, Man TK, Gurusiddappa S, Phillips MT, Hicks MJ, Gaikwad A, et al. 2010. Cell-specific gene expression in Langerhans cell histiocytosis lesions reveals a distinct profile compared with epidermal Langerhans cells. *J Immunol* **184:** 4557–4567. doi:10.4049/jimmunol.0902336

Andrasiak I, Rybka J, Wrobel T. 2018. Response to the therapy in hairy cell leukemia: Systematic review and meta-analysis. *Clin Lymphoma Myeloma Leuk* **18:** 392–399.e3. doi:10.1016/j.clml.2018.03.011

Andrulis M, Lehners N, Capper D, Penzel R, Heining C, Huellein J, Zenz T, von Deimling A, Schirmacher P, Ho AD, et al. 2013. Targeting the *BRAF* V600E mutation in multiple myeloma. *Cancer Discov* **3:** 862–869. doi:10.1158/2159-8290.CD-13-0014

Arcaini L, Zibellini S, Boveri E, Riboni R, Rattotti S, Varettoni M, Guerrera ML, Lucioni M, Tenore A, Merli M, et al. 2012. The *BRAF* V600E mutation in hairy cell leukemia and other mature B-cell neoplasms. *Blood* **119:** 188–191. doi:10.1182/blood-2011-08-368209

Arceci RJ. 1999. The histiocytoses: The fall of the Tower of Babel. *Eur J Cancer* **35:** 747–767; discussion 767–749. doi:10.1016/S0959-8049(99)00039-8

Arceci RJ, Brenner MK, Pritchard J. 1998. Controversies and new approaches to treatment of Langerhans cell histiocytosis. *Hematol Oncol Clin North Am* **12:** 339–357. doi:10.1016/S0889-8588(05)70514-1

Arons E, Suntum T, Stetler-Stevenson M, Kreitman RJ. 2009. VH4-34^{+} hairy cell leukemia, a new variant with poor prognosis despite standard therapy. *Blood* **114:** 4687–4695. doi:10.1182/blood-2009-01-201731

Arribas AJ, Rinaldi A, Chiodin G, Kwee I, Mensah AA, Cascione L, Rossi D, Kanduri M, Rosenquist R, Zucca E, et al. 2019. Genome-wide promoter methylation of hairy cell leukemia. *Blood Adv* **3:** 384–396. doi:10.1182/bloodadvances.2018024059

Badalian-Very G, Vergilio JA, Degar BA, MacConaill LE, Brandner B, Calicchio ML, Kuo FC, Ligon AH, Stevenson

KE, Kehoe SM, et al. 2010. Recurrent *BRAF* mutations in Langerhans cell histiocytosis. *Blood* **116:** 1919–1923. doi:10.1182/blood-2010-04-279083

Basso K, Liso A, Tiacci E, Benedetti R, Pulsoni A, Foa R, Di Raimondo F, Ambrosetti A, Califano A, Klein U, et al. 2004. Gene expression profiling of hairy cell leukemia reveals a phenotype related to memory B cells with altered expression of chemokine and adhesion receptors. *J Exp Med* **199:** 59–68. doi:10.1084/jem.20031175

Berres ML, Lim KP, Peters T, Price J, Takizawa H, Salmon H, Idoyaga J, Ruzo A, Lupo PJ, Hicks MJ, et al. 2014. *BRAF*-V600E expression in precursor versus differentiated dendritic cells defines clinically distinct LCH risk groups. *J Exp Med* **211:** 669–683. doi:10.1084/jem.20130977

Bhatia A, Ulaner G, Rampal R, Hyman DM, Abdel-Wahab O, Durham BH, Dogan A, Ozkaya N, Lacouture ME, Hajdenberg J, et al. 2018. Single-agent dabrafenib for *BRAF*^{V600E}-mutated histiocytosis. *Haematologica* **103:** e177–e180. doi:10.3324/haematol.2017.185298

Bohn JP, Wanner D, Steurer M. 2017. Ibrutinib for relapsed refractory hairy cell leukemia variant. *Leuk Lymphoma* **58:** 1224–1226. doi:10.1080/10428194.2016.1239262

Borys D, Nystrom L, Song A, Lomasney LM. 2016. Erdheim–Chester disease with appendicular skeletal, renal and pleural involvement responding to Zelboraf (*BRAF* inhibitor) treatment: Case report. *Skeletal Radiol* **45:** 1397–1402. doi:10.1007/s00256-016-2431-6

Bouroncle BA, Wiseman BK, Doan CA. 1958. Leukemic reticuloendotheliosis. *Blood* **13:** 609–630. doi:10.1182/blood.V13.7.609.609

Broadbent V, Egeler RM, Nesbit ME Jr. 1994. Langerhans cell histiocytosis—Clinical and epidemiological aspects. *Br J Cancer Suppl* **23:** S11–S16.

Brown NA, Furtado LV, Betz BL, Kiel MJ, Weigelin HC, Lim MS, Elenitoba-Johnson KS. 2014. High prevalence of somatic *MAP2K1* mutations in *BRAF* V600E-negative Langerhans cell histiocytosis. *Blood* **124:** 1655–1658. doi:10.1182/blood-2014-05-577361

Brown RA, Kwong BY, McCalmont TH, Ragsdale B, Ma L, Cheung C, Rieger KE, Arber DA, Kim J. 2015. *ETV3-NCOA2* in indeterminate cell histiocytosis: Clonal translocation supports sui generis. *Blood* **126:** 2344–2345. doi:10.1182/blood-2015-07-655530

Burotto M, Stetler-Stevenson M, Arons E, Zhou H, Wilson W, Kreitman RJ. 2013. Bendamustine and rituximab in relapsed and refractory hairy cell leukemia. *Clin Cancer Res* **19:** 6313–6321. doi:10.1158/1078-0432.CCR-13-1848

Byrd JC, Furman RR, Coutre SE, Burger JA, Blum KA, Coleman M, Wierda WG, Jones JA, Zhao W, Heerema NA, et al. 2015. Three-year follow-up of treatment-naive and previously treated patients with CLL and SLL receiving single-agent ibrutinib. *Blood* **125:** 2497–2506. doi:10.1182/blood-2014-10-606038

Cai J, Huang X, Yin M, Pan C, Song L, Zhan Z, Chen J, Gao Y, Tang J, Li Y, et al. 2019. A novel fusion gene PLEKHA6-NTRK3 in Langerhans cell histiocytosis. *Int J Cancer* **144:** 117–124. doi:10.1002/ijc.31636

Carapeti M, Aguiar RC, Goldman JM, Cross NC. 1998. A novel fusion between MOZ and the nuclear receptor coactivator TIF2 in acute myeloid leukemia. *Blood* **91:** 3127–3133. doi:10.1182/blood.V91.9.3127

Chakraborty R, Hampton OA, Shen X, Simko SJ, Shih A, Abhyankar H, Lim KP, Covington KR, Trevino L, Dewal N, et al. 2014. Mutually exclusive recurrent somatic mutations in *MAP2K1* and *BRAF* support a central role for ERK activation in LCH pathogenesis. *Blood* **124:** 3007–3015. doi:10.1182/blood-2014-05-577825

Chakraborty R, Burke TM, Hampton OA, Zinn DJ, Lim KP, Abhyankar H, Scull B, Kumar V, Kakkar N, Wheeler DA, et al. 2016. Alternative genetic mechanisms of *BRAF* activation in Langerhans cell histiocytosis. *Blood* **128:** 2533–2537. doi:10.1182/blood-2016-08-733790

Chakraborty R, Hampton OA, Abhyankar H, Zinn DJ, Grimes A, Skull B, Eckstein O, Mahmood N, Wheeler DA, Lopez-Terrada D, et al. 2017. Activating *MAPK1* (ERK2) mutation in an aggressive case of disseminated juvenile xanthogranuloma. *Oncotarget* **8:** 46065–46070. doi:10.18632/oncotarget.17521

Chang KTE, Tay AZE, Kuick CH, Chen H, Algar E, Taubenheim N, Campbell J, Mechinaud F, Campbell M, Super L, et al. 2019. ALK-positive histiocytosis: An expanded clinicopathologic spectrum and frequent presence of *KIF5B-ALK* fusion. *Mod Pathol* **32:** 598–608. doi:10.1038/s41379-018-0168-6

Chester W. 1930. Über lipoidgranulomatose. *Virchows Arch Pathol Anat Physiol Klin Med* **279:** 561–602. doi:10.1007/BF01942684

Chihara D, Kantarjian H, O'Brien S, Jorgensen J, Pierce S, Faderl S, Ferrajoli A, Poku R, Jain P, Thompson P, et al. 2016. Long-term durable remission by cladribine followed by rituximab in patients with hairy cell leukaemia: Update of a phase II trial. *Br J Haematol* **174:** 760–766. doi:10.1111/bjh.14129

Chikwava K, Jaffe R. 2004. Langerin (CD207) staining in normal pediatric tissues, reactive lymph nodes, and childhood histiocytic disorders. *Pediatr Dev Pathol* **7:** 607–614. doi:10.1007/s10024-004-3027-z

Christian HA. 1919. Defects in membranous bones, exophthalmos and diabetes insipidus. An unusual syndrome of dyspituitarism—A clinical study. *Contrib Med Biol Res* **1:** 390.

Chung SS, Kim E, Park JH, Chung YR, Lito P, Teruya-Feldstein J, Hu W, Beguelin W, Monette S, Duy C, et al. 2014. Hematopoietic stem cell origin of *BRAF*V600E mutations in hairy cell leukemia. *Sci Transl Med* **6:** 238ra271.

Clipson A, Wang M, de Leval L, Ashton-Key M, Wotherspoon A, Vassiliou G, Bolli N, Grove C, Moody S, Escudero-Ibarz L, et al. 2015. *KLF2* mutation is the most frequent somatic change in splenic marginal zone lymphoma and identifies a subset with distinct genotype. *Leukemia* **29:** 1177–1185. doi:10.1038/leu.2014.330

Cohen-Aubart F, Emile JF, Maksud P, Galanaud D, Idbaih A, Chauvet D, Amar Y, Benameur N, Amoura Z, Haroche J. 2014. Marked efficacy of vemurafenib in suprasellar Erdheim–Chester disease. *Neurology* **83:** 1294–1296. doi:10.1212/WNL.0000000000000832

Cohen Aubart F, Emile JF, Carrat F, Charlotte F, Benameur N, Donadieu J, Maksud P, Idbaih A, Barete S, Hoang-Xuan K, et al. 2017. Targeted therapies in 54 patients with Erdheim–Chester disease, including follow-up after interruption (the LOVE study). *Blood* **130:** 1377–1380. doi:10.1182/blood-2017-03-771873

Cohen Aubart F, Emile JF, Maksud P, Galanaud D, Cluzel P, Benameur N, Aumaitre O, Amoura Z, Haroche J. 2018. Efficacy of the MEK inhibitor cobimetinib for wild-type *BRAF* Erdheim–Chester disease. *Br J Haematol* **180:** 150–153. doi:10.1111/bjh.14284

Cohen-Aubart F, Emile JF, Carrat F, Helias-Rodzewicz Z, Taly V, Charlotte F, Cluzel P, Donadieu J, Idbaih A, Barete S, et al. 2018. Phenotypes and survival in Erdheim–Chester disease: Results from a 165-patient cohort. *Am J Hematol* **93:** E114–E117. doi:10.1002/ajh.25055

Cornet E, Delmer A, Feugier P, Garnache-Ottou F, Ghez D, Leblond V, Levy V, Maloisel F, Re D, Zini JM, et al. 2014. Recommendations of the SFH (French Society of Haematology) for the diagnosis, treatment and follow-up of hairy cell leukaemia. *Ann Hematol* **93:** 1977–1983. doi:10.1007/s00277-014-2140-y

Crispo F, Notarangelo T, Pietrafesa M, Lettini G, Storto G, Sgambato A, Maddalena F, Landriscina M. 2019. *BRAF* inhibitors in thyroid cancer: Clinical impact, mechanisms of resistance and future perspectives. *Cancers (Basel)* **11:** 1388. doi:10.3390/cancers11091388

da Costa CE, Szuhai K, van Eijk R, Hoogeboom M, Sciot R, Mertens F, Björgvinsdóttir H, Debiec-Rychter M, de Krijger RR, Hogendoorn PC, et al. 2009. No genomic aberrations in Langerhans cell histiocytosis as assessed by diverse molecular technologies. *Genes Chromosomes Cancer* **48:** 239–249. doi:10.1002/gcc.20634

Dearden CE, Else M, Catovsky D. 2011. Long-term results for pentostatin and cladribine treatment of hairy cell leukemia. *Leuk Lymphoma* **52** (Suppl 2)**:** 21–24. doi:10.3109/10428194.2011.565093

Degar BA, Rollins BJ. 2009. Langerhans cell histiocytosis: Malignancy or inflammatory disorder doing a great job of imitating one? *Dis Model Mech* **2:** 436–439. doi:10.1242/dmm.004010

Deguchi K, Ayton PM, Carapeti M, Kutok JL, Snyder CS, Williams IR, Cross NC, Glass CK, Cleary ML, Gilliland DG. 2003. MOZ-TIF2-induced acute myeloid leukemia requires the MOZ nucleosome binding motif and TIF2-mediated recruitment of CBP. *Cancer Cell* **3:** 259–271. doi:10.1016/S1535-6108(03)00051-5

Destombes P. 1965. [Adenitis with lipid excess, in children or young adults, seen in the Antilles and in Mali. (4 cases)]. *Bull Soc Pathol Exot Filiales* **58:** 1169–1175.

Diamond EL, Abdel-Wahab O, Pentsova E, Borsu L, Chiu A, Teruya-Feldstein J, Hyman DM, Rosenblum M. 2013. Detection of an *NRAS* mutation in Erdheim–Chester disease. *Blood* **122:** 1089–1091. doi:10.1182/blood-2013-02-482984

Diamond EL, Dagna L, Hyman DM, Cavalli G, Janku F, Estrada-Veras J, Ferrarini M, Abdel-Wahab O, Heaney ML, Scheel PJ, et al. 2014. Consensus guidelines for the diagnosis and clinical management of Erdheim–Chester disease. *Blood* **124:** 483–492. doi:10.1182/blood-2014-03-561381

Diamond EL, Durham BH, Haroche J, Yao Z, Ma J, Parikh SA, Wang Z, Choi J, Kim E, Cohen-Aubart F, et al. 2016. Diverse and targetable kinase alterations drive histiocytic neoplasms. *Cancer Discov* **6:** 154–165. doi:10.1158/2159-8290.CD-15-0913

Diamond EL, Subbiah V, Lockhart AC, Blay JY, Puzanov I, Chau I, Raje NS, Wolf J, Erinjeri JP, Torrisi J, et al. 2018. Vemurafenib for *BRAF* V600–mutant Erdheim–Chester disease and Langerhans cell histiocytosis: Analysis of data from the histology-independent, phase 2, open-label VE-BASKET study. *JAMA Oncol* **4:** 384–388. doi:10.1001/jamaoncol.2017.5029

Diamond EL, Durham BH, Ulaner GA, Drill E, Buthorn J, Ki M, Bitner L, Cho H, Young RJ, Francis JH, et al. 2019. Efficacy of MEK inhibition in patients with histiocytic neoplasms. *Nature* **567:** 521–524. doi:10.1038/s41586-019-1012-y

Dietrich S, Glimm H, Andrulis M, von Kalle C, Ho AD, Zenz T. 2012. *BRAF* inhibition in refractory hairy-cell leukemia. *N Engl J Med* **366:** 2038–2040. doi:10.1056/NEJMc1202124

Dietrich S, Hüllein J, Lee SC, Hutter B, Gonzalez D, Jayne S, Dyer MJ, Oleś M, Else M, Liu X, et al. 2015. Recurrent *CDKN1B* (p27) mutations in hairy cell leukemia. *Blood* **126:** 1005–1008. doi:10.1182/blood-2015-04-643361

Donadieu J, Pritchard J. 1999. Langerhans cell histiocytosis-400 BC. *Med Pediatr Oncol* **33:** 520.

Durham BH. 2019. Molecular characterization of the histiocytoses: Neoplasia of dendritic cells and macrophages. *Semin Cell Dev Biol* **86:** 62–76. doi:10.1016/j.semcdb.2018.03.002

Durham BH, Diamond EL, Abdel-Wahab O. 2016. Histiocytic neoplasms in the era of personalized genomic medicine. *Curr Opin Hematol* **23:** 416–425. doi:10.1097/MOH.0000000000000256

Durham BH, Getta B, Dietrich S, Taylor J, Won H, Bogenberger JM, Scott S, Kim E, Chung YR, Chung SS, et al. 2017a. Genomic analysis of hairy cell leukemia identifies novel recurrent genetic alterations. *Blood* **130:** 1644–1648. doi:10.1182/blood-2017-01-765107

Durham BH, Roos-Weil D, Baillou C, Cohen-Aubart F, Yoshimi A, Miyara M, Papo M, Hélias-Rodzewicz Z, Terrones N, Ozkaya N, et al. 2017b. Functional evidence for derivation of systemic histiocytic neoplasms from hematopoietic stem/progenitor cells. *Blood* **130:** 176–180. doi:10.1182/blood-2016-12-757377

Durham BH, Lopez Rodrigo E, Picarsic J, Abramson D, Rotemberg V, De Munck S, Pannecoucke E, Lu SX, Pastore A, Yoshimi A, et al. 2019. Activating mutations in CSF1R and additional receptor tyrosine kinases in histiocytic neoplasms. *Nat Med* **25:** 1839–1842. doi:10.1038/s41591-019-0653-6

Else M, Dearden CE, Matutes E, Forconi F, Lauria F, Ahmad H, Kelly S, Liyanage A, Ratnayake V, Shankari J, et al. 2011. Rituximab with pentostatin or cladribine: An effective combination treatment for hairy cell leukemia after disease recurrence. *Leuk Lymphoma* **52** (Suppl. 2)**:** 75–78. doi:10.3109/10428194.2011.568650

Else M, Dearden CE, Catovsky D. 2015. Long-term follow-up after purine analogue therapy in hairy cell leukaemia. *Best Pract Res Clin Haematol* **28:** 217–229. doi:10.1016/j.beha.2015.09.004

Emile JF, Diamond EL, Hélias-Rodzewicz Z, Cohen-Aubart F, Charlotte F, Hyman DM, Kim E, Rampal R, Patel M, Ganzel C, et al. 2014. Recurrent *RAS* and *PIK3CA* mutations in Erdheim–Chester disease. *Blood* **124:** 3016–3019. doi:10.1182/blood-2014-04-570937

Emile J, Abla O, Fraitag S, Horne A, Haroche J, Donadieu J, Emile J, Abla O, Fraitag S, Horne A, et al. 2016. Revised classification of histiocytoses and neoplasms of the macrophage-dendritic cell lineages. *Blood* **127:** 2672–2681. doi:10.1182/blood-2016-01-690636

Estrada-Veras JI, O'Brien KJ, Boyd LC, Dave RH, Durham B, Xi L, Malayeri AA, Chen MY, Gardner PJ, Alvarado-Enriquez JR, et al. 2017. The clinical spectrum of Erdheim–Chester disease: An observational cohort study. *Blood Adv* **1:** 357–366. doi:10.1182/bloodadvances.2016001784

Falini B, Martelli MP, Tiacci E. 2016. *BRAF* V600E mutation in hairy cell leukemia: From bench to bedside. *Blood* **128:** 1918–1927. doi:10.1182/blood-2016-07-418434

Farber S. 1941. The nature of "solitary or eosinophilic granuloma" of bone. *Am J Pathol* **17:** 84–102.

Fatobene G, Haroche J, Hélias-Rodzwicz Z, Charlotte F, Taly V, Ferreira AM, Abdo ANR, Rocha V, Emile JF. 2018. *BRAF* V600E mutation detected in a case of Rosai–Dorfman disease. *Haematologica* **103:** e377–e379. doi:10.3324/haematol.2018.190934

Favara BE, Feller AC, Pauli M, Jaffe ES, Weiss LM, Arico M, Bucsky P, Egeler RM, Elinder G, Gadner H, et al. 1997. Contemporary classification of histiocytic disorders. The WHO committee on histiocytic/reticulum cell proliferations. Reclassification working group of the histiocyte society. *Med Pediatr Oncol* **29:** 157–166.

Forconi F, Sozzi E, Cencini E, Zaja F, Intermesoli T, Stelitano C, Rigacci L, Gherlinzoni F, Cantaffa R, Baraldi A, et al. 2009. Hairy cell leukemias with unmutated *IGHV* genes define the minor subset refractory to single-agent cladribine and with more aggressive behavior. *Blood* **114:** 4696–4702. doi:10.1182/blood-2009-03-212449

Gadner H, Minkov M, Grois N, Pötschger U, Thiem E, Aricò M, Astigarraga I, Braier J, Donadieu J, Henter JI, et al. 2013. Therapy prolongation improves outcome in multisystem Langerhans cell histiocytosis. *Blood* **121:** 5006–5014. doi:10.1182/blood-2012-09-455774

Garces S, Medeiros LJ, Patel KP, Li S, Pina-Oviedo S, Li J, Garces JC, Khoury JD, Yin CC. 2017. Mutually exclusive recurrent *KRAS* and *MAP2K1* mutations in Rosai–Dorfman disease. *Mod Pathol* **30:** 1367–1377. doi:10.1038/modpathol.2017.55

Gomez Perdiguero E, Klapproth K, Schulz C, Busch K, Azzoni E, Crozet L, Garner H, Trouillet C, de Bruijn MF, Geissmann F, et al. 2015. Tissue-resident macrophages originate from yolk-sac-derived erythro-myeloid progenitors. *Nature* **518:** 547–551. doi:10.1038/nature13989

Grever MR, Abdel-Wahab O, Andritsos LA, Banerji V, Barrientos J, Blachly JS, Call TG, Catovsky D, Dearden C, Demeter J, et al. 2017. Consensus guidelines for the diagnosis and management of patients with classic hairy cell leukemia. *Blood* **129:** 553–560. doi:10.1182/blood-2016-01-689422

Grois NG, Favara BE, Mostbeck GH, Prayer D. 1998. Central nervous system disease in Langerhans cell histiocytosis. *Hematol Oncol Clin North Am* **12:** 287–305. doi:10.1016/S0889-8588(05)70511-6

Grois N, Fahrner B, Arceci RJ, Henter JI, McClain K, Lassmann H, Nanduri V, Prosch H, Prayer D, Histiocyte Society CNS LCH Study Group. 2010. Central nervous system disease in Langerhans cell histiocytosis. *J Pediatr* **156:** 873–881.e1. doi:10.1016/j.jpeds.2010.03.001

Guyot-Goubin A, Donadieu J, Barkaoui M, Bellec S, Thomas C, Clavel J. 2008. Descriptive epidemiology of childhood Langerhans cell histiocytosis in France, 2000–2004. *Pediatr Blood Cancer* **51:** 71–75. doi:10.1002/pbc.21498

Hand A. 1893. Polyuria and tuberculosis. *Arch Pediatr* **10:** 673–675.

Haroche J, Abla O. 2015. Uncommon histiocytic disorders: Rosai–Dorfman, juvenile xanthogranuloma, and Erdheim–Chester disease. *Hematology Am Soc Hematol Educ Program* **2015:** 571–578. doi:10.1182/asheducation-2015.1.571

Haroche J, Charlotte F, Arnaud L, von Deimling A, Hélias-Rodzewicz Z, Hervier B, Cohen-Aubart F, Launay D, Lesot A, Mokhtari K, et al. 2012. High prevalence of *BRAF* V600E mutations in Erdheim–Chester disease but not in other non-Langerhans cell histiocytoses. *Blood* **120:** 2700–2703. doi:10.1182/blood-2012-05-430140

Haroche J, Cohen-Aubart F, Emile JF, Arnaud L, Maksud P, Charlotte F, Cluzel P, Drier A, Hervier B, Benameur N, et al. 2013. Dramatic efficacy of vemurafenib in both multisystemic and refractory Erdheim-Chester disease and Langerhans cell histiocytosis harboring the *BRAF* V600E mutation. *Blood* **121:** 1495–1500. doi:10.1182/blood-2012-07-446286

Haroche J, Cohen-Aubart F, Emile JF, Maksud P, Drier A, Tolédano D, Barete S, Charlotte F, Cluzel P, Donadieu J, et al. 2015. Reproducible and sustained efficacy of targeted therapy with vemurafenib in patients with *BRAF*^{V600E}-mutated Erdheim–Chester disease. *J Clin Oncol* **33:** 411–418. doi:10.1200/JCO.2014.57.1950

Haroche J, Cohen-Aubart F, Rollins BJ, Donadieu J, Charlotte F, Idbaih A, Vaglio A, Abdel-Wahab O, Emile JF, Amoura Z. 2017. Histiocytoses: Emerging neoplasia behind inflammation. *Lancet Oncol* **18:** e113–e125. doi:10.1016/S1470-2045(17)30031-1

Héritier S, Saffroy R, Radosevic-Robin N, Pothin Y, Pacquement H, Peuchmaur M, Lemoine A, Haroche J, Donadieu J, Emile JF. 2015. Common cancer-associated *PIK3CA* activating mutations rarely occur in Langerhans cell histiocytosis. *Blood* **125:** 2448–2449. doi:10.1182/blood-2015-01-625491

Héritier S, Hélias-Rodzewicz Z, Chakraborty R, Sengal AG, Bellanné-Chantelot C, Thomas C, Moreau A, Fraitag S, Allen CE, Donadieu J, et al. 2017. New somatic *BRAF* splicing mutation in Langerhans cell histiocytosis. *Mol Cancer* **16:** 115. doi:10.1186/s12943-017-0690-z

Héritier S, Barkaoui MA, Miron J, Thomas C, Moshous D, Lambilliotte A, Mazingue F, Kebaili K, Jeziorski E, Plat G, et al. 2018. Incidence and risk factors for clinical neurodegenerative Langerhans cell histiocytosis: A longitudinal cohort study. *Br J Haematol* **183:** 608–617. doi:10.1111/bjh.15577

Holderfield M, Deuker MM, McCormick F, McMahon M. 2014. Targeting RAF kinases for cancer therapy: *BRAF*-mutated melanoma and beyond. *Nat Rev Cancer* **14:** 455–467. doi:10.1038/nrc3760

Hyman DM, Puzanov I, Subbiah V, Faris JE, Chau I, Blay JY, Wolf J, Raje NS, Diamond EL, Hollebecque A, et al. 2015. Vemurafenib in multiple nonmelanoma cancers with *BRAF* V600 mutations. *N Engl J Med* **373:** 726–736. doi:10.1056/NEJMoa1502309

Jallades L, Baseggio L, Sujobert P, Huet S, Chabane K, Callet-Bauchu E, Verney A, Hayette S, Desvignes JP, Salgado D, et al. 2017. Exome sequencing identifies recurrent *BCOR* alterations and the absence of *KLF2*, *TNFAIP3* and *MYD88* mutations in splenic diffuse red pulp small B-cell lymphoma. *Haematologica* **102:** 1758–1766. doi:10.3324/haematol.2016.160192

Jebaraj BM, Kienle D, Bühler A, Winkler D, Dohner H, Stilgenbauer S, Zenz T. 2013. *BRAF* mutations in chronic lymphocytic leukemia. *Leuk Lymphoma* **54:** 1177–1182. doi:10.3109/10428194.2012.742525

Kansal R, Quintanilla-Martinez L, Datta V, Lopategui J, Garshfield G, Nathwani BN. 2013. Identification of the V600D mutation in Exon 15 of the *BRAF* oncogene in congenital, benign Langerhans cell histiocytosis. *Genes Chromosomes Cancer* **52:** 99–106. doi:10.1002/gcc.22010

Kreitman RJ, Wilson W, Calvo KR, Arons E, Roth L, Sapolsky J, Zhou H, Raffeld M, Stetler-Stevenson M. 2013. Cladribine with immediate rituximab for the treatment of patients with variant hairy cell leukemia. *Clin Cancer Res* **19:** 6873–6881. doi:10.1158/1078-0432.CCR-13-1752

Kreitman RJ, Dearden C, Zinzani PL, Delgado J, Karlin L, Robak T, Gladstone DE, le Coutre P, Dietrich S, Gotic M, et al. 2018. Moxetumomab pasudotox in relapsed/refractory hairy cell leukemia. *Leukemia* **32:** 1768-1777. doi:10.1038/s41375-018-0210-1

Laman JD, Leenen PJ, Annels NE, Hogendoorn PC, Egeler RM. 2003. Langerhans-cell histiocytosis 'insight into DC biology'. *Trends Immunol* **24:** 190–196. doi:10.1016/S1471-4906(03)00063-2

Lampert F. 1998. Langerhans cell histiocytosis. Historical perspectives. *Hematol Oncol Clin North Am* **12:** 213–219. doi:10.1016/S0889-8588(05)70506-2

Lee LH, Gasilina A, Roychoudhury J, Clark J, McCormack FX, Pressey J, Grimley MS, Lorsbach R, Ali S, Bailey M, et al. 2017. Real-time genomic profiling of histiocytoses identifies early-kinase domain *BRAF* alterations while improving treatment outcomes. *JCI Insight* **2:** e89473.

Leeksma AC, Taylor J, Wu B, Gardner JR, He J, Nahas M, Gonen M, Alemayehu WG, Te Raa D, Walther T, et al. 2019. Clonal diversity predicts adverse outcome in chronic lymphocytic leukemia. *Leukemia* **33:** 390–402. doi:10.1038/s41375-018-0215-9

Letterer E. 1924. Aleukämische Retikulose ein Beitrag zu den Proliferativen Erkraukungen des Retikuloendothelial Apparates. *Frankfurt Z Pathol* **50:** 377–393.

Lichtenstein L. 1953. Histiocytosis X: Integration of eosinophilic granuloma of bone," Letterer–Siwe disease," and "Schuller–Christian disease" as related manifestations of a single nosologic entity. *Arch Pathol* **56:** 84–102.

Lohr JG, Stojanov P, Carter SL, Cruz-Gordillo P, Lawrence MS, Auclair D, Sougnez C, Knoechel B, Gould J, Saksena G, et al. 2014. Widespread genetic heterogeneity in multiple myeloma: Implications for targeted therapy. *Cancer Cell* **25:** 91–101. doi:10.1016/j.ccr.2013.12.015

Maitre E, Bertrand P, Maingonnat C, Viailly PJ, Wiber M, Naguib D, Salaun V, Cornet E, Damaj G, Sola B, et al. 2018. New generation sequencing of targeted genes in the classical and the variant form of hairy cell leukemia highlights mutations in epigenetic regulation genes. *Oncotarget* **9:** 28866–28876. doi:10.18632/oncotarget.25601

Maitre E, Cornet E, Troussard X. 2019. Hairy cell leukemia: 2020 update on diagnosis, risk stratification, and treatment. *Am J Hematol* **94:** 1413–1422. doi:10.1002/ajh.25653

Mass E, Jacome-Galarza CE, Blank T, Lazarov T, Durham BH, Ozkaya N, Pastore A, Schwabenland M, Chung YR, Rosenblum MK, et al. 2017. A somatic mutation in erythro-myeloid progenitors causes neurodegenerative disease. *Nature* **549:** 389–393. doi:10.1038/nature23672

McClain KL, Natkunam Y, Swerdlow SH. 2004. Atypical cellular disorders. *Hematology* **2004:** 283–296. doi:10.1182/asheducation-2004.1.283

McDonagh J, McDonagh J. 1912. A contribution to our knowledge of the naevo-xantho-endotheliomata. *Br J Dermatol* **24:** 85–99. doi:10.1111/j.1365-2133.1912.tb16720.x

Merad M, Manz MG, Karsunky H, Wagers A, Peters W, Charo I, Weissman IL, Cyster JG, Engleman EG. 2002. Langerhans cells renew in the skin throughout life under steady-state conditions. *Nat Immunol* **3:** 1135–1141. doi:10.1038/ni852

Mesquita B, Lopes P, Rodrigues A, Pereira D, Afonso M, Leal C, Henrique R, Lind GE, Jeronimo C, Lothe RA, et al. 2013. Frequent copy number gains at 1q21 and 1q32 are associated with overexpression of the ETS transcription factors *ETV3* and *ELF3* in breast cancer irrespective of molecular subtypes. *Breast Cancer Res Treat* **138:** 37–45. doi:10.1007/s10549-013-2408-2

Milne P, Bigley V, Bacon CM, Néel A, McGovern N, Bomken S, Haniffa M, Diamond EL, Durham BH, Visser J, et al. 2017. Hematopoietic origin of Langerhans cell histiocytosis and Erdheim–Chester disease in adults. *Blood* **130:** 167–175. doi:10.1182/blood-2016-12-757823

Nelson DS, Quispel W, Badalian-Very G, van Halteren AG, van den Bos C, Bovée JV, Tian SY, Van Hummelen P, Ducar M, MacConaill LE, et al. 2014. Somatic activating ARAF mutations in Langerhans cell histiocytosis. *Blood* **123:** 3152–3155. doi:10.1182/blood-2013-06-511139

Nelson DS, van Halteren A, Quispel WT, van den Bos C, Bovée JV, Patel B, Badalian-Very G, van Hummelen P, Ducar M, Lin L, et al. 2015. *MAP2K1* and *MAP3K1* mutations in Langerhans cell histiocytosis. *Genes Chromosomes Cancer* **54:** 361–368. doi:10.1002/gcc.22247

Nezelof C, Basset F. 2001. From histiocytosis X to Langerhans cell histiocytosis: A personal account. *Int J Surg Pathol* **9:** 137–146. doi:10.1177/106689690100900208

Nezelof C, Basset F, Rousseau M. 1973. Histiocytosis X histogenetic arguments for a Langerhans cell origin. *Biomedicine* **18:** 365–371.

Nordmann TM, Juengling FD, Recher M, Berger CT, Kalbermatten D, Wicki A, Paasinen-Sohns A, Cathomas G, Tzankov A, Daikeler T. 2017. Trametinib after disease reactivation under dabrafenib in Erdheim–Chester disease with both *BRAF* and *KRAS* mutations. *Blood* **129:** 879–882. doi:10.1182/blood-2016-09-740217

O'Malley DP, Agrawal R, Grimm KE, Hummel J, Glazyrin A, Dim DC, Madhusudhana S, Weiss LM. 2015. Evidence of *BRAF* V600E in indeterminate cell tumor and interdigitating dendritic cell sarcoma. *Ann Diagn Pathol* **19:** 113–116. doi:10.1016/j.anndiagpath.2015.02.008

Ozkaya N, Rosenblum MK, Durham BH, Pichardo JD, Abdel-Wahab O, Hameed MR, Busam KJ, Travis WD, Diamond EL, Dogan A. 2018. The histopathology of Erdheim–Chester disease: A comprehensive review of a molecularly characterized cohort. *Mod Pathol* **31:** 581–597. doi:10.1038/modpathol.2017.160

Ozono S, Inada H, Nakagawa SI, Ueda K, Matsumura H, Kojima S, Koga H, Hashimoto T, Oshima K, Matsuishi T. 2011. Juvenile myelomonocytic leukemia characterized by cutaneous lesion containing Langerhans cell histiocytosis-like cells. *Int J Hematol* **93:** 389–393. doi:10.1007/s12185-011-0787-x

Papaemmanuil E, Gerstung M, Bullinger L, Gaidzik VI, Paschka P, Roberts ND, Potter NE, Heuser M, Thol F, Bolli N, et al. 2016. Genomic classification and prognosis in acute myeloid leukemia. *N Engl J Med* **374:** 2209–2221. doi:10.1056/NEJMoa1516192

Pettirossi V, Santi A, Imperi E, Russo G, Pucciarini A, Bigerna B, Schiavoni G, Fortini E, Spanhol-Rosseto A, Sportoletti P, et al. 2015. *BRAF* inhibitors reverse the unique molecular signature and phenotype of hairy cell leukemia and exert potent antileukemic activity. *Blood* **125:** 1207–1216. doi:10.1182/blood-2014-10-603100

Piva R, Deaglio S, Famà R, Buonincontri R, Scarfò I, Bruscaggin A, Mereu E, Serra S, Spina V, Brusa D, et al. 2015. The Krüppel-like factor 2 transcription factor gene is recurrently mutated in splenic marginal zone lymphoma. *Leukemia* **29:** 503–507. doi:10.1038/leu.2014.294

Poret N, Fu Q, Guihard S, Cheok M, Miller K, Zeng G, Quesnel B, Troussard X, Galiègue-Zouitina S, Shelley CS. 2015. CD38 in hairy cell leukemia is a marker of poor prognosis and a new target for therapy. *Cancer Res* **75:** 3902–3911. doi:10.1158/0008-5472.CAN-15-0893

Raje N, Chau I, Hyman DM, Ribrag V, Blay JY, Tabernero J, Elez E, Wolf J, Yee AJ, Kaiser M, et al. 2018. Vemurafenib in patients with relapsed refractory multiple myeloma harboring $BRAF^{V600}$ mutations: A cohort of the histology-independent VE-BASKET Study. *JCO Precis Oncol* **2:** 1–9. doi:10.1200/PO.18.00070

Rezk SA, Spagnolo DV, Brynes RK, Weiss LM. 2008. Indeterminate cell tumor: A rare dendritic neoplasm. *Am J Surg Pathol* **32:** 1868–1876. doi:10.1097/PAS.0b013e31818593d6

Rosai J, Dorfman RF. 1969. Sinus histiocytosis with massive lymphadenopathy. A newly recognized benign clinicopathological entity. *Arch Pathol* **87:** 63–70.

Rosai J, Dorfman RF. 1972. Sinus histiocytosis with massive lymphadenopathy: A pseudolymphomatous benign disorder. Analysis of 34 cases. *Cancer* **30:** 1174–1188. doi:10.1002/1097-0142(197211)30:5<1174::AID-CNCR2820300507>3.0.CO;2-S

Sadeghi N, Li HC. 2018. MRD-negative complete remission in relapsed refractory hairy cell leukemia with bendamustine and obinutuzumab. *Ann Hematol* **97:** 723–724. doi:10.1007/s00277-017-3219-z

Sarvaria A, Topp Z, Saven A. 2016. Current therapy and new directions in the treatment of hairy cell leukemia: A review. *JAMA Oncol* **2:** 123–129. doi:10.1001/jamaoncol.2015.4134

Satoh T, Smith A, Sarde A, Lu HC, Mian S, Trouillet C, Mufti G, Emile JF, Fraternali F, Donadieu J, et al. 2012. B-RAF mutant alleles associated with Langerhans cell histiocytosis, a granulomatous pediatric disease. *PLoS One* **7:** e33891. doi:10.1371/journal.pone.0033891

Schüller A. 1915. Über eigenartige schädeldefekte im jugendalter. *Fortschr Röntgenstr* **23:** 1916.

Senechal B, Elain G, Jeziorski E, Grondin V, Patey-Mariaud de Serre N, Jaubert F, Beldjord K, Lellouch A, Glorion C, Zerah M, et al. 2007. Expansion of regulatory T cells in patients with Langerhans cell histiocytosis. *PLoS Med* **4:** e253. doi:10.1371/journal.pmed.0040253

Shalem O, Sanjana NE, Hartenian E, Shi X, Scott DA, Mikkelson T, Heckl D, Ebert BL, Root DE, Doench JG, et al. 2014. Genome-scale CRISPR–Cas9 knockout screening in human cells. *Science* **343:** 84–87. doi:10.1126/science.1247005

Shanmugam V, Margolskee E, Kluk M, Giorgadze T, Orazi A. 2016. Rosai–Dorfman disease harboring an activating KRAS K117N missense mutation. *Head Neck Pathol* **10:** 394–399. doi:10.1007/s12105-016-0709-6

Siwe SA. 1933. Die reiticuloendotheliose—ein neues krankheitsbild unter den hepatosphlenomegalien. *Eur J Pediatr* **55:** 212–247.

Stålemark H, Laurencikas E, Karis J, Gavhed D, Fadeel B, Henter JI. 2008. Incidence of Langerhans cell histiocytosis in children: A population-based study. *Pediatr Blood Cancer* **51:** 76–81. doi:10.1002/pbc.21504

Strehl S, Nebral K, Konig M, Harbott J, Strobl H, Ratei R, Struski S, Bielorai B, Lessard M, Zimmermann M, et al. 2008. *ETV6-NCOA2*: A novel fusion gene in acute leukemia associated with coexpression of T-lymphoid and myeloid markers and frequent *NOTCH1* mutations. *Clin Cancer Res* **14:** 977–983. doi:10.1158/1078-0432.CCR-07-4022

Sumegi J, Streblow R, Frayer RW, Dal Cin P, Rosenberg A, Meloni-Ehrig A, Bridge JA. 2010. Recurrent t(2;2) and t(2;8) translocations in rhabdomyosarcoma without the canonical *PAX-FOXO1* fuse *PAX3* to members of the nuclear receptor transcriptional coactivator family. *Genes Chromosomes Cancer* **49:** 224–236.

Swerdlow SH, Campo E, Harris NL, Jaffe ES, Pileri SA, Stein H, Thiele J. 2017. *WHO classification of tumours of haematopoietic and lymphoid tissues, revised 4th ed.* International Agency for Research on Cancer, Lyon.

Taylor J, Pavlick D, Yoshimi A, Marcelus C, Chung SS, Hechtman JF, Benayed R, Cocco E, Durham BH, Bitner L, et al. 2018. Oncogenic TRK fusions are amenable to inhibition in hematologic malignancies. *J Clin Invest* **128:** 3819–3825. doi:10.1172/JCI120787

Techavichit P, Sosothikul D, Chaichana T, Teerapakpinyo C, Thorner PS, Shuangshoti S. 2017. *BRAF* V600E mutation in pediatric intracranial and cranial juvenile xanthogranuloma. *Hum Pathol* **69:** 118–122. doi:10.1016/j.humpath.2017.04.026

Thompson PA, Ravandi F. 2017. How I manage patients with hairy cell leukaemia. *Br J Haematol* **177:** 543–556. doi:10.1111/bjh.14524

Tiacci E, Trifonov V, Schiavoni G, Holmes A, Kern W, Martelli MP, Pucciarini A, Bigerna B, Pacini R, Wells VA, et al. 2011. *BRAF* mutations in hairy-cell leukemia. *N Engl J Med* **364:** 2305–2315. doi:10.1056/NEJMoa1014209

Tiacci E, Park JH, De Carolis L, Chung SS, Broccoli A, Scott S, Zaja F, Devlin S, Pulsoni A, Chung YR, et al. 2015. Targeting mutant *BRAF* in relapsed or refractory hairy-cell leukemia. *N Engl J Med* **373:** 1733–1747. doi:10.1056/NEJMoa1506583

Trunzer K, Pavlick AC, Schuchter L, Gonzalez R, McArthur GA, Hutson TE, Moschos SJ, Flaherty KT, Kim KB, Weber JS, et al. 2013. Pharmacodynamic effects and mechanisms of resistance to vemurafenib in patients with metastatic melanoma. *J Clin Oncol* **31:** 1767–1774. doi:10.1200/JCO.2012.44.7888

Tschernitz S, Flossbach L, Bonengel M, Roth S, Rosenwald A, Geissinger E. 2014. Alternative *BRAF* mutations in *BRAF* V600E-negative hairy cell leukaemias. *Br J Haematol* **165:** 529–533. doi:10.1111/bjh.12735

Vaglio A, Diamond EL. 2017. Erdheim–Chester disease: The "targeted" revolution. *Blood* **130:** 1282–1284. doi:10.1182/blood-2017-07-795054

Veyssier-Belot C, Cacoub P, Caparros-Lefebvre D, Wechsler J, Brun B, Remy M, Wallaert B, Petit H, Grimaldi A, Wechsler B, et al. 1996. Erdheim–Chester disease. Clinical and radiologic characteristics of 59 cases. *Medicine (Baltimore)* **75:** 157–169. doi:10.1097/00005792-199605000-00005

Wander SA, Hasserjian RP, Oduro K, Glomski K, Nardi V, Cote GM, Graubert TA, Brunner AM, Chen YBA, Fathi AT. 2017. Combined targeted therapy for *BRAF*-mutant, treatment-related acute myeloid leukemia. *JCO Precis Oncol* **1:** 1–7. doi:10.1200/PO.16.00032

Wang L, Motoi T, Khanin R, Olshen A, Mertens F, Bridge J, Dal Cin P, Antonescu CR, Singer S, Hameed M, et al. 2012. Identification of a novel, recurrent *HEY1-NCOA2* fusion in mesenchymal chondrosarcoma based on a genome-wide screen of exon-level expression data. *Genes Chromosomes Cancer* **51:** 127–139. doi:10.1002/gcc.20937

Waterfall JJ, Arons E, Walker RL, Pineda M, Roth L, Killian JK, Abaan OD, Davis SR, Kreitman RJ, Meltzer PS. 2014. High prevalence of MAP2K1 mutations in variant and IGHV4-34-expressing hairy-cell leukemias. *Nat Genet* **46:** 8–10. doi:10.1038/ng.2828

Weitzman S, Jaffe R. 2005. Uncommon histiocytic disorders: The non-Langerhans cell histiocytoses. *Pediatr Blood Cancer* **45:** 256–264. doi:10.1002/pbc.20246

Wellbrock C, Karasarides M, Marais R. 2004. The RAF proteins take centre stage. *Nat Rev Mol Cell Biol* **5:** 875–885. doi:10.1038/nrm1498

Whittaker SR, Theurillat JP, Van Allen E, Wagle N, Hsiao J, Cowley GS, Schadendorf D, Root DE, Garraway LA. 2013. A genome-scale RNA interference screen implicates NF1 loss in resistance to RAF inhibition. *Cancer Discov* **3:** 350–362. doi:10.1158/2159-8290.CD-12-0470

Wood GS, Hu CH, Beckstead JH, Turner RR, Winkelmann RK. 1985. The indeterminate cell proliferative disorder: Report of a case manifesting as an unusual cutaneous histiocytosis. *J Dermatol Surg Oncol* **11:** 1111–1119. doi:10.1111/j.1524-4725.1985.tb01399.x

Xi L, Arons E, Navarro W, Calvo KR, Stetler-Stevenson M, Raffeld M, Kreitman RJ. 2012. Both variant and IGHV4-34-expressing hairy cell leukemia lack the *BRAF* V600E mutation. *Blood* **119:** 3330–3332. doi:10.1182/blood-2011-09-379339

Zarnegar S, Durham BH, Khattar P, Shukla NN, Benayed R, Lacouture ME, Lavi E, Lyden DC, Diamond EL, Dunkel IJ, et al. 2018. Novel activating *BRAF* fusion identifies a recurrent alternative mechanism for ERK activation in pediatric Langerhans cell histiocytosis. *Pediatr Blood Cancer* **65:** e26699. doi:10.1002/pbc.26699

Non-Hodgkin Lymphomas: Malignancies Arising from Mature B Cells

Jennifer Shingleton, Jie Wang, Carolyn Baloh, Tushar Dave, Nicholas Davis, Lanie Happ, Othmane Jadi, Rachel Kositsky, Xiang Li, Cassandra Love, Razvan Panea, Qiu Qin, Anupama Reddy, Naina Singhi, Eileen Smith, Devang Thakkar, and Sandeep S. Dave

Department of Medicine and Center for Genomic and Computational Biology, Duke Cancer Institute, Duke University, Durham, North Carolina 27707, USA

Correspondence: Sandeep.dave@duke.edu

Non-Hodgkin lymphomas (NHLs) are a diverse group of entities, both clinically and molecularly. Here, we review the evolution of classification schemes in B-cell lymphoma, noting the now standard WHO classification system that is based on immune cell-of-origin and molecular phenotypes. We review how lymphomas arise throughout the B-cell development process as well as the molecular and clinical features of prominent B-cell lymphomas. We provide an overview of the major progress that has occurred over the past decade in terms of our molecular understanding of these diseases. We discuss treatment options available and focus on a number of the diverse research tools that have been employed to improve our understanding of these diseases. We discuss the problem of heterogeneity in lymphomas and anticipate that the near future will bring significant advances that provide a measurable impact on NHL outcomes.

Non-Hodgkin lymphomas (NHLs) are cancers that arise predominantly from mature B lymphocytes, white blood cells responsible for humoral immunity. These malignancies are common, affecting nearly 75,000 new patients each year in the United States alone. Lymphomas represent a striking degree of diversity in molecular origins and clinical behavior. Efforts to classify lymphomas were initially developed based on the recognition of the varying clinical aggressiveness of the disease. This early classification ("Working Formulation" [Robb-Smith 1982]) has since been supplanted by more biological approaches that have culminated in the now standard, but still evolving, World Health Organization (WHO) classification that is guided by immune cell lineage (Swerdlow et al. 2017).

B-cell development sets the stage for the acquisition of a number of different genetic alterations that result in a tumor with a stage-specific immunophenotype, including cell surface markers and a gene expression profile that reflects the normal cell of origin. This resemblance to the normal cell of origin in lymphoid development serves as the foundation for the WHO classification of lymphomas.

Cite this article as *Cold Spring Harb Perspect Med* doi: 10.1101/cshperspect.a034843

Here, we describe our current understanding of the pathogenesis, underlying biology, and clinical treatment of NHLs.

LYMPHOCYTE DEVELOPMENT AND LYMPHOMAGENESIS

Although lymphomas can arise from either B or T cells, the vast majority of lymphomas arise from B cells. B cells undergo a complex and well-regulated program of development beginning in the bone marrow before terminally differentiating into mature effector cells following antigen stimulation (Fig. 1). In the bone marrow, the earliest progenitor B cells begin to undergo rearrangement of the immunoglobulin gene locus, giving rise to a unique antigen-binding B-cell receptor (BCR) comprised of heavy and light peptide chains that both contain variable and constant regions. The variable region of the heavy chain locus (IGH) is composed of variable (V), diversity (D), and joining (J) segments, whereas the variable regions of the light chain loci (IGK and IGL) contain only V and J segments. During B-cell differentiation, a random assortment of V, D, and J segments is chosen in each pre-B cell, which leads a BCR repertoire size on the order of 10^{10}. Certain lymphomas show preferential selection of particular V(D)J segments. For instance, in particular, mucosa-associated lymphoid tissue (MALT) lymphomas frequently manifest identical V segments, whereas certain V(D)J recombinations are preferentially selected in B-cell chronic lymphocytic leukemias (B-CLLs) (Fais et al. 1998; Widhopf and Kipps 2001; Zucca and Bertoni 2004; Ghiotto et al. 2006). These data point to the role of particular antigens, including autoantibodies, in the development of these lymphomas.

Following initial recognition of a foreign antigen by the BCR, B-cell immunoglobulin genes undergo somatic hypermutation (SHM) in lymphoid tissue germinal centers (GCs) (Di Noia and Neuberger 2007). The process of SHM refines the affinity of the antibodies produced by B cells and further increases the antibody repertoire. The diversity of antibodies created during SHM is caused by direct mutagenesis of nucleotides in the variable region by the enzyme AID, encoded by *AICDA* (activation-induced cytidine deaminase) (Maul and Gearhart 2010). The SHM status of malignant cells in a tumor can be an additional indicator of the stage of B-cell maturation of the lymphoma cell of origin.

In parallel, at different stages of development, B-lineage cells express one of nine constant region gene segments corresponding to different immunoglobulin heavy chain isotypes with various effector functions. Only IgM is expressed in immature B cells. As B cells mature, they gain the ability to produce either IgM or IgD through alternative splicing mechanisms directed by AID. Upon activation, B cells in the GC undergo class switch recombination (CSR), which brings additional *IG* variable regions into proximity with one of the constant region gene segments to produce IgG, IgA, or IgE (Li et al. 2004).

The rearrangements associated with BCR formation in the GC can go awry and result in powerful oncogenic signals that transform B cells. Indeed, a majority of B-cell lymphomas arise from GC B cells. For instance, Burkitt lymphoma is associated with a translocation of the *MYC* gene to one of the *IG* loci, dysregulating the *MYC* gene more than 100-fold, a scale that makes Burkitt lymphoma one of the fastest growing tumors (Molyneux et al. 2012). Likewise, *BCL2* is commonly deregulated in GC B-cell-derived lymphomas including follicular lymphoma and diffuse large B-cell lymphomas (Takata et al. 2014; Reddy et al. 2017; Chapuy et al. 2018; Schmitz et al. 2018).

CLASSIFICATION OF B-CELL LYMPHOMAS

Lymphomas can be broadly divided into four categories: B-cell lymphomas, T-cell lymphomas, cutaneous lymphomas, and lymphomas related to transplant and immunodeficiency. This section describes these categories and the most common lymphoma types in each category (summarized in Table 1).

As discussed above, the nature of the GC reaction leaves B cells vulnerable to genetic alterations that lead to lymphoma. The morphological, antigen-expression, and genetic features of each B-cell lymphoma subtype often mirror

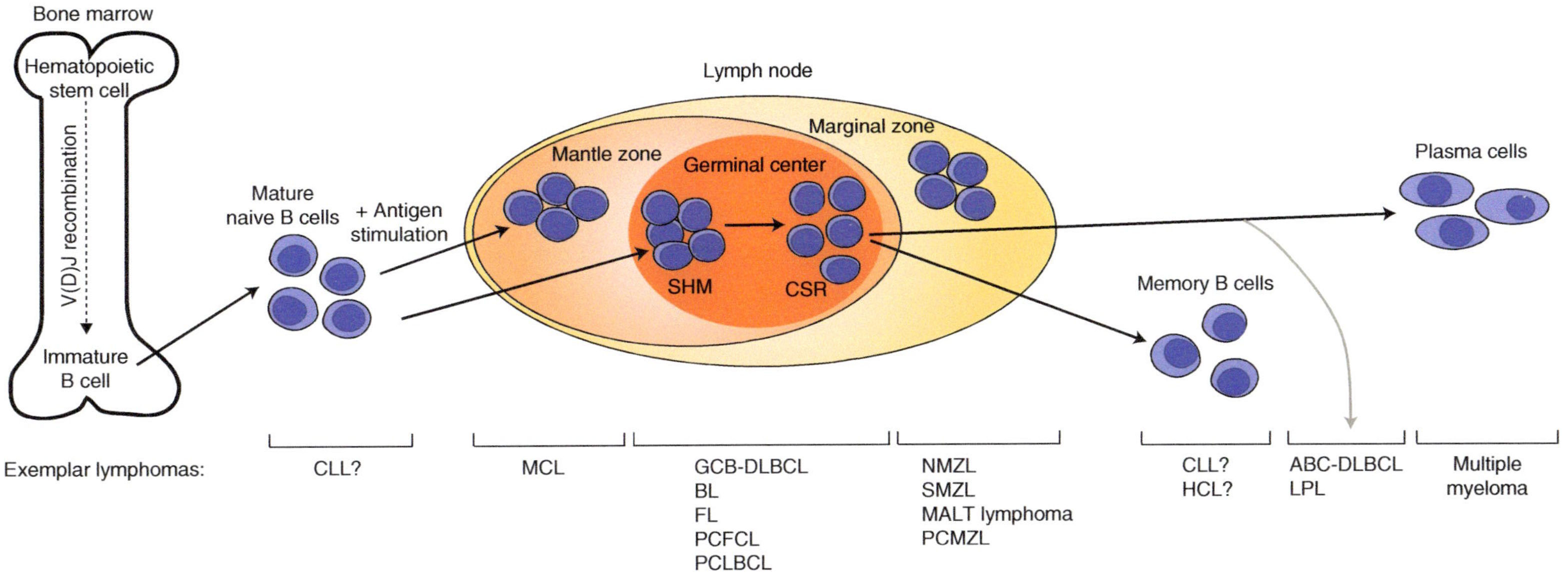

Figure 1. B-cell development. Progenitor B cells undergo V(D)J recombination in the bone marrow before exiting at the immature B-cell stage. Upon antigen stimulation, mature B cells undergo somatic hypermutation (SHM) and class-switch recombination (CSR) in the germinal center before undergoing terminal differentiation into plasma or memory B cells. Examples of lymphomas that can arise at each B-cell stage are noted. HSC, hematopoietic stem cell; CLL, chronic lymphocytic leukemia; MCL, mantle cell lymphoma; GCB-DLBCL, germinal center B-cell diffuse large B-cell lymphoma; BL, Burkitt lymphoma; FL, follicular lymphoma; PCFCL, primary cutaneous follicle center lymphoma; PCLBCL, primary cutaneous large B-cell lymphoma; NMZL, nodal marginal zone lymphoma; SMZL, splenic marginal zone lymphoma; MALT, mucosa-associated lymphoid tissue; PCMZL, primary cutaneous marginal zone lymphoma; HCL, hairy cell leukemia; ABC-DLBCL, activated B-cell like DLBCL; LPL, lymphoplasmacytic lymphoma.

Table 1. The genetic features of B-cell lymphoma

Type	Recurrent translocations (if known)	Recurrently mutated genes (if known)
Pre-germinal center origin		
B-cell prolymphocytic leukemia (B-PLL)	t(8;14)(MYC/IGH), t(2;8)(IGK/MYC), t(8;22)(MYC/IGL)	*MYC, TP53*
Mantle cell lymphoma	t(11;14)(CCND1/IGH), t(2;11)(IGK/CCND1), t(11;22)(CCND1/IGL), t(8;14)(MYC/IGH), t(3;14)(BCL6/IGH)	*ATM, CCND1, KMT2D, NOTCH1/2, TP53*
Germinal center origin		
Burkitt lymphoma	t(8;14)(MYC/IGH), t(2;8)(IGK/MYC), t(8;22)(MYC/IGL)	*MYC, ID3, DDX3X, TP53, TCF3, CCND3, RHOA, SMARCA4, ARID1A*
Diffuse large B-cell lymphoma (DLBCL), NOS	BCL2, BCL6, and MYC rearrangements	*EZH2, SGK1, GNA13, MYD88, ETV6, CD78B*
Follicular lymphoma	t(14;18)(IGH/BCL2)	*BCL2, KMT2D, EZH2, BCL6, CREBBP, EP300, FAS, MEF2B*
Follicular lymphoma (pediatric type)	None	*TNFRSF14, MAP2K1*
High-grade B-cell lymphoma with MYC and BCL2 and/or BCL6 rearrangements	MYC, BCL2, and/or BCL6 rearrangements	*TP53, MYD88, ID3*
Primary diffuse large B-cell lymphoma of the CNS	IG genes, BCL6 and MYC rearrangements	*MYD88, CD79B, INPP5D, CBL, BLNK, CARD11, MALT1, BCL2*
Post-germinal center origin		
ALK-positive large B-cell lymphoma	t(2;17)(ALK/CLTC), t(2;5)(ALK/NPM), ALK rearrangements with SQSTM1, SEC31A	
Chronic lymphocytic leukemia (CLL)/Small lymphocytic lymphoma (SLL)	t(14;18)(IGH/BCL2), t(14;19)(IGH/BCL3)	*NOTCH1, SF3B1, TP53, ATM, BIRC3, POT1, MYD88*
Extranodal marginal zone lymphoma of mucosa-associated lymphoid tissue (MALT lymphoma)	t(11;18)(BIRC3/MALT1), t(14;18)(IGH/MALT1), t(1;14)(BCL10/IGH), t(3;14)(FOXP1/IGH)	*MYD88*
Hairy cell leukemia	None	*BRAF, MAP2K1*
Hairy cell leukemia variant		*TP53, MAP2K1*
Lymphoplasmacytic lymphoma (LPL)/Waldenstrom's macroglobulinemia (WM)	None	*MYD88, CXCR4, ARID1A, TP53, CD79B, KMT2D, MYBBP1A*
Nodal marginal zone lymphoma	None	
Plasmablastic lymphoma	MYC rearrangements with IG genes	
Primary effusion lymphoma	None	*BCL6*

Continued

Table 1. *Continued*

Type	Recurrent translocations (if known)	Recurrently mutated genes (if known)
Splenic marginal zone lymphoma	t(14;18)(IGH/BCL2), t(11;14)(CCND1/IGH), t(11;18)(BIRC3/MALT1), t(14;18)(IGH/MALT1), t(1;14)(BCL10/IGH), t(2;7)(IGK/CDK6)	*NOTCH2, KLF2*
Cutaneous lymphomas		
Primary cutaneous diffuse large B-cell lymphoma, leg-type	t(3;14)(BCL6/IGH), t(8;14)(MYC/IGH)	*MYD88, CARD11, CD78B, TNFAIP3*
Primary cutaneous follicle center lymphoma	t(14;18)(IGH/BCL2)	*CDKN2A, CDKN2B*
Unknown origin		
High-grade B-cell lymphoma, NOS	None	
Intravascular large B-cell lymphoma		
Large B-cell lymphoma with IRF4 rearrangement	t(6;14)(IRF4/IGH), t(3;14)(BCL6/IGH)	*TP53*
Primary mediastinal (thymic) large B-cell lymphoma	MHC CIIA rearrangements with PDL1/2, PDL1/2 rearrangements	*SOCS1, STAT6, PTPN1, BCL6, ITPKB, MFHAS1, XPO1*
Splenic diffuse red pulp small B-cell lymphoma	t(9;14)(PAX5/IGH)	*TP53, CCND3, NOTCH1, MAP2K1, BRAF, SF3B1*
T-cell/histiocyte-rich large B-cell lymphoma		

Major B-cell lymphoma subtypes grouped by cell of origin with characteristic translocations and recurrently mutated genes. NOS, Not otherwise specified; CNS, central nervous system; ALK, anaplastic lymphoma kinase.

that of their normal cell of origin and are used as diagnostic markers.

Pre-GC B-Cell-Derived Lymphomas

Before entering germinal centers, (the pre-GC stage), B cells are primed for antigen exposure and migration. Such "naive" B cells often reside in the mantle zone of lymph nodes. These cells can transition from the mantle zone to germinal centers and sometimes back to the mantle zone. Mantle cell lymphoma (MCL) develops from such cells (Bertoni and Ponzoni 2007). This lymphoma is often associated with gastrointestinal and extranodal involvement. The genetic aspects that define MCL include t(11;14) translocation of the *CCND1* gene to the IGH locus, high *SOX11* expression, and mutations in *ATM*, *KMT2C*, *NOTCH1*, and *TP53* (Rimokh et al. 1994; Ek et al. 2008; Kridel et al. 2012; Zhang et al. 2014). Interestingly, chronic lymphocytic leukemias (CLLs) can arise from pre- or post-GC cells, evidenced by patterns of somatic hypermutation, giving rise to distinct subgroups ("mutated" and "unmutated" CLL) that respond at different rates to standard chemotherapy. Genes across many pathways are recurrently mutated including *MYD88*, *NOTCH1*, and *MAPK1* (Puente et al. 2011).

GC B-Cell-Derived Lymphomas

The GC represents the most vulnerable stage for the oncogenic transformation of B cells and is where a majority of B-cell lymphomas arise. These include the two most common forms of lymphoma: diffuse large B-cell lymphoma (DLBCL) and follicular lymphoma (FL), in addition to Burkitt lymphoma (BL) and others (Fig. 2). DLBCL comprises at least two subtypes arising from either GC B cells (GCB-DLBCL) or activated B cells (ABC-DLBCL), which likely arise from a pre- or post-GC stage associated with differentiation to plasma cells (Lenz et al.

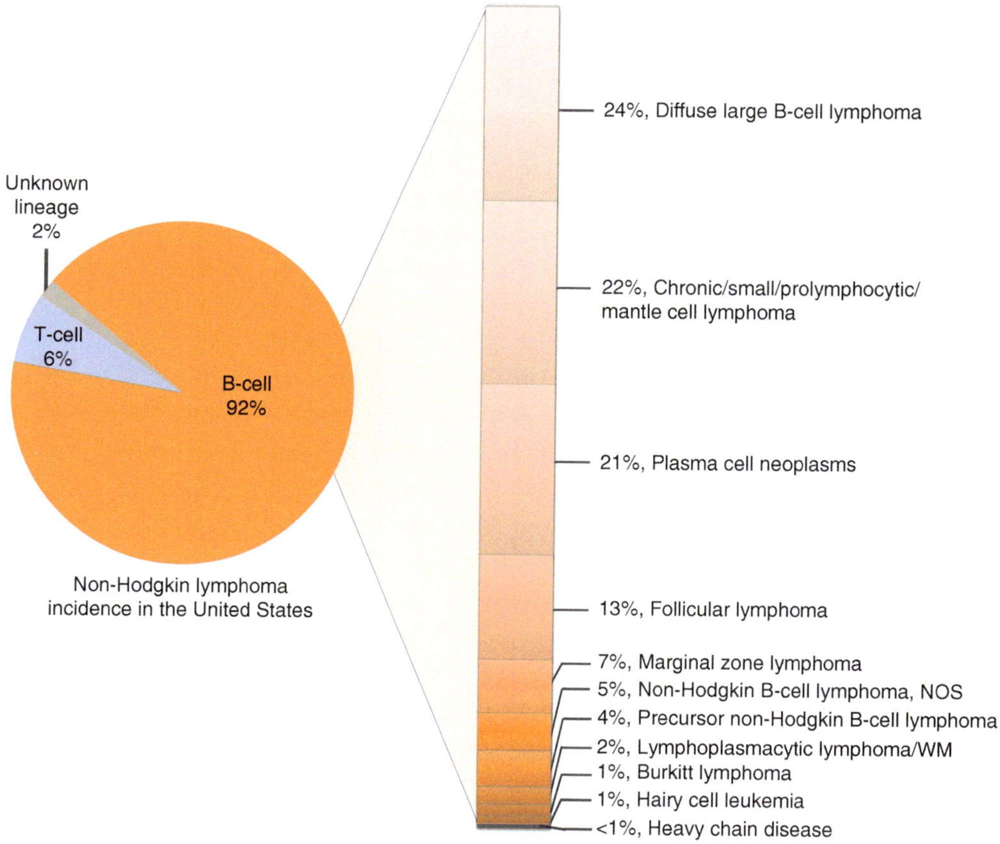

Figure 2. Incidence of B-cell non-Hodgkin lymphomas. NOS, Not otherwise specified; WM, Waldenström's macroglobulinemia.

2008). DLBCLs commonly manifest mutations in *KMT2D*, *SPEN*, *PIM1*, and *CREBBP*. Mutations in *EZH2*, *SGK1*, and *GNA13* are associated with the GCB subtype, whereas mutations in *MYD88*, *ETV6*, and *CD79B* are associated with the ABC subtype (Morin et al. 2013; Zhang et al. 2013). A proportion of cases also present with chromosomal rearrangements involving *BCL2*, *BCL6*, or *MYC*, which are termed "double-hit" or "triple-hit" lymphomas and are associated with a poorer prognosis.

Follicular lymphoma can be an indolent disease that can transforms into DLBCL. The hallmark translocation observed in >90% of follicular lymphomas is t(14;18) translocation of the *BCL2* gene to the *IGH* locus (Cleary and Sklar 1985). Commonly mutated genes in follicular lymphoma include *BCL2*, *KMT2D*, *CREBBP*, *GNA13*, and *EZH2* (Okosun et al. 2014).

BL arises from GC cells and is comprised of three subtypes: sporadic, endemic (associated with EBV), and immunosuppression-associated (associated with HIV). BL is highly aggressive and can present in extranodal sites depending on the subtype. BLs present with hallmark t(8;14), t(2;8), or t(8;22) translocations of the *MYC* gene to the *IGH*, *IGK*, or *IGL* promoter sites, respectively (Taub et al. 1982). Commonly mutated genes include *MYC*, *ID3*, *DDX3X*, and *TP53* (Love et al. 2012; Richter et al. 2012; Schmitz et al. 2012).

Post-GC and Marginal Zone B-Cell-Derived Lymphomas

Differentiated B cells that do not develop into plasma cells or memory B cells either undergo apoptosis or migrate to the mantle zone and

Cite this article as *Cold Spring Harb Perspect Med* doi: 10.1101/cshperspect.a034843

marginal zones. These B cells may later differentiate into plasma cells or monocytoid B cells. Three types of lymphomas with distinct clinical behaviors arise from these B cells; they include nodal and splenic marginal zone lymphomas (NMZLs and SMZLs, respectively), and MALT lymphoma. NMZL manifests as peripheral lymphadenopathy in the head and neck lymph nodes. SMZL presents with splenomegaly with bone marrow involvement and can be associated with autoimmune thrombocytopenia or anemia. MALT lymphoma involvement is observed in the stomach, ocular adnexa, or thyroid, with involvement of multiple extranodal sites observed. Although there is no hallmark translocation, t(14;18) (*IGH-MALT1*) leads to deregulation of *MALT1* and is found in ocular adnexa, orbit, and salivary gland sites (Clark et al. 1992). The t(3;14) translocation (*FOXP1-IGH*) is associated with deregulation of *FOXP1* and is found in thyroid, ocular adnexa, orbit, and skin (Streubel et al. 2005).

Plasma cells represent terminally differentiated post-GC B cells. Multiple myeloma is the malignancy that arises from plasma cells. There are likely intermediate B-cell stages between the GC B cells and plasma cells as there are at least two distinct malignancies that are characterized by expression profiles intermediate between these cell types. First, WM or lymphoplasmacytic lymphoma (LPL) is derived from cells with plasmacytic differentiation. These cells may arise from memory B cells that can undergo differentiation to plasma cells outside GCs. Most WM cases have a mutation in genes in the B-cell receptor pathway including *MYD88*, *CXCR4*, and *CD79B* (Treon et al. 2012; Hunter et al. 2014). A subset of DLBCLs, ABC DLBCLs, arise from cells with an intermediate expression of genes that distinguish GC cells from plasma cells (Wright et al. 2003).

Primary Cutaneous Lymphoma

Primary cutaneous B-cell lymphoma (CBCL) is characterized by its sole localization in the skin at the time of diagnosis. CBCL consists of indolent types including primary cutaneous marginal zone B-cell lymphoma (PCMZL, 30% of cases) and primary cutaneous follicle center lymphoma (PCFCL, 48% of cases), and intermediate aggressive types such as primary cutaneous diffuse large B-cell lymphoma (PCLBCL, 20% of cases) (Willemze et al. 2005). These lymphomas are mainly derived from mature GC B cells. PCMZL arises as a tumor of marginal zone cells, lymphoplasmacytoid cells, and plasma cells on the trunk or extremities. PCFCL is characterized by centrocytes and centroblasts in a follicular or diffuse pattern on the head or truck. PCLBCL is characterized by skin lesions, mostly on the legs. These "leg-type" PCLBCLs resemble DLBCLs that arise from lymph nodes in terms of their cell of origin (Pham-Ledard et al. 2017). However, the origins of the immune cells that give rise to cutaneous lymphomas remain obscure.

Immunodeficiency-Related Lymphomas

Immunodeficiency diseases, both primary diseases caused by a genetic defect (PIDDs) and secondary, are associated with a 10-fold increased risk of lymphoma compared to the general population (Mayor et al. 2018). This increased lymphoma risk may be due to increased susceptibility to viral illness (including Epstein–Barr virus [EBV]), defective immune surveillance, DNA repair defects, tumor-suppressor gene defects, iatrogenic effects, or chronic inflammation (Gangemi et al. 2015; Mortaz et al. 2016). Ataxia telangiectasia, a disorder of DNA repair with mutations in *ATM*, has the highest rate of malignancy (mostly lymphoma) among PIDDs (Mortaz et al. 2016). Interestingly, *ATM* is also frequently mutated in a number of different lymphomas including DLBCL and CLL. Common variable immunodeficiency, Wiskott–Aldrich syndrome, and severe combined immunodeficiency (SCID) are other PIDDs associated with a higher risk for lymphomas. Lymphomas in PIDD patients are often associated with poorer outcomes than those without PIDDs.

HIV-AIDS, which results in immunodeficiency from the selective depletion of $CD4^+$ helper T cells, is known to have an increased incidence of NHL and Hodgkin lymphoma compared to the general U.S. population (Seaberg et al. 2010). The most common types of NHL seen in this population include DLBCL and BL (Meister et al. 2018). Additional types of NHL include Burkitt-like lymphoma, extranodal MALT lymphoma, peripheral T-cell lymphoma (PTCL), primary effusion/body cavity lymphoma, plasmablastic lymphoma of the oral cavity, and polymorphic B-cell lymphoma (Rubinstein et al. 2014). An important mechanism in AIDS-related lymphoma development is chronic infection with EBV and/or HHV8 leading to chronic B-cell stimulation and production of a monoclonal B-cell population. EBV infection is associated with DLBCL (30%), plasmablastic DLBCL (90%), and primary effusion/body cavity lymphoma (100%). HHV8 infection is associated with 50% of plasmablastic lymphomas of the oral cavity. A patient's risk of lymphoma and response to therapy are correlated with the CD4 cell count, viral load, infections, and treatment with combination antiretroviral therapy (Meister et al. 2018).

Another state of secondary immunodeficiency is that which occurs as a result of iatrogenic immunosuppression to protect the graft after a solid organ or hematopoietic stem cell transplant (HSCT). Posttransplant lymphoproliferative disorders (PTLDs) comprise 20% of all cancers that occur after solid organ transplantation and are rare complications of HSCT (Nagle et al. 2017). Most cases of PTLD are due to EBV infection (either following primary EBV infection or reactivation of a previous infection), although PTLD can occur without the presence of EBV (Martinez and Krams 2017; Nagle et al. 2017). Iatrogenic immunosuppression allows EBV-induced B-cell proliferation and PTLD development (Martinez and Krams 2017). The main risk factors for PTLD include EBV status of the recipient and the degree of immunosuppression, specifically T-cell suppression. Therefore, treatment involves the reduction of immune suppression (Nagle et al. 2017). It may also involve the addition of the anti-CD20 antibody rituximab to control the proliferating B cells. There is no accepted system for determining prognosis, although tumor monoclonality, EBV negativity, and graft involvement are thought to predict a poorer outcome.

THERAPEUTIC APPROACHES IN B-CELL LYMPHOMA

Therapeutic Approaches and Promising Clinical Trials

For the clinician, the initial general therapeutic approach for the management of lymphoma is determined by the aggressiveness of disease and treatment intent. This guiding principle goes back to the original attempts to classify lymphoma (Working Formulation) that classified non-Hodgkin lymphomas as low-, intermediate-, or high-grade solely based on morphological and clinical characteristics of the disease (Robb-Smith 1982). Indolent, or slow-growing lymphomas (CLL, FL, and others), are generally considered incurable; the goal is to control the disease and prevent complications like organ dysfunction, cytopenias, malignant effusions, and symptoms attributable to the disease. In the absence of these problems, active observation is often pursued. In contrast, aggressive lymphomas (BL, DLBCL, PTCLs, etc.) are treated with curative intent. Here, multi-agent chemotherapy regimens are employed up front for several cycles with the goal of obtaining a complete response.

Lymphoma is a systemic disease. Although lymphocytes are exquisitely sensitive to radiation, radiation therapy is generally used in patients with localized disease in conjunction with chemotherapy and/or immunotherapy. Palliative radiation for relief of symptoms caused by bulky tumors remains an effective, if short-lived, therapy for patients.

Although aggressive B-cell lymphomas generally respond well to multi-agent chemotherapy, the complete response rate is far less in aggressive T-cell lymphomas, in which relapses are also more common. Therefore, some clinicians opt to give high-dose chemotherapy with autologous stem cell transplant upon attaining first complete remission in aggressive T-cell lymphomas, although there are no randomized data to support this practice.

The approach to subsequent line treatment of lymphoma is also largely guided by the intent to cure versus palliate. In large B-cell lymphomas and Hodgkin lymphomas that have relapsed or are refractory to first-line treatment, second-line multi-agent chemotherapy is given, and if response is attained, high-dose chemotherapy followed by autologous stem cell transplantation is considered standard of care. This approach offers the best chance for long-term remission in second-line treatment. With each subsequent relapse, the chance for long-term complete remission with chemotherapy decreases, and alternative small-molecule inhibitors, targeted agents, and cellular or immunotherapies may be used, even as the intent may not be to attempt a cure. In indolent and aggressive lymphomas alike, the optimal sequence of subsequent line therapies is not defined and is chosen based on urgency for disease control, toxicity profile, and patient or physician preference.

The current WHO classification of lymphoma integrates immunohistochemical and molecular characteristics of disease in addition to clinical and morphologic features. For example, molecular features like *MYC*, *BCL2*, and *BCL6* translocations are associated with particularly aggressive disease, informing up-front treatment decisions while providing prognostic information as long-term remissions are difficult to obtain. Many clinicians tend to use more aggressive chemotherapy regimens, particularly in patients whose tumors manifest two or more translocations ("double hit") simultaneously.

Determination of cell of origin in aggressive B-cell lymphomas by the Hans algorithm may provide the clinician some biological basis for selecting a subsequent line therapy for a given patient, although the optimal treatment for any given molecular subtype of lymphoma remains to be defined. Therefore, there is ample room for consideration of clinical trial options in the up-front treatment of high-risk disease or subsequent treatment of refractory disease. Outside of clinical trials, novel approaches using immune checkpoint blockade and chimeric antigen receptor modified T cells are appropriate in the relapsed or refractory setting after failing two lines of systemic therapy.

Chemotherapy

The most common treatment for NHL continues to be combination chemotherapy. Many of the compounds used in these therapies leverage the cytotoxic stress of DNA damage in the rapidly proliferating cancer cells in order to preferentially eliminate them. Alkylating agents (e.g., cyclophosphamide) and platins (e.g., cisplatin) form DNA cross-links that exploit the impaired ability of cancer cells to repair and replicate DNA with these genetic lesions. Purine analogs (e.g., fludarabine) act both as an antimetabolite of purines and as a DNA synthesis inhibitor once integrated into DNA. Pyrimidine antimetabolites (cytarabine) act in a similar manner to inhibit DNA synthesis at the incorporated base. Other antimetabolites (e.g., methotrexate) target folate metabolism that is required for the production of DNA/RNA bases and thymidylates (Rajagopalan et al. 2002). Anthracycline compounds (e.g., doxorubicin) intercalate into DNA, preventing topoisomerase II progression as well as evicting histones from transcriptionally active regions of the genome (Pommier et al. 2010; Pang et al. 2013). Vinca alkaloids (e.g., vincristine) are also effective in many lymphomas, inhibiting microtubule formation and thus disrupting mitosis. Many combination therapies for lymphoid neoplasms contain a corticosteroid agent (e.g., prednisone) that leverages the immunomodulating effects of the glucocorticoid pathway within the tumor cells.

Patients with NHL are typically treated with a combination of these chemotherapeutic agents. Common treatment regimens include CHOP (cyclophosphamide, doxorubicin, vincristine, and prednisone) and EPOCH (etoposide, prednisone, vincristine, cyclophosphamide, and doxorubicin). Escalated regimens for refractory or aggressive tumors include hyper-CVAD (cyclophosphamide, vincristine, doxorubicin, dexamethasone, methotrexate, and cytarabine) and DHAP (dexamethasone, cytarabine, and cisplatin). Many chemotherapy regimens are augmented with rituximab and/or targeted immunotherapy. Rituximab is an anti-CD20 monoclonal antibody that, when administered in conjunction with chemotherapy, is an effective component of curative standard care for B-cell lymphoma patients (>85% of all NHL patients) (Weiner 2010). Rituximab induces killing of $CD20^+$ cells via multiple mechanisms including complement-mediated cytotoxicity and antibody-dependent cell-mediated cytotoxicity.

Brentuximab is an anti-CD30 antibody that is administered conjugated to a chemotherapeutic drug via protease-cleavable linker (Bhatt et al. 2013). This complex, brentuximab vedotin, can be used to treat some T-cell lymphomas in conjunction with CHOP or as an alternative treatment if lymphoma persists after utilizing other treatment options. Upon binding the CD30 antigen, brentuximab vedotin is internalized and transported to lysosomes, where the chemotherapeutic agent is released and binds to tubulin, causing cell cycle arrest and apoptosis.

Although these standard therapies are effective for a majority of patients, drug resistance and disease relapse in the remaining patients lead to poor clinical outcomes. Drug resistance can be intrinsic, treatment-acquired, or tumor microenvironment–mediated (for review, see Camicia et al. 2015). Major avenues of therapy resistance that arise via these mechanisms involve up-regulation of anti-apoptotic proteins (e.g., BCL2), down-regulation of pro-apoptotic factors (e.g., BAX), and down-regulation or mutation of drug targets (e.g., CD20). Disease relapse can arise from a clone that diverged either early or late from the dominant clone. Alterations that mediate immune evasion have been associated with relapse (Jiang et al. 2014). Resistant patients and the extreme side effects of treatment call for new, more effective treatment options to be added to the current treatment regimens.

Targeted Therapies

One of the promising avenues of targeted therapies in NHL is targeting endogenous and altered signaling pathways within the tumor. Recurrent genetic alterations indicate critical genes and pathways that drive the disease. Targeting these critical pathways with small molecules deprives the cancer cells of required signaling without the global off-target effects of other chemotherapy types such as genotoxic agents (Fig. 3).

There are several notable signaling pathways that are shared to differing degrees by NHLs. These include the JAK-STAT pathway, which is critical for lymphoid cell formation and differentiation and is a primary driver of activating signaling via cytokines (Liao et al. 2011). Constitutive STAT3/STAT5 activation is a feature of a number of different lymphoid malignancies (Migone et al. 1995; Buettner et al. 2002). JAK2 inhibition with ruxolitinib is currently in clinical trials in a number of lymphomas (Lee et al. 2018).

The major signaling networks in both B and T cells are modulated by surface immunoglobulin receptors that, once activated, generate powerful signaling cascades that induce growth, proliferation, and differentiation. The natural function of these immune cells requires an ability to rapidly divide upon antigen stimulation and then recede upon antigen clearance. Activation of the B-cell receptor (BCR) pathway is critical in B-cell neoplasms as it circumvents poised apoptosis of the unstimulated state (Lam et al. 1997). The BCR pathway contains a series of critical kinase nodes (SYK, PI3K, CD79A, and BTK) that are essential for proper BCR activation and have become important therapeutic targets (Seda and Mraz 2015). The Bruton's tyrosine kinase (BTK) inhibitor ibrutinib was shown to be effective in MCL and CLL, but other B-cell malignancies have not been as responsive, suggesting that more refined drugs or different signaling nodes should be targeted in these cases. Upstream in the signaling cascade, SYK has also been a target to disrupt tonic BCR signaling that drives lymphoma. Fostamatinib was developed as a potent SYK inhibitor and has shown response in a variety of NHL patients. The efficacy of these types of drugs demonstrate a path for disrupting the tonic endogenous growth signals that sustain lymphoma.

Further down the signaling cascade, both the B- and T-cell receptors signal through PI3K and NF-κB. Dysregulation of the PI3K pathway has been described in several lymphoid malignancies including Hodgkin lymphoma, MCL, and FL (Psyrri et al. 2009; Meadows et al. 2012; Yahiaoui et al. 2014). Idelalisib, a potent PI3Kδ inhibitor, was shown to be effective in preclinical

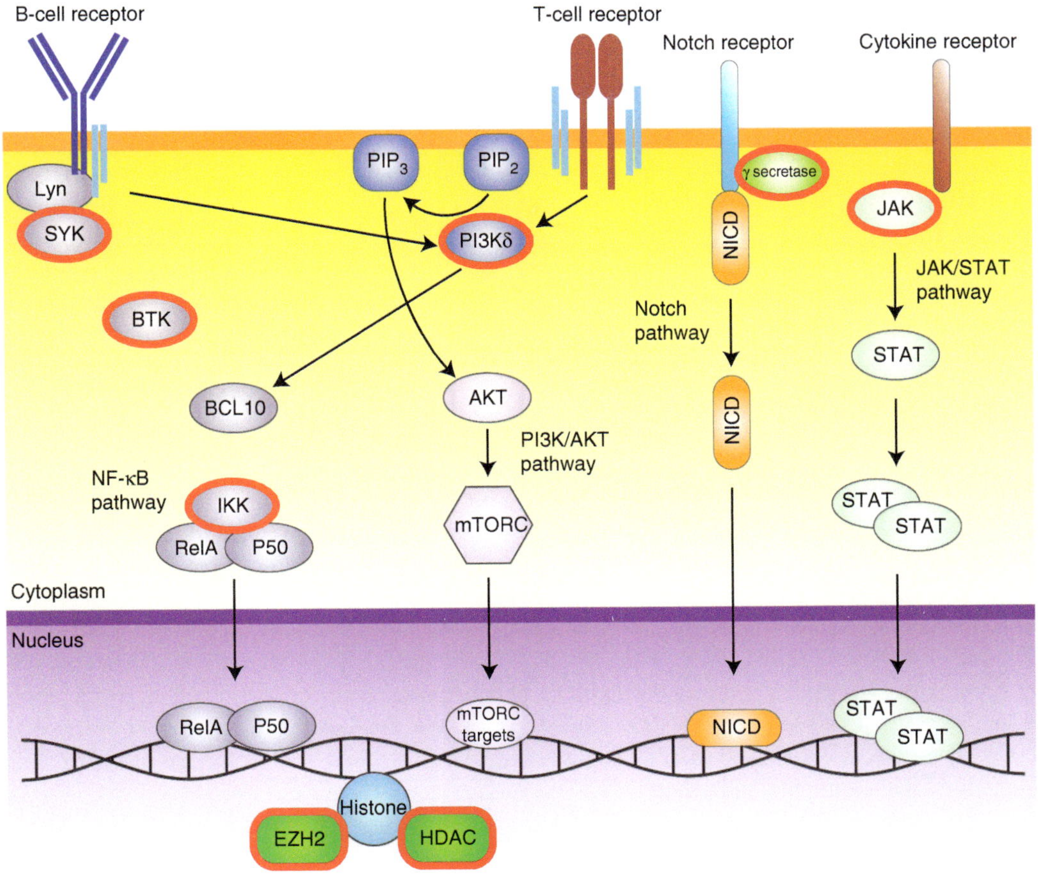

Figure 3. Targetable signaling pathways in non-Hodgkin lymphoma. Targetable nodes with clinically available small molecule inhibitors are ringed in red. BCR, B-cell receptor; SYK, spleen tyrosine kinase; BTK, Bruton's tyrosine kinase; PI3Kδ, phosphoinositide 3-kinases delta; NICD, Notch intracellular domain; JAK, Janus kinase; IKK, IκB kinase; HDAC, histone deacetylase.

models at not only reducing tonic BCR signaling, but also modulating the tumor microenvironment to be less tumor-supporting (Hoellenriegel et al. 2011). As a monotherapy, idelalisib was very effective in refractory patients; however, in combination, serious side effects halted further trials. DLBCL has been shown to be NF-κB-dependent, with mutations in genes such as *CARD11* leading to constitutive NF-κB activation, making these related nodes attractive targets for targeted therapies (Davis et al. 2001; Milhollen et al. 2010; Staudt 2010).

Notch pathway mutations and dysregulation have been observed in many lymphoma subtypes, including DLBCL, SMZL, FL, MCL, and PTCL (Karube et al. 2014). Many of these changes involve loss of the PEST domain that regulates NOTCH degradation, leading to increased protein half-life and thus activity and related downstream signaling. The major targetable component of this pathway is γ-secretase; however, no clinical trials focused on lymphoma have been performed thus far.

The histone methyltransferase EZH2 is recurrently mutated in both DLBCL and FL (Morin et al. 2010; Bodor et al. 2011; Béguelin et al. 2016; Reddy et al. 2017). Interestingly, *EZH2* mutations are largely gain-of-function alterations that impair the normal course of B-cell differentiation. In particular, the Y641 amino acid is a hotspot for missense mutations that result in increased levels of H3K27me3. A recent phase 1 trial of the inhibitor tazemetostat exhibited promising clinical response in patients with relapsed or refractory B-cell lymphomas (Italiano et al. 2018). EZH2 inhibitors might also be combined with HDAC inhibitors to relieve transcriptional repression of key target genes (Lue et al. 2019).

Whereas targeted therapies offer the ability to single out specific pathways that lymphomas rely on for growth and cell death escape, there is much to learn about translating the genetic and experimental findings into effective therapies. Unraveling the genetics provides a critical first step to this understanding.

Immunotherapy

Immunotherapy presents a highly promising new method for treating lymphomas. Immunotherapy consists of multiple approaches, chiefly (1) checkpoint inhibitor therapy, (2) chimeric antigen receptor (CAR) T-cell therapy, and (3) bispecific T-cell engager (BiTE) therapy.

Checkpoint inhibitor therapy targets proteins found on the surface of T cells or antigen-presenting cells that act to dampen T-cell activity in a normal immune response. Although this approach has proven to be effective in solid tumors and in Hodgkin lymphoma, the results in NHL have been disappointing. Ongoing work will help delineate the potential application of these therapies.

On the other hand, CARs are genetically engineered immune receptors that consist of a single peptide–containing V-heavy chain and V-light chain segments connected to an intracellular signaling chain. T cells are expanded from peripheral blood mononuclear cells (PBMCs) collected from patients, then transduced to express CARs targeting a tumor-associated antigen (TAA) of choice. One of the most widely used and most effective TAAs is CD19, which is widely expressed on NHLs. Early CAR T-cell clinical trials have demonstrated a striking degree of efficacy in patients, even as further advancements are needed to improve efficacy and reduce toxicity.

BiTE therapy also seeks to promote T-cell activity against tumor cells. As their name implies, BiTE antibodies bind two antigens simultaneously, generally the CD3 component of the T-cell receptor and a tumor antigen, resulting in T-cell activation and target cell lysis. To date, BiTE antibodies targeting CD19 (blinatumomab) and CD20 (e.g., mosunetuzumab) have been developed to treat B-cell malignancies. Blinatumomab is approved for relapsed/refractory acute lymphoblastic leukemia, but the severity of side effects, short half-life, and the advent of anti-CD19 CAR-T therapy have hindered its widespread adoption in NHL (Bacac et al. 2018; Yu et al. 2019). CD20-targeting BiTE antibodies with longer half-lives are still in early phases of investigation, although results have been promising (Chu et al. 2014; Sun et al. 2015; Schuster et al. 2019).

Much work is still needed in understanding the appropriate duration, intensity, and sequencing of different approaches in the appropriately risk-stratified patients with NHLs.

MODELING LYMPHOMAS

Preclinical models of cancer are essential tools that have furthered our understanding of the disease. These models allow for investigation of tumor biology and disease progression, evaluation of drug targets, and development of effective treatment strategies. There are currently three main approaches to model lymphomas, each representing a different set of trade-offs in recapitulating the complete tumor phenotypes: cell lines, patient-derived xenograft models (PDXs), and genetically engineered mouse models (GEMMs) (Fig. 4).

Cancer cell lines are derived by in vitro immortalization of lymphoma patient–derived tumor cells. As such, cancer cell lines represent the complete genotype of the tumor, in a way that is hard to achieve in engineered models. Many established lymphoma cell lines have well-characterized genetic alterations and cytogenetics, providing a platform to assess various genomic pathways. They allow for rapid and economical testing of therapeutic approaches and predictions of treatment efficacy. Cell lines, however,

Cite this article as *Cold Spring Harb Perspect Med* doi: 10.1101/cshperspect.a034843

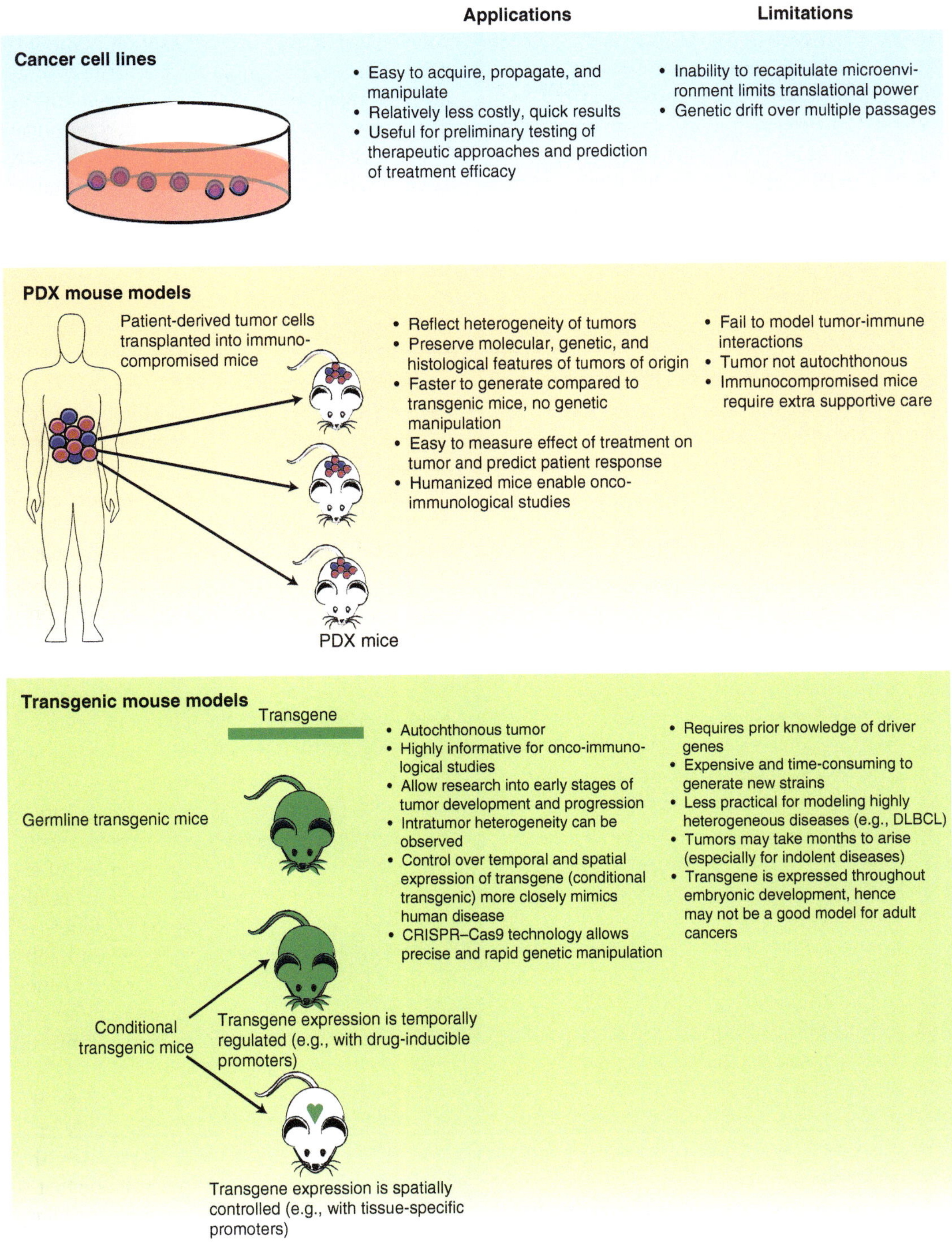

Figure 4. Lymphoma models. Cell culture, patient-derived xenograft (PDX), and transgenic mouse models are used to model lymphomas in the research and clinical settings.

have a limited ability to translate findings to clinical practice because of their unregulated growth outside a normal tumor microenvironment, which can result in genetic divergence from the primary tumors of origin. Cell lines also lack the ability to model interactions with the surrounding stroma normally present within the microenvironment, which currently can only be replicated in vivo.

Some of these limitations are overcome in PDX mouse models, which are generated by implanting patient-derived tumor cells into immunocompromised mice. Propagation of PDXs does not require in vitro manipulation and has been shown to maintain the same biological, genetic, and histopathological features as the tumor of origin (Zhang et al. 2017). As such, PDXs have been used to predict drug response in patients and for confirming in vitro findings. Transplanted cells may take up to several months to engraft after implantation, and supportive care is needed for the maintenance of immunocompromised mice. Nevertheless, xenografts can be generated more rapidly than transgenic mice. A major drawback of xenografts is that due to the compromised immune system of host mice, treatment strategies such as immunotherapy cannot be evaluated. This limitation has spurred the development of humanized mice in which human hematopoietic stem progenitor cells (HSPCs) are co-transplanted with genetically manipulated cells or tumor cells into immunocompromised mice (Choi et al. 2018). These human HSPCs repopulate the host immune system, enabling investigations into tumor-immune system interactions. Although generation of humanized mice can be more time-consuming and expensive than traditional xenograft models, they may be more informative as they closely recapitulate the human disease and allow study of the tumor microenvironment.

Generation of GEMMs primarily involves introduction of "knock-out" mutations or "knock-in" of target genes into immunocompetent mice to study loss of function and gain of function, respectively. Germline transgenic mice express the transgene at all developmental stages and in all tissues. However, such systems may not accurately model adult cancers and may lead to embryonic lethality. Incorporation of specific gene-regulatory elements, such as drug-inducible and cell/tissue-specific promoters, allows for temporal or tissue-specific control of transgene expression. The advent of CRISPR–Cas9 technology has improved generation of in vivo models. CRISPR–Cas9 allows more rapid introduction of gene mutations in mouse zygotes, especially in situations with multiple target genes of interest (Wang et al. 2013; Aida et al. 2015). CRISPR–Cas9 editing also allows the mutated gene to remain under the control of its endogenous promoter. Newly developed Cas9 base editors allow investigators to make precise nucleotide changes and model hotspot or intergenic point mutations (Zafra et al. 2018). As the CRISPR–Cas9 toolbox expands, investigators will have more tools with which to model hematologic malignancies with increasing accuracy.

THE "HETEROGENEITY PROBLEM" IN LYMPHOMA

In spite of steady progress over the past decades in our understanding of the biology of lymphomas, the frontline therapies for most lymphomas have remained unchanged. A major reason for the lack of progress in these cancers is the biologic heterogeneity that underlies each lymphoma type. This problem is exemplified in the most common lymphoma, DLBCL.

DLBCLs have been extensively characterized to identify molecular subgroups and genomic correlates of prognosis following standard therapy. Gene expression profiling has revealed many competing approaches for classification (Kuze et al. 2000; Ando et al. 2002; Lossos et al. 2003; Rimsza et al. 2004; Hans et al. 2005; Natkunam et al. 2008)—two of the most widely cited include those based on cell of origin (Alizadeh et al. 2000) and those based on host response, B-cell receptor, and tumor metabolic states (Monti et al. 2005). The clinical application of these approaches has remained limited, even a decade after their initial description.

The advent of next-generation sequencing has provided a powerful approach to incorporate genetic alterations into prognostic models

Table 2. Recently published next-generation sequencing (NGS) studies of diffuse large B-cell lymphoma (DLBCL)

References	Reddy et al. 2017	Schmitz et al. 2018	Chapuy et al. 2018
Number of samples	1001	574	304
Paired tumor/normal samples	401	0	167
Percentage FFPE samples	95%	0%	50%
Data types	Exome-seq, RNA-seq, CRISPR screen	Exome-seq, RNA-seq, aCGH	Exome-seq, targeted sequencing
Survival time	Overall survival	Overall survival, progression-free survival	Progression-free survival
Predictor type	Survival predictor	Supervised clustering	Supervised clustering
Number of subgroups	3	4	5

FFPE, formalin-fixed paraffin-embedded; aCGH, array comparative genomic hybridization.

and subgroups. More than 100 genetic drivers have been described in DLBCL, with the average tumor comprising five to 10 distinct events simultaneously. Thus, no two patients appear to manifest identical sets of mutations, confounding our ability to subgroup patients and presenting daunting power calculations for samples needed to effectively discern the prognostic effects of diverse mutations.

The relatively high prevalence of DLBCL has enabled several landmark studies that used complementary approaches to understand the heterogeneity underlying survival differences in DLBCL (Table 2). There are two distinct approaches to genomic survival modeling in cancers including lymphoma. The first approach treats survival as a continuous variable that is modeled on individual mutations and critical expression features (e.g., MYC, BCL2, and cell of origin). The second approach treats survival as a reflection of underlying discrete subgroups with characteristic alterations that have distinct survival outcomes. The latter approach is particularly attractive because it enables us to consider such subgroups as the minimal entity to focus on for disease modeling and therapeutic targeting.

The first approach of treating survival as a continuous variable was utilized in a study of 1001 patients with DLBCL that showed that combinatorial blending of different genomic features generated very strong effects on overall patient survival. The second approach of treating survival as a function of distinct subgroups of genetic alterations was adopted by two different studies summarized in Table 2. Both studies were based on highly supervised approaches to analysis with somewhat different assumptions with relatively little overlap in the subgroups described between the two studies. The first study described five subgroups that collectively describe all 304 patients (i.e., no unclassified cases). The second study described four subgroups that collectively comprised fewer than one-half the patients with the remainder being unclassified. These subgroups offer a different window into DLBCL biology by highlighting mutually exclusive genetic events. Importantly, these described subgroups are themselves heterogeneous. Existing survival factors such as BCL2, MYC, cell of origin, EBV status, and many others remain prognostic within these subgroups, suggesting considerable molecular and clinical heterogeneity within these subgroups.

Interestingly, the issue of clinical and genetic heterogeneity has been studied in acute myeloid leukemia (AML) in large studies (Papaemmanuil et al. 2016; Gerstung et al. 2017). These studies have demonstrated that survival is better understood as a large set of combinatorial effects, rather than a few dominant subgroups. It appears that, in terms of overall survival, DLBCL shares this critical feature with AML. Ultimately, the utility of all survival models can only be established clinically.

CONCLUSION

Lymphomas collectively represent the fourth most common group of cancers and are a leading cause of cancer mortality. B-cell lymphomas represent a strikingly diverse group of malignancies that are best understood in the context of lineage. Recent work has given us greater insight into the molecular composition of these tumors. The coming years hold great promise for translating that knowledge into better clinical outcomes.

ACKNOWLEDGMENTS

The authors gratefully acknowledge support from the Lymphoma Research Foundation and the National Institutes of Health.

REFERENCES

Aida T, Chiyo K, Usami T, Ishikubo H, Imahashi R, Wada Y, Tanaka KF, Sakuma T, Yamamoto T, Tanaka K. 2015. Cloning-free CRISPR/Cas system facilitates functional cassette knock-in in mice. *Genome Biol* **16:** 87. doi:10.1186/s13059-015-0653-x

Alizadeh AA, Eisen MB, Davis RE, Ma C, Lossos IS, Rosenwald A, Boldrick JC, Sabet H, Tran T, Yu X, et al. 2000. Distinct types of diffuse large B-cell lymphoma identified by gene expression profiling. *Nature* **403:** 503–511. doi:10.1038/35000501

Ando T, Suguro M, Hanai T, Kobayashi T, Honda H, Seto M. 2002. Fuzzy neural network applied to gene expression profiling for predicting the prognosis of diffuse large B-cell lymphoma. *Jpn J Cancer Res* **93:** 1207–1212. doi:10.1111/j.1349-7006.2002.tb01225.x

Bacac M, Colombetti S, Herter S, Sam J, Perro M, Chen S, Bianchi R, Richard M, Schoenle A, Nicolini V, et al. 2018. CD20-TCB with obinutuzumab pretreatment as next-generation treatment of hematologic malignancies. *Clin Cancer Res* **24:** 4785–4797.

Béguelin W, Teater M, Gearhart MD, Calvo Fernández MT, Goldstein RL, Cárdenas MG, Hatzi K, Rosen M, Shen H, Corcoran CM, et al. 2016. EZH2 and BCL6 cooperate to assemble CBX8-BCOR complex to repress bivalent promoters, mediate germinal center formation and lymphomagenesis. *Cancer Cell* **30:** 197–213. doi:10.1016/j.ccell.2016.07.006

Bertoni F, Ponzoni M. 2007. The cellular origin of mantle cell lymphoma. *Int J Biochem Cell Biol* **39:** 1747–1753. doi:10.1016/j.biocel.2007.04.026

Bhatt S, Ashlock BM, Natkunam Y, Sujoy V, Chapman JR, Ramos JC, Mesri EA, Lossos IS. 2013. CD30 targeting with brentuximab vedotin: a novel therapeutic approach to primary effusion lymphoma. *Blood* **122:** 1233–1242. doi:10.1182/blood-2013-01-481713

Bodor C, O'Riain C, Wrench D, Matthews J, Iyengar S, Tayyib H, Calaminici M, Clear A, Iqbal S, Quentmeier H, et al. 2011. EZH2 Y641 mutations in follicular lymphoma. *Leukemia* **25:** 726–729.

Buettner R, Mora LB, Jove R. 2002. Activated STAT signaling in human tumors provides novel molecular targets for therapeutic intervention. *Clin Cancer Res* **8:** 945–954.

Camicia R, Winkler HC, Hassa PO. 2015. Novel drug targets for personalized precision medicine in relapsed/refractory diffuse large B-cell lymphoma: a comprehensive review. *Mol Cancer* **14:** 207.

Chapuy B, Stewart C, Dunford AJ, Kim J, Kamburov A, Redd RA, Lawrence MS, Roemer MGM, Li AJ, Ziepert M, et al. 2018. Molecular subtypes of diffuse large B cell lymphoma are associated with distinct pathogenic mechanisms and outcomes. *Nat Med* **24:** 679–690. doi:10.1038/s41591-018-0016-8

Choi Y, Lee S, Kim K, Kim SH, Chung YJ, Lee C. 2018. Studying cancer immunotherapy using patient-derived xenografts (PDXs) in humanized mice. *Exp Mol Med* **50:** 99. doi:10.1038/s12276-018-0115-0

Chu TW, Yang J, Zhang R, Sima M, Kopecek J. 2014. Cell surface self-assembly of hybrid nanoconjugates via oligonucleotide hybridization induces apoptosis. *ACS Nano* **8:** 719–730.

Clark HM, Jones DB, Wright DH. 1992. Cytogenetic and molecular studies of t(14;18) and t(14;19) in nodal and extranodal B-cell lymphoma. *J Pathol* **166:** 129–137. doi:10.1002/path.1711660208

Cleary ML, Sklar J. 1985. Nucleotide sequence of a t(14;18) chromosomal breakpoint in follicular lymphoma and demonstration of a breakpoint-cluster region near a transcriptionally active locus on chromosome 18. *Proc Natl Acad Sci* **82:** 7439–7443. doi:10.1073/pnas.82.21.7439

Davis RE, Brown KD, Siebenlist U, Staudt LM. 2001. Constitutive nuclear factor κB activity is required for survival of activated B cell–like diffuse large B cell lymphoma cells. *J Exp Med* **194:** 1861–1874. doi:10.1084/jem.194.12.1861

Di Noia JM, Neuberger MS. 2007. Molecular mechanisms of antibody somatic hypermutation. *Annu Rev Biochem* **76:** 1–22. doi:10.1146/annurev.biochem.76.061705.090740

Ek S, Dictor M, Jerkeman M, Jirström K, Borrebaeck CA. 2008. Nuclear expression of the non-B-cell lineage Sox11 transcription factor identifies mantle cell lymphoma. *Blood* **111:** 800–805. doi:10.1182/blood-2007-06-093401

Fais F, Ghiotto F, Hashimoto S, Sellars B, Valetto A, Allen SL, Schulman P, Vinciguerra VP, Rai K, Rassenti LZ, et al. 1998. Chronic lymphocytic leukemia B cells express restricted sets of mutated and unmutated antigen receptors. *J Clin Invest* **102:** 1515–1525. doi:10.1172/JCI3009

Gangemi S, Allegra A, Musolino C. 2015. Lymphoproliferative disease and cancer among patients with common variable immunodeficiency. *Leuk Res* **39:** 389–396. doi:10.1016/j.leukres.2015.02.002

Gerstung M, Papaemmanuil E, Martincorena I, Bullinger L, Gaidzik VI, Paschka P, Heuser M, Thol F, Bolli N, Ganly P. 2017. Precision oncology for acute myeloid leukemia using a knowledge bank approach. *Nat Genet* **49:** 332–340. doi:10.1038/ng.3756

Ghiotto F, Fais F, Albesiano E, Sison C, Valetto A, Gaidano G, Reinhardt J, Kolitz JE, Rai K, Allen SL, et al. 2006. Similarities and differences between the light and heavy chain Ig variable region gene repertoires in chronic lymphocytic leukemia. *Mol Med* **12:** 300–308. doi:10.2119/2006-00080.Ghiotto

Hans CP, Weisenburger DD, Greiner TC, Chan WC, Aoun P, Cochran GT, Pan Z, Smith LM, Lynch JC, Bociek RG. 2005. Expression of PKC-β or cyclin D2 predicts for inferior survival in diffuse large B-cell lymphoma. *Mod Pathol* **18:** 1377–1384. doi:10.1038/modpathol.3800434

Hoellenriegel J, Meadows SA, Sivina M, Wierda WG, Kantarjian H, Keating MJ, Giese N, O'Brien S, Yu A, Miller LL, et al. 2011. The phosphoinositide 3′-kinase delta inhibitor, CAL-101, inhibits B-cell receptor signaling and chemokine networks in chronic lymphocytic leukemia. *Blood* **118:** 3603–3612. doi:10.1182/blood-2011-05-352492

Hunter ZR, Xu L, Yang G, Zhou Y, Liu X, Cao Y, Manning RJ, Tripsas C, Patterson CJ, Sheehy P, et al. 2014. The genomic landscape of Waldenström macroglobulinemia is characterized by highly recurring MYD88 and WHIM-like CXCR4 mutations, and small somatic deletions associated with B-cell lymphomagenesis. *Blood* **123:** 1637–1646. doi:10.1182/blood-2013-09-525808

Italiano A, Soria JC, Toulmonde M, Michot JM, Lucchesi C, Varga A, Coindre JM, Blakemore SJ, Clawson A, Suttle B, et al. 2018. Tazemetostat, an EZH2 inhibitor, in relapsed or refractory B-cell non-Hodgkin lymphoma advanced solid tumours: a first-in-human, open-label, phase 1 study. *Lancet Oncol* **19:** 649–659.

Jiang Y, Redmond D, Nie K, Eng KW, Clozel T, Martin P, Tan LH, Melnick AM, Tam W, Elemento O. 2014. Deep sequencing reveals clonal evolution patterns mutation events associated with relapse in B-cell lymphomas. *Genome Biol* **15:** 432.

Karube K, Martínez D, Royo C, Navarro A, Pinyol M, Cazorla M, Castillo P, Valera A, Carrió A, Costa D, et al. 2014. Recurrent mutations of *NOTCH* genes in follicular lymphoma identify a distinctive subset of tumours. *J Pathol* **234:** 423–430. doi:10.1002/path.4428

Kridel R, Meissner B, Rogic S, Boyle M, Telenius A, Woolcock B, Gunawardana J, Jenkins C, Cochrane C, Ben-Neriah S, et al. 2012. Whole transcriptome sequencing reveals recurrent *NOTCH1* mutations in mantle cell lymphoma. *Blood* **119:** 1963–1971. doi:10.1182/blood-2011-11-391474

Kuze T, Nakamura N, Hashimoto Y, Sasaki Y, Abe M. 2000. The characteristics of Epstein–Barr virus (EBV)-positive diffuse large B-cell lymphoma: comparison between EBV^+ and EBV^- cases in Japanese population. *Jpn J Cancer Res* **91:** 1233–1240. doi:10.1111/j.1349-7006.2000.tb00909.x

Lam KP, Kühn R, Rajewsky K. 1997. In vivo ablation of surface immunoglobulin on mature B cells by inducible gene targeting results in rapid cell death. *Cell* **90:** 1073–1083. doi:10.1016/S0092-8674(00)80373-6

Lee S, Shah T, Yin C, Hochberg J, Ayello J, Morris E, van de Ven C, Cairo MS. 2018. Ruxolitinib significantly enhances in vitro apoptosis in Hodgkin lymphoma and primary mediastinal B-cell lymphoma and survival in a lymphoma xenograft murine model. *Oncotarget* **9:** 9776–9788.

Lenz G, Wright GW, Emre NC, Kohlhammer H, Dave SS, Davis RE, Carty S, Lam LT, Shaffer AL, Xiao W, et al. 2008. Molecular subtypes of diffuse large B-cell lymphoma arise by distinct genetic pathways. *Proc Natl Acad Sci* **105:** 13520–13525. doi:10.1073/pnas.0804295105

Li Z, Woo CJ, Iglesias-Ussel MD, Ronai D, Scharff MD. 2004. The generation of antibody diversity through somatic hypermutation and class switch recombination. *Genes Dev* **18:** 1–11. doi:10.1101/gad.1161904

Liao W, Lin JX, Leonard WJ. 2011. IL-2 family cytokines: new insights into the complex roles of IL-2 as a broad regulator of T helper cell differentiation. *Curr Opin Immunol* **23:** 598–604. doi:10.1016/j.coi.2011.08.003

Lossos IS, Alizadeh AA, Rajapaksa R, Tibshirani R, Levy R. 2003. HGAL is a novel interleukin-4–inducible gene that strongly predicts survival in diffuse large B-cell lymphoma. *Blood* **101:** 433–440. doi:10.1182/blood-2002-06-1931

Love C, Sun Z, Jima D, Li G, Zhang J, Miles R, Richards KL, Dunphy CH, Choi WW, Srivastava G, et al. 2012. The genetic landscape of mutations in Burkitt lymphoma. *Nat Genet* **44:** 1321–1325. doi:10.1038/ng.2468

Lue JK, Prabhu SA, Liu Y, Gonzalez Y, Verma A, Mundi PS, Abshiru N, Camarillo JM, Mehta S, Chen EI, et al. 2019. Precision targeting with EZH2 HDAC inhibitors in epigenetically dysregulated lymphomas. *Clin Cancer Res* **25:** 5271–5283.

Martinez OM, Krams SM. 2017. The immune response to Epstein–Barr virus and implications for posttransplant lymphoproliferative disorder. *Transplantation* **101:** 2009–2016. doi:10.1097/TP.0000000000001767

Maul RW, Gearhart PJ. 2010. AID and somatic hypermutation. *Adv Immunol* **105:** 159–191. doi:10.1016/S0065-2776(10)05006-6

Mayor PC, Eng KH, Singel KL, Abrams SI, Odunsi K, Moysich KB, Fuleihan R, Garabedian E, Lugar P, Ochs HD, et al. 2018. Cancer in primary immunodeficiency diseases: Cancer incidence in the United States Immune Deficiency Network Registry. *J Allergy Clin Immunol* **141:** 1028–1035. doi:10.1016/j.jaci.2017.05.024

Meadows SA, Vega F, Kashishian A, Johnson D, Diehl V, Miller LL, Younes A, Lannutti BJ. 2012. PI3Kδ inhibitor, GS-1101 (CAL-101), attenuates pathway signaling, induces apoptosis, and overcomes signals from the microenvironment in cellular models of Hodgkin lymphoma. *Blood* **119:** 1897–1900. doi:10.1182/blood-2011-10-386763

Meister A, Hentrich M, Wyen C, Hübel K. 2018. Malignant lymphoma in the HIV-positive patient. *Eur J Haematol* **101:** 119–126. doi:10.1111/ejh.13082

Migone TS, Lin JX, Cereseto A, Mulloy JC, O'Shea JJ, Franchini G, Leonard WJ. 1995. Constitutively activated Jak-STAT pathway in T cells transformed with HTLV-I. *Science* **269:** 79–81. doi:10.1126/science.7604283

Milhollen MA, Traore T, Adams-Duffy J, Thomas MP, Berger AJ, Dang L, Dick LR, Garnsey JJ, Koenig E, Langston SP, et al. 2010. MLN4924, a NEDD8-activating enzyme inhibitor, is active in diffuse large B-cell lymphoma models: rationale for treatment of NF-κB-dependent lymphoma. *Blood* **116:** 1515–1523. doi:10.1182/blood-2010-03-272567

Molyneux EM, Rochford R, Griffin B, Newton R, Jackson G, Menon G, Harrison CJ, Israels T, Bailey S. 2012. Burkitt's lymphoma. *Lancet* **379:** 1234–1244. doi:10.1016/S0140-6736(11)61177-X

Monti S, Savage KJ, Kutok JL, Feuerhake F, Kurtin P, Mihm M, Wu B, Pasqualucci L, Neuberg D, Aguiar RC, et al. 2005. Molecular profiling of diffuse large B-cell lymphoma identifies robust subtypes including one characterized by host inflammatory response. *Blood* **105:** 1851–1861. doi:10.1182/blood-2004-07-2947

Morin RD, Johnson NA, Severson TM, Mungall AJ, An J, Goya R, Paul JE, Boyle M, Woolcock BW, Kuchenbauer F, et al. 2010. Somatic mutations altering EZH2 (Tyr641) in follicular diffuse large B-cell lymphomas of germinal-center origin. *Nat Genet* **42:** 181–185.

Morin RD, Mungall K, Pleasance E, Mungall AJ, Goya R, Huff RD, Scott DW, Ding J, Roth A, Chiu R, et al. 2013. Mutational and structural analysis of diffuse large B-cell lymphoma using whole-genome sequencing. *Blood* **122:** 1256–1265. doi:10.1182/blood-2013-02-483727

Mortaz E, Tabarsi P, Mansouri D, Khosravi A, Garssen J, Velayati A, Adcock IM. 2016. Cancers related to immunodeficiencies: update and perspectives. *Front Immunol* **7:** 365. doi:10.3389/fimmu.2016.00365

Nagle SJ, Reshef R, Tsai DE. 2017. Posttransplant lymphoproliferative disorder in solid organ and hematopoietic stem cell transplantation. *Clin Chest Med* **38:** 771–783. doi:10.1016/j.ccm.2017.08.001

Natkunam Y, Farinha P, Hsi ED, Hans CP, Tibshirani R, Sehn LH, Connors JM, Gratzinger D, Rosado M, Zhao S. 2008. LMO2 protein expression predicts survival in patients with diffuse large B-cell lymphoma treated with anthracycline-based chemotherapy with and without rituximab. *J Clin Oncol* **26:** 447–454. doi:10.1200/JCO.2007.13.0690

Okosun J, Bödör C, Wang J, Araf S, Yang CY, Pan C, Boller S, Cittaro D, Bozek M, Iqbal S, et al. 2014. Integrated genomic analysis identifies recurrent mutations and evolution patterns driving the initiation and progression of follicular lymphoma. *Nat Genet* **46:** 176–181. doi:10.1038/ng.2856

Pang B, Qiao X, Janssen L, Velds A, Groothuis T, Kerkhoven R, Nieuwland M, Ovaa H, Rottenberg S, van Tellingen O, et al. 2013. Drug-induced histone eviction from open chromatin contributes to the chemotherapeutic effects of doxorubicin. *Nat Commun* **4:** 1908. doi:10.1038/ncomms2921

Papaemmanuil E, Gerstung M, Bullinger L, Gaidzik VI, Paschka P, Roberts ND, Potter NE, Heuser M, Thol F, Bolli N. 2016. Genomic classification and prognosis in acute myeloid leukemia. *N Engl J Med* **374:** 2209–2221. doi:10.1056/NEJMoa1516192

Pham-Ledard A, Prochazkova-Carlotti M, Deveza M, Laforet MP, Beylot-Barry M, Vergier B, Parrens M, Feuillard J, Merlio JP, Gachard N. 2017. Molecular analysis of immunoglobulin variable genes supports a germinal center experienced normal counterpart in primary cutaneous diffuse large B-cell lymphoma, leg-type. *J Dermatol Sci* **88:** 238–246. doi:10.1016/j.jdermsci.2017.07.008

Pommier Y, Leo E, Zhang H, Marchand C. 2010. DNA topoisomerases and their poisoning by anticancer and antibacterial drugs. *Chem Biol* **17:** 421–433. doi:10.1016/j.chembiol.2010.04.012

Psyrri A, Papageorgiou S, Liakata E, Scorilas A, Rontogianni D, Kontos CK, Argyriou P, Pectasides D, Harhalakis N, Pappa V, et al. 2009. Phosphatidylinositol 3′-kinase catalytic subunit α gene amplification contributes to the pathogenesis of mantle cell lymphoma. *Clin Cancer Res* **15:** 5724–5732. doi:10.1158/1078-0432.CCR-08-3215

Puente XS, Pinyol M, Quesada V, Conde L, Ordóñez GR, Villamor N, Escaramis G, Jares P, Beà S, González-Díaz M, et al. 2011. Whole-genome sequencing identifies recurrent mutations in chronic lymphocytic leukaemia. *Nature* **475:** 101–105. doi:10.1038/nature10113

Rajagopalan PT, Zhang Z, McCourt L, Dwyer M, Benkovic SJ, Hammes GG. 2002. Interaction of dihydrofolate reductase with methotrexate: ensemble and single-molecule kinetics. *Proc Natl Acad Sci* **99:** 13481–13486. doi:10.1073/pnas.172501499

Reddy A, Zhang J, Davis NS, Moffitt AB, Love CL, Waldrop A, Leppa S, Pasanen A, Meriranta L, Karjalainen-Lindsberg ML, et al. 2017. Genetic and functional drivers of diffuse large B cell lymphoma. *Cell* **171:** 481–494.e15. doi:10.1016/j.cell.2017.09.027

Richter J, Schlesner M, Hoffmann S, Kreuz M, Leich E, Burkhardt B, Rosolowski M, Ammerpohl O, Wagener R, Bernhart SH, et al. 2012. Recurrent mutation of the *ID3* gene in Burkitt lymphoma identified by integrated genome, exome and transcriptome sequencing. *Nat Genet* **44:** 1316–1320. doi:10.1038/ng.2469

Rimokh R, Berger F, Bastard C, Klein B, French M, Archimbaud E, Rouault JP, Santa Lucia B, Duret L, Vuillaume M, et al. 1994. Rearrangement of CCND1 (BCL1/PRAD1) 3′ untranslated region in mantle-cell lymphomas and t(11q13)-associated leukemias. *Blood* **83:** 3689–3696. doi:10.1182/blood.V83.12.3689.3689

Rimsza LM, Roberts RA, Miller TP, Unger JM, LeBlanc M, Braziel RM, Weisenberger DD, Chan WC, Muller-Hermelink HK, Jaffe ES. 2004. Loss of MHC class II gene and protein expression in diffuse large B-cell lymphoma is related to decreased tumor immunosurveillance and poor patient survival regardless of other prognostic factors: A follow-up study from the Leukemia and Lymphoma Molecular Profiling Project. *Blood* **103:** 4251–4258. doi:10.1182/blood-2003-07-2365

Robb-Smith AH. 1982. U.S. National Cancer Institute working formulation of non-Hodgkin's lymphomas for clinical use. *Lancet* **320:** 432–434. doi:10.1016/S0140-6736(82)90454-8

Rubinstein PG, Aboulafia DM, Zloza A. 2014. Malignancies in HIV/AIDS: from epidemiology to therapeutic challenges. *AIDS* **28:** 453–465. doi:10.1097/QAD.0000000000000071

Schmitz R, Young RM, Ceribelli M, Jhavar S, Xiao W, Zhang M, Wright G, Shaffer AL, Hodson DJ, Buras E, et al. 2012. Burkitt lymphoma pathogenesis and therapeutic targets from structural and functional genomics. *Nature* **490:** 116–120. doi:10.1038/nature11378

Schmitz R, Wright GW, Huang DW, Johnson CA, Phelan JD, Wang JQ, Roulland S, Kasbekar M, Young RM, Shaffer AL, et al. 2018. Genetics and pathogenesis of diffuse large B-cell lymphoma. *N Engl J Med* **378:** 1396–1407. doi:10.1056/NEJMoa1801445

Schuster SJ, Bartlett NL, Assouline S, Yoon SS, Bosch F, Sehn LH, Cheah CY, Shadman M, Gregory GP, Ku M, et al. 2019. Mosunetuzumab induces complete remissions in poor prognosis non-Hodgkin lymphoma patients, including those who are resistant to or relapsing after chimeric antigen receptor T-cell (CAR-T) therapies, is active in treatment through multiple lines. *Blood* **134:** 6.

Seaberg EC, Wiley D, Martínez-Maza O, Chmiel JS, Kingsley L, Tang Y, Margolick JB, Jacobson LP. 2010. Cancer incidence in the multicenter AIDS Cohort Study before and during the HAART era: 1984 to 2007. *Cancer* **116:** 5507–5516. doi:10.1002/cncr.25530

Seda V, Mraz M. 2015. B-cell receptor signalling and its crosstalk with other pathways in normal and malignant cells. *Eur J Haematol* **94:** 193–205. doi:10.1111/ejh.12427

Staudt LM. 2010. Oncogenic activation of NF-κB. *Cold Spring Harb Perspect Biol* **2:** a000109. doi:10.1101/cshperspect.a000109

Streubel B, Vinatzer U, Lamprecht A, Raderer M, Chott A. 2005. T(3;14)(p14.1;q32) involving IGH and FOXP1 is a novel recurrent chromosomal aberration in MALT lymphoma. *Leukemia* **19:** 652–658. doi:10.1038/sj.leu.2403644

Sun LL, Ellerman D, Mathieu M, Hristopoulos M, Chen X, Li Y, Yan X, Clark R, Reyes A, Stefanich E, et al. 2015. Anti-CD20/CD3 T cell–dependent bispecific antibody for the treatment of B cell malignancies. *Sci Transl Med* **7:** 287ra270.

Swerdlow SHCE, Harris NL, Jaffe ES, Pileri SA, Stein H, Thiele J, ed. 2017. *WHO classification of tumours of haematopoietic and lymphoid tissues*, revised 4th ed. International Agency for Research on Cancer, Lyon.

Takata K, Miyata-Takata T, Sato Y, Yoshino T. 2014. Pathology of follicular lymphoma. *J Clin Exp Hematop* **54:** 3–9. doi:10.3960/jslrt.54.3

Taub R, Kirsch I, Morton C, Lenoir G, Swan D, Tronick S, Aaronson S, Leder P. 1982. Translocation of the c-myc gene into the immunoglobulin heavy chain locus in human Burkitt lymphoma and murine plasmacytoma cells. *Proc Natl Acad Sci* **79:** 7837–7841. doi:10.1073/pnas.79.24.7837

Treon SP, Xu L, Yang G, Zhou Y, Liu X, Cao Y, Sheehy P, Manning RJ, Patterson CJ, Tripsas C, et al. 2012. MYD88 L265P somatic mutation in Waldenström's macroglobulinemia. *N Engl J Med* **367:** 826–833. doi:10.1056/NEJMoa1200710

Wang H, Yang H, Shivalila CS, Dawlaty MM, Cheng AW, Zhang F, Jaenisch R. 2013. One-step generation of mice carrying mutations in multiple genes by CRISPR/Cas-mediated genome engineering. *Cell* **153:** 910–918. doi:10.1016/j.cell.2013.04.025

Weiner GJ. 2010. Rituximab: mechanism of action. *Semin Hematol* **47:** 115–123. doi:10.1053/j.seminhematol.2010.01.011

Widhopf GF II, Kipps TJ. 2001. Normal B cells express *51p1*-encoded Ig heavy chains that are distinct from those expressed by chronic lymphocytic leukemia B cells. *J Immunol* **166:** 95–102. doi:10.4049/jimmunol.166.1.95

Willemze R, Jaffe ES, Burg G, Cerroni L, Berti E, Swerdlow SH, Ralfkiaer E, Chimenti S, Diaz-Perez JL, Duncan LM, et al. 2005. WHO-EORTC classification for cutaneous lymphomas. *Blood* **105:** 3768–3785. doi:10.1182/blood-2004-09-3502

Wright G, Tan B, Rosenwald A, Hurt EH, Wiestner A, Staudt LM. 2003. A gene expression-based method to diagnose clinically distinct subgroups of diffuse large B cell lymphoma. *Proc Natl Acad Sci* **100:** 9991–9996. doi:10.1073/pnas.1732008100

Yahiaoui OI, Nunès JA, Castanier C, Devillier R, Broussais F, Fabre AJ, Naimi D, Bouabdallah R, Olive D, Xerri L. 2014. Constitutive AKT activation in follicular lymphoma. *BMC Cancer* **14:** 565. doi:10.1186/1471-2407-14-565

Yu J, Wang W, Huang H. 2019. Efficacy safety of bispecific T-cell engager (BiTE) antibody blinatumomab for the treatment of relapsed/refractory acute lymphoblastic leukemia and non-Hodgkin's lymphoma: a systemic review and meta-analysis. *Hematology* **24:** 199–207.

Zafra MP, Schatoff EM, Katti A, Foronda M, Breinig M, Schweitzer AY, Simon A, Han T, Goswami S, Montgomery E, et al. 2018. Optimized base editors enable efficient editing in cells, organoids and mice. *Nat Biotechnol* **36:** 888–893. doi:10.1038/nbt.4194

Zhang J, Grubor V, Love CL, Banerjee A, Richards KL, Mieczkowski PA, Dunphy C, Choi W, Au WY, Srivastava G, et al. 2013. Genetic heterogeneity of diffuse large B-cell lymphoma. *Proc Natl Acad Sci* **110:** 1398–1403. doi:10.1073/pnas.1205299110

Zhang J, Jima D, Moffitt AB, Liu Q, Czader M, Hsi ED, Fedoriw Y, Dunphy CH, Richards KL, Gill JI, et al. 2014. The genomic landscape of mantle cell lymphoma is related to the epigenetically determined chromatin state of normal B cells. *Blood* **123:** 2988–2996. doi:10.1182/blood-2013-07-517177

Zhang L, Nomie K, Zhang H, Bell T, Pham L, Kadri S, Segal J, Li S, Zhou S, Santos D, et al. 2017. B-cell lymphoma patient-derived xenograft models enable drug discovery and are a platform for personalized therapy. *Clin Cancer Res* **23:** 4212–4223. doi:10.1158/1078-0432.CCR-16-2703

Zucca E, Bertoni F. 2004. *MALT lymphomas.* Landes Bioscience, Georgetown, TX.

Biology and Molecular Pathogenesis of Mature T-Cell Lymphomas

José R. Cortés[1] and Teresa Palomero[1,2]

[1]Institute for Cancer Genetics, [2]Department of Pathology and Cell Biology, Columbia University Irving Medical Center, New York, New York 10032, USA

Correspondence: tp2151@columbia.edu

Peripheral T-cell lymphomas (PTCLs) constitute a highly heterogeneous group of hematological diseases with complex clinical and molecular features consistent with the diversity of the T-cell type from which they originate. In the past several years, the systematic implementation of high-throughput genomic technologies for the analysis of T-cell malignancies has supported an exponential progress in our understanding of the genetic drivers of oncogenesis and unraveled the molecular complexity of these diseases. Recent findings have helped redefine the classification of T-cell malignancies and provided novel biomarkers to improve diagnosis accuracy and analyze the response to therapy. In addition, multiple novel targeted therapies including small-molecule inhibitors, antibody-based approaches, and immunotherapy have shown promising results in early clinical analysis and have the potential to completely change the way T-cell malignancies have been treated traditionally.

Peripheral T-cell lymphomas (PTCLs) are a heterogeneous group of highly aggressive malignant hematologic tumors that arise from clonal proliferation of mature post-thymic T cells (Gaulard and de Leval 2014). PTCLs account for ~15% of all non-Hodgkin lymphomas and cover almost 30 different entities (Swerdlow et al. 2016). Compared with B-cell lymphomas, PTCLs are less common, are more difficult to diagnose and classify, are more aggressive, and have inferior outcomes with current treatments. Indeed, with rare exceptions, the prognosis for PTCL is dismal, with survival rates in the 20%–30% range at 5 years (Savage 2008). T-cell lymphomas are also less understood in terms of their normal T-cell counterparts, and until recently, most subtypes lacked defined drivers that could potentially be targeted for the development of precision therapies. Interestingly, the incidence of PTCL, which generally affects the elderly population, has been consistently increasing over the past decades, but unfortunately, this increase has not been accompanied by improvements in survival (Weisenburger et al. 2011).

However, over the past few years, genomic and transcriptomic studies have substantially advanced our understanding of the molecular subtyping of PTCL and facilitated the identifi-

Cite this article as *Cold Spring Harb Perspect Med* doi: 10.1101/cshperspect.a035402

cation of molecular vulnerabilities in these tumors, opening the field for the development of tailored therapies targeting specific driver genetic alterations that will hopefully be translated into better clinical outcomes.

CLASSIFICATION AND MOLECULAR ETIOLOGY OF T-CELL LYMPHOMA

The fourth edition of the World Health Organization (WHO) classification established the guidelines for classification of hematopoietic and lymphoid tumors in 2008, with a major revision published in 2016 primarily to address several major advances in the field with significant clinical and biological implications in patient management (Swerdlow et al. 2016). Many of these changes are the result of genomic studies, including analysis of Gene Expression Profile (GEP) and characterization of the genetic landscape of T-cell and natural killer (NK)-cell neoplasms. This revised classification of the lymphoid neoplasms included the addition of a number of provisional entities highlighted in Table 1. In this review, we will describe the most frequent subtypes of PTCL, as well as the most common genetic aberrations identified for each subgroup.

Table 1. Classification of mature T and NK neoplasms according to WHO 2016 revision

Angioimmunoblastic T-cell lymphoma
Peripheral T-cell lymphoma, NOS
*Follicular T-cell lymphoma**
Nodal peripheral T-cell lymphoma with TFH phenotype*
Anaplastic large-cell lymphoma, ALK$^+$
Anaplastic large-cell lymphoma, ALK$^-$*
*Breast implant-associated anaplastic large-cell lymphoma**
T-cell prolymphocytic leukemia
T-cell large granular lymphocytic leukemia
Chronic lymphoproliferative disorder of NK cells
Aggressive NK-cell leukemia
Systemic EBV$^+$ T-cell lymphoma of childhood*
Hydroa vacciniforme–like lymphoproliferative disorder*
Adult T-cell leukemia/lymphoma
Extranodal NK/T-cell lymphoma, nasal type
Enteropathy-associated T-cell lymphoma
Monomorphic epitheliotropic intestinal T-cell lymphoma*
*Indolent T-cell lymphoproliferative disorder of the GI tract**
Hepatosplenic T-cell lymphoma
Subcutaneous panniculitis-like T-cell lymphoma
Mycosis fungoides
Sézary syndrome
Primary cutaneous CD30$^+$ T-cell lymphoproliferative disorders
Lymphomatoid papulosis
Primary cutaneous anaplastic large cell lymphoma
Primary cutaneous γδ T-cell lymphoma
Primary cutaneous CD8$^+$ aggressive epidermotropic cytotoxic T-cell lymphoma
*Primary cutaneous acral CD8$^+$ T-cell lymphoma**
*Primary cutaneous CD4$^+$ small/medium T-cell lymphoproliferative disorder**

Data adapted from Swerdlow et al. 2016.

Provisional entities are listed in *italics* and changes from the 2008 classification are indicated by asterisks (*). Entities that will be discussed in this review are shown in **bold**.

(NK) Natural killer, (NOS) not otherwise specified, (TFH) T-follicular helper, (ALK) anaplastic lymphoma kinase, (EBV) Epstein–Barr virus, (GI) gastrointestinal.

ANGIOIMMUNOBLASTIC T-CELL LYMPHOMA

Angioimmunoblastic T-cell lymphoma (AITL) is the second most common PTCL subtype worldwide and the most frequent subtype in the Western world, where it represents >30% of PTCL cases (Federico et al. 2013). AITL develops with a unique pathobiology and clinical presentation including a chronically activated immune system with frequent hypergammaglobulinemia and autoimmune features (Lunning and Vose 2017). AITL is characterized by the presence of clonal $CD4^+$ neoplastic T cells, a highly reactive tumor microenvironment, and clonal expansions affecting the B-cell compartment, frequently positive for Epstein–Barr virus (EBV) (Zhou et al. 2007). Initial gene expression profiling studies contributed to establish T follicular helper (TFH) cells as the cell of origin in AITL (de Leval et al. 2007), based on a characteristic expression of TFH markers in the malignant T cells. Indeed, the differential diagnosis criteria for AITL requires the concurrent presence of at least two TFH markers, including PD-1, CXCR5, ICOS, BCL6, CXCL13, CD10, and SAP, to confirm the diagnosis of AITL.

Genetic alterations affecting epigenetic regulators, including *TET2*, *DNMT3A*, and *IDH2*, are one of the hallmarks of AITL (Cortés and Palomero 2016). The ten-eleven translocation 2 (TET2) encodes a 2-oxoglutarate/$Fe2^+$–dependent oxygenase that participates in the epigenetic control of gene expression by catalyzing the oxidation of DNA 5-methylcytosine to 5-hydroxymethylcytosine (Tahiliani et al. 2009; Ito et al. 2010; Cimmino et al. 2011). First identified as a tumor suppressor in myeloid malignancies (Abdel-Wahab et al. 2009; Delhommeau et al. 2009), multiple studies have shown a high prevalence of loss-of-function mutations in TET2 in PTCLs particularly in AITL (~50%) and PTCL-not otherwise specified (NOS) (~40%), in which they are frequently identified as an initial event in the process of transformation (Couronné et al. 2012; Palomero et al. 2014; Sakata-Yanagimoto et al. 2014; Yoo et al. 2014) and are associated with worse outcome (Lemonnier et al. 2012). In a recent study, analysis of *TET2* mutations and *TCR* rearrangements in AITL and PTCL-NOS cases demonstrated the presence of biclonal populations derived from a common TET2 mutant progenitor, suggestive of parallel tumor evolution from common hematopoietic progenitor pool (Yao et al. 2020). Loss of *Tet2* has been associated with enhanced hematopoietic stem cell (HSC) self-renewal and an increased HSC pool (Moran-Crusio et al. 2011). Moreover, *TET2* mutations are frequently found in the blood of healthy elderly individuals, a condition termed clonal hematopoiesis of indeterminate potential (CHIP), and are associated with increased risk for developing a hematologic malignancy (Busque et al. 2012; Steensma 2018; Steensma and Ebert 2020). The relative high frequency of clonal hematopoiesis in otherwise healthy individuals indicates that these initial TET2 mutations are not sufficient for transformation; however, mutant premalignant cells can fully transform into diverse malignancies upon acquisition of secondary genetic hits.

DNMT3A encodes a DNA methyltransferase that controls cytosine methylation and is recurrently affected by loss-of-function mutations in 10%–40% of AITL patients. Mutations in DNMT3A are considered an initial event in the process of transformation and interestingly frequently co-occur with *TET2* mutations (Cortés and Palomero 2016). Indeed, cooperation between loss-of-function mutations in *Dnmt3a* and *Tet2* has been shown to lead to malignant transformation in mouse models (Scourzic et al. 2016).

Finally, IDH2 is a metabolic mitochondrial enzyme involved in the generation of 2-oxoglutarate that is specifically mutated in 30%–40% of AITL patients (Cortés and Palomero 2016). Mutant *IDH2* forms have a neomorphic enzymatic activity leading instead to the generation of 2-hydroxyglutarate, an oncometabolite that antagonizes the activity the TET family of enzymes (Cortés and Palomero 2016). AITL is the only PTCL subgroup in which *IDH2* mutations are found, and, remarkably, they occur almost exclusively in position R172 (R172K, R172S) (Cairns et al. 2012), which is associated with increased production of 2-HG compared to other IDH2 mutant alleles. Although mutations in

TET2 and IDH2 are also present in myeloid malignancies, where they are mutually exclusive, AITLs frequently present co-occurring mutations in *IDH2* and *TET2* (Cortés and Palomero 2016). Interestingly, IDH2 mutations in AITL are presumed to constitute a secondary hit and might refine the differentiation of the premalignant clones. Indeed, the co-occurrence of TET2 inactivation and IDH2 mutations is associated with a potential cooperative effect in the regulation of the expression of TFH specific genes, leading to a more polarized TFH signature than achieved by the presence of TET2 mutations alone (Wang et al. 2015a).

Gene expression profiling studies have proposed that AITL tumors may be driven by increased T-cell receptor signaling. Consistently, genomic studies have uncovered the presence of highly recurrent mutations affecting T-cell receptor–initiated signaling pathways, including the frequent mutations in the small GTPase *RHOA*, as well as genetic alterations affecting *VAV1*, *PLCG1*, *CD28*, and the tyrosine kinase *FYN* (Vallois et al. 2016).

A central role of RHOA in the pathogenesis of AITL is supported by the identification of a recurrent, highly prevalent heterozygous missense *RHOA G17V* mutation detected in up to 70% of the patients with AITLs (Fig. 1; Palomero et al. 2014; Sakata-Yanagimoto et al. 2014; Yoo et al. 2014). The presence of the *RHOA* G17V mutation is highly specific of AITL and has become a molecular diagnostic determinant for this PTCL subgroup. Clinical studies have even suggested that the presence of *RHOA* G17V could be associated with worse prognosis (Nagao et al. 2016; Ondrejka et al. 2016). Mutations in *RHOA* G17V generally co-occur with mutations in epigenetic regulators, being most frequently associated with loss-of-function mutations in TET2. Mutations in

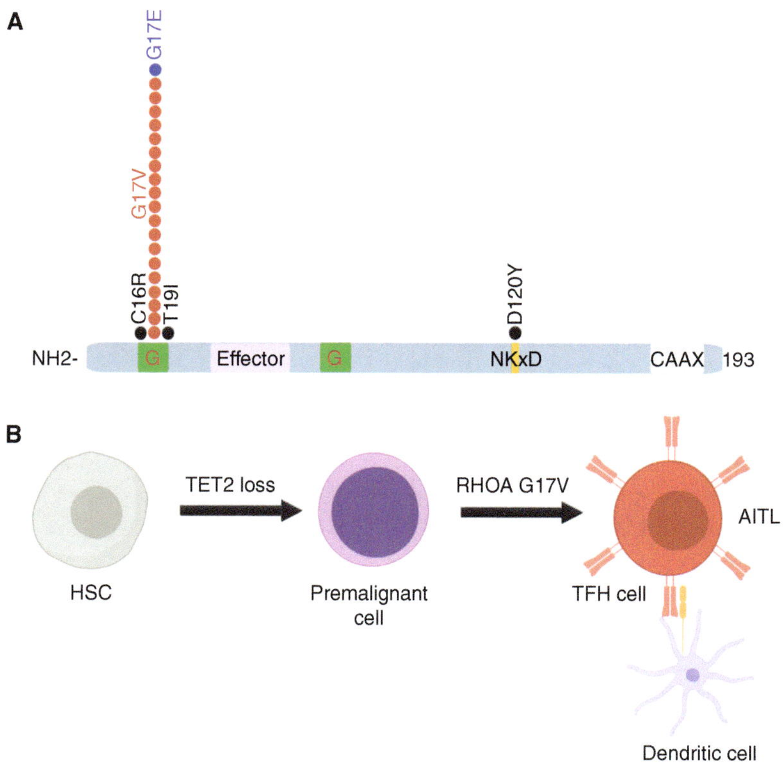

Figure 1. Schematic (*A*) representation of the RHOA mutations identified in AITL and model for process of malignant transformation leading to AITL (*B*). (*A*, Adapted from Palomero et al. 2014, courtesy of Springer/Nature © 2014; *B*, adapted from Cortés et al. 2018, with permission from Elsevier © 2018.)

RHOA G17V act as dominant negatives interfering with the signaling initiated by wild-type RHOA (Palomero et al. 2014). Recent studies using engineered mouse models demonstrated that expression of *Rhoa* G17V in $CD4^+$ T cells induces increased proliferation and TFH-cell specification (Cortés et al. 2018; Ng et al. 2018). Notably, the combination of *Tet2* loss and expression of *Rhoa* G17V is sufficient to induce AITL development (Cortés et al. 2018). This result supports a multistep model for AITL development in which loss-of-function mutations in epigenetics factors in early hematopoietic progenitors will be an initiating event in the process of transformation, inducing the generation of multipotent premalignant clones. Upon acquisition of a second hit in *RHOA* G17V, premalignant cells differentiate toward TFH cells and induce development of AITL (Fig. 1). Both TFH lineage specification and AITL development downstream of RHOA G17V depend on the activation of the ICOS/PI3K/mTOR signaling pathway and are sensitive to PI3K inhibitors (Cortés et al. 2018).

Mutations in *VAV1* have been identified in up to 10% of AITL and PTCL-NOS patients. *VAV1* encodes a hematopoietic-specific Rho family-specific guanine exchange factor (Bustelo 2000). Genomic alterations in *VAV1* in PTCL include a recurrent in-frame deletion mutation (*VAV1* Δ778–786) generated by alternative splicing mechanism as well as multiple *VAV1* gene fusions affecting the carboxy-terminal domain of VAV1 that lead to its constitutive activation (Abate et al. 2017). Alterations in *RHOA* and *VAV1* are mutually exclusive, suggesting they could be affecting the same genetic pathway (Fujisawa et al. 2018).

Recurrent mutations in *CD28*, a major costimulatory molecule for the T-cell receptor (TCR), have also been described in AITL (Rohr et al. 2015). PTCL-associated *CD28* mutations affect the D124 and T195 residues and increase ligand–receptor interaction and signal transduction. Notably, CD28-mutated AITL patients have inferior survival compared to nonmutated cases (Rohr et al. 2015). Finally, recurrent activating mutations in FYN, a SRC family kinase, have been found in ~3% of PTCL-NOS and AITL cases (Palomero et al. 2014).

Similar genomic aberrations to the ones identified in AITL have been described for follicular T-cell lymphoma and nodal peripheral T-cell lymphoma with TFH phenotype (see Table 1). This has led to the grouping of these two provisional entities with AITL. All three groups share similar gene expression patterns, TFH-associated immunophenotypic markers, and genetic abnormalities; however, despite their common TFH phenotype, these diseases have differing clinical and pathological features and, as such, remain distinct entities within the classification (Swerdlow et al. 2016).

PTCL-NOS

PTCL-NOS includes mature T-cell lymphoma cases that cannot unequivocally be assigned to other subtypes, making this group highly heterogeneous and poorly understood. PTCL-NOS is the most common entity in mature T-cell neoplasms; however, the diagnosis of PTCL-NOS has decreased in recent years because of the introduction of molecular profiling that allows for better lymphoma classification.

The characterization of the molecular landscape of PTCL-NOS has identified the presence of frequent mutations epigenetic regulators, including *KMT2C* and *KMT2D*, *KDM6A*, *ARID1B*, *SETD1B*, *CREBBP* and *ARID2* as well as *TET2* and *DNMT3A*, which are likely associated with the TFH-like group (Palomero et al. 2014). Also, genes involved in signaling pathways are frequent targets of alterations in PTCL-NOS, including genes in the NF-κB and TCR signaling pathways such as *TNFAIP3*, *APC*, *CHD8*, *ZAP70*, *NF1*, *TNFRSF14*, *TRAF3*, and *VAV1* (Palomero et al. 2014; Abate et al. 2017; Watatani et al. 2019). Recent analysis of a large PTCL-NOS cohort has identified additional altered genes, such as *YTHDF2*, a RNA methyl transferase, and *PD-1* (Watatani et al. 2019). More interestingly, a previously undescribed molecular subtype characterized by TP53 and/or CDKN2A mutations and deletions, has been identified associated with worse prognosis, chromosomal instability, and altered immune evasion (Watatani et al. 2019), suggesting a driver role for TP53 in PTCL-NOS (Watatani et al. 2019).

Gene expression profiling in PTCL-NOS has identified two distinct molecular subgroups characterized by the differential high expression of *TBX21* or *GATA3*, two key regulators of Th1 and Th2 cell differentiation (Iqbal et al. 2014; Wang et al. 2015a). Although the precise mechanisms that lead to the increased expression of these master regulators are unknown, they might be related to different cells of origin. More importantly, these groups are associated with different clinical behavior and response to therapy, with expression of *GATA3* being linked to worse outcome (Iqbal et al. 2014).

ANAPLASTIC LARGE-CELL LYMPHOMAS

Anaplastic large cell lymphoma (ALCL) includes several subtypes of aggressive lymphoid neoplasms with similar histologic characteristics but distinct genomic features. The latest WHO classification contains two systemic ALCL entities: ALK^- ALCL and ALK^+ ALCL (Swerdlow et al. 2016) in addition to a primarily cutaneous form of ALCL, (cALCL), more closely related to ALK^- ALCL, and a new provisional category, breast implant–associated ALCL (BIALCL) (Swerdlow et al. 2016). The neoplastic cells are typically large with abundant cytoplasm and characteristic horseshoe nuclei shapes and characterized by strong expression of CD30 and negative for TCR (Shustov and Soma 2019). Despite the lack of expression of surface TCR, ALCLs are classified as T-cell lymphoma because of their peripheral presentation and the presence of TCR rearrangements that are detectable in the tumor cells at the molecular level that are supportive of a T-cell origin. Interestingly, data from murine models suggests that transformation could be initiated in early thymocytes, before TCR β-rearrangement, and although TCR is still required for thymic egress and development of peripheral murine tumors, down-regulation of the TCR would be required to complete lymphomagenesis. This model is consistent with the characteristics of TCR rearrangements in human ALCL, which are often aberrant and would not be permissive for survival during thymic development (Malcolm et al. 2016)

ALK^+ ALCL is generally diagnosed in younger individuals of Western origin with slight male predominance (Ferreri et al. 2012). ALK^+ ALCL constitutes also the most frequent mature aggressive lymphoma within the pediatric population. Moreover, it is also the PTCL subtype with the best overall outcome (Savage 2008). ALK^+ ALCL is associated with the presence of chromosomal translocations that lead to the constitutive activation of ALK, a receptor tyrosine kinase, being the most frequent t(2;5) translocation (nucleophosmin [NPM]-ALK). ALK translocations lead to increased activation of ERK/MAPK, JAK/STAT, and PI3K signaling pathways. Moreover, ALK fusion-mediated activation of STAT3 has been shown to be required for the maintenance of the transformed phenotype in ALK^+ ALCL (Chiarle et al. 2005). ALK fusions constitutively activate VAV1 and VAV3 in ALCL, increasing RAC1 and CDC42 activity, down-regulating the Wiskott–Aldrich syndrome protein (WASP) and WASP-interacting protein (WIP) tumor suppressors and promoting lymphoma survival (Choudhari et al. 2016; Menotti et al. 2019).

ALK^- ALCL patients are generally older and associated with a worse outcome (Ferreri et al. 2013). Molecular events affecting DUSP22 and TP63 have been reported to be mutually exclusive and predictors of survival outcomes, with expression of DUSP22 associated with a favorable prognosis and TP63 being an unfavorable marker. Recurrent translocations and loss of TP53 and PRDM1/BLIMP1 have also been proved to have a pathogenic role associated with less favorable outcomes (Boi et al. 2013; Parrilla Castellar et al. 2014). In addition, very frequent activating mutations in the JAK/STAT pathways, more specifically in *JAK1* and *STAT3*, have been identified in almost 20% of ALK-ALCL (Crescenzo et al. 2015). Recurrent gene translocations linked to JAK/STAT pathway activation, including NCOR2-ROS1, NFkB2-ROS1, and different fusions affecting the TYK2 kinase, have also been identified (Crescenzo et al. 2015). This suggests that activation of STAT3 is a common mechanism of malignant transformation in ALCL, independently of ALK status, and provides a genetic rationale for the

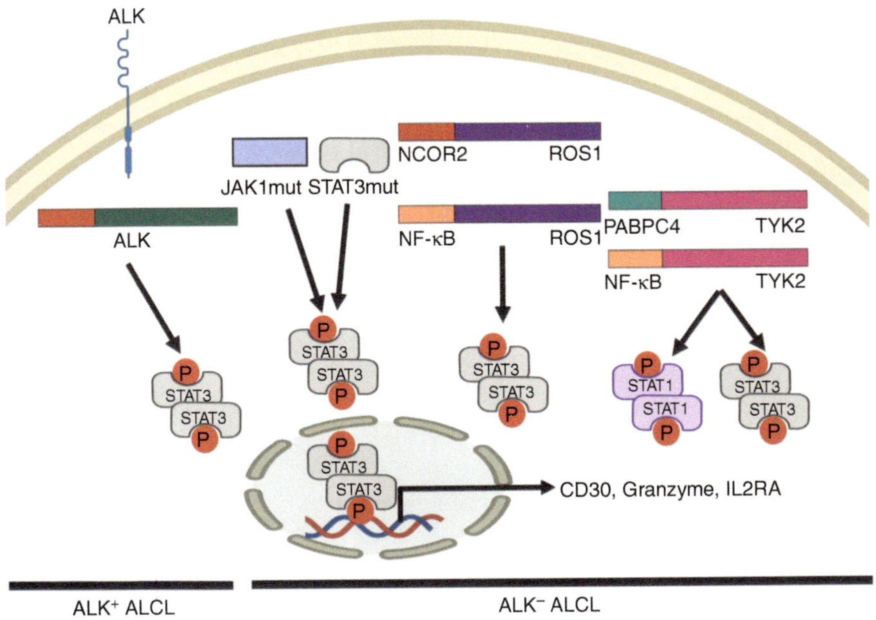

Figure 2. Recurrent mutations and kinase fusions in anaplastic large cell lymphoma (ALCL) converge to induce oncogenic STAT3 activation in ALK$^+$ and ALK$^-$ ALCL subtypes. (Figure was created from data adapted from Crescenzo et al. 2015.)

morphologic and phenotypic similarities between ALK$^+$ and ALK$^-$ ALCL (Fig. 2).

Finally, there is a novel provisional category, BIALCL, arising in association with prolonged exposure to breast implants, for which the factors leading to progression still remain to be determined (Miranda et al. 2014; Laurent et al. 2016).

ADULT T-CELL LEUKEMIA/LYMPHOMA

Adult T-cell leukemia/lymphoma (ATLL) is a mature T-cell lymphoma derived from the transformation of regulatory T cells and associated with the infection by the human T-cell lymphotropic virus type 1 (HTLV-1) (Bangham and Toulza 2011). In ATLL pathogenesis, viral products such as *Tax* and *HBZ* have important roles in oncogenic transformation (Giam and Semmes 2016). However, although the *Tax* gene, a nonstructural gene on the HTLV-1 genome, appears to play a critical role in transformation initiation, it is not critical to sustain tumor cell growth, and it is frequently no longer expressed in transformed cells. *HBZ* is one of the few genes consistently overexpressed in most ATLL cases (Bazarbachi et al. 2011). Interestingly, <5% of HTLV1-infected individuals will eventually develop ATLL and only after a long latency (Giam and Semmes 2016); thus, other factors are required for transformation in a multistep process that might involve viral and epigenetic mechanisms in conjunction with acquired genomic alterations. ATLL is geographically restricted to those regions where HTLV-1 is endemic, including Japan, Central and South America, the Caribbean, and certain regions in western Africa. In this regard, the introduction of preventative approaches to reduce the spread of HTLV1 infection could have a significant impact on the incidence of ATLL.

Four different clinical presentations of ATLL have been described: acute, lymphomatous, chronic, and smoldering (Matutes 2007). The acute presentation is the most common and severe, being associated with the worst prognosis. Malignant cells have a classical nuclear morphology resembling a cloverleaf, and might express CD30. In most cases, ATLL cells express CD3, CD4, and CD25, and lack CD7, whereas in 10%–15% of cases, there is expression of CD4 and CD8. The cell of origin of ATLL cells is hypothesized to be regulatory T cells based on the expression of FoxP3 in some tumor cells; however, the assignment remains controversial (Malcolm et al. 2016). ATLL cells are also characterized by high expression of CCR4 and CCR7 chemokine receptors, which are involved in ATLL cell migration and infiltration of lymphoid organs and skin (Ohshima 2015).

Analyses of large patient cohorts using next-generation sequencing approaches have delineated the molecular landscape of ATLL and identified recurrent somatic mutations and genetic aberrations affecting multiple elements of the TCR-NF-κB signaling pathways (Kataoka et al. 2015). Thus, gain-of-function mutations and focal amplifications leading to constitutive activation of this pathway have been identified in proximal (*CD28, PLCG1, VAV1, RHOA* and *FYN*) and distal (*PRKCB* and *CARD11*) elements within the TCR-NF-κB pathway. Fusions involving CD28 such as CTLA4-CD28 and ICOS-CD28 are also recurrent. Mutations or deletions involving p16 and *p53* tumor suppressors are common and generally associated with disease progression (Yamada and Kamihira 2005). Frequent mutations affecting CCR4 and CCR7 receptors, mostly involving truncation of the carboxy-terminal domains have been described. These mutations interfere with ligand-induced receptor internalization, leading to enhanced activation of downstream PI3K/AKT signaling (Kataoka et al. 2015). Finally, missense mutations affecting the NOTCH1 receptor have also been described in 30% of ATLL patients. The mutations affect the PEST domain of the NOTCH1 protein preventing the FBXW7-mediated degradation of NOTCH (Pancewicz et al. 2010). Interestingly, FBXW7 is also found mutated in 25% of ATLL (Yeh et al. 2016)

Several key transcription factors in lymphocyte activation and homeostasis are also recurrently mutated in ATLL. Thus, focal amplifications and frequent mutations in *IRF4*, a major downstream target of NF-κB, confer gain-of-function activity to the mutated protein. *GATA3*, required for T-cell differentiation, is affected by nonsense and frameshift mutations distributed throughout the coding regions that result in dominant negative isoforms, whereas *IKZF2* is frequently affected by intragenic deletions in more than one-third of ATLL patients, leading to abnormally spliced shorter forms that act as dominant negatives and have oncogenic activity in vivo.

Last, molecules associated with immune surveillance, such as *HLA-A/B, CD58,* and *FAS*, are recurrently affected by loss-of-function mutations. Structural variations that truncate the PD-L1 3′-untranslated region leading to its overexpression are also frequent (Kataoka et al. 2019). Interestingly, expression of PD-L1 in ATLL cells has been correlated with a poor prognosis (Miyoshi et al. 2016). This might be of relevance in the context of ATLL immunotherapy, considering recent reports describing rapid disease progression in ATLL patients receiving PD-1 inhibitor therapy (Ratner et al. 2018).

NK/T-CELL LYMPHOMA

Natural killer/T-cell lymphoma (NKTCL) is an aggressive type of non-Hodgkin lymphoma characterized by a clonal proliferation of NK T cells. It most commonly affects the upper respiratory and digestive tracts although sometimes it involves extranasal tissues such as the skin, gastrointestinal tract, soft tissues, and testis (de Mel et al. 2019b,a). NKTCL is most prevalent in Asians and the Native American populations of Mexico, Central America, and South America (Haverkos et al. 2016).

NKTCL is commonly associated with EBV viral infection (Suzuki 2014; Chaudhary et al. 2015; Komabayashi et al. 2017), although little is known about the genomic and transcriptomic profiles of EBV in NKTCL. Sequence variations of LMP1, a key latent protein with abilities to promote cell proliferation and inhibit cell apoptosis in NKTCL, have been demonstrated (Ito et al. 2014). It has been suggested that the role of LMP1 in NK and T cells is to increase the sensitivity of the infected cell to the growth-promoting effects of IL-2.

Activation of the JAK/STAT pathway plays a prominent role in the pathogenesis of NKTCL, and up-regulation of IL2, IL10, and IFNGR1 are frequent events in NKTCL. JAK3-activating mutations promoting cytokine-independent STAT activation and enhancing NKTCL cell proliferation have also been described (Koo et al. 2012; Sim et al. 2017). Increased JAK/STAT signaling induces up-regulation of MYC and its interacting proteins (Huang et al. 2018); as well as phosphorylation of EZH2, a component of the Polycomb repressive complex 2 (PRC2), resulting in the up-regulation of genes involved in cell cycle regulation, DNA replication, invasiveness, and stemness (Yan et al. 2016).

In addition to the multiple modalities of JAK/STAT dysregulation in NKTCL, mutations in genes related to epigenetic modification are also common in NKTCL, including genes associated with histone methylation (KMT2D), histone acetylation (EP300), histone deubiquitination (ASXL3), and chromatin remodeling (ARID1A) (Choi et al. 2016).

ENTEROPATHY-ASSOCIATED T-CELL LYMPHOMAS

Enteropathy-associated T-cell lymphomas derive from the transformation of small intestinal intraepithelial lymphocytes (Chander et al. 2018). The most recent PTCL classification distinguishes between enteropathy-associated lymphoma closely linked to celiac disease (EATL, previously named EATL, type I) and monomorphic epitheliotropic intestinal T-cell lymphoma (MEITL, previously named EATL type II) (Swerdlow et al. 2016).

EATL is a rare entity usually associated to elderly individuals of Northern European descent (Delabie et al. 2011) and is a known complication of celiac disease, an autoimmune disorder characterized by gluten intolerance (Chander et al. 2018). Most EATLs were believed to arise from the neoplastic transformation of thymus-derived cytotoxic intraepithelial TCRαβ$^+$ T cells; however, recent reports have also suggested an origin of a subset of EATLs from intraepithelial TCRγδ$^+$ T cells (Chander et al. 2018). Recurrent activating mutations in members of the JAK/STAT pathway, including JAK1 and STAT3, have been recently described in EATL (Roberti et al. 2016; Moffitt et al. 2017), which suggests deregulation of cytokine signaling to be an early event in lymphomagenesis.

MEITL is less common than EATL, shows no association with celiac disease, and occurs worldwide (Roberti et al. 2016). In the majority of the cases, MEITL neoplastic cells are derived from γδ T cells, although there are also exceptions (Chan et al. 2011; Swerdlow et al. 2016). Recurrent alterations in SETD2 are the hallmark of MEITL, being detected in >90% of patients (Roberti et al. 2016). Additional mutations in other epigenetic regulators including CREBBP, ARID1, EP300, and EZH2 were also found at lower frequencies. Also recurrent were mutations affecting the JAK/STAT signaling pathway, including STAT5 and JAK3 (Kucuk et al. 2015; Nairismägi et al. 2016), the MAPK pathway (including BRAF, KRAS, and NRAS) and TP53 (Roberti et al. 2016).

HEPATOSPLENIC T-CELL LYMPHOMA

Hepatosplenic T-cell lymphoma (HSTCL) derives from nonactivated cytotoxic T cells. This rare entity is found in younger male patients, sometimes associated with chronic immunosuppression (Shi and Wang 2015). HSTCL primarily affects the liver, spleen, and frequently the bone marrow and is characterized by the expansion of malignant medium-sized T cells expressing cytotoxic markers (including T1A1$^+$ and granzyme M$^+$) and killer immunoglobulin receptors (Kirs) (Yabe et al. 2018). The most common HSCTL type is derived from γ/δ T cells with a small percentage derived from α/β T cells (Shi and Wang 2015; Swerdlow et al. 2016), although both subtypes are otherwise clinically and genetically similar. The most frequent mutations identified in HSCTL affect chromatin-modifier genes such as the SETD2 tumor suppressor, INO80, and ARID1B, in addition to recurrent activating mutations affecting elements of the JAK/STAT pathway, predominantly *STAT5B* and less often *STAT3*, and PIK3CD (Nicolae et al. 2014; McKinney et al. 2017)

CUTANEOUS T-CELL LYMPHOMAS

Cutaneous T-cell lymphomas (CTCLs) are characterized by the presence of skin-homing CD4$^+$ malignant T cells. Although current models place the origin of mature cutaneous T-cell lymphomas from memory T cells in the periphery, there have also been reports of quiescent cancer precursor cells residing in bone marrow, which secondarily migrate to the skin producing clinically apparent cutaneous lymphoma lesions (Gniadecki et al. 2003; Hamrouni et al. 2019). Mycosis fungoides (MF) and Sézary syndrome (SS) are two major subtypes of CTCL, constituting 75% of the cases diagnosed as CTCL (Devata and Wilcox 2016). MF cases with limited skin involvement have a generally good prognosis; however, advanced skin involvement, presence of characteristic Sézary cells in peripheral blood and/or lymph node, and organ infiltration are associated with dismal outcomes.

Multiple genomic studies to define the mutational landscape of CTCL have demonstrated the existence of a marked genomic heterogeneity (Vaqué et al. 2014; Choi et al. 2015; da Silva Almeida et al. 2015; Ungewickell et al. 2015; Wang et al. 2015b). Common driver genetic lesions include mutations and copy number alterations affecting cell cycle regulators (*CDKN1B*), chromatin-modifying genes (*ARID1A, ARID5B, SMARCC1, DNMT3A*, and *TET2*), DNA damage response genes, and immune evasion genes, as well as genes involved in T-cell signaling, migration, and differentiation (including a recurrent mutation in *RHOA* N117I of unknown significance). Frequent mutations and chromosomal deletions affecting TP53 have been identified in >50% of the patients with CTCL (Chang et al. 2018). Genomic analysis of CTCL found recurrent gain-of-function mutations and amplifications affecting the JAK/STAT pathway, including *JAK1, JAK3, STAT3*, and *STAT5B*, resulting in the hyperactivation of this signaling pathway. In addition, the NF-κB pathway is frequently targeted by somatic mutations in CTCL, including *PLCG1, CARD11, TNFRSF1B*, and recently *RLTPR*, a scaffolding protein that strongly upregulates the NF-κB signaling (Park et al. 2017). The convergence of diverse mutations on this pathway, generally mutually exclusive, highlights the role of NF-κB signaling in CTCL lymphomagenesis and supports the potential therapeutic role for NF-κB inhibitors.

NOVEL THERAPEUTIC APPROACHES FOR THE TREATMENT OF MATURE T-CELL LYMPHOMAS

The current standard of care for mature T-cell lymphomas is based on traditional chemotherapy with an induction therapy using a combination of cyclophosphamide, doxorubicin, vincristine, and prednisone (CHOP) followed by stem cell transplant after first remission. Unfortunately, this therapeutic approach only achieves survival rates of 40%–50% and prognosis remains dismal for most of the PTCL subtypes (Lue et al. 2017). CHOP-based approaches are specifically ineffective in ATLL patients, who present low response rates with frequent relapses and short survival. In this specific group, antiretroviral treatment, combining zidovudine (AZT) and interferon alpha (IFN-α), appears to be an option for first-line therapy (Bazarbachi et al. 2010).

The increased understanding of the biology of PTCL achieved during the past few years has supported an exponential rise in the development of novel targeted therapies in PTCL that are generally better tolerated and in multiple instances have achieved very significant responses (Table 2; Fig. 3). Most of these agents have been tested as second-line salvage therapies in relapsed/refractory PTCL and their efficacy has been mostly analyzed as single agents although a variety of clinical trials focused on novel drug combinations are also ongoing (Ma et al. 2018).

In general, PTCL exhibits a marked epigenetic dysregulation that supports the use of epigenetic modifiers including inhibitors of histone deacetylases (HDACs) and hypomethylating agents for the treatment of this disease.

Two widely used hypomethylating agents are decitabine (5-aza-2′-deoxycytidine) and 5-aza-cytidine, cytidine antimetabolite analogs that incorporate into DNA and inhibit DNA methyltransferases, resulting in hypomethyla-

 Cite this article as *Cold Spring Harb Perspect Med* doi: 10.1101/cshperspect.a035402

Table 2. Targeted therapies for PTCL: Small molecules, antibodies, and immune checkpoint inhibitors targeting molecular pathways

Small molecules	Inhibitors
Vorinostat	Histone deacetylases (HDACs)
Romidepsin	
Belinostat	
Chidamide	
Pralatrexate	Dihydrofolate reductase
Decitabine (5-aza-2′-deoxycytidine)	DNA methyltransferases
5-aza-cytidine	
Duvelisib	PI3 kinases
Copanlisib	
Tenalisib	
Bortezomib	Blocks IκB degradation and NF-κB translocation by targeting 26S proteasome
Carfilzomib	20S proteasome
Ixazomib	Proteasome subunit beta type-5 (PSMB5)
Everolimus	Targets FK506 binding protein-12 (FKBP-12) inhibiting mTORC1
Crizotinib	Tyrosine kinase receptors: anaplastic lymphoma kinase (ALK), hepatocyte growth factor receptor (HGFR)
Antibodies	
Mogamulizumab	CCR4 chemokine receptor
Brentuximab vedotin	CD30 (TNFRSF8)
Hu5F9-G4	CD47
TTI-621	
Immune checkpoint inhibitors	
Nivolumab	PD-L1
Durvalumab	
Pembrolizumab	PD-1

tion of DNA. Initial case reports demonstrated a positive outcome for AITL patients treated with 5-aza-cytidine (Cheminant et al. 2015; Saillard et al. 2016) and a clinical trial with relapsed PTCL patients resulted in 53% overall response rate (ORR) and 75% ORR when only AITL patients were analyzed (Saillard et al. 2016).

HDAC inhibitors constitute a class of small-molecule inhibitors that activate gene expression by inhibiting HDAC activity. Although initially being considered as "epigenetic modifiers" with a predominant role in chromatin remodeling via histone acetylation, HDACis have been shown to exert wider more pleiotropic effects in tumor cells associated with acetylation of nonhistone proteins and regulation of DNA repair (O'Connor et al. 2014). Interestingly, HDACis have been particularly effective for the treatment of PTCL, and several have been approved by the U.S. Federal Drug Administration (FDA) including vorinostat (Duvic et al. 2007; Olsen et al. 2007), romidepsin (Piekarz et al. 2011; Coiffier et al. 2012, 2014; Maruyama et al. 2017b), and belinostat (Foss et al. 2015) with an additional HDACi, chidamide, being approved in China (Shi et al. 2017). Challenges remain to better define the patients that will respond to HDACi, identify the mechanisms of resistance, and leverage the effectiveness of epigenetic modifiers alone and in combination. Indeed, a recent clinical trial combining oral 5-azacytidine and romidepsin exhibited marked activity in patients with PTCL in a phase I clinical trial, with overall and complete response rates of 73% and 55%, respectively, in patients with T-cell lymphoma (O'Connor et al. 2019).

Pralatrexate is an antifolate that works by inhibiting dihydrofolate reductase, leading to

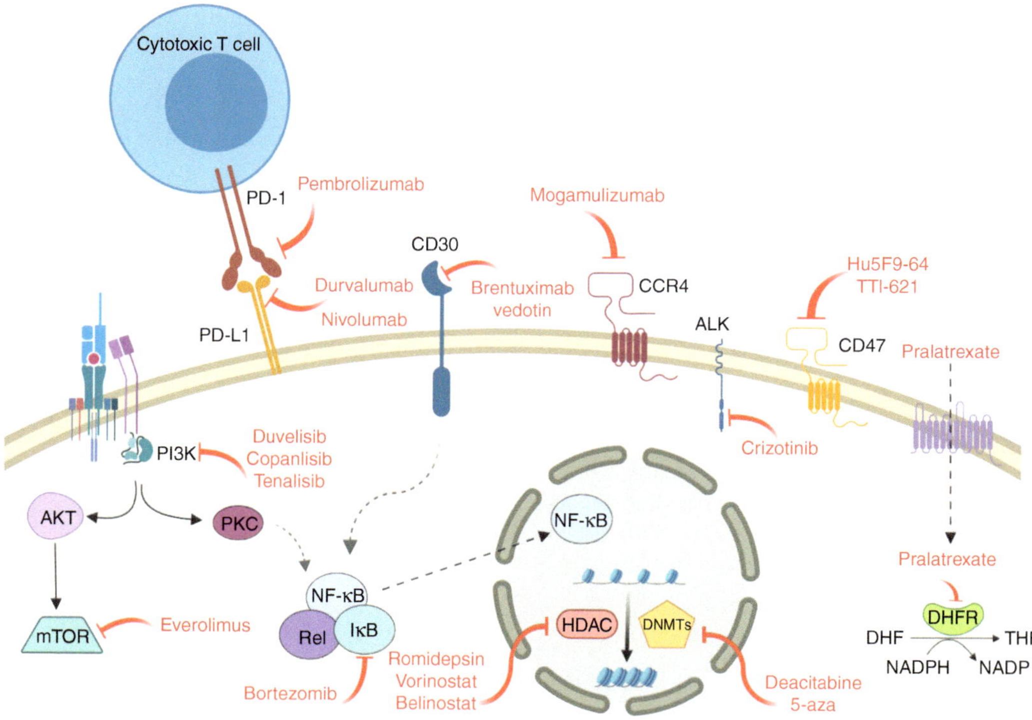

Figure 3. Relevant molecular pathways in PTCL amenable to therapeutic intervention using targeted therapies.

depletion of tetrahydrofolate with the subsequent inhibition of pyrimidines synthesis and tumor growth. Palatrexate was FDA-approved in 2009 after two independent clinical trials reported a 29%–45% response rate (O'Connor et al. 2011; Maruyama et al. 2017a).

The PI3 K/AKT signaling pathway is frequently activated in PTCL and pharmacologic inhibition of the PI3 K/AKT pathway has been extensively studied in preclinical models and has shown efficacy in T-cell malignancies (Cortés et al. 2018). Currently, several PI3 K inhibitors, including duvelisib (Horwitz et al. 2018), copanlisib (Dreyling et al. 2017), and tenalisib (Ito et al. 2019) with differential affinity for the different PI3 K subunits, are being tested in T-cell malignancies, where they are thought to mediate both cell autonomous effects on tumor cells and immune-mediated effects because of their activity on the tumor microenvironment (Horwitz et al. 2018).

Bortezomib is a proteasome inhibitor that blocks degradation of IκB and the proteolytic processing of p105, thereby inhibiting NF-κB nuclear translocation (Wang et al. 2014). In mature lymphomas, the use of bortezomib led to an ORR of 67% in 15 patients with CTCL when used as single agent. In a phase II study in combination with CHOP in newly diagnosed PTCL cases, the drug combination achieved an 76% ORR (Kim et al. 2012). Newer proteasome inhibitors, including carfilzomib and ixazomib, are currently being tested in clinical trials for the treatment of relapsed PTCL in the context of drug combinations.

Everolimus, a derivative of rapamycin that inhibits the mTOR pathways, achieved an ORR of 44% as a single agent in relapsed or refractory lymphomas (Witzig et al. 2015), and a more recent phase II study with a combination of everolimus plus CHOP demonstrated an increased efficacy over CHOP alone (Kim et al. 2016).

Considering the prevalence of mutations affecting the JAK/STAT pathway in multiple subtypes of PTCL, treatment with small-molecule inhibitors targeting this pathway could have potential relevance for the treatment of PTCL. Recently, the JAK3 inhibitor tofacitinib has achieved hematologic responses in a phase I trial in TGL, whereas the dual SYK/JAK inhibitor cerdulatinib has also been studied in a phase II trial on relapsed PTCL achieving a 35% overall response (Ng and Jacobsen 2019). Similarly, dasatinib, a multikinase inhibitor that targets members of the Src family of intracellular tyrosine kinases, has shown promising results for the treatment of AITL in a phase I trial, probably because of its inhibitory effect on the deregulated TCR signaling characteristic of this tumors (Nguyen et al. 2020)

Finally, crizotinib, a small-molecule inhibitor of the ALK tyrosine kinase, has been markedly successful in patients with ALK-positive ALCL, for whom treatment with crizotinib induced a 91% response rate (Gambacorti Passerini et al. 2014). Crizotinib is currently being evaluated in additional clinical trials directed both at pediatric and adult populations. Additional ALK inhibitors are being considered as next-line therapy, anticipating the potential development of resistances to crizotinib (Sharma et al. 2018).

Development of immunotherapeutic approaches has become a major interest in the field of T-cell malignancies. Promising results have been obtained with the use of monoclonal antibodies, immune checkpoint inhibitors and CAR-T-cell therapies. Mogamulizumab, a humanized monoclonal antibody directed against the CCR4 chemokine receptor that is highly expressed in ATLL and CTCL subtypes (Ishida et al. 2003; Hristov et al. 2011), has demonstrated efficacy in patients with CCR4-positive ATLL, PTCL, and CTCL (Yamamoto et al. 2010; Ishida et al. 2012; Duvic et al. 2015; Kim et al. 2018). The results from the phase III clinical trial on CTCL patients demonstrated an overall response rate of 28% (Kim et al. 2018), leading to the approval of mogamulizumab by the FDA for the treatment of patients with ATLL and CTCL. Brentuximab vedotin is an antibody-drug conjugate that contains the microtubule-disrupting agent mono-methylauristatin E (MMAE) linked to an anti-CD30 monoclonal antibody. CD30 is highly expressed on activated T cells as well as ALCL and at variable levels in other PTCL subtypes (Onaindia et al. 2016). Initial studies with anti-CD30 unconjugated antibodies have failed to show significant clinical responses (Ansell et al. 2007; Duvic et al. 2009); however, results from a phase II clinical trial using the MMAE-conjugated form showed impressive responses in ALCL (Pro et al. 2012) with a ORR of 86% and achievement of long-term remission. Significant improvement was also observed in $CD30^+$ CTCL (Prince et al. 2017). However, clinical responses in PTCL-NOS or AITL were modest (Horwitz et al. 2014; Lamarque et al. 2016) and likely due to the variability in CD30 expression (Bossard et al. 2014). A different approach to target CD30 has been demonstrated with the development of AFM13, a bispecific chimeric antibody containing an anti CD16A domain to recruit NK T cells linked to an anti CD30 domain, which achieved partial responses in the initial studies in refractory lymphoma (Rothe et al. 2015) and is currently being tested on patients with $CD30^+$ lymphomas with cutaneous involvement.

Finally, different antibody molecules targeting CD47, a ubiquitous membrane protein that binds to SIRPα inhibiting macrophage phagocytosis and allowing escape from immune surveillance, are currently being studied in clinical trials. Inhibition of the CD47-SIRPα interaction results in activation of innate immunity and promotion of cancer cell destruction by macrophages. Hu5F9-G4, a humanized anti-CD47 blocking antibody (Liu et al. 2018), and TTI-621, a fusion protein containing the CD47 binding domain of human SIRPα and linked to the Fc region of IgG1 with enhanced antitumor activity, are two examples of CD47 targeting molecules under investigation. In an ongoing phase I study in CTCL patients, intratumoral injections of TTI-621 led to decreased tumor size (Folkes et al. 2018).

The past few years have witnessed an increased effort toward the implementation of immunotherapy approaches for the treatment of lymphoid malignancies. Blocking antibodies targeting CTLA-4, PD-L1, and PD-1 immune checkpoints have resulted in the development of highly effective antitumor responses in solid tumors; however, their indication for the treatment of mature T-cell malignancies remains controversial. Although multiple trials are testing the effect of checkpoint inhibitors in PTCL, including nivolumab (Lesokhin et al. 2016), pembrolizumab (Kwong et al. 2017a,b), and durvalumab (Heyman and Yang 2018), recent reports have also described a role for *PD-1* as a tumor suppressor in T-cell lymphomagenesis and demonstrated that *Pd-1* deletion in mouse models leads to highly aggressive lymphoma (Wartewig et al. 2017). Similarly, expansion of malignant clones and oncogenic activation of the TCR pathways have described associated to checkpoint inhibitor therapy in ATLL (Ratner et al. 2018). These results, together with the variable efficacy of checkpoint inhibitors in different PTCL subtypes, suggest that immunotherapy targeting of PD-1 needs to be carefully evaluated for disease stage, composition of the tumor microenvironment, PD-1 genetic deletions, and TCR oncogenic alterations prior to treatment.

Modulating the immune system to eliminate tumor cells using CAR-T-cell-based cellular therapies has proven successful for the treatment of lymphoid malignancies, especially for patients with refractory or relapsed B-cell malignancies. However, treating T-cell malignancies has proven to be challenging endeavor because of the shared expression of many targetable antigens between normal and malignant T cells. This shared antigenicity can cause fratricide in CAR-transduced T cells, inhibiting their proliferation and viability, and in the clinic may also result in eradication of normal peripheral T cells leading to severe immunodeficiency and other serious side effects. Despite these caveats, significant progress has been made on the identification of targetable antigens and development of cell-based therapies for T-cell leukemia and lymphoma. CD30 represents an attractive and validated target for antibody-based therapies and its expression is generally restricted to lymphoma cells. CAR-T cells targeting CD30 have shown potent antilymphoma activity in preclinical studies in various tumor models (Hombach et al. 1999). In addition, recent success in targeting a constant region of the TCR beta chain (TRBC1) could prove relevant for the treatment of PTCL (Maciocia et al. 2017).

CLOSING REMARKS

In the past few years, multiple studies have led to an increased understanding of the pathogenesis and molecular classification of PTCL. High-throughput studies have achieved a deeper understanding of the underlying disease biology and led to improved diagnostic accuracy based on the molecular classification of PTCL. The identification of novel therapeutic vulnerabilities has induced a significant shift in the clinical management of these diseases because of the introduction of targeted agents. The success of epigenetic drugs in PTCL, specifically of HDACi and hypomethylating agents, supports leveraging their use alone and in combination for the treatment of this disease. Many challenges and opportunities for improvement remain, including identification of biomarkers of response to targeted therapies, characterization of mechanisms of resistance, and development of successful combination therapies for the treatment of PTCL.

In addition, continuous progress toward the understanding of the mechanisms that drive T-cell oncogenesis, generation of animal models, and patient-derived xenografts for the experimental therapeutics and implementation of immunotherapy approaches will be instrumental to improve survival for mature T-cell malignancies.

ACKNOWLEDGMENTS

The authors thank Dr. Adolfo Ferrando and Dr. Laura Belver for their insightful comments and their contribution to the editing of the manuscript. J.R.C. is a recipient of a Postdoctoral fellowship from the Lady Tata Research Foundation. T.P. is supported by National Institutes of Health (NIH) grants 1R01 CA197945-01 and U01 CAZ43073. J.R.C. and T.P. designed and wrote the manuscript.

Conflict-of-interest disclosure: T.P. is the recipient of a research grant from Kura Technologies.

REFERENCES

Abate F, da Silva-Almeida AC, Zairis S, Robles-Valero J, Couronne L, Khiabanian H, Quinn SA, Kim MY, Laginestra MA, Kim C, et al. 2017. Activating mutations and translocations in the guanine exchange factor VAV1 in peripheral T-cell lymphomas. *Proc Natl Acad Sci* **114:** 764–769. doi:10.1073/pnas.1608839114

Abdel-Wahab O, Mullally A, Hedvat C, Garcia-Manero G, Patel J, Wadleigh M, Malinge S, Yao J, Kilpivaara O, Bhat R, et al. 2009. Genetic characterization of TET1, TET2, and TET3 alterations in myeloid malignancies. *Blood* **114:** 144–147. doi:10.1182/blood-2009-03-210039

Ansell SM, Horwitz SM, Engert A, Khan KD, Lin T, Strair R, Keler T, Graziano R, Blanset D, Yellin M, et al. 2007. Phase I/II study of an anti-CD30 monoclonal antibody (MDX-060) in Hodgkin's lymphoma and anaplastic large-cell lymphoma. *J Clin Oncol* **25:** 2764–2769. doi:10.1200/JCO.2006.07.8972

Bangham CR, Toulza F. 2011. Adult T cell leukemia/lymphoma: $FoxP3^+$ cells and the cell-mediated immune response to HTLV-1. *Adv Cancer Res* **111:** 163–182. doi:10.1016/B978-0-12-385524-4.00004-0

Bazarbachi A, Plumelle Y, Carlos Ramos J, Tortevoye P, Otrock Z, Taylor G, Gessain A, Harrington W, Panelatti G, Hermine O. 2010. Meta-analysis on the use of zidovudine and interferon-alfa in adult T-cell leukemia/lymphoma showing improved survival in the leukemic subtypes. *J Clin Oncol* **28:** 4177–4183. doi:10.1200/JCO.2010.28.0669

Bazarbachi A, Suarez F, Fields P, Hermine O. 2011. How I treat adult T-cell leukemia/lymphoma. *Blood* **118:** 1736–1745. doi:10.1182/blood-2011-03-345702

Boi M, Rinaldi A, Kwee I, Bonetti P, Todarò M, Tabbò F, Piva R, Rancoita PM, Matolcsy A, Timar B, et al. 2013. *PRDM1*/BLIMP1 is commonly inactivated in anaplastic large T-cell lymphoma. *Blood* **122:** 2683–2693. doi:10.1182/blood-2013-04-497933

Bossard C, Dobay MP, Parrens M, Lamant L, Missiaglia E, Haioun C, Martin A, Fabiani B, Delarue R, Tournilhac O, et al. 2014. Immunohistochemistry as a valuable tool to assess CD30 expression in peripheral T-cell lymphomas: High correlation with mRNA levels. *Blood* **124:** 2983–2986. doi:10.1182/blood-2014-07-584953

Busque L, Patel JP, Figueroa ME, Vasanthakumar A, Provost S, Hamilou Z, Mollica L, Li J, Viale A, Heguy A, et al. 2012. Recurrent somatic *TET2* mutations in normal elderly individuals with clonal hematopoiesis. *Nat Genet* **44:** 1179–1181. doi:10.1038/ng.2413

Bustelo XR. 2000. Regulatory and signaling properties of the Vav family. *Mol Cell Biol* **20:** 1461–1477. doi:10.1128/MCB.20.5.1461-1477.2000

Cairns RA, Iqbal J, Lemonnier F, Kucuk C, de Leval L, Jais JP, Parrens M, Martin A, Xerri L, Brousset P, et al. 2012. *IDH2* mutations are frequent in angioimmunoblastic T-cell lymphoma. *Blood* **119:** 1901–1903. doi:10.1182/blood-2011-11-391748

Chan JK, Chan AC, Cheuk W, Wan SK, Lee WK, Lui YH, Chan WK. 2011. Type II enteropathy-associated T-cell lymphoma: A distinct aggressive lymphoma with frequent γδ T-cell receptor expression. *Am J Surg Pathol* **35:** 1557–1569. doi:10.1097/PAS.0b013e318222dfcd

Chander U, Leeman-Neill RJ, Bhagat G. 2018. Pathogenesis of enteropathy-associated T cell lymphoma. *Curr Hematol Malig Rep* **13:** 308–317. doi:10.1007/s11899-018-0459-5

Chang LW, Patrone CC, Yang W, Rabionet R, Gallardo F, Espinet B, Sharma MK, Girardi M, Tensen CP, Vermeer M, et al. 2018. An integrated data resource for genomic analysis of cutaneous T-cell lymphoma. *J Invest Dermatol* **138:** 2681–2683. doi:10.1016/j.jid.2018.06.176

Chaudhary RK, Bhatt VR, Vose JM. 2015. Management of extranodal natural killer/T-cell lymphoma, nasal type. *Clin Lymphoma Myeloma Leuk* **15:** 245–252. doi:10.1016/j.clml.2014.12.014

Cheminant M, Bruneau J, Kosmider O, Lefrere F, Delarue R, Gaulard P, Radford I, Derrieux C, Hermine O, Lemonnier F. 2015. Efficacy of 5-azacytidine in a *TET2* mutated angioimmunoblastic T cell lymphoma. *Br J Haematol* **168:** 913–916. doi:10.1111/bjh.13170

Chiarle R, Simmons WJ, Cai H, Dhall G, Zamo A, Raz R, Karras JG, Levy DE, Inghirami G. 2005. Stat3 is required for ALK-mediated lymphomagenesis and provides a possible therapeutic target. *Nat Med* **11:** 623–629. doi:10.1038/nm1249

Choi J, Goh G, Walradt T, Hong BS, Bunick CG, Chen K, Bjornson RD, Maman Y, Wang T, Tordoff J, et al. 2015. Genomic landscape of cutaneous T cell lymphoma. *Nat Genet* **47:** 1011–1019. doi:10.1038/ng.3356

Choi S, Go JH, Kim EK, Lee H, Lee WM, Cho CS, Han K. 2016. Mutational analysis of extranodal NK/T-cell lymphoma using targeted sequencing with a comprehensive cancer panel. *Genomics Inform* **14:** 78–84. doi:10.5808/GI.2016.14.3.78

Choudhari R, Minero VG, Menotti M, Pulito R, Brakebusch C, Compagno M, Voena C, Ambrogio C, Chiarle R. 2016. Redundant and nonredundant roles for Cdc42 and Rac1 in lymphomas developed in NPM-ALK transgenic mice. *Blood* **127:** 1297–1306. doi:10.1182/blood-2015-11-683052

Cimmino L, Abdel-Wahab O, Levine RL, Aifantis I. 2011. TET family proteins and their role in stem cell differentiation and transformation. *Cell Stem Cell* **9:** 193–204. doi:10.1016/j.stem.2011.08.007

Coiffier B, Pro B, Prince HM, Foss F, Sokol L, Greenwood M, Caballero D, Borchmann P, Morschhauser F, Wilhelm M, et al. 2012. Results from a pivotal, open-label, phase II study of romidepsin in relapsed or refractory peripheral T-cell lymphoma after prior systemic therapy. *J Clin Oncol* **30:** 631–636. doi:10.1200/JCO.2011.37.4223

Coiffier B, Pro B, Prince HM, Foss F, Sokol L, Greenwood M, Caballero D, Morschhauser F, Wilhelm M, Pinter-Brown L, et al. 2014. Romidepsin for the treatment of relapsed/refractory peripheral T-cell lymphoma: pivotal study update demonstrates durable responses. *J Hematol Oncol* **7:** 11. doi:10.1186/1756-8722-7-11

Cortés JR, Palomero T. 2016. The curious origins of angioimmunoblastic T-cell lymphoma. *Curr Opin Hematol* **23:** 434–443. doi:10.1097/MOH.0000000000000261

Cortés JR, Ambesi-Impiombato A, Couronné L, Quinn SA, Kim CS, da Silva Almeida AC, West Z, Belver L, Martin MS, Scourzic L, et al. 2018. *RHOA G17 V* induces T follicular helper cell specification and promotes lymphomagenesis. *Cancer Cell* **33:** 259–273.e7. doi:10.1016/j.ccell.2018.01.001

Couronné L, Bastard C, Bernard OA. 2012. *TET2* and *DNMT3A* mutations in human T-cell lymphoma. *N Engl J Med* **366:** 95–96. doi:10.1056/NEJMc1111708

Crescenzo R, Abate F, Lasorsa E, Tabbo F, Gaudiano M, Chiesa N, Di Giacomo F, Spaccarotella E, Barbarossa L, Ercole E, et al. 2015. Convergent mutations and kinase fusions lead to oncogenic STAT3 activation in anaplastic large cell lymphoma. *Cancer Cell* **27:** 516–532. doi:10.1016/j.ccell.2015.03.006

da Silva Almeida AC, Abate F, Khiabanian H, Martinez-Escala E, Guitart J, Tensen CP, Vermeer MH, Rabadan R, Ferrando A, Palomero T. 2015. The mutational landscape of cutaneous T cell lymphoma and Sezary syndrome. *Nat Genet* **47:** 1465–1470. doi:10.1038/ng.3442

de Leval L, Rickman DS, Thielen C, Reynies A, Huang YL, Delsol G, Lamant L, Leroy K, Brière J, Molina T, et al. 2007. The gene expression profile of nodal peripheral T-cell lymphoma demonstrates a molecular link between angioimmunoblastic T-cell lymphoma (AITL) and follicular helper T (TFH) cells. *Blood* **109:** 4952–4963. doi:10.1182/blood-2006-10-055145

Delabie J, Holte H, Vose JM, Ullrich F, Jaffe ES, Savage KJ, Connors JM, Rimsza L, Harris NL, Müller-Hermelink K, et al. 2011. Enteropathy-associated T-cell lymphoma: Clinical and histological findings from the international peripheral T-cell lymphoma project. *Blood* **118:** 148–155. doi:10.1182/blood-2011-02-335216

Delhommeau F, Dupont S, Della Valle V, James C, Trannoy S, Massé A, Kosmider O, Le Couedic JP, Robert F, Alberdi A, et al. 2009. Mutation in *TET2* in myeloid cancers. *N Engl J Med* **360:** 2289–2301. doi:10.1056/NEJMoa081 0069

de Mel S, Hue SS, Jeyasekharan AD, Chng WJ, Ng SB. 2019a. Molecular pathogenic pathways in extranodal NK/T cell lymphoma. *J Hematol Oncol* **12:** 33. doi:10.1186/s13045-019-0716-7

de Mel S, Tan JZ, Jeyasekharan AD, Chng WJ, Ng SB. 2019b. Transcriptomic abnormalities in Epstein Barr virus associated T/NK lymphoproliferative disorders. *Front Pediatr* **6:** 405. doi:10.3389/fped.2018.00405

Devata S, Wilcox RA. 2016. Cutaneous T-cell lymphoma: A review with a focus on targeted agents. *Am J Clin Dermatol* **17:** 225–237. doi:10.1007/s40257-016-0177-5

Dreyling M, Morschhauser F, Bouabdallah K, Bron D, Cunningham D, Assouline SE, Verhoef G, Linton K, Thieblemont C, Vitolo U, et al. 2017. Phase II study of copanlisib, a PI3 K inhibitor, in relapsed or refractory, indolent or aggressive lymphoma. *Ann Oncol* **28:** 2169–2178. doi:10.1093/annonc/mdx289

Duvic M, Talpur R, Ni X, Zhang C, Hazarika P, Kelly C, Chiao JH, Reilly JF, Ricker JL, Richon VM, et al. 2007. Phase 2 trial of oral vorinostat (suberoylanilide hydroxamic acid, SAHA) for refractory cutaneous T-cell lymphoma (CTCL). *Blood* **109:** 31–39. doi:10.1182/blood-2006-06-025999

Duvic M, Reddy SA, Pinter-Brown L, Korman NJ, Zic J, Kennedy DA, Lorenz J, Sievers EL, Kim YH. 2009. A phase II study of SGN-30 in cutaneous anaplastic large cell lymphoma and related lymphoproliferative disorders. *Clin Cancer Res* **15:** 6217–6224. doi:10.1158/1078-0432.CCR-09-0162

Duvic M, Pinter-Brown LC, Foss FM, Sokol L, Jorgensen JL, Challagundla P, Dwyer KM, Zhang X, Kurman MR, Ballerini R, et al. 2015. Phase 1/2 study of mogamulizumab, a defucosylated anti-CCR4 antibody, in previously treated patients with cutaneous T-cell lymphoma. *Blood* **125:** 1883–1889. doi:10.1182/blood-2014-09-600924

Federico M, Rudiger T, Bellei M, Nathwani BN, Luminari S, Coiffier B, Harris NL, Jaffe ES, Pileri SA, Savage KJ, et al. 2013. Clinicopathologic characteristics of angioimmunoblastic T-cell lymphoma: Analysis of the international peripheral T-cell lymphoma project. *J Clin Oncol* **31:** 240–246. doi:10.1200/JCO.2011.37.3647

Ferreri AJ, Govi S, Pileri SA, Savage KJ. 2012. Anaplastic large cell lymphoma, ALK-positive. *Crit Rev Oncol Hematol* **83:** 293–302. doi:10.1016/j.critrevonc.2012.02.005

Ferreri AJ, Govi S, Pileri SA, Savage KJ. 2013. Anaplastic large cell lymphoma, ALK-negative. *Crit Rev Oncol Hematol* **85:** 206–215. doi:10.1016/j.critrevonc.2012.06.004

Folkes AS, Feng M, Zain JM, Abdulla F, Rosen ST, Querfeld C. 2018. Targeting CD47 as a cancer therapeutic strategy: The cutaneous T-cell lymphoma experience. *Curr Opin Oncol* **30:** 332–337. doi:10.1097/CCO.0000000000000468

Foss F, Advani R, Duvic M, Hymes KB, Intragumtornchai T, Lekhakula A, Shpilberg O, Lerner A, Belt RJ, Jacobsen ED, et al. 2015. A Phase II trial of Belinostat (PXD101) in patients with relapsed or refractory peripheral or cutaneous T-cell lymphoma. *Br J Haematol* **168:** 811–819. doi:10.1111/bjh.13222

Fujisawa M, Sakata-Yanagimoto M, Nishizawa S, Komori D, Gershon P, Kiryu M, Tanzima S, Fukumoto K, Enami T, Muratani M, et al. 2018. Activation of RHOA-VAV1 signaling in angioimmunoblastic T-cell lymphoma. *Leukemia* **32:** 694–702. doi:10.1038/leu.2017.273

Gambacorti Passerini C, Farina F, Stasia A, Redaelli S, Ceccon M, Mologni L, Messa C, Guerra L, Giudici G, Sala E, et al. 2014. Crizotinib in advanced, chemoresistant anaplastic lymphoma kinase-positive lymphoma patients. *J Natl Cancer Inst* **106:** djt378. doi:10.1093/jnci/djt378

Gaulard P, de Leval L. 2014. The microenvironment in T-cell lymphomas: Emerging themes. *Semin Cancer Biol* **24:** 49–60. doi:10.1016/j.semcancer.2013.11.004

Giam CZ, Semmes OJ. 2016. HTLV-1 infection and adult T-cell leukemia/lymphoma--A tale of two proteins: Tax and HBZ. *Viruses* **8:** 161. doi:10.3390/v8060161

Gniadecki R, Lukowsky A, Rossen K, Madsen HO, Thomsen K, Wulf HC. 2003. Bone marrow precursor of extranodal T-cell lymphoma. *Blood* **102:** 3797–3799. doi:10.1182/blood-2003-03-0899

Hamrouni A, Fogh H, Zak Z, Ødum N, Gniadecki R. 2019. Clonotypic diversity of the T-cell receptor corroborates the immature precursor origin of cutaneous T-cell lymphoma. *Clin Cancer Res* **25:** 3104–3114. doi:10.1158/1078-0432.CCR-18-4099

Haverkos BM, Pan Z, Gru AA, Freud AG, Rabinovitch R, Xu-Welliver M, Otto B, Barrionuevo C, Baiocchi RA, Rochford R, et al. 2016. Extranodal NK/T cell lymphoma, nasal type (ENKTL-NT): An update on epidemiology, clinical presentation, and natural history in North American and European cases. *Curr Hematol Malig Rep* **11:** 514–527. doi:10.1007/s11899-016-0355-9

Heyman B, Yang Y. 2018. New developments in immunotherapy for lymphoma. *Cancer Biol Med* **15:** 189–209. doi:10.20892/j.issn.2095-3941.2018.0037

Hombach A, Heuser C, Sircar R, Tillmann T, Diehl V, Pohl C, Abken H. 1999. Characterization of a chimeric T-cell receptor with specificity for the Hodgkin's lymphoma-associated CD30 antigen. *J Immunother* **22:** 473–480. doi:10.1097/00002371-199911000-00001

Horwitz SM, Advani RH, Bartlett NL, Jacobsen ED, Sharman JP, O'Connor OA, Siddiqi T, Kennedy DA, Oki Y. 2014. Objective responses in relapsed T-cell lymphomas with single-agent brentuximab vedotin. *Blood* **123:** 3095–3100. doi:10.1182/blood-2013-12-542142

Horwitz SM, Koch R, Porcu P, Oki Y, Moskowitz A, Perez M, Myskowski P, Officer A, Jaffe JD, Morrow SN, et al. 2018. Activity of the PI3K-δ,γ inhibitor duvelisib in a phase 1 trial and preclinical models of T-cell lymphoma. *Blood* **131:** 888–898. doi:10.1182/blood-2017-08-802470

Hristov AC, Vonderheid EC, Borowitz MJ. 2011. Simplified flow cytometric assessment in mycosis fungoides and Sézary syndrome. *Am J Clin Pathol* **136:** 944–953. doi:10.1309/AJCP09OTJOYAVZZK

Huang L, Liu D, Wang N, Ling S, Tang Y, Wu J, Hao L, Luo H, Hu X, Sheng L, et al. 2018. Integrated genomic analysis identifies deregulated JAK/STAT-MYC-biosynthesis axis in aggressive NK-cell leukemia. *Cell Res* **28:** 172–186. doi:10.1038/cr.2017.146

Iqbal J, Wright G, Wang C, Rosenwald A, Gascoyne RD, Weisenburger DD, Greiner TC, Smith L, Guo S, Wilcox RA, et al. 2014. Gene expression signatures delineate biological and prognostic subgroups in peripheral T-cell lymphoma. *Blood* **123:** 2915–2923. doi:10.1182/blood-2013-11-536359

Ishida T, Utsunomiya A, Iida S, Inagaki H, Takatsuka Y, Kusumoto S, Takeuchi G, Shimizu S, Ito M, Komatsu H, et al. 2003. Clinical significance of CCR4 expression in adult T-cell leukemia/lymphoma: Its close association with skin involvement and unfavorable outcome. *Clin Cancer Res* **9:** 3625–3634.

Ishida T, Joh T, Uike N, Yamamoto K, Utsunomiya A, Yoshida S, Saburi Y, Miyamoto T, Takemoto S, Suzushima H, et al. 2012. Defucosylated anti-CCR4 monoclonal antibody (KW-0761) for relapsed adult T-cell leukemia-lymphoma: A multicenter phase II study. *J Clin Oncol* **30:** 837–842. doi:10.1200/JCO.2011.37.3472

Ito S, D'Alessio AC, Taranova OV, Hong K, Sowers LC, Zhang Y. 2010. Role of Tet proteins in 5mC to 5hmC conversion, ES-cell self-renewal and inner cell mass specification. *Nature* **466:** 1129–1133. doi:10.1038/nature09303

Ito T, Kawazu H, Murata T, Iwata S, Arakawa S, Sato Y, Kuzushima K, Goshima F, Kimura H. 2014. Role of latent membrane protein 1 in chronic active Epstein–Barr virus infection–derived T/NK-cell proliferation. *Cancer Med* **3:** 787–795. doi:10.1002/cam4.256

Ito Y, Makita S, Tobinai K. 2019. Development of new agents for peripheral T-cell lymphoma. *Expert Opin Biol Ther* **19:** 197–209. doi:10.1080/14712598.2019.1572746

Kataoka K, Nagata Y, Kitanaka A, Shiraishi Y, Shimamura T, Yasunaga J, Totoki Y, Chiba K, Sato-Otsubo A, Nagae G, et al. 2015. Integrated molecular analysis of adult T cell leukemia/lymphoma. *Nat Genet* **47:** 1304–1315. doi:10.1038/ng.3415

Kataoka K, Miyoshi H, Sakata S, Dobashi A, Couronné L, Kogure Y, Sato Y, Nishida K, Gion Y, Shiraishi Y, et al. 2019. Frequent structural variations involving programmed death ligands in Epstein–Barr virus–associated lymphomas. *Leukemia* **33:** 1687–1699. doi:10.1038/s41375-019-0380-5

Kim SJ, Yoon DH, Kang HJ, Kim JS, Park SK, Kim HJ, Lee J, Ryoo BY, Ko YH, Huh J, et al. 2012. Bortezomib in combination with CHOP as first-line treatment for patients with stage III/IV peripheral T-cell lymphomas: A multicentre, single-arm, phase 2 trial. *Eur J Cancer* **48:** 3223–3231. doi:10.1016/j.ejca.2012.06.003

Kim SJ, Shin DY, Kim JS, Yoon DH, Lee WS, Lee H, Do YR, Kang HJ, Eom HS, Ko YH, et al. 2016. A phase II study of everolimus (RAD001), an mTOR inhibitor plus CHOP for newly diagnosed peripheral T-cell lymphomas. *Ann Oncol* **27:** 712–718. doi:10.1093/annonc/mdv624

Kim YH, Bagot M, Pinter-Brown L, Rook AH, Porcu P, Horwitz SM, Whittaker S, Tokura Y, Vermeer M, Zinzani PL, et al. 2018. Mogamulizumab versus vorinostat in previously treated cutaneous T-cell lymphoma (MAVORIC): An international, open-label, randomised, controlled phase 3 trial. *Lancet Oncol* **19:** 1192–1204. doi:10.1016/S1470-2045(18)30379-6

Komabayashi Y, Kishibe K, Nagato T, Ueda S, Takahara M, Harabuchi Y. 2017. Circulating Epstein-Barr virus–encoded micro-RNAs as potential biomarkers for nasal natural killer/T-cell lymphoma. *Hematol Oncol* **35:** 655–663. doi:10.1002/hon.2360

Koo GC, Tan SY, Tang T, Poon SL, Allen GE, Tan L, Chong SC, Ong WS, Tay K, Tao M, et al. 2012. *Janus kinase 3*-activating mutations identified in natural killer/T-cell lymphoma. *Cancer Discov* **2:** 591–597. doi:10.1158/2159-8290.CD-12-0028

Kucuk C, Hu X, Jiang B, Klinkebiel D, Geng H, Gong Q, Bouska A, Iqbal J, Gaulard P, McKeithan TW, et al. 2015. Global promoter methylation analysis reveals novel candidate tumor suppressor genes in natural killer cell lymphoma. *Clin Cancer Res* **21:** 1699–1711. doi:10.1158/1078-0432.CCR-14-1216

Kwong YL, Chan TSY, Tan D, Kim SJ, Poon LM, Mow B, Khong PL, Loong F, Au-Yeung R, Iqbal J, et al. 2017a. PD1 blockade with pembrolizumab is highly effective in relapsed or refractory NK/T-cell lymphoma failing L-asparaginase. *Blood* **129:** 2437–2442. doi:10.1182/blood-2016-12-756841

Kwong YL, Lopes D, Khong PL. 2017b. Low-dose pembrolizumab induced remission in patients with refractory classical Hodgkin lymphoma. *Br J Haematol* **176:** 131–132. doi:10.1111/bjh.13920

Lamarque M, Bossard C, Contejean A, Brice P, Parrens M, Le Gouill S, Briere J, Bouabdallah R, Canioni D, Tilly H, et al. 2016. Brentuximab vedotin in refractory or relapsed peripheral T-cell lymphomas: The French named patient program experience in 56 patients. *Haematologica* **101:** e103–e106. doi:10.3324/haematol.2015.135400

Laurent C, Delas A, Gaulard P, Haioun C, Moreau A, Xerri L, Traverse-Glehen A, Rousset T, Quintin-Roue I, Petrella T, et al. 2016. Breast implant-associated anaplastic large cell lymphoma: Two distinct clinicopathological variants with different outcomes. *Ann Oncol* **27:** 306–314. doi:10.1093/annonc/mdv575

Lemonnier F, Couronné L, Parrens M, Jaïs JP, Travert M, Lamant L, Tournillac O, Rousset T, Fabiani B, Cairns RA, et al. 2012. Recurrent *TET2* mutations in peripheral T-cell lymphomas correlate with T_{FH}-like features and adverse clinical parameters. *Blood* **120:** 1466–1469. doi:10.1182/blood-2012-02-408542

Lesokhin AM, Ansell SM, Armand P, Scott EC, Halwani A, Gutierrez M, Millenson MM, Cohen AD, Schuster SJ, Lebovic D, et al. 2016. Nivolumab in patients with relapsed or refractory hematologic malignancy: Preliminary results of a Phase Ib Study. *J Clin Oncol* **34:** 2698–2704. doi:10.1200/JCO.2015.65.9789

Liu B, Guo H, Xu J, Qin T, Guo Q, Gu N, Zhang D, Qian W, Dai J, Hou S, et al. 2018. Elimination of tumor by CD47/PD-L1 dual-targeting fusion protein that engages innate and adaptive immune responses. *MAbs* **10:** 315–324. doi:10.1080/19420862.2017.1409319

Lue JK, Kress A, Amengual JE. 2017. Therapeutic options for aggressive T-cell lymphomas. *Curr Hematol Malig Rep* **12:** 269–281. doi:10.1007/s11899-017-0389-7

Lunning MA, Vose JM. 2017. Angioimmunoblastic T-cell lymphoma: The many-faced lymphoma. *Blood* **129:** 1095–1102. doi:10.1182/blood-2016-09-692541

Ma H, Davarifar A, Amengual JE. 2018. The future of combination therapies for peripheral T cell lymphoma (PTCL). *Curr Hematol Malig Rep* **13:** 13–24. doi:10.1007/s11899-018-0432-3

Maciocia PM, Wawrzyniecka PA, Philip B, Ricciardelli I, Akarca AU, Onuoha SC, Legut M, Cole DK, Sewell AK, Gritti G, et al. 2017. Targeting the T cell receptor β-chain constant region for immunotherapy of T cell malignancies. *Nat Med* **23:** 1416–1423. doi:10.1038/nm.4444

Malcolm TI, Villarese P, Fairbairn CJ, Lamant L, Trinquand A, Hook CE, Burke GA, Brugières L, Hughes K, Payet D, et al. 2016. Anaplastic large cell lymphoma arises in thymocytes and requires transient TCR expression for thymic egress. *Nat Commun* **7:** 10087. doi:10.1038/ncomms10087

Maruyama D, Nagai H, Maeda Y, Nakane T, Shimoyama T, Nakazato T, Sakai R, Ishikawa T, Izutsu K, Ueda R, et al. 2017a. Phase I/II study of pralatrexate in Japanese patients with relapsed or refractory peripheral T-cell lymphoma. *Cancer Sci* **108:** 2061–2068. doi:10.1111/cas.13340

Maruyama D, Tobinai K, Ogura M, Uchida T, Hatake K, Taniwaki M, Ando K, Tsukasaki K, Ishida T, Kobayashi N, et al. 2017b. Romidepsin in Japanese patients with relapsed or refractory peripheral T-cell lymphoma: A phase I/II and pharmacokinetics study. *Int J Hematol* **106:** 655–665. doi:10.1007/s12185-017-2286-1

Matutes E. 2007. Adult T-cell leukaemia/lymphoma. *J Clin Pathol* **60:** 1373–1377. doi:10.1136/jcp.2007.052456

McKinney M, Moffitt AB, Gaulard P, Travert M, De Leval L, Nicolae A, Raffeld M, Jaffe ES, Pittaluga S, Xi L, et al. 2017. The genetic basis of hepatosplenic T-cell lymphoma. *Cancer Discov* **7:** 369–379. doi:10.1158/2159-8290.CD-16-0330

Menotti M, Ambrogio C, Cheong TC, Pighi C, Mota I, Cassel SH, Compagno M, Wang Q, Dall'Olio R, Minero VG, et al. 2019. Wiskott–Aldrich syndrome protein (WASP) is a tumor suppressor in T cell lymphoma. *Nat Med* **25:** 130–140. doi:10.1038/s41591-018-0262-9

Miranda RN, Aladily TN, Prince HM, Kanagal-Shamanna R, de Jong D, Fayad LE, Amin MB, Haideri N, Bhagat G, Brooks GS, et al. 2014. Breast implant-associated anaplastic large-cell lymphoma: Long-term follow-up of 60 patients. *J Clin Oncol* **32:** 114–120. doi:10.1200/JCO.2013.52.7911

Miyoshi H, Kiyasu J, Kato T, Yoshida N, Shimono J, Yokoyama S, Taniguchi H, Sasaki Y, Kurita D, Kawamoto K, et al. 2016. PD-L1 expression on neoplastic or stromal cells is respectively a poor or good prognostic factor for adult T-cell leukemia/lymphoma. *Blood* **128:** 1374–1381. doi:10.1182/blood-2016-02-698936

Moffitt AB, Ondrejka SL, McKinney M, Rempel RE, Goodlad JR, Teh CH, Leppa S, Mannisto S, Kovanen PE, Tse E, et al. 2017. Enteropathy-associated T cell lymphoma subtypes are characterized by loss of function of SETD2. *J Exp Med* **214:** 1371–1386. doi:10.1084/jem.20160894

Moran-Crusio K, Reavie L, Shih A, Abdel-Wahab O, Ndiaye-Lobry D, Lobry C, Figueroa ME, Vasanthakumar A, Patel J, Zhao X, et al. 2011. *Tet2* loss leads to increased hematopoietic stem cell self-renewal and myeloid transformation. *Cancer Cell* **20:** 11–24. doi:10.1016/j.ccr.2011.06.001

Nagao R, Kikuti YY, Carreras J, Kikuchi T, Miyaoka M, Matsushita H, Kojima M, Ando K, Sakata-Yanagimoto M, Chiba S, et al. 2016. Clinicopathologic analysis of angioimmunoblastic T-cell lymphoma with or without *RHOA* G17 V mutation using formalin-fixed paraffin-embedded sections. *Am J Surg Pathol* **40:** 1041–1050. doi:10.1097/PAS.0000000000000651

Nairismägi ML, Tan J, Lim JQ, Nagarajan S, Ng CC, Rajasegaran V, Huang D, Lim WK, Laurensia Y, Wijaya GC, et al. 2016. JAK-STAT and G-protein-coupled receptor signaling pathways are frequently altered in epitheliotropic intestinal T-cell lymphoma. *Leukemia* **30:** 1311–1319. doi:10.1038/leu.2016.13

Ng SY, Jacobsen ED. 2019. Peripheral T-cell lymphoma: Moving toward targeted therapies. *Hematol Oncol Clin North Am* **33:** 657–668. doi:10.1016/j.hoc.2019.04.002

Ng SY, Brown L, Stevenson K, deSouza T, Aster JC, Louissaint A, Weinstock DM. 2018. *RhoA G17 V* is sufficient to induce autoimmunity and promotes T cell lymphomagenesis in mice. *Blood* **132:** 935–947.

Nguyen TB, Sakata-Yanagimoto M, Fujisawa M, Nuhat ST, Miyoshi H, Nannya Y, Hashimoto K, Fukumoto K, Bernard OA, Kiyoki Y, et al. 2020. Dasatinib is an effective treatment for angioimmunoblastic T-cell lymphoma. *Cancer Res* doi: 10.1158/0008-5472.CAN-19-2787.

Nicolae A, Xi L, Pittaluga S, Abdullaev Z, Pack SD, Chen J, Waldmann TA, Jaffe ES, Raffeld M. 2014. Frequent *STAT5B* mutations in γδ hepatosplenic T-cell lymphomas. *Leukemia* **28:** 2244–2248. doi:10.1038/leu.2014.200

O'Connor OA, Pro B, Pinter-Brown L, Bartlett N, Popplewell L, Coiffier B, Lechowicz MJ, Savage KJ, Shustov AR, Gisselbrecht C, et al. 2011. Pralatrexate in patients with relapsed or refractory peripheral T-cell lymphoma: Results from the pivotal PROPEL study. *J Clin Oncol* **29:** 1182–1189. doi:10.1200/JCO.2010.29.9024

O'Connor OA, Bhagat G, Ganapathi K, Pedersen MB, D'Amore F, Radeski D, Bates SE. 2014. Changing the paradigms of treatment in peripheral T-cell lymphoma: From biology to clinical practice. *Clin Cancer Res* **20:** 5240–5254. doi:10.1158/1078-0432.CCR-14-2020

O'Connor OA, Falchi L, Lue JK, Marchi E, Kinahan C, Sawas A, Deng C, Montanari F, Amengual JE, Kim HA, et al.

2019. Oral 5-azacytidine and romidepsin exhibit marked activity in patients with PTCL: A multicenter phase 1 study. *Blood* **134:** 1395–1405. doi:10.1182/blood.2019001285

Ohshima K. 2015. Molecular pathology of adult T-cell leukemia/lymphoma. *Oncology* **89:** 7–15. doi:10.1159/000431058

Olsen EA, Kim YH, Kuzel TM, Pacheco TR, Foss FM, Parker S, Frankel SR, Chen C, Ricker JL, Arduino JM, et al. 2007. Phase IIb multicenter trial of vorinostat in patients with persistent, progressive, or treatment refractory cutaneous T-cell lymphoma. *J Clin Oncol* **25:** 3109–3115. doi:10.1200/JCO.2006.10.2434

Onaindia A, Martínez N, Montes-Moreno S, Almaraz C, Rodríguez-Pinilla SM, Cereceda L, Revert JB, Ortega C, Tardio A, González L, et al. 2016. CD30 expression by B and T cells: A frequent finding in angioimmunoblastic T-cell lymphoma and peripheral T-cell lymphoma-not otherwise specified. *Am J Surg Pathol* **40:** 378–385. doi:10.1097/PAS.0000000000000571

Ondrejka SL, Grzywacz B, Bodo J, Makishima H, Polprasert C, Said JW, Przychodzen B, Maciejewski JP, Hsi ED. 2016. Angioimmunoblastic T-cell lymphomas with the *RHOA* p.Gly17Val mutation have classic clinical and pathologic features. *Am J Surg Pathol* **40:** 335–341. doi:10.1097/PAS.0000000000000555

Palomero T, Couronné L, Khiabanian H, Kim MY, Ambesi-Impiombato A, Perez-Garcia A, Carpenter Z, Abate F, Allegretta M, Haydu JE, et al. 2014. Recurrent mutations in epigenetic regulators, *RHOA* and *FYN* kinase in peripheral T cell lymphomas. *Nat Genet* **46:** 166–170. doi:10.1038/ng.2873

Pancewicz J, Taylor JM, Datta A, Baydoun HH, Waldmann TA, Hermine O, Nicot C. 2010. Notch signaling contributes to proliferation and tumor formation of human T-cell leukemia virus type 1-associated adult T-cell leukemia. *Proc Natl Acad Sci* **107:** 16619–16624. doi:10.1073/pnas.1010722107

Park J, Yang J, Wenzel AT, Ramachandran A, Lee WJ, Daniels JC, Kim J, Martinez-Escala E, Amankulor N, Pro B, et al. 2017. Genomic analysis of 220 CTCLs identifies a novel recurrent gain-of-function alteration in RLTPR (p. Q575E). *Blood* **130:** 1430–1440. doi:10.1182/blood-2017-02-768234

Parrilla Castellar ER, Jaffe ES, Said JW, Swerdlow SH, Ketterling RP, Knudson RA, Sidhu JS, Hsi ED, Karikehalli S, Jiang L, et al. 2014. ALK-negative anaplastic large cell lymphoma is a genetically heterogeneous disease with widely disparate clinical outcomes. *Blood* **124:** 1473–1480. doi:10.1182/blood-2014-04-571091

Piekarz RL, Frye R, Prince HM, Kirschbaum MH, Zain J, Allen SL, Jaffe ES, Ling A, Turner M, Peer CJ, et al. 2011. Phase 2 trial of romidepsin in patients with peripheral T-cell lymphoma. *Blood* **117:** 5827–5834. doi:10.1182/blood-2010-10-312603

Prince HM, Kim YH, Horwitz SM, Dummer R, Scarisbrick J, Quaglino P, Zinzani PL, Wolter P, Sanches JA, Ortiz-Romero PL, et al. 2017. Brentuximab vedotin or physician's choice in CD30-positive cutaneous T-cell lymphoma (ALCANZA): An international, open-label, randomised, phase 3, multicentre trial. *Lancet* **390:** 555–566. doi:10.1016/S0140-6736(17)31266-7

Pro B, Advani R, Brice P, Bartlett NL, Rosenblatt JD, Illidge T, Matous J, Ramchandren R, Fanale M, Connors JM, et al. 2012. Brentuximab vedotin (SGN-35) in patients with relapsed or refractory systemic anaplastic large-cell lymphoma: Results of a phase II study. *J Clin Oncol* **30:** 2190–2196. doi:10.1200/JCO.2011.38.0402

Ratner L, Waldmann TA, Janakiram M, Brammer JE. 2018. Rapid progression of adult T-cell leukemia-lymphoma after PD-1 inhibitor therapy. *N Engl J Med* **378:** 1947–1948. doi:10.1056/NEJMc1803181

Roberti A, Dobay MP, Bisig B, Vallois D, Boéchat C, Lanitis E, Bouchindhomme B, Parrens MC, Bossard C, Quintanilla-Martinez L, et al. 2016. Type II enteropathy-associated T-cell lymphoma features a unique genomic profile with highly recurrent *SETD2* alterations. *Nat Commun* **7:** 12602. doi:10.1038/ncomms12602

Rohr J, Guo S, Huo J, Bouska A, Lachel C, Li Y, Simone PD, Zhang W, Gong Q, Wang C, et al. 2015. Recurrent activating mutations of CD28 in peripheral T-cell lymphomas. *Leukemia* **30:** 1062–1070. doi:10.1038/leu.2015.357

Rothe A, Sasse S, Topp MS, Eichenauer DA, Hummel H, Reiners KS, Dietlein M, Kuhnert G, Kessler J, Buerkle C, et al. 2015. A phase 1 study of the bispecific anti-CD30/CD16A antibody construct AFM13 in patients with relapsed or refractory Hodgkin lymphoma. *Blood* **125:** 4024–4031. doi:10.1182/blood-2014-12-614636

Saillard C, El Cheikh J, Granata A, Coso D, Schiano JM, Bouabdallah R, Blaise D, Charrier N, Broussais F. 2016. Histone deacetylase inhibitor abexinostat (S78454/PCI-24781) as a successful approach in a case of refractory peripheral angio-immunoblastic T-cell lymphoma, as a bridge to reduced intensity conditioning haplo-identical allogenic stem cell transplant. *Leuk Lymphoma* **57:** 714–716. doi:10.3109/10428194.2015.1061190

Sakata-Yanagimoto M, Enami T, Yoshida K, Shiraishi Y, Ishii R, Miyake Y, Muto H, Tsuyama N, Sato-Otsubo A, Okuno Y, et al. 2014. Somatic *RHOA* mutation in angioimmunoblastic T cell lymphoma. *Nat Genet* **46:** 171–175. doi:10.1038/ng.2872

Savage KJ. 2008. Peripheral T-cell lymphomas: An historical perspective. *Hematology Am Soc Hematol Educ Program* 271. doi:10.1182/asheducation-2008.1.271

Scourzic L, Couronné L, Pedersen MT, Della Valle V, Diop M, Mylonas E, Calvo J, Mouly E, Lopez CK, Martin N, et al. 2016. $DNMT3A^{R882H}$ mutant and *Tet2* inactivation cooperate in the deregulation of DNA methylation control to induce lymphoid malignancies in mice. *Leukemia* **30:** 1388–1398. doi:10.1038/leu.2016.29

Sharma GG, Mota I, Mologni L, Patrucco E, Gambacorti-Passerini C, Chiarle R. 2018. Tumor resistance against ALK targeted therapy—Where it comes from and where it goes. *Cancers (Basel)* **10:** 62.

Shi Y, Wang E. 2015. Hepatosplenic T-cell lymphoma: A clinicopathologic review with an emphasis on diagnostic differentiation from other T-cell/natural killer-cell neoplasms. *Arch Pathol Lab Med* **139:** 1173–1180. doi:10.5858/arpa.2014-0079-RS

Shi Y, Jia B, Xu W, Li W, Liu T, Liu P, Zhao W, Zhang H, Sun X, Yang H, et al. 2017. Chidamide in relapsed or refractory peripheral T cell lymphoma: A multicenter real-world study in China. *J Hematol Oncol* **10:** 69. doi:10.1186/s13045-017-0439-6

Shustov A, Soma L. 2019. Anaplastic large cell lymphoma: Contemporary concepts and optimal management. *Cancer Treat Res* **176:** 127–144. doi:10.1007/978-3-319-99716-2_6

Sim SH, Kim S, Kim TM, Jeon YK, Nam SJ, Ahn YO, Keam B, Park HH, Kim DW, Kim CW, et al. 2017. Novel *JAK3*-activating mutations in extranodal NK/T-cell lymphoma, nasal type. *Am J Pathol* **187:** 980–986. doi:10.1016/j.ajpath.2017.01.004

Steensma DP. 2018. Clinical consequences of clonal hematopoiesis of indeterminate potential. *Blood Adv* **2:** 3404–3410. doi:10.1182/bloodadvances.2018020222

Steensma DP, Ebert BL. 2020. Clonal hematopoiesis as a model for premalignant changes during aging. *Exp Hematol* **83:** 48–56. doi:10.1016/j.exphem.2019.12.001

Suzuki R. 2014. Pathogenesis and treatment of extranodal natural killer/T-cell lymphoma. *Semin Hematol* **51:** 42–51. doi:10.1053/j.seminhematol.2013.11.007

Swerdlow SH, Campo E, Pileri SA, Harris NL, Stein H, Siebert R, Advani R, Ghielmini M, Salles GA, Zelenetz AD, et al. 2016. The 2016 revision of the World Health Organization classification of lymphoid neoplasms. *Blood* **127:** 2375–2390. doi:10.1182/blood-2016-01-643569

Tahiliani M, Koh KP, Shen Y, Pastor WA, Bandukwala H, Brudno Y, Agarwal S, Iyer LM, Liu DR, Aravind L, et al. 2009. Conversion of 5-methylcytosine to 5-hydroxymethylcytosine in mammalian DNA by MLL partner TET1. *Science* **324:** 930–935. doi:10.1126/science.1170116

Ungewickell A, Bhaduri A, Rios E, Reuter J, Lee CS, Mah A, Zehnder A, Ohgami R, Kulkarni S, Armstrong R, et al. 2015. Genomic analysis of mycosis fungoides and Sézary syndrome identifies recurrent alterations in TNFR2. *Nat Genet* **47:** 1056–1060. doi:10.1038/ng.3370

Vallois D, Dobay MP, Morin RD, Lemonnier F, Missiaglia E, Juilland M, Iwaszkiewicz J, Fataccioli V, Bisig B, Roberti A, et al. 2016. Activating mutations in genes related to TCR signaling in angioimmunoblastic and other follicular helper T-cell-derived lymphomas. *Blood* **128:** 1490–1502. doi:10.1182/blood-2016-02-698977

Vaqué JP, Gómez-López G, Monsálvez V, Varela I, Martínez N, Pérez C, Domínguez O, Graña O, Rodríguez-Peralto JL, Rodríguez-Pinilla SM, et al. 2014. PLCG1 mutations in cutaneous T-cell lymphomas. *Blood* **123:** 2034–2043. doi:10.1182/blood-2013-05-504308

Wang H, Guan F, Chen D, Dou QP, Yang H. 2014. An analysis of the safety profile of proteasome inhibitors for treating various cancers. *Expert Opin Drug Saf* **13:** 1043–1054. doi:10.1517/14740338.2014.939953

Wang C, McKeithan TW, Gong Q, Zhang W, Bouska A, Rosenwald A, Gascoyne RD, Wu X, Wang J, Muhammad Z, et al. 2015a. *IDH2*^{R172} mutations define a unique subgroup of patients with angioimmunoblastic T-cell lymphoma. *Blood* **126:** 1741–1752. doi:10.1182/blood-2015-05-644591

Wang L, Ni X, Covington KR, Yang BY, Shiu J, Zhang X, Xi L, Meng Q, Langridge T, Drummond J, et al. 2015b. Genomic profiling of Sézary syndrome identifies alterations of key T cell signaling and differentiation genes. *Nat Genet* **47:** 1426–1434. doi:10.1038/ng.3444

Wartewig T, Kurgyis Z, Keppler S, Pechloff K, Hameister E, Öllinger R, Maresch R, Buch T, Steiger K, Winter C, et al. 2017. PD-1 is a haploinsufficient suppressor of T cell lymphomagenesis. *Nature* **552:** 121–125. doi:10.1038/nature24649

Watatani Y, Sato Y, Miyoshi H, Sakamoto K, Nishida K, Gion Y, Nagata Y, Shiraishi Y, Chiba K, Tanaka H, et al. 2019. Molecular heterogeneity in peripheral T-cell lymphoma, not otherwise specified revealed by comprehensive genetic profiling. *Leukemia* **33:** 2867–2883. doi:10.1038/s41375-019-0473-1

Weisenburger DD, Savage KJ, Harris NL, Gascoyne RD, Jaffe ES, MacLennan KA, Rüdiger T, Pileri S, Nakamura S, Nathwani B, et al. 2011. Peripheral T-cell lymphoma, not otherwise specified: A report of 340 cases from the International Peripheral T-cell Lymphoma Project. *Blood* **117:** 3402–3408. doi:10.1182/blood-2010-09-310342

Witzig TE, Reeder C, Han JJ, LaPlant B, Stenson M, Tun HW, Macon W, Ansell SM, Habermann TM, Inwards DJ, et al. 2015. The mTORC1 inhibitor everolimus has antitumor activity in vitro and produces tumor responses in patients with relapsed T-cell lymphoma. *Blood* **126:** 328–335. doi:10.1182/blood-2015-02-629543

Yabe M, Miranda RN, Medeiros LJ. 2018. Hepatosplenic T-cell lymphoma: A review of clinicopathologic features, pathogenesis, and prognostic factors. *Hum Pathol* **74:** 5–16. doi:10.1016/j.humpath.2018.01.005

Yamada Y, Kamihira S. 2005. Inactivation of tumor suppressor genes and the progression of adult T-cell leukemia-lymphoma. *Leuk Lymphoma* **46:** 1553–1559. doi:10.1080/10428190500244217

Yamamoto K, Utsunomiya A, Tobinai K, Tsukasaki K, Uike N, Uozumi K, Yamaguchi K, Yamada Y, Hanada S, Tamura K, et al. 2010. Phase I study of KW-0761, a defucosylated humanized anti-CCR4 antibody, in relapsed patients with adult T-cell leukemia-lymphoma and peripheral T-cell lymphoma. *J Clin Oncol* **28:** 1591–1598. doi:10.1200/JCO.2009.25.3575

Yan J, Li B, Lin B, Lee PT, Chung TH, Tan J, Bi C, Lee XT, Selvarajan V, Ng SB, et al. 2016. EZH2 phosphorylation by JAK3 mediates a switch to noncanonical function in natural killer/T-cell lymphoma. *Blood* **128:** 948–958. doi:10.1182/blood-2016-01-690701

Yao WQ, Wu F, Zhang W, Chuang SS, Thompson JS, Chen Z, Zhang SW, Clipson A, Wang M, Liu H, et al. 2020. Angioimmunoblastic T-cell lymphoma contains multiple clonal T-cell populations derived from a common *TET2* mutant progenitor cell. *J Pathol* **250:** 346–357. doi:10.1002/path.5376

Yeh CH, Bellon M, Pancewicz-Wojtkiewicz J, Nicot C. 2016. Oncogenic mutations in the FBXW7 gene of adult T-cell leukemia patients. *Proc Natl Acad Sci* **113:** 6731–6736. doi:10.1073/pnas.1601537113

Yoo HY, Sung MK, Lee SH, Kim S, Lee H, Park S, Kim SC, Lee B, Rho K, Lee JE, et al. 2014. A recurrent inactivating mutation in *RHOA* GTPase in angioimmunoblastic T cell lymphoma. *Nat Genet* **46:** 371–375. doi:10.1038/ng.2916

Zhou Y, Attygalle AD, Chuang SS, Diss T, Ye H, Liu H, Hamoudi RA, Munson P, Bacon CM, Dogan A, et al. 2007. Angioimmunoblastic T-cell lymphoma: Histological progression associates with *EBV* and *HHV6B* viral load. *Br J Haematol* **138:** 44–53. doi:10.1111/j.1365-2141.2007.06620.x

Biological and Translational Considerations regarding the Recent Therapeutic Successes and Upcoming Challenges for Multiple Myeloma

Constantine S. Mitsiades[1,2]

[1]Department of Medical Oncology, Dana-Farber Cancer Institute, Boston, Massachusetts 02215, USA

[2]Department of Medicine, Harvard Medical School, Broad Institute of MIT & Harvard, Boston, Massachusetts 02215, USA

Correspondence: Constantine_Mitsiades@dfci.harvard.edu

Even though multiple myeloma (MM) is still considered incurable, the therapeutic management of this disease has undergone a major transformation over the last two decades, with several new classes of therapeutics and diverse options for their combined use in many different regimens that have contributed to major improvement in overall survival of patients. This review discusses key themes underlying the pharmacological and immune-based therapies that represent the cornerstones of this progress. A major part of the clinical progress achieved by these classes' therapeutics has depended on the targeting of molecular pathways with distinct or preferential roles for the biology of plasma cells—normal or malignant—and the ability of many of these agents to be incorporated into combination regimens that exhibit enhanced antimyeloma responses, without precipitating acceptable levels of toxicity. This review also discusses why these advances have not yet translated into curative outcomes and how these remaining barriers could be overcome.

Multiple myeloma (MM) is a plasma cell neoplasia that represents the second most commonly diagnosed hematologic neoplasia in the western world (Kyle and Rajkumar 2004; Palumbo and Anderson 2011; Cowan et al. 2018). During the last 20 years, major progress has been achieved in the therapeutic management of this disease. For instance, the median overall survival of patients increased from ~2–3 yr in the late 1990s to >6 yr for patients diagnosed during the time frame of 2006–2010 (Kumar et al. 2014). There is optimism that the median overall survival could reach or exceed 10 years based on data relevant to patient cohorts diagnosed after 2015. In spite of this major therapeutic progress, MM is still considered incurable and the development of novel therapeutic approaches to bridge the gap toward a cure is still necessary.

Many comprehensive review articles in the literature have focused on the biological basis (Barwick et al. 2019), pathophysiological features (Pawlyn and Davies 2019), and clinical aspects of MM, including diagnosis (Gavriatopoulou et al. 2018), prognostication (Rajkumar 2020), treatment (Chim et al. 2018; Kaufman

Cite this article as *Cold Spring Harb Perspect Med* doi: 10.1101/cshperspect.a034900

2019; Leng et al. 2019; Manasanch 2019; Sidana and Manasanch 2019), disease monitoring (Manasanch 2019; Sidana and Manasanch 2019; Baffour et al. 2020), and supportive care. Readers are encouraged to refer to these or other comprehensive articles for more in-depth analysis on the respective topics, with the additional note that the therapeutic management of MM, exactly because of its rapid ongoing progress, represents a continuously moving landscape, which in recent years has outpaced the ability to capture this progress in the literature. The main goal of this current review is to present some key considerations regarding the underlying reasons that facilitated this major and still ongoing therapeutic progress in this disease. In addition, this review discusses some concepts explaining why this progress has not yet translated into curative outcomes and outlines possible implications of these considerations for current and future basic and bench-to-bedside research for MM. Given that some of these challenges are not unique to MM but are also shared by other currently incurable subtypes of other hematologic malignancies, it is hoped that this review will stimulate a broader understanding about these concepts across the hematologic neoplasias discussed in this series of reviews.

THERAPEUTIC PROGRESS IN MM THROUGH DEVELOPMENT OF NOVEL THERAPEUTIC CLASSES

The development of thalidomide (Singhal et al. 1999) and bortezomib (Orlowski et al. 2002; Richardson et al. 2003, 2005) as the first members of their therapeutic classes (CRBN-binding agents and proteasome inhibitors, respectively) arguably constitutes the first major inflection points in the therapeutic progress in MM. The subsequent development of additional members for the respective drug classes (lenalidomide [CC-5013, IMID-3] [Richardson et al. 2002; Mitsiades and Mitsiades 2004; Dimopoulos et al. 2007; Weber et al. 2007], pomalidomide [CC-4047, IMID-1] [Miguel et al. 2013; Richardson et al. 2013] as thalidomide derivatives; carfilzomib [O'Connor et al. 2009; Alsina et al. 2012; Jakubowiak et al. 2012; Siegel et al. 2012; Stewart et al. 2015; Dimopoulos et al. 2016a, 2017; Orlowski et al. 2019] and ixazomib [Moreau et al. 2016; Krishnan et al. 2018] as proteasome inhibitors) further extended in a nonincremental manner the therapeutic impact of these new classes of therapeutics. During this last decade, another major inflection point was the development of several monoclonal antibodies, including the CS1/SLAMF7-targeting elotuzumab (Lonial et al. 2015) and the CD38-targeting antibodies daratumumab (Lokhorst et al. 2015; Dimopoulos et al. 2016b; Palumbo et al. 2016; Mateos et al. 2018; Facon et al. 2019) and isatuximab (Martin et al. 2017; Mikhael et al. 2019, 2020; Dimopoulos et al. 2020). In addition, BCMA (*TNFRSF17*) has already emerged as a major therapeutic target for MM, with promising results in clinical trials for several different classes of therapeutics that target BCMA, including chimeric antigen receptor T (CAR-T) cells (Madduri et al. 2019; Raje et al. 2019; Yan et al. 2019), antibody drug conjugates (ADCs) (Panowski et al. 2019; Popat et al. 2019, 2020; Trudel et al. 2019a; Lonial et al. 2020), or bispecific antibodies as T-cell engagers (Topp et al. 2016, 2018; Seckinger et al. 2017; Dilillo et al. 2018; Einsele et al. 2019; Li et al. 2019; Frerichs et al. 2020). In addition, the histone deacetylase inhibitor panobinostat (LBH-589) is U.S. Federal Drug Administration (FDA)-approved (for use in combination with bortezomib) (San-Miguel et al. 2013, 2014; Manasanch et al. 2018), whereas promising clinical results have been reported with the use of venetoclax, especially in MM patients with the t(11;14) translocation (Kaufman et al. 2017, 2019a,b; Kumar et al. 2017; Harrison et al. 2019). For some of these therapeutics (e.g., panobinostat), the extent of their use remains relatively limited. For others, especially anti-CD38 antibodies, their pronounced clinical activity has already had a major impact on MM therapeutic management: Given their relatively recent introduction (first FDA approval of daratumumab in 2015) in the therapeutic armamentarium, it may take several more years of follow-up to fully appreciate the impact of this therapeutic class on patient outcomes. On aggregate, though, the therapeutic management of MM in 2020 bears no resemblance to the limited options available approximately 20 years ago, when the therapeutic management of MM was predominantly based on glucocorticoids, alkylating agents (in standard doses or as high-dose melphalan with hematopoietic stem cell transplant), and anthracyclines.

How were all these novel classes of therapeutics capable of transforming the therapeutic landscape of MM? From the standpoint of clinical efficacy, when each of these therapeutic classes was being first developed, they exhibited pronounced rates, depth, and durability of clinical responses in patients who had been previously exposed to and developed resistance/refractoriness to all previously available therapeutic classes, including their combinations. For instance, the early development of thalidomide was hallmarked by substantial single-agent activity in patients refractory to all previously available therapeutic agents of the prethalidomide era (Singhal et al. 1999). Bortezomib demonstrated early on that that activity in MM patients was relapsed/refractory to prethalidomide era treatments, but also to thalidomide itself (Richardson et al. 2002, 2003, 2005). Next-generation members of the thalidomide derivative class also demonstrated activity in sizable fractions of patients who were refractory to earlier members of the class (e.g., lenalidomide activity in thalidomide-refractory cases [Richardson et al. 2002, 2006], pomalidomide activity in lenalidomide-refractory patients) (Richardson et al. 2013, 2014a, 2017; Ichinohe et al. 2015). Daratumumab, also demonstrated, even as a single agent, clinical activity in a substantial proportion of patients who were refractory to all previously available therapeutic classes and combinations thereof (Plesner et al. 2012a,b; Lokhorst et al. 2015).

THE SIGNIFICANCE OF INCORPORATING NOVEL THERAPEUTIC CLASSES INTO COMBINATION REGIMENS FOR MM

The significance of combination regimens for the therapeutic progress in MM cannot be overstated. The single-agent activity demonstrated by these aforementioned novel agents (even in many patients who were refractory to all previously available therapies) solidified the notion that these novel agents should be included in the therapeutic armamentarium for MM. It can be argued though that a larger and more lasting impact of these agents was related to their ability to be introduced in safe and efficacious combination regimens with other established or recently developed anti-MM agents. Many of these combinations were associated with enhancement (in some cases very pronounced) of the rates, depth, and durability of clinical responses, without precipitation of unmanageable new toxicities.

As a testament to the value of bench-to-bedside research in MM, some of these combinations were informed by and heavily relied on conceptual frameworks established from preclinical studies that suggested supra-additive/synergistic interactions between the anti-MM activity of these therapeutics (Mitsiades et al. 2002a,b,c, 2003, 2004). Importantly, in several cases the enhanced anti-MM activity of these combinations could not have been readily predicted based on the original rationale for preclinical and clinical development of the respective single agents. A prominent example of this concept is the combination of proteasome inhibitors with thalidomide derivatives. When the first in vitro experiments combining these drug classes were reported (Mitsiades et al. 2002c), the observed enhancement of activity of the combination compared to the single agents was initially met with skepticism or indifference. The latter reactions were perhaps fueled by the perception that these two drug classes were clinically incompatible: For thalidomide derivatives, their clinical activity was largely attributed at that time to cell-nonautonomous effects on activation of immune effector cells or the MM-associated neoangiogenesis in the bone marrow, whereas in the early days of clinical development of proteasome inhibitors, a concern existed that their activity would be immunosuppressive. It was thus unclear to many in the MM field how combining a potentially immunosuppressive (proteasome inhibitors) with a presumed immunostimulatory (thalidomide derivatives) drug class would be clinically beneficial. Despite this early skepticism, the clinical development of these combinations moved forward and produced striking clinical activity (Richardson et al. 2009, 2010, 2014b), including responses in relapsed/refractory MM patients who were not responding any more to multiple different combination regimens that were available at that time, including regimens that incorporated a proteasome inhibitor or a thalidomide/lenalidomide (but not both classes). The doublet of a proteasome inhibitor and a thalidomide derivative (or a triplet with the addition of dexamethasone) was applied clinically in the form of their combination with dexamethasone (the RVD regimen) (Attal et al. 2017) and became a major backbone of MM therapy for many years, but has also progressed to several additional forms of it: Proteasome inhibitor–thalidomide derivative combinations have evolved to include other next-generation members of the respective classes (e.g., carfilzomib-lenalidomide-dexamethasone [KRD regimen] [Jakubowiak et al. 2012; Stewart et al. 2015]; ixazomib-lenalidomide-dexamethasone [IRD regimen]) and, very importantly, addition to these backbone regimens of recently developed monoclonal antibodies (e.g., daratumumab-RVD [Lin et al. 2017; Voorhees et al. 2017, 2020; Chari et al. 2019], daratumumab-KRD [Jakubowiak et al. 2017; Usmani et al. 2017; Costa et al. 2019]; daratumumab-IRD [Kumar et al. 2018]; isatuximab-KRD [Weisel et al. 2019]). It can be argued that, notwithstanding its own single-agent activity, the incorporation of daratumumab to the backbone of proteasome inhibitors and thalidomide derivatives builds on and further extends the therapeutic impact of the original doublet.

MOST NOVEL THERAPEUTIC CLASSES AND COMBINATION REGIMENS DRIVING THERAPEUTIC PROGRESS IN MM TARGET THE "PLASMA CELL BIOLOGY" OF MM CELLS

Although the major impact of these combination regimens on the therapeutic progress in MM is tangible, what has been less appreciated is why these therapeutic classes developed in the last 20 years have been so amenable to so many safe and effective combination regimens. An even broader question is how have all these seemingly different classes of therapeutics been able to have such profound impact on the therapeutic management of a disease such as MM? This question becomes even more intriguing if one considers that many of these therapeutics have relatively limited, if any, therapeutic applications in other diseases beyond MM (or other related plasma cell malignancies). Indeed, the clinical applications of proteasome inhibitors are primarily restricted to MM and other plasma cell dyscrasias (e.g., amyloidosis [Kastritis et al. 2007; Reece et al. 2009; Treon 2009; Sanchorawala et al. 2011; Palladini et al. 2020] or Wahlstrom's macroglobulinemia [Mitsiades et al. 2003; Dimopoulos et al. 2005; Goy et al. 2005; Chen et al. 2007; Treon et al. 2007]) and to some extent mantle cell lymphoma. Thalidomide derivatives have had activity as monotherapy with, for example, lenalidomide in 5q- MDS (Krönke et al. 2015) (whereas the approval of lenalidomide for treatment of follicular lymphoma or marginal zone lymphoma involves combinations with rituximab), but MM remains the predominant context of clinical use of these agents. Although it is hoped that daratumumab or isatuximab will have extensive therapeutic applications in neoplasias beyond MM, so far this is also the dominant therapeutic setting for these antibodies. Moreover, notwithstanding the excitement about the impact of BCMA-targeting therapies in MM, the highly restricted expression of the surface molecule in normal or malignant plasma cells (Hatzoglou et al. 2000; Claudio et al. 2002; Novak et al. 2004) raises the possibility that the therapeutic impact of BCMA-targeting approaches may also turn out to be primarily focused on plasma cell neoplasias, with limited roles in neoplasias derived from other lineages.

These considerations raise the plausible unifying explanation for the major, but relatively MM/plasma cell disorder–focused, impact of all these different therapeutic classes—namely, the notion that these therapies may actually target the malignant plasma cells of MM, not because they are malignant, but because they are plasma cells. This conceptual framework was first vocalized by Boise et al. (Boise et al. 2014;

Barwick et al. 2019), who proposed that the anti-MM activity of proteasome inhibitors and thalidomide derivatives reflected the distinct roles if these classes of therapeutics on both malignant and normal plasma cells, compared to (normal or malignant) cells from other lineages, including earlier stages of B-cell differentiation. More broadly, Boise et al. reasoned that the biological behavior of MM cells is governed by the aggregate impact of their plasma cell identity and the cancer-related (e.g., genetic, epigenetic) defects they harbor and that proteasome inhibitors or thalidomide derivatives largely target the former and far less so the latter aspect of MM cell biology. This concept (aka lineage dependency), often referred to as the "Tao of Myeloma" (Boise et al. 2014), presents many features that fit both the biological and clinical features of the disease. Importantly, since its original inception, additional biological and clinical data (including the clinical development of anti-CD38 antibodies or therapeutic strategies against BCMA) have come to support and extend this view of MM and its therapeutic vulnerabilities.

On aggregate, we now know that all the major classes of anti-MM therapeutics developed over the last two decades are targeting biological processes that are far more critical for the biology of plasma cells than other lineages and/or engage targets with distinct biological consequences in MM compared to other tumor types or normal tissues. In the case of proteasome inhibitors, a broadly accepted construct is that MM cells, similarly to normal plasma cells, are more vulnerable to endoplasmic reticulum stress because of their high quantity of immunoglobulin production and the substantial amounts of misfolded proteins that are generated through this process (Obeng et al. 2006; Bianchi et al. 2009): Endoplasmic reticulum–associated degradation (ERAD) of misfolded proteins involves their translocation from the ER to the cytosol and requires intact proteasome function. Consequently, the substantial decrease (but not complete abrogation) of proteasome activity conferred by bortezomib or other proteasome inhibitors has been proposed to have selectively more pronounced impact on MM cells compared to other neoplasias (Mitsiades 2015). Thalidomide and its derivatives bind to the E3 ligase CRBN and cause it to recognize the transcription factors IKZF1 and IKZF3 as neomorphic substrates, triggering their ubiquitination and eventually degradation (Krönke et al. 2014; Lu et al. 2014). These two transcription factors support proliferation and survival of MM cells, but exhibit different roles in other hematopoietic malignancies. For instance, loss of IKZF1 is associated with lymphoid blast crisis of chronic-phase chronic myeloid leukemia (CML) (Mullighan et al. 2008; Iacobucci et al. 2009). IKZF1 suppresses IL-2 production and functional activation of T cells (Gandhi et al. 2014; O'Brien et al. 2014). These distinct roles of IKZF1 on the proliferative capacity of MM cells versus T cells could explain how thalidomide derivatives may be suppressing proliferation in MM cells, but stimulating it in T cells. Because IKZF1 and IKZF3 are generally not expressed in the overwhelming majority of non-hematopoietic tissues, this could conceivably contribute to the generally manageable profile of adverse events for this therapeutic class. CD38 exhibits restricted expression in hematopoietic tissues, primarily in different stages of B-cell differentiation, and especially high levels among plasma cells. BCMA is also exhibiting preferentially high expression in plasma cells—normal or malignant—compared to other hematopoietic cell types or solid tissues (Claudio et al. 2002; O'Connor et al. 2004; Carpenter et al. 2013). Collectively, these considerations support the notion that all major therapeutic classes that have shaped the therapeutic landscape of MM during the last two decades exhibit relatively selective therapeutic impact in this disease (compared to most other neoplasias) because they target molecules and biological processes that are preferentially more important for plasma cells—malignant or normal—compared to other tissue types. It is plausible that these considerations also explain in part why these therapeutic classes are amenable to many different safe and effective combination regimens: As most of these therapeutics have a far less pronounced impact on the function of other tissues (if they are expressed at all) beyond normal or malignant plasma cells, their combinations are unlikely to lead to broad-spectrum synergistic toxicities, but apparently do cause more than additive suppression of molecular networks critical for the survival and proliferation of MM cells.

The Challenge of Targeting the "Cancer Cell Biology" Aspect of MM Cells

An important aspect of the MM/plasma cell–selective nature of the targets and biological processes that are being perturbed by the recently developed anti-MM agents is the notion that the clinical success of these agents cannot be readily attributed to direct targeting of genes/proteins that are recurrently mutated in MM. It is indeed notable that despite extensive characterization of the mutational landscape of MM during the last 10 years using next-generation sequencing approaches (Chapman et al. 2011; Egan et al. 2012; Walker et al. 2012; Andrulis et al. 2013; Bolli et al. 2014; Lohr et al. 2014; Melchor et al. 2014; Cifola et al. 2015; Vikova et al. 2019; Ziccheddu et al. 2020), very few of the recurrently mutated MM genes represent druggable events. In addition, no immediate connection can be made between those recurrent gene perturbations and the therapeutic applications of the major therapeutic classes that emerged in MM during the last two decades. For example, there is no direct link between recurrent mutations in genes for proteasome pathway members or endoplasmic reticulum stress regulators and the activity of proteasome inhibitors in this disease. Interestingly, even for those few "druggable" mutational events identified recurrently (though infrequently) in MM patients, their respective inhibitors have not been able to achieve major clinical impact in this disease. For example, BRAF mutations have been reported in ~5%–8% of newly diagnosed MM patients (Chapman et al. 2011; Bolli et al. 2014), and early clinical studies suggested intriguing clinical activities in specific case series of patients harboring those mutations (Andrulis et al. 2013). However, the extent and duration of these responses appear to be less pronounced than those observed in other types of BRAF-mutant neoplasias (Hyman et al. 2015), suggesting that the dependence of BRAF-mutant MM cells on this activated oncogene is more attenuated compared to their solid tumor counterparts. More broadly, existing or investigational therapeutics directly target only a minority of mutations recurrently present in MM patients. In addition, genes recurrently dysregulated in MM include many prominent genes that generally do not have available direct and selective targeted therapies, including p53, N-Ras, or K-RAS (with the exception of G12C mutations, which are detected very rarely in myeloma [Chapman et al. 2011] or other hematologic malignancies), and c-myc. Notably, as MM patients progress through successive lines of therapies, the rates of genomic lesions involving these genes also exhibit gradual increase (Avet-Loiseau et al. 2007; Bolli et al. 2014), to the point that MM patients who are refractory to currently available therapies tend to harbor in their tumor cells these and other genetic lesions in patterns that do not appear qualitatively different from those observed in different types of solid tumors or in other hematologic malignancies (Mitsiades Laboratory, unpubl. observations).

In fact, the inability of the therapeutic classes developed over the last 20 years to provide curative outcomes for MM, even when used in combination(s), may again reflect the notion that they are the targeting the "plasma cell biology" aspect of the MM cells, but not the "cancer cell biology" side of MM cells, and especially those key "undruggable" (for MM and other neoplasias) lesions that are responsible for the eventual demise of patients in both MM and beyond. For this reason, and despite their successes so far, it is plausible that MM/plasma cell–specific pharmacological and antibody-based therapies may perhaps be intrinsically unable, on their own, to achieve curative outcomes for the large majority of MM patients, because of their inability to control the "cancer biology" side of MM cells.

Development of novel therapies that effectively target the dysregulation of p53, Ras mutations, or c-Myc has been a challenging task for solid tumors, but also blood cancers, for many years. Although some progress has been achieved (e.g., preclinical development of BET bromodomain inhibitors to target MYC function or expression [Delmore et al. 2011] or

 Cite this article as *Cold Spring Harb Perspect Med* doi: 10.1101/cshperspect.a034900

the recent studies of KRAS G12C inhibitors for select solid tumors [Janes et al. 2018; Canon et al. 2019; Molina-Arcas et al. 2019]), these therapeutic challenges remain to be addressed not just for MM, but across neoplasias. Until some of these challenges are addressed, it is likely that combinations of pharmacological agents will continue facing major hurdles toward the goal of providing curative outcomes for MM. This may partly explain why it has been both appropriate and necessary for the MM field to intensify its efforts for develop immune-based therapies against this disease, as an approach that can overcome the challenges of targeting pathways disrupted by the mutational events of MM patients and potentially complement the targeting of the "plasma cell biology component" of the MM cell.

IMMUNOLOGICAL TARGETING OF MM: A "NEW," YET FAMILIAR, FRONTIER

The development of immune-based therapies has been a long-standing goal for the field of MM, for several reasons. First, for many years it has been hoped that reversing the immunoparesis associated with MM would not only attenuate the infectious complications associated with MM (Jacobson and Zolla-Pazner 1986) but also directly contribute to better control of the disease itself (Cook and Campbell 1999). Even in the context of monoclonal gammopathy of undetermined significance (MGUS), which precedes MM, T-cell exhaustion (Bailur et al. 2019) and increased numbers of immunosuppressive regulatory T cells (Feyler et al. 2009) are detected. Progression to symptomatic MM is also linked with additional immune dysregulation including further increases in regulatory T cells and proinflammatory Th17 cells (Dhodapkar et al. 2008; Feyler et al. 2009; Prabhala et al. 2010), loss of antigen-specific T-cell function, loss of BM stem-like /resident memory T cells (TRMs) (Bailur et al. 2019), and increased detection of terminally differentiated T cells, as well as dysregulation of dendritic cell (DC) function (Ratta et al. 2002; Brimnes et al. 2006; Racanelli et al. 2010). This complex picture of T-cell dysfunction in MM, combined with the successful clinical application of T-cell-directed therapies in other neoplasias during the last decade, created legitimate optimism that similar approaches can be leveraged therapeutically for MM. Second, for many years, it was hoped that, similarly to the development of rituximab approximately two decades ago for $CD20^{+}$ lymphomas, MM would also become a prototypical tumor type for the development of monoclonal antibody–based therapies, especially given that MM cells express a series of distinct surface markers that could conceivably facilitate their selective targeting. Finally, before the more recent development of antibody-based therapies or T-cell-directed immune approaches for MM, the hope for major clinical applications of anti-MM immunotherapy was fueled by the clinical success of thalidomide derivatives: Because these agents exhibited "immunomodulatory" effects and achieved clinical activity in MM, it was perceived that these two properties were linked and therefore provided hope that the underlying immunoparesis of MM could be reversible and that MM could be the focus of a more extensive application of diverse form immunotherapies. It is now understood that thalidomide derivatives have a major cell-autonomous effect on CRBN-mediated degradation of IKZF1 and IKZF3, and perhaps the "immunomodulatory" properties of thalidomide derivatives may make a less pronounced contribution to the anti-MM activity of this drug class than initially hypothesized. Nevertheless, the overall therapeutic principle of restoring T-cell function in MM is now well-supported by the exciting clinical progress of several T-cell-dependent immune oncologic therapies, including cell-based therapies (e.g., chimeric antigen receptor T cells), bispecific antibodies with T-cell engager activity (BiTEs), and the overall trajectory of clinical studies involving the DC-MM fusion vaccines and immune checkpoint inhibitors.

The impact of monoclonal antibody–based therapies on MM management has already been profound. The anti-CD38 antibody daratumumab has arguably become a backbone agent for the treatment of MM: After initial documentation of its single-agent anti-MM activity in patients that were relapsed/refractory to previously established therapeutics (Lokhorst et al. 2015), daratumumab is now routinely incorporated into diverse combination regimens with other established therapeutics, including thalidomide derivatives, proteasome inhibitors, or their combination (as outlined in earlier sections of this review). Isatuximab, another anti-CD38 antibody, was also recently FDA-approved (Attal et al. 2019), also exhibits pronounced anti-MM activity, and is expected to be a recurrent partner in diverse combination regimens. Elotuzumab, a monoclonal antibody targeting the surface glycoprotein SLAMF7/CS-1, is also approved in combination with lenalidomide and dexamethasone for MM patients with relapsed disease; we have received at least one line with prior therapy (Lonial et al. 2015). Mechanistically, these antibodies are considered to elicit their anti-MM effects through a variety of processes including complement-dependent cytotoxicity (CDC), antibody-dependent cellular cytotoxicity (ADCC), or antibody-dependent cellular phagocytosis (ADCP) (as reviewed in Palumbo and Sonneveld 2015; Weisel 2016; Campbell et al. 2018; van de Donk and Usmani 2018; Franssen et al. 2020). Daratumumab and isatuximab have also been proposed to induce MM cell death in a manner that involves Fc-γ receptor–mediated cross-linking in the case of daratumumab, whereas it is independent of cross-linking for isatuximab (van de Donk and Usmani 2018; Franssen et al. 2020).

Notably, anti-CD38 antibodies have been proposed to target negative regulators of the immune response including $CD38^+$ regulatory T cells, regulatory B cells, and myeloid-derived suppressor cells (MDSCs) (Krejcik et al. 2016). The precise contribution of in vivo targeting of these immunosuppressive cell populations on the clinical activity of the anti-CD38 antibodies remains to be fully determined, but this concept of indirect targeting of the tumor cell population through engagement of $CD38^+$ immunoregulatory cells has also been explored (either alone [e.g., in clinical trial NCT03473730] or in combination with checkpoint inhibitors [e.g., NCT03023423 and NCT03098550]) in patients with solid tumors that do not express CD38. It is notable that both CD38 and SLAMF7/CS1 are expressed in natural killer (NK) cells, raising intriguing questions about the impact of these two classes of antibodies on NK-cell function. For elotuzumab, it has been proposed that, because the intracellular domain of SLAMF7/CS1 interacts with different adaptor proteins in MM versus NK cells, the binding of elotuzumab on SLAMF7 elicits different downstream signaling events that are antiproliferative in MM cells but stimulatory for NK cells (Tassi and Colonna 2005; Collins et al. 2013; Guo et al. 2015). NK cells are an important component of the mechanisms of action of daratumumab, but also susceptible to its effect in vitro, whereas in the clinical setting, peripheral blood NK-cell numbers exhibit rapid, reversible, and dose-dependent decrease after daratumumab treatment (Casneuf et al. 2017, 2020). Notably this decrease in peripheral blood NK cell counts was not associated with decreased response rates, shorter progression-free survival, nor increased rates of infectious or other adverse events (Casneuf et al. 2017), suggesting that more research will be needed to further clarify the impact of this daratumumab-induced NK-cell reduction on clinical outcomes. More broadly, the great clinical progress achieved with monoclonal antibodies, especially those targeting CD38, is expected to lead to further efforts to understand the complex biological effects of these agents on MM cells, but also on different types of nonmalignant immune cell populations that may also express these surface markers.

In parallel with the clinical successes of daratumumab and other monoclonal antibodies, two additional exciting areas of progress in MM have involved the development of CAR-T cells (e.g., Brudno et al. 2018; Cohen et al. 2019; Raje et al. 2019) and of ADCs (Panowski et al. 2019; Popat et al. 2019, 2020; Trudel et al. 2019a; Lonial et al. 2020). For both of these modalities, the most pronounced progress in MM has been achieved through targeting of the B-cell maturation antigen (BCMA), in view of its nearly universal expression (despite variable intensity) on the surface of MM cells and the relatively restricted expression of this antigen on normal or malignant plasma cells (O'Connor et al. 2004). So far, the clinical trials with different types of anti-BCMA CAR-T cells have demonstrated variable, but high, response rates (e.g., ~60%–90% overall response rates in patients with refractory MM receiving >10^8 CAR-T cells), including substantial fraction of patients who have complete remissions with negative minimal residual disease (MRD) testing (Brudno et al. 2018; Raje et al. 2019 and as reviewed in Cho et al. 2018; Adaniya et al. 2019; Cohen 2019; Cohen et al. 2020; Shah et al. 2020). Building on this encouraging early clinical experience, important ongoing research seeks to optimize the long-term impact of CAR-T cell uses in MM therapy. For instance, a key goal will be to improve the durability of responses and the progression-free survival of patients receiving CAR-T cells: Currently these outcomes appear to be variable, with more favorable results observed in less heavily pretreated patients (as reviewed in Adaniya et al. 2019; Cohen 2019; Cohen et al. 2020; Shah et al. 2020). A substantial proportion of patients with aggressive disease who have been leukapheresed for the manufacturing of CAR-T cells end up not receiving them because of rapid disease progression (Cohen et al. 2019; Raje et al. 2019). Similar to other applications of CAR-T cells in other hematologic malignancies, cytokine release syndrome or neurotoxicity is observed frequently, but is usually responsive to anti-IL-6 receptor monoclonal antibody tocilizumab (for cytokine release syndrome) or glucocorticoids (for neurotoxicity) (Brudno et al. 2018; Raje et al. 2019). Collectively, future uses of CAR-T cells in MM are expected to benefit from development of off-the-shelf allogeneic CAR-T cell products (Sommer et al. 2019); the development of more rapid manufacturing procedures (Ghassemi et al. 2018); the deployment of CAR-T cells against new targets (Smith et al. 2019), combinations of targets (Yan et al. 2019), or bi-epitopic CAR-T cells (Xu et al. 2019); and a better understanding of the optimal time point(s) in the course of the disease when these CAR-T cells should be deployed.

ADCs involve a monoclonal antibody conjugated with a cytotoxic small molecule ("payload") through a specialized chemical linker: Upon binding to the respective antigen on the surface of target cells, the ADC/antigen complex is internalized, leading to payload release and cytotoxic cell death. The concept of ADCs as an approach to selectively deliver cytotoxic compounds to tumor cells while sparing normal tissues has been examined for many years, but has gained particular traction in recent years given the successful clinical development of several ADCs that were FDA-approved for other lymphoid malignancies (e.g., brentuximab vedotin [Younes et al. 2012], inotuzumab ozogamicin [Kantarjian et al. 2016], moxetumomab pasudotox [Kreitman et al. 2018; Short et al. 2018], and polatuzumab vedotin [Morschhauser et al. 2019]). Belantamab mafodotin (GSK2857916) is humanized anti-BCMA IgG1 monoclonal antibody conjugated to monomethyl auristatin F (MMAF, mafodotin) via a noncleavable linker (Anderson et al. 2016; Dettman et al. 2018; Popat et al. 2018, 2020; Trudel et al. 2018, 2019a,b; Bonello et al. 2020; Shah et al. 2020) and is currently the most advanced ADC in terms of clinical development for MM. The clinical studies of the belantamab mafodotin have documented clinical activity in patients with relapsed/refractory MM, including partial responses or better in ~60% of patients treated at the recommended phase II dose of a phase I trial that enrolled patients with progressive disease following stem cell transplant, alkylators, proteasome inhibitors, and immunomodulators (Trudel et al. 2018). The safety profile from that study was notable for corneal events (including blurry vision, dry eyes, or photophobia) in 58% of patients, with a manageable profile of hematologic adverse events and no evidence of cytokine release syndrome or neurotoxicity. Other ADCs currently in development also target BCMA (Singh et al. 2018; Lee et al. 2020) or other targets including FcRH5 (Stewart et al. 2019) or CS1 (Vij et al. 2020).

An exciting area of major recent developments for the MM field involves bispecific antibodies/antibody constructs engineered to engage simultaneously the endogenous T cells (via binding to CD3) and tumor cells (through binding to a tumor-associated surface antigen). These BiTEs present several advantageous features, as they can facilitate activation of T cells;

enable their close proximity to the tumor cells; do not require ex vivo T-cell manipulation; extended manufacturing process, peptide antigen presentation, or lymphodepletion; and function independently of the major histocompatibility antigens and T-cell-receptor sequences of the patient (Slaney et al. 2018; Cohen et al. 2019). Similarly to CAR-T cells, bispecific antibodies are associated with serial killing of the tumor cells by the T cells (as reviewed in Slaney et al. 2018; Cohen et al. 2019) and can be associated with cytokine release syndrome and neurotoxicity, whereas, distinctly from CAR-T cells, repeat administration (including continuous intravenous infusion regimens) may be needed for those BiTEs (including AMG420) that have short serum half-life because of their two single-chain variable domains connected by a short linker (Slaney et al. 2018). Among the diverse bispecific antibodies/antibody constructs that are currently being developed against BCMA or other targets (e.g., CD38, FcRH5, GPRC5D) (as reviewed in Slaney et al. 2018; Cohen 2019), some are now incorporating an Fc domain, to recapitulate at least some IgG-like aspects of this molecule—for example, to increase the half-life, enable intermittent dosing and potentially subcutaneous administration, or facilitate Fc-mediated effector functions (Fan et al. 2015; Velasquez et al. 2018). More clinical data may be needed to determine whether the prolonged half-life of these Fc-containing BiTEs might also lead to prolonged side effects. It is has been postulated, based on studies in acute lymphoblastic leukemia (ALL), that the antitumor activity of BiTEs is affected by the quality of the endogenous T-cell repertoire in patients (Zugmaier et al. 2015): Projecting this experience to the MM setting suggests that perhaps this therapeutic class of bispecific T-cell engagers may be optimally placed during the earlier phase(s) of the MM disease continuum, during which the endogenous T-cell quality may conceivably be in a healthier state. Overall, BiTEs represent an extremely active and promising area of research, with many potential opportunities for the MM field.

Unlike the progress with monoclonal antibodies, CAR-T cells, ADCs, or BiTEs, and in contrast to many other neoplasias, immune checkpoint inhibitors have not yet established a clear role in the therapeutic management of MM. Even though the anti-PD 1 monoclonal antibody nivolumab documented no significant single-agent activity in relapsed/refractory MM (Lesokhin et al. 2016), the combination of different combinations of the anti-PD 1 antibody pembrolizumab plus a thalidomide derivative and dexamethasone documented overall response rates of 44% and 60% in relapsed/refractory MM patients (Badros et al. 2017; Mateos et al. 2019a). Despite the enthusiasm created by these phase I-II combination studies, two subsequent phase III clinical trials focusing on these pembrolizumab-based combinations in newly diagnosed or relapsed/refractory MM were suspended because of higher rates (compared to the control arm) of grade 3 or higher immune-related adverse events/death, without substantial improvements in response rates (Mateos et al. 2019b; Usmani et al. 2019). The results of these studies delayed further development of other immune checkpoint inhibitors in MM. However, PD-1 or PDL-1 inhibitors remain the focus of active research in MM. A critical question is why immune checkpoint inhibitors have not been successful in MM, either as single agents or in combination with thalidomide derivatives. Part of the answer may be related to observations that the dysfunctional clonal T cells in MM exhibit, as their predominant feature, immune senescence, and not exhaustion (as they have low expression of PD1 and CTLA4) (Suen et al. 2016), which could explain at least in part the suboptimal outcomes with PD1 targeting and could also suggest the need for other immunostimulatory strategies. Consistent with this direction, there is also active interest in MM for agonistic antibodies that engage costimulatory receptors (e.g., CD137/4-1BB, OX40) (e.g., as in Guillerey et al. 2019).

An important common denominator between the more successful or promising immunotherapeutic approaches for MM (monoclonal antibodies, CAR-T cells, ADCs, or BiTEs) is the fact that they leverage the surface expression of antigens with relatively plasma cell/MM–restricted expression: Consistent with the concept of the "Tao of MM," the immunotherapy approaches that have documented the most promising results in this disease so far are distinct from the immune checkpoint inhibitors that have been highly successful in other neoplasias, perhaps because patient-derived MM cells typically exhibit modest levels of mutational burden and that are generally lower than those neoplasias that are highly responsive to checkpoint inhibition (Alexandrov et al. 2013). In contrast, daratumumab, CAR-T cells, and BiTEs have so far leveraged the high levels of CD38 and BCMA on the surface of MM cells, which conceivably allows these therapies to spare the overwhelming majority of normal lineages (and, in the case of daratumumab, perhaps suppress those immunoregulatory cell populations that express CD38) while achieving potent and selective targeting of the tumor cell population.

FUTURE DIRECTIONS

Although MM remains incurable, the major success achieved over the last two decades in its therapeutic management has been based on concepts that have apparently not yet been saturated: Based on data from preclinical functional genomics studies (de Matos Simoes et al. 2019), it appears that the MM field has only began to "scratch the surface" of the spectrum of genes and molecular pathways that are preferentially critical for MM cells compared to (normal or malignant) cells from other lineages, suggesting that there will be additional pharmacologically tractable targets that may be developed for therapeutic interventions in this disease in the near future. Similarly, in regard to immune-based therapies against MM, beyond BCMA or CD38, there are several other surface antigens with high levels of expression in plasma cells/MM cells, but limited expression in any other tissues: These targets are already or are expected in the near future to be the basis for additional monoclonal antibodies, CAR-T cells, or BiTEs, which may help further improve the outcome for this disease. At the same time, it is hoped that more improvements in our understanding about the "cancer cell biology" of MM cells will enable their therapeutic targeting in a manner that will hopefully bring us closer to curative outcomes for the majority of patients with MM.

REFERENCES

Adaniya SPS, Cohen AD, Garfall AL. 2019. Chimeric antigen receptor T cell immunotherapy for multiple myeloma: A review of current data and potential clinical applications. *Am J Hematol* **94:** S28–S33. doi:10.1002/ajh.25428

Alexandrov LB, Nik-Zainal S, Wedge DC, Aparicio SA, Behjati S, Biankin AV, Bignell GR, Bolli N, Borg A, Børresen-Dale AL, et al. 2013. Signatures of mutational processes in human cancer. *Nature* **500:** 415–421. doi:10.1038/nature12477

Alsina M, Trudel S, Furman RR, Rosen PJ, O'Connor OA, Comenzo RL, Wong A, Kunkel LA, Molineaux CJ, Goy A. 2012. A phase I single-agent study of twice-weekly consecutive-day dosing of the proteasome inhibitor carfilzomib in patients with relapsed or refractory multiple myeloma or lymphoma. *Clin Cancer Res* **18:** 4830–4840. doi:10.1158/1078-0432.CCR-11-3007

Anderson LD, Cavet J, Cohen AD, Degenhardt YY, Ellis CE, Germaschewski F, Lendvai N, Libby E, Opalinska J, Popat R, et al. 2016. A phase I study of GSK2857916, a BCMA-directed monoclonal antibody conjugated to microtubule-disrupting agent in patients with relapsed, refractory multiple myeloma and other BCMA-expressing hematologic malignancies. *Cancer Res* **76**. doi:10.1158/1538-7445.AM2016-CT034

Andrulis M, Lehners N, Capper D, Penzel R, Heining C, Huellein J, Zenz T, von Deimling A, Schirmacher P, Ho AD, et al. 2013. Targeting the BRAF V600E mutation in multiple myeloma. *Cancer Discov* **3:** 862–869. doi:10.1158/2159-8290.CD-13-0014

Attal M, Lauwers-Cances V, Hulin C, Leleu X, Caillot D, Escoffre M, Arnulf B, Macro M, Belhadj K, Garderet L, et al. 2017. Lenalidomide, bortezomib, and dexamethasone with transplantation for myeloma. *N Engl J Med* **376:** 1311–1320. doi:10.1056/NEJMoa1611750

Attal M, Richardson PG, Rajkumar SV, San-Miguel J, Beksac M, Spicka I, Leleu X, Schjesvold F, Moreau P, Dimopoulos MA, et al. 2019. Isatuximab plus pomalidomide and low-dose dexamethasone versus pomalidomide and low-dose dexamethasone in patients with relapsed and refractory multiple myeloma (ICARIA-MM): A randomised, multicentre, open-label, phase 3 study. *Lancet* **394:** 2096–2107. doi:10.1016/S0140-6736(19)32556-5

Avet-Loiseau H, Attal M, Moreau P, Charbonnel C, Garban F, Hulin C, Leyvraz S, Michallet M, Yakoub-Agha I, Garderet L, et al. 2007. Genetic abnormalities and survival in multiple myeloma: The experience of the Intergroupe Francophone du Myélome. *Blood* **109:** 3489–3495. doi:10.1182/blood-2006-08-040410

Badros A, Hyjek E, Ma N, Lesokhin A, Dogan A, Rapoport AP, Kocoglu M, Lederer E, Philip S, Milliron T, et al. 2017. Pembrolizumab, pomalidomide, and low-dose dexamethasone for relapsed/refractory multiple myeloma. *Blood* **130:** 1189–1197. doi:10.1182/blood-2017-03-775122

Baffour FI, Glazebrook KN, Kumar SK, Broski SM. 2020. Role of imaging in multiple myeloma. *Am J Hematol* **95:** 966–977. doi:10.1002/ajh.25846.

Bailur JK, McCachren SS, Doxie DB, Shrestha M, Pendleton K, Nooka AK, Neparidze N, Parker TL, Bar N, Kaufman JL, et al. 2019. Early alterations in stem-like/resident T cells, innate and myeloid cells in the bone marrow in preneoplastic gammopathy. *JCI Insight* **5:** e127807. doi:10.1172/jci.insight.12780.

Barwick BG, Gupta VA, Vertino PM, Boise LH. 2019. Cell of origin and genetic alterations in the pathogenesis of multiple myeloma. *Front Immunol* **10:** 1121. doi:10.3389/fimmu.2019.01121

Bianchi G, Oliva L, Cascio P, Pengo N, Fontana F, Cerruti F, Orsi A, Pasqualetto E, Mezghrani A, Calbi V, et al. 2009. The proteasome load versus capacity balance determines apoptotic sensitivity of multiple myeloma cells to proteasome inhibition. *Blood* **113:** 3040–3049. doi:10.1182/blood-2008-08-172734

Boise LH, Kaufman JL, Bahlis NJ, Lonial S, Lee KP. 2014. The Tao of myeloma. *Blood* **124:** 1873–1879. doi:10.1182/blood-2014-05-578732

Bolli N, Avet-Loiseau H, Wedge DC, Van Loo P, Alexandrov LB, Martincorena I, Dawson KJ, Iorio F, Nik-Zainal S, Bignell GR, et al. 2014. Heterogeneity of genomic evolution and mutational profiles in multiple myeloma. *Nat Commun* **5:** 2997. doi:10.1038/ncomms3997

Bonello F, Mina R, Boccadoro M, Gay F. 2020. Therapeutic monoclonal antibodies and antibody products: Current practices and development in multiple myeloma. *Cancers (Basel)* **12:** 15. doi:10.3390/cancers12010015

Brimnes MK, Svane IM, Johnsen HE. 2006. Impaired functionality and phenotypic profile of dendritic cells from patients with multiple myeloma. *Clin Exp Immunol* **144:** 76–84. doi:10.1111/j.1365-2249.2006.03037.x

Brudno JN, Maric I, Hartman SD, Rose JJ, Wang M, Lam N, Stetler-Stevenson M, Salem D, Yuan C, Pavletic S, et al. 2018. T cells genetically modified to express an anti-B-cell maturation antigen chimeric antigen receptor cause remissions of poor-prognosis relapsed multiple myeloma. *J Clin Oncol* **36:** 2267–2280. doi:10.1200/JCO.2018.77.8084

Campbell KS, Cohen AD, Pazina T. 2018. Mechanisms of NK cell activation and clinical activity of the therapeutic SLAMF7 antibody, elotuzumab in multiple myeloma. *Front Immunol* **9:** 2551. doi:10.3389/fimmu.2018.02551

Canon J, Rex K, Saiki AY, Mohr C, Cooke K, Bagal D, Gaida K, Holt T, Knutson CG, Koppada N, et al. 2019. The clinical KRAS(G12C) inhibitor AMG 510 drives anti-tumour immunity. *Nature* **575:** 217–223. doi:10.1038/s41586-019-1694-1

Carpenter RO, Evbuomwan MO, Pittaluga S, Rose JJ, Raffeld M, Yang S, Gress RE, Hakim FT, Kochenderfer JN. 2013. B-cell maturation antigen is a promising target for adoptive T-cell therapy of multiple myeloma. *Clin Cancer Res* **19:** 2048–2060. doi:10.1158/1078-0432.CCR-12-2422

Casneuf T, Xu XS, Adams HC, Axel AE, Chiu C, Khan I, Ahmadi T, Yan X, Lonial S, Plesner T, et al. 2017. Effects of daratumumab on natural killer cells and impact on clinical outcomes in relapsed or refractory multiple myeloma. *Blood Adv* **1:** 2105–2114. doi:10.1182/bloodadvances.2017006866

Casneuf T, Adams HC, van de Donk NWCJ, Abraham Y, Bald J, Vanhoof G, Van der Borght K, Smets T, Foulk B, Nielsen KC, et al. 2020. Deep immune profiling of patients treated with lenalidomide and dexamethasone with or without daratumumab. *Leukemia* doi:10.1038/s41375-020-0855-4.

Chapman MA, Lawrence MS, Keats JJ, Cibulskis K, Sougnez C, Schinzel AC, Harview CL, Brunet JP, Ahmann GJ, Adli M, et al. 2011. Initial genome sequencing and analysis of multiple myeloma. *Nature* **471:** 467–472. doi:10.1038/nature09837

Chari A, Voorhees PM, Kaufman JL, Laubach J, Sborov DW, Reeves B, Rodriguez C, Silbermann R, Costa LJ, Anderson JR LD, et al. 2019. Daratumumab plus lenalidomide, bortezomib, and dexamethasone (D-RVd) improves depth of response in transplant-eligible newly diagnosed multiple myeloma: GRIFFIN primary analysis. *Am J Hematol* **94:** S31.

Chen CI, Kouroukis CT, White D, Voralia M, Stadtmauer E, Stewart AK, Wright JJ, Powers J, Walsh W, Eisenhauer E, et al. 2007. Bortezomib is active in patients with untreated or relapsed Waldenström's macroglobulinemia: A phase II study of the National Cancer Institute of Canada Clinical Trials Group. *J Clin Oncol* **25:** 1570–1575. doi:10.1200/JCO.2006.07.8659

Chim CS, Kumar SK, Orlowski RZ, Cook G, Richardson PG, Gertz MA, Giralt S, Mateos MV, Leleu X, Anderson KC. 2018. Management of relapsed and refractory multiple myeloma: Novel agents, antibodies, immunotherapies and beyond. *Leukemia* **32:** 252–262. doi:10.1038/leu.2017.329

Cho SF, Anderson KC, Tai YT. 2018. Targeting B cell maturation antigen (BCMA) in multiple myeloma: Potential uses of BCMA-based immunotherapy. *Front Immunol* **9:** 1821. doi:10.3389/fimmu.2018.01821

Cifola I, Lionetti M, Pinatel E, Todoerti K, Mangano E, Pietrelli A, Fabris S, Mosca L, Simeon V, Petrucci MT, et al. 2015. Whole-exome sequencing of primary plasma cell leukemia discloses heterogeneous mutational patterns. *Oncotarget* **6:** 17543–17558. doi:10.18632/oncotarget.4028

Claudio JO, Masih-Khan E, Tang H, Gonçalves J, Voralia M, Li ZH, Nadeem V, Cukerman E, Francisco-Pabalan O, Liew CC, et al. 2002. A molecular compendium of genes expressed in multiple myeloma. *Blood* **100:** 2175–2186. doi:10.1182/blood-2002-01-0008

Cohen AD. 2019. Myeloma: Next generation immunotherapy. *Hematology Am Soc Hematol Educ Program* **2019:** 266–272. doi:10.1182/hematology.2019000068

Cohen AD, Garfall AL, Stadtmauer EA, Melenhorst JJ, Lacey SF, Lancaster E, Vogl DT, Weiss BN, Dengel K, Nelson A, et al. 2019. B cell maturation antigen-specific CAR T cells are clinically active in multiple myeloma. *J Clin Invest* **129:** 2210–2221. doi:10.1172/JCI126397

Cohen AD, Raje N, Fowler JA, Mezzi K, Scott EC, Dhodapkar MV. 2020. How to train your T cells: Overcoming immune dysfunction in multiple myeloma. *Clin Cancer Res* **26:** 1541–1554. doi:10.1158/1078-0432.CCR-19-2111

Collins SM, Bakan CE, Swartzel GD, Hofmeister CC, Efebera YA, Kwon H, Starling GC, Ciarlariello D, Bhaskar S, Briercheck EL, et al. 2013. Elotuzumab directly enhances NK cell cytotoxicity against myeloma via CS1 ligation:

Evidence for augmented NK cell function complementing ADCC. *Cancer Immunol Immunother* **62:** 1841–1849. doi:10.1007/s00262-013-1493-8

Cook G, Campbell JD. 1999. Immune regulation in multiple myeloma: The host–tumour conflict. *Blood Rev* **13:** 151–162. doi:10.1054/blre.1999.0111

Costa LJ, Chhabra S, Godby KN, Medvedova E, Cornell RF, Hall AC, Silbermann RW, Innis-Shelton R, Dhakal B, Deldiaquez D, et al. 2019. Daratumumab, carfilzomib, lenalidomide and dexamethasone (Dara-KRd) induction, autologous transplantation and post-transplant, response-adapted, measurable residual disease (MRD)-based Dara-Krd consolidation in patients with newly diagnosed multiple myeloma (NDMM). *Blood* **134:** 860.

Cowan AJ, Allen C, Barac A, Basaleem H, Bensenor I, Curado MP, Foreman K, Gupta R, Harvey J, Hosgood HD, et al. 2018. Global burden of multiple myeloma: A systematic analysis for the global burden of disease study 2016. *JAMA Oncol* **4:** 1221–1227. doi:10.1001/jamaoncol.2018.2128

de Matos Simoes R, Shirasaki R, Downey-Kopyscinski SL, Matthews G, Yiguo H, Sheffer M, Dhimolea E, Dashevsky O, Gandolfi S, Dempster J, et al. 2019. Systematic characterization of genes representing preferential molecular vulnerabilities for myeloma cells compared to other neoplasias—Implications for the biology and therapeutic targeting of myeloma. *Blood* **134:** 4407. doi:10.1182/blood-2019-130901

Delmore JE, Issa GC, Lemieux ME, Rahl PB, Shi J, Jacobs HM, Kastritis E, Gilpatrick T, Paranal RM, Qi J, et al. 2011. BET bromodomain inhibition as a therapeutic strategy to target c-Myc. *Cell* **146:** 904–917. doi:10.1016/j.cell.2011.08.017

Dettman EJ, Rigat F, Albert J, Barnard R, Birchler M, Deghenhardt Y, DeWall S, Gaye B, He Z, Liu V, et al. 2018. Expression of myeloma cell and soluble B-cell maturation antigen (BCMA) in relapsed and refractory multiple myeloma patients treated with GSK2857916 in BMA117159. *Blood* **132:** 1977. doi:10.1182/blood-2018-99-115200

Dhodapkar KM, Barbuto S, Matthews P, Kukreja A, Mazumder A, Vesole D, Jagannath S, Dhodapkar MV. 2008. Dendritic cells mediate the induction of polyfunctional human IL17-producing cells (Th17-1 cells) enriched in the bone marrow of patients with myeloma. *Blood* **112:** 2878–2885. doi:10.1182/blood-2008-03-143222

Dilillo DJ, Olson K, Mohrs K, Meagher TC, Bray K, Sineshchekova O, Startz T, Retter M, Godin S, Delfino F, et al. 2018. REGN5458, a bispecific BCMAxCD3 T cell engaging antibody, demonstrates robust in vitro and in vivo anti-tumor efficacy in multiple myeloma models, comparable to that of BCMA CAR T cells. *Blood* **132:** 1944. doi:10.1182/blood-2018-99-112500

Dimopoulos MA, Anagnostopoulos A, Kyrtsonis MC, Castritis E, Bitsaktsis A, Pangalis GA. 2005. Treatment of relapsed or refractory Waldenstrom's macroglobulinemia with bortezomib. *Haematologica* **90:** 1655–1658.

Dimopoulos M, Spencer A, Attal M, Prince HM, Harousseau J-L, Dmoszynska A, Miguel JS, Hellmann A, Facon T, Foà R, et al. 2007. Lenalidomide plus dexamethasone for relapsed or refractory multiple myeloma. *N Engl J Med* **357:** 2123–2132. doi:10.1056/NEJMoa070594

Dimopoulos MA, Moreau P, Palumbo A, Joshua D, Pour L, Hájek R, Facon T, Ludwig H, Oriol A, Goldschmidt H, et al. 2016a. Carfilzomib and dexamethasone versus bortezomib and dexamethasone for patients with relapsed or refractory multiple myeloma (ENDEAVOR): A randomised, phase 3, open-label, multicentre study. *Lancet Oncol* **17:** 27–38. doi:10.1016/S1470-2045(15)00464-7

Dimopoulos MA, Oriol A, Nahi H, San-Miguel J, Bahlis NJ, Usmani SZ, Rabin N, Orlowski RZ, Komarnicki M, Suzuki K, et al. 2016b. Daratumumab, lenalidomide, and dexamethasone for multiple myeloma. *N Engl J Med* **375:** 1319–1331. doi:10.1056/NEJMoa1607751

Dimopoulos MA, Goldschmidt H, Niesvizky R, Joshua D, Chng WJ, Oriol A, Orlowski RZ, Ludwig H, Facon T, Hajek R, et al. 2017. Carfilzomib or bortezomib in relapsed or refractory multiple myeloma (ENDEAVOR): An interim overall survival analysis of an open-label, randomised, phase 3 trial. *Lancet Oncol* **18:** 1327–1337. doi:10.1016/S1470-2045(17)30578-8

Dimopoulos MA, Leleu X, Moreau P, Richardson PG, Liberati AM, Harrison SJ, Prince HM, Ocio EM, Assadourian S, Campana F, et al. 2020. Isatuximab plus pomalidomide and dexamethasone in relapsed/refractory multiple myeloma patients with renal impairment: ICARIA-MM subgroup analysis. *Leukemia* doi:10.1038/s41375-020-0868-2

Egan JB, Shi CX, Tembe W, Christoforides A, Kurdoglu A, Sinari S, Middha S, Asmann Y, Schmidt J, Braggio E, et al. 2012. Whole-genome sequencing of multiple myeloma from diagnosis to plasma cell leukemia reveals genomic initiating events, evolution, and clonal tides. *Blood* **120:** 1060–1066. doi:10.1182/blood-2012-01-405977

Einsele H, Düll J, Zugmaier G, Attal M, Moreau P, Langer C, Krönke J, Facon T, Salnikov A, Lesley R, et al. 2019. The anti-BCMA bispecific T-cell engager (BiTE®) molecule AMG 420 induced MRD-negative complete responses in R/R multiple myeloma in a FIH study. *Clin Lymphoma Myeloma Leuk* **19:** E18–E19. doi:10.1016/j.clml.2019.09.026

Facon T, Kumar S, Plesner T, Orlowski RZ, Moreau P, Bahlis N, Basu S, Nahi H, Hulin C, Quach H, et al. 2019. Daratumumab plus lenalidomide and dexamethasone for untreated myeloma. *N Engl J Med* **380:** 2104–2115. doi:10.1056/NEJMoa1817249

Fan G, Wang Z, Hao M, Li J. 2015. Bispecific antibodies and their applications. *J Hematol Oncol* **8:** 130. doi:10.1186/s13045-015-0227-0

Feyler S, von Lilienfeld-Toal M, Jarmin S, Marles L, Rawstron A, Ashcroft AJ, Owen RG, Selby PJ, Cook G. 2009. $CD4^+CD25^+FoxP3^+$ regulatory T cells are increased whilst $CD3^+CD4^-CD8^-\alpha\beta TCR^+$ double negative T cells are decreased in the peripheral blood of patients with multiple myeloma which correlates with disease burden. *Br J Haematol* **144:** 686–695. doi:10.1111/j.1365-2141.2008.07530.x

Franssen LE, Stege CAM, Zweegman S, van de Donk N, Nijhof IS. 2020. Resistance mechanisms towards CD38-directed antibody therapy in multiple myeloma. *J Clin Med* **9:** 1195. doi:10.3390/jcm9041195

Frerichs KA, Broekmans MEC, Soto JAM, van Kessel B, Heymans MW, Holthof LC, Verkleij CPM, Boominathan R, Baidya B, Sendicki J, et al. 2020. Preclinical activity of

JNJ-7957, a novel BCMA×CD3 bispecific antibody for the treatment of multiple myeloma, is potentiated by daratumumab. *Clin Cancer Res* **26:** 2203–2215. doi:10.1158/1078-0432.CCR-19-2299

Gandhi AK, Kang J, Havens CG, Conklin T, Ning Y, Wu L, Ito T, Ando H, Waldman MF, Thakurta A, et al. 2014. Immunomodulatory agents lenalidomide and pomalidomide co-stimulate T cells by inducing degradation of T cell repressors Ikaros and Aiolos via modulation of the E3 ubiquitin ligase complex CRL4^{CRBN}. *Br J Haematol* **164:** 811–821. doi:10.1111/bjh.12708

Gavriatopoulou M, Musto P, Caers J, Merlini G, Kastritis E, van de Donk N, Gay F, Hegenbart U, Hajek R, Zweegman S, et al. 2018. European myeloma network recommendations on diagnosis and management of patients with rare plasma cell dyscrasias. *Leukemia* **32:** 1883–1898. doi:10.1038/s41375-018-0209-7

Ghassemi S, Nunez-Cruz S, O'Connor RS, Fraietta JA, Patel PR, Scholler J, Barrett DM, Lundh SM, Davis MM, Bedoya F, et al. 2018. Reducing *ex vivo* culture improves the antileukemic activity of chimeric antigen receptor (CAR) T cells. *Cancer Immunol Res* **6:** 1100–1109. doi:10.1158/2326-6066.CIR-17-0405

Goy A, Younes A, McLaughlin P, Pro B, Romaguera JE, Hagemeister F, Fayad L, Dang NH, Samaniego F, Wang M, et al. 2005. Phase II study of proteasome inhibitor bortezomib in relapsed or refractory B-cell non-Hodgkin's lymphoma. *J Clin Oncol* **23:** 667–675. doi:10.1200/JCO.2005.03.108

Guillerey C, Nakamura K, Pichler AC, Barkauskas D, Krumeich S, Stannard K, Miles K, Harjunpää H, Yu Y, Casey M, et al. 2019. Chemotherapy followed by anti-CD137 mAb immunotherapy improves disease control in a mouse myeloma model. *JCI Insight* **4:** e125932.

Guo H, Cruz-Munoz ME, Wu N, Robbins M, Veillette A. 2015. Immune cell inhibition by SLAMF7 is mediated by a mechanism requiring src kinases, CD45, and SHIP-1 that is defective in multiple myeloma cells. *Mol Cell Biol* **35:** 41–51. doi:10.1128/MCB.01107-14

Harrison S, Cavo M, De la Rubia J, Popat R, Gasparetto C, Hungria VTM, Salwender H, Suzuki K, Kim I, Moreau P, et al. 2019. T(11;14) and high *BCL2* expression are predictive biomarkers of response to venetoclax in combination with bortezomib and dexamethasone in patients with relapsed/refractory multiple myeloma: Biomarker analyses from the Phase 3 Bellini Study. *Blood* **134:** 142. doi:10.1182/blood-2019-126094

Hatzoglou A, Roussel J, Bourgeade MF, Rogier E, Madry C, Inoue J, Devergne O, Tsapis A. 2000. TNF receptor family member BCMA (B cell maturation) associates with TNF receptor-associated factor (TRAF) 1, TRAF2, and TRAF3 and activates NF-κ B, elk-1, c-Jun N-terminal kinase, and p38 mitogen-activated protein kinase. *J Immunol* **165:** 1322–1330. doi:10.4049/jimmunol.165.3.1322

Hyman DM, Puzanov I, Subbiah V, Faris JE, Chau I, Blay JY, Wolf J, Raje NS, Diamond EL, Hollebecque A, et al. 2015. Vemurafenib in multiple nonmelanoma cancers with *BRAF* V600 mutations. *N Engl J Med* **373:** 726–736. doi:10.1056/NEJMoa1502309

Iacobucci I, Storlazzi CT, Cilloni D, Lonetti A, Ottaviani E, Soverini S, Astolfi A, Chiaretti S, Vitale A, Messa F, et al. 2009. Identification and molecular characterization of recurrent genomic deletions on 7p12 in the *IKZF1* gene in a large cohort of *BCR-ABL1*-positive acute lymphoblastic leukemia patients: On behalf of Gruppo Italiano Malattie Ematologiche dell'Adulto Acute Leukemia Working Party (GIMEMA AL WP). *Blood* **114:** 2159–2167. doi:10.1182/blood-2008-08-173963

Ichinohe T, Kuroda Y, Okamoto S, Matsue K, Iida S, Sunami K, Komeno T, Suzuki K, Ando K, Taniwaki M, et al. 2015. A multicenter phase 2 study of pomalidomide plus dexamethasone in patients with relapsed and refractory multiple myeloma: The Japanese MM-011 trial. *Exp Hematol Oncol* **5:** 11. doi:10.1186/s40164-016-0040-7

Jacobson DR, Zolla-Pazner S. 1986. Immunosuppression and infection in multiple myeloma. *Semin Oncol* **13:** 282–290.

Jakubowiak AJ, Dytfeld D, Griffith KA, Lebovic D, Vesole DH, Jagannath S, Al-Zoubi A, Anderson T, Nordgren B, Detweiler-Short K, et al. 2012. A phase 1/2 study of carfilzomib in combination with lenalidomide and low-dose dexamethasone as a frontline treatment for multiple myeloma. *Blood* **120:** 1801–1809. doi:10.1182/blood-2012-04-422683

Jakubowiak AJ, Chari A, Lonial S, Weiss BM, Comenzo RL, Wu K, Khokhar NZ, Wang J, Doshi P, Usmani SZ. 2017. Daratumumab (DARA) in combination with carfilzomib, lenalidomide, and dexamethasone (KRd) in patients (pts) with newly diagnosed multiple myeloma (MMY1001): An open-label, phase 1b study. *J Clin Oncol* **35:** 8000. doi:10.1200/JCO.2017.35.15_suppl.8000

Janes MR, Zhang J, Li LS, Hansen R, Peters U, Guo X, Chen Y, Babbar A, Firdaus SJ, Darjania L, et al. 2018. Targeting KRAS mutant cancers with a covalent G12C-specific inhibitor. *Cell* **172:** 578–589.e17. doi:10.1016/j.cell.2018.01.006

Kantarjian HM, DeAngelo DJ, Stelljes M, Martinelli G, Liedtke M, Stock W, Gökbuget N, O'Brien S, Wang K, Wang T, et al. 2016. Inotuzumab ozogamicin versus standard therapy for acute lymphoblastic leukemia. *N Engl J Med* **375:** 740–753. doi:10.1056/NEJMoa1509277

Kastritis E, Anagnostopoulos A, Roussou M, Toumanidis S, Pamboukas C, Migkou M, Tassidou A, Xilouri I, Delibasi S, Psimenou E, et al. 2007. Treatment of light chain (AL) amyloidosis with the combination of bortezomib and dexamethasone. *Haematologica* **92:** 1351–1358. doi:10.3324/haematol.11325

Kaufman JL. 2019. Roundtable: How I treat a newly diagnosed patient with high-risk myeloma. *Hematology Am Soc Hematol Educ Program* **2019:** 120–124. doi:10.1182/hematology.2019000015

Kaufman JL, Gasparetto CJ, Mikhael J, Moreau P, Touzeau C, Vij R, Facon T, Pegourie B, Benboubker L, Boise LH, et al. 2017. Phase 1 study of venetoclax in combination with dexamethasone as targeted therapy for t(11;14) relapsed/refractory multiple myeloma. *Blood* **130:** 3131. doi:10.1182/blood.V130.Suppl_1.3131.3131

Kaufman J, Gasparetto C, Mikhael J, Moreau P, Touzeau C, Vij R, Facon T, Pegourie B, Benboubker L, Boise L, et al. 2019a. Venetoclax monotherapy and combined with dexamethasone as targeted therapy for relapsed/refractory t(11;14) multiple myeloma. *Br J Haematol* **185:** 182–183.

Kaufman JL, Gasparetto C, Schjesvold FH, Moreau P, Touzeau C, Facon T, Boise LH, Alzate S, Macartney T, Pesko J, et al. 2019b. Phase I/II study evaluating the safety and efficacy of venetoclax in combination with dexamethasone as targeted therapy for patients with t(11;14) relapsed/refractory multiple myeloma. *Blood* **134:** 926. doi:10.1182/blood-2019-125871

Kreitman RJ, Tallman MS, Robak T, Coutre S, Wilson WH, Stetler-Stevenson M, FitzGerald DJ, Santiago L, Gao G, Lanasa MC, et al. 2018. Minimal residual hairy cell leukemia eradication with moxetumomab pasudotox: Phase 1 results and long-term follow-up. *Blood* **131:** 2331–2334. doi:10.1182/blood-2017-09-803072

Krejcik J, Casneuf T, Nijhof IS, Verbist B, Bald J, Plesner T, Syed K, Liu K, van de Donk NWCJ, Weiss BM, et al. 2016. Daratumumab depletes $CD38^+$ immune regulatory cells, promotes T-cell expansion, and skews T-cell repertoire in multiple myeloma. *Blood* **128:** 384–394. doi:10.1182/blood-2015-12-687749

Krishnan A, Kapoor P, Palmer JM, Tsai NC, Kumar S, Lonial S, Htut M, Karanes C, Nathwani N, Rosenzweig M, et al. 2018. Phase I/II trial of the oral regimen ixazomib, pomalidomide, and dexamethasone in relapsed/refractory multiple myeloma. *Leukemia* **32:** 1567–1574. doi:10.1038/s41375-018-0038-8

Krönke J, Udeshi ND, Narla A, Grauman P, Hurst SN, McConkey M, Svinkina T, Heckl D, Comer E, Li X, et al. 2014. Lenalidomide causes selective degradation of IKZF1 and IKZF3 in multiple myeloma cells. *Science* **343:** 301–305. doi:10.1126/science.1244851

Krönke J, Fink EC, Hollenbach PW, MacBeth KJ, Hurst SN, Udeshi ND, Chamberlain PP, Mani DR, Man HW, Gandhi AK, et al. 2015. Lenalidomide induces ubiquitination and degradation of CK1α in del(5q) MDS. *Nature* **523:** 183–188. doi:10.1038/nature14610

Kumar SK, Dispenzieri A, Lacy MQ, Gertz MA, Buadi FK, Pandey S, Kapoor P, Dingli D, Hayman SR, Leung N, et al. 2014. Continued improvement in survival in multiple myeloma: Changes in early mortality and outcomes in older patients. *Leukemia* **28:** 1122–1128. doi:10.1038/leu.2013.313

Kumar S, Kaufman JL, Gasparetto C, Mikhael J, Vij R, Pegourie B, Benboubker L, Facon T, Amiot M, Moreau P, et al. 2017. Efficacy of venetoclax as targeted therapy for relapsed/refractory t(11;14) multiple myeloma. *Blood* **130:** 2401–2409. doi:10.1182/blood-2017-06-788786

Kumar SK, Kapoor P, Laplant B, Muchtar E, Buadi FK, Gonsalves WI, Dingli D, Go RS, Warsame R, Kourelis T, et al. 2018. Phase 2 trial of ixazomib, lenalidomide, dexamethasone and daratumumab in patients with newly diagnosed multiple myeloma. *Blood* **132:** 304. doi:10.1182/blood-2018-99-111065

Kyle RA, Rajkumar SV. 2004. Multiple myeloma. *N Engl J Med* **351:** 1860–1873. doi:10.1056/NEJMra041875

Lee HC, Raje NS, Landgren O, Upreti VV, Wang J, Avilion AA, Hu X, Rasmussen E, Mgarmchamnanrith G, Fujii H, et al. 2020. Letter phase 1 study of the anti-BCMA antibody-drug conjugate AMG 224 in patients with relapsed/refractory multiple myeloma. *Leukemia* doi:10.1038/s41375-020-0834-9

Leng S, Bhutani D, Lentzsch S. 2019. How I treat a refractory myeloma patient who is not eligible for a clinical trial. *Hematology Am Soc Hematol Educ Program* **2019:** 125–136. doi:10.1182/hematology.2019000016

Lesokhin AM, Ansell SM, Armand P, Scott EC, Halwani A, Gutierrez M, Millenson MM, Cohen AD, Schuster SJ, Lebovic D, et al. 2016. Nivolumab in patients with relapsed or refractory hematologic malignancy: Preliminary results of a Phase Ib Study. *J Clin Oncol* **34:** 2698–2704. doi:10.1200/JCO.2015.65.9789

Li C, Mei H, Hu Y, Guo T. 2019. A bispecific CAR-T cell therapy targeting BCMA and CD38 for relapsed/refractory multiple myeloma: Updated results from a phase 1 dose-climbing trial. *Blood* **134:** 930. doi:10.1182/blood-2019-130340

Lin T, Hydutsky L, Parros H, Murphy S, Pei H, Londhe A, Ukropec J, Qi M, Lutska Y, Sharma M. 2017. Phase 2 randomized study of daratumumab (dara), lenalidomide (R), bortezomib (V), and dexamethasone (d; Dara-RVd) vs. RVd in patients (pts) with newly diagnosed multiple myeloma (MM) eligible for high-dose therapy (HDT) and autologous stem cell transplantation (ASCT). *Ann Oncol* **28:** v355–v371. doi:10.1093/annonc/mdx373.

Lohr JG, Stojanov P, Carter SL, Cruz-Gordillo P, Lawrence MS, Auclair D, Sougnez C, Knoechel B, Gould J, Saksena G, et al. 2014. Widespread genetic heterogeneity in multiple myeloma: Implications for targeted therapy. *Cancer Cell* **25:** 91–101. doi:10.1016/j.ccr.2013.12.015

Lokhorst HM, Plesner T, Laubach JP, Nahi H, Gimsing P, Hansson M, Minnema MC, Lassen U, Krejcik J, Palumbo A, et al. 2015. Targeting CD38 with daratumumab monotherapy in multiple myeloma. *N Engl J Med* **373:** 1207–1219. doi:10.1056/NEJMoa1506348

Lonial S, Dimopoulos M, Palumbo A, White D, Grosicki S, Spicka I, Walter-Croneck A, Moreau P, Mateos MV, Magen H, et al. 2015. Elotuzumab therapy for relapsed or refractory multiple myeloma. *N Engl J Med* **373:** 621–631. doi:10.1056/NEJMoa1505654

Lonial S, Lee HC, Badros A, Trudel S, Nooka AK, Chari A, Abdallah AO, Callander N, Lendvai N, Sborov D, et al. 2020. Belantamab mafodotin for relapsed or refractory multiple myeloma (DREAMM-2): A two-arm, randomised, open-label, phase 2 study. *Lancet Oncol* **21:** 207–221. doi:10.1016/S1470-2045(19)30788-0

Lu G, Middleton RE, Sun H, Naniong MV, Ott CJ, Mitsiades CS, Wong KK, Bradner JE, Kaelin WG Jr. 2014. The myeloma drug lenalidomide promotes the cereblon-dependent destruction of Ikaros proteins. *Science* **343:** 305–309. doi:10.1126/science.1244917

Madduri D, Usmani SZ, Jagannath S, Singh I, Zudaire E, Yeh T-M, Allred AJ, Banerjee A, Goldberg JD, Schecter JM, et al. 2019. Results from CARTITUDE-1: A phase 1b/2 study of JNJ-4528, a CAR-T cell therapy directed against B-cell maturation antigen (BCMA), in patients with relapsed and/or refractory multiple myeloma (R/R MM). *Blood* **134:** 577. doi:10.1182/blood-2019-121731

Manasanch EE. 2019. What to do with minimal residual disease testing in myeloma. *Hematology Am Soc Hematol Educ Program* **2019:** 137–141. doi:10.1182/hematology.2019000080

Manasanch EE, Shah JJ, Lee HC, Weber DM, Thomas SK, Amini B, Feng L, Berkova Z, Hildebrandt M, Orlowski RZ. 2018. Bortezomib, lenalidomide, and dexamethasone with panobinostat for front-line treatment of patients with multiple myeloma who are eligible for transplantation: A phase 1 trial. *Lancet Haematol* **5:** e628–e640. doi:10.1016/S2352-3026(18)30174-1

Martin T, Baz R, Benson DM, Lendvai N, Wolf J, Munster P, Lesokhin AM, Wack C, Charpentier E, Campana F, et al. 2017. A phase 1b study of isatuximab plus lenalidomide and dexamethasone for relapsed/refractory multiple myeloma. *Blood* **129:** 3294–3303. doi:10.1182/blood-2016-09-740787

Mateos MV, Dimopoulos MA, Cavo M, Suzuki K, Jakubowiak A, Knop S, Doyen C, Lucio P, Nagy Z, Kaplan P, et al. 2018. Daratumumab plus bortezomib, melphalan, and prednisone for untreated myeloma. *N Engl J Med* **378:** 518–528. doi:10.1056/NEJMoa1714678

Mateos MV, Orlowski RZ, Ocio EM, Rodríguez-Otero P, Reece D, Moreau P, Munshi N, Avigan DE, Siegel DS, Ghori R, et al. 2019a. Pembrolizumab combined with lenalidomide and low-dose dexamethasone for relapsed or refractory multiple myeloma: Phase I KEYNOTE-023 study. *Br J Haematol* **186:** E117–E121. doi:10.1111/bjh.15946

Mateos MV, Blacklock H, Schjesvold F, Oriol A, Simpson D, George A, Goldschmidt H, Larocca A, Chanan-Khan A, Sherbenou D, et al. 2019b. Pembrolizumab plus pomalidomide and dexamethasone for patients with relapsed or refractory multiple myeloma (KEYNOTE-183): A randomised, open-label, phase 3 trial. *Lancet Haematol* **6:** E459–E469. doi:10.1016/S2352-3026(19)30110-3

Melchor L, Brioli A, Wardell CP, Murison A, Potter NE, Kaiser MF, Fryer RA, Johnson DC, Begum DB, Hulkki Wilson S, et al. 2014. Single-cell genetic analysis reveals the composition of initiating clones and phylogenetic patterns of branching and parallel evolution in myeloma. *Leukemia* **28:** 1705–1715. doi:10.1038/leu.2014.13

Miguel JS, Weisel K, Moreau P, Lacy M, Song K, Delforge M, Karlin L, Goldschmidt H, Banos A, Oriol A, et al. 2013. Pomalidomide plus low-dose dexamethasone versus high-dose dexamethasone alone for patients with relapsed and refractory multiple myeloma (MM-003): A randomised, open-label, phase 3 trial. *Lancet Oncol* **14:** 1055–1066. doi:10.1016/S1470-2045(13)70380-2

Mikhael J, Richardson P, Usmani SZ, Raje N, Bensinger W, Karanes C, Campana F, Kanagavel D, Dubin F, Liu Q, et al. 2019. A phase 1b study of isatuximab plus pomalidomide/dexamethasone in relapsed/refractory multiple myeloma. *Blood* **134:** 123–133. doi:10.1182/blood-2019-02-895193

Mikhael J, Richter J, Vij R, Cole C, Zonder J, Kaufman JL, Bensinger W, Dimopoulos M, Lendvai N, Hari P, et al. 2020. A dose-finding phase 2 study of single agent isatuximab (anti-CD38 mAb) in relapsed/refractory multiple myeloma. *Leukemia* doi:10.1038/s41375-020-0857-2

Mitsiades CS. 2015. Therapeutic landscape of carfilzomib and other modulators of the ubiquitin-proteasome pathway. *J Clin Oncol* **33:** 782–785. doi:10.1200/JCO.2014.55.5748

Mitsiades CS, Mitsiades N. 2004. CC-5013 (Celgene). *Curr Opin Investig Drugs* **5:** 635–647.

Mitsiades N, Mitsiades CS, Poulaki V, Chauhan D, Fanourakis G, Gu X, Bailey C, Joseph M, Libermann TA, Treon SP, et al. 2002a. Molecular sequelae of proteasome inhibition in human multiple myeloma cells. *Proc Natl Acad Sci* **99:** 14374–14379. doi:10.1073/pnas.202445099

Mitsiades N, Mitsiades CS, Poulaki V, Chauhan D, Richardson PG, Hideshima T, Munshi N, Treon SP, Anderson KC. 2002b. Biologic sequelae of nuclear factor-κB blockade in multiple myeloma: Therapeutic applications. *Blood* **99:** 4079–4086. doi:10.1182/blood.V99.11.4079

Mitsiades N, Mitsiades CS, Poulaki V, Hideshima T, Munshi N, Treon SP, Anderson KC. 2002c. Apoptotic signaling induced by immunomodulatory thalidomide analogs in human multiple myeloma cells: Therapeutic implications. *Blood* **99:** 4525–4530. doi:10.1182/blood.V99.12.4525

Mitsiades N, Mitsiades CS, Richardson PG, Poulaki V, Tai YT, Chauhan D, Fanourakis G, Gu X, Bailey C, Joseph M, et al. 2003. The proteasome inhibitor PS-341 potentiates sensitivity of multiple myeloma cells to conventional chemotherapeutic agents: Therapeutic applications. *Blood* **101:** 2377–2380. doi:10.1182/blood-2002-06-1768

Mitsiades CS, Mitsiades NS, McMullan CJ, Poulaki V, Shringarpure R, Hideshima T, Akiyama M, Chauhan D, Munshi N, Gu X, et al. 2004. Transcriptional signature of histone deacetylase inhibition in multiple myeloma: Biological and clinical implications. *Proc Natl Acad Sci* **101:** 540–545. doi:10.1073/pnas.2536759100

Molina-Arcas M, Moore C, Rana S, van Maldegem F, Mugarza E, Romero-Clavijo P, Herbert E, Horswell S, Li LS, Janes MR, et al. 2019. Development of combination therapies to maximize the impact of KRAS-G12C inhibitors in lung cancer. *Sci Transl Med* **11:** eaaw7999. doi:10.1126/scitranslmed.aaw7999

Moreau P, Masszi T, Grzasko N, Bahlis NJ, Hansson M, Pour L, Sandhu I, Ganly P, Baker BW, Jackson SR, et al. 2016. Oral Ixazomib, lenalidomide, and dexamethasone for multiple myeloma. *N Engl J Med* **374:** 1621–1634. doi:10.1056/NEJMoa1516282

Morschhauser F, Flinn IW, Advani R, Sehn LH, Diefenbach C, Kolibaba K, Press OW, Salles G, Tilly H, Chen AI, et al. 2019. Polatuzumab vedotin or pinatuzumab vedotin plus rituximab in patients with relapsed or refractory non-Hodgkin lymphoma: Final results from a phase 2 randomised study (ROMULUS). *Lancet Haematol* **6:** e254–e265. doi:10.1016/S2352-3026(19)30026-2

Mullighan CG, Miller CB, Radtke I, Phillips LA, Dalton J, Ma J, White D, Hughes TP, Le Beau MM, Pui CH, et al. 2008. *BCR-ABL1* lymphoblastic leukaemia is characterized by the deletion of Ikaros. *Nature* **453:** 110–114. doi:10.1038/nature06866

Novak AJ, Darce JR, Arendt BK, Harder B, Henderson K, Kindsvogel W, Gross JA, Greipp PR, Jelinek DF. 2004. Expression of BCMA, TACI, and BAFF-R in multiple myeloma: A mechanism for growth and survival. *Blood* **103:** 689–694. doi:10.1182/blood-2003-06-2043

Obeng EA, Carlson LM, Gutman DM, Harrington WJ Jr, Lee KP, Boise LH. 2006. Proteasome inhibitors induce a terminal unfolded protein response in multiple myeloma cells. *Blood* **107:** 4907–4916. doi:10.1182/blood-2005-08-3531

O'Brien S, Thomas RM, Wertheim GB, Zhang F, Shen H, Wells AD. 2014. Ikaros imposes a barrier to $CD8^+$ T cell differentiation by restricting autocrine IL-2 production. *J Immunol* **192:** 5118–5129. doi:10.4049/jimmunol.1301992

O'Connor BP, Raman VS, Erickson LD, Cook WJ, Weaver LK, Ahonen C, Lin LL, Mantchev GT, Bram RJ, Noelle RJ. 2004. BCMA is essential for the survival of long-lived bone marrow plasma cells. *J Exp Med* **199:** 91–98. doi:10.1084/jem.20031330

O'Connor OA, Stewart AK, Vallone M, Molineaux CJ, Kunkel LA, Gerecitano JF, Orlowski RZ. 2009. A phase 1 dose escalation study of the safety and pharmacokinetics of the novel proteasome inhibitor carfilzomib (PR-171) in patients with hematologic malignancies. *Clin Cancer Res* **15:** 7085–7091. doi:10.1158/1078-0432.CCR-09-0822

Orlowski RZ, Stinchcombe TE, Mitchell BS, Shea TC, Baldwin AS, Stahl S, Adams J, Esseltine DL, Elliott PJ, Pien CS, et al. 2002. Phase I trial of the proteasome inhibitor PS-341 in patients with refractory hematologic malignancies. *J Clin Oncol* **20:** 4420–4427. doi:10.1200/JCO.2002.01.133

Orlowski RZ, Moreau P, Niesvizky R, Ludwig H, Oriol A, Chng WJ, Goldschmidt H, Yang Z, Kimball AS, Dimopoulos M. 2019. Carfilzomib-dexamethasone versus bortezomib-dexamethasone in relapsed or refractory multiple myeloma: Updated overall survival, safety, and subgroups. *Clin Lymphoma Myeloma Leuk* **19:** 522–530.e1. doi:10.1016/j.clml.2019.04.018

Palladini G, Kastritis E, Maurer MS, Zonder J, Minnema MC, Wechalekar AD, Jaccard A, Lee HC, Bumma N, Kaufman JL, et al. 2020. Daratumumab plus CyBorD for patients with newly diagnosed AL amyloidosis: Safety run-in results of ANDROMEDA. *Blood* **136:** 71–80. doi:10.1182/blood.2019004460

Palumbo A, Anderson K. 2011. Multiple myeloma. *N Engl J Med* **364:** 1046–1060. doi:10.1056/NEJMra1011442

Palumbo A, Sonneveld P. 2015. Preclinical and clinical evaluation of elotuzumab, a SLAMF7-targeted humanized monoclonal antibody in development for multiple myeloma. *Expert Rev Hematol* **8:** 481–491. doi:10.1586/17474086.2015.1053866

Palumbo A, Chanan-Khan A, Weisel K, Nooka AK, Masszi T, Beksac M, Spicka I, Hungria V, Munder M, Mateos MV, et al. 2016. Daratumumab, bortezomib, and dexamethasone for multiple myeloma. *N Engl J Med* **375:** 754–766. doi:10.1056/NEJMoa1606038

Panowski SH, Kuo TC, Zhang Y, Chen A, Geng T, Aschenbrenner L, Kamperschroer C, Pascua E, Chen W, Delaria K, et al. 2019. Preclinical efficacy and safety comparison of CD3 bispecific and ADC modalities targeting BCMA for the treatment of multiple myeloma. *Mol Cancer Ther* **18:** 2008–2020. doi:10.1158/1535-7163.MCT-19-0007

Pawlyn C, Davies FE. 2019. Toward personalized treatment in multiple myeloma based on molecular characteristics. *Blood* **133:** 660–675. doi:10.1182/blood-2018-09-825331

Plesner T, Lokhorst H, Gimsing P, Nahi H, Lisby S, Richardson PG. 2012a. Daratumumab, a CD38 monoclonal antibody in patients with multiple myeloma—Data from a dose-escalation phase I/II study. *Blood* **120:** 73. doi:10.1182/blood.V120.21.73.73

Plesner T, Lokhorst HM, Gimsing P, Nahi H, Lisby S, Richardson PGG. 2012b. Daratumumab, a CD38 mab, for the treatment of relapsed/refractory multiple myeloma patients: Preliminary efficacy data from a multicenter phase I/II study. *J Clin Oncol* **30:** 8019. doi:10.1200/jco.2012.30.15_suppl.8019

Popat R, Trudel S, Lendvai N, Popat R, Voorhees PM, Reeves B, Libby EN, Richardson PG, Anderson LD, Sutherland HJ, et al. 2018. Targeting B-cell maturation antigen (BCMA) with GSK2857916 antibody-drug conjugate provides durable responses in patients (PTS) with heavily-pretreated relapsed/refractory multiple myeloma (RRMM): Preliminary results from study BMA117159. *Haematologica* **103:** 30.

Popat R, Warcel D, O'Nions J, Cowley A, Smith S, Yong K, Esposti SD. 2019. Durability of response and characterisation of corneal events with extended follow-up after belantamab mafodotin monotherapy for patients with relapsed/refractory multiple myeloma. *Clinical Lymphoma Myeloma & Leukemia* **19:** E150. doi:10.1016/j.clml.2019.09.250

Popat R, Warcel D, O'Nions J, Cowley A, Smith S, Tucker WR, Yong K, Esposti SD. 2020. Characterization of response and corneal events with extended follow-up after belantamab mafodotin (GSK2857916) monotherapy for patients with relapsed multiple myeloma: A case series from the first-time-in-human clinical trial. *Haematologica* **105:** E261–E263. doi:10.3324/haematol.2019.235937

Prabhala RH, Pelluru D, Fulciniti M, Prabhala HK, Nanjappa P, Song W, Pai C, Amin S, Tai YT, Richardson PG, et al. 2010. Elevated IL-17 produced by T_H17 cells promotes myeloma cell growth and inhibits immune function in multiple myeloma. *Blood* **115:** 5385–5392. doi:10.1182/blood-2009-10-246660

Racanelli V, Leone P, Frassanito MA, Brunetti C, Perosa F, Ferrone S, Dammacco F. 2010. Alterations in the antigen processing-presenting machinery of transformed plasma cells are associated with reduced recognition by $CD8^+$ T cells and characterize the progression of MGUS to multiple myeloma. *Blood* **115:** 1185–1193. doi:10.1182/blood-2009-06-228676

Raje N, Berdeja J, Lin Y, Siegel D, Jagannath S, Madduri D, Liedtke M, Rosenblatt J, Maus MV, Turka A, et al. 2019. Anti-BCMA CAR T-cell therapy bb2121 in relapsed or refractory multiple myeloma. *N Engl J Med* **380:** 1726–1737. doi:10.1056/NEJMoa1817226

Rajkumar SV. 2020. Multiple myeloma: 2020 update on diagnosis, risk-stratification and management. *Am J Hematol* **95:** 548–567. doi:10.1002/ajh.25791

Ratta M, Fagnoni F, Curti A, Vescovini R, Sansoni P, Oliviero B, Fogli M, Ferri E, Della Cuna GR, Tura S, et al. 2002. Dendritic cells are functionally defective in multiple myeloma: The role of interleukin-6. *Blood* **100:** 230–237. doi:10.1182/blood.V100.1.230

Reece DE, Sanchorawala V, Hegenbart U, Merlini G, Palladini G, Fermand JP, Vescio RA, Liu X, Elsayed YA, Cakana A, et al. 2009. Weekly and twice-weekly bortezomib in patients with systemic AL amyloidosis: Results of a phase 1 dose-escalation study. *Blood* **114:** 1489–1497. doi:10.1182/blood-2009-02-203398

Richardson PG, Schlossman RL, Weller E, Hideshima T, Mitsiades C, Davies F, LeBlanc R, Catley LP, Doss D, Kelly K, et al. 2002. Immunomodulatory drug CC-5013 overcomes drug resistance and is well tolerated in patients with relapsed multiple myeloma. *Blood* **100:** 3063–3067. doi:10.1182/blood-2002-03-0996

Richardson PG, Barlogie B, Berenson J, Singhal S, Jagannath S, Irwin D, Rajkumar SV, Srkalovic G, Alsina M, Alexanian R, et al. 2003. A phase 2 study of bortezomib in relapsed, refractory myeloma. *N Engl J Med* **348:** 2609–2617. doi:10.1056/NEJMoa030288

Richardson PG, Sonneveld P, Schuster MW, Irwin D, Stadtmauer EA, Facon T, Harousseau JL, Ben-Yehuda D, Lonial S, Goldschmidt H, et al. 2005. Bortezomib or high-dose dexamethasone for relapsed multiple myeloma. *N Engl J Med* **352:** 2487–2498. doi:10.1056/NEJMoa043445

Richardson PG, Blood E, Mitsiades CS, Jagannath S, Zeldenrust SR, Alsina M, Schlossman RL, Rajkumar SV, Desikan KR, Hideshima T, et al. 2006. A randomized phase 2 study of lenalidomide therapy for patients with relapsed or relapsed and refractory multiple myeloma. *Blood* **108:** 3458–3464. doi:10.1182/blood-2006-04-015909

Richardson PG, Weller E, Jagannath S, Avigan DE, Alsina M, Schlossman RL, Mazumder A, Munshi NC, Ghobrial IM, Doss D, et al. 2009. Multicenter, phase I, dose-escalation trial of lenalidomide plus bortezomib for relapsed and relapsed/refractory multiple myeloma. *J Clin Oncol* **27:** 5713–5719. doi:10.1200/JCO.2009.22.2679

Richardson PG, Weller E, Lonial S, Jakubowiak AJ, Jagannath S, Raje NS, Avigan DE, Xie W, Ghobrial IM, Schlossman RL, et al. 2010. Lenalidomide, bortezomib, and dexamethasone combination therapy in patients with newly diagnosed multiple myeloma. *Blood* **116:** 679–686. doi:10.1182/blood-2010-02-268862

Richardson PG, Siegel D, Baz R, Kelley SL, Munshi NC, Laubach J, Sullivan D, ALsina M, Schlossman R, Ghobrial IM, et al. 2013. Phase 1 study of pomalidomide MTD, safety, and efficacy in patients with refractory multiple myeloma who have received lenalidomide and bortezomib. *Blood* **121:** 1961–1967. doi:10.1182/blood-2012-08-450742

Richardson PG, Siegel DS, Vij R, Hofmeister CC, Baz R, Jagannath S, Chen C, Lonial S, Jakubowiak A, Bahlis N, et al. 2014a. Pomalidomide alone or in combination with low-dose dexamethasone in relapsed and refractory multiple myeloma: A randomized phase 2 study. *Blood* **123:** 1826–1832. doi:10.1182/blood-2013-11-538835

Richardson PG, Xie W, Jagannath S, Jakubowiak A, Lonial S, Raje NS, Alsina M, Ghobrial IM, Schlossman RL, Munshi NC, et al. 2014b. A phase 2 trial of lenalidomide, bortezomib, and dexamethasone in patients with relapsed and relapsed/refractory myeloma. *Blood* **123:** 1461–1469. doi:10.1182/blood-2013-07-517276

Richardson PG, Hofmeister CC, Raje NS, Siegel DS, Lonial S, Laubach J, Efebera YA, Vesole DH, Nooka AK, Rosenblatt J, et al. 2017. Pomalidomide, bortezomib and low-dose dexamethasone in lenalidomide-refractory and proteasome inhibitor-exposed myeloma. *Leukemia* **31:** 2695–2701. doi:10.1038/leu.2017.173

Sanchorawala V, Quillen K, Sloan JM, Andrea NT, Seldin DC. 2011. Bortezomib and high-dose melphalan conditioning for stem cell transplantation for AL amyloidosis: A pilot study. *Haematologica* **96:** 1890–1892. doi:10.3324/haematol.2011.049858

San-Miguel JF, Richardson PG, Günther A, Sezer O, Siegel D, Bladé J, LeBlanc R, Sutherland H, Sopala M, Mishra KK, et al. 2013. Phase Ib study of panobinostat and bortezomib in relapsed or relapsed and refractory multiple myeloma. *J Clin Oncol* **31:** 3696–3703. doi:10.1200/JCO.2012.46.7068

San-Miguel JF, Hungria VT, Yoon SS, Beksac M, Dimopoulos MA, Elghandour A, Jedrzejczak WW, Günther A, Nakorn TN, Siritanaratkul N, et al. 2014. Panobinostat plus bortezomib and dexamethasone versus placebo plus bortezomib and dexamethasone in patients with relapsed or relapsed and refractory multiple myeloma: A multicentre, randomised, double-blind phase 3 trial. *Lancet Oncol* **15:** 1195–1206. doi:10.1016/S1470-2045(14)70440-1

Seckinger A, Delgado JA, Moser S, Moreno L, Neuber B, Grab A, Lipp S, Merino J, Prosper F, Emde M, et al. 2017. Target expression, generation, preclinical activity, and pharmacokinetics of the BCMA-T cell bispecific antibody EM801 for multiple myeloma treatment. *Cancer Cell* **31:** 396–410. doi:10.1016/j.ccell.2017.02.002

Shah N, Chari A, Scott E, Mezzi K, Usmani SZ. 2020. B-cell maturation antigen (BCMA) in multiple myeloma: Rationale for targeting and current therapeutic approaches. *Leukemia* **34:** 985–1005. doi:10.1038/s41375-020-0734-z

Short NJ, Kantarjian H, Jabbour E, Cortes JE, Thomas DA, Rytting ME, Daver N, Alvarado Y, Konopleva M, Kebriaei P, et al. 2018. A phase I study of moxetumomab pasudotox in adults with relapsed or refractory B-cell acute lymphoblastic leukaemia. *Br J Haematol* **182:** 442–444. doi:10.1111/bjh.14806

Sidana S, Manasanch E. 2019. Evidence-based minireview: Does achieving MRD negativity after initial therapy improve prognosis for high-risk myeloma patients? *Hematology Am Soc Hematol Educ Program* **2019:** 142–147. doi:10.1182/hematology.2019000075

Siegel DS, Martin T, Wang M, Vij R, Jakubowiak AJ, Lonial S, Trudel S, Kukreti V, Bahlis N, Alsina M, et al. 2012. A phase 2 study of single-agent carfilzomib (PX-171-003-A1) in patients with relapsed and refractory multiple myeloma. *Blood* **120:** 2817–2825. doi:10.1182/blood-2012-05-425934

Singh RK, Jones RJ, Hong S, Shirzai F, Wang F, Wang H, Kuiatse I, Pahl A, Orlowski RZ. 2018. HDP101, a novel B-cell maturation antigen (BCMA)-targeted antibody conjugated to alpha-amanitin, is active against myeloma with preferential efficacy against pre-clinical models of deletion 17p. *Blood* **132:** 593.

Singhal S, Mehta J, Desikan R, Ayers D, Roberson P, Eddlemon P, Munshi N, Anaissie E, Wilson C, Dhodapkar M, et al. 1999. Antitumor activity of thalidomide in refractory multiple myeloma. *N Engl J Med* **341:** 1565–1571. doi:10.1056/NEJM199911183412102

Slaney CY, Wang P, Darcy PK, Kershaw MH. 2018. CARs versus BiTEs: A comparison between T cell-redirection strategies for cancer treatment. *Cancer Discov* **8:** 924–934. doi:10.1158/2159-8290.CD-18-0297

Smith EL, Harrington K, Staehr M, Masakayan R, Jones J, Long TJ, Ng KY, Ghoddusi M, Purdon TJ, Wang X, et al. 2019. GPRC5D is a target for the immunotherapy of multiple myeloma with rationally designed CAR T cells. *Sci Transl Med* **11:** eaau7746. doi:10.1126/scitranslmed.aau7746

Sommer C, Boldajipour B, Kuo TC, Bentley T, Sutton J, Chen A, Geng T, Dong H, Galetto R, Valton J, et al. 2019.

Preclinical evaluation of allogeneic CAR T cells targeting BCMA for the treatment of multiple myeloma. *Mol Ther* **27:** 1126–1138. doi:10.1016/j.ymthe.2019.04.001

Stewart AK, Rajkumar SV, Dimopoulos MA, Masszi T, Špička I, Oriol A, Hájek R, Rosiñol L, Siegel DS, Mihaylov GG, et al. 2015. Carfilzomib, lenalidomide, and dexamethasone for relapsed multiple myeloma. *N Engl J Med* **372:** 142–152. doi:10.1056/NEJMoa1411321

Stewart AK, Krishnan AY, Singhal S, Boccia RV, Patel MR, Niesvizky R, Chanan-Khan AA, Ailawadhi S, Brumm J, Mundt KE, et al. 2019. Phase I study of the anti-FcRH5 antibody-drug conjugate DFRF4539A in relapsed or refractory multiple myeloma. *Blood Cancer J* **9:** 17. doi:10.1038/s41408-019-0178-8

Suen H, Brown R, Yang S, Weatherburn C, Ho PJ, Woodland N, Nassif N, Barbaro P, Bryant C, Hart D, et al. 2016. Multiple myeloma causes clonal T-cell immunosenescence: Identification of potential novel targets for promoting tumour immunity and implications for checkpoint blockade. *Leukemia* **30:** 1716–1724. doi:10.1038/leu.2016.84

Tassi I, Colonna M. 2005. The cytotoxicity receptor CRACC (CS-1) recruits EAT-2 and activates the PI3 K and phospholipase Cγ signaling pathways in human NK cells. *J Immunol* **175:** 7996–8002. doi:10.4049/jimmunol.175.12.7996

Topp MS, Attal M, Langer C, Moreau P, Facon T, Düll J, Hebraud B, Gomez-Roca C, Munzert G, Gracien E, et al. 2016. Phase 1 dose-escalation study of BI 836909, an anti-BCMA bi-specific 1-cell engager, in relapsed and for refractory multiple myeloma (RRMM). *J Clin Oncol* **34.** doi:10.1200/JCO.2016.34.15-suppl.TPS8067

Topp MS, Düll J, Zugmaier G, Attal M, Moreau P, Langer C, Kroenke J, Facon T, Einsele E, Munzert G. 2018. Treatment with AMG 420, an anti-B-cell maturation antigen (BCMA) bispecific T-cell engager (BiTE®) antibody construct, induces minimal residual disease (MRD) negative complete responses in relapsed and/or refractory (R/R) multiple myeloma (MM) patients: Results of a first-in-human (FIH) phase I dose escalation study. *Blood* **132:** 1010. doi:10.1182/blood-2018-99-109769

Treon SP. 2009. How I treat Waldenström macroglobulinemia. *Blood* **114:** 2375–2385. doi:10.1182/blood-2009-05-174359

Treon SP, Hunter ZR, Matous J, Joyce RM, Mannion B, Advani R, Cook D, Songer J, Hill J, Kaden BR, et al. 2007. Multicenter clinical trial of bortezomib in relapsed/refractory Waldenstrom's macroglobulinemia: Results of WMCTG Trial 03-248. *Clin Cancer Res* **13:** 3320–3325. doi:10.1158/1078-0432.CCR-06-2511

Trudel S, Lendvai N, Popat R, Voorhees PM, Reeves B, Libby EN, Richardson PG, Anderson LD, Sutherland HJ, Yong K, et al. 2018. Targeting B-cell maturation antigen with GSK2857916 antibody-drug conjugate in relapsed or refractory multiple myeloma (BMA117159): A dose escalation and expansion phase 1 trial. *Lancet Oncol* **19:** 1641–1653. doi:10.1016/S1470-2045(18)30576-X

Trudel S, Nooka A, Fecteau D, Talekar M, Jewell RC, Williams D, Evans J, Opalinska J. 2019a. DREAMM 4: A phase I/II single-arm open-label study to explore safety and clinical activity of belantamab mafodotin (GSK2857916) administered in combination with pembrolizumab in patients with relapsed/refractory multiple myeloma (RRMM). *Ann Oncol* **30:** v447. doi:10.1093/annonc/mdz251.039.

Trudel S, Lendvai N, Popat R, Voorhees PM, Reeves B, Libby EN, Richardson PG, Hoos A, Gupta I, Bragulat V, et al. 2019b. Antibody-drug conjugate, GSK2857916, in relapsed/refractory multiple myeloma: An update on safety and efficacy from dose expansion phase I study. *Blood Cancer J* **9:** 37. doi:10.1038/s41408-019-0196-6

Usmani SZ, Chari A, Lonial S, Weiss B, Comenzo RL, Wu K, Khokhar NZ, Wang J, Doshi P, Jakubowiak A. 2017. An open-label, phase 1B study (MMY1001) of daratumumab combined with carfilzomib, lenalidomide, and dexamethasone (KRD) in patients with newly diagnosed multiple myeloma (MM). *Haematologica* **102:** 269.

Usmani SZ, Schjesvold F, Oriol A, Karlin L, Cavo M, Rifkin RM, Yimer HA, LeBlanc R, Takezako N, McCroskey RD, et al. 2019. Pembrolizumab plus lenalidomide and dexamethasone for patients with treatment-naive multiple myeloma (KEYNOTE-185): A randomised, open-label, phase 3 trial. *Lancet Haematol* **6:** E448–E458. doi:10.1016/S2352-3026(19)30109-7

van de Donk N, Usmani SZ. 2018. CD38 Antibodies in multiple myeloma: Mechanisms of action and modes of resistance. *Front Immunol* **9:** 2134. doi:10.3389/fimmu.2018.02134

Velasquez MP, Bonifant CL, Gottschalk S. 2018. Redirecting T cells to hematological malignancies with bispecific antibodies. *Blood* **131:** 30–38. doi:10.1182/blood-2017-06-741058

Vij R, Nath R, Afar DEH, Mateos MV, Berdeja JG, Raab MS, Guenther A, Martínez-López J, Jakubowiak AJ, Leleu X, et al. 2020. First-in-human phase I study of ABBV-838, an antibody-drug conjugate targeting SLAMF7/CS1 in patients with relapsed and refractory multiple myeloma. *Clin Cancer Res* **26:** 2308–2317. doi:10.1158/1078-0432.CCR-19-1431

Vikova V, Jourdan M, Robert N, Requirand G, Boireau S, Bruyer A, Vincent L, Cartron G, Kelin B, Elemento O, et al. 2019. Comprehensive characterization of the mutational landscape in multiple myeloma cell lines reveals potential drivers and pathways associated with tumor progression and drug resistance. *Theranostics* **9:** 540–553. doi:10.7150/thno.28374

Voorhees PM, Costa LJ, Reeves B, Nathwani N, Rodriguez C, Lutska Y, Hydutsky L, Pei H, Ukropec J, Qi M, et al. 2017. Interim safety analysis of a phase 2 randomized study of daratumumab (Dara), lenalidomide (R), bortezomib (V), and dexamethasone (d; Dara-Rvd) vs. Rvd in patients (Pts) with newly diagnosed multiple myeloma (MM) eligible for high-dose therapy (HDT) and autologous stem cell transplantation (ASCT). *Blood* **130:** 1879. doi:10.1182/blood.V130.Suppl_1.1879.1879

Voorhees PM, Kaufman JL, Laubach JP, Sborov DW, Reeves B, Rodriguez C, Chari A, SIlbermann R, Costa LJ, Anderson LD, et al. 2020. Depth of response to daratumumab (DARA), lenalidomide, bortezomib, and dexamethasone (RVd) improves over time in patients (pts) with transplant-eligible newly diagnosed multiple myeloma (NDMM): Griffin Study Update. *Blood* **134:** 691. doi:10.1182/blood-2019-123465

Walker BA, Wardell CP, Melchor L, Hulkki S, Potter NE, Johnson DC, Fenwick K, Kozarewa I, Gonzalez D, Lord CJ, et al. 2012. Intraclonal heterogeneity and distinct molecular mechanisms characterize the development of t(4;14) and t(11;14) myeloma. *Blood* **120:** 1077–1086. doi:10.1182/blood-2012-03-412981

Weber DM, Chen C, Niesvizky R, Wang M, Belch A, Stadtmauer EA, Siegel D, Borrello I, Rajkumar SV, Chanan-Khan AA, et al. 2007. Lenalidomide plus dexamethasone for relapsed multiple myeloma in North America. *N Engl J Med* **357:** 2133–2142. doi:10.1056/NEJMoa070596

Weisel K. 2016. Spotlight on elotuzumab in the treatment of multiple myeloma: The evidence to date. *Onco Targets Ther* **9:** 6037–6048. doi:10.2147/OTT.S94531

Weisel K, Asemissen AM, Schieferdecker A, Besemer B, Zago M, Mann C, Lutz R, Benner A, Tichy D, Bokemeyer C, et al. 2019. Isatuximab, carfilzomib, lenalidomide and dexamethasone (I-KRd) in front-line treatment of high-risk multiple myeloma: Results of the Safety Run-In cohort in the phase II, multicenter GMMG-CONCEPT trial. *Clinical Lymphoma Myeloma & Leukemia* **19:** E17.

Xu J, Chen LJ, Yang SS, Sun Y, Wu W, Liu YF, Xu J, Zhuang Y, Zhang W, Weng XQ, et al. 2019. Exploratory trial of a biepitopic CAR T-targeting B cell maturation antigen in relapsed/refractory multiple myeloma. *Proc Natl Acad Sci* **116:** 9543–9551. doi:10.1073/pnas.1819745116

Yan Z, Cao J, Cheng H, Qiao J, Zhang H, Wang Y, Shi M, Lan J, Fei X, Jin L, et al. 2019. A combination of humanised anti-CD19 and anti-BCMA CAR T cells in patients with relapsed or refractory multiple myeloma: A single-arm, phase 2 trial. *Lancet Haematol* **6:** E521–E529. doi:10.1016/S2352-3026(19)30115-2

Younes A, Gopal AK, Smith SE, Ansell SM, Rosenblatt JD, Savage KJ, Ramchandren R, Bartlett NL, Cheson BD, de Vos S, et al. 2012. Results of a pivotal phase II study of brentuximab vedotin for patients with relapsed or refractory Hodgkin's lymphoma. *J Clin Oncol* **30:** 2183–2189. doi:10.1200/JCO.2011.38.0410

Ziccheddu B, Biancon G, Bagnoli F, De Philippis C, Maura F, Rustad EH, Dugo M, Devecchi A, De Cecco L, Sensi M, et al. 2020. Integrative analysis of the genomic and transcriptomic landscape of double-refractory multiple myeloma. *Blood Adv* **4:** 830–844. doi:10.1182/bloodadvances.2019000779

Zugmaier G, Gökbuget N, Klinger M, Viardot A, Stelljes M, Neumann S, Horst HA, Marks R, Faul C, Diedrich H, et al. 2015. Long-term survival and T-cell kinetics in relapsed/refractory ALL patients who achieved MRD response after blinatumomab treatment. *Blood* **126:** 2578–2584. doi:10.1182/blood-2015-06-649111

Index

F

I

J

K

L